Method for conversion of mg to mEq/L (or to mmole/L)

mg = milligram
gm = gram
ml = milliliter
1 ml = 1.000027 cc
dl = deciliter = 100 ml
mmole = millimole

$$\text{mEq/L (milliequivalents per liter)} = \frac{\text{mg/L}}{\text{equivalent weight}}$$

$$\text{Equivalent weight} = \frac{\text{atomic weight}}{\text{valence of element}}$$

For example: A sample of blood serum contains 10 mg of Ca in 1 dl (100 ml). The valence of Ca is 2, and the atomic weight is 40. The equivalent weight of Ca is therefore 40 ÷ 2, or 20. The milliequivalents of Ca per liter are 10 (mg/dl) × 10 (dl/l) ÷ 20, or 5 mEq/L.

$$\text{mM/L} = \frac{\text{mg/L}}{\text{molecular weight}}$$ vol % (volumes percent) = mM/L × 2.24 for a gas whose properties approach that of an ideal gas, such as oxygen or nitrogen.
For carbon dioxide the factor is 2.226.

Temperature (Fahrenheit [F] to centigrade [C])

°F	°C	°F	°C	°F	°C	°F	°C
95.0	35.0	98.0	36.7	101.0	38.3	104.0	40.0
95.2	35.1	98.2	36.8	101.2	38.4	104.2	40.1
95.4	35.2	98.4	36.9	101.4	38.6	104.4	40.2
95.6	35.3	98.6	37.0	101.6	38.7	104.6	40.3
95.8	35.4	98.8	37.1	101.8	38.8	104.8	40.4
96.0	35.6	99.0	37.2	102.0	38.9	105.0	40.6
96.2	35.7	99.2	37.3	102.2	39.0	105.2	40.7
96.4	35.8	99.4	37.4	102.4	39.1	105.4	40.8
96.6	35.9	99.6	37.6	102.6	39.2	105.6	40.9
96.8	36.0	99.8	37.7	102.8	39.3	105.8	41.0
97.0	36.1	100.0	37.8	103.0	39.4	106.0	41.1
97.2	36.2	100.2	37.9	103.2	39.6	106.2	41.2
97.4	36.3	100.4	38.0	103.4	39.7	106.4	41.3
97.6	36.4	100.6	38.1	103.6	39.8	106.6	41.4
97.8	36.6	100.8	38.2	103.8	39.9	106.8	41.6

Note: °C = (°F − 32) × 5⁄9. Centigrade temperature equivalents rounded to one decimal place by adding 0.1 when second decimal place is 5 or greater.
The metric system replaces the term *centigrade* with *Celsius* (the inventor of the scale).

Manual of Neonatal Care

Manual of Neonatal Care

Third Edition

Joint Program in Neonatology
Harvard Medical School
Beth Israel Hospital
Brigham and Women's Hospital
Children's Hospital
Boston

Edited by
John P. Cloherty, M.D.,
and Ann R. Stark, M.D.

Foreword by
Merton Bernfield, M.D.
Clement A. Smith Professor of Pediatrics and Professor of Anatomy and Cellular Biology, Harvard Medical School; Director, Joint Program in Neonatology, Beth Israel Hospital, Brigham and Women's Hospital, and Children's Hospital, Boston

Little, Brown and Company
Boston/Toronto/London

Third Edition

Third Printing April 1993

Library of Congress Catalog Card No.
91-60067

ISBN 0-316-14762-1

Printed in the United States of America

SEM

To Laura, Gregory, Maryann, Joan, Danny, Tommy, Anne, David, Ann, and Peter

Contents

Contributing Authors

Angela M. Bader, M.D.
Assistant Professor of Anesthesia, Harvard Medical School; Staff Anesthesiologist, Brigham and Women's Hospital, Boston

Diana W. Bianchi, M.D.
Assistant Professor of Pediatrics, Harvard Medical School; Attending Neonatologist and Geneticist, Joint Program in Neonatology, Beth Israel Hospital, Brigham and Women's Hospital, and Children's Hospital, Boston

Brian S. Bradley, M.S., M.D.
Clinical Assistant Professor of Pediatrics and Communicable Diseases, University of Michigan Medical School, Ann Arbor; Staff Neonatologist, Department of Pediatrics, Henry Ford Hospital, Detroit (former Fellow in Joint Program in Neonatology)

John P. Cloherty, M.D.
Associate Clinical Professor of Pediatrics, Harvard Medical School; Associate Neonatologist, Joint Program in Neonatology, Beth Israel Hospital, Brigham and Women's Hospital, and Children's Hospital, Boston

William D. Cochran, M.D.
Associate Clinical Professor in Pediatrics, Harvard Medical School; Associate Neonatologist, Joint Program in Neonatology, Beth Israel Hospital, Brigham and Women's Hospital, and Children's Hospital; Physician-in-Charge, Special Care Nursery, Beth Israel Hospital, Boston

F. Sessions Cole, M.D.
Assistant Professor of Pediatrics, Harvard Medical School; Associate Neonatologist, Joint Program in Neonatology, Beth Israel Hospital, Brigham and Women's Hospital, Children's Hospital, Boston

Jonathan H. Cronin, M.D.
Instructor in Pediatrics, Harvard Medical School; Associate Neonatologist, Joint Program in Neonatology, Beth Israel Hospital, Brigham and Women's Hospital, and Children's Hospital, Boston

Jean B. Crouch, M.P.H., R.D.
Nutrition Support Service, Brigham and Women's Hospital, Boston

Joan C. Downey, M.D., M.P.H.
Instructor in Pediatrics, Washington University School of Medicine; Instructor in Pediatrics, Division of Newborn Medicine, St. Louis Children's Hospital, St. Louis (former Fellow in Joint Program in Neonatology)

Jeanne W. Driscoll, M.S., R.N., C.S.
Private Practice in Psychotherapy; Vice President, Lifecycle Products, Inc., Newton, Massachusetts

Eric C. Eichenwald, M.D.
Instructor in Pediatrics, Harvard Medical School; Associate Neonatologist, Joint Program in Neonatology, Beth Israel Hospital, Brigham and Women's Hospital, and Children's Hospital, Boston

Michael F. Epstein, M.D.
Associate Professor of Pediatrics, Harvard Medical School; Vice President for Medical Affairs, Children's Hospital, Boston

Margaret Flanagan-Everett, M.D.
Instructor in Pediatrics, Harvard Medical School; Associate Neonatologist, Joint Program in Neonatology, Beth Israel Hospital, Brigham and Women's Hospital, Children's Hospital, Boston

Michael Fant, M.D., Ph.D.
Assistant Professor of Pediatrics, University of Texas Southwestern Medical Center at Dallas Southwestern Medical School; Staff Neonatologist, Parkland Memorial Hospital and St. Paul Hospital, Dallas (former Fellow in Joint Program in Neonatology)

James Filiano, M.D.
Clinical Instructor in Neurology, Harvard Medical School; Assistant Neurologist, Children's Hospital, Boston

Alan M. Fujii, M.D.
Instructor in Pediatrics, Harvard Medical School; Associate Neonatologist, Joint Program in Neonatology, Beth Israel Hospital, Brigham and Women's Hospital, Children's Hospital, Boston; Director, Special Care Nursing, Winchester Hospital, Winchester

Allen M. Goorin, M.D.
Assistant Professor in Pediatrics, Harvard Medical School; Hematology-Oncology, Children's Hospital and Brigham and Women's Hospital, Boston

Michael F. Greene, M.D.
Associate Professor, Department of Obstetrics and Gynecology, Harvard Medical School; Director, Maternal-Fetal Medicine, Brigham and Women's Hospital, Boston

Paul P. Griffin, M.D.
Professor of Orthopaedic Surgery, Medical University of South Carolina; Attending Physician, Department of Orthopaedic Surgery, Medical University Hospital, Charleston (former Chief of Orthopedics, Children's Hospital, Boston)

Nicholas G. Guerina, M.D., Ph.D.
Instructor in Pediatrics, Harvard Medical School; Associate in Infectious Diseases, Children's Hospital; Associate Neonatologist, Joint Program in Neonatology, Beth Israel Hospital, Brigham and Women's Hospital, and Children's Hospital, Boston

Susan Hall Guttentag, M.D.
Fellow in Newborn Medicine, Joint Program in Neonatology, Beth Israel Hospital, Brigham and Women's Hospital, and Children's Hospital, Boston

Rogers G. Howell II, M.D.
Former Instructor in Pediatrics, Harvard Medical School; Former Fellow in Neonatology, Joint Program in Neonatology, Beth Israel Hospital, Brigham and Women's Hospital, and Children's Hospital, Boston; Chief, Neonatology Service, Thirteenth Air Force Medical Center, Clark Air Base, Philippines

John P. Hubbell, Jr., M.D.
Assistant Clinical Professor, Emeritus, of Pediatrics, Harvard Medical School; Director, Normal Newborn Nurseries, Brigham and Women's Hospital, Boston

Julie R. Ingelfinger, M.D.
Associate Professor of Pediatrics, Harvard Medical School; Co-Chief, Pediatric Nephrology, Massachusetts General Hospital, Boston

Lawrence C. Kaplan, M.D.
Assistant Professor of Pediatrics, University of Connecticut School of Medicine, Farmington; Director, Disabled Child Care Program, Department of Pediatrics, Newington Children's Hospital, Newington, Connecticut (former Chief, Birth Defects Clinic, Children's Hospital, Boston)

James R. Kasser, M.D.
Assistant Professor of Orthopedic Surgery, Harvard Medical School; Associate Chief of Orthopedic Surgery, Children's Hospital, Boston

Sherwin V. Kevy, M.D.
Associate Professor of Pediatrics, Harvard Medical School; Director of Transfusion Service, Children's Hospital, Boston

Stella Kourembanas, M.D.
Assistant Professor of Pediatrics, Harvard Medical School; Associate Neonatologist, Joint Program in Neonatology, Beth Israel Hospital, Brigham and Women's Hospital, and Children's Hospital, Boston

Karl Kuban, M.D.
Assistant Professor of Neurology, Harvard Medical School; Assistant in Neurology, Children's Hospital, Boston

Gretchen Lawhon, R.N., M.S.N.	Doctoral Student, University of Washington School of Nursing, Seattle; Former Neonatal Clinical Nurse Specialist, and Assistant Director, Neonatal Individualized Developmental Care and Assessment Program, Brigham and Women's Hospital, Boston
Harvey Levy, M.D.	Associate Professor of Neurology, Harvard Medical School; Senior Associate in Medicine, Children's Hospital, Boston
Helen G. Liley, M.B., Ch.B.	Instructor in Pediatrics, Harvard Medical School; Associate Neonatologist, Joint Program in Neonatology, Beth Israel Hospital, Brigham and Women's Hospital, and Children's Hospital, Boston
James E. Lock, M.D.	Associate Professor of Pediatrics, Harvard Medical School; Chief of Clinical Cardiology, Children's Hospital, Boston
Denise Poirier Maguire, R.N.C., M.S.	Nurse Manager, Special Care Nursery, Beth Israel Hospital, Boston
Celeste M. Marx, Pharm.D.	Assistant Professor of Pediatrics, Case Western Reserve School of Medicine; Section of Pediatric Pharmacology, Division of Pediatric Emergency Medicine, Rainbow Babies and Children's Hospital, Cleveland (previously Director of Drug Information Center, Brigham and Women's Hospital, Boston)
Karen R. McAlmon, M.D.	Instructor in Pediatrics, Harvard Medical School; Associate in Joint Program in Neonatology, Beth Israel Hospital, Brigham and Women's Hospital, and Children's Hospital, Boston
Marie C. McCormick, M.D., Sc.D.	Associate Professor of Pediatrics, Harvard Medical School; Director, Infant Follow-up Program of The Joint Program in Neonatology, Children's Hospital, Boston
Alexandra Melzar, R.N.C., B.S.	Staff Nurse, Brigham and Women's Hospital, Boston
John M. North, M.D.	Neonatologist, Department of Pediatrics, The Fairfax Hospital, Falls Church, Virginia (former Fellow in Joint Program in Neonatology)

Gerard W. Ostheimer, M.D.	Associate Professor of Anesthesia, Harvard Medical School; Vice Chairman, Department of Anesthesia, Brigham and Women's Hospital, Boston
Richard B. Parad, M.D.	Instructor in Pediatrics, Harvard Medical School; Associate Neonatologist, Joint Program in Neonatology, Beth Israel Hospital, Brigham and Women's Hospital, and Children's Hospital, Boston
DeWayne M. Pursley, M.D.	Instructor in Pediatrics, Harvard Medical School; Associate Neonatologist, Joint Program in Neonatology, Beth Israel Hospital, Brigham and Women's Hospital, and Children's Hospital, Boston
Douglas Richardson, M.D., M.B.A.	Instructor in Pediatrics, Harvard Medical School; Attending Neonatologist, Joint Program in Neonatology, Beth Israel Hospital, Brigham and Women's Hospital, and Children's Hospital, Boston
Steven A. Ringer, M.D., Ph.D.	Instructor in Pediatrics, Harvard Medical School; Medical Director, Newborn Intensive Care Unit, Brigham and Women's Hospital; Associate Neonatologist, Joint Program in Neonatology, Beth Israel Hospital, Brigham and Women's Hospital, and Children's Hospital, Boston
Lewis P. Rubin, M.D.	Assistant Professor of Pediatrics, Division of Biology and Medicine, Brown University Program in Medicine; Staff Neonatologist, Women and Infants Hospital, Providence (former Associate Neonatologist, Joint Program in Neonatology)
Mary Deming Scott, M.D.	Instructor in Pediatrics, Harvard Medical School; Assistant in Medicine, Children's Hospital, Boston
E. Manning Sears, M.D.	Instructor in Pediatrics, Harvard Medical School; Senior Pediatrician, Brigham and Women's Hospital; Associate in Newborn Medicine, Children's Hospital, Boston

Charles F. Simmons, Jr., M.D.	Assistant Professor of Pediatrics, Harvard Medical School; Associate Neonatologist, Joint Program in Neonatology, Beth Israel Hospital, Brigham and Women's Hospital, and Children's Hospital, Boston
Stephanie J. Skoolicas, A.D.N., R.N.C.	Senior Staff Nurse, Neonatal Intensive Care Unit, Children's Hospital, Boston
Evan Y. Snyder, M.D., Ph.D.	Instructor in Neurology (Neonatology), Harvard Medical School; Associate Neonatologist, Joint Program in Neonatology, Beth Israel Hospital, Brigham and Women's Hospital, and Children's Hospital; Assistant in Neurology, Children's Hospital, Boston
Ann R. Stark, M.D.	Associate Professor of Pediatrics, Harvard Medical School; Medical Director, Newborn Intensive Care Unit, Children's Hospital; Chairman of NICU Directors, Joint Program in Neonatology, Beth Israel Hospital, Brigham and Women's Hospital, and Children's Hospital, Boston
Cheryl A. Stoukides, Pharm.D.	Clinical Assistant Professor of Pharmacy, University of Rhode Island; Director, Drug Information Center of University of Rhode Island, Roger Williams Medical Center, Providence (former Director of Drug Information Center, Brigham and Women's Hospital, Boston)
John S. Torday, Ph.D.	Assistant Professor of Pediatrics (Physiology), Harvard Medical School; Director, Fetal Lung Maturity Laboratory, Brigham and Women's Hospital, Boston
Linda J. Van Marter, M.D., M.P.H.	Instructor in Pediatrics, Harvard Medical School; Associate Neonatologist, Beth Israel Hospital, Brigham and Women's Hospital, Children's Hospital, Boston

Foreword

Birth initiates the progression of independent life events that each of us experiences. For some infants, the initial events take place in a newborn intensive care unit, an alien environment for the infant and for most other members of society, including many physicians who care for children. This *Manual* provides clearly defined, practical, and proven approaches to the major problems affecting these infants. The success of the prior two editions attests to its capacity to improve the clinical care given in this environment. We are indebted to the faculty and fellows of the Joint Program in Neonatology of Harvard Medical School and especially to John P. Cloherty and Ann R. Stark for their leadership in crafting this tool for the care of sick newborns.

Neonatal medicine is a young discipline and its practitioners can be justifiably proud of their accomplishments. Substantive improvements in the United States in infant mortality, beginning in the late 1960s, can be linked directly to the introduction of intensive medical care for newborns. The changes in practice in newborn nurseries were followed by changes in obstetric practice directed toward evaluation of the fetus and by the introduction of regionalized perinatal care. These successful efforts led to the increasingly aggressive application of medical technology in nurseries and to the publication in 1980 of the *Manual of Neonatal Care.*

The care of ill newborns has evolved rapidly since the appearance of the first edition of this *Manual.* Advances in reproductive and developmental biology, in prenatal assessment of the fetus, and in respiratory, fluid, and nutritional support technology have provided newly potent means of improving the survival of smaller and sicker infants. There has been a concomitant increase in the human and financial costs of these improvements. We place new emphasis on according these infants a moral and social status that can influence their care and that often imposes ethical concerns. We ask more frequently whether the resources expended in the care of these infants might be better expended in the prevention of these births, especially in communities where a disproportionate number of these infants are born.

Medical care for the ill newborn is changing at a rapid pace. Infant deaths in the United States due to immaturity—once the preeminent problem in the nursery—are now exceeded by deaths arising from malformations. Scrutiny of the consequences of the medical interventions in the nursery continues to revamp once standard practices. We expect care to continue to improve in the future because the explosion in new knowledge of the biology of developing organisms has yet to be felt in our intensive care nurseries.

Much of the improvement in infant mortality rates and in the quality of survivors of intensive care nurseries has come from research. Although the Joint Program in Neonatology is committed to providing the best possible medical care to newborns, as can be seen in the pages of this *Manual,* it is equally devoted to expanding knowledge relevant to the newborn and to training future leaders in newborn medicine. Our research and training focus on two areas—developmental biology and perinatal epidemiology—because we believe that optimal care in the future will require in-depth understanding of both the molecular physiology of developing cells and the clinically significant behavior of pregnant women and their infants.

Our fellows in training acquire credentials in both the clinical and scientific bases of newborn medicine. They are the initial judges of the approaches to care outlined here and they have contributed to this *Manual* in many ways, most importantly by challenging us continually to ask more incisive questions and to generate more complete answers.

Merton Bernfield, M.D.

Preface

The third edition of the *Manual of Neonatal Care* of the Joint Program in Neonatology (JPN) builds on the two previous editions (1980, 1985) and updates our current practice in perinatal and neonatal medicine. The JPN, which has grown to 23 attending neonatologists and 16 fellows, is responsible for over 16,000 newborns delivered annually at the Beth Israel Hospital (BIH) and the Brigham and Women's Hospital (BWH, formerly the Boston Lying-In Hospital and the Boston Hospital for Women). We care for these infants in the Special Care Nursery at the BIH and the Newborn Intensive Care Unit (NICU) and Regular Nurseries of BWH. Because these patients are inborn, the obstetricians and neonatologists cooperate closely in providing prenatal and intrapartum care. The BWH and the BIH are referral centers for women with pregnancies complicated by maternal illness, fetal problems, and anticipated neonatal problems. This prenatal and perinatal experience is reflected in the chapters on Maternal Diabetes, Maternal-Fetal Thyroid Disorders, Infection, Fetal Assessment, Identifying the High Risk Newborn, Resuscitation in the Delivery Room, Neural Tube Defects, and Genetic Issues Presenting in the Nursery. The close involvement with families in an inborn hospital population is reflected in the chapters on Breast-Feeding, Developmentally Supportive Interventions, and Maternal Use of Drugs During Pregnancy and Lactation. In addition, through our NICU at Children's Hospital, members of the JPN provide transport and care for critically ill newborns born at other hospitals throughout New England. In this capacity we provide telephone consultation to many obstetricians, pediatricians, and nurses at community hospitals in the area. Many of the infants seen in this outborn population have problems such as perinatal encephalopathy, cardiac disease, extreme prematurity, respiratory disorders, malformations, and metabolic defects. As a result of our experience, we have developed practical approaches to common problems that affect neonates in a major perinatal center; these approaches are outlined in the *Manual*.

The *Manual* is organized into four parts: Maternal and Fetal Problems; Neonatal Problems; Procedures; and Appendixes, which discuss medications used during pregnancy, breast-feeding, and in the neonatal period. We have outlined our current approaches to these problems and procedures, although we recognize that many areas of controversy exist and often there is more than one approach to a problem. We have added new chapters on Developmentally Supportive Interventions, Decision Making and Ethical Dilemmas, and Auditory and Ophthalmologic Evaluation. The chapters on Infection, Genetics Issues Presenting in the Nursery, Chronic Lung Disease, Congenital Heart Disease, Shock, Blood Products Used in the Newborn, Metabolic Problems, and Drugs Used in Pregnancy and Lactation have been expanded. All other chapters have been extensively revised and updated.

For their efforts on behalf of the care of the newborns and the training of physicians interested in newborn medicine, we are indebted to Clement Smith, Mary Ellen Avery, Merton Bernfield, H. William Taeusch, Jr., William D. Cochran, Barry T. Smith,

Stewart Clifford, and Nicholas M. Nelson. We also thank the parents, nurses, medical students, house officers, fellows, and members of the neonatal and obstetric staff for their constructive suggestions. For their editorial assistance and advice, we thank Executive Editor, Susan F. Pioli; Senior Editorial Assistant, Karen Oberheim; Production Editor, Karen Feeney; Production Supervisor, Lou Bruno; and the rest of the staff of Little, Brown and Company, Boston.

J.P.C.
A.R.S.

Acknowledgments

The authors thank Margarita Rosado for her extraordinary effort in typing the manuscript. We thank Julie Reid, Mardy Murphy, and Coral Amarteifio for their administrative help in organization and secretarial assistance. We express appreciation to our many local and national colleagues for contributing chapters in the manual or for permission to use data, illustrations, or tables.

Fellows of the Joint Program in Neonatology (1989–90): Joan C. Downey, M.D.; Eric G. Eichenwald, M.D.; Margaret Flanagan Everett, M.D.; Jeffery Garland, M.D.; James Gray, M.D.; Susan Hall Guttentag, M.D.; Kenneth Huttner, M.D.; Kenneth Kupke, M.D.; David Ma, M.D.; Virginia Nichols, M.D.; James Pellegrini, M.D.; DeWayne M. Pursley, M.D.; Istvan Seri, M.D.; Jane Stewart, M.D.; and Miles Tsuji, M.D.

Special thanks go to the following people, who are not listed as contributing authors but who assisted in preparing previous editions, reviewed the present edition, or helped to make this work possible.

Mary Ellen Avery, M.D.
Merton Bernfield, M.D.
Stewart Clifford, M.D.
Ann Colangelo, R.N.
Willa Drummond, M.D.
Frederic D. Frigoletto, M.D.
Donald C. Fyler, M.D.
Luke Gillespie, M.D.
Donald Goldmann, M.D.
Angelyn Konugres, Ph.D.
Thomas Kulick, M.D.
Kenneth McIntosh, M.D.
Alexander S. Nadas, M.D.
Mark Phillippe, M.D.
Istvan Seri, M.D.
Richard Slavin, R.R.T.
Barry T. Smith, M.D.
Clement Smith, M.D.
H. William Taeusch, Jr., M.D.
Joseph Volpe, M.D.

We also offer grateful acknowledgment to all the nurses, residents, parents, and babies who provide the source and measure of usefulness of the information contained in this book.

Maternal and Fetal Problems

Notice. The indications and dosages of all drugs in this book have been recommended in the medical literature and conform to the practices of the general medical community. The medications described do not necessarily have specific approval by the Food and Drug Administration for use in the diseases and dosages for which they are recommended. The package insert for each drug should be consulted for use and dosage as approved by the FDA. Because standards for usage change, it is advisable to keep abreast of revised recommendations, particularly those concerning new drugs.

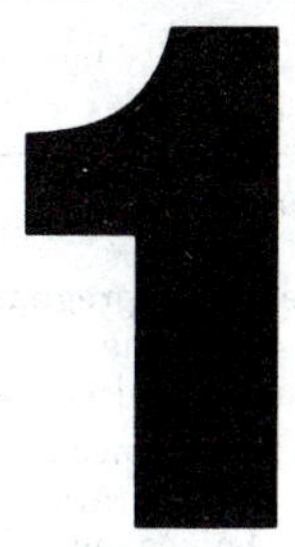

Metabolic Disorders

Maternal Diabetes

John P. Cloherty and
Michael F. Epstein

The recent reduction in perinatal mortality and morbidity in infants of diabetic mothers (IDMs) has been due to improvements in medical and obstetric care of mothers and advances in the care of newborns. One of the major causes of this improvement has been the prolongation of diabetic pregnancies, and the ability to assess pulmonary maturity in the fetus which has reduced the incidence of respiratory distress syndrome (RDS) in IDMs. Infants of mothers with severe renal and vascular disease are often delivered because of maternal problems (hypertension, renal failure) or fetal distress. These infants are more likely to have such complications as asphyxia, respiratory distress syndrome, jaundice, and poor feeding.

Before the delivery of the IDMs, there should be clear communication among specialists in medicine, obstetrics, and pediatrics so that problems can be anticipated. Areas that should be discussed are (1) outcome of previous pregnancies, (2) gestational age and fetal assessment, (3) control of diabetes during pregnancy, (4) present maternal diabetic and medical state, (5) maternal hemoglobin A_1 (HbA_1) levels in pregnancy, (6) results of fetal monitoring for malformations or distress, (7) fetal size, (8) evidence for pulmonary maturity, and (9) monitoring during labor.

I. **Classification.** Mothers with diabetes are classified according to White's classification (Table 1-1). There is a relationship between perinatal outcome and White class [8]. The risk of complications is minimal in gestational diabetes, although macrosomia and neonatal hypoglycemia are sometimes seen. The most difficult maternal, fetal, and neonatal problems occur in women with renal, cardiac, or retinal disease. Class F disease (renal) has an adverse affect on fetal outcome. It is associated with the necessity for early delivery. Class H (cardiac disease) is associated with maternal death. Retinopathy may progress during pregnancy.

II. **Maternal-fetal problems**

   A. **Fertility.** Diabetic women appear to have normal fertility.

   B. **Abortions.** There is no increase in the spontaneous abortion rate in early pregnancy in **well-controlled** diabetic pregnancies as compared with nondiabetic pregnancies. The spontaneous abortion rate in nondiabetic pregnancy is 16 percent. Women with poor diabetic control in pregnancy had a significantly increased incidence of spontaneous abortion [1,4,17].

   C. **Problems during pregnancy and delivery** [7]

      1. In the first half of pregnancy, metabolism is anabolic. Hypoglycemia and ketonuria are common. The nausea and vomiting seen in any pregnancy may make control difficult. Moderate hypoglycemia not associated with hypotension may not be harmful to the fetus.

      2. In the second trimester, the **insulin requirement** increases. This in-

Table 1-1. White's classification of maternal diabetes (revised*)

Gestational diabetes (GD):	Diabetes not known to be present before pregnancy Abnormal glucose tolerance test in pregnancy
GD diet	Euglycemia maintained by diet alone
GD insulin	Diet alone insufficient; insulin required
Class A:	Chemical diabetes; glucose intolerance prior to pregnancy; treated by diet alone; rarely seen Prediabetes; history of large babies more than kg or unexplained stillbirths after 28 weeks.
Class B:	Insulin-dependent; onset after 20 years of age; duration less than 10 years
Class C:	C_1: Onset at 10 to 19 years of age C_2: Duration 10 to 19 years
Class D:	D_1: Onset before 10 years of age D_2: Duration 20 years D_3: Calcification of vessels of the leg (macrovascular disease) D_4: Benign retinopathy (microvascular disease) D_5: Hypertension (not preeclampsia)
Class F:	Nephropathy with over 500 mg per day of proteinuria
Class R:	Proliferative retinopathy or vitreous hemorrhage
Class RF:	Criteria for both classes R and F coexist
Class G:	Many reproductive failures
Class H:	Clinical evidence of arteriosclerotic heart disease
*Class T:	Prior renal transplantation

Note: All classes below A require insulin. Classes R, F, RF, H, and T have no criteria for age of onset or duration of disease but usually occur in long-term diabetes.
Source: Modified from Hare, J. W. Gestational Diabetes. In *Diabetes Complicating Pregnancy: The Joslin Clinic Method.* New York: Alan R. Liss, 1989. Chap. 3.

creased requirement is sometimes associated with **ketoacidosis,** which may result in high fetal mortality.

3. In the third trimester, a major problem is **sudden, unexpected fetal death.** Such deaths are sometimes associated with ketoacidosis, preeclampsia, or maternal vascular disease of the decidua and myometrium but many are unexplained. The incidence of this problem has decreased during the past 10 years with the use of tests of fetal well-being, but still occurs occasionally.
4. In the third trimester, class F mothers may have anemia, hypertension and decreased renal function. Class H women have a great risk of myocardial failure with infarction. Class R women have a risk of neovascularization, vitreous hemorrhage, or retinal detachment; their infants are usually delivered by cesarean section.
5. Fetal macrosomia and enlargement of the cord and placenta may be seen in gestational diabetics and in class A, B, C, and some D diabetic pregnancies [12]. Macrosomia increases the potential for difficult delivery, obstetric trauma, or primary cesarean section.
6. In diabetic women with vascular disease (especially class F), there is an increased risk of in utero growth retardation (20 percent) [10]. Th

growth retardation is associated with a small infarcted placenta, decreased uteroplacental perfusion, decreased urinary estriols, and increased incidence of in utero fetal death, fetal distress, neonatal complications, and poor outcome. Hypertension in pregnancy is the largest cause of premature delivery and thus of respiratory distress syndrome in our patient population [3].

7. Many diabetic pregnancies are associated with **polyhydramnios.** Although this is usually not a sign of significant fetal anomaly (as it is in nondiabetic pregnancies), it may be associated with premature rupture of membranes, early cord prolapse, or abruptio placentae. Women with the best metabolic control have the least polyhydramnios.
8. The **placenta** has extramedullary hematopoiesis in diabetic pregnancies, and this observation may be helpful in the postpartum investigation of the cause of late stillbirths.

III. Pregnancy management [7,12]

A. Diabetic women should be educated about the need to gain metabolic control of their diabetes before conception. This control may decrease the incidence of major congenital anomalies. Good control throughout the pregnancy will improve the perinatal outcome. All pregnant patients should have a screening test for gestational diabetes (GD). If they have GD or class A diabetes, they should be managed by diet to keep their fasting plasma glucose level below 105 mg/dl and their postprandial plasma glucose level below 120 mg/dl. If these goals are not reached by dietary therapy, then insulin should be used. Oral agents should not be used because they cross the placenta and may be associated with severe neonatal hypoglycemia if used near the time of birth [31]. Gestational diabetics who can maintain fasting plasma glucose levels under 105 mg/dl and 2-hour postprandial blood sugar levels under 120 mg/dl on a diabetic diet should be followed with weekly blood sugar determinations because 15 percent of them will eventually require insulin in pregnancy. If gestational diabetics are maintained on diet alone, they do not appear to be at risk for stillbirth. If they develop an insulin requirement, required insulin in the past, or have preeclampsia or a past history of stillbirth, they should be treated as any other insulin-requiring diabetic. Diabetics who require insulin should maintain fasting plasma glucose levels of less than 105 mg/dl and postprandial levels of less than 120 mg/dl. This will require home monitoring of capillary blood glucose, urine glucose, and acetone levels several times a day along with multiple daily injections of insulin. Hemoglobin A_1 (HbA_1) is measured to assess control over a longer period of time.

B. At the first prenatal visit, a complete medical history is obtained and a thorough physical examination is done. The estimated date of conception is determined by history of last menstrual period and ultrasound. Besides the usual prenatal tests, the following studies are done: glycosylated hemoglobin (HbA_1), thyroid function studies, a 24-hour urine for total protein and creatinine clearance, and an ophthalmologic evaluation. The mother should begin a comprehensive diabetes education program that stresses the importance of good glycemic control to reduce perinatal morbidity and mortality. Mothers in poor metabolic control at this visit or at any time should be admitted for regulation.

C. At the next visit, the mother's situation is reviewed and her diabetic control is assessed. She is informed about the risks of congenital malformations in diabetic women in relationship to her glycemic control as measured by her level of glycoslated hemoglobin (see sec. **V.F**).

D. In the second trimester, anticipate an increasing insulin requirement to avoid ketoacidosis, which is associated with fetal death. Measure maternal serum alpha-fetoprotein at 16 to 18 weeks (see Chaps. 3 and 21). Diabetic pregnancies are associated with a lower maternal serum alpha-fetoprotein level than nondiabetic pregnancies [18]. Do fetal ultrasonography at 18 weeks to rule out anomalies and to confirm the duration of the pregnancy. This examination, when performed by experienced personnel, will diagnose most (95 percent) major anomalies of the central nervous system, heart, skeleton, ga trointestinal tract, and urinary tract [5]. Monitor hematocrit, renal functic blood pressure, diabetic control, and fetal growth.

E. The problems in the third trimester are fetal demise, premature delivery, a macrosomia. In the third trimester there is also usually a rise in insulin quirement until 34 to 36 weeks. The mother must be monitored for glycem control, polyhydramnios, preeclampsia, premature labor, and decreasing nal function. The fetus must be monitored for well-being, size, and pulmona maturity. Repeat ultrasonography at 26 to 28 weeks, and start weekly nc stress tests (NSTs) or oxytocin challenge tests (OCT). Mothers with proble may need to start this monitoring at 26 weeks. Before 30 weeks, the OCT probably more reliable than the NST. In the Joslin Pregnancy Clinic wi careful maternal care and fetal monitoring there have been only two une plained, unanticipated fetal deaths after a normal nonstress test or oxytoc challenge test since 1976 (about 1000 patients) [7]. This is still a significa potential problem, and results such as these can only be obtained with mu meticulous effort.

Amniocentesis is performed at 38 weeks for measurement of the lecithi sphingomyelin (L/S) ratio and saturated phosphatidylcholine (SPC) level, u less there are fetal or maternal reasons to deliver earlier. In our laborato in nondiabetic pregnancies with an L/S ratio greater than 2:1, there is a percent incidence of respiratory distress syndrome (RDS); with an SI greater than 500 μg/dl, there is a 1 percent incidence (see Tests for Pulmona Surfactant in Chap. 13). There are many reports of RDS in IDMs with L ratios greater than 2:1 [11]. The level of L/S and SPC considered "mature" an IDM should depend on the experience of the local laboratory. In our hc pital, 10 percent of IDMs with L/S ratios between 2.0 and 3.5:1.0 have RD and 1 percent of IDMs with L/S ratios greater than 3.5:1.0 have RDS. An SI level of 500 μg/dl is usually considered mature in non-IDMs; in our hospit however, 11 percent of IDMs with SPC levels between 501 and 1000 μg/dl h RDS, and 1 percent of IDMs with SPC levels over 1000 μg/dl had RDS. In t 244 diabetic pregnancies from which these data are taken, none had RDS both the SPC level was greater than 1000 μg/dl and the L/S ratio was ov 3.5:1.0 (Table 1-2). More recent data are shown in Table 1-3. We thus consid a fetus of a diabetic mother to have mature indices when the L/S ratio is ov 3.5 and the SPC level is over 1000 μg/dl. The tables give the risk of RDS that the risks of a premature delivery can be properly evaluated. Diabe pregnancies requiring insulin should continue to 38 to 39 weeks as long as (there are no maternal contraindications and (2) there is evidence of fet growth and well-being. This practice will result in more vaginal deliverie more mature babies, and a lower perinatal mortality and morbidity [11], b cause the increased incidence of RDS in IDMs is not seen in term infants b rather in premature infants (Fig. 1-1). The time of delivery is decided in ea case by an assessment of maternal health and of the relative fetal and ne natal risks as judged by gestational age, pulmonary maturity, and tests fetal growth and well-being. Mothers with vascular complications (e. White's class F) who have proteinuria of over 400 mg per day in the first ha of their pregnancy without a urinary tract infection and who have elevat blood pressure and a creatinine clearance under 90 ml/min will often requi hospitalization at 26 weeks' gestation for bed rest and antihypertensive me ication. They are the group at greatest risk for uncontrollable hypertensi and decreasing renal function and are most likely to have fetuses with intr uterine growth retardation and fetal distress, leading to early delivery. T perinatal survival (after 24 weeks' gestation) in this group is about 85 to percent [10,12]. More recent data (after 24 weeks' gestation) from the Josl Clinic show no increased mortality but more prematurity and low bir weights [8]. There are still fetal losses in the second trimester. These mothe have an increased risk of intrapartum fetal distress, cesarean section, pe natal asphyxia, and RDS. If there are no fetal or maternal problems, insuli

Table 1-2. Lecithin-sphingomyelin ratio, saturated phosphatidylcholine level, and respiratory distress syndrome in infants of diabetic mothers at the Boston Hospital for Women 1977–1980

SPC level, μg/dl	L/S ratio			Mild, moderate, or severe RDS/total
	<2.0 : 1.0	2.0–3.4 : 1	≥3.5 : 1.0	
Not done	0/1	0/12	0/13	0/26 (0%)
≤500	6/6	1/9	1/2	8/17 (47%)
501–1000	0/2	3/20	1/15	4/37 (11%)
>1000	0/0	2/22	0/142	2/164 (1.2%)
Total (RDS)	6/9 (67%)	6/63 (10%)	2/172 (1.2%)	14/244 (5.7%)

Key: SPC = saturated phosphatidylcholine; L/S = lecithin/sphingomyelin; RDS = respiratory distress syndrome.

Table 1-3. Lecithin-sphingomyelin (L/S) ratio, saturated phosphatidylcholine (SPC) level, and RDS in infants born to mothers with insulin-requiring diabetes mellitus antedating pregnancy at the Brigham and Women's Hospital between January 1, 1983 and June 30, 1988. Samples were all obtained within 72 hours of delivery.

		Insulin-dependent diabetics L/S to delivery internal ≤ 72 hours			
L/S		SPC level, μg/dl	No RDS	RDS	Percent
≥3.5		≥1000	255	0	0
—		≥1000	288	1	0.3
≥3.5		—	285	1	0.3
2.0–3.4	and	≥1000	31	1	3.1
2.0–3.4	and	500–999	25	4	13.8
—		500–999	52	7	11.9
2.0–3.4		—	57	5	8.1

Source: From Greene, M. F., Torday, J., Wilson, M., and Richardson, D. Abstract presented at the Annual Meeting of the Society of Perinatal Obstetricians, New Orleans, La., February 1989.

requiring diabetics are delivered at 38 to 39 weeks' gestation after pulmonary maturity is documented.

Emergency delivery may be necessary even in the face of pulmonary immaturity because of maternal problems such as hypertension, decreasing renal function, and preeclampsia or because of poor fetal growth or evidence of fetal distress. Because of the difficulty in controlling the maternal diabetes while waiting for an effect, we usually do not use steroids to accelerate fetal pulmonary maturity unless the L/S ratio is less than 2:1, the SPC level is less than 500 μg/dl, and the patient is at very high risk to deliver in the following 7 days. This policy is usually followed at Brigham and Women's Hospital (BWH), but other centers may not follow it. The route of delivery is selected based on the usual obstetric indications. If the infant appears large based on clinical and ultrasonographic examination (>4000 gm), cesarean section is usually indicated because of the risk of shoulder dystocia. Prolongation of ges-

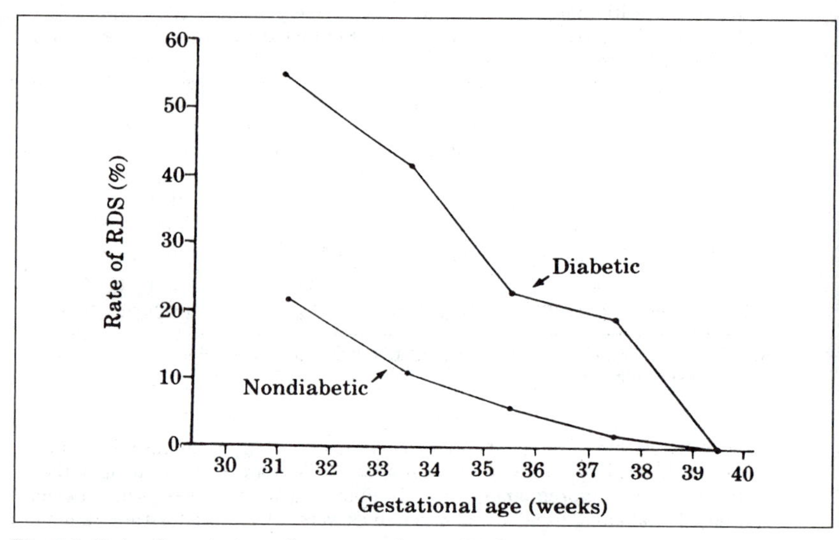

Fig. 1-1. Rate of respiratory distress syndrome (RDS) versus gestational age in nondiabetic and diabetic pregnancies at the Boston Hospital for Women from 1958–1968. (Reprinted with permission from M. Robert, Association between maternal diabetes and the respiratory distress syndrome in the newborn. *N. Engl. J. Med.* 294: 357, 1976.)

tation beyond 38 weeks does not increase the incidence of dystocia and birth trauma [11]. In labor, the maternal blood glucose level is kept around 120 mg/dl, and fetal well-being is assessed by electronic monitoring and measurement of fetal scalp pH. About 25 percent of diabetic women undergo primary cesarean section because of fetal distress in labor. Because of failure in induction, dystocia, or fetal distress in labor in our insulin-requiring diabetics, 47 percent undergo primary cesarean section. Twenty-five percent have repeat cesarean section, and 28 percent have vaginal delivery. The delivery should be planned in cooperation with a pediatrician who is informed about the mother's status and the infant's maturity. The pediatrician should be present in the delivery room and should be able to care for the infant's problems.

IV. Evaluation of the infant

A. The **evaluation** of the infant in the delivery room begins **prior to the actual delivery.** Immediately before opening the amniotic sac at the time of cesarean section, the obstetrician can obtain a sterile sample of amniotic fluid for culture, Gram stain, L/S ratio determination, shake test, or SPC determination when indicated.

B. Once the baby has been delivered, a careful assessment made on the basis of the Apgar score should indicate the need for any resuscitative efforts. The infant should be dried well and placed under a heat source, with careful attention paid to clearing the airway of mucus. The stomach is not suctioned at this point because of the risk of reflex bradycardia and apnea with pharyngeal stimulation. In the delivery room, a screening physical examination for major congenital anomalies should be performed, and the placenta also should be examined. A specimen of cord blood should be obtained for glucose determination in anticipation of the reactive hypoglycemia associated with hyperglycemia at delivery. Cord pH also should be measured (see Chap. 5).

C. In the nursery, the initial care involves the simultaneous provision of what is needed to support the infant while making a continuous evaluation of the infant. This includes providing warmth, suction, and oxygen as needed, while checking vital signs (heart rate, temperature, respiratory rate, perfusion, color, and blood pressure). The presence of cyanosis should make one consider cardiac disease, respiratory distress syndrome (RDS), transient tachypnea of the newborn (TTN), or polycythemia. A careful examination should be done for the presence of anomalies because of the 6 to 9 percent incidence of major congenital anomalies in IDM [14]. Special attention should be paid to the brain, heart, kidneys, and skeletal system. Reports indicate that IDMs have a 47 percent risk of significant hypoglycemia, a 22 percent risk of hypocalcemia, a 19 percent risk of hyperbilirubinemia, and a 34 percent risk of polycythemia [11]; therefore, the following studies are performed:

1. **Blood glucose** levels are checked at 1, 2, 3, 6, 12, 24, 26, and 48 hours. Glucose is measured with Chemstrip B-G (Bio-Dynamics, BMC, Indianapolis, Indiana). Readings under 40 mg/dl should be checked rapidly by a clinical laboratory or by Ames eyetone instrument (Ames Company, Division of Miles Laboratories, Inc., Elkhart, Indiana).
2. **Hematocrit** levels are checked at 1 and 24 hours.
3. **Calcium** levels are checked if the baby appears jittery or is sick for any reason (see sec. **V.C**).
4. **Bilirubin** levels are checked if the baby appears jaundiced.

The infant is fed PO or is given IV glucose by 1 hour of age (see sec. **V.B**). Every effort is made to involve the parents in the care of the infant as soon as possible.

V. Specific problems frequently observed in IDMs

A. Respiratory distress. In a study of pregnancies from 1958 to 1968, IDMs had an approximately sixfold increased risk of HMD compared with infants of nondiabetic mothers of the same gestational age, independent of the method of delivery [22] (Figs. 1-1 and 1-2). With changes in the management of pregnant

Fig. 1-2. Rate of respiratory distress syndrome (RDS) versus gestational age according to route of delivery: vaginal (pelvic) or cesarean section (C/S). (Reprinted with permission from M. Robert, Association between maternal diabetes and the respiratory distress syndrome in the newborn. *N. Engl. J. Med.* 294: 357, 1976.)

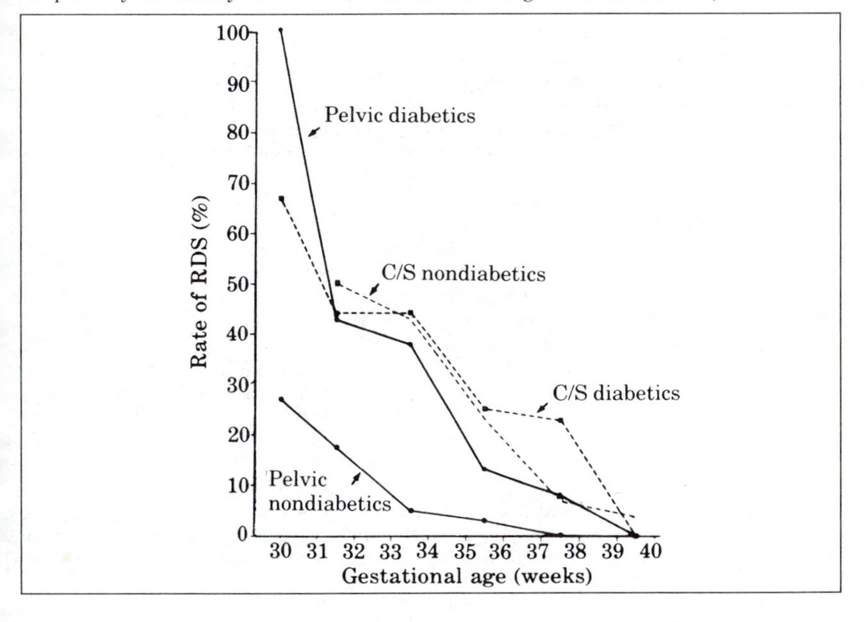

diabetics resulting in longer gestations and more vaginal deliveries, the incidence of respiratory distress syndrome (RDS) in IDMs has fallen from 28 percent in 1950–1960 [9] to 8 percent in 1975–1976 [11] to 5.7 percent in 1983–1984 [5]. Since the major difference in the incidence of RDS between diabetics and nondiabetics is in infants before 37 weeks of gestation, the longer gestations allowed by better in utero surveillance and the more accurate prediction of pulmonary maturity have had a marked influence on the reduction of RDS in IDMs. Most of the deaths from RDS are infants under 37 weeks' gestation who were delivered by cesarean section because of fetal distress or maternal indications. Delayed lung maturation in IDMs occurs because hyperinsulinemia may block cortisol induction of lung maturation. Other causes of respiratory distress that may be present in IDMs are cardiac or pulmonary anomalies (4 percent) [11], hypertrophic cardiomyopathy (1 percent) [6], transient tachypnea of the newborn, and polycythemia. Pneumonia, pneumothorax, and pneumonic and diaphragmatic hernias should be considered in the differential diagnosis. The following studies should be done in infants with respiratory distress:

1. **Gastric aspirate** should be obtained during the first hour of life, after the baby has been stabilized. A polyethylene catheter with a mucous trap is used. The gastric aspirate is used for two tests:
   a. **Gram stain** for polymorphonuclear leukocytes and bacteria.
   b. **Gastric aspirate** shake test to assess the amount of pulmonary surfactant in the newborn's lungs (see Tests for Pulmonary Surfactant in Chap. 13).
2. **Chest roentgenogram** to evaluate aeration, presence of infiltrates, cardiac size and position, and the presence of pneumothorax.
3. **Blood gases** are determined with the use of radial artery puncture or by the capillary method to evaluate gas exchange and the presence of right-to-left shunts.
4. **Electrocardiogram, blood pressure measurements,** and an **echocardiogram** should be done if hypertrophic cardiomyopathy or a cardiac anomaly is thought to be present.
5. **Cultures** should be taken from gastric aspirate, urine, and blood. Spinal fluid examination and culture should be included if the infant's condition allows. The differential diagnosis and management of respiratory disorders is discussed in Chapter 13.

B. **Hypoglycemia.** Hypoglycemia is defined as a blood glucose level under 30 mg/dl in any infant, regardless of gestational age and whether associated with symptoms or not.

1. The **incidence** of hypoglycemia in IDMs is from 30 to 40 percent [11]. The onset is frequently within 1 to 2 hours of age and is most common in macrosomic infants.
2. The **pathogenesis** of the neonatal hypoglycemia in IDMs is explained by the maternal hyperglycemia–fetal hyperinsulinism hypothesis of Pederson. The correlation between fetal macrosomia, elevated HbA_1 in maternal and cord blood, and neonatal hypoglycemia, as well as between elevated cord blood c-peptide or immunoreactive insulin levels and hypoglycemia, suggests that control of maternal blood sugar in the last trimester may decrease the incidence of neonatal hypoglycemia in IDMs [13,19,24]. Some studies have shown less neonatal hypoglycemia if the maternal blood sugar level is in the normal range at delivery. Mothers should not receive large doses of glucose before or at delivery because this may stimulate an insulin response in the hyperinsulinemic offspring. (From 1977 to 1980 at the Boston Hospital for Women, the mean blood sugar levels of diabetic mothers at delivery were 300, 276, 120, and 140 mg/dl for each year, respectively. There was no change in the incidence of neonatal hypoglycemia.) We attempt to keep the maternal blood sugar level at delivery around 120 mg/dl. Hypoglycemia in small-for-

gestational-age (SGA) infants born to mothers with vascular disease may be due to inadequate glycogen stores; it may present later (e.g., at 12 to 24 hours of age). Other factors that may cause hypoglycemia in IDMs are decreased catecholamine and glycogen secretion as well as inadequate substrate mobilization (diminished hepatic glucose production and decreased oxygenation of fatty acids).

3. **Symptoms.** If IDMs have symptoms from hypoglycemia, they usually are quiet and lethargic rather than jittery. Other symptoms such as apnea, tachypnea, respiratory distress, hypotonia, shock, cyanosis, and seizures may occur. If symptoms are present, the infant is probably at greater risk for sequelae than if asymptomatic. The significance of **hypoglycemia without symptoms** is unclear, but conservative management to maintain the blood sugar level in the normal range appears to be indicated.
4. **Diagnosis.** Blood glucose level is measured at birth and at 1, 2, 3, 6, 12, 24, and 48 hours. It is measured more often if the infant is symptomatic, if the infant has had a low blood glucose level, and to see the response to therapy. We use Chemstrip B-G for screening and the laboratory for confirmation (see Chap. 24).
5. **Treatment**
   a. **Asymptomatic infants with normal blood glucose levels**
      (1) In our nursery, we begin to feed "well" IDMs by bottle or gavage with dextrose 10% (5 ml/kg body weight) at or before 1 hour of age. Infants less than 2 kg should not be given oral feedings; they should have parenteral dextrose starting in the first hour of life. Larger infants can be fed hourly for three or four feedings until the blood sugar determinations are stable. The feedings can then be given every 2 hours and later every 3 hours; as the interval between feedings increases, the volume is increased.
      (2) If the infant feeds successfully by 12 hours of age and the blood sugar level is normal, he or she should be given 20 cal per 30 ml of formula, with extra dextrose added as needed. This method of rapid oral feeding will prevent or correct the hypoglycemia in most "well" IDMs.
      (3) If by 2 hours of age the blood glucose level is low (under 30 mg/dl) despite feeding, or if feedings are not tolerated, as indicated by large volumes retained in the stomach, parenteral treatment is indicated to raise the blood glucose level.
   b. **Symptomatic infants, infants with a low blood glucose level** after an enteral feed, **sick infants,** or **infants less than 2 kg in weight**
      (1) The basic element in treatment is **IV glucose administration.** This must be done through a reliable route.
         (a) Administration of IV glucose is usually by peripheral veins. These sites are free of the infectious and thrombotic complications of central catheters. Peripheral lines may be difficult to place in obese IDMs, and sudden interruption of the infusion may cause a reactive hypoglycemia in these hyperinsulinemic infants. Use of an indwelling peripheral venous catheter will eliminate the latter problem. In emergency situations with symptomatic babies, we have utilized umbilical venous catheters placed in the inferior vena cava until a stable peripheral line is placed.
         (b) **Specific treatment** is determined by the baby's condition. If the infant is in distress (e.g., seizure or respiratory compromise), 0.5 to 1.0 gm glucose per kilogram of body weight is given by an IV push of 2 to 4 ml/kg 25% dextrose in water (D/W) at a rate of 1 ml/min. For example, a 4-kg infant would receive 8 to 16 ml of 25% D/W over 8 to 16 minutes. This is followed by a continuous infusion of dextrose at a rate of 4 to

8 mg glucose per kilogram of body weight per minute. The concentration of dextrose in the IV fluid will depend on the total daily fluid requirement. For example, on day 1, the usual fluid intake is 65 ml/kg, or 0.045 ml/kg per minute. Therefore, 10% D/W would provide 4.5 mg glucose per kilogram per minute, and 15% D/W would provide 6.75 mg glucose per kilogram per minute. In other words, 10% D/W at a standard IV fluid maintenance rate usually supplies sufficient glucose to raise the blood glucose level above 30 mg/dl. The concentration of dextrose and the infusion rates, however, are increased as necessary to maintain the blood glucose in the normal range.

Another method is to give 200 mg of glucose per kilogram of body weight (2 ml/kg of 10% dextrose) over 2 to 3 minutes. This is followed by a maintenance drip of 6 to 8 mg of glucose per kilogram per minute (10% dextrose at 80 to 120 ml/kg per day) (see Chap. 24).

(c) **Treatment of the asymptomatic infant.** If the infant does not have symptoms but has a blood glucose level in the hypoglycemic range, an initial push of concentrated sugar should **not** be given. (This is to avoid a hyperinsulinemic response.) Rather, an initial infusion of 5 to 10 ml 10% D/W at 1 ml/min is followed by the continuous infusion of glucose at 4 to 8 mg/kg per minute. Blood glucose levels must be carefully monitored at frequent intervals, after beginning IV glucose infusions, to be certain of adequate treatment of the hypoglycemia as well as to avoid hyperglycemia and the risk of osmotic diuresis and dehydration.

(d) **Parenteral sugar should never be abruptly discontinued** because of the risk of a reactive hypoglycemia. As oral feeding progresses, the rate of the infusion can be decreased gradually, and the concentration of glucose infused can be reduced by using 5% D/W. It is particularly important to measure blood glucose levels during this process of tapering the IV infusion.

(e) Since the hypoglycemia of most IDMs responds to the preceding treatment, unresponsiveness or persistence (over 48 hours) should cause a search for other problems (e.g., infection, islet cell tumor). Hydrocortisone (5 mg/kg per day IM in two divided doses) has occasionally been helpful. In our experience, other drugs (epinephrine, diazoxide, or growth hormone) have not been necessary in the treatment of the hypoglycemia of IDMs.

(f) In a **hypoglycemic infant,** if difficulty is experienced in achieving vascular access, we have administered crystalline glucagon IM or SQ (300 μg/kg to a maximum dose of 1.0 mg). This will cause a rapid rise in blood glucose levels in large IDMs who have good glycogen stores, although it is not reliable in the smaller infants of maternal classes D, E, F, and others. This rise in blood glucose level may last 2 to 3 hours and is useful until parenteral glucose can be administered.

C. **Hypocalcemia** (calcium level <7 mg/dl; see Hypocalcemia, Hypercalcemia, and Hypomagnesemia in Chap. 24) is found in 22 percent of IDMs [11]. It is not related to hypoglycemia [11]. Hypocalcemia may be caused by a delay in the usual postnatal rise of parathyroid hormone (PTH). Other factors in IDMs may be vitamin D antagonism at the intestine from elevated cortisol and hyperphosphatemia from tissue catabolism. There is no evidence of elevated serum calcitonin concentrations in these infants in the absence of prematurity or asphyxia [23]. Other causes of hypocalcemia such as asphyxia and prematurity may be seen in IDMs. The nadir in calcium levels occurs between 24 and 72 hours, and between 20 and 50 percent of IDMs will become hypocalcemic as defined by a total serum calcium level under 7 mg/dl. Hypocalcemia in "well" IDMs will usually resolve without treatment. We do not routinely measure serum calcium levels in "well" asymptomatic IDMs. Infants who are sick for any reason—prematurity, asphyxia, infection, respiratory distress—or IDMs with symptoms of lethargy, jitteriness, or seizures should have their serum calcium level measured. If the infant has symptoms that coexist with a low calcium level, has an illness that will delay onset of calcium regulation, or is unable to feed, treatment with calcium may be necessary (see Chap. 24). Hypomagnesemia should be considered as a cause of hypocalcemia in IDMs because the hypocalcemia may not respond until the hypomagnesemia is treated.

D. **Polycythemia** (see Chap. 18) is common in IDMs [2]. In infants who are small for gestational age, polycythemia may be related to placental insufficiency which causes hypoxia and increased erythropoietin. In IDMs it also may be due to reduced oxygen delivery secondary to elevated glycosylated hemoglobin in both maternal and fetal serum. If there was fetal distress, there may be a shift of blood from the placenta to the fetus. Management is discussed in Chapter 18.

E. **Jaundice.** Hyperbilirubinemia (bilirubin >15 mg/dl) is seen with increased frequency in IDMs. Bilirubin levels over 16 mg/dl were seen in 19 percent of IDMs at the Brigham and Women's Hospital (BWH) [11]. Bilirubin production is increased in IDMs as compared with infants of nondiabetic mothers. Insulin causes increased erythropoietin. When measurement of carboxyhemoglobin production is used as an indicator of increased heme turnover, IDMs are found to have increased production as compared with controls. There may be decreased red blood cell life span because of less deformable red blood cell membranes, possibly related to glycosylation of the red blood cell membrane. This mild hemolysis is compensated for but may result in increased bilirubin production. Other factors that may account for the increased jaundice are prematurity, impairment of the hepatic conjugation of bilirubin, and an increased enterohepatic circulation of bilirubin. Infants born to well-controlled diabetic mothers have less problems with hyperbilirubinemia. The increasing gestational age of IDMs at delivery has contributed to the decreased incidence of hyperbilirubinemia [25]. Hyperbilirubinemia in IDMs is diagnosed and treated as in any other infant (see Chap. 15).

F. **Congenital anomalies** are found more frequently in IDMs than in infants of nondiabetic mothers.

1. **Incidence.** In a series of 150 IDMs in 1976 and 1977 from the Boston Hospital for Women (BHW), 9 percent had major anomalies, and anomalies accounted for 50 percent of the perinatal mortality [11]. As mortality from other causes such as prematurity, stillbirth, asphyxia, and RDS falls, malformations become the major cause of perinatal mortality in IDMs. Infants of diabetic fathers showed the same incidence of anomalies as the normal population; consequently, the maternal environment may be the important factor. Most studies show a 6 to 9 percent incidence of major anomalies in IDMs [1,2,4,7,14,16,19]. This is threefold to fivefold greater than the rate of major congenital malformations in the general population (see Chap. 11). The usual major anomaly rate for the general population is 2 percent. The types of anomalies seen in IDMs involve the central nervous system (anencephaly, meningocele syndrome, holoprosencephaly), the cardiac, vertebral, skeletal, and renal systems, situs inversus, and the caudal regression syndrome (sacral agenesis). The central nervous system and cardiac anomalies make up two-thirds of the malformations seen in IDMs. Although there is a general increase in the anom-

aly rate in IDMs, no anomaly is specific for IDMs, although half of all cases of caudal regression syndrome are seen in IDMs.

2. In a study of 116 IDMs at the Brigham and Women's Hospital (BWH) in 1981, there was a positive correlation between poor control of diabetes in early pregnancy (as measured by maternal HbA_1c levels) and major congenital anomalies in offspring of these pregnancies [14]. This finding suggests that good metabolic control before conception and in the first 3 months of pregnancy may decrease the incidence of major congenital anomalies. There have been several other studies correlating good metabolic control of diabetes as measured by maternal glycohemoglobin values in early pregnancy with decreased incidence of anomalies in offspring [20,30]. A recent multicenter study of IDMs compared outcomes in 347 diabetics who were full participants in a rigid control program from early pregnancy, 279 diabetics coming for care in late pregnancy, and 389 nondiabetic pregnancies [15,16]. Major malformation rates were 4.9 percent in the full participants, 9.0 percent in the late entrants, and 2.1 percent in the controls. There were no significant differences in the home glucose results from weeks 5 to 12 in the mothers of the malformed or normal infants. Nor were there any significant differences in levels of glycosylated hemoglobin or frequency of hypoglycemic episodes in the mothers of the malformed and normal infants. Of note, diabetic women coming for early care had fewer infants with malformations than those coming late for care. This study could not show a correlation between hyperglycemia, elevated glycosylated hemoglobin levels, and malformations in women who prospectively opted for rigorous control of diabetes. The authors felt that some, but not all, malformations can be prevented by good control of blood sugar and that more subtle means are needed to identify the teratogenic mechanisms in IDMs. There were only a few diabetic women in both the full-participant and late-entry groups who had glycosylated hemoglobin levels as high as those seen in references 14, 20, and 30. Thus most of the women in this study had rather good control of diabetes in pregnancy.

   A more recent study measured the relationship between hemoglobin A_1 in the first trimester and spontaneous abortions and major malformations in 303 insulin-requiring diabetics. The range of diabetic control was broader than in the preceding study. The risk for spontaneous abortion was 12.4 percent with first-trimester HbA_1 under 9.3 percent and 37.5 with HbA_1 over 14.3 percent. The risk for major malformations was 3 percent with HbA_1 under 9.3 percent and 40 percent with HbA_1 over 14.4 percent. The risks were high with poor control in the first trimester but reasonable (4 percent) with "acceptable" control [4].

3. Because of the high incidence of malformations in IDMs, an ultrasound examination should be performed in early pregnancy (see secs. **III.C, D**). Maternal alpha-fetoprotein (AFP) also should be measured (see Chaps. 3 and 21). The newborn should have a careful physical examination to diagnose any anomalies that were missed by intrauterine surveillance.

G. **Poor feeding** is a major problem in these infants. It occurred in 37 percent of a series of 150 IDMs at the BWH [11]. Sometimes poor feeding is related to prematurity, respiratory distress, or other problems; however, it is often present in the absence of other problems. In our most recent experience (unpublished), it was found in 17 percent of class B to D IDMs and in 31 percent of class F IDMs. Infants born to class F diabetic mothers are often premature. There was no difference in the incidence of poor feeding in large-for-gestational-age (LGA) infants versus appropriate-for-gestational-age (AGA) infants and no relation to polyhydramnios. Poor feeding is a major reason for prolongation of hospital stay and parent-infant separation.

H. **Macrosomia,** defined as a birth weight over the 90th percentile or over 4000 gm, may be associated with an increased incidence of primary cesarean section or obstetric trauma such as fractured clavicle, Erb's palsy, or phrenic nerve palsy due to shoulder dystocia. The incidence of macrosomia was 36 percent in a series from the BHW in 1975–1976 [11]. It was 28 percent at the BWH in 1983–1984 [5]. An association was found between elevated maternal blood sugars in the last trimester and macrosomia. There also was an association between hyperinsulinemia in IDMs and macrosomia and between macrosomia and hypoglycemia [24]. Macrosomia is not usually seen in infants born to mothers with class F diabetes. Better control of maternal diabetes in the third trimester should be associated with less macrosomia, resulting in less trauma and a lower primary cesarean section rate.

I. **Myocardial dysfunction.** Transient hypertrophic subaortic stenosis resulting from ventricular septal hypertrophy in IDMs has been reported frequently [6]. The infants may present with congestive heart failure, poor cardiac output, and cardiomegaly. This cardiomyopathy may complicate the management of other illnesses such as RDS. The diagnosis is made by echocardiography, which will show hypertrophy of the ventricular septum, the right anterior ventricular wall, and the left posterior ventricular wall in the absence of chamber dilation. Cardiac output decreases with increasing septal thickness [26].

Most symptoms resolve by 2 weeks of age. The septal hypertrophy resolves by 4 months of age. In the series by Walther, 18 of 42 (43 percent) IDMs had hypertrophic cardiomyopathy; 7 of the 18 were symptomatic [26]. Most infants will respond to supportive care. Digitalis and other intropic drugs are contraindicated unless myocardial dysfunction is seen on echocardiography. Propranolol is the most useful drug [29]. The differential diagnosis of myocardial dysfunction due to diabetic cardiomyopathy of the newborn includes (1) postasphyxial cardiomyopathy, (2) myocarditis, (3) endocardial fibroelastosis, (4) glycogen storage disease of the heart, and (5) aberrant left coronary artery coming off the pulmonary artery. There is some evidence that good control of diabetes in pregnancy may reduce the severity of hypertrophic cardiomyopathy.

J. **Renal vein thrombosis.** Renal vein thrombosis may occur in utero or postpartum. Intrauterine and postnatal diagnosis may be made by ultrasound examination. Postnatal presentation may be as hematuria, flank mass, hypertension, or embolic phenomena. Most renal vein thrombosis can be managed conservatively, allowing preservation of renal tissue (see Chaps. 26 and 27).

K. **Small left colon syndrome.** Small left colon syndrome presents as generalized abdominal distension because of inability to pass meconium. Meconium is obtained by passage of a rectal catheter. An enema performed with meglumine diatrizoate (Gastrograffin) will make the diagnosis and often results in evacuation of the colon. The infant should be well hydrated before Gastrograffin is used. The infant may have some problems with passage of a stool in the first week of life, but this usually resolves after treatment with half-normal saline enemas (5 ml/kg) and glycerine suppositories.

L. **Perinatal survival.** Despite all these problems, the diabetic woman has a 95 percent chance to bear a healthy child if she is willing to participate in a program of pregnancy management and surveillance in a modern perinatal center. In 147 IDMs over 24 weeks of gestation born to mothers who required insulin at the BHW in 1976–1977, the perinatal mortality was 34 in 1000 [11]. Between 1977 and 1980 at the same center, the perinatal mortality of infants born to women with class B, C, D, H, or R diabetes was 20 in 1000 (unpublished). In the earlier series, 24 infants born to class F diabetic women had a perinatal mortality of 125 in 1000 [10]. More recent data at the BWH do not show an increased perinatal mortality in pregnancies complicated by class F diabetes as compared with other insulin-requiring diabetics. There is, however, increased morbidity [8].

In a more recent series of 215 IDMs at the BWH from 1983 to 1984, the total perinatal mortality from 24 weeks of gestation to 28 days postpartum was 28 in 1000. There was one intrauterine demise of a singleton near term [5]. Thus perinatal survival is encouragingly good and results from advances in medical, obstetrical, and neonatal treatment. More infants are born healthy than ever before, and if ill, more survive [7].

M. Risk of insulin-dependent diabetes in offspring of diabetic parents. Infants born to an insulin-dependent diabetic father have a 6 percent risk of having insulin-dependent diabetes by age 20. In infants born to an insulin-dependent mother, the risk is 1.3 percent [27]. This difference may be due to some effect on the fetal immune system that makes the offspring of the diabetic mother more resistant to the development of diabetes [28].

References

Maternal Diabetes

1. Coustan, D. R. *N. Engl. J. Med.* 319: 1663, 1988.
2. Gabbe, S. G., and Oh, W. (Eds.). *Infant of the Diabetic Mother. Report of the 93rd Ross Conference on Pediatric Research.* Columbus, Ohio: Ross Laboratories, 1986.
3. Greene, M. F., et al. *Am. J. Obstet. Gynecol.* 1989.
4. Greene, M. F., et al. *Teratology* 39: 225, 1989.
5. Greene, M. F. Personal communication, 1988.
6. Gutgesell, H. P., et al. *Circulation* 61: 441, 1980.
7. Hare, J. W. (Ed.). *Diabetes Complicating Pregnancy.* New York: Alan R. Liss, 1989.
8. Hare, J. W. *Diabetes* 37(1): 250A, 1988.
9. Hubbell, J. P. *Med. Clin. North Am.* 49: 1035, 1965.
10. Kitzmiller, J. *Am. J. Obstet. Gynecol.* 141: 741, 1981.
11. Kitzmiller, J. L. *Am. J. Obstet. Gynecol.* 131: 560, 1978.
12. Kitzmiller, J. L., Cloherty, J. P., and Graham, C. A. Management of Diabetes and Pregnancy. In G. P. Kozak (Ed.), *Clinical Diabetes Mellitus.* Philadelphia: Saunders, 1982.
13. Krip, M. *J. Pediatr.* 103: 603, 1983.
14. Miller, E. M. *N. Engl. J. Med.* 304: 1331, 1981.
15. Mills, J. C. Diabetes in early pregnancy study. *Diabetes* 36(1): 5A, 1987.
16. Mills, J. L. *N. Engl. J. Med.* 318: 671, 1988.
17. Mills, J. L., et al. *N. Engl. J. Med.* 319: 1617, 1988.
18. Milunsky, A. *Am. J. Obstet. Gynecol.* 142: 1030, 1982.
19. Pedersen, J. *The Pregnant Diabetic and Her Newborn,* 2d Ed. Baltimore: Williams & Wilkins, 1971.
20. Reid, M., et al. *Br. Med. J.* 289: 1001, 1984.
21. Reller, M. D. *J. Pediatr.* 106: 86, 1985.
22. Robert, M. *N. Engl. J. Med.* 294: 357, 1976.
23. Schedewie, H. K., and Fisher, D. A. Perinatal Mineral Homeostasis. In D. Tulchinsky and K. J. Ryan (Eds.), Maternal-Fetal Endocrinology. Philadelphia: Saunders, 1980.
24. Sosenko, I. R. *N. Engl. J. Med.* 301: 859, 1979.
25. Stevenson, D. K. Bilirubin Metabolism in the Infant of the Diabetic Mother: An Overview. In S. G. Gabbe and W. Oh (Eds.), *Infant of the Diabetic Mother: Report of 93rd Ross Conference on Pediatric Research.* Columbus, Ohio: Ross Laboratories, 1986. P. 109.
26. Walther, F. J. *J. Pediatr.* 107: 109, 1985.
27. Warram, J. H. *N. Engl. J. Med.* 311: 149, 1984.
28. Warram, J. H. *Diabetes* 37: 1328, 1988.
29. Way, G. L. *J. Pediatr.* 95: 1020, 1979.
30. Ylinen, K. *Br. Med. J.* 289: 345, 1984.
31. Zucker, P. *Pediatrics* 42: 824, 1968.

Maternal-Fetal Thyroid Disorders

Mary Deming Scott

I. Thyroid metabolism in pregnancy [13]. During pregnancy, alterations occur in many of the function tests used to evaluate the thyroid, primarily because of an estrogen-induced increase in maternal thyroid-binding globulin (TBG). Concentrations of free thyroxine (free T_4), thyroxine production rate, and thyroid-stimulating hormone (TSH) remain constant, but radioactive iodine uptake (RAIU), basal metabolic rate, response to thyrotropin-releasing hormone (TRH), T_4, and total triiodothyronine (T_3) are all elevated.

The placenta is relatively impermeable to T_4, T_3, reverse T_3, and TSH. TRH and thyroid-stimulating immunoglobulins (TSIs) may cross the placenta [2].

II. Maternal hyperthyroidism [3,13]. Graves' disease complicates 1 in 2000 pregnancies. Thioamides should be used in the lowest possible doses to achieve maternal control [50 to 100 mg per day of propylthiouracil (PTU)]. PTU crosses the placenta, as do iodides and thyroid-stimulating immunoglobulins, and the fetus may be goitrous and hypothyroid or may have neonatal thyrotoxicosis. PTU-induced neonatal goiter (maternal dose of 100 to 200 mg per day) is rarely obstructive [2,3], and the resulting fetal hypothyroidism is usually mild and transient [4], with no intellectual deficits reported [2,3]. Since maternal hypothyroidism is poorly tolerated by the fetus, mothers should be kept mildly thyrotoxic, and TSIs should be measured in mothers with Graves' disease near term [32]. If TSIs are present, the newborn should be closely watched for neonatal thyrotoxicosis. Propranolol treatment of the parturient is poorly tolerated by the fetus. It depresses the infant and may cause growth retardation, impaired responses to anoxia, bradycardia, and hypoglycemia [14]. Because some PTU is excreted in human milk, breast-feeding cannot be recommended until large-scale studies confirm its safety [3].

III. Neonatal hyperthyroidism [2,3,14,24,29,32]. Infants born to mothers with Graves' disease may be hyperthyroid at birth because of the transplacental passage of TSIs or may be euthyroid owing to maternal PTU. As the effects of maternal thioamides disappear, infants may become thyrotoxic. Transplacentally acquired TSI may exert effects for as long as 12 weeks [6]. The thyrotoxic newborn may have low birth weight, microcephaly, irritability, tachycardia, goiter, vomiting, diarrhea, organomegaly, and failure to gain despite hyperphagia. Diagnosis is confirmed by measuring TSI, T_4, free T_4, and T_3.

A. Supportive treatment, including optimal nutrition, may be all that is required in this self-limited disorder. In unusual cases, PTU (5 to 10 mg/kg per day) or methimazole (0.5 to 1.0 mg/kg per day) may be used, as well as Lugol's solution, (1 drop tid). Lugol's solution [aqueous solution of iodine (also known as Strong iodine solution)] contains 4.5 to 5.5 gm elemental iodine and 9.5 to 10.5 gm potassium iodine per deciliter. If there is no response, the dose of Lugol's solution may be increased by 25 to 100 percent until a response occurs. Propranolol (2 mg/kg per day in three divided doses) may be used in refractory cases to reduce sympathetic stimulation, as manifested by severe tachycardia and cardiac failure [29].

IV. Neonatal goiter. Goiter in a newborn indicates inherited hypothyroidism, maternal ingestion of iodine for asthma or thyroid disease, maternal PTU use, or neonatal hyperthyroidism. Hemangiomas or lymphangiomas of the thyroid should be included in the differential diagnosis. Iodine-induced goiter may cause airway problems at birth [12]. Neonatal goiter from maternal iodine therapy will resolve over 2 to 3 months. Resolution may be speeded by treatment with thyroxine in the doses used for congenital hypothyroidism. T_4, TSH, and T_3 determinations should be obtained prior to treatment to exclude permanent metabolic defects in T_4 synthesis.

V. Congenital hypothyroidism [30]

A. Thyroid embryogenesis occurs during the first 12 weeks of gestation. Iodothyronines are made by 9 to 11 weeks, and TSH and T_4 become measurable. The neuroendocrine-thyroid axis continues to mature until term, particularly with regard to autoregulation of T_4 synthesis. Birth results in a 30-minute peak in TSH and in release of T_4. TSH declines to less than 20 μU/ml by age 3 days in term and premature infants. Mean T_4 in cord blood is 11 to 12 μg/dl, rises to 16 μg/dl by 24 to 36 hours, and falls thereafter. T_3 rises more rapidly owing to abrupt increases in $T_4 \rightarrow T_3$ peripheral conversion. TSH, T_3, and T_4 responses are blunted in preterm infants [9,10]. Mean T_4 was 8.9 μg/dl in a group of premature infants; the mean for full-term infants was 11 μg/dl. Twenty percent of premature infants have T_4 levels below 6 μg/dl on screening [20].

B. Incidence and etiology of congenital hypothyroidism. Screening programs [23] have shown the incidence of congenital hypothyroidism to be 1 in 3500 newborns in the United States. The causes of congenital hypothyroidism are as follows:

1. **Permanent conditions** (incidence is 1 in 3500 live births):
   a. **Thyroid dysgenesis** (aplasia, hypoplasia, or ectopic) is usually sporadic, but some familial cases have been described. The female-to-male ratio is 2:1 (no goiter, low T_4, elevated TSH).
   b. **Autosomal recessive disorders of thyroid hormone synthesis** constitute 10 to 15 percent of the cases of primary congenital hypothyroidism. The disorders should be suspected when there is a family history of thyroid disease or when there is parental consanguinity. These disorders may involve any of the enzymatic steps in thyroid synthesis (goiter, low T_4, elevated TSH).
   c. **TSH deficiency** has an incidence of 1 in 110,000 births. In hypothalamic TSH deficiency there may be a normal or prolonged TSH response to thyrotropin releasing hormone (TRH). In pituitary TSH deficiency there is low TSH and a low TSH response to TRH (no goiter, low T_4).
   d. **Thyroid gland unresponsiveness to TSH** is rare [31] (no goiter, high TSH, low T_4).
   e. **Peripheral unresponsiveness to thyroid hormone** has not been identified in the newborn (mild goiter, high T_4, high TSH, systemic symptoms of hypothyroidism).
   f. **Thyroid binding globulin (TBG) deficiency** has an incidence of 1 in 11,000 births, a male-to-female ratio of 9:1, and is inherited as an X chromosome–linked trait (no goiter, low T_4 and T_3, low TBG, normal free T_4 and T_3, normal TSH, normal response to TRH, euthyroid).
2. **Transient conditions** are found in 1 to 2 percent of newborns and in up to 15 percent of premature infants [9,21].
   a. **Low T_4, normal TSH, and normal TBG** is found in 1 in 6000 infants ($T_4 < 6$ μg/dl, TSH < 20 μU/ml, low or normal free T_4, normal response to TRH). These values usually return to normal in 1 to 4 months. Development appears normal. The condition appears most often in premature infants and may be due to a delay in maturation of the pituitary-thyroid axis, stress, or perinatal exposure of iodine. Preterm hypothyroxinemia affects 11 percent of infants of 34 to 36 weeks' gestation and 53 percent of infants 28 to 30 weeks' gestation. Eight symptomatic premature infants (jaundice, lethargy, constipation, edema, hoarse cry) have been treated with resolution of symptoms within 10 days. Thyroxine was stopped when the infants were 3 to 9 months old, and none had persistent hypothyroidism [26]. Large premature infants who have respiratory distress syndrome (RDS) have a higher than expected incidence of congenital hypothyroidism. This may be related to the effects of thyroid hormone on the synthesis of surfactant [16,17,19].

b. **High TSH and normal T_3 and T_4** is found in 1 in 20,000 infants. Values usually return to normal by 9 months of age [8].

c. **Low T_4 and high TSH** (transient hypothyroidism) is found in 1 in 50,000 to 1 in 150,000 infants [8]. This disorder is usually classified and treated as primary hypothyroidism until a trial off therapy is given at age 3 years. This disorder has been seen in infants who are stressed, in those who had pre- or perinatal exposure to PTU or iodine, and in those who had transplacentally passed antibodies due to maternal Hashimoto's thyroiditis [20] or maternal thyroid-simulating hormone-binding inhibitor immunoglobulins [11,33]. Immaturity of thyroid iodine organification enzymes also has been reported as a cause of transient hypothyroidism [28].

d. **Low T_3 syndrome** may be seen in euthyroid sick infants. They have low T_3 and normal reverse T_3 (rT_3) owing to the effect of illness on thyroid metabolism.

e. **High T_4 and low TSH** (transient neonatal hyperthyroidism) may be seen in infants born to mothers with Graves' disease and is due to transplacental passage of TSIs.

C. **Symptoms and laboratory diagnosis of hypothyroidism.** Symptoms of primary hypothyroidism are usually absent in the first weeks of life. Poor temperature control, mottling, poor tone, feeding difficulties due to lethargy, and jaundice (due to delayed glucuronyl-transferase maturation) are all **early signs.** A hoarse cry, constipation, dry skin, decreased activity, hypothermia, umbilical hernia, and enlarged tongue are all **late signs.** Palpable goiters are unusual except with inherited defects in thyroid synthesis and maternal PTU treatment. Retarded ossification of the tibial and femoral epiphyses as well as maturational delay in the calvarium (large posterior fontanelle) should be looked for. T_4 and TSH screening is now being done along with phenylketonuria (PKU) screening tests in most states in the United States. Physicians are notified of abnormal results within 2 weeks. T_4 levels of less than 6 μg/dl on day 4 and TSH levels greater than 20 μU/ml are diagnostic. T_3 levels may be normal or low. Screening programs miss 1 case of hypothyroidism for every 590,000 infants screened. Forty-five percent of those missed are due to laboratory error, with another 14 percent due to improper specimen collection and 16 percent due to poor follow-up. Ten percent never have an initial specimen sent. Hospital transfers, sick neonates, and home deliveries require extra vigilance to be sure screening is accomplished [18]. Eleven percent are due to biologic variants (initial normal T_4 or low T_4 with normal TSH). In all cases, the diagnosis was clinically suspected by 3 weeks of age. All infants under 1 month of age in whom the diagnosis is suspected clinically should be rescreened even if initial values are normal. An iodine-123 scan will show iodine metabolism and will identify ectopic tissue with a comparatively low total-body radiation dose. The iodine-123 scan enables genetic counseling to be given to parents [17].

D. **Treatment and prognosis of hypothyroidism** [30]. New England infants with congenital hypothyroidism (who were detected by screening since 1967 and treated) have had normal mean IQs and IQ distributions when examined at 3 to 4 years of age [26], and a similarly aged group of Canadian infants have mean global IQs above 100 [15]. Treatment should be initiated with 0.025 mg per day (10 μg/kg) of L-thyroxine, and the dose should be increased by 0.012 mg every 2 weeks until the TSH level is <20 μU/ml and the T_4 level is 10 to 15 μg/dl. Doses during the first year of life range between 0.025 and 0.075 mg per day. Doses must be adjusted in each infant based on frequent determinations of T_4 and TSH levels. The T_4 level should be raised to 9 to 10 μg/dl by 2 weeks and to 12 μg/dl by 4 weeks. The T_4 level should be maintained at 12 μg/dl for the first year of life and above 10 μg/dl after that. The TSH level should be kept under 5 μU/ml [15,20,21,22,26]. Ten percent of infants with congenital hypothyroidism will need T_4 levels of 14 to 16 μg/dl to return TSH levels to normal.

Infants with transient hypothyroidism (low T_4, elevated TSH) must be treate as primary hypothyroidism patients until it is certain they have only tran sient disease. All infants being treated for congenital hypothyroidism shoul have a brief trial off medication between 3 and 4 years of age to see if the have transient disease. The question of whether T_4 supplementation of th premature infant with low T_4 and normal TSH levels (<30 weeks' gestatio or 1000 gm) might improve outcome has not been settled [8,26]. One recen study [5] suggests no benefit. The present opinion of the New England Hy pothyroid Collaborative is that there is no benefit to routine T_4 supplemen tation of these premature infants (see subsec. **B.2.a**).

VI. Maternal hypothyroidism. Mothers with acquired juvenile or adult hypothyroid ism have usually delivered normal babies. Untreated maternal hypothyroidisn results in an increased frequency of first-trimester abortions and intrauterin growth retardation, and one study suggests intellectual function may be slightl lower in children whose mothers' hypothyroidism was inadequately treated i pregnancy [13,25].

VII. Maternal thyroiditis. Thyroiditis is **familial** in that 15 to 25 percent of affecte patients have relatives with thyroiditis or other immune disorders. This form o immunologic thyroidectomy renders many teenagers and adult women hypothy roid. Maternal antithyroid antibodies freely cross the placenta and are secrete in breast milk. Transient hypothyroidism has been described in infants who hav transplacental passage of antithyroid antibodies from mothers with Hashimoto' thyroiditis [11,21]. An association between cretinism and maternal thyroi autoimmunization has been reported [1].

References

Maternal-Fetal Thyroid Disorders

1. Blizzard, R. M. *N. Engl. J. Med.* 263: 327, 160.
2. Burrow, G. N. *N. Engl. J. Med.* 298: 150, 1978.
3. Burrow, G. N. *N. Engl. J. Med.* 298: 150, 1978.
4. Cheron, R. G. *N. Engl. J. Med.* 304: 525, 1981.
5. Choudhry, P. *Pediatrics* 73: 301, 1984.
6. DiGeorge, A. M., and Lischner, H. W. Endocrine Disorders. In E. R. Steihm anc V. A. Fulginiti (Eds.), *Immunologic Disorders in Infants and Children.* Philadel phia: Saunders, 1980. P. 589.
7. Dussault, J. H. *J. Pediatr.* 96: 385, 1980.
8. Dussault, J. H., et al. Regional Screening for Congenital Hypothyroidism: Re sults of Screening One Million North American Infants with Filter Paper Spo T_4-TSH. In G. N. Burrow and J. H. Dussault (Eds.), *Neonatal Thyroid Screening* New York: Raven Press, 1980. Pp. 155–165.
9. Erenberg, A. *Pediatr. Clin. North Am.* 29: 1205, 1982.
10. Fisher, D. A. *N. Engl. J. Med.* 304: 702, 1981.
11. Francis, G., and Riley, W. *Am. J. Dis. Child.* 141: 1081, 1987.
12. Galina, M. P. *N. Engl. J. Med.* 267: 1124, 1962.
13. Gibson, M., and Tulchinsky, D. The Maternal Thyroid. In D. Tulchinsky an K. D. Ryan (Eds.), *Maternal-Fetal Endocrinology.* Philadelphia: Saunders, 1980 Chap. 7.
14. Gladstone, G. R. *Pediatrics* 86: 962, 1975.
15. Glorieux, J. *J. Pediatr.* 102: 19, 1983.
16. Hadeed, A. *J. Pediatr.* 68: 491, 1981.
17. Heyman, S. *J. Pediatr.* 101: 571, 1982.
18. Holtzman, C., et al. *Pediatrics* 78: 553, 1986.
19. Klein, A. H. *Pediatrics* 63: 380, 1979.
20. Klein, R. Z. *New England Congenital Hypothyroidism Collaborative Newsletter* 305 South Street, Jamaica Plain, Mass. 02130, October 1982.

21. Klein, R. Z. *New England Congenital Hypothyroidism Collaborative Newsletter.* 305 South Street, Jamaica Plain, Mass. 02130, April 1982.
22. Klein, R. Z. *New England Congenital Hypothyroidism Collaborative Newsletter.* Department of Maternal and Child Health, Dartmouth Medical School, Hanover, N.H. 03756, August 1988.
23. LaFranchi, S. Hypothyroidism: Congenital and Acquired. In: S. A. Kaplan (Ed.), *Clinical Pediatric and Adolescent Endocrinology.* Philadelphia: Saunders, 1982.
24. MacGillivray, M. H. *Clin. Perinatol.* 2: 15, 1975.
25. Man, E. B. *Am. J. Obstet. Gynecol.* 125: 949, 1976.
26. Mercado, M., et al. *Clin. Pediatr.* 26: 343, 1987.
27. New England Congenital Hypothyroidism Collaborative. *Lancet* 2:1095, 1981.
28. Nose, O., et al. *J. Pediatr.* 108: 573, 1986.
29. Pemberton, P. J. *Arch. Dis. Child.* 49: 813, 1974.
30. Sobel, E. H., et al. *Pediatr. Rev.* 11: 15, 1989.
31. Stanbury, J. H., Aiginger, P., and Harbison, M. D. Familial Goiter and Related Disorders. In L. DeGroot et al. (Eds.), *Endocrinology.* New York: Grune & Stratton, 1979. Pp. 523–539.
32. Solomon, D. H. *N. Engl. J. Med.* 304: 538, 1981.
33. Takasu, N., et al. *J. Clin. Endocrinol. Metab.* 59(1): 142, 1984.

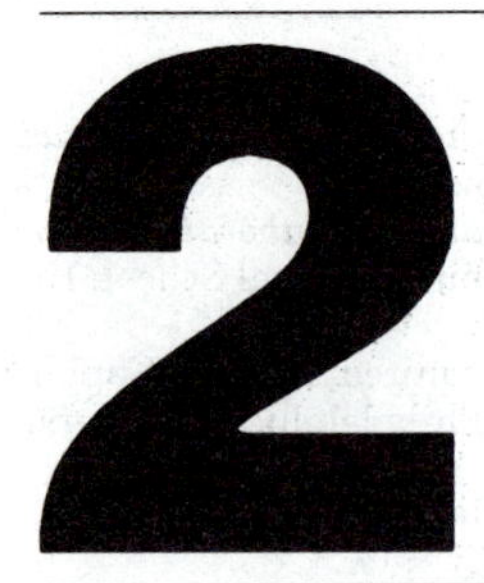

Drug Abuse and Withdrawal

Margaret Flanagan-Everett

I. **Maternal narcotic addiction** [1,2,11,39]. Ten thousand heroin-dependent babies are born in the United States every year. Many narcotic-addicted mothers in the United States are in methadone treatment programs. Narcotic addiction should be considered in women who have had no prenatal care, who want to leave the hospital shortly after delivery, who have signs of addiction (e.g., needle marks, hepatitis), or who demand medication frequently and in large doses while they are in the hospital.

   A. **All** women should be asked **directly** during pregnancy about drug use, including tobacco, alcohol, marijuana, opiates, cocaine, benzodiazepams, amphetamines, PCP, barbiturates, other prescription medications, and over-the-counter preparations. Women who use one drug tend to use another [25].

   B. Drug-addicted mothers are at increased risk for sexually transmitted diseases, hepatitis, and AIDS, especially if they are involved in IV drug use or prostitution. The HIV seropositivity rate in childbearing IV drug addicts is currently 30 percent [8].

   C. **Pregnant drug addicts** may be unsure of their dates, and many usual parameters of fetal maturity and well-being may be unreliable. The fetus may be symmetrically small for gestational age (SGA), and there may be delayed bony maturation of the fetus.

   D. **Narcan** (naloxone) should **never** be given to infants born to mothers with narcotic addiction because it may precipitate immediate withdrawal.

   E. A good review of this subject is found in reference 11.

II. **Withdrawal in the infant.** Signs of acute narcotic withdrawal usually begin in 24 to 48 hours, depending on the time of the last dose and the presence of other drugs, but symptoms may not appear until 3 to 4 days [30,45,56]. Table 2-1 shows the reported withdrawal symptoms in newborns after maternal drug ingestion. A screen of the mother's and infant's blood and urine may be useful. **Cocaine** is the most common drug causing problems in our nurseries. Heroin is less commonly seen as compared with 5 years ago.

   A. **The severity of withdrawal** depends on the drugs used. Withdrawal from opiates plus cocaine or amphetamine (polydrug abuse) is much more severe than from methadone, which is more severe than from other opiates alone or cocaine alone [48].

   B. **Methadone** causes withdrawal symptoms in about 75 percent of babies [20,55], although symptoms are mild in infants born to women maintained on less than 20 mg per day [4]. With higher methadone doses, withdrawal may be severe and prolonged. Some have late withdrawal, which may be of two types:

      1. **Symptoms** appear shortly after birth, improve, and then recur at 2 to 4 weeks.
      2. No symptoms are seen at birth, but they develop 2 to 3 weeks later. These infants will have the usual signs of **withdrawal,** but may also give a history of a sudden, tremendous increase in appetite.
      3. The infants of methadone-addicted mothers have a lower birth weight, length, and head circumference [10,22] than control infants.

4. Head circumference may not be normal by 2 years [11]. Some studies show deficits in motor skills at 18 months [20,55], but others blame low socioeconomic status and environment rather than narcotic addiction [38,41].
5. Other sequelae include abnormal interactive behavior and state control [43], poor auditory and visual orientation responses [10], poor motor control [10], decreased quiet sleep [52], abstinence-associated seizures [23], hyperactivity, a persistent Moro reflex [15], abnormal pneumograms [64], and a five- to tenfold increased incidence of sudden infant death syndrome (SIDS) [20].

C. **Differential diagnosis.** Hypoglycemia, hypocalcemia, hypomagnesemia, sepsis, meningitis, and infectious diarrhea must be considered, even if the diagnosis of drug-addicted mother is certain.

III. **Treatment.** The treatment goal should be an infant who is not irritable, has no vomiting or diarrhea, can sleep between feedings, and yet is not heavily sedated.

A. **Symptomatic treatment.** Forty percent of infants who have symptoms of drug withdrawal can be treated without medication. Using medication may prolong hospitalization. Symptomatic care includes holding, rocking, decreasing stimulation, swaddling, waterbeds [49], and providing frequent, small feedings of a hypercaloric formula (24 cal per 30 ml). Infants having severe symptoms may need IV fluids.

B. **Medication.** Infants who do not respond to symptomatic treatment will need medication. The decision to start medication should be based on some **objective** measurement of symptoms recorded on a **withdrawal scoring sheet,** such as that shown in Figure 2-1. All oral and parenteral medications have additives that may not have been well studied in the newborn. Package inserts should be reviewed so that the physician is aware of other ingredients that are being given with the primary medication. The goal is to stop symptoms and keep the infant comfortable but not sedated. Once the desired effect has been achieved, the dose can be slowly tapered until it is discontinued. The infant should then be observed for 2 or 3 days before discharge. The current recommended pharmacotherapies for narcotic addiction are diluted tincture of opium and phenobarbital. Previous recommendations are also included in the following list.

1. **Diluted tincture of opium (DTO).** This narcotic is our treatment of choice for narcotic withdrawal. Advantages are that it is a pharmacologic replacement, controls all symptoms, impairs suck the least, and contains few additives. Disadvantages are a relatively slow withdrawal, continued exposure to narcotics, and short shelf life. A 10% solution of tincture of opium USP (Laudanum) is equal to morphine 1.0%. This is diluted 25-fold with sterile water to a concentration and potency equal to that of paregoric (0.4 mg/ml of morphine). This dilution is stable for 2 weeks. The stock solution of tincture of opium should not be kept near the patient care area because of the possibility of the stronger mixture being given in error. The diluted mixture should be called **neonatal opium solution,** as suggested in the Neonatal Drug Withdrawal Statement of the American Academy of Pediatrics' Committee on Drugs [2]. The dose is 0.05 ml/kg or 2 drops per kilogram q4–6h. The dose is increased by 2 drops (or 0.05 ml/kg) at the end of each 4-hour period until the desired response is achieved.
   a. Some babies will need medication more often than q4h. Once an adequate dose has been found, it can be tapered by 10 percent daily.
   b. The length of treatment is 1 to 6 weeks.
   c. Side effects include sleepiness and constipation. Colace has been used to treat constipation.
   d. Overdosage may cause narcosis, which is manifest by decreased reflexes and poor Moro reflex, suck, grasp, and response to pain. More profound narcosis is manifest by hypotonia, obtundation, coma, a respiratory rate under 20, irregular shallow respiration, apnea, brady-

Table 2-1. Reported withdrawal syndromes in newborns after maternal drug ingestion

	Lethargy	Poor state control	Fever	Diaphoresis	Tachycardia	Tachypnea	Cyanosis	High-pitched cry	Altered sleeping	Tremors	Hypotonicity	Hypertonicity	Hyperreflexia	Increased suck	Ineffective suck	Irritability	Jitteriness	Seizures	Nasal congestion	Sneezing/yawning	Ravenous appetite	Vomiting	Excessive regurgitation	Diarrhea	Weight loss	Abdominal distention	Onset	Duration
Narcotics																												
Heroin [28,44]			X	X	X	X		X	X	X		X	X	X		X	X	X	X	X	X	X	X	X	X		1–144 h	7–20 days
Methadone [19,55]			X	X	X	X		X	X	X		X	X	X		X	X	X	X	X	X	X	X	X	X		1–14 days	20–45 days
Propoxyphene				X	X	X		X		X		X	X	X		X	X	X	X		X	X		X	±		3–20 h	56 h–6 days
Pentazocine [21] plus tripelennamine					X	X		X		X	X	X		X		X	X	X		X		X		X		X		
("T's and Blues")						X		X					X		X	X	X											
Codeine			X							X		X	X		X	X	X					X		X			0.5–30 h	4–17 days
Sedatives																												
Barbiturates				X				±	X	X	X	X	X		X	X	X	X		X	X	X	X	X	X		0.5 h–14 days	11 days–6 mos.
Butalbital [49] (Fiorinal, Esgic)															X	X	X	?	X								2 days	24 days
Chlordiazepoxide										X						X											21 days	37 days

Diazepam					X	X				X		X	X	X		X						X		X	2–6 h	10 days–6 weeks
Diphenhydramine									X												X				5 days	10 days–5 weeks
Ethanol [30,50,51,60]					X				X		X				X	X	X		±				±	X	6–12 h	
Ethchlorvynol (Placidyl) (plus propoxyphene plus diazepam)					X					X				X	X	X				X	X				24 h	9–10 days
Glutethimide (plus heroin)			X		X		X		X		X	X			X								X		8 h	45 days
Hydroxyzine (Vistaril) (600 mg/day plus Pb)					X		X		X			X		X	X	X	X								15 min	156 h
Stimulants																										
Methamphetamine	X	X					X				X				X				X							5–24 h
Phencyclidine [9,18,24]										X	X	X				X					X		X		18–20 h	18 days–2 mos.
Cocaine	X	X					X	X	X		X	X	X	X			X	X	X							1–3 days
Antidepressants																										
Tricyclics			X	X	X	X			X	X	X	X		X	X	X	X								5–12 h	96 h–30 days
Antipsychotics																										
Phenothiazines							X		X		X	X	X	X	X	X								X	21 days	>11 days–4 mos.

Key: X = symptom usually present; ± = symptom may be present, but not always; Pb = phenobarbital.

DATE: ________

SYSTEM	SIGNS AND SYMPTOMS	SCORE	AM						PM						COMMENTS
CENTRAL NERVOUS SYSTEM DISTURBANCES	Excessive High-pitched (OR Other) Cry Continuous High-pitched (OR Other) Cry	2 3													Daily Weight:
	Sleeps < 1 Hour After Feeding Sleeps < 2 Hours After Feeding Sleeps < 3 Hours After Feeding	3 2 1													
	Hyperactive Moro Reflex Markedly Hyperactive Moro Reflex	2 3													
	Mild Tremors Disturbed Moderate-Severe Tremors Disturbed	1 2													
	Mild Tremors Undisturbed Moderate-Severe Tremors Undisturbed	3 4													
	Increased Muscle Tone	2													
	Excorlation (Specify Area): ________	1													
	Myoclonic Jerks	3													
	Generalized Convulsions	5													
METABOLIC/VASOMOTOR/RESPIRATORY DISTURBANCES	Sweating	1													
	Fever < 101 (99-100.8° F./37.2-38.2° C) Fever > 101 (38.4° C. and Higher)	1 2													
	Frequent Yawning (> 3-4 times/interval)	1													
	Mottling	1													
	Nasal Stuffiness	1													
	Sneezing (> 3-4 times/interval)	1													
	Nasal Flaring	2													
	Respiratory Rate > 60/Min. Respiratory Rate > 50/Min. with Retractions	1 2													

Guidelines for the use of neonatal abstinence scoring system

1. Record time of scoring (end of observation interval).
2. Give points for all behaviors or symptoms observed during the scoring interval, even though they may not be present at the time of recording. (For example, if the baby was diaphoretic at 11 A.M. and is "scored" at noon, when he or she is not, the baby still gets the "sweating" point.)
3. Awaken the baby to test reflexes. Calm before assessing muscle tone, respirations, or Moro reflex. Many of the signs of hunger can appear the same as withdrawal. Appearance after feeding gives a good idea of muscle activity.
4. Count respirations for a full minute. Always take temperature at the same site. The temperatures on the sheet are *rectal* levels; an axillary temperature that is 2 degrees cooler may also indicate withdrawal.
5. Do not give points for perspiration if it occurs due to swaddling.
6. A startle reflex should not be substituted for the Moro reflex.

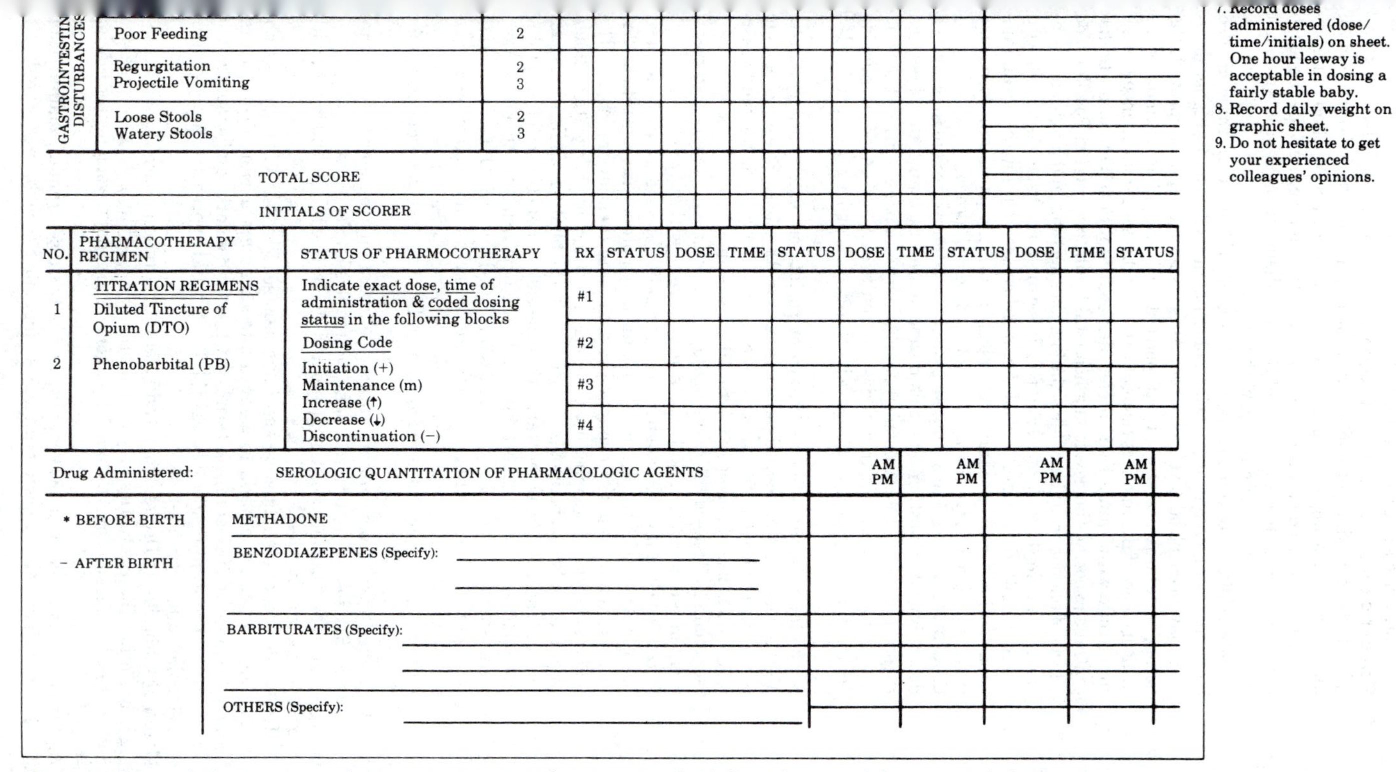

GASTROINTESTINAL DISTURBANCES															
	Poor Feeding	2													
	Regurgitation Projectile Vomiting	2 3													
	Loose Stools Watery Stools	2 3													
TOTAL SCORE															
INITIALS OF SCORER															

7. Record doses administered (dose/time/initials) on sheet. One hour leeway is acceptable in dosing a fairly stable baby.
8. Record daily weight on graphic sheet.
9. Do not hesitate to get your experienced colleagues' opinions.

NO.	PHARMACOTHERAPY REGIMEN	STATUS OF PHARMOCOTHERAPY	RX	STATUS	DOSE	TIME	STATUS	DOSE	TIME	STATUS	DOSE	TIME	STATUS
	TITRATION REGIMENS	Indicate exact dose, time of administration & coded dosing status in the following blocks	#1										
1	Diluted Tincture of Opium (DTO)		#2										
2	Phenobarbital (PB)	Dosing Code Initiation (+) Maintenance (m)	#3										
		Increase (↑) Decrease (↓) Discontinuation (−)	#4										

Drug Administered:	SEROLOGIC QUANTITATION OF PHARMACOLOGIC AGENTS	AM PM	AM PM	AM PM	AM PM
* BEFORE BIRTH	METHADONE				
− AFTER BIRTH	BENZODIAZEPENES (Specify):				
	BARBITURATES (Specify):				
	OTHERS (Specify):				

Fig. 2-1. Neonatal abstinence syndrome assessment and treatment. Guidelines for use of the neonatal abstinence scoring system are also included. (Adapted from L. P. Finnigan et al., A Scoring System for Evaluation and Treatment of Neonatal Abstinence Syndrome: A New Clinical and Research Tool. In P. L. Morselli, S. Garattini, and F. Sereni (Eds.), *Basic and Therapeutic Aspects of Perinatal Pharmacology*. New York: Raven Press, 1975.)

cardia, or hypothermia. If this occurs, stop the medication until the abstinence scores are over 8.

2. **Paregoric** contains opium 0.4%, equivalent to morphine 0.04% (0.4 mg/ml). It also contains anise oil, benzoic acid, camphor, and glycerine in an alcohol base. Dosing and tapering is as in diluted tincture of opium. Paregoric is often used because of its availability and long shelf life. Because of the unknown effects of many of the ingredients in paregoric, we do not use it for treatment of narcotic withdrawal.
3. **Phenobarbital** (5 to 8 mg/kg per day) is given IM or PO in three divided doses and is tapered over 2 weeks. Some infants will require higher doses and may need blood levels checked. After symptoms have improved, the dosage should be decreased by 10 percent each day. Phenobarbital is the drug of choice if the infant is thought to be withdrawing from phenobarbital. In narcotic withdrawal, some prefer phenobarbital to DTO in order to discontinue exposing the developing neonatal brain to narcotics. Possible side effects of phenobarbital include sedation, poor sucking, and heightened sensitivity to pain. Long-term use in febrile seizures has been associated with lower IQ [26]. It does not control the diarrhea seen with withdrawal. Phenobarbital elixir may contain 20% alcohol, and the parenteral form may contain propylene glycol, ethyl alcohol, and benzyl alcohol.
4. **Chlorpromazine** (1.5 to 3.0 mg/kg per day) is administered in four divided doses, initially IM, then PO; this dose is maintained for 2 to 4 days and then is tapered as tolerated q2–4 days. Chlorpromazine controls the vomiting and diarrhea seen in withdrawal, but because of unacceptable side effects, including tardive dyskinesia, this drug is no longer recommended by us.
5. **Methadone** should not be used until more data on toxicity are available. Methadone has a prolonged plasma half-life (24 hours). Since methadone is excreted in breast milk, methadone-treated mothers should not breastfeed. Doses used have been 0.5 to 1.0 mg q4–8h.
6. **Morphine** in doses of 0.1 to 0.2 mg/kg has been used in emergency treatment of seizures or shock due to acute narcotic withdrawal.
7. **Diazepam (Valium).** Although not recommended by us, diazepam has been used in doses of 0.1 to 0.3 mg/kg IM until symptoms are controlled. The dose is then halved, then changed to q12h, and then lowered again. The major side effect is respiratory depression. The sodium benzoate included in parenteral diazepam may interfere with the binding of bilirubin to albumin. The manufacturer warns that the safety and efficacy of injectable diazepam have not been established in the newborn (see Appendix A).
8. **Lorazepam** is often used for sedation by itself or with DTO. The parenteral preparation of lorazepam contains benzyl alcohol, polyethylene glycol, and propylene glycol. Limited data is available about its use in newborns. This may decrease the amount of DTO needed (see Appendix A for dose).
9. In withdrawal from nonnarcotic drugs, medication treatment is symptomatic. Phenobarbital or lorazepam is often used for sedation.

C. There must be close monitoring of fluid and electrolyte intake and losses, with replacement as needed.

D. Use of the **narcotic abstinence scoring sheet** (see Fig. 2-1) will help to establish some **objective criteria to wean the medications.** Irritability, tremors, and disturbance of sleeping patterns may last for 6 months and should not be a reason for continuing medication [65]. The general approach to management is displayed in Figure 2-2.

IV. **Maternal Addiction to Drugs Other Than Narcotics.** Infants born to mothers using drugs other than narcotics may be symptomatic (see Table 2-1). Cocaine was detected in the urine of more than 10 percent of pregnant women in a Florida study [12].

A. **Cocaine** has a potent anorexic effect and may cause prenatal malnutrition [17]. In infants, the following congenital anomalies have been reported: cardiac anomalies, skull defects [7], genitourinary malformations [13], and "prune belly" syndrome [6,13]. A low threshold for cardiac evaluation and renal ultrasound may be indicated.

1. **Cocaine and amphetamines** are associated with an increased rate of spontaneous abortion, placental abruption, fetal distress, meconium staining, low Apgar scores, prematurity, growth retardation, and microcephaly [7,14,15,18,32,48,57,67]. Perinatal cerebral infarctions [16] and necrotizing enterocolitis [35,62] have been reported. Cocaine causes maternal hypertension and placental vasoconstriction with diminished uterine blood flow and fetal hypoxia, which may be responsible for these findings [66].
2. Cocaine addicted infants do not exhibit classic narcotic withdrawal symptoms [57] (see Table 2-1). Cocaine exposed neonates have been shown to have depression of interactive behavior with poor organizational response, increased tremulousness, irritability, state lability, poor consolability [14,15] transiently abnormal EEG's and visual evoked potentials [21,24], visual dysfunction [21], and retinal changes [36]. The effect of cocaine may be by blocking the reuptake of neurotransmitters at presynaptic terminals. Medical treatment of symptoms is rarely needed. Phenobarbital or lorazepam are used in our nurseries (see Appendix A).
3. Cocaine exposed infants may be at a very high risk for SIDS [15]. Long-term disabilities such as attention deficits, concentration difficulties, abnormal play patterns, and flat, apathetic moods have been reported [54]. Convulsions have been seen both in infants of breastfeeding mothers using cocaine [9,18], and in infants exposed to passive crack smoke inhalation [5].

B. **Phencyclidine.** Infants of PCP-abusing mothers are of normal size but show more lability of state and poorer consolability than all other drug-exposed newborns [10,19]. Reports of infants born to chronic PCP users have shown cerebral palsy, neonatal depression, behavioral abnormalities, and facial dysmorphogenesis [31].

C. **Marijuana.** Evidence suggests that heavy marijuana use in pregnancy is associated with a fetal alcohol–like syndrome characterized by tremulousness, intrauterine growth retardation, facial dysmorphogenesis, and lower birth weight [34,67]. Marijuana may cause the segregation of chromosomes during somatic cell division, leading to aneuploidy [63].

D. **Ethanol.** Teratogenic studies are confounded by other risk factors, but no safe level of ethanol use in pregnancy has been established. Consumption of more than one to two drinks daily has been associated with a significant decrease in birth weight [43]. Features of **fetal alcohol syndrome** (FAS) are microcephaly, in utero growth retardation, short palpebral fissures, midfacial hypoplasia, flattened philtrum, thin vermilion border, micrognathia, renal anomalies, cardiac anomalies, and mental retardation [33,47,50,51,59].

E. **Tobacco.** Smoking by mothers is associated with **smaller babies** and an increase in perinatal risks, with lower Apgar scores, increased abruption, placental insufficiency, and prematurity [29,37]. Birth weights less than 2500 gm are twice as common in smokers, with an average of a 160-gm reduction in birth weight per pack of cigarettes smoked per day [58]. There are no reported congenital anomalies.

F. **Benzodiazepine.** A recent report suggests that benzodiazepine is a possible human teratogen [40].

G. **Diagnostic tests.** When drug withdrawal is a possibility, examinations of specimens of maternal and newborn urine and screening for toxic substances in the serum may be helpful. Screening done after withdrawal symptoms are evident may be negative [1,28,42]. Sometimes drugs administered during labor cause confusion in interpretation of the screen. The length of time that drugs are present in urine after use varies with the drug. Some examples are cocaine, 1 to 3 days; heroin or PCP, 2 to 4 days; and marijuana, 2 to 5 days, occasionally up to 10 days [1]. Some hospitals screen for cocaine in cases of preterm labor, placental abruption, or precipitous delivery [46].

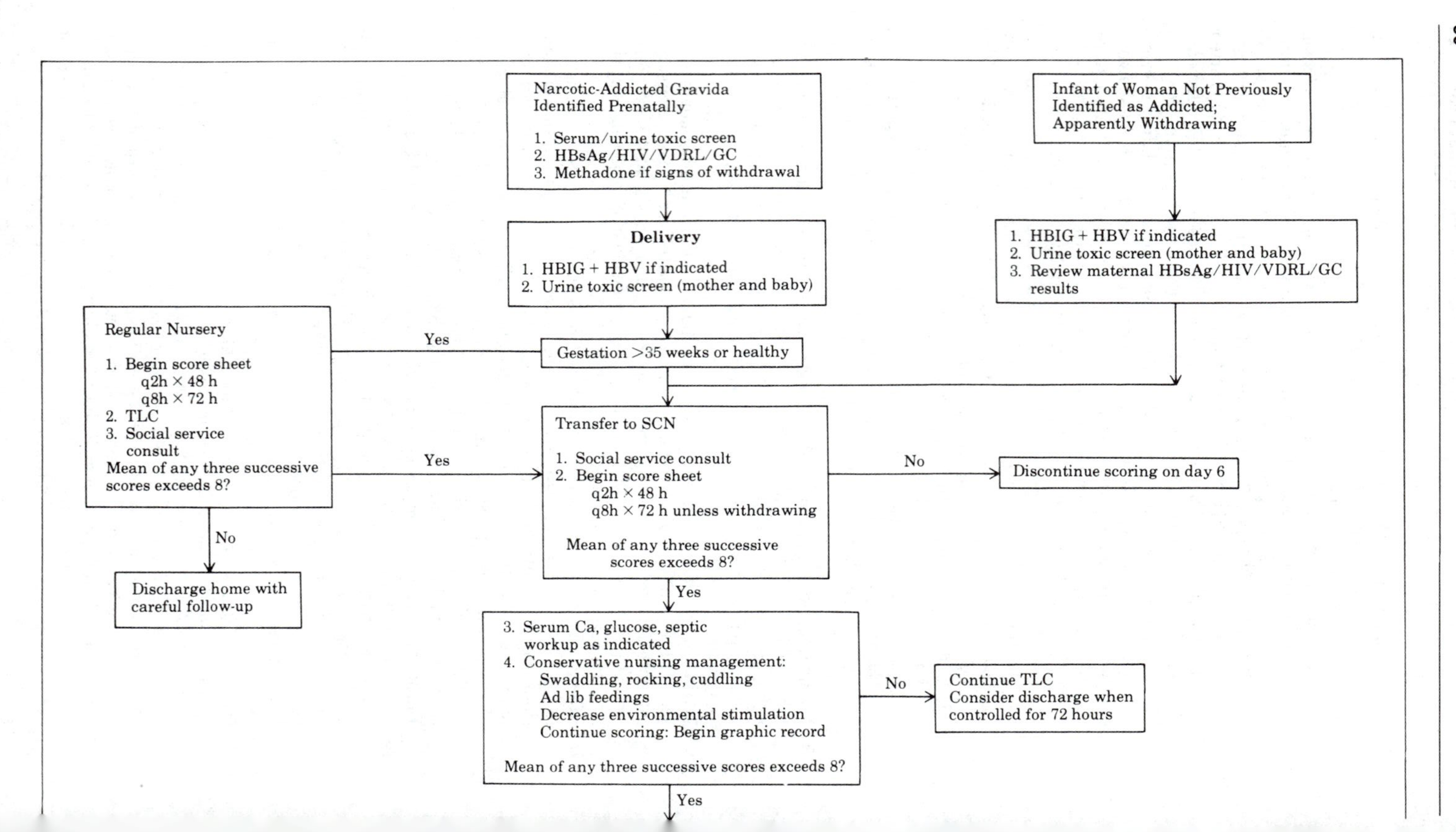
Narcotic-Addicted Gravida Identified Prenatally
1. Serum/urine toxic screen
2. HBsAg/HIV/VDRL/GC
3. Methadone if signs of withdrawal
Infant of Woman Not Previously Identified as Addicted; Apparently Withdrawing
Delivery
1. HBIG + HBV if indicated
2. Urine toxic screen (mother and baby)
1. HBIG + HBV if indicated
2. Urine toxic screen (mother and baby)
3. Review maternal HBsAg/HIV/VDRL/GC results
Regular Nursery
1. Begin score sheet
q2h × 48 h
q8h × 72 h
2. TLC
3. Social service consult
Mean of any three successive scores exceeds 8?
Yes
Gestation >35 weeks or healthy
Yes
Transfer to SCN
1. Social service consult
2. Begin score sheet
q2h × 48 h
q8h × 72 h unless withdrawing
Mean of any three successive scores exceeds 8?
No
Discontinue scoring on day 6
No
Discharge home with careful follow-up
Yes
3. Serum Ca, glucose, septic workup as indicated
4. Conservative nursing management:
Swaddling, rocking, cuddling
Ad lib feedings
Decrease environmental stimulation
Continue scoring: Begin graphic record
Mean of any three successive scores exceeds 8?
No
Continue TLC
Consider discharge when controlled for 72 hours
Yes

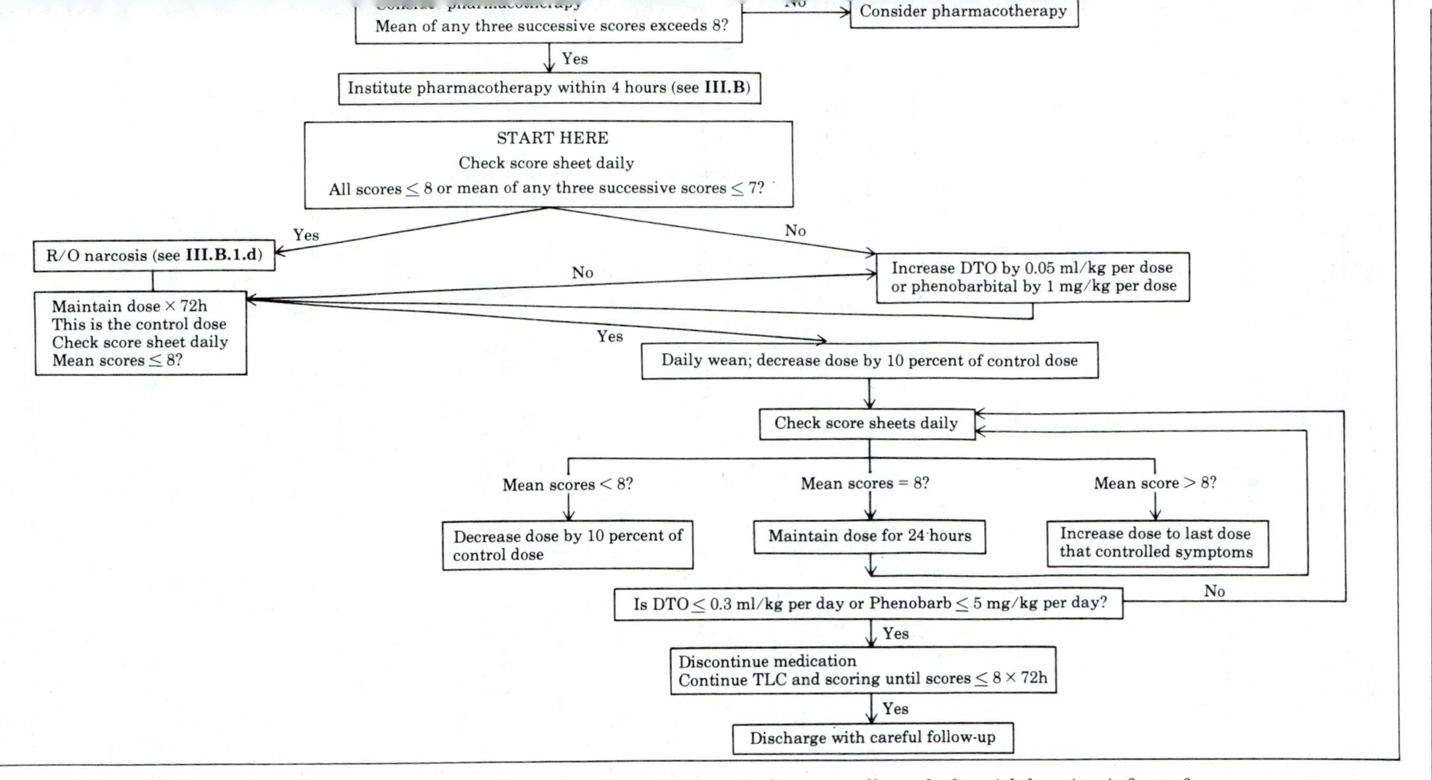

Fig. 2-2. General approach to management of a narcotic-addicted gravida identified antenatally and of a withdrawing infant of a woman not previously identified as addicted (HBsAG = hepatitis B surface antigen; VDRL = veneral disease research laboratory; TLC = tender, loving care; DTO = diluted tincture of opium; RR = respiratory rate; HR = heart rate; GC = gonorrhea; HBIG = hepatitis B immune globulin; HBV = hepatitis B vaccine; HIV = human immunodeficiency virus; SCN = special care nursery).

H. **Treatment** of infants withdrawing from drugs other than narcotics is usually supportive care. If a drug is to be used, phenobarbital is probably safest. The references should be checked for specific suggestions.

V. **Disposition.** The major problems with these children are proper disposition and follow-up.

A. The risk factors to be considered before sending infants home with their mothers are listed below. Studies show a high incidence of abuse and violence in the childhood and current lives of drug-abusing pregnant women. This, along with their own drug use and chaotic lifestyles, places them at risk for inadequate parenting [53]. These factors may be more important in the eventual outcome for the child than the kind or amount of drug the mother is using.

1. **Maternal age.** Risk increases inversely with age.
2. **Length of drug use.** Risk increases with length of usage.
3. **Presence in drug program.** Presence by court order or voluntarily because of concern for infant.
4. **Drug use while on methadone.**
5. **Home situation.**
6. **Ability to care for other children.**
7. **Health of the mother,** especially if she has AIDS. In the Boston area, 20 percent of intravenous-drug-using mothers have a positive blood test for HIV.

B. These infants are difficult to care for even in the best of situations. They will be irritable, have poor sleeping patterns, and will try the patience of their caretakers. They are at increased risk for child abuse and for **sudden infant death syndrome (SIDS)** [11,20,55,60,61,65]. Infants of HIV-positive mothers should be followed closely because of their **increased risk of AIDS** [3].

C. Coordination of plans with local social service agencies, drug treatment centers, and the courts (if necessary) is essential for proper follow-up and disposition. Many states have laws requiring that infants who show signs of withdrawal be reported as battered children [44].

References

1. American Academy of Pediatrics, Substance abuse: A guide for health professionals. Schonberg, S. K. (ed.), Elk Grove Village, IL:AAP, 1988. P. 55.
2. American Academy of Pediatrics. Neonatal drug withdrawal statement of the AAP Committee on Drugs. *Pediatrics* 72: 895, 1983.
3. American Academy of Pediatrics. *Pediatrics* 82: 941, 1988.
4. Bashore, R. A., et al. *West J. Med.* 134: 506, 1981.
5. Bateman, D. A., et al. *Am. J. Dis. Child.* 143: 25, 1989.
6. Bingol, N., et al. *Am. J. Hum. Genet.* 39: 147A, 1986.
7. Bingol, N., et al. *J. Pediatr.* 110: 93, 1987.
8. Centers for Disease Control. *MMWR* 36: 801, 1987.
9. Chaney, N. E. *J. Pediatr.* 172: 134, 1988.
10. Chasnoff, I. J. *Neurobehavioral Toxicology and Teratology* 8: 357, 1986.
11. Chasnoff, I. J. *Ped. in Rev.* 9: 273, 1988.
12. Chasnoff, I. J. *N. Engl. J. Med.* 322: 1202, 1990.
13. Chasnoff, I. J. *Teratology* 37: 201, 1988.
14. Chasnoff, I. J. *N. Engl. J. Med.* 313: 666, 1985.
15. Chasnoff, I. J. *Neurotoxicology and Teratology* 9: 291, 1987.
16. Chasnoff, I. J. *J. Pediatr.* 108: 456, 1986.
17. Chasnoff, I. J., et al. Cocaine babies. *Special Currents.* Ross Laboratories, Columbus, OH, 1989.
18. Chasnoff, I. J. *Pediatrics* 80: 836, 1987.
19. Chasnoff, I. J., et al. *Dev. Pharmacol. Ther.* 6: 404, 1983.
20. Chavez, C. J., et al. *J. Pediatr.* 95: 407, 1979.
21. Dixon, *Ped. Res.* 21: 359A, 1987.

22. Doberczak, T. M., et al. *Am. J. Dis. Child.* 141: 1163, 1987.
23. Doberczak, T. M., et al. *Arch. Neurol.* 45: 649, 1988.
24. Doberczak, T. M. *J. Pediatr.* 113: 354, 1988.
25. Edelin, K. C., et al. *Obstet. Gynecol.* 71: 399, 1988.
26. Farwell, J. R., et al. *N. Engl. J. Med.* 322: 364, 1990.
27. Finnigan, L. P., et al. A scoring system for evaluation and treatment of the neonatal abstinence syndrome: A new clinical and research tool. In Morselli, P. L., Garattini, S., and Sereni, F. (eds.), *Basic and Therapeutic Aspects of Perinatal Pharmacology.* New York: Raven Press, 1975.
28. Frank, D. A., et al. *Pediatrics* 82: 888, 1988.
29. Garn, S. M., et al. *Am. J. Dis. Child.* 135: 503, 1981.
30. Glass, L. *Pediatr. Ann.* 4: 384, 1975.
31. Golden N. L., et al. *Pediatrics* 65: 18, 1980.
32. Hadeed, A. J., et al. *Pediatrics* 84: 205, 1989.
33. Hanson, J. W. *J.A.M.A.* 235: 1458, 1976.
34. Hingson, R., et al. *Pediatrics* 70: 539, 1982.
35. Hoyme, H. E., et al. *Pediatrics* 85: 743, 1990.
36. Isenberg, S. J., et al. *Am. J. Opth.* 103: 211, 1987.
37. Johnston, C. *Clin. Toxicol.* 18: 189, 1981.
38. Kaltenbach, K., et al. *Neurotoxicity and Teratology* 9: 311, 1987.
39. Koop, G. E., et al. Maternal addiction. *Special Currents.* Ross Laboratories, Columbus, OH, 1990.
40. Laegreid, L., et al. *J. Pediatr.* 114: 126, 1989.
41. Lifschitz, M. H., et al. *Pediatrics* 75: 269, 1985.
42. MacKenzie, R. G., et al. *Clin. N. Am.* 34: 423, 1987.
43. Mills, J. L., et al. *J.A.M.A.* 252: 1875, 1985.
44. Morris, R. A., Sorderegger, T. B. *Neurotoxicology and Teratology* 8: 363, 1986.
45. Neumann, L. L. *Clin. Perinatol.* 2: 99, 1975.
46. Ney, J. A. et al. *Am. J. Obstet. Gynecol.* 162: 1562, 1990.
47. Nichols, M. M. *Am. J. Dis. Child.* 113: 714, 1967.
48. Oro, A. S., and Dixon, S. D. *J. Pediatr.* 111: 571, 1987.
49. Oro, A. S., and Dixon, S. D. *Am. J. Dis. Child.* 142: 186, 1988.
50. Ouellette, E. M., et al. *N. Engl. J. Med.* 297: 528, 1977.
51. Pierog, S. J. *Pediatrics* 90: 630, 1977.
52. Pinto, F., et al. *Drug and Alcohol Dependence* 21: 43, 1988.
53. Regan, D. O., et al. *Neurotoxicology and Teratology* 9: 315, 1987.
54. Rodning, C., et al. *Neurotoxicology* 10: 629, 1989.
55. Rosen, T. S. *J. Pediatr.* 101: 192, 1982.
56. Rothstein, P., et al. *Pediatr. Clin. N. Am.* 21: 307, 1974.
57. Ryan, L., et al. *Neurotoxicology and Teratology* 9: 295, 1987.
58. Sexton, J. S., et al. *J.A.M.A.* 251: 911, 1984.
59. Smith, D. W. The fetal alcohol syndrome. In Smith, D. W. (ed.), *Recognizable Patterns of Human Malformations.* Philadelphia: Saunders, 1982, p. 414.
60. Stimmel, B., et al. Electrocardiographic changes in heroin, methadone, and multiple drug abuse: A postulated mechanism of sudden death in narcotic addicts. (Program funded by New York State Narcotics Addiction Control Commission) *National Conference of Methadone Treatment Proceedings.* 1: 706, 1973.
61. Strauss, M. E. *J. Pediatr.* 89: 842, 1976.
62. Telsey, A. M., et al. *Clin. Pediatr.* 27: 547, 1988.
63. The Surgeon General's warning on marijuana, *MMWR* 31: 428, 1982.
64. Ward, S. L., et al. *Am. J. Dis. Child.* 140: 1015, 1986.
65. Wilson, G. S. *Am. J. Dis. Child.* 126: 457, 1973.
66. Woods, J. R., Jr., et al. *J.A.M.A.* 257: 957, 1987.
67. Zuckerman, B., et al. *N. Engl. J. Med.* 320: 762, 1989.

Fetal Assessment

Michael F. Greene

The human embryo and fetus are particularly inaccessible to study by the methods that are routinely applied after birth. For this reason, progress in fetal assessment has been rather slow. Recent technical advances have greatly facilitated our ability to study the human fetus with little or no risk to the fetus. The techniques that involve essentially no risk to the fetus are indirect and therefore entail greater degrees of imprecision than would be tolerable with direct examination. More precise information can be obtained by several new methods of direct examination, but these pose a small but significant threat to the fetus.

The questions that we need to ask and our ability to answer them change with gestational age. The following specific aspects of fetal assessment will be discussed: (1) gestational age, (2) functional maturity, (3) fetal growth, (4) fetal well-being, and (5) specific fetal diseases.

I. **Gestational age assessment** with a reasonable degree of precision is important for several reasons. First, elective obstetrical interventions such as amniocentesis for chromosomal or biochemical studies or elective repeat cesarean section must be timed appropriately. Second, when premature delivery is inevitable, the gestational age of the fetus is important for counseling the parents with regard to prognosis and may influence the management of labor and delivery. Third, to judge the adequacy of fetal growth at any point in gestation, it is necessary to know the age of the gestation. And finally, correct interpretation of the results of fetal functional tests is based on knowledge of gestational age. As will be further discussed later, a nonreactive nonstress test in a known 33-week gestation that is 28-week size carries a totally different implication than the same result in a 28-week gestation.

   A. **Clinical estimate** of gestational age through careful history of the last menstrual period is usually accurate for women with regular, ovulatory menstrual cycles not using hormonal contraception. A recording of the basal body temperature from the cycle during which conception occurred is also very accurate and particularly helpful when menstrual periods have been somewhat irregular. These historical data, when accompanied by physical examination early in pregnancy, the date of quickening (first observation of fetal activity), and the date when the fetal heart is first heard with a stethoscope, are the traditional criteria for estimating gestational age [2]. If the patient is unable to remember the date of her last menstrual period, or if any of these other criteria cannot be met, then it becomes helpful to have an objective laboratory estimate of the gestational age.

   B. **Laboratory estimates** of gestational age have been made by measuring various biochemical or cytologic parameters in serum or amniotic fluid. All these techniques have generally been replaced by ultrasonic estimation of gestational age.

   C. **Ultrasonic imaging devices** are now in common use. All operate by placing a transducer in contact with the patient through an acoustic coupling medium of oil or gel. The transducer emits very high frequency (generally 2 to 6.5 million cycles per second) sound waves that are transmitted through the tissues and are reflected back to the trandsucer from interfaces of differing acoustic densities. The sound waves are emitted in very brief (1 microsecond) pulses so that the trandsucer actually spends most of its time (999 microseconds) "listening" for echoes. The reflected sound waves are picked up by the transducer, transformed back into electrical signals, and assembled into an image on a cathode-ray tube. This image may then be permanently recorded.

1. **During the first trimester,** the gestational age can be estimated by measuring the crown-rump length of the embryo. Prior to approximately 5 weeks of menstrual age, the gestation is visible only as a fluid-filled gestational sac. By 5½ weeks, however, a small embryo, or "fetal pole," can be seen and usually a beating heart can be identified. Measurement of the crown-rump length from 5 to 12 weeks of gestation can provide an estimate of the gestational age accurate to within 3 to 5 days [26]. This is the most accurate ultrasonic gestational age assessment available. The higher the frequency of the sound waves used in imaging, the better is the resolution of the structures being imaged, but the poorer is the penetration of the tissues. The recent introduction of a very high frequency (6.5 MHz) transducer that can be introduced into the vagina and placed directly against the lower uterine segment has permitted very detailed examination of the first-trimester embryo.
2. **During the second and third trimesters,** measurements of the biparietal diameter (BPD) of the fetal skull and the fetal femur length are useful in estimating gestational age. Strict criteria must be observed in making and measuring the cross-sectional images through the fetal head in order to ensure accuracy. Nonetheless, due to biologic variability in fetal growth and head shape, the accuracy with which the gestational age can be estimated decreases with increasing gestational age. For measurements made at 16 weeks of gestation, the variation is ±10 to 11 days; at 27 to 28 weeks, it is ±14 days; and at 29 to 40 weeks, the variation is ±21 days [27]. The length of the calcified fetal femur can be measured and may be useful in cross-checking BPD measurements. Femur length may provide a significantly more accurate estimate of gestational age in the third trimester than the BPD, with an error of only 5 days at 25 to 35 weeks and 6 days at 40 weeks [32]. Under circumstances where the BPD may be technically difficult to measure, e.g., a deeply engaged fetal head, or where there is pathologic anatomy of the fetal head, e.g., hydrocephalus, the femur length may be the only accurate measurement available. Other indications for ultrasound examinations during pregnancy are listed in Table 3-1.
3. **Routine ultrasound examination** for all pregnant women (universal screening) has been suggested and is practiced in some European countries. Proposed advantages of universal screening include reliable documentation of gestational age and early identification of many major congenital malformations. Potential benefits that might accrue include a reduction in the incidence of inductions of labor for the indication of "post dates," a reduction in the incidence of iatrogenic prematurity, improved detection of intrauterine growth retardation, and improved outcome for multiple gestations. Some of these goals have been realized in randomized, controlled trials [30] in Europe. A very large randomized, controlled trial is in progress in the United States.

II. **Functional maturity** of the lungs is the most critical variable in determining neonatal survival in the otherwise normal infant. A number of physical and biochemical tests can be performed on amniotic fluid to determine pulmonary maturity (see Chap. 13). Several tests of fetal well-being (IV) depend on the functional maturity of the fetal nervous system. Efforts to establish a timetable of fetal central nervous system functional maturity, however, are still underway.

III. **Fetal size and growth rate abnormalities** may have important implications for perinatal care (see Chap. 9). Intrauterine growth retardation (IUGR) may reflect chronic deficiencies in supplies of oxygen or nutrients to the fetus or conditions intrinsic to the fetus. It is important to identify fetuses that are chronically malnourished or oxygen-deprived for several reasons. First, their risk of mortality

Table 3-1. Indications for pelvic ultrasound examination during pregnancy

To assess gestational age:
Menstrual dates uncertain
Clinical sizing not compatible with menstrual dates
Clinical sizing not reliable owing to obesity, known or suspected uterine fibroids, or advanced gestational age
To confirm menstrual dates in a pregnancy where possible complications are anticipated
To assess fetal growth
To diagnose fetal demise
To evaluate the source of bleeding in the third trimester
To rule out gestational trophoblastic neoplasm
At the time of amniocentesis or other intrauterine procedure
To evaluate the fetus for anomalies
To confirm the presence of and evaluate a coexisting pelvic mass
To assess fetal well-being
To rule out ectopic gestation
To evaluate a fetal dysrhythmia
To evaluate an abnormal serum alpha-fetoprotein level
To diagnose fetal presentation

both prior to the onset of labor and intrapartum is increased severalfold. It therefore necessary to monitor the well-being of these fetuses carefully, and may be desirable to intervene early to obtain optimal perinatal survival. Secon these newborns are at increased risk for such immediate complications as hyp glycemia, hypocalcemia, polycythemia, and pulmonary hemorrhage [13]. Ident fication of such at-risk fetuses would alert the neonatologist to the possibility problems and permit delivery to occur at an appropriately equipped facility. Pro lems intrinsic to the fetus that can cause growth retardation include congenit malformations, chromosomal abnormalities (such as trisomies), and congenit infections (such as CMV or rubella). Antenatal diagnosis of malformed or infect fetuses is important so that appropriate surgical or isolation facilities can be in mediately available to care for these babies. Prior knowledge that a fetus is a fected with a malformation (e.g., anencephaly) or chromosomal imbalance (e.g trisomy 13) that is incompatible with life might influence the management labor and delivery. The identification of IUGR should be considered a clinic finding rather than a diagnosis per se. Since there can be many causes of IUG its identification makes no implication regarding its etiology.

Unusually large fetal size also can result from pathologic conditions in the moth and can have implications for perinatal management.

A. Definition of IUGR. There is not universal agreement as to how IUGR shou be defined. Commonly used definitions have classified fetuses weighing le than two standard deviations below the mean or less than the third centile less than the tenth centile for gestational age as IUGR [10]. This is furth complicated by the fact that the actual values for these criteria will vary fro population to population depending on the genetic background, the socioec nomic status distribution, and such environmental factors as elevation abo sea level at which the population lives. Furthermore, if our real goal is identify fetuses that are in danger of being physiologically compromised, may be necessary to be more liberal in our definition, e.g., fifteenth or twe tieth centile, so as not to miss compromised fetuses. In the United States day, the most commonly used standard is that of Brenner et al. [5], which the tenth centile of a sea-level, mixed racial and socioeconomic status U. population.

B. Diagnosis. The clinical diagnosis of poor fetal growth has historically been difficult, with only one-half to one-third of all growth-retarded fetuses detected antepartum. Although the experience with ultrasound diagnosis of IUGR has not been perfect, ultrasound is more sensitive than clinical diagnosis alone. If a patient is suspected clinically of having IUGR or is at risk for IUGR because of maternal factors, serial ultrasound examinations may be helpful. A variety of one-, two-, and three-dimensional parameters such as head diameters or circumferences, abdominal cross-sectional areas, head-abdomen ratios, and estimated fetal weights have been measured or calculated to attempt to predict IUGR. Amniotic fluid volume estimation also has been advocated as a more physiologic measure [18]. Since infants may be small-for-dates by being short but well nourished, of normal height but malnourished, or both malnourished and short, no single parameter measured by ultrasound has been entirely satisfactory in predicting IUGR. It is likely that a composite "growth profile" compiled from a variety of measurements and repeated serially during pregnancy will provide the greatest sensitivity and specificity in diagnosing IUGR [7].

C. Two broad categories of IUGR have been described. These are somewhat stereotypic but are advantageous to keep in mind as long as one does not become blinded by them.

1. The **early onset,** or **symmetrical,** type of IUGR is thought to result from an insult that begins relatively early in pregnancy, prior to 28 weeks. It results in a baby whose head and body are proportionately sized. The ponderal index (weight for height) is normal. Very severe maternal vascular disease with hypertension and renal disease, for example, could cause this pattern. This pattern is also commonly seen with congenital malformations or chromosomal abnormalities.
2. **Late onset,** or **asymmetrical** or **head-sparing,** IUGR begins after 28 weeks. The head seems relatively large for the body size. The ponderal index is low, and the infant seems relatively long and "scrawny." Another term used to describe this pattern is **late flattening,** because the growth trajectory will follow a normal centile line initially and then "fall off" the curve late in gestation. Milder maternal hypertension or systemic disease may be etiologic, and poor maternal weight gain may be an associated finding.

D. Macrosomic fetuses (greater than 4000 gm) are at increased risk of shoulder dystocia and traumatic birth injury. Conditions such as maternal diabetes mellitus, "post dates" pregnancy, and maternal obesity are associated with an increased incidence of macrosomia and birth trauma. Accurate prediction of weight in these large fetuses could help to identify those at increased risk for birth injury. Unfortunately, efforts to use a variety of measurements and formulas have met with only modest success[4] in predicting macrosomia.

IV. The assessment of fetal well-being has been a major focus of recent efforts to improve perinatal outcome. As discussed earlier, poor fetal growth may indicate chronic fetal compromise, but evidence of acute compromise must be sought through other means. These techniques are divided between antepartum fetal evaluation and intrapartum fetal evaluation.

A. Antepartum tests of fetal well-being can be divided into biochemical and biophysical tests. Recent years have generally seen a shift in emphasis from the biochemical (endocrine) to the biophysical studies. **Biophysical tests** of fetal well-being require a certain degree of neurophysiologic maturity on the part of the fetus being tested. Since this maturity increases progressively with advancing gestational age, it is important not to attempt to apply these tests to fetuses that are too young to respond appropriately. These tests are designed to evaluate fetuses in the third trimester.

1. **Fetal movement** monitoring may be the simplest method of fetal assessment. Clinically, this can be done very easily by asking the patient to lie quietly on her left side for an hour at her convenience each day. The patient then notes each perceived fetal movement during that hour and re-

cords it in a diary. Although a patient does not perceive all fetal move ments that might be noted by continuous ultrasound observation, she wi record enough of them to be meaningful. Electromechanical strain gauge that record fetal movements that distort the maternal abdominal wa have been used experimentally but are not commercially available.

Fetuses normally have a sleep-wake cycle. They are not continuously ac tive, but there is a diurnal variation at least in the mother's perception c fetal activity. Active periods tend to average 30 to 40 minutes in lengtl Periods of inactivity greater than 1 hour are unusual in a healthy fetu and should alert the physician to the possibility of fetal compromis Further fetal evaluation to ensure fetal well-being might be indicate [24].

2. **The nonstress test (NST)** has become the most popular means of fet evaluation [14]. This popularity is due to several factors: First, it is sim ple to perform. Second, it is less time consuming than the contractio stress test. Third, it involves no discomfort for the patient. Fourth, it en tails no actual or theoretical risks from induced contractions. There ar therefore, no contraindications to the NST. And finally, extensive expe rience with the NST has shown it to be quite reliable.

   The principle upon which the NST is based is that fetal activity is accom panied by a reflex acceleration in the fetal heart rate. This reflex require a degree of fetal maturity that is generally reached by about 32 weeks (gestation. Failure to find these accelerations in a mature fetus is pr sumptive evidence of fetal hypoxia that has depressed the central nervou system to the point where this reflex is no longer functioning.

   The test is performed by placing the patient on a fetal heart rate monit through either a Doppler ultrasound device or skin-surface electrodes o the maternal abdomen. Uterine activity is also recorded either through simple tocodynamometer, palpation by trained test personnel, or the p tient's report of activity. The test result may be reactive, nonreactive c inadequate. A number of different sets of criteria have been proposed f a **reactive** test [15]. A conservative set of criteria would be as follows: (heart rate between 120 and 160, (2) normal beat-to-beat variability (beats per minute), and (3) four accelerations of at least 15 beats per mi ute lasting for not less than 15 seconds each within a 20-minute perio A **nonreactive** test is one that fails to meet these criteria. If an adequa fetal heart tracing cannot be established for any reason, the test wou be considered **inadequate.**

   A reactive test is reassuring. The risk that a fetus with a reactive te would die within the week following the test is approximately 3 in 10([9]. Generally, a nonreactive test would be repeated either later the san day or early the next day. Following two consecutive nonreactive NST consideration would usually be given to delivering the fetus. If immedia delivery is not desirable owing to prematurity or induction of labor likely to fail in the face of an unfavorable cervix and continuation of tl pregnancy is preferred, then reassurance of fetal well-being must sought. This could be done through either a contraction stress test (s **I.V.A.3**) or a biophysical profile (see **I.V.A.3**). It is difficult to obtain da to indicate exactly what would happen if consistently nonreactive NS were ignored because intervention usually occurs. There is no questi that the incidence of fetal distress in labor following a nonreactive N is substantially higher than that following a reactive NST. The majori of labors that follow nonreactive NSTs, however, are not marked by fet distress. The NST, therefore, predicts fetal well-being more reliably th it predicts fetal distress.

3. **The contraction stress test (CST)** was originally developed as a provo ative test for fetal well-being. It has largely been replaced in primary su veillance by the NST. Its main role at present is as a backup or confi matory test in cases where the NST is not reassuring.

The principle upon which the CST is based is different from that of the NST. During uterine contractions, the pressure generated within the uterus and transmitted through the placenta can equal or exceed the pressure with which the intervillous space is perfused by the maternal circulation. When this happens, perfusion of the intervillous space is momentarily reduced or shut off. A healthy fetoplacental unit has sufficient respiratory reserve to tolerate this momentary reduction in oxygen supply without any change in physiology. Under a variety of pathologic circumstances, however, respiratory reserve may be so compromised that this momentary reduction in oxygen supply may produce fetal hypoxia. When the fetal myocardium experiences hypoxia, its contraction rate slows in a characteristic way in association with uterine contractions. The deceleration of the fetal heart rate begins 15 to 30 seconds after onset of the contraction, its nadir is reached after the peak of the contraction, and the heart rate does not return to baseline until after the contraction is over. This pattern of heart rate deceleration is known as a **late deceleration** because of its relationship to the uterine contraction. Synonyms are **type II deceleration** or **deceleration of uteroplacental insufficiency (UPI).**

The test is conducted by monitoring the fetal heart rate and uterine contractions with a fetal monitor as described earlier for a NST. After 30 minutes, if uterine contractions have spontaneously occurred and last 40 to 60 seconds each and at a frequency of three within a 10-minute interval, the CST is completed and evaluated as described below. If there are no spontaneous contractions, then they must be induced. This can be done with intravenous oxytocin, in which case the test is called an **oxytocin challenge test (OCT).** Recently, several investigators have described good success with inducing contractions simply by stimulating the patient's nipples manually.

A CST is **positive** if late decelerations are consistently seen in association with contractions. A CST is **negative** if there are at least three contractions of at least 40 seconds each within a 10-minute period with no late decelerations. A CST is **suspicious** if there are occasional or inconsistent late decelerations. If contractions are stimulated to occur more frequently than every 2 minutes or last longer than 90 seconds, this is an unreasonable stress, and even if late decelerations are seen, they would be difficult to interpret. Such a test would be a **hyperstimulated test** and would not be evaluable. An **unsatisfactory test** is one in which either contractions cannot be stimulated or a satisfactory fetal heart rate tracing cannot be obtained.

A negative CST, like a reactive NST, is very reassuring. The chance that a fetus will die within a week of a negative CST is probably about 0.4 per 1000. If a positive CST follows a nonreactive NST, however, the risk of stillbirth is 88 per 1000, and the risk of neonatal mortality is also 88 per 1000 [8]. One-third of patients with a positive CST will require cesarean section for persistent late decelerations in labor.

4. **The biophysical profile** is a method of fetal assessment that combines the nonstress test with a variety of parameters determined by real-time ultrasound examination. The most widely used method is that of Manning [19], which assigns a score of 0 or 2 for the absence or presence of each of the following: a reactive nonstress test, adequate amniotic fluid volume, fetal breathing movements, fetal activity, and normal fetal musculoskeletal tone. The clinical course of action is then determined by the total score. Reassuring tests (8 to 10) are repeated at weekly intervals. Less reassuring results (4 to 6) should be repeated promptly (later the same day). Frankly ominous testing (0 to 2) should prompt delivery except under extraordinary circumstances. The likelihood that a fetus will die in utero within 1 week of a reassuring test is about the same as that for a negative CST, approximately 0.6 to 0.7 per 1000 [20,21].

5. **Doppler** studies of fetal umbilical artery blood flow velocity provide indirect evidence of placental function. Poorly functioning placentas with extensive vasospasm and/or infarction have increased resistance to flow through the placental circulation that is particularly noticeable in diastole. Thus a decreased velocity of flow may indicate reduced placental function. Recent studies [25] have shown an increased ratio of systolic to diastolic flow and/or absence of diastolic flow to be a sensitive predictor of IUGR but not of acute fetal distress. Reversed flow during diastole is seen very rarely but is a reliable indicator of severe and acute fetal distress [31].

B. **Intrapartum assessment** of fetal well-being is an integral part of the management of labor.

1. **Continuous electronic fetal monitoring (EFM)** is widely used for this purpose. Fetal monitors simultaneously record both the fetal heart rate and the activity of the uterus during labor.

a. The **fetal heart rate (FHR)** can be monitored in one of three ways.

(1) **Ultrasound** waves can be reflected from the fetal heart valves or ventricular walls that are moving toward and away from the transducer. The fetal heart rate can then be calculated by the monitor.

(2) **Surface electrodes** placed on the maternal abdomen can record the maternal and fetal ECG, and the circuitry in the monitor can pick out and display the fetal ECG selectively.

(3) The most direct, accurate, and reliable method, however, is to place a small **electrode** just into the skin of the fetal presenting part to record the fetal ECG directly. This requires rupture of the fetal membranes. The standard spiral electrode penetrates only 2 mm into the fetal skin. When properly placed in the fetal scalp, it is associated with a very low risk of fetal injury. Approximately 4 percent of monitored babies will develop a mild infection at the electrode site, and most respond to local cleansing. Very rarely is any specific therapy or systemic antibiotic necessary for a scalp abscess or cellulitis.

b. **Uterine activity** can be recorded either from outside the maternal abdomen or within the uterus.

(1) A **tocodynamometer** is a strain gauge that can be strapped to the maternal abdomen. When the uterus contracts, the strain gauge is depressed and records the activity. This device is capable of recording the timing and duration of contractions and their crude relative intensity. It is subject to a number of artifacts from a variety of sources (especially maternal and fetal movement and obesity) and cannot quantitatively record intrauterine pressure.

(2) The **intrauterine pressure catheter** can be inserted into the uterus following rupture of the fetal membranes to directly and quantitatively record the pressure developed with each contraction. This is particularly helpful in prolonged or difficult labors, especially in obese patients, although it is not routinely necessary in all laboring patients. Invasive monitoring is associated with an increased incidence of chorioamnionitis and postpartum maternal infection.

c. **Parameters** of the monitoring record that are evaluated include the following:

(1) **Baseline rate** is normally between 120 and 160 beats per minute. Baseline bradycardia may result from congenital heart block associated with fetal congenital heart malformation or maternal systemic lupus erythematosus. Tachycardia may result from maternal fever or chorioamnionitis or fetal dysrhythmia with or without fetal congestive heart failure.

(2) **Beat-to-beat variability** is continuously recorded on the heart rate tracing from a calculation of the heart rate from each RR interval. The heart rate of a healthy, awake fetus is constantly varied from beat to beat by the autonomic nervous system. This normal variability is 5 to 10 beats per minute. Reduced beat-to-beat variability may result from fetal CNS depression due to hypoxia, fetal sleep, fetal immaturity, or maternal narcotic or sedative use.

(3) **Accelerations** of the fetal heart rate during labor are reassuring, as they are during NST.

(4) **Decelerations** of the fetal heart rate may be benign or ominous depending on their characteristic shape and timing in relation to uterine contractions. The patterns are defined as follows:

(a) **Early, type I, or head-compression decelerations** are symmetrical in shape and closely mirror uterine contractions in time of onset, duration, and time of termination. They usually occur in the company of good beat-to-beat variability. The fetal heart rate may slow to 60 to 80 beats per minute before returning to baseline. These decelerations are more commonly seen late in labor when the fetal head is compressed within the bony pelvis and vagina, especially with maternal valsalva. The deceleration is largely due to parasympathetic outflow in response to head compression. This is a benign pattern, not indicative of fetal hypoxia.

(b) **Late, type II, or uteroplacental insufficiency (UPI) decelerations** are asymmetrical with a longer decelerative phase and a shorter return to baseline. The fall in fetal heart rate begins 10 to 30 seconds after the onset of the contraction and does not return to baseline until after the contraction is over. A fall in the heart rate of only 10 to 20 beats per minute below the baseline rate (even though still within the normal range 120 to 160) is significant. Late decelerations indicate fetal hypoxia. With increasingly severe hypoxia: (1) the beat-to-beat variability will be lost, (2) the decelerations will last longer, (3) they will begin sooner following the onset of a contraction, (4) they will take longer to return to baseline following the end of the contraction, and (5) the absolute minimum rate to which the fetal heart slows will be lower [11]. The mechanism of heart rate slowing is probably multifactorial, involving hypoxic depression of both the CNS and the myocardium. Repetitive late decelerations demand action. Shifting the mother to the left lateral decubitus position to relieve aortocaval compression or administration of intravenous fluids may improve maternal hypotension. Administration of O_2 to the mother may be helpful. If these measures fail, then a fetal scalp pH determination (see subsec. **B.2**) should be done.

(c) **Variable, type III, or cord-pattern decelerations** are variable in their shape on the monitor tracing and with respect to their timing in relation to contractions. This pattern occurs occasionally in a high percentage of otherwise normal monitored labors. They would be a cause for concern if they were severe (down to a rate of 60 beats per minute and/or lasting for 60 seconds or more), associated with poor beat-to-beat variability, or mixed with late decelerations. In this case, reassurance of fetal well-being with a scalp pH determination should be sought. This pattern may result from compression of the cord, especially if it is wrapped around the neck or if a loop is compressed between the cervix and the presenting part. A shift in maternal or fetal position or both will often cause this pattern to resolve.

2. **A fetal scalp blood sample** for pH determination can be obtained using a long, cone-shaped vaginal speculum, a long-handled lancet that makes a 2 × 2 mm laceration in the fetal scalp, and long heparinized capillary tubes. Ready access to a micro blood gas analysis machine is necessary. Whenever possible, a suspicion of fetal distress raised by the monitor tracing should be confirmed or dismissed by fetal scalp pH. The fetal pH is usually approximately 0.04 pH units below the maternal pH. A scalp pH above 7.25 is considered normal during labor. A pH between 7.20 and 7.25 is worrisome and should be followed quickly with another pH determination. Generally, a pH of 7.20 or less would suggest significant fetal hypoxia and prompt delivery.
3. **A fetal scalp pH electrode** that can be attached to the fetus to give continuous readings of the tissue pH is under development. It is not in wide use yet due to technical problems with placement and reliability.
4. **A fetal scalp transcutaneous pO_2 monitor** is also under development. This is the same device used in the neonatal intensive care unit (see Chap. 13). There are still practical problems in attempting to attach the probe to the hairy fetal scalp through the long, narrow maternal vagina.
5. **The value and clinical consequences** of intrapartum electronic fetal heart rate monitoring have been called into question by a number of investigators [23]. The observations that the introduction of nearly universal electronic fetal heart rate monitoring has not significantly reduced the incidence of perinatal asphyxia and that it has been associated, at least temporally, with a dramatic rise in the cesarean section rate have led to several large prospective, randomized trials of such monitoring in low-risk patients [16,17]. These have failed to show a reduction in perinatal mortality or asphyxia with electronic monitoring. They have shown that the incidence of operative delivery, i.e., cesarean section and forceps delivery, is increased in the electronic monitoring group. Accordingly, the American College of Obstetrics and Gynecology has recently issued a statement to the effect that electronic fetal heart rate monitoring is not obligatory and that careful auscultation of the fetal heart rate during labor is adequate to ensure fetal well-being.

V. **Testing for specific fetal diseases** can be accomplished through the use of several diagnostic techniques.

A. **Maternal serum** levels of **alpha-fetoprotein (AFP)** can be measured as a screening test for a variety of fetal conditions. Such testing is only a screening technique, because most abnormal values are associated with normal fetuses. An abnormal result is an indication for further investigation and does not mean that a definite problem exists. This must be explained carefully to patients about to enter the process of screening to avoid much needless concern.

Early in embryonic life, AFP is the main serum protein of the developing fetus. It is produced first in the yolk sac and later in the liver. As development progresses, more serum albumin is produced and AFP production declines. Maternal serum AFP levels normally rise very rapidly during the second trimester. Interpretation of the values, therefore, requires accurate knowledge of the gestational age at which the specimen was obtained [1].

1. **High maternal serum AFP** levels are associated with a large number of fetal abnormalities, as listed in Table 3-2. The initial report of a high maternal serum AFP level, however, should prompt a repetition of the test and an ultrasound examination to confirm the gestational age of the fetus and to survey for anomalies. After dating errors, miscarriages, and multiple gestations have been ruled out as potential causes of the elevated maternal serum AFP level, then an amniocentesis may be appropriate to further evaluate the fetus. The most common malformations found in association with high maternal serum AFP values are open neural tube defects (NTDs) (see Chap. 21).

Table 3-2. Conditions associated with elevated maternal serum AFP levels

Anencephaly	Necrosis of fetal liver secondary to herpesvirus infection
Congenital nephrosis	Nuchal bleb
Duodenal atresia	Omphalocele
Encephalocele	Rh isoimmune disease
Esophageal atresia	Sacrococcygeal teratoma
Fetal blood contamination	Spontaneous abortion
Fetal death	Trisomy 13
Gastroschisis	Turner syndrome with cystic hygroma
Hydrocephalus	Twins (AFP increased in maternal serum; amniotic fluid AFP usually normal)
Meckel's syndrome	Urinary obstruction
Myelomeningocele	

Source: From Greene, M. F., Fencl, M., et al. Biochemical Aspects of Pregnancy. In N. W. Teitz (Ed.), *Textbook of Clinical Chemistry*. Philadelphia: Saunders, 1986. P. 1745.

2. **Low maternal serum AFP** levels have been associated with Down syndrome. Using the combination of maternal age and the maternal serum AFP value, a more specific estimate of the patient's risk of carrying a Down fetus can be made than by using age alone [22]. This information can then be used by the patient to decide whether she wants cytogenetic studies to definitely rule out Down syndrome (see Chap. 11).

B. **Amniotic fluid** can be obtained by amniocentesis (see Chap. 11). Both the liquid phase and the cellular elements have proven very useful for the diagnosis of a large number of fetal disorders.

The safety of amniocentesis at around 16 weeks has been evaluated by a number of large studies. The major risk of amniocentesis is for spontaneous abortion immediately following the procedure. Initial estimates of the risk were made prior to the modern practice of continuous ultrasonic guidance of a small-gauge needle. Recent estimates of the risk of spontaneous abortion following amniocentesis by an experienced operator are approximately 1 in 350 [29].

Traditionally, amniocenteses for cytogenetic studies were done at 16 weeks' gestation for two reasons. First, prior to the era of real-time ultrasonic guidance, fluid could not reliably be obtained by "blind" stick much earlier than 16 weeks. Second, the incidence of failure to grow the cells from fluid rose with decreasing gestational age. Real-time ultrasound guidance has made it possible to routinely obtain fluid as early as 12 weeks' gestation, and advances in the laboratory have made it possible to reliably grow the cells from 12-week samples. Many centers are now offering amniocentesis at 12 weeks and are studying its safety.

1. **The liquid phase** contains a variety of proteins, enzymes, and other substances, only a few of which have found diagnostic value.
   a. **Alpha-fetoprotein (AFP)** is found in elevated quantities in amniotic fluid (AF) as a consequence of a variety of congenital malformations. Measurement of AFP levels in AF in conjunction with a careful ultrasound examination is the next step in the evaluation of an elevated serum AFP level.
   b. **Acetylcholinesterase (AChE)** is also found in AF in abnormally high concentrations in association with open NTDs and omphalocele. In addition, isomers not normally found in AF are found there in the presence of NTDs. Amniotic fluid AChE is normally evaluated in cases of suspected NTD.

c. **Bilirubin** is normally found in AF in small amounts that decrease toward term. In cases of isoimmune hemolysis, the level of bilirubin in the AF is elevated. This elevation is proportional to the degree of hemolysis and is a useful adjunct in evaluating affected pregnancies. The bilirubin is measured spectrophotometrically as the ΔOD_{450} (see Chap. 15).

2. **The cellular elements** of AF may be used to diagnose a variety of chromosomal and genetic disorders (see Chap. 11). The cells in the AF are desquamated from a variety of fetal surfaces, including amnion, skin, and the tracheobronchial tree. Only a small percentage of these cells are viable or capable of dividing, but they can be cultured to produce large numbers of actively growing and dividing cells for necessary studies.
   a. **Karyotyping** of cultured AF cells is the most commonly performed test on fetal cells. The most common reason to do the karyotyping is to detect Down syndrome or other trisomies that occur with increasing frequency with increasing maternal age. History of a previous trisomic infant or a known balanced translocation in either parent also would be an indication for karyotype analysis of the fetus. Karyotyping reliably determines the fetal sex early in pregnancy, which is useful in counseling a patient with regard to her risk in families with known X-linked disorders that are not definitively diagnosable (e.g., X-linked hydrocephalus).
   b. **Biochemical and enzymatic assays** can be performed on the cultured cells to detect a wide variety of inborn errors of metabolism [28]. The enzyme deficiencies responsible for the sphingolipidoses, glycogenoses, and mucopolysaccharidoses, as well as Lesch-Nyhan syndrome and others, have been demonstrated. The biochemical abnormalities associated with a number of the aminoacidurias as well as such varied diseases as porphyria and Menke's disease have been demonstrated.
   c. **DNA analysis** by means of recombinant DNA technology is rapidly replacing standard biochemical and enzymatic techniques for a number of reasons [3]. First, it is not necessary to study the expression of the biochemical abnormality in any particular cell line. For example, it was formerly necessary to obtain fetal blood to analyze for hemoglobin S and A to diagnose sickle-cell disease. By recombinant DNA technology, however, any fetal cells can be studied because all cells contain the same DNA complement even if they do not express it. Second, it is not necessary to understand the biochemical abnormality responsible for the disease in question. Recently, the diagnosis of Huntington's chorea has been achieved through a large family study of linkage analysis between the Huntington's gene and a closely linked polymorph.

      As more endonucleases are found, larger DNA probe libraries are developed, and more polymorphic DNA regions are discovered, the entire human genome should theoretically be definable.

C. **Fetal blood** has, until very recently, been all but inaccessible for diagnostic purposes.
   1. **Percutaneous umbilical blood sampling (PUBS)** is the most exciting advance in fetal assessment of this decade. Accidental needle puncture of the umbilical cord at the time of amniocentesis had always been carefully avoided because it was thought to be associated with a high risk of fetal death. Daffos [6] showed that a small needle could be intentionally guided into the cord vessels under ultrasound with little risk of fetal morbidity or mortality. The revelation that fetal blood is relatively readily accessible in this way has permitted major advances in prenatal diagnosis and treatment of a number of disorders. Some of the more important specific applications to date have included the following:
      a. Diagnosis and treatment of fetal anemia due to isoimmune hemolysis (see Chap. 15).

b. Diagnosis of fetal toxoplasmosis infection (see Chap. 12).
c. Diagnosis and treatment of fetal thrombocytopenia due to maternal idiopathic thrombocytopenia purpura (ITP) or isoimmune destruction (see Chap. 19).
d. Diagnosis of fetal distress by pH measurement.
e. Rapid chromosome analysis from lymphocytes on occasions when major malformations have been diagnosed in the third trimester.
f. Diagnosis of nonimmune fetal hydrops (see Chap. 15).

D. **Chorionic villus sampling (CVS)** is the technique of obtaining a small quantity of placental tissue for diagnostic purposes. The greatest utility of this technique is in the first trimester. Placental "biopsies" in the third trimester have also been described, but PUBS makes them unnecessary. There has been tremendous interest in this technique in recent years, with intensive investigations into the safest techniques for obtaining the specimens. The most commonly used technique in the United States is to introduce a 1.5-mm-diameter cathether through the cervix at 9 to 11 completed weeks of gestation. The catheter is guided by means of ultrasound to the placenta, where suction is applied and a specimen is aspirated into a syringe. The tissue is then examined immediately to confirm that an adequate quantity of villi has been obtained, and the decidua clinging to the villi is stripped away. Alternatively, villi can be aspirated through an 18-gauge needle introduced through the maternal abdominal wall and directed into the placenta. The fetal tissue can then be processed for karyotyping, biochemical and enzymatic assays, or DNA analysis. CVS offers three major advantages over amniocentesis. First, sufficient numbers of mitoses are present in the villi that direct preparations can be made for karyotyping without first culturing the specimens. This yields very rapid diagnosis. Second, a relatively large quantity of actively growing tissue is obtained that is often sufficient for direct biochemical or enzymatic analysis. If culture is necessary, relatively large numbers of cells grow quickly. Finally, the entire process of prenatal diagnosis and, if necessary, pregnancy termination can be completed early in pregnancy, when the termination procedure is safer and less emotionally traumatic. At present, the safety of the procedure is still a concern. Data indicate that the transcervical CVS procedure–related spontaneous abortion rate of approximately 2 percent is higher than that for amniocentesis. Whether this can be improved with experience and technical refinements remains to be seen. A large mulitcenter trial in the United States has recently been completed and reported. These results confirm that the risk of procedure related loss for CVS is still somewhat higher than amniocentesis at 16 weeks.

References

1. Adams, M. J., Jr. *Am. J. Obstet. Gynecol.* 148: 241, 1984.
2. Anderson, J. F. *Am. J. Obstet. Gynecol.* 139: 173, 1981.
3. Antonarakis, S. E. *J. Pediatr.* 100: 845, 1982.
4. Benson, C. B. *Am. J. Obstet. Gynecol.* 156: 441, 1987.
5. Brenner, W. E. *Am. J. Obstet. Gynecol.* 126: 555, 1976.
6. Daffos, F. *Am. J. Obstet. Gynecol.* 153: 655, 1985.
7. Deter, R. L., Hadlock, F. P., and Harrist, R. B. Evaluation of Normal Fetal Growth and the Detection of Intrauterine Growth Retardation. In P. W. Callen (Ed.), *Ultrasonography in Obstetrics and Gynecology.* Philadelphia: Saunders, 1983. P. 113.
8. Freeman, R. K. *Am. J. Obstet. Gynecol.* 143: 771, 1982.
9. Freeman, R. K. *Am. J. Obstet. Gynecol.* 143: 778, 1982.
10. Frigoletto, F. D. Jr. *Clin. Obstet. Gynecol.* 20: 915, 1977.
11. Gimovsky, M. L. *Clin. Perinatol.* 9: 313, 1982.
12. Greene, M. F., Fencl, M. deM., and Tulchinsky, D. Biochemical Aspects of Preg-

nancy. In N. W. Tietz (Ed.), *Textbook of Clinical Chemistry*. Philadelphia: Saunders, 1986. P. 1745.

13. Jones, M. D. *Am. J. Obstet. Gynecol.* 127: 540, 1977.
14. Keegan, K. A. *Am. J. Obstet. Gynecol.* 136: 75, 1980.
15. Knuppel, R. A. *J. Reprod. Med.* 27: 120, 1982.
16. Leveno, K. J. *N. Engl. J. Med.* 315: 615, 1986.
17. MacDonald, D. *Am. J. Obstet. Gynecol.* 152: 524, 1985.
18. Manning, F. A. *Am. J. Obstet. Gynecol.* 139: 254, 1981.
19. Manning, F. A. *Am. J. Obstet. Gynecol.* 140: 289, 1981.
20. Manning, F. A. *Am. J. Obstet. Gynecol.* 151: 343, 1985.
21. Manning, F. A. *Am. J. Obstet. Gynecol.* 157: 880, 1987.
22. Palomaki, G. E. *Am. J. Obstet. Gynecol.* 156: 460, 1987.
23. Prentice, A. *Lancet* 2: 1375, 1987.
24. Rayburn, W. F. *Clin. Perinatol.* 9: 231, 1982.
25. Reuwer, P. J. H. M. *Lancet* 2: 415, 1987.
26. Robinson, H. P. *Br. J. Obstet. Gynaecol.* 82: 702, 1975.
27. Sabbagha, R. E. *Obstet. Gynecol.* 52: 420, 1978.
28. Stephenson, S. R. *Am. J. Obstet. Gynecol.* 141: 319, 1981.
29. Verjaal, M. *Prenat. Diagn.* 1: 173, 1981.
30. Waldenstrom, U. *Lancet* 2: 585, 1988.
31. Woo, J. S. K. *J. Ultrasound Med.* 6: 291, 1987.
32. Yeh, M. N. *Am. J. Obstet. Gynecol.* 144: 519, 1982.

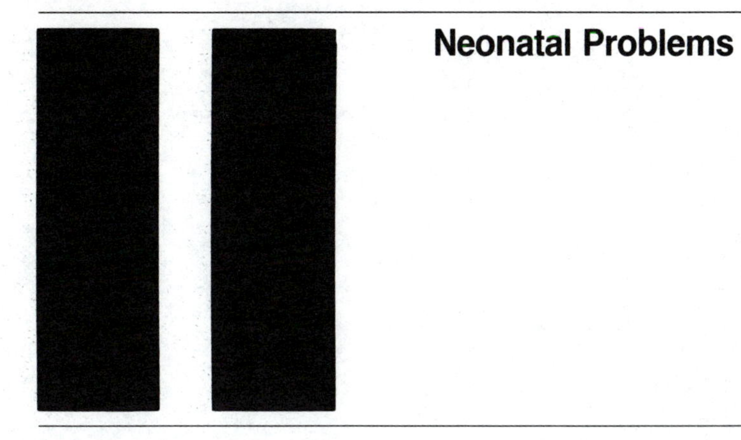

Neonatal Problems

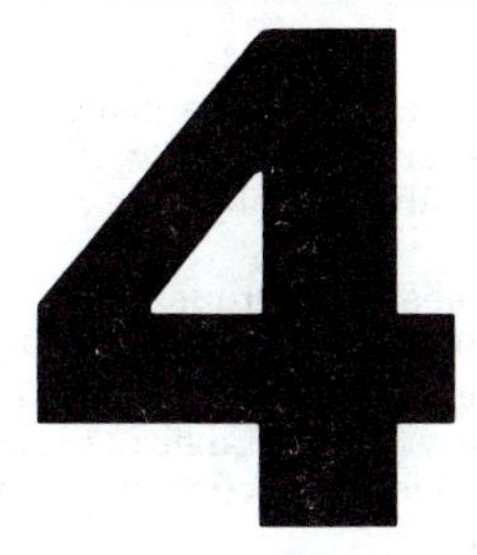

Obstetric and Neonatal Anesthesia

Angela M. Bader and
Gerard W. Ostheimer

I. **Goals of Obstetric Anesthesia.** Of continuing concern to obstetricians, anesthesiologists, and pediatricians are the effects of maternally administered drugs on the fetus and the newborn. This chapter presents an overview of the drugs and techniques commonly used for pain relief during labor and delivery.

A. **The ideal therapeutic program** would have the following characteristics:
1. Relief of maternal pain
2. No interference with the normal forces of labor
3. Preservation of maternal homeostatic mechanisms
4. Preservation of maternal awareness and participation
5. Minimal fetal drug exposure
6. No interference with normal neonatal adjustments to extrauterine life
7. No additional risk to an already compromised mother, fetus, or neonate

B. **Modern anesthetic agents and techniques attempt to approach these goals** [16,19]. Anesthetic effects on mother and fetus depend on the agent, dosage, route and time of administration, and presence of medical or obstetric complications.

II. **Drugs and techniques in obstetric analgesia and anesthesia**

A. **Anesthesia practices at the Brigham and Women's Hospital (BWH) in 1988–1989**
1. **For vaginal delivery** (76.0 percent of deliveries).
   a. Continuous lumbar epidural block (55.2 percent)
   b. Spinal anesthesia (0.6 percent)
   c. Local anesthesia (31.7 percent) or no anesthesia (12.4 percent)
   d. General anesthesia (0.03 percent)
2. **For cesarean delivery** (24.0 percent of deliveries)
   a. Epidural anesthesia (52.8 percent)
   b. Spinal anesthesia (38.5 percent)
   c. General anesthesia (8.7 percent)

B. **Systemic analgesia and sedation for labor**
1. **Narcotics.** The primary form of systemic pain relief. Most commonly used are meperidine (Demerol), butorphanol (Stadol), nalbuphine (Nubain), and fentanyl (Sublimaze).
2. **Tranquilizers**—phenothiazines (Phenergan, Vistaril) or benzodiazapines (Valium)
3. **Sedative-hypnotics** such as barbiturates are no longer popular because of prolonged neonatal depressant effects [4].

C. **Inhalation analgesia for delivery.** Inhalation analgesia is not recommended because of the risk of maternal aspiration.

D. **General anesthesia**
1. **Intravenous agents**—thiopental or ketamine
2. **Inhalation anesthetics**—nitrous oxide with halothane, enflurane, or isoflurane
3. **Neuromuscular blockers**—succinylcholine or curare-like agents
4. In the doses currently used, no significant fetal effects have been demonstrated. However, all inhalational agents equilibrate across the pla-

centa, and after 15 minutes, the fetus is essentially under general anesthesia. Therefore, all infants born after cesarean delivery with general anesthesia need oxygen by mask to prevent diffusion hypoxia as the inhalational agents are excreted.

E. Conduction (regional) anesthesia with local anesthetic drugs

1. **For labor only. Paracervical block:** Local anesthetic is injected lateral to cervix. This method is rarely used because of the relatively high incidence of fetal bradycardia. Because of the proximity of the fetal head to the site of injection, there is also a risk of accidental fetal injection and local anesthetic intoxication.
2. **For delivery only**
   - **a.** Spinal or subarachnoid block ("saddle block")
   - **b.** Pudendal nerve block
   - **c.** Infiltration of the perineum
3. **For labor and delivery**
   - **a.** Lumbar epidural block
   - **b.** Caudal block is rarely used because of the larger drug doses needed and the difficulty extending sensory level should cesarean delivery be required.

F. At BWH, with 24-hour in-house anesthesia service, **epidural anesthesia** is commonly used for **vaginal delivery.** For **cesarean delivery, regional anesthesia** is used when possible to avoid complications of endotracheal intubation. **General anesthesia** is used in **emergencies** where speed is essential and where regional anesthesia is contraindicated (maternal blood loss, coagulopathy). Fathers are permitted to attend both vaginal and cesarean deliveries, except when general anesthesia is administered.

III. Potential causes of anesthesia-related complications [16,19]

A. Maternal effects

1. **Alterations of maternal ventilation**
   - **a. Central respiratory depression (e.g., due to narcotics).** Agonist/antagonist agents such as butorphanol and nalbuphine may offer some advantage because of the ceiling effect for respiratory depression.
   - **b. Respiratory obstruction.** Aspiration of gastric contents into the lungs may occur when a patient is given general anesthesia (Mendelson's syndrome). All obstetric patients receive clear antacids (0.3 *M* sodium citrate or its equivalent) if any anesthetic is administered. Endotracheal intubation is mandatory after rapid intravenous induction of anesthesia.
   - **c. Hyperventilation.** Very low maternal arterial carbon dioxide tension ($PaCO_2$) is associated with low fetal arterial oxygen tension (PaO_2) and increased base deficit.
2. **Alterations in maternal circulation**
   - **a. Hypotension** is frequently associated with the sympathetic blockade that accompanies spinal or epidural block. Hypotension is aggravated by positional effects.
   - **b. Positional effects.** The supine position with the gravid uterus produces aortocaval compression (supine hypotensive syndrome). Labor should progress with the patient on her side or tilted to the left. Cesarean delivery should be performed with the patient tilted to the left. Maternal hypotension is associated with decreased placental blood flow and fetal hypoxia. Prevention or treatment is by fluid infusion and position change. Ephedrine is the vasopressor of choice because of minimal effects on uterine blood flow [10].
3. **Toxic effects of local anesthetics.** High maternal systemic levels may cause convulsions, asphyxia, and cardiovascular depression. The capability for resuscitation is mandatory whenever regional anesthesia is used.

4. **Effects of anesthesia on uterine activity**
   a. **Inhalation anesthetics** (halothane, enflurane, isoflurane) decrease uterine contractility.
   b. **Local anesthetics** and epinephrine-containing local anesthetic solutions in the doses used are believed to have little effect on uterine activity.

B. **Fetal effects.** All the commonly used drugs cross the placenta in varying degrees. Placental transfer is by simple diffusion according to Fick's law.
   1. **Direct fetal effects.** Some drugs (e.g., atropine, diazepam, butorphanol) cause alterations in fetal heart rate patterns that may not be associated with fetal asphyxia. Loss of variability has been associated with diazepam, and narcotics have been associated with a sinusoidal fetal heart rate pattern [3,17].
   2. **Unintentional direct intrafetal injection** of local anesthetic has been reported with paracervical and caudal blocks. A syndrome of apnea, bradycardia, and opisthotonus has been associated with local anesthetic intoxication. Flaccidity or convulsions may occur. Needle marks may be found on the infant's scalp. In these infants, local anesthetic concentrations were found to be greater in gastric secretions and in urine than in blood. Treatment consists of supportive measures and includes gastric lavage and promotion of urinary excretion as well as exchange transfusion [7,12].

C. **Neonatal effects**
   1. **Respiratory depression.** Morphine and meperidine are believed to cause a dose-related neonatal respiratory depression [24]. Because the metabolites of meperidine also have a respiratory depressant effect, less neonatal respiratory depression is seen when delivery occurs less than 1 hour or more than 4 hours after IM injection of meperidine [20]. Respiratory depressant effects are reversible with naloxone administration (see Chap. 5).
   2. **Thermoregulation.** Diazepam (Valium) impairs neonatal response to cold stress [9].
   3. **Neurobehavioral effects.** Sophisticated tests of neurologic and behavioral function in the newborn, such as the Brazelton and Scanlon examinations, have been developed [16,19]. These tests suggest that maternal analgesia and anesthesia may have subtle neonatal effects whose clinical significance is not yet established.
      a. These effects are largely dose-related and are particularly marked with systemic medication, such as narcotics, barbiturates, and diazepam [4,9,20,24].
      b. Bupivacaine, lidocaine, and chloroprocaine are the primary agents used for epidural anesthesia. Adverse effects on neurobehavior have not been seen with bupivacaine or chloroprocaine. For lidocaine, some studies show a decrease in motor tone for the first few hours of life; other studies do not confirm these results. At present, since the clinical significance of any alterations is not known, all three drugs appear safe for epidural use when used properly [6].

D. **Anesthesia interaction with medical or obstetric complications.** The goal is the provision of maternal analgesia or anesthesia without further compromise to mother or fetus. Areas of concern include the following:
   1. **Uteroplacental insufficiency** may be associated with fetal distress, intrauterine growth retardation, and fetal acidosis. An already acidotic fetus may accumulate local anesthetic, and this may aggravate cardiovascular depression [5].
   2. **Toxemia.** It is important to avoid hypotension in the face of placental vascular insufficiency. Maternal treatment with large doses of magnesium sulfate may cause neonatal hypermagnesemia with flaccidity, hyporeflexia, ileus, and hypoventilation [15].

3. **Diabetes.** Regional anesthesia can be safely used in diabetic mothers if fluid status is carefully evaluated and hypotension is avoided [11]. The goal is to keep maternal blood sugar levels in the normal range to prevent rebound hypoglycemia in the neonate after delivery.
4. **Abnormal presentation.** Regional anesthesia is associated with good fetal outcome in breech deliveries and with twins [16,19].
5. **Obesity.** Maternal obesity presents difficulties with administration of either regional or general anesthesia. The anesthesiologist is particularly concerned with potential difficulties with endotracheal intubation and will frequently recommend early institution of epidural anesthesia [16,19].

IV. **Specific anesthetic techniques** [16,19]

A. **Spinal anesthesia** is used at BWH in 0.6 percent of vaginal deliveries and 38.5 percent of cesarean deliveries.

1. **Advantages of spinal anesthesia**
   a. It is **rapid** and **efficient.**
   b. There is **minimal fetal drug exposure** and no adverse fetal effects if hypotension is avoided.
   c. The patient remains **conscious.**
   d. There is **good muscle relaxation** of the abdomen and perineum.
2. **Disadvantages of spinal anesthesia**
   a. **Hypotension** may occur secondary to sympathetic blockade. Significant hypotension is associated with fetal acidosis.
   b. It is **less controllable** than epidural block in terms of duration and extent.
   c. **Dural puncture headache** may occur (an incidence of about 5 percent even when a 26-gauge needle is used).
3. **Bupivacaine** (0.75% in 8.25% dextrose) is the agent most commonly used for spinal anesthesia at BWH.

B. **Lumbar epidural block** is used in 55.2 percent of vaginal deliveries and in 52.8 percent of cesarean deliveries at BWH.

1. **Advantages of epidural anesthesia**
   a. It is **effective** for both labor and delivery.
   b. The patient is **conscious.**
   c. It is **controllable** and can be individualized; a catheter inserted in the lumbar epidural space allows reinjection of local anesthetic as required.
2. **Disadvantages of epidural anesthesia**
   a. Fetal and maternal drug exposure is much greater than with spinal anesthesia because of the **larger doses required.** Because of the higher maternal systemic levels, the possibility of local anesthetic toxic reactions exists.
   b. Administration is more **time consuming.**
   c. **Hypotension** may occur as with spinal anesthesia (see above).
   d. Unintentional **dural puncture** may occur (1.5 percent incidence).
3. **Local anesthetic agents for epidural block**
   a. **Bupivacaine** (Marcaine) is long acting and has low blood levels, a low fetal-maternal concentration ratio, a short half-life in neonatal blood, and no known neurobehavioral effects in the newborn. During labor, this drug can be given in low concentrations and can be combined with epidural narcotics to provide effective analgesia and minimize the motor block. Maternal toxic levels have been associated with arrhythmias and cardiac arrest [14].
   b. **Chloroprocaine** (Nesacaine) has a more rapid onset and is shorter acting. It is rapidly destroyed by plasma pseudocholinesterase and has little fetal exposure and no known neonatal neurobehavioral effects. Previous concerns about neurotoxicity [18] have been alleviated by a new formulation of this agent.
   c. **Lidocaine** (Xylocaine) is an intermediate-acting agent. Because of the

relatively greater degree of motor block, it is usually reserved for cesarean or forceps delivery.

C. **Pudendal nerve block or local infiltration of the perineum**
   1. **Advantages**
      a. **Simple** to perform.
      b. The mother is **conscious.**
      c. There are **few reported complications** or side effects.
   2. **Disadvantages.** These methods are not as effective as epidural or spinal anesthesia.

D. **General anesthesia** is not offered for normal, uncomplicated vaginal delivery at BWH, but it is used in 8.7 percent of cesarean deliveries.
   1. **Advantages of general anesthesia**
      a. **Speed**
      b. **Controllability**
   2. **Disadvantages**
      a. **Complications** of endotracheal intubation may occur.
      b. Maternal awareness may occur.
      c. The fetus is exposed to the anesthetic agents used (see sec. **II**).
      d. **Hyperventilation** may occur with possible uterine vasoconstriction and adverse effects on the fetus.
      e. There is an increased incidence of low Apgar scores if the induction-to-delivery interval is prolonged.

V. **Perinatal pharmacology.** The following is a listing of some of the factors that influence drug action and pharmacokinetics in the perinatal period:

A. **Maternal factors**
   1. Physiologic changes of pregnancy and parturition
   2. Altered drug sensitivity
   3. Drug distribution in the mother (effects of uterine blood flow and protein binding)

B. **Placental factors**
   1. Uterine and umbilical blood flow
   2. Drug diffusion (effects of lipid solubility, ionization, and protein binding)

C. **Fetal factors**
   1. Fetal circulation ("first pass" effect in the fetal liver)
   2. Protein binding
   3. Altered tissue permeabilities and affinities
   4. Drug biotransformation
   5. Excretion and presence in amniotic fluid

D. **Neonatal factors**
   1. Physiologic changes at birth
   2. Developmental age and stage of maturation
   3. Reduced esterase activity
   4. Plasma protein binding
      a. Reduced protein concentration
      b. High concentrations of bilirubin and free fatty acids
      c. Increased apparent volume of drug distribution
   5. Drug distribution
      a. Changing pattern of regional blood flows
      b. Relatively greater brain and liver mass
      c. Lower myelin content of brain
      d. Higher total-body water and extracellular-intracellular water ratio
      e. Scanty adipose tissue
   6. Biotransformation
      a. Immaturity of certain hepatic enzyme systems
      b. Enzyme induction or inhibition
   7. Reduced renal function

VI. **Use of anesthetic agents in the neonate** [27]. In the past, some physicians avoided using analgesic or anesthetic agents in neonates because of beliefs that neonates do not have sufficiently mature cortical function to recall painful experiences and that neonates undergoing surgery are too unstable to justify the risk of an anesthetic. There is an increasing body of evidence that neonates demonstrate physiologic responses to surgical procedures similar to those of adults and that neonatal cortical function may be greater than previously thought [1,13,23,25]. The American Academy of Pediatrics and the American Society of Anesthesiology now advocate that local or systemic pharmacologic agents can be safely administered to provide analgesia and anesthesia to neonates [8]. In the sick neonate, the usual anesthetic guidelines for treatment of high-risk, potentially unstable patients are applicable.

A. **Local anesthetics** in appropriate doses can be used for peripheral procedures such as circumcision or chest tube insertion [21,22,25]. Lidocaine (0.5–1%) or bupivacaine (0.25–0.5%) can be used. Because of the immaturity of neonatal systems, the maximum anesthetic dose used should not exceed 50 percent of the suggested maximum dose for older children and adults [21]. The suggested maximum doses vary with the type of block performed and whether epinephrine is added to the local anesthetic. A textbook of anesthesia should be consulted for the specific block used [21]. Rough guidelines for maximum doses in older children are 5 mg/kg of lidocaine with 1:200,000 epinephrine and 2 mg/kg of bupivacaine with or without epinephrine. The length of anesthesia ranges from about 1 hour with plain lidocaine to over 4 hours for bupivacaine with epinephrine. Do not use epinephrine with local anesthesia for circumcision (see Chap. 8).

B. **Fentanyl** can be used for analgesia and anesthesia in the neonate. Low doses can be given and titrated as needed [2,26]. Adverse effects can be reversed with naloxone. Fentanyl in increments of 2.5 μg/kg has been used during surgery in infants. A total dose of at least 10 μg/kg is generally required for surgical anesthesia. Analgesia lasts about 2 hours after an IV bolus of fentanyl. For continuous analgesia, a drip of 5 μg/kg per hour can be administered intravenously. Fentanyl in high doses may be associated with chest wall rigidity. Fentanyl should only be given in a setting where support of respiration is immediately available. Chronic use of Fentanyl is associated with drug dependence in the newborn.

References

1. Anand, K. *N. Engl. J. Med.* 317: 1321, 1987.
2. Anand, K. *Lancet* 1(8524): 62, 1987.
3. Angel, J. *Am. J. Obstet. Gynecol.* 149: 465, 1984.
4. Brazelton, T. B. *Am. J. Psych.* 126: 95, 1970.

4A. Brown, T. C. K. Blockade for Pediatric Surgery. In *Neural Blockade,* J. B. Lippincott, Philadelphia, 1988.

5. Brown, W. *Obstet. Gynecol.* 48: 27, 1976.
6. Chantigian, R. C. and G. W. Ostheimer Effect of maternally administered drugs on the Fetus and Newborn. In A. Mulinksy (Ed.), *Advances in Perinatal Medicine.* Plenum Medicine Book Co., New York, 1986. P. 181.
7. Chase, D. *J. Pediatr.* 90: 127, 1977.
8. Committee on Fetus and Newborn, American Academy of Pediatrics. *Pediatrics* 80: 446, 1987.
9. Cree, J. *Br. Med. J.* 4: 251, 1973.
10. Datta, S. *Anesthesiology* 56: 68, 1982.
11. Datta, S. *Anesthesiology* 47: 272, 1977.
12. Dodson, W. *J. Pediatr.* 86: 624, 1975.
13. Holve, R. *Clin. Pediatr.* (Phila.) 22: 813, 1983.
14. Kotelko, D. *Anesthesiology* 60: 10, 1984.
15. Lipsitz, P. *Pediatrics* 47: 501, 1971.
16. Ostheimer, G. W. (Ed.). *Manual of Obstetric Anesthesia.* New York: Churchill-Livingstone, 1984.

17. Petrie, R. *Semin. Perinatol.* 2: 147, 1978.
18. Ravindran, R. *Anesth. Analg.* 61: 279, 1982.
19. Shnider, S. (Ed.) *Anesthesia for Obstetrics.* Baltimore: Williams & Wilkins, 1987.
20. Shnider, S. *Am. J. Obstet. Gynecol.* 89: 1009, 1964.
21. Singler, R. Pediatric Regional Anesthesia. In G. A. Gregory (Ed.), *Pediatric Anesthesia.* New York: Churchill-Livingstone, 1983. Chap. 16.
22. Stang, H. *J.A.M.A.* 1259: 1507, 1988.
23. Vacanti, J. *J. Pediatr. Surg.* 19: 672, 1984.
24. Way, W. *Clin. Pharmacol. Ther.* 6: 454, 1965.
25. Williamson, P. *Pediatrics* 71: 36, 1983.
26. Yaster, M. *Anesthesiology* 66: 433, 1987.
27. Yaster, M. *J. Pediatr.* 111: 394, 1987.

Resuscitation in the Delivery Room

Michael F. Epstein

I. **General principles.** A person skilled in resuscitation of the newborn should be present at the delivery of all high-risk infants [6,16]. To perform optimally, one must become as comfortable as possible in the delivery room atmosphere and develop a routine of evaluation and resuscitation that can be carried out systematically. There is no time for indecision, yet an incorrect decision can be tragic. Successful performance in this situation involves knowledge of perinatal physiology and principles of resuscitation, mastery of technical skills, and the ability to interact successfully with delivery room physicians and nurses.

A. **Physiologic factors.** Resuscitation efforts in the delivery room are designed to aid the newborn in his or her efforts to accomplish the necessary physiologic changes in the transition from fetal to neonatal life. These respiratory and circulatory changes must be accomplished rapidly and effectively in the first minutes after delivery or survival is jeopardized. The physiologic changes that occur are related primarily to expansion of the lungs, establishment of effective air exchange, and termination of the right-to-left circulatory shunts that are normally present during fetal life. The critical time for these physiologic changes is during the first several breaths, which result in lung expansion and elevation of the partial pressure of oxygen (PO_2) in both the alveoli and the arterial circulations. Once the PO_2 has been elevated from the fetal levels of approximately 25 mmHg to the level of 50 to 70 mmHg after delivery, there is (1) a decrease in pulmonary vascular resistance, (2) a decrease in the right-to-left shunting by way of the ductus arteriosus, (3) an increase in venous return to the left atrium, (4) a rise in left atrial pressure, and (5) a cessation of right-to-left shunt through the foramen ovale. The result is a conversion from fetal to transitional and, finally, to neonatal circulation pattern. Adequate systemic arterial oxygenation results from perfusion of well-expanded and well-ventilated lungs.

B. **Goals of resuscitation.** Resuscitation efforts are directed toward the following:

1. Expansion of the lungs by clearing the upper airway and ensuring a patent route to the trachea.
2. Increasing the arterial PO_2 by providing adequate alveolar ventilation, with added oxygen if necessary.
3. Supporting adequate cardiac output.
4. Ensuring that oxygen consumption by the neonate is minimized by reducing heat losses in the immediate postpartum period.

II. **Preparation**

A. **Perinatal conditions associated with high-risk deliveries.** In most cases the obstetrician should notify the pediatrician well in advance of the actual birth of the infant. The pediatrician then has the opportunity to review the history of the pregnancy and the events leading to the high-risk delivery. Knowledge of maternal history will help the pediatrician prepare for the specific problems that may be encountered. The following prepartum and intrapartum events indicate that an individual skilled in resuscitation should be present at a delivery [5].

1. **Fetal distress as evident by**
   a. Serious abnormalities of fetal heart rate, e.g., sustained bradycardia
   b. Scalp pH $\leq$ 7.20
2. **Fetal disease or potentially serious conditions**
   a. Thick meconium in amniotic fluid
   b. Prematurity ($\leq$36 weeks), postmaturity (>42 weeks), low birth weight (<2.0 kg), or large birth weight (>4.5 kg).
   c. Major congenital anomalies detected antenatally
   d. Hydrops
   e. Multiple births
   f. Cord prolapse
3. **Labor and delivery conditions**
   a. Significant vaginal bleeding
   b. Midforceps delivery
   c. Abnormal presentation
   d. Prolonged, unusual, or difficult labor

B. The following conditions do not require a skilled resuscitator to be present but require the availability of such a person for assessment and triage.
   1. **Neonatal conditions**
      (a) Unexpected congenital anomalies
      (b) Respiratory distress
      (c) Unanticipated neonatal depression, Apgar score of <6 at 5 minutes
   2. **Maternal conditions**
      (a) Signs of maternal infection:
         (1) Maternal fever
         (2) Membranes ruptured for >24 hours
         (3) Foul-smelling amniotic fluid
         (4) History of sexually transmitted disease
      (b) Maternal illness or conditions
         (1) Diabetes mellitus
         (2) Rh sensitization or other isoimmunization
         (3) Chronic hypertension or pregnancy-induced hypertension
         (4) Renal, endocrine, pulmonary, or cardiac disease
         (5) Substance or alcohol abuse

C. Equipment. The necessary equipment must be present and operating properly. Each delivery room should be equipped with the following:
1. **Radiant warmer** with procedure table or bed. Additional heat lamps for warming the very-low-birth-weight infant are also useful.
2. **Oxygen source** with adjustable flowmeter and adequate length of tubing. Humidifier and warmer are desirable, although not essential.
3. Flow-through **anesthesia bag** with adjustable pop-off valve capable of delivering 100% oxygen.
4. **Face mask(s)** of appropriate size.
5. **Stethoscope** with infant- or premature-sized head.
6. **Emergency box** containing:
   a. Laryngoscope with no. 0 and no. 1 blades
   b. Extra batteries
   c. Uniform diameter endotracheal tubes (2.5-, 3.0-, and 3.5-mm internal diameters), two each
   d. Drugs, including epinephrine (1:10,000), sodium bicarbonate (0.50 mEq/ml), naloxone, albumin 5%, and NaCl 0.9%
   e. Umbilical catheterization tray and no. 3.5 and no. 5 French catheters.
   f. Syringes (1.0, 3.0, 5.0, 10.0, and 20.0 ml), needles (18 to 25 gauge), T-connectors, and stopcocks
7. Transport incubator and battery-operated heat source and portable oxygen supply should be available if the delivery room and nursery are not in close proximity.

8. There is no consensus regarding equipment to continuously monitor cardiopulmonary status in the delivery room. Standard leads for cardiac monitors and transcutaneous oxygen monitors are either difficult to apply effectively or take too much time to stabilize for accurate readings. Recent studies of oximeters provide hope that useful data regarding oxygen saturation as well as heart rate may be immediately available in a noninvasive, relatively inexpensive, and easily applied technique [13].

D. **Preparation of equipment.** On arriving in the delivery room, one must make certain that the transport incubator is plugged in, warming up, and equipped with a full oxygen tank. In the delivery room, the specialist should introduce himself or herself to the obstetrician and anesthesiologist, the mother (if she is awake), and the father (if he is present). While obtaining the history from the obstetrician and anesthesiologist, the following should be done:

1. Make sure the radiant warmer is on and dry blankets are available.
2. Turn on the oxygen source and ensure an adequate flow (5–8 l/min) to fill the bag.
3. Check the anesthesia bag for pop-off control and adequate flow. Be sure to have the proper-sized mask.
4. Make sure the laryngoscope light is bright and has an appropriate blade (no. 1 for full-term infants, no. 0 for premature infants).
5. Set out an endotracheal tube of the appropriate size for the expected birth weight (3.5 mm for full-term infants, 3.0 mm for premature infants over 1250 gm, and 2.5 mm for smaller infants).
6. If the potential clinical situation so indicates:
   a. Set up an umbilical catheterization tray for venous catheterization.
   b. Draw up sodium bicarbonate (0.5 mEq/ml solution, 1:10,000 epinephrine, and isotonic saline for catheter flush solution).
   c. Make sure that other potentially necessary drugs are present and ready for administration.

E. **Universal precautions.** In some urban areas, as many as 2.5 percent of all pregnant women are HIV-positive. Clearly, the delivery room is a setting where the risk of blood exposure is inevitable. Therefore, we practice universal precautions in the delivery room or birthing room by wearing caps, masks, goggles or glasses, gloves, and gowns. These precautions are maintained until the cord is cut and the baby is dried and wrapped.

III. **Delivery.** During the delivery, attention should be paid to the type and duration of anesthesia, amount of maternal bleeding, previously unrecognized problems such as meconium in the amniotic fluid or nuchal cord, and degree of placental transfusion.

A. **Once the infant is born,** a continual process of evaluation and resuscitation begins. When the infant is born,

1. Place the baby on the warming table.
2. Suction the mouth and oropharynx, and then the nares thoroughly with a suction bulb. If thick meconium (not just stained fluid) is present, suctioning of the oropharynx and trachea before the onset of respiration is indicated (see sec. **IV** and Meconium Aspiration in Chap. 13).
3. Dry the infant, especially the head and face, which comprise nearly 20 percent of body surface area.
4. Determine heart rate, respiration, tone, color, and response to stimulation (Apgar score) (see Table 5-1).
5. On the basis of this immediate assessment, observe and aid the baby's airway clearance and temperature maintenance or continue further resuscitation.

B. **Apgar score.** The Apgar score [2] consists of the total points assigned to five objective signs in the newborn. The five objective signs are evaluated and given a score of 0, 1, or 2. Scores at 1 and 5 minutes after birth are usually noted in the chart. If the 5-minute score is ≤ 6, the score should continue to be noted at 5-minute intervals until it is greater than 6 (see Table 5-1). A score of 10 indicates an infant in perfect condition, but this is quite unusual, be-

Table 5-1. Apgar scoring system

	Score		
Sign	0	1	2
Heart rate	Absent	Under 100 beats per minute	Over 100 beats per minute
Respiratory effort	Absent	Slow (irregular)	Good crying
Muscle tone	Limp	Some flexion of extremities	Active motion
Reflex irritability	No response	Grimace	Cough or sneeze
Color	Blue, pale	Pink body, blue extremities	All pink

Source: From Apgar, V. A proposal for a new method of evaluation of the newborn infant. *Anesth. Analg.* 32: 260, 1953.

cause most babies have some degree of acrocyanosis. The scoring, if done properly, yields the following information:

1. **One-minute Apgar score.** This score generally correlates with umbilical cord blood pH and is an index of intrapartum asphyxia. Babies with a score of 0 to 4 have been shown to have a significantly lower pH, higher partial pressure of carbon dioxide ($PaCO_2$), and lower buffer base than those whose Apgar score is greater than 7. One group of babies in whom a low Apgar *may* not indicate severe asphyxia is the very-low-birth-weight (VLBW) infant. Apgar scores of 0 to 3 have been reported in as many as 50 percent of 25- to 26-week gestation infants who have had a cord pH of greater than 7.25. A VLBW infant with a low Apgar score cannot be assumed to be severely asphyxiated. Nonetheless, such an infant should be resuscitated actively and will usually respond more promptly and to less invasive measures than the baby whose low Apgar accurately reflects acidemia.
2. **Apgar scores beyond 1 minute** are reflective of the child's changing condition and the adequacy of the resuscitative efforts. Persistence of a low Apgar score indicates that further therapeutic efforts are needed. The most common therapeutic error is failure to adequately inflate and ventilate the lungs. Failure to achieve a good seal with the mask, incorrect placement of the endotracheal tube, and most frequently, inadequate peak inspiratory pressure applied to the bag are correctable problems that should be addressed if the Apgar score fails to rise as resuscitation proceeds.

   The more prolonged the period of severe depression (i.e., Apgar score $\leq$ 3), the more likely is an abnormal long-term neurologic outcome. Nevertheless, many babies with prolonged depression (>15 minutes) are normal in follow-up. Moreover, most babies with long-term motor abnormalities such as cerebral palsy have not had periods of neonatal depression after birth [9] (see Perinatal Asphyxia in Chap. 21).

C. **Sequence of intervention.** The institution and sequence of resuscitative efforts are determined by the condition of the baby as evaluated by using the Apgar system. Adjustments in the level and intensity of efforts should be made continuously based on changes in this score. Caution must be taken not to be too vigorous in intervening when infants are making adequate progress by their own efforts. There are the risks of laryngospasm and cardiac arrhythmias from overly vigorous suctioning or of pneumothorax from overly vigorous bagging. Experience is the best guide to determining the measures that are indicated, and judgment based on the Apgar score is the best guide to achieving that experience successfully.

1. **No asphyxia (Apgar score of 8 to 10).** These scores are found in over 90 percent of all term babies by 1 minute after delivery.

a. Dry and place the infant under the warmer; suction upper airway with a bulb syringe. Evaluate for a full 5 minutes to be sure that hypoventilation does not occur. Make every effort to maintain body temperature, and avoid invasive maneuvers during the initial period of stabilization.

b. Cordero and Hon [7] investigated the effect of nasopharyngeal stimulation by a suction catheter on the heart rate of the newborn and found that deep pharyngeal stimulation may cause arrhythmias that are probably of vagal origin. We routinely use a suction bulb rather than a catheter to avoid deep pharyngeal and glottic stimulation, and only rarely have we observed such complications.

c. **Gastric aspiration** should **not** be done in the first few minutes of life in order to avoid causing any arrhythmias from nasopharyngeal or glottic stimulation; by 5 minutes after delivery, the neonate has become more stable and will tolerate passage of a nasogastric tube. All patients in the study by Cordero and Hon tolerated this procedure without bradycardia after 5 minutes of age.

2. **Mild asphyxia (Apgar score of 5 to 7).** Infants with Apgar scores of 5 to 7 are only mildly depressed. They generally have a normal heart rate and require only stimulation and oxygen. The goal is to induce the baby to take a spontaneous breath to achieve lung expansion and establish a **functional residual capacity (FRC).**

   a. **Stimulation.** Gentle slapping of the feet or rubbing of the back is all the stimulation needed for the newborn. More vigorous stimulation or manipulation has no therapeutic value and is potentially harmful.

   b. **Oxygen.** An oxygen-enriched atmosphere may easily be provided by gently placing the mask, connected to a flow-through anesthesia bag, above the baby's face. An Ambu-type, self-inflating bag has no oxygen flow unless pressure is applied and the valve is thereby opened. Therefore, the self-inflating bag is not useful in this situation. The goal is to elevate arterial PO_2 by making each breath deliver more oxygen to the alveoli. This is unnecessary in the preceding group of babies (Apgar scores of 8 to 10), in whom adequate respiratory efforts have sufficed to achieve adequate oxygenation.

3. **Moderate asphyxia (Apgar score of 3 to 4).** If the heart rate falls below 100 beats per minute despite stimulation and facial oxygen, bag and mask ventilation should be started. The critical determinants of adequate bag and mask ventilation are the use of a mask of appropriate size, correct application of the mask to the infant's face, correct positioning of the infant's head, adequate flow through the bag, and adequate inspiratory pressure. The initial breath after delivery should be delivered at a pressure of 30 to 40 cm H_2O. This will result in the establishment of functional residual capacity (FRC), and subsequent inflations will be effective at lower inspiratory pressures [4,14,23]. The inspiratory pressures should be reduced to 15 to 20 cm H_2O, except in infants with known or suspected disease leading to decreased pulmonary compliance. In that case, inspiratory pressures of 20 to 40 cm H_2O may be required. A rate of 40 breaths per minute should be used and the infant should be continually reassessed.

   Although these moderately asphyxiated infants are acidotic at birth, they are generally able to correct their respiratory acidosis spontaneously once respiration is established. This process may take up to several hours, but unless the pH remains less than 7.25, acidosis does not need further treatment.

4. **Severe asphyxia (Apgar score of 0 to 2).** These infants require immediate and vigorous resuscitation (see Fig. 5-1). This process requires at least three trained people working together swiftly and efficiently. A plan should be established prior to delivery of the infant so that each person knows what is his or her primary responsibility.

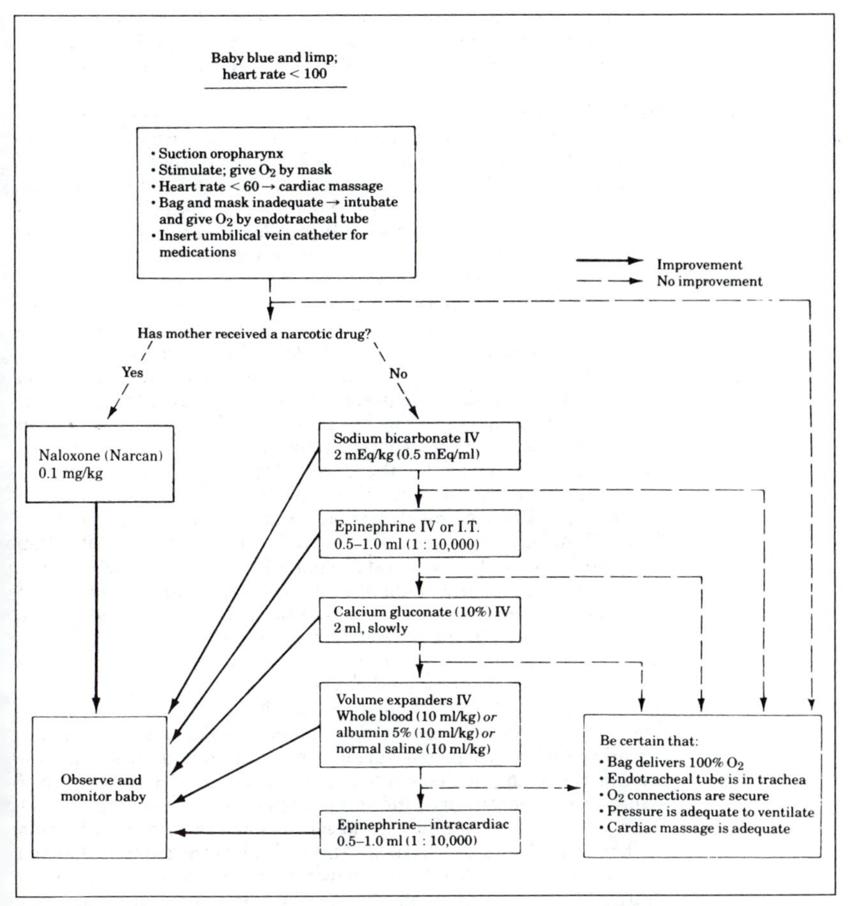

Fig. 5-1. Flow sheet for resuscitation of the newborn. (Adapted from Perinatal Continuing Education Program, University of Virginia. Courtesy of J. Kattwinkel.)

a. The **principles of newborn resuscitation** are the same as those for adult resuscitation:
   (1) **Airway management**
   (2) **Breathing**
   (3) **Circulation** (i.e., adequate cardiac output to maintain cerebral oxygenation)
   (4) **Drugs**

b. **Ventilation.** In most cases, once the airway is cleared, bag and mask ventilation is adequate.
   (1) **Adequacy of ventilation** is assessed by observing chest-wall motion at the cephalad portions of the thorax and listening for equal breath sounds laterally over the right and left hemithoraces at the midaxillary lines. The infant should be ventilated at a rate of 40 breaths per minute using the minimum pressure (usually 15 to 20 cm H_2O) that will move the chest and produce audible breath sounds. Infants with respiratory distress syndrome (RDS), pulmonary hypoplasia, or ascites may require higher pressures. The

most important measure of adequacy of ventilation is the infant's response. If, despite good air entry, the heart rate fails to increase and color remains poor, the baby needs to be intubated (see Chap. 39).

(2) Intubation should be accomplished rapidly by a skilled person (pediatrician, obstetrician, anesthetist, nurse, or respiratory therapist). The heart rate should increase to over 100 beats per minute, and color should rapidly improve with adequate ventilation. This skill can be readily learned and maintained through practice utilizing one of several commercially available models or through the humane use of ketamine-anesthetized kittens [11].

The key to intubation is to correctly position the baby and the laryngoscope and to know the anatomic landmarks. If the baby's chin, sternum, and genitalia are all lined up in a single plane, and if the laryngoscope handle and blade are placed in that plane, the intubator can only be seeing one of four anatomic landmarks: from cephalad to caudad, the posterior tongue, the epiglottis, the larynx, or the esophagus. The key to successful intubation is to be in the right plane and to know whether the landmark being observed is cephalad or caudad to the larynx. With correct identification of location, the intubator can make the adjustment of several millimeters in the position of the blade and locate the vocal cords.

c. Circulation. If, after intubation and 15 to 30 seconds of ventilation with 100% oxygen, the heart rate remains below 60 beats per minute, cardiac massage should be instituted. The best technique is to stand at the foot of the infant and place both thumbs at the junction of the middle and lower thirds of the sternum, with the fingers wrapped around and supporting the back [21]. Compress the sternum 120 times per minute. Determine the effectiveness of massage by palpating the femoral or brachial pulse or umbilical cord.

The best techniques for ensuring adequate cardiac output and, specifically, cerebral perfusion during resuscitation of adults and children as well as infants have recently been reviewed [18]. Advocates of simultaneous ventilation and chest compression have shown that mean aortic pressure and carotid blood flow are increased by this method. The theoretical basis for this finding is the concept that the heart is not compressed during conventional cardiopulmonary resuscitation (CPR) in adults and, therefore, is not a pump. Rather, chest compression increases intrathoracic pressure on all chest contents. This pressure is transmitted differentially to the extrathoracic arteries and veins, leading to forward flow during compression. During relaxation, pressure is higher in the extrathoracic veins than in the intrathoracic veins, and cardiac return occurs.

These observations have been well documented in dogs and in adults during monitored resuscitations. Their relevance to the newborn remains unclear. Since sternal compression by the fingers-encircling method almost certainly directly compresses the heart of the newborn, any added benefit of simultaneous ventilation and compression would be small. Moreover, the more rapid rates for both ventilation and compression used in newborns make the specific relationship of timing of these two activities more theoretical than practical.

At this time, there appears to be no grounds on which to alter the traditional approach to cardiac compression and ventilation in the newborn [20].

d. Medication. If, by 3 to 5 minutes after delivery, a heart rate of more than 100 beats per minute has not been achieved despite adequate ventilation with 100% oxygen, it is essential to correct acidosis and to provide the myocardium with glucose. It is often necessary to provide chronotropic and inotropic agents. The drugs used in resuscitation, along with their indications and dosages, are listed in Table 5-2 [3,17]. The goal of medication is to provide substrate and stimulation for the heart so that the heart can provide oxygen and nutrients to the brain.

(1) The most accessible route for administering medication to the neonate in the delivery room is by cannulation of the umbilical vein (see Chap. 39). Cannulation can be done rapidly and aseptically. Although the saline-filled catheter can be advanced into the inferior vena cava (i.e., 8 to 10 cm), in 60 to 70 percent of babies, the catheter may become wedged in an undesirable or dangerous location, e.g., hepatic, portal, or pulmonary vein. Therefore, insertion of the cannula approximately 1 to 2 cm past the abdominal wall to the point of easy blood return is safest prior to the injection of drugs. If the catheter rests in the ductus venosus, it is important to flush all medications through the catheter, because there is no flow through this vessel after cord separation.

(2) **Initial drug therapy** is designed to correct acidosis and to provide glucose as a substrate for myocardial metabolism. In the severely asphyxiated neonate, 2 to 4 mEq sodium bicarbonate per kilogram of body weight may be necessary to correct a documented acidosis (Fig. 5-2). This amount of **bicarbonate** may be administered as 4 to 8 ml/kg of **0.5 mEq/ml** sodium bicarbonate mixed with an equal volume of 25% dextrose in water administered over 2 to 4 minutes through the umbilical vein. Give dextrose 0.5 gm to 1.0 gm/kg (2 to 4 mg/kg of 25% solution). Continuing bradycardia is an indication for **epinephrine** administration. A dose of 0.1-0.3 ml/kg (up to 1.0 ml) of a 1:10,000 epinephrine solution should be given through the umbilical venous catheter and flushed into the central circulation. When access to the central circulation is difficult or delayed, consideration should be given to delivering epinephrine by means of the endotracheal tube for transpulmonary absorption. Studies in asphyxiated animals support the rapid absorption and action of endotracheally administered epinephrine to increase the heart rate and arterial blood pressure even in the presence of severe acidosis [8,16]. Case reports attest to the same effect in newborn infants, although larger experiences and controlled studies are lacking [12]. Nevertheless, it appears that intratracheal installation of 0.1 to 0.2 ml/kg of 1:10,000 epinephrine diluted 1:1 with sterile water is more rapid and safer than an attempt at intracardiac administration.

Since there are potential risks as well as benefits for all of the medications in Table 5-2, the use of drugs administered by means of the umbilical vein should be reserved for those babies in whom bradycardia persists despite adequate oxygen delivery and ventilation. If an adequate airway has been established, adequate ventilation has been achieved, and the heart rate exceeds 100 beats per minute, the infant is best moved to the neonatal intensive care unit, where careful physical examination and determination of blood pressure, heart rate, arterial blood gases, and chest radiographic appearance will more clearly identify the further need for specific interventions.

(3) **Volume expansion.** If, after oxygenation and correction of acidosis, blood pressure is low and peripheral perfusion is poor, volume expansion with albumin 5%, packed red blood cells, or whole blood may be indicated (see sec. **IV.B**). Volume expansion should be carried out cautiously in babies in whom asphyxial myocardial damage rather than hypovolemia may be the cause of the hypotension. It is important to use the appropriate gestational age–

Table 5-2. Drugs for resuscitation (see Appendix A) [3,17]

Drug or other form of therapy	How supplied	Dosage	Indication
Epinephrine	1 : 10,000 or 1 : 1000	0.1–0.3 ml/kg up to 1.0 ml of 1 : 10,000 solution injected into the umbilical vein or into the endotracheal tube	Asystole or severe bradycardia
Sodium bicarbonate	2.4 mEq/5 ml or 44 mEq/50 ml; the 44 mEq/50 ml (but not the 2.4 mEq/5 ml) should be diluted 1 : 1 with 10–25% D/W	2–4 mEq/kg (base excess × weight × 0.3), then repeat prn	Metabolic acidosis
Naloxone (Narcan) [1]	0.4 or 1.0 mg/ml (best to use 0.4 mg/ml)	0.1 mg/kg (including prematures) give IV, IM, or intratracheal in delivery room; dose may be repeated in 5 minutes; if after 2 or 3 doses no improvement is observed, discontinue naloxone; if there is initial reversal, the dose may have to be repeated at 1- to 2-hour intervals, depending on amount of and time interval since the last dose of narcotic: *do not use in infants born to narcotic-addicted mothers because it may precipitate acute withdrawal syndrome*	Narcotic depression
Dopamine	40 mg/ml	5–10 μg/kg per minute as needed to maintain blood pressure (dilute 1 ml with 100 ml 5% D/W)	Low cardiac output
Cardioversion		1 W/s per kilogram of body weight; maximum of 10 W/s	Ventricular fibrillation, paroxysmal atrial tachycardia (PAT)
Dextrose	10% or 25% solution	0.5–1 gm/kg of 25% solution (2.0–4.0 ml/kg) IV	Hypoglycemia
Plasma, Ringer's lactate, or whole blood		10–20 ml/kg	Blood loss, hypotension, volume depletion
Albumin	25% or 5% solution	1 gm/kg; dilute 25% solution to 5% (4 ml + 16 ml saline) for volume expansion; infuse over 10 minutes	Same as above

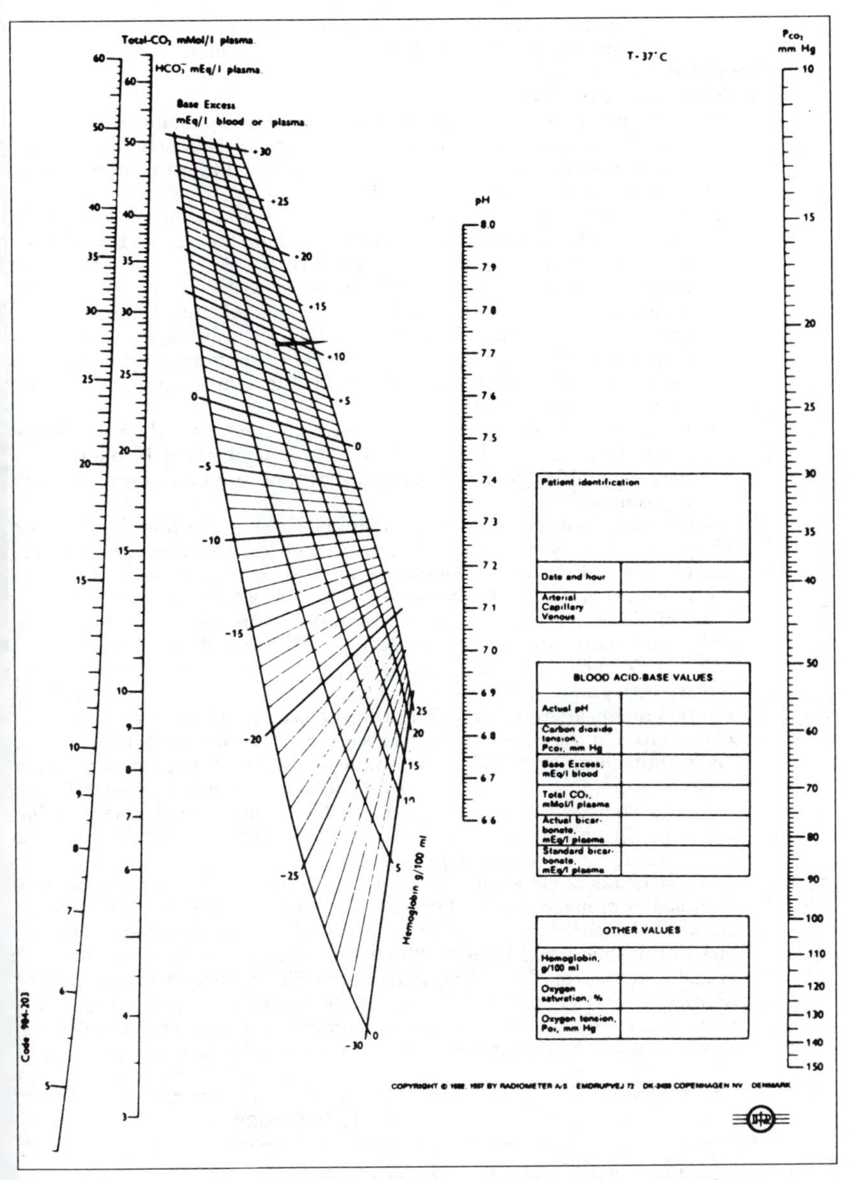

Fig. 5-2. Siggaard-Anderson alignment nomogram. This nomogram is used to determine the amount of bicarbonate (mEq HCO_3^- per liter of blood or plasma). It is reproduced for illustrative purposes only and as such cannot be used in actual laboratories for hospital work. (From O. Siggaard-Anderson, Blood acid-base alignment nomogram. *Scand. J. Clin. Lab. Invest.* 15(Suppl. 70): 1, 1963. Radiometer Reprint AS21. Copyright © 1962 by Radiometer A/S, Copenhagen, Denmark.)

and the birth weight–related blood pressure norms to determine the adequacy of volume status [22] (see Chap. 16).

IV. Special situations

A. Meconium aspiration

1. If the infant is born through thick, particulate meconium, the trachea must be suctioned (see Chap. 13). The obstetrician should suction the mouth and pharynx with a suction catheter or bulb syringe after delivery of the head and before breathing begins [6].
2. Following completion of the delivery, the infant should immediately be handed to the pediatrician, who should intubate the trachea and aspirate meconium, before the first breath if possible. Even if the infant has gasped, some meconium may still be removed with direct tracheal suction in many cases. New devices have been manufactured that have an adapter at one end that fits a suction catheter and an adapter at the other end that fits the endotracheal tube [3]. The resuscitator should be careful not to use suction techniques that could allow self-contamination with blood or vaginal contents.
3. In infants at risk of meconium aspiration syndrome who show initial respiratory distress, care should be taken at all times in the delivery room and NICU to provide adequate oxygen to prevent even transient hypoxemia.

B. Shock. Some infants present with pallor and shock in the delivery room (see Chaps. 6 and 16). Shock may result from a significant intrapartum blood loss due to placental separation, fetal-maternal hemorrhage, avulsion of the umbilical cord from the placenta, vasa or placenta previa, incision through an anterior placenta at cesarean section, twin-twin transfusion, or rupture of an abdominal viscus (liver or spleen) during a difficult delivery. These infants will be pale, tachycardic (over 180 beats per minute), tachypneic, and hypotensive with poor capillary filling and weak pulses. After stabilization of respiration and heart rate, immediate transfusion with O-negative packed red blood cells and 5% albumin may be necessary. A volume of 20 ml/kg can be given through an umbilical venous catheter. If clinical improvement is not seen, causes of further blood loss should be sought, and more vigorous blood and colloid replacement should be continued. It is important to remember that the hematocrit may be normal immediately after delivery if the blood loss was acute during the intrapartum period.

If a blood bank is not available, autologous blood from the placenta may be obtained by prepping the fetal surface of the placenta with Betadine and using a sterile needle and syringe that have been rinsed with heparin [10]. The risk of transmission of hepatitis B, HIV, or other infectious agents by blood transfusion from mother to baby must be considered when choosing a method of acute volume expansion. Although all these agents can cross the placenta and lead to antenatal infection, direct inoculation of maternal blood will certainly increase the risk of neonatal exposure and infection.

References

1. American Academy of Pediatrics. *Pediatrics* 83: 803, 1989.
2. Apgar, V. *Anesth. Analg.* 32: 260, 1953.
3. Bloom, R. S., and Cropley, C. *Textbook of Neonatal Resuscitation.* American Heart Association and American Academy of Pediatrics. Dallas, Texas: American Heart Association, 1987.
4. Boon, A. W. *J. Pediatr.* 95: 1031, 1979.
5. Braun, A. W., and Cefalo, R. C. (Eds.). Perinatal Care Services. In *Guidelines for Perinatal Care,* 2d Ed. American Academy of Pediatrics, American College of Obstetricians and Gynecologists, 1988. Pp. 73–80.
6. Carson, B. S. *Am. J. Obstet. Gynecol.* 126: 712, 1976.

7. Cordero, L. *J. Pediatr.* 78: 441, 1971.
8. Elam, J. O. The Intrapulmonary Route for CPR Drugs. In P. Safar (Ed.), *Advances in Cardiopulmonary Resuscitation.* New York: Springer-Verlag, 1977. Pp. 132–140.
9. Freeman, J. M., and Nelson, K. B. *Pediatrics* 82: 240, 1988.
10. Golden, S. M. *J. Pediatr.* 97: 810, 1980.
11. Jennings, P. B. *Pediatrics* 53: 283, 1974.
12. Lindemann, R. *Acta Paediatr. Scand.* 73: 210, 1984.
13. Maxwell, L. B., et al. *Clin. Pediatr.* 26: 18, 1987.
14. Milner, A. D., Vyas, H., and Hopkin, I. E. *Br. Med. J.* 289: 1563, 1984.
15. Primhak, R. A., Herber, S. M., Whincup, G., and Milner, R. D. *Br. Med. J.* 289: 16, 1984.
16. Redding, J. S. Drug Therapy During Cardiac Arrest. In P. Safar (Ed.), *Advances in Cardiopulmonary Resuscitation.* New York: Springer-Verlag, 1977. Pp. 113–117.
17. Roberts, R. J., et al. *Pediatrics* 81: 462, 1988.
18. Rogers, M. *Pediatrics* 71: 655, 1983.
19. Siggaard-Anderson, O. *Scand. J. Clin. Lab. Invest.* 12: 177, 1960.
20. Standards and guidelines for cardiopulmonary resuscitation and emergency cardiac care. *J.A.M.A.* 255: 2905, 1986.
21. Todres, I. D. *J. Pediatr.* 86: 781, 1975.
22. Versmold, H. T. *Pediatrics* 67: 607, 1981.
23. Vyas, H. *J. Pediatr.* 99: 635, 1981.

Shock

Stella Kourembanas

I. **Background.** Shock is an acute, complex pathophysiologic state of circulatory dysfunction that results in insufficient oxygen and nutrient delivery to satisfy the requirements of the tissue beds.

II. **Etiology of shock**

A. **Hypovolemia.** Decreased circulating blood volume is the most common cause of shock in the neonate (see Chap. 16). This decrease in blood volume can result from whole blood, plasma, or extravascular fluid loss due to the following:

1. Placental hemorrhage as in abruptio placentae or placenta previa
2. Fetal to maternal hemorrhage (diagnosed by Kleihauer-Betke test of mother's blood for presence of fetal red blood cells)
3. Twin-to-twin transfusion
4. Intracranial hemorrhage
5. Intraabdominal bleeding due to liver laceration from gastrointestinal surgery or due to a traumatic breech delivery (Necrotizing enterocolitis or other causes of peritonitis can result in excessive plasma loss.)
6. Massive pulmonary hemorrhage
7. Disseminated intravascular coagulation due to sepsis or other severe coagulation abnormalities
8. Plasma loss into the extravascular compartment seen with low oncotic pressure states or capillary leak syndrome as in sepsis
9. Excessive extravascular fluid losses seen with dehydration from insensible water loss or inappropriate diuresis commonly seen in the very premature infant.

B. **Distributive causes.** Abnormalities of distribution of blood flow can cause inadequate tissue perfusion. This may occur as a result of increased venous capacitance, vasomotor paralysis from pharmacologic agents, or shunting past capillary beds. Etiologies of maldistribution of blood flow include

1. **Sepsis.** The precise mechanisms underlying circulatory dysfunction in septic shock are not clear. They include a combination of factors such as direct depressing effect of microbial products on the cardiovascular system as well as release of other vasoactive agents such as serotonin, prostaglandins, histamine, and endorphins resulting in peripheral vasodilatation and relative hypovolemia.
2. **Drugs.** Agents that decrease vascular tone include muscle relaxants and anesthetics. Vancomycin has been reported to cause acute circulatory failure in newborn infants [5].

C. **Cardiogenic shock.** Although an infant's myocardium normally exhibits good contractility, various insults in the perinatal period, congenital cardiac abnormalities, or arrhythmias can result in heart failure.

1. Intrapartum asphyxia can cause poor contractility and papillary muscle dysfunction with tricuspid regurgitation resulting in low cardiac output.
2. Myocardial dysfunction can occur secondary to infectious agents (bacterial or viral) and to metabolic abnormalities such as hypoglycemia. In addition, cardiomyopathy can be seen in infants of diabetic mothers (IDMs) with or without hypoglycemia (see Chap. 1).

3. Obstruction to blood flow and resultant decreased cardiac output can be seen with a variety of congenital heart defects. These include

a. Inflow obstructions (see Chap. 14)

(1) Total anomalous pulmonary venous drainage

(2) Cor triatriatum

(3) Tricuspid atresia

(4) Mitral atresia

(5) Acquired inflow obstruction can occur from intravascular air or thrombotic embolus or from increased intrathoracic pressure with high airway pressures, pneumothorax, pneumomediastinum, or pneumopericardium.

b. Outflow obstructions

(1) Pulmonary stenosis or atresia

(2) Aortic stenosis or atresia

(3) Hypertrophic subaortic stenosis seen in IDMs with resultant compromised left ventricular outflow, particularly when cardiotonic agents (see below) are used.

(4) Coarctation of the aorta or interrupted aortic arch.

(5) Arrhythmias also can compromise cardiac output. Supraventricular arrhythmias, as in paroxysmal atrial tachycardia, are most commonly seen and, if prolonged, can precipitate cardiogenic shock.

II. Pathophysiology of circulatory failure

A. Hypovolemic shock. In the compensated phases of hypovolemic shock, central venous pressure (CVP) and urine output are decreased with tachycardia and increased systemic vascular resistance. In the very premature infant, however, acute hypotension with bradycardia can occur without a preceding period of tachycardia.

B. Cardiogenic shock. In contrast to hypovolemic shock, intrinsic compensatory mechanisms can have deleterious effects in patients with cardiogenic shock. Increased vascular resistance will maintain adequate blood supply to vital organs but also will increase left ventricular afterload and hence cardiac work. Decreased renal perfusion from low cardiac output will result in sodium and water retention causing increased central blood volume, increased left ventricular pressure and volume, and therefore pulmonary edema, with hypoxia and acidosis further compromising cardiac function. Tachycardia, hypotension, oliguria, and acidosis dominate the picture of cardiogenic shock.

C. Distributive shock. Distributive shock presents initially with a hyperdynamic state of tachycardia and normal blood pressure and urine output with bounding pulses. The arteriovenous oxygen saturation difference, if measured, would be narrow. Eventually, cardiogenic shock ensues with hypotension, tachycardia, acidosis, and hypoxemia.

III. Clinical presentation. In addition to hypotension and tachycardia (except in the very premature infant, see Hypovolemic shock above), the syndrome of shock is manifested by pallor and poor skin perfusion; cool extremities; irritability, lethargy, or coma; and decreased urine output. Organ dysfunction will occur because of inadequate blood flow and oxygen supply to tissues, and cellular metabolism will become predominantly anaerobic with the production of lactic and pyruvic acid. The presence of a metabolic acidosis often indicates an inadequate circulation. The consequences of inadequate organ perfusion are as follows:

A. Brain—irritability, lethargy, coma, and seizures

B. Heart—decreased cardiac output and increased pulmonary blood volume

C. Lungs—release of vasoactive substances, pulmonary edema, and decreased compliance

D. Gut—mucosal dysfunction, diarrhea, sepsis, hemorrhage, and perforation

E. Kidneys—reduced glomerular filtration rate (GFR) and urinary output, loss of renal tubular epithelium, uremia, electrolyte abnormalities, and hypotension

IV. Treatment. Therapy always begins with ensuring a patent airway, assessing ventilation, and providing supplemental oxygen. Heart rate, blood pressure, and oxygenation should be monitored continuously. A volume infusion of 10 ml/kg normal saline or 5% albumin-saline solution will help establish the cause. In the case of low blood volume, this will be therapeutic, at least temporarily, until the underlying etiology of hypovolemia is corrected.

A. Measurement of central venous pressure (CVP) will help with the management. CVP is measured by placement of a catheter with its tip in the right atrium or intrathoracic superior or inferior vena cava. The catheter can be placed by insertion through the umbilical vein or percutaneously by means of the external or internal jugular or subclavian vein. In many infants, maintaining CVP at 5 to 8 mmHg with volume infusions is associated with improvement in cardiac output. If CVP is greater than 5 to 8 mmHg, additional volume will usually not be helpful. CVP is influenced by noncardiac factors such as ventilator pressures, and by cardiac factors, such as tricuspid valve function. Both noncardiac and cardiac factors may affect the interpretation and usefulness of CVP determinations.

B. Cardiac output can be improved by increasing both heart rate and stroke volume. Negative inotropic factors such as hypoxia, acidosis, hypoglycemia, and other metabolic derangements should be corrected. **Sodium bicarbonate** infusion at a dose of 1 to 2 mEq/kg stat. is indicated for treating metabolic acidosis when the pH falls below 7.20, provided there is adequate ventilation ($PCO_2 < 40$ mmHg). Further bicarbonate infusion can be administered if the pH remains low. In addition, hypocalcemia frequently occurs in infants who are in circulatory failure, especially after administration of large amounts of solutions containing albumin, and this must be corrected. The effect of calcium in this setting is frequently a positive inotropic response. Calcium gluconate 10% (1 ml/kg) can be infused slowly intravenously on an empiric basis or after measurement of the ionized calcium level (see Chap. 24).

C. Positive inotropic agents. In addition to correcting the metabolic disturbances, positive inotropic agents should be used to increase cardiac output.

1. **Sympathomimetic amines** [9]. Sympathomimetic amines are very commonly used in infants. The advantages of these agents include rapidity of onset, the ability to control dosage, and ultrashort half-lives (Table 6-1).
   a. **Dopamine** [2,3]. Dopamine is a precursor of norepinephrine and activates delta, beta, and alpha receptors in a dose-dependent fashion. At very low doses, 2 to 4 μg/kg per minute, its clinical effect is principally renal and splanchnic vasodilation with a decrease in systemic vascular resistance and no effect on heart rate in the full-term infant. In the intermediate range, 5 to 20 μg/kg per minute, dopamine has moderate positive inotropic action (beta-1) and some systemic vascular (beta-2) effects. At high doses, greater than 20 μg/kg per minute it acts similar to norepinephrine, with significant alpha vasoconstrictor effects. The increased cardiac output depends on myocardial norepinephrine stores.
   b. **Dobutamine** [6]. Dobutamine is a synthetic catecholamine that acts by direct stimulation of cardiac alpha-1 and B-1 receptors. It has been widely used in adults to increase cardiac contractility, but there has been little experience in children. In adults, its inotropic effects, unlike dopamine, are independent of cardiac catecholamine stores, and it increases cardiac output with minimal tachycardia. In a series of 10 infants 9 hours to 7 weeks old who had low cardiac output unresponsive to other cardiotonic drugs, dobutamine (2 to 12 μg/kg per minute) improved symptoms 67 to 100 percent [8]. Driscoll et al. [1 also have reported increased cardiovascular function in children in response to dobutamine. Dobutamine is indicated in the newborn infant at doses of 5 to 15 μg/kg per minute to increase cardiac contractility through stimulation of alpha-1 and B-1 adrenoreceptors in the myocardium with little effect on heart rate or systemic vascular resistance. It is often used with dopamine to maximally increase cardiac

Table 6-1. Sympathomimetic amines (see Appendix A)

Agent	Dose range	Comments
Dopamine*	2–4 μg/kg per minute (renal effect) 5–20 μg/kg per minute (beta effect) >20 gm/kg per minute (alpha effect)	Splanchnic and renal vasodilator; may be used with dobutamine or isoproterenol; increasing doses produce more alpha effect
Dobutamine	5–15 μg/kg per minute (cardiac alpha-1 and beta-1 effect)	Strong inotropic agent with less heart rate effect; maintains systemic vascular resistance
Isoproterenol	0.05–1.0 μg/kg per minute (beta effect)	Strong inotropic and chronotropic agent; peripheral vasodilator; reduces preload; may "steal" renal blood flow

*Effects may be seen at lower doses in premature infants.

output and to avoid very high infusion rates of dopamine (>20 μg/kg per minute) with the accompanying severe vasoconstrictive effect.

c. **Isoproterenol** [9]. Isoproterenol is used at doses of 0.05 to 1.0 μg/kg per minute and is a pure beta-agonist that affects both beta-1 and beta-2 receptors, thus causing bronchodilation and cardiac stimulation. It causes intense chronotropism and lowering of systemic and pulmonary vascular resistance. Adequate blood volume needs to be maintained.

d. **Epinephrine and norepinephrine** are not first-line drugs in cardiac failure in the newborn. Effective in increasing systemic vascular resistance, they are more useful in low perfusion states due to such factors as endotoxemia.

2. **Other agents**

a. **Corticosteroids** have been used in septic shock, but their efficacy remains controversial. Studies in adults have shown at best a transient reversal of shock in response to steroids without an improvement in overall survival [7].

b. **Naloxone.** Endorphins and other endogenous opiates appear to have roles as mediators in various forms of shock. Several reports [4] have described the use of naloxone, a specific opiate antagonist, at doses of 0.3 mg/kg in patients with refractory hypotension secondary to sepsis with variable results. At this time, further well-designed studies need to be undertaken before naloxone can be routinely used to treat shock.

References

1. Driscoll, D. J. *Am. J. Cardiol.* 43: 581, 1979.
2. Driscoll, D. J. *J. Pediatr.* 92(2): 309, 1978.
3. Driscoll, D. J. *J. Thorac. Cardiovasc. Surg.* 78: 765, 1979.
4. Groeger, J. S. *Crit. Care Med.* 11(8): 650, 1983.
5. Lacouture, P. G. *J. Pediatr.* 111(4): 615, 1987.
6. Ruffolo, R. R. *Am. J. Med. Sci.* 294: 244, 1987.
7. Sprung, C. L. *N. Engl. J. Med.* 311(18): 1137, 1984.
8. Ward, R. M. *Pediatr. Res.* 15: 686, 1981.
9. Zaritsky, A. *J. Pediatr.* 105(3): 341, 1984.

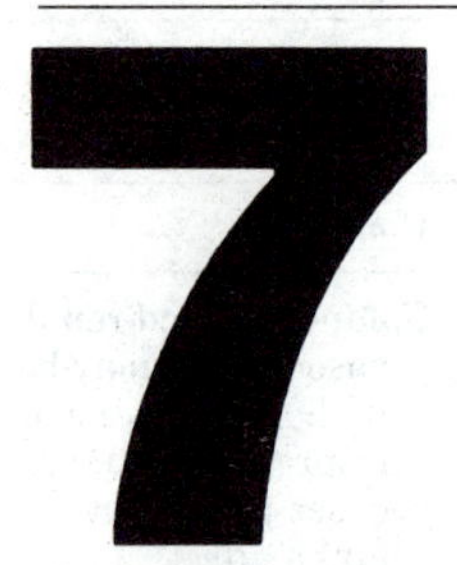

History and Physical Examination of the Newborn

William D. Cochran

I. **History.** The family, maternal, paternal, pregnancy, and perinatal history should be reviewed. The important aspects of this history are found in Table 7-1 [7].

II. **Physical examination.** Regarding the "normal" newborn, at no other time is more information obtained from the general overall visual and auditory appraisal of a naked infant and less information obtained from a "careful" organ examination. Certain parts of a routine examination are almost worthless when applied to newborn infants (e.g., percussion of the chest). Although no statistics are available, the first routine newborn examination probably reveals more abnormalities than any other routine examination done. With experience, the examiner should be able to perform the following steps of evaluation in a normal newborn in 5 to 7 minutes, if no abnormality is found.

A. **General examination.** At the initial examination, attention should be directed to determine (1) whether any congenital anomalies are present, (2) whether the infant has made a successful transition from "water breathing" to "air breathing," (3) to what extent gestation, labor, delivery, analgesics, or anesthetics have affected the infant, and (4) whether he or she has any sign of infection or metabolic disease that was unsuspected.

1. The baby should be naked during the examination. **Warm** infants and young children have the delightful characteristic of being happier naked than clothed, and advantage should be taken of this fact. Naked newborns are easily chilled, however, so they should not be kept uncovered for periods of more than a minute or two at a time unless they are in or under a warming device. A general appraisal of a naked newborn allows one to assess more quickly whether any major anomalies are present, whether jaundice or meconium staining is present, and whether the infant is having trouble making the adjustment to breathing air rather than water. At least half of all infants exhibit jaundice, although usually only when it peaks on the third or fourth day of life. Jaundice, if noted, usually means the bilirubin level is at least 5 mg/dl.

2. Since the nurses or obstetrician will often have already discovered more obvious anomalies, such as a cleft palate and lip or imperforate anus, this examination is more likely to pick up abnormalities of the heart, abdomen, or hips. It is usually wise to examine infants in the order listed below in subsections **B** to **K** because they will be quieter at the beginning, when you need their cooperation. If the infant being examined is crying or fretful, pacify the baby by letting him or her suck a nipple.

B. **Cardiorespiratory system**

1. **Color.** An infant's color is probably the single most important index of the function of the cardiorespiratory system. "Good" color in Caucasian infants means a reddish pink hue all over, except for possible cyanosis of the hands, feet, and occasionally the lips (acrocyanosis). The mucous membranes of dark-skinned babies are more reliable indicators of cyanosis than the skin. Infants of diabetic mothers are pinker than average, and "post mature" infants are paler.

2. **Respiratory rate** is usually between 40 and 60 breaths per minute. All infants are **periodic** rather than regular breathers, and premature in-

fants are more so than full-term infants. Thus they may breathe at a fairly regular rate for a minute or so and then have a short period of no breathing at all (usually 5 to 10 seconds). **Apnea,** often defined as periods of no breathing, during which an infant's color changes from normal reddish pink to grades of cyanosis, is not a normal phenomenon, whereas periodic breathing is. Apnea is thus an abnormal prolongation of periodic breathing (see Chap. 13).

3. In a warm infant there should be no expiratory grunting and little or no flaring of the alae nasae. When crying, infants (especially the more premature infants) exhibit mild chest retraction, which is largely sternal and subdiaphragmatic; if unaccompanied by grunting, it may be considered normal. As a general rule, if the infant has good color and appears in no respiratory distress, it is of no further benefit to percuss the chest.
4. **Auscultation** is rarely helpful when an infant is pink and breathing, without retractions or grunting, at a rate of less than 60 breaths per minute. Unless an infant has severe central nervous system (CNS) depression as well, significant respiratory disease in the absence of tachypnea is rare. Rales, decreased heart sounds or breath sounds, or asymmetry of breath sounds is occasionally found in the asymptomatic infant and may reveal occult disease that is confirmed by chest roentgenography.
5. The **heart** should be examined, with the limitations of this examination kept in mind. The examiner should observe precordial activity, rate, rhythm, the quality of the heart sounds, and the presence or absence of murmurs.

   a. If the infant is crying, a pacifier or nipple should be offered to quiet the baby. If these fail, pick up and cuddle the baby, listening to the heart while you hold him or her. Not only is it worthless to try to examine the heart of a fussy or crying infant, but it is also very frustrating. When the baby is peaceful, the rate, rhythm, and presence of murmurs can be determined much more easily.
   b. It should be determined whether the heart is on the right or left side. This is best done by auscultation, but it can be confirmed occasionally by palpation.
   c. The **heart rate** is normally between 120 and 160 beats per minute. It varies with changes in the infant's activity, being faster when he or she is crying, active, or breathing rather rapidly and appreciably slower when the baby has periods of slow breathing and is quiet. To some, this physiologic slowing provides a very important indicator that there is no significant stress on the heart. An occasional term or postterm infant may, at rest, have a heart rate well below 100. In a normal infant, the heart rate will increase when the baby is stimulated.
   d. **Murmurs** mean less in the newborn period than at any other time. Infants can have extremely serious heart anomalies without any murmurs. On the other hand, a closing ductus arteriosus may cause a murmur that, in retrospect, is only transient, but at the time is very loud, worrisome, and misleading. Gallop sounds may be an ominous finding, while the presence of a split S2 may be reassuring.
   e. If there is any question on the basis of auscultation and observation that the heart is abnormally placed, abnormally large, or overactive, a **chest roentgenogram** is the best means of providing a more accurate assessment. Distant heart sounds, especially if accompanied by respiratory symptoms, are often secondary to pneumothorax or pneumomediastinum.
   f. The **femoral pulses** should be felt for, although often they feel quite weak in the first day or two. Dorsalis pedis pulses may be substituted. If there is doubt about the femoral pulses by discharge, the blood pressure in the legs should be checked.

Table 7-1. Important aspects of maternal and perinatal history

Family History

Inherited diseases (e.g., metabolic disorders, hemophilia, cystic fibrosis, polycystic kidneys, history of perinatal deaths)

Maternal History

Age
Blood type
Transfusions
Blood group sensitization
Chronic maternal illness
Hypertension
Renal disease
Cardiac disease
Bleeding disorders
Sexually-transmitted disease
Herpes
Diabetes
Infertility
Recent infections or exposures

Previous Pregnancies—Problems and Outcome

Abortions
Fetal demise
Neonatal deaths
Prematurity
Postmaturity
Malformations
Respiratory distress syndrome
Jaundice
Apnea

Drug History

Medications
Drug abuse
Alcohol
Tobacco

Current Pregnancy

Probable gestational age
Quickening (16–18 weeks)
Fetal heart heard with fetoscope (18–20 weeks)
Results of any fetal testing (e.g., amniocentesis, ultrasound, estriols, monitoring of and tests of fetal lung maturity)
Preeclampsia
Bleeding
Trauma
Infection
Surgery
Polyhydramnios
Oligohydramnios

Table 7-1 (continued)

Current Pregnancy (continued)
Glucocorticoids
Labor suppressant
Antibiotics
Labor and Delivery
Presentation
Onset of labor
Rupture of membranes
Duration of labor
Fever
Fetal monitoring
Amniotic fluid (blood, meconium, volume)
Analgesic
Anesthesia
Maternal oxygenation and perfusion
Method of delivery
Initial delivery room assessment (shock, asphyxia, trauma, anomalies, temperature, infection)
Apgar scores
Resuscitation
Placental examination

C. **Abdomen.** The abdominal examination of a newborn infant differs from that of older infants in that observation can again be utilized to a greater advantage.

1. Since strong abdominal musculature does not develop until several months after birth, the anterior abdominal organs (i.e., the liver, spleen, or bowel) can often be seen through the abdominal wall, especially in thin or premature infants. The edge of the liver is occasionally seen, and intestinal patterning is easily visible. Asymmetry due to congenital anomalies or masses often is first appreciated by observation only.
2. When palpating the abdomen, start with gentle pressure or gentle stroking of the abdomen from lower to upper quadrants to reveal the edges of an otherwise unsuspected enlarged liver or spleen. Try to appreciate the soft mushiness when palpating over the intestine compared with the firmer feel over the liver or other organs or masses. The normal newborn liver extends 2.0 to 2.5 cm below the costal margin. The spleen is usually not palpable. Remember, there can be situs inversus.
3. Once the abdomen is observed and gently palpated, **deep palpation** is possible, not only because of the lack of abdominal musculature, but also because there is no food and little air in the intestine. Abnormal, absent, or misplaced kidneys and other deep masses should now be felt for. Only during the first 1 to 2 days of life is it possible for the kidneys to be routinely palpated with relative ease and reliability (see Chap. 27).

D. **Genitalia and rectum**

1. The external genitalia of a full-term newborn infant are quite different from those of slightly older infants and even differ from those of a premature infant.
   a. **Male**
      (1) The male almost invariably has a marked **phimosis.**

(2) The **scrotum** is often quite large, since it is an embryonic analogue of the labia of the female and therefore has responses to maternal hormones.

(3) **Hydroceles** are not uncommon, but unless they are communicating types, they will disappear in time without being the forerunner of an inguinal hernia.

(4) The **testes** should be palpated, and the epididymis and vas should be identified. The testis is best found by running a finger from the internal ring down on either side of the upper shaft of the penis, thus pushing and trapping the testis in the scrotum. The testes should be the same size; they should be neither too soft nor too hard, and they should not appear blue (one of the signs of torsion) through the skin of the scrotum.

(5) If present, the degree of **hypospadias** should be noted.

(6) The length and width of the penis should be noted (see Chap. 26). Torsion of the penis is seen in 1.5 percent of normal males [2].

b. **Female**

(1) Female genitalia at term are most noticeable for their enlarged **labia majora.**

(2) Occasionally, a **mucosal tag** from the wall of the vagina is noted.

(3) A **discharge** from the vagina, usually creamy white in color and consistency, is commonly found and, on occasion, is replaced after the second day by pseudomenses.

(4) The **labia** should always be spread, and cysts of the vaginal wall, an inperforate hymen, or other less common anomalies should be sought.

2. The **anus** and **rectum** should be checked carefully for patency, position, and size (normal 10 mm in diameter) [4]. Occasionally, large fistulas are mistaken for a normal anus, but if one checks carefully, it will be noted that a fistula will be either anterior or posterior to the usual location of a normal anus.

E. **Skin** (see Chap. 29). The epidermis of the skin of a newborn (especially a premature infant) is amazingly thin; therefore, the oxygenated capillary blood makes it very pink. The common abnormalities of the skin include tiny **milia** on the nose (plugged sweat glands), unusually brown-pigmented nevi scattered around any area of the body, and what are referred to as **mongolian spots.** These mongolian spots are bluish, often quite large areas most commonly on the back, buttocks, or thighs that fade slightly as the weeks go by.

Occasionally at birth, although much more common in the next day or two, **erythema toxicum** may be noted. These papular lesions with an erythematous base are found more on the trunk than on the extremities and fade away without treatment by 1 week of age. Occasionally, their profusion is alarming. Jaundice should be noted, if present.

F. Palpable **lymph nodes** are found in about one-third of normal neonates. They are usually under 12 mm in diameter and are often found in the inguinal, cervical, and occasionally the axillary area [1].

G. **Extremities, spine, and joints** (see Chap. 23).

1. **Extremities.** Anomalies of the digits (too few, too many, syndactyly, or abnormal placement), club feet, and hip dislocation are the common deviations from normal. Because of fetal positioning, many infants have forefoot adduction, tibial bowing, or even tibial torsion. Forefoot adduction, if correctable with passive motion on the part of the examiner, will correct itself in a matter of days and should be no cause for concern. Mild degrees of tibial bowing or torsion are also normal.

2. To check for **hip dislocation** (if present, remember that the head of the femur will most often have been displaced superiorly and posteriorly), place the infant's legs in the frogleg position. With the third finger on the greater trochanter and the thumb and index finger holding the knee, attempt to relocate the femoral head in the acetabulum by pushing upward

away from the mattress with the third finger and toward the mattress and laterally with the thumb at the knee. If there has been a dislocation, a distinct upward movement of the femoral head will be felt as it relocates in the acetabulum. Hip "clicks," possible due to movement of the ligamentum teres in the acetabulum, are much more common than dislocated hips (hip "clunks") and are not a cause for concern.

3. **Back.** The infant should be turned over and held face down on your hand. The back, especially in the lower lumbar and sacral areas, should be examined. Special care should be taken to look for pilonidal sinus tracts and small soft midline swellings over the back that might indicate a small meningocele or other anomaly.

H. Head, neck, and mouth

1. **Head**
   a. The average full-term **head circumference** is 33 to 38 cm.
   b. The infant's **skull** should be inspected for cuts or bruises due to either forcep application or fetal monitor leads and laterally for erosions from the bony spines of the maternal pelvis.
   c. **Caput succedaneum** (edema of the scalp from labor pressure) should be checked to see if there are underlying beginning cephalohematomas; these usually do not become "full blown" until the third or fourth day.
   d. **Mobility of the suture lines** will rule out **craniosynostosis.** Mobility of sutures is checked by putting each thumb on opposite sides of the suture and then pushing in alternately while feeling for motion.
   e. The degree of **molding of the skull bones** themselves should be noted, and it may be considerable. Usually, this molding will subside within 5 days.
   f. Occasional infants have **craniotabes,** a soft Ping-Pong ball effect of the skull bones (usually the parietal bones). It is most often found in postpartum dysmature infants. If present, craniotabes is usually only an incidental finding that disappears in a matter of days, even if marked at birth.
   g. **Fontanelles.** As long as the head circumference is within normal limits and there is motion of the suture lines, one need pay little attention to the size (large or small) of the fontanelles. Very large fontanelles reflect a delay in ossification of bones and may be associated with hypothyroidism (see Maternal-Fetal Thyroid Disorders in Chap. 1), trisomy syndromes, in utero malnutrition, hypophosphatasia, rickets, and osteogenesis imperfecta [5].
2. The **neck** should be checked for range of motion, goiter, and thyroglossal or branchial arch sinus tracks. Occasionally, a marked asymmetry of the neck is noted with a deep concavity on one side. Although the uninitiated might interpret this as possible agenesis of a muscle or even of a muscle group, it is most commonly due to persistent fetal posture with the head tilted to one side **(asynclitism)**. This is most easily confirmed by noting that the mandibular gum line is not parallel to the maxillary line, further evidence of unequal pressure on the jaw as a result of the head's being held tilted in utero for a period of time.
3. The **mouth** should be checked, and one should especially ensure that there are neither hard nor soft palatal clefts, no gum clefts, and no deciduous teeth present. Rarely, cysts appear on the gum or under the tongue. **Epstein's pearls** (small white inclusion cysts clustered about the midline at the juncture or the hard and soft palate) are a normal finding.

I. Neurologic examination. Much has been written about the neurologic examination of the newborn, but more will have to be learned before it becomes an accurate evaluation—especially one with prognostic significance—when done on the first day of life. Surely a carefully performed, detailed neurologic examination will reveal more than a superficial one, but the extra information obtained from such a detailed examination usually is not worthwhile. Senior members of any large hospital will be able to recall the case of an infant with hydranencephaly or some similar gross internal neurologic lesion that was completely missed by rather careful neurologic testing only to be picked up later by the valuable procedure of transillumination.

1. Probably the most reliable information that can be obtained quickly from a neurologic evaluation is gained while handling the infant during the preceding parts of the physical examination. With experience, the examiner is able to carry out at least two examinations concurrently, that is, the examinations of organ and physiologic systems and a simultaneous neurologic evaluation. Symmetry of movement and posturing, body tone, and response to being handled and disturbed (i.e., crying appropriately and quieting appropriately) can all be evaluated while other parts of the body are being tested.
2. The amount of crying should be carefully noted as well as whether it is high-pitched or not. When the baby is crying, seventh nerve weaknesses should be looked for (the affected side of the mouth does not pull down). Erb's palsy, if present, will usually be revealed by lack of motion of the arm; the arm will lie beside the body in repose rather than being normally flexed with the fist near the mouth. In general, it is a waste of time to check the sucking and rooting reflexes and the knee-jerk reflex if all other parts of the neurologic assessment have been normal.
3. The essentials of a neurologic examination (beyond the knowledge acquired while carrying out the other components of the physical examination) may be covered by doing the following: Put your index fingers in the infant's palms and obtain the plantar grasp. When you have obtained this, hold the infant's fingers between your thumb and forefinger and raise the infant's body by pulling him or her to a sitting position. Note the degrees of head lag and head control; however, a crying infant often throws his or her head back in anger. The baby should be held in a sitting position and the trunk moved forward and back enough to test head control again. Now let the trunk and head slowly fall back toward the mattress. If you wish to test the Moro reflex, just before the baby's head touches the mattress, pull your fingers quickly from his or her grasp, thus allowing the infant to fall back the rest of the way. Usually the Moro reflex will result. Sucking and rooting can be checked by using a nipple. Touching the upper lip laterally will cause most infants to turn toward the touch and open their mouth; the hungrier and more vigorous the infant, the more intense is the rooting response. Placing a nipple in the infant's mouth will then initiate a sucking response.
4. **Stepping (and placing)** are probably reflexes of fetal importance. Stepping may possibly represent the genetic wisdom of the fetus to turn himself or herself from the more dangerous breech position to vertex. This stepping can be elicited by holding the infant upright with his or her feet on the mattress and then leaning the baby way forward. This forward motion often sets off a slow alternate stepping action. Occasionally, an infant will not perform this reflex.
5. The complete **behavioral examination** is more dependent on infant-examiner interaction. Much of it depends on the infant's state of sleepiness or wakefulness, whether the baby has just been fed or not, and to a degree, on the analgesia and anesthesia used during delivery. One part of the examination that might be of special interest is eye opening, which is brought on when the infant is sucking or being held vertically. Most mothers are interested in seeing their baby's eyes (possibly a further "bonding" phenomenon). Nature has thus "responded" by concentrating open-eyed periods to times when the mother is likely to be present (nursing or holding her baby vertically). Some infants will be noted to "alert" and listen when they are spoken to in a pleasant voice. Almost all infants enjoy being cuddled. If some of these behavioral responses cannot be elicited, they may indicate either temporary or permanent problems. The

more detailed behavioral examination also involves habituation to repeated stimuli of various sorts (noxious and otherwise) and will not be discussed here [3].

J. Head circumference and length. These measurements are usually the final parts of the examination. The head circumference of a full-term (38- to 40-week) infant of normal weight (2.7 to 3.6 kg, or 6 to 8 pounds) is usually between 33 and 38 cm (13 and 15 inches). The length of such an infant is 48 to 53 cm (19 to 21 inches).

K. Eye examination [6]. In the first 3 days of newborn life, puffy eyelids sometimes preclude examining the eyes at all. On the third day, usually the day of discharge, the eyes can and should be examined for the presence of scleral hemorrhages, conjunctival exudate, iris coloring, and pupillary size, equality, and centering. The red reflex should be obtained, and cataracts should be looked for. Glaucoma is manifest by a large cloudy cornea. The normal cornea in an infant at birth measures less than 10.5 mm in horizontal diameter.

L. Discharge examination. At discharge, the infant should be reexamined with the following points considered:

1. **Heart**—development of murmur, cyanosis, or failure
2. **CNS**—fullness of fontanelles, sutures, activity
3. **Abdomen**—any masses previously missed, stools, urine output
4. **Skin**—jaundice, pyoderma
5. **Cord**—infection
6. **Infection**—any signs of sepsis
7. **Feeding**—spitting, vomiting, distension, weight gain, dehydration
8. **Maternal competence** to provide adequate care

M. Follow-up (see Chap. 37).

References

1. Bamji, M., et al. *Pediatrics* 78: 573, 1986.
2. Ben-Ari, J., et al. *J. Urol.* 135: 521, 1985.
3. Brazelton, T. B. *Clin. Dev. Med.* 50: 1, 1973.
4. El-Haddao, M., et al. *Pediatrics* 76: 927, 1985.
5. Faix, R. G. *J. Pediatr.* 100: 304, 1982.
6. Nelson, L. B. *Pediatric Ophthalmology* Philadelphia: Saunders, 1984.
7. Scanlon, J. W. *A System of Newborn Physical Examination.* Baltimore: University Park Press, 1979.

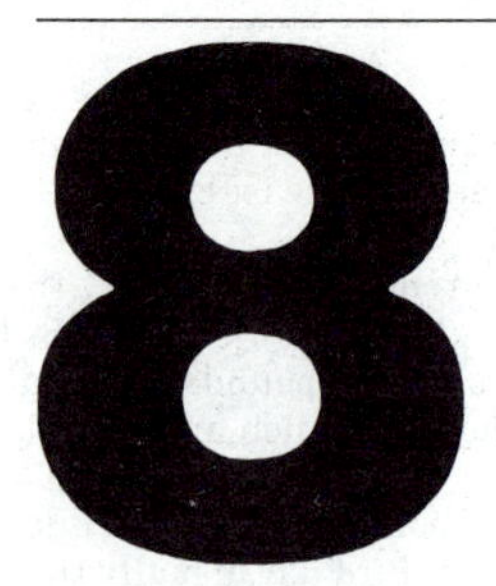

Nursery Care of the Well Newborn

E. Manning Sears

I. Initial period [5,7]

A. Protective gloves are worn when one handles newborns who have not bee bathed.

B. Stabilize temperature with warming lights or an incubator if necessary (defe initial skin care until stable).

C. Observe for

1. Respiratory distress
2. Poor color
   - a. **Pallor**—shock, anemia
   - b. **Plethora** (see Chap. 18)
   - c. **Cyanosis** other than acrocyanosis
3. Diaphoresis
4. Jitteriness. Check blood glucose level by Dextrostix: If below 25 mg/dl give dextrose 5% in water and recheck (see Chap. 24).
5. Hypotonia
6. Hypertonia
7. Malformations (major and minor)
8. Classify as large for gestational age, appropriate for gestational age, o small for gestational age (see Chap. 9).
9. Babies are no longer footprinted; instead, bracelets are used fo identification.

D. Skin care. The skin should be examined for signs of trauma that may serv as an entry site for infection. The best method for routine skin care is dry ski care. This method reduces heat loss, diminishes trauma, and does not expos the newborn to agents with possible side effects.

1. Sterile cotton sponges soaked with fresh tap water are used to remov blood and meconium from the head and face, or a nonmedicated soap in single-use container can be used, followed with water. Unless the rest o the baby is very soiled, there is no reason to wash him or her. There i also no reason to remove the vernix caseosa. During the rest of the infant' hospital stay, the baby can be cleaned as required with fresh water or soa and water.
2. If the nursery is having problems with ***Staphylococcus aureus* infec tions,** a hexachlorophene soap may be used for bathing until the epidemi has passed. Hexachlorophene may be absorbed through intact skin and i potentially toxic to neonates. Many antiseptic compounds have been use to prevent infection and colonization in neonates. They usually are al absorbed through neonatal skin and are associated with changes in bac terial flora on the neonatal skin.
3. **Skin abrasions** may be an entry point for infection and should be care fully cleaned with soap and water. The use of topical antibiotics on abra sions of neonatal skin may be reasonable in infants who will only be i the hospital a few days. Use of topical antibiotics in nurseries for routin skin care in infants who have prolonged hospitalization has been associ ated with the emergence of multiple antibiotic-resistant organisms in th nursery. These medications should be used for specific indications.

E. **Cord care.** We use a plastic cord clamp (double-grip umbilical cord clamp, Hollister, Inc., Libertyville, Illinois), which is removed 48 hours after birth. There are several methods of cord care, and no single method has proved superior in the prevention of colonization and infection. Alcohol helps drying of the cord and, although used by us, has not been conclusively shown to prevent colonization and infection. We have occasionally used topical antibiotic ointments (bacitracin, neomycin) as part of an attack on an epidemic of neonatal *S. aureus* skin infection. Triple dye (2.29 gm crystal violet mixed with enough water to make 1 liter) also has been used, but not by us. The absorption and toxicity of these agents have not been well studied.

F. **Initial physician's examination** should take place no later than 24 hours after birth, sooner if problems are reported (see Chap. 9). The physician should pay attention to areas that may have been missed in the routine delivery room, maternal, or nursery evaluation. These areas are the eyes, palate, heart, abdomen, and hips. Not all future dislocations of the hip are detectable in the newborn period.

G. **Eye care** (see Chap. 12).

H. **Vitamin K** is used to prevent hemorrhagic disease of the newborn. Administer 0.5-1.0 mg vitamin K_1 oxide (phytonadione) during the first hour of life.

II. **Subsequent care**

A. **Weight.** Check the infant's weight daily.

Note: Compare weight with gestational age. If the infant is large for gestational age or small for gestational age, there is an increased risk of complications (see Chaps. 1, 9, 11, 12, 24). Check maternal history for cigarette and alcohol use or other drug abuse and maternal weight gain.

B. Record stools, urine, and axillary temperature at least every 8 hours. Pulse and respiration should be recorded every 8 hours in infants with any risk factors for infection or pulmonary or cardiac disease. One-third of newborns admitted to newborn intensive care nurseries were considered healthy at birth.

C. **Feeding** (see Chap. 30)

1. **Breast-feeding** is preferred if there are no contraindications. Begin as soon as possible (see Chap. 31).

a. **Contraindications** to breast-feeding include

(1) **Chronic illness**

(a) Active untreated tuberculosis (see Chap. 12)

(b) ? Maternal hepatitis B (controversial) (see Chap. 12)

(c) ? Active maternal cytomegaloviral disease (see Chap. 12)

(d) ? Herpes simplex. Breast-feeding is permitted if the mother prevents the infant from having contact with the lesion and if she washes her hands carefully (see Chap. 12).

(2) **Maternal medications**—alcohol, drugs (see Appendix C and Chap. 2)

(3) **Phenylketonuria (PKU),** galactosemia, and some other inborn errors of metabolism (see Chap. 24).

(4) **Breast milk jaundice.** Only 1 to 2 percent of infants require temporary interruption (see Chap. 15).

III. **Visiting**

A. Healthy family members

B. Other adults

Note: During unusual viral epidemics, visiting may need to be curtailed.

IV. **Education**

A. **Daily classes** for mothers on feeding and home care

B. **Booklets** on care of the healthy newborn [3]

C. Special **pamphlets** on child care [5,6]

D. **Circumcision.** There is much dispute about the justification for nonritual neonatal circumcision. After much discussion, the following policy has been agreed on in our nurseries:

1. There is no absolute medical indication for the routine circumcision of

newborns. This policy is currently under review and will be modified if data demonstrate the value of the procedure [1]. The Academy of Pediatrics has stated that circumcision "has potential medical benefits and advantages as well as disadvantages and risks," but it has not recommended routine circumcision.

2. The pros and cons of circumcision should be discussed with the parents prior to birth of the child [1,6,7].
3. Adequate lifelong penile hygiene should be defined.
4. Infants who have problems that may make lifelong penile hygiene difficult (e.g., mental retardation) should probably be circumcised.
5. It is impossible to be dogmatic about the value of circumcision because of the many variables, such as race, social and economic status, education, and climate, that make a large, prospective, long-term study difficult to do.
6. If circumcision is to be done, it should not be performed during the stabilization period just after birth. It should be done at least 12 to 24 hours later with meticulous technique by well-trained personnel.
   a. **Advantages** [12]
      (1) Ease of cleanliness
      (2) Custom of 80 percent of American males [13]
      (3) Prevention of paraphimosis, phimosis, and balanitis
      (4) Prevention of squamous cell cancer. Cancer of the penis is usually found only in uncircumcised men. It is a rare cancer in uncircumcised men (0.7 to 0.9 per 100,000 men in the United States) **if proper hygiene is practiced.** In populations with poor hygiene, the incidence is 3 to 6 per 100,000. Human papillomavirus has been implicated in the development of penile cancer. Poor hygiene, lack of circumcision, and some sexually transmitted diseases all correlate with penile cancer.
      (5) Prevention of cervical cancer in females (not supported by recent studies). There is a correlation between carcinoma of the cervix and sexually transmitted diseases, multiple sexual partners, and intercourse at an early age.
      (6) Prevention of need for later circumcision. Five percent of uncircumcised males may need to be circumcised. Conversely, 95 percent will never require the procedure.
      (7) Recent retrospective studies show an increased incidence of urinary tract infection in the first year of life in uncircumcised infants as compared with circumcised infants. If these studies are repeated and are generally true, a positive benefit for circumcision must be recognized [8,17,18].
      (8) Possible decreased incidence of sexually transmitted disease [1,16].
   b. **Disadvantages** [12]
      (1) **Pain** may be relieved by penile nerve block with lidocaine HC1 1% without epinepherine in a total dose of 3 to 4 mg/kg [14]. Circumferential anesthesia may be hazardous. Local anesthesia adds an element of risk. Data on its use have not been collected in a large number of cases. The Academy of Pediatrics states that local anesthesia may reduce the physiologic response to neonatal circumcision, but it has its own inherent risks. More data should be obtained from large, controlled series before advocating local anesthesia as an integral part of newborn circumcision.
      (2) **Risks of surgery.** There is a 0.2 to 0.6 percent complication rate [1].
         (a) Hemorrhage
         (b) Infection
         (c) Surgical trauma (partial amputation, denudation) [13]
         (d) Late complications—meatal stenosis or ulceration

(3) **Expense**—hospital and physicians fees [4]

c. The final decision about circumcision should be made by informed parents. Do not perform circumcision if the infant has hypospadias or chordee of the penis.

V. Laboratory procedures

A. Cord blood—save for 2 weeks

1. Uses

a. To perform a blood type and Coombs' test on infants born to Rh-negative mothers

b. To perform a blood type and Coombs' test if jaundice is noted within 24 hours of age

Note: Routine typing of O-positive mothers has been discontinued at the Brigham and Women's Hospital (see Chap. 15).

c. Serologic test for syphilis if not performed prepartum on mother

d. Later screening for viral or toxoplasmosis infection

e. Screening for sickle cell disease or other hemoglobinopathies as indicated [14]

B. Metabolic disease screening [10]. Blood is collected on the third day of life to screen for metabolic disorders such as hypothyroidism, PKU, galactosemia, and disorders of leucine and methionine metabolism. Infants discharged at or before 24 hours of age should have a follow-up sample done after 4 days of age. Infants born with major medical problems who are transferred to other institutions may be missed on neonatal metabolic screening. We get a sample prior to transfer from our institution and remind the receiving institution to get another sample. Infants with galactosemia who are fed lactose-free formulas from birth will be missed on a newborn screen for galactosemia if serum galactose level is used as the marker. See Maternal-Fetal Thyroid Disorders (Chap. 1) and Inborn Errors of Metabolism (Chap. 24). A review of causes of missed cases of metabolic diseases is found in reference 8.

C. Newborns in Massachusetts are screened for toxoplasmosis, sickle cell disease, and congenital adrenyl hyperplasia with blood from the metabolic screen (see page 456).

D. Follow-up hearing tests for special-risk newborns [11] (see Chap. 38.)

E. A general reference on newborn screening for various diseases such as PKU, hypothyroidism, galactosemia, sickle-cell disease, thalassemia, hemocystinuria, maple syrup urine disease, biotinidase deficiency, cystic fibrosis and muscular dystrophy is reference 2.

VI. Plan for discharge

A. Final examination by physician or pediatric nurse-practitioner is done the day before or the day of discharge.

B. Provide copies of initial and discharge summaries to parents or send them to physician or clinic rendering follow-up care.

C. If in doubt that infant will receive proper follow-up care, refer to a social service agency.

D. If special follow-up care is indicated, such as hearing screening, inform parents and put note on discharge summary.

E. Infant is taken to transport vehicle by nurse or other responsible hospital person.

F. Infant should be taken home only in vehicle having appropriate infant car seat. The infant should **not** be carried on the mother's lap.

G. In these days of early discharges, parents should be informed about jaundice, skin infections, and other problems that may not manifest themselves until the fourth or fifth day of life.

References

1. American Academy of Pediatrics. *Pediatrics* 84: 388, 1989.
2. American Academy of Pediatrics. *Pediatrics* 83: 449, 1989.

3. Brown, M. D. *Pediatrics* 80: 215, 1987.
4. Cadman, D. *Can. Med. Assoc. J.* 131: 1353, 1984.
5. Caravella, S. J. *Pediatrics* 80: 1, 1987.
6. *Caring for Your Newborn.* Corporate Communications, Brigham and Women's Hospital, 75 Francis Street, Boston, Mass. 02115.
7. Frigoletto, F. D., and Little, G. A. (Eds.). *Guidelines for Perinatal Care,* 2d Ed. Elk Grove Village, Ill.: American Academy of Pediatrics and American Academy of Obstetricians and Gynecologists, 1988.
8. Herzog, L. W. *Am. J. Dis. Child.* 143: 349, 1989.
9. Holtzman, C. *Pediatrics* 78: 553, 1986.
10. *Protecting Your Baby* (Form MD-12-100M.8.79-152155). The Commonwealth of Massachusetts Department of Public Health, State Laboratory Institute, 305 South Street, Jamaica Plain, Mass. 02130.
11. *Screening and Hearing Evaluation Program for Infants and Toddlers.* Massachusetts Department of Public Health 80M-7-83:173396, 80 Boylston Street, Room 742, Boston, Mass. 02116.
12. Thompson, H. C. *Am. J. Dis. Child.* 137: 939, 1983.
13. Sotolong, J. R. *J. Urol.* 133: 102, 1985.
14. Stang, H. J. *JAMA* 259: 1507, 1988.
15. Vichinsky, E., et al. *Pediatrics* 81: 749, 1988.
16. Thompson, H. C. *Am. J. Dis. Child.* 137: 939, 1983.
17. Wiswell, T. E. *Pediatrics* 75: 901, 1985.
18. Wiswell, T. E. *Pediatrics* 79: 338, 1987.

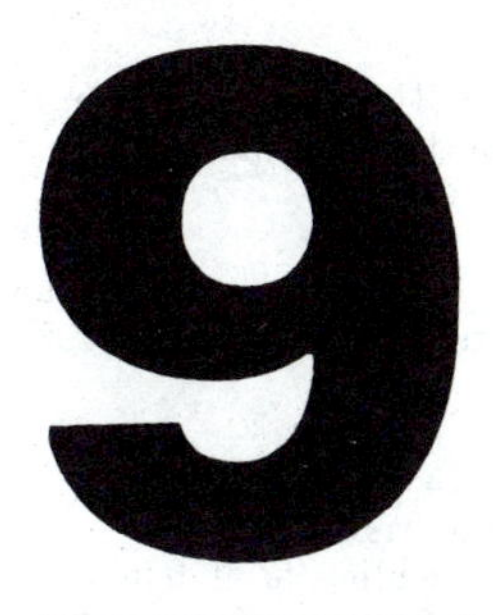

Identifying the High-Risk Newborn and Evaluating Gestational Age, Prematurity, Postmaturity, Large-for-Gestational-Age, and Small-for-Gestational-Age Infants

DeWayne M. Pursley
and John P. Cloherty

I. High-risk newborn. Certain conditions are associated with high-risk newborns [41]; the nursery staff should be made aware of these problems so as to anticipate difficulties.

Note: Cord blood and placentas should be saved for all problem newborns, including infants transferred from elsewhere as well as those born in the hospital. Many times an elusive diagnosis such as toxoplasmosis or cytomegalic inclusion viral disease will be made on pathologic examination of the placenta.

The following conditions are associated with high-risk newborns:

A. Maternal conditions	**Associated risk in fetus and neonate**
1. Maternal age over 40	Chromosomal abnormalities, small for gestational age (SGA)
2. Maternal age under 16	Prematurity, preeclampsia, child abuse
3. Poverty	Prematurity, infection, SGA
4. Infertility	Low birth weight, congenital anomalies, increased perinatal mortality
5. Smoking	SGA, increased perinatal mortality
6. Drug or alcohol abuse	SGA, fetal alcohol syndrome, withdrawal syndrome, sudden infant death syndrome
7. Diabetes	Stillbirth, respiratory distress syndrome, congenital anomalies, hypoglycemia
8. Thyroid disease	Goiter, hypothyroidism, hyperthyroidism
9. Renal disease	SGA, stillbirth
10. Urinary tract infection	Prematurity, sepsis
11. Heart or lung disease	SGA, stillbirth, prematurity
12. Hypertension (chronic or preeclampsia)	SGA, asphyxia, stillbirth, prematurity
13. Anemia	SGA, asphyxia, stillbirth, prematurity, hydrops
14. Isoimmunization (red cell antigens)	Stillbirth, anemia, jaundice
15. Isoimmunization (platelets)	Stillbirth, bleeding
16. Thrombocytopenia	Stillbirth, bleeding
17. Polyhydramnios	Anomalies (anencephaly, gastrointestinal obstruction, renal disease, goiter)
18. Low urinary estriols	SGA, stillbirth
19. Bleeding in early pregnancy	Prematurity, stillbirth
20. Bleeding in third trimester	Anemia, stillbirth
21. Premature rupture of membranes, fever, infection	Infection

22. TORCH infections	See TORCH infections (Chap. 12)
23. Past history of infant with jaundice, respiratory distress syndrome (RDS), or anomalies	Same in this pregnancy
24. Maternal medications (e.g., steroids, antimetabolites, antithyroid medications, reserpine, salicylates)	See individual medication package inserts and see index
25. Poor diet	Slightly SGA, fetal wasting in severe malnutrition
26. Hyperthermia	Fetal anomalies, fetal demise
27. Trauma	Fetal demise, prematurity
B. Fetal conditions	**Associated risk in fetus and neonate**
1. Multiple birth	Prematurity, twin transfusion syndrome, asphyxia, trauma
2. Poor fetal growth	Fetal demise, stillbirth, asphyxia, congenital anomalies, hypoglycemia
3. Excessive fetal size	Malformations, trauma, hypoglycemia
4. Abnormal fetal position	Trauma, hemorrhage, malformation
5. Abnormality of fetal heart rate or rhythm	Asphyxia, congestive heart failure, heartblock, hydrops
6. Acidosis	Asphyxia, RDS
7. Decreased activity	Fetal demise, stillbirth, asphyxia
8. Polyhydramnios	Anencephaly, central nervous system (CNS) disorders, neuromuscular disorders, problems with swallowing (e.g., agnathia, esophageal atresia, cord around neck), chylothorax, diaphragmatic hernia, omphalocele, gastroschisis, trisomy, tumors, hydrops, isoimmunization, anemia, cardiac failure, in utero infection, inability to concentrate urine, maternal diabetes
9. Oligohydramnios	Poor fetal growth, placental insufficiency, postmaturity, intrauterine death, intrapartum distress, renal agenesis, pulmonary hypoplasia, deformations
C. Conditions of labor and delivery	**Associated risk in fetus and neonate**
1. Premature labor	Respiratory distress, asphyxia, infection
2. Labor occurring 2 weeks or more after term	Stillbirth, asphyxia, meconium aspiration (see sec. **VI**)
3. Maternal fever	Infection
4. Rapid labor	Trauma, intracranial hemorrhage (ICH)
5. Long labor	Asphyxia, stillbirth, trauma
6. Abnormal presentation	Trauma, asphyxia
7. Uterine tetany	Asphyxia
8. Meconium-stained amniotic fluid	Asphyxia, meconium aspiration syndrome, stillbirth, persistent pulmonary hypertension
9. Prolapsed cord	Asphyxia, ICH
10. Maternal hypotension	Asphyxia, stillbirth

11. Cesarean section	RDS, transient tachypnea of the newborn (TTN), blood loss
12. Analgesia and anesthesia	Respiratory depression, hypotension, hypothermia
13. Placental anomalies	Risk to newborn
a. Small placenta	SGA
b. Large placenta	Hydrops, maternal diabetes
c. Torn placenta	Blood loss
d. Vasa praevia	Blood loss
D. Immediate neonatal conditions	**Associated risk in fetus and neonate**
1. Prematurity	RDS, ICH, infection
2. Low 1-minute Apgar score	RDS, asphyxia, ICH
3. Low 5-minute Apgar score	Developmental delay
4. Pallor or shock	Blood loss
5. Foul smell of amniotic fluid or membranes	Infection
6. Small for gestational age	See sec. **IV**
7. Postmaturity	See sec. **VI**

II. Gestational age estimation and birth weight classification [3,8,17,36,55]

A. An attempt should be made to classify infants by gestational age [27]. Gestational age may be assessed by the following:

1. Obstetric information (see Chap. 3)

a. Date of last menstrual period. The estimated date of confinement (EDC) can be quickly calculated by McDonald's rule: Add 7 days and subtract 3 months. The accuracy of menstrual dating is quite variable, however, especially in anticipated preterm and postterm deliveries [32].

b. Date of early clinical and ultrasonic examination during pregnancy. In the absence of multiple gestation, molar pregnancy, and various structural abnormalities, uterine size is an accurate predictor of the EDC. An ultrasonagraphic estimate based on biparietal diameter, femur length, head circumference, and/or abdominal circumference is considered quite accurate provided it is obtained prior to 20 weeks' gestation [9,47,50].

c. Date of first recorded fetal activity. "Quickening" is first felt at approximately 16 to 18 weeks.

d. Date of first recorded fetal heart sounds. These are first detected at approximately 10 to 12 weeks by ultrasonic Doppler and by about 20 weeks by fetoscope.

2. Newborn information can be obtained by use of the modified Dubowitz examination [2], as in Figures 9-1 and 9-2. There are, however, limitations to this method, especially in small and sick newborns.

3. The degree of prematurity can be estimated by examination of the anterior vascular capsule of the lens in the first 24 to 48 hours [24] (Fig. 9-3).

4. Infants are **classified** as [51,54]:

a. Preterm (<37 weeks).

b. Term (37–41$^{6}/_{7}$ weeks).

c. Postterm (42 weeks or more).

B. Although there is no universal agreement on birth weight classification, the commonly accepted definitions are (11) as follows:

1. Normal birth weight (NBW)—2500 gm or more

2. Very low birth weight (VLBW)—<1500 gm

3. Low birth weight (LBW)—<2500 gm. Infants of low birth weight are further classified by maturity and appropriateness for gestational age as follows:

a. Those who are premature and are appropriate size for gestational age (**preterm AGA**)

b. Those who are premature but whose weight is still small for gestational age (**preterm SGA**)

NEUROMUSCULAR MATURITY

	0	1	2	3	4	5
Posture						
Square Window (Wrist)	90°	60°	45°	30°	0°	
Arm Recoil	180°		100°-180°	90°-100°	< 90°	
Popliteal Angle	180°	160°	130°	110°	90°	< 90°
Scarf Sign						
Heel to Ear						

PHYSICAL MATURITY

	0	1	2	3	4	5
SKIN	gelatinous red, trans-parent	smooth pink, visible veins	superficial peeling & or rash, few veins	cracking pale area, rare veins	parchment, deep cracking, no vessels	leathery, cracked, wrinkled
LANUGO	none	abundant	thinning	bald areas	mostly bald	
PLANTAR CREASES	no crease	faint red marks	anterior transverse crease only	creases ant. 2/3	creases cover entire sole	
BREAST	barely percept.	flat areola, no bud	stippled areola, 1–2 mm bud	raised areola, 3–4 mm bud	full areola, 5–10 mm bud	
EAR	pinna flat, stays folded	sl. curved pinna, soft with slow recoil	well-curv. pinna, soft but ready recoil	formed & firm with instant recoil	thick cartilage, ear stiff	
GENITALS Male	scrotum empty, no rugae		testes descend-ing, few rugae	testes down, good rugae	testes pendulous, deep rugae	
GENITALS Female	prominent clitoris & labia minora		majora & minora equally prominent	majora large, minora small	clitoris & minora completely covered	

Gestation by Dates ________ wks

Birth Date ________ Hour ________ am pm

APGAR ________ 1 min ________ 5 min

MATURITY RATING

Score	Wks
5	26
10	28
15	30
20	32
25	34
30	36
35	38
40	40
45	42
50	44

SCORING SECTION

	1st Exam=X	2nd Exam=O
Estimating Gest Age by Maturity Rating	______ Weeks	______ Weeks
Time of Exam	Date ______ am Hour ______ pm	Date ______ am Hour ______ pm
Age at Exam	______ Hours	______ Hours
Signature of Examiner	______ M.D.	______ M.D.

Fig. 9-1. Sample of a form used to estimate gestational age by evaluation of various aspects of maturity. The scoring was developed by Ballard, Kazmaier, and Driver [1]. (Reproduced with permission from a form developed by Jacob L. Kay, M.D., Seton Medical Center, Austin, Texas, with Mead Johnson & Co., Evansville, Indiana.)

c. Those who are term and small for gestational age (**term SGA**)

III. **Prematurity** [19,29,39]. A **preterm neonate** is any neonate whose birth occurs through the end of the last day of the thirty-seventh week (259th day) following onset of the last menstrual period.

A. **Incidence.** Approximately 9 percent of all U.S. births are premature, and almost 2 percent of U.S. infants are less than 32 weeks' gestation [45]. In smaller segments of the U.S. population, demographics play a major role in the prevalence of prematurity.

B. **Etiology.** Most premature deliveries occur for unknown reasons. Premature (and, in many cases, LBW) delivery occurs in association with the following conditions [26]:

1. **Low socioeconomic status (SES),** whether measured by family income, educational level, residency, social class, or occupation, is associated with higher rates of premature delivery.
2. **Black women** experience more than twice the rate of premature delivery

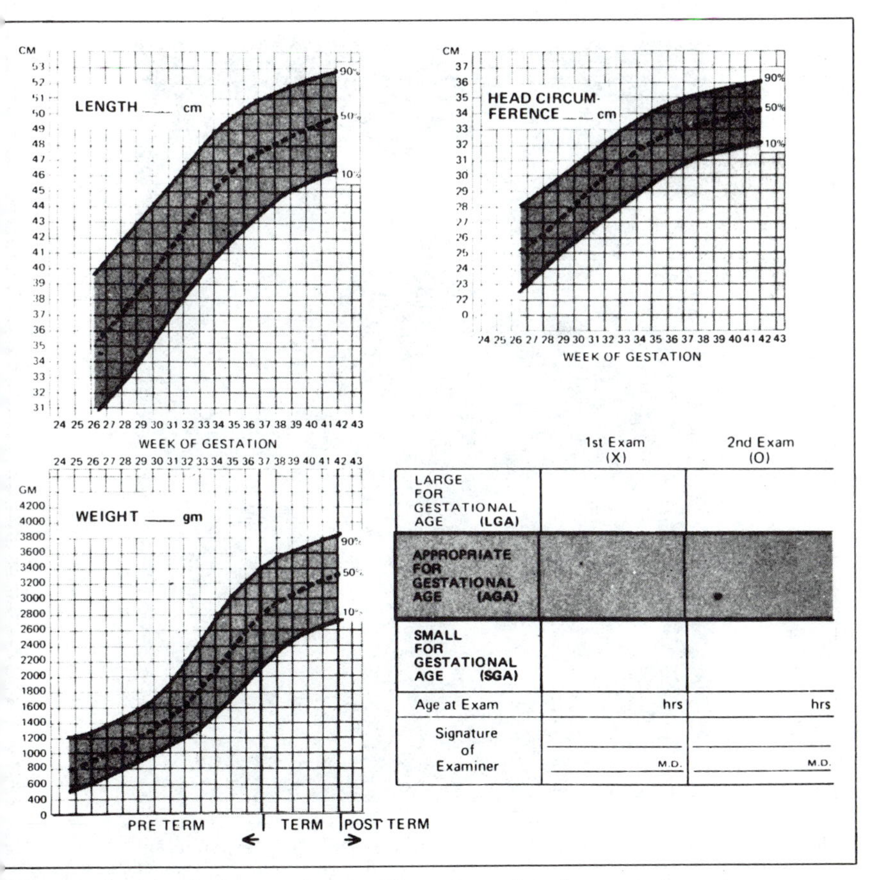

Fig. 9-2. Sample of a form used to classify newborns based on maturity and intrauterine growth. (Reproduced with permission from a form developed by Jacob L. Kay, M.D., Seton Medical Center, Austin, Texas, with Mead Johnson & Co., Evansville, Indiana.)

than white women, giving birth to almost a third of all premature infants [45].

3. **Malnutrition** before pregnancy and poor nutritional intake during pregnancy have a negative impact on fetal weight gain.
4. **Women under age 16 or over 35** are more likely to deliver LBW infants than their counterparts—a more significant factor in white births than in black births.
5. **Increased maternal activity** that requires long periods of standing or other substantial amounts of physical stress is probably associated with intrauterine growth retardation and prematurity. In mothers from higher socio-economic groups who have access to good medical care, this is not a significant problem.
6. **Smoking** is associated with a reduction in birth weight of offspring in the range of 150 to 250 gm [53].
7. **Acute or chronic maternal illness,** such as urinary tract infection, hypertension or preeclampsia, diabetes, and maternal pulmonary or cardiac disease, is associated with early delivery.

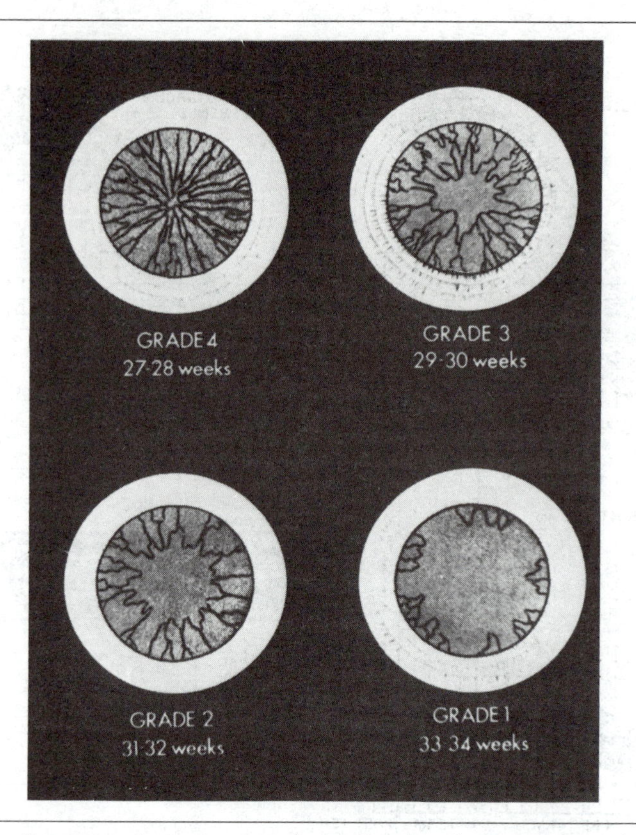

Fig. 9-3. Grading system for assessment of gestational age by examination of the anterior vascular capsule of the lens. (Reproduced with permission from H. M. Hittner et al., Assessment of gestational age by examination of the anterior capsule of the lens. *J. Pediatr.* 91: 455, 1977.)

8. **Multiple-gestation births** occur before 37 weeks about 50 percent of the time. Because birth weight–specific mortality is no higher in multiple-gestation infants compared with singletons, the higher rate of neonatal mortality in these infants is primarily related to their higher rates of prematurity [42].
9. **Prior poor birth outcome** is the single strongest predictor of poor birth outcome. A premature first birth is the best predictor of a preterm second birth [26].
10. **Obstetric factors** such as polyhydramnios, uterine malformations (such as double uterus), uterine trauma, vaginal bleeding (e.g., placenta previa, abruptio placentae), incompetent cervix (sometimes associated with exposure of the mother to diethystilbesterol in her own gestation), premature rupture of membranes, and amnionitis are also important contributors to prematurity.
11. **Fetal conditions** such as erythroblastosis, fetal distress, or poor fetal growth may require early delivery.
12. **Inadvertent early delivery,** by induced labor or repeat cesarean section,

because of an incorrect estimate of gestational age, is another potential cause of prematurity.

C. **Problems of prematurity** [10]. These problems, which are related to difficulty in extrauterine adaptation due to immaturity of organ systems, are mentioned here but are considered in greater detail in other chapters.

1. **Respiratory.** Premature infants may have difficulty adapting to air breathing. This may at first appear as perinatal depression in the delivery room (see Chap. 5). Respiratory distress syndrome (RDS) may occur because of surfactant deficiency (see Chap. 13), and apnea may occur because of immaturity of mechanisms for the control of breathing (see Chap. 13). Premature infants are also at risk for bronchopulmonary dysplasia, Wilson-Mikity disease, and chronic pulmonary insufficiency.
2. **Neurologic.** Premature infants are at risk for acute neurologic problems such as intracranial hemorrhage and perinatal depression (see Chap. 21).
3. **Cardiovascular.** Premature infants may be subject to hypotension due to hypovolemia (blood or fluid loss is exaggerated by their small size) or cardiac dysfunction and/or vasodilation due to sepsis. A patent ductus arteriosus is a common problem that may result in congestive heart failure (see Chap. 14).
4. **Hematologic** problems, especially anemia resulting from a more profound physiologic nadir, peri- or postnatal blood loss, or iatrogenic causes, are seen frequently (see Chaps. 16 and 17). Infants with hyperbilirubinemia need special attention because low levels of bilirubin may be toxic to the nervous system of very immature infants (see Chap. 15).
5. **Nutritional.** Feeding problems are often significant. Prematures require specific attention to the type, amount, and route of feeding (see Chap. 30).
6. **Gastrointestinal** problems can be quite significant. Prematurity is the single greatest risk factor for necrotizing enterocolitis (see Chap. 28).
7. **Metabolic** problems, especially disorders in glucose and calcium metabolism, are more common in premature infants [especially those who are malnourished, sick, or who have emerged from an abnormal uterine environment (see Chap. 24).
8. **Renal.** The immature kidney is characterized by a low glomerular filtration rate and an inability to handle water, solute, and acid loads; these characteristics make fluid and electrolyte management difficult (see Chap. 26).
9. **Temperature regulation.** Premature infants are especially susceptible to hypothermia and hyperthermia, and they require strict attention to their environment (see Chap. 32).
10. **Immunologic.** Because of deficiencies in both humoral and cellular immune response, premature infants are at greater risk for infection than are full-term infants.
11. **Ophthalmologic.** Retinopathy of prematurity may develop in the immature retina (see Chap. 38).

D. **Management of the premature infant**

1. **Immediate postnatal management**
   a. **Delivery** in a hospital equipped and staffed to care for this type of infant is most important. The risk to the very premature or sick preterm infant is greatly increased by transfer and by the lack of necessary early care.
   b. **Resuscitation and stabilization** begin with appropriate planning and require the immediate availability of qualified personnel and equipment. Anticipation and prevention of problems should be the major thrust, rather than reaction to problems already present. Adequate oxygen delivery and maintenance of proper temperature control are the immediate postnatal goals (see Chap. 5).
2. **Neonatal management**
   a. **Thermal regulation** should be directed toward achieving a neutral thermal zone, i.e., the environmental temperature at which oxygen

consumption is minimal yet sufficient to maintain the body temperature. For the small preterm infant, this will require either an overhead radiant warmer (with the advantages of infant accessibility and rapid temperature response) or a closed incubator (with the advantages of diminished insensible water loss and barrier to infection) (see Chap. 32).

b. **Oxygen therapy and assisted ventilation** may be necessary in the preterm infant to maintain adequate oxygenation. Oxygen may be delivered by increasing ambient O_2 concentration (for mild and transient pulmonary disease), through continuous positive airway pressure (CPAP) by means of nasal prongs, a nasopharyngeal tube, or an endotracheal tube (for infants whose primary blood gas abnormality is hypoxia alone, such as RDS), or through intermittent positive-pressure ventilation (see Chap. 13).

c. **Patent ductus arteriosus** most often requires only conservative management with adequate oxygenation, fluid restriction, and possibly intermittent diuretic use. In more symptomatic cases, a prostaglandin antagonist, such as indomethacin, may be necessary. In the most symptomatic infants, surgical ligation may be necessary if medical treatment fails (see Chap. 14).

d. **Fluid and electrolyte therapy** must account for potentially high insensible water loss while avoiding overhydration and maintaining normal glucose and plasma electrolyte concentrations (see Chap. 24).

e. **Nutrition,** which may be limited by the inability of many preterm infants to suck and swallow effectively or to tolerate enteral feedings, may require gavage feeding or parenteral nutrition (see Chap. 30).

f. **Hyperbilirubinemia,** which is inevitable in the smallest of preterm infants, can usually be managed effectively by careful monitoring of bilirubin levels and judicious use of phototherapy. In the most severe cases, exchange transfusion may be necessary to avoid kernicterus (see Chap. 15).

g. **Infection** should always be considered after preterm delivery. Broad-spectrum antibiotics should be begun when suspicion of infection is strong. Antistaphyloccal antibiotics should be considered in VLBW infants who have undergone multiple procedures or have remained for long periods in the hospital and thus are at increased risk of nosocomial infection (see Chap. 12).

h. **Immunization** against diphtheria, pertussis, tetanus (DPT), and oral polio vaccine (OPV) should be administered in full doses to premature infants based on their chronologic age (i.e., weeks after birth), not their postconceptional age [5,49]. When a preterm (or term) infant is in the nursery 2 months after birth, DPT should be administered. Pertussis vaccine usually should be withheld from infants who have evidence of central nervous system damage [15]. OPV should be administered at discharge to avoid the risk of cross-infection in the nursery. OPV should not be given to immunocompromised infants. The infants should be given inactivated polio vaccine (IPU).

E. **Survival of premature infants** [6,21,23]. Figure 9-4 and Tables 9-1 and 9-2 show the survival rates of infants of various birth weights admitted to the neonatal intensive care units of Beth Israel Hospital, Brigham and Women's Hospital, and The Children's Hospital (Joint Program in Neonatology) in 1987 and 1988. **Admission** is defined as death or admission for more than 24 hours. Admission criteria include prematurity less than 35 weeks, respiratory distress, major congenital anomalies, and perinatal depression. Infants requiring observation or stabilization and admitted for less than 24 hours (**triage infants**) are not included in this analysis. The inborn population, from which the Brigham and Women's Hospital and Beth Israel Hospital infants are drawn, represents approximately 30,000 births. These hospitals serve residents of the urban and suburban Boston area as well as high-risk maternal

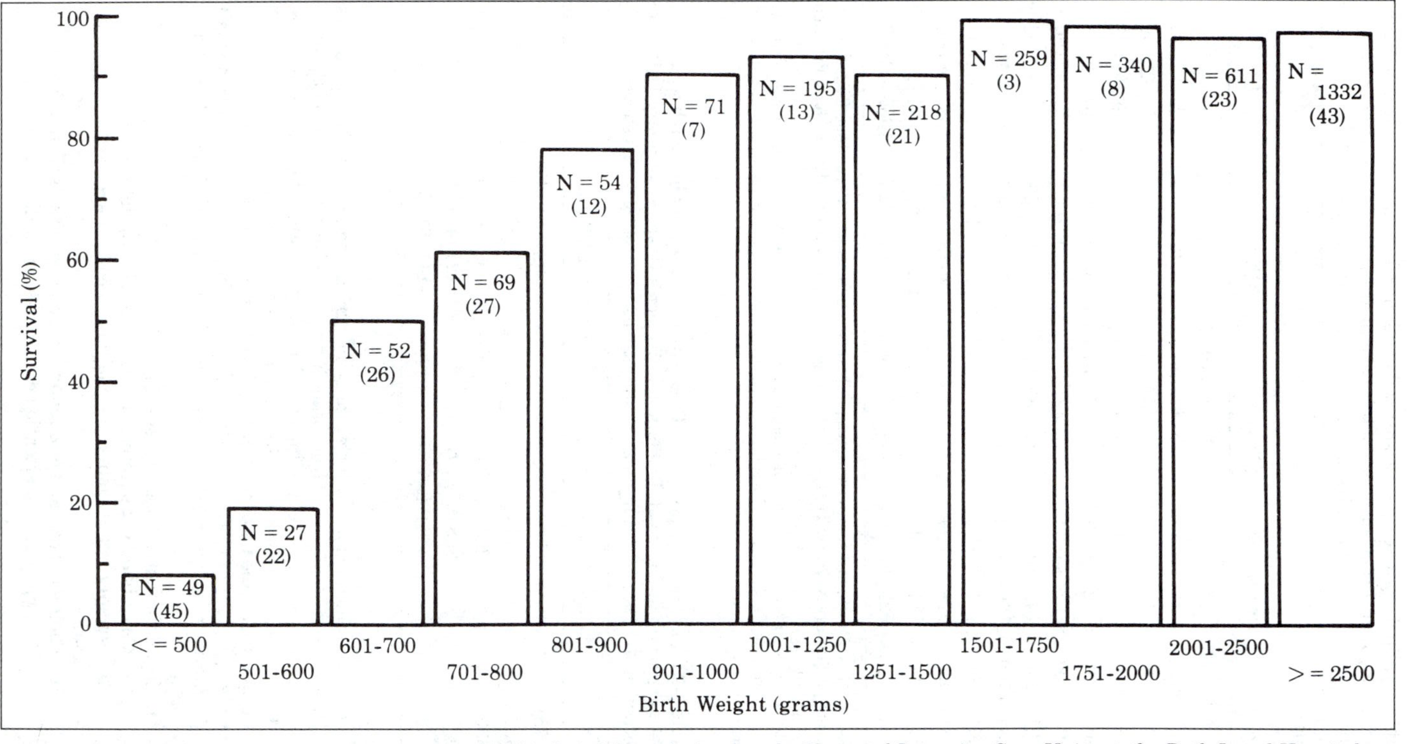

Fig. 9-4. Survival rate of premature infants of various birth weights admitted to the Neonatal Intensive Care Units at the Beth Israel Hospital, Brigham and Women's Hospital, and The Children's Hospital (Joint Program in Neonatology) in 1987 and 1988. Gestational age was 24 weeks or more. Deaths are listed in parentheses. N = total admissions in each birth weight category. Deaths are in parentheses. Note: Admission is defined as death or admission for more than 24 hours.

Table 9-1. Birth weight–specific survival of admitted infants, neonatal intensive care units, Joint Program in Neonatology, January 1, 1987 to December 31, 1988: Total number of admissions (deaths), percent survival

Birth weight (gm)	BWH	TCH	BIH	All JPN
<500	35 (34) 3%	5 (3) 40%	9 (8) 11%	49 (45) 8%
501–600	22 (18) 18%	3 (2) 33%	2 (2) 0%	27 (22) 19%
601–700	42 (18) 57%	5 (3) 40%	5 (5) 0%	52 (26) 50%
701–800	39 (21) 46%	7 (5) 29%	3 (1) 67%	69 (27) 61%
801–900	42 (9) 79%	7 (3) 57%	5 (0) 100%	54 (12) 78%
901–1000	62 (5) 92%	7 (2) 71%	2 (0) 100%	71 (7) 90%
1001–1250	142 (9) 94%	31 (3) 90%	22 (1) 95%	195 (13) 93%
1251–1500	159 (13) 92%	27 (3) 89%	32 (5) 84%	218 (21) 90%
1501–1750	181 (3) 98%	29 (0) 100%	49 (0) 100%	259 (3) 99%
1751–2000	228 (3) 99%	42 (2) 95%	70 (3) 96%	340 (8) 98%
2001–2500	381 (12) 97%	108 (7) 94%	122 (4) 97%	611 (23) 96%
>2500	620 (12) 98%	469 (27) 94%	243 (4) 98%	1332 (43) 97%

Key: BWH = Brigham and Women's Hospital Neonatal Intensive Care Unit; BIH = Beth Israel Special Care Nursery; TCH = The Children's Hospital, 7 North; JPN = Joint Program in Neonatology.
Note: *Admission* is defined as death or admission for more than 24 hours. Admission criteria include prematurity less than 35 weeks, respiratory distress, major congenital anomalies, and perinatal depression.

Table 9-2. Very low birth weight (≤1500 gm) and extremely low birth weight (≤1000 gm) infant survival, Brigham and Women's Hospital, January 1, 1987 to December 31, 1988: Total number of admissions (deaths), percent survival

Year	≤1500 gm	≤1000 gm
1975	99 (44) 56%	42 (32) 24%
1982	177 (39) 78%	66 (27) 60%
1983	208 (53) 75%	100 (40) 60%
1987	258 (55) 79%	121 (47) 61%
1988	312 (72) 77%	141 (58) 59%

referrals from other areas of New England. Infants admitted to The Children's Hospital were transferred from other hospitals in New England and the eastern United States. The leveling off of VLBW survival in the 1980s (see Table 9-2) has been witnessed in other perinatal centers [21,60].

F. **Long-term problems of prematurity.** The premature infant is vulnerable to a wide spectrum of morbidity. Although severe impairment occurs in a small population of survivors, the prevalence of the lesser morbidities is less clearly defined [1].

1. **Developmental disability** (see Chap. 37)
   a. **Major handicaps** (cerebral palsy, mental retardation)
   b. **Sensory impairments** (hearing loss, visual impairment) (see Chap. 38)
   c. **Minimal cerebral dysfunction** (language disorders, learning disability, hyperactivity, attention deficits, behavior disorders)

2. **Retinopathy of prematurity** (see Chap. 38)
3. **Chronic lung disease** (see Chap. 13)
4. **Poor growth** [20] (see Chap. 37)
5. **Increased rates of postneonatal illness and rehospitalization** [43]
6. **Increased frequency of congenital anomalies** [39]
7. **Increased risk of child abuse and neglect** [33]

IV. Infants who are small for gestational age (SGA) (see Chap. 3) [16,38,51,55]

A. Definition. There is no uniform definition of SGA, although most reports define this as two standard deviations below the mean for gestational age or as below the tenth percentile. Numerous "normal birth curves" have been defined using studies of large populations of infants (see Fig. 9-2) [58].

B. Etiology [25,28]. It is estimated that one-third of LBW infants are SGA. There is an association of the following factors with SGA infants:

1. **Maternal factors**
   - **a.** Maternal age
   - **b.** Parity
   - **c.** Race
   - **d.** Infertility
   - **e.** Previous spontaneous abortions
   - **f.** Unwed state
   - **g.** Underweight mother
   - **h.** Poor maternal weight gain in pregnancy
   - **i.** Working during pregnancy [44] (see **III.5**)
   - **j.** High altitude (Fig. 9-5) [40].
   - **k.** Teratogens such as alcohol, drugs, and radiation
   - **l.** Chronic maternal disease
   - **m.** Anything that may interfere with placental flow and oxygenation, including:
     - **(1)** Heart disease
     - **(2)** Renal disease
     - **(3)** Hypertension [7]
     - **(4)** Smoking
     - **(5)** Sickle-cell disease
     - **(6)** Pulmonary disease
     - **(7)** Collagen-vascular disease
     - **(8)** Diabetes—classes D, E, F, and R
     - **(9)** Preeclampsia
     - **(10)** Postmaturity
     - **(11)** Multiple gestation
     - **(12)** Uterine anomalies
2. **Placental lesions**
   - **a.** Secondary to maternal vascular disease
   - **b.** Multiple gestation
   - **c.** Malformations
   - **d.** Tumor
3. **Fetal factors**
   - **a. Constitutional**—normal, genetically small infant
   - **b. Chromosomal abnormality,** especially the trisomies and Turner syndrome
   - **c. Malformations,** especially abnormalities of CNS and skeletal system
   - **d. Congenital infection,** especially rubella (60 percent of these infants are SGA) and CMV (40 percent of these infants are SGA) [48] (see Chap. 12)
   - **e. Multiple gestation**

C. Management of the SGA infant

1. **During pregnancy** (see Chap. 3)
   - **a. Identification, evaluation, and monitoring.** Determination of the cause of poor fetal growth should be attempted when intrauterine

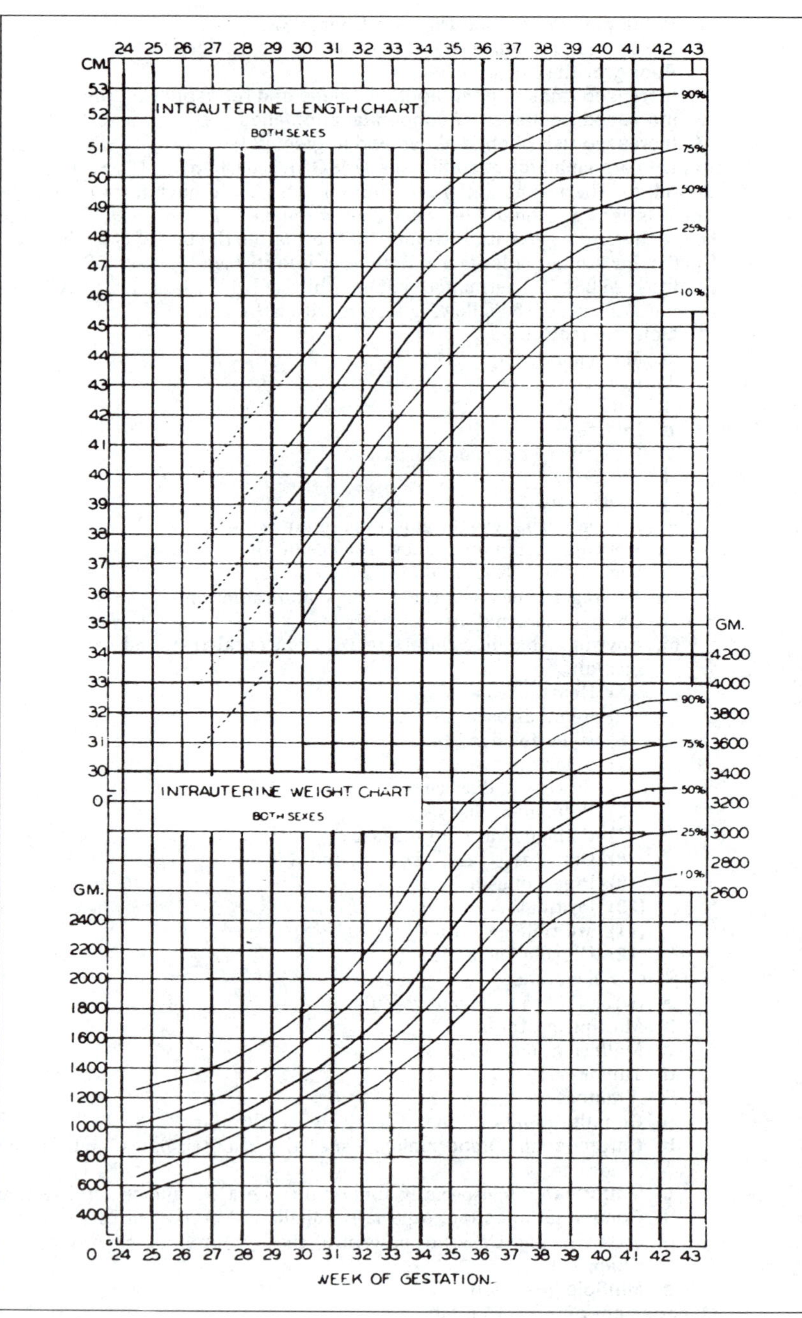

Fig. 9-5. These data represent infants born in Denver at an altitude of 1 mile above sea level. (From L. O. Lubchenco et al., Intrauterine growth in length and head circumference as estimated from live born birth weight data at 24 to 42 weeks of gestation. *Pediatrics* 37: 403, 1966.)

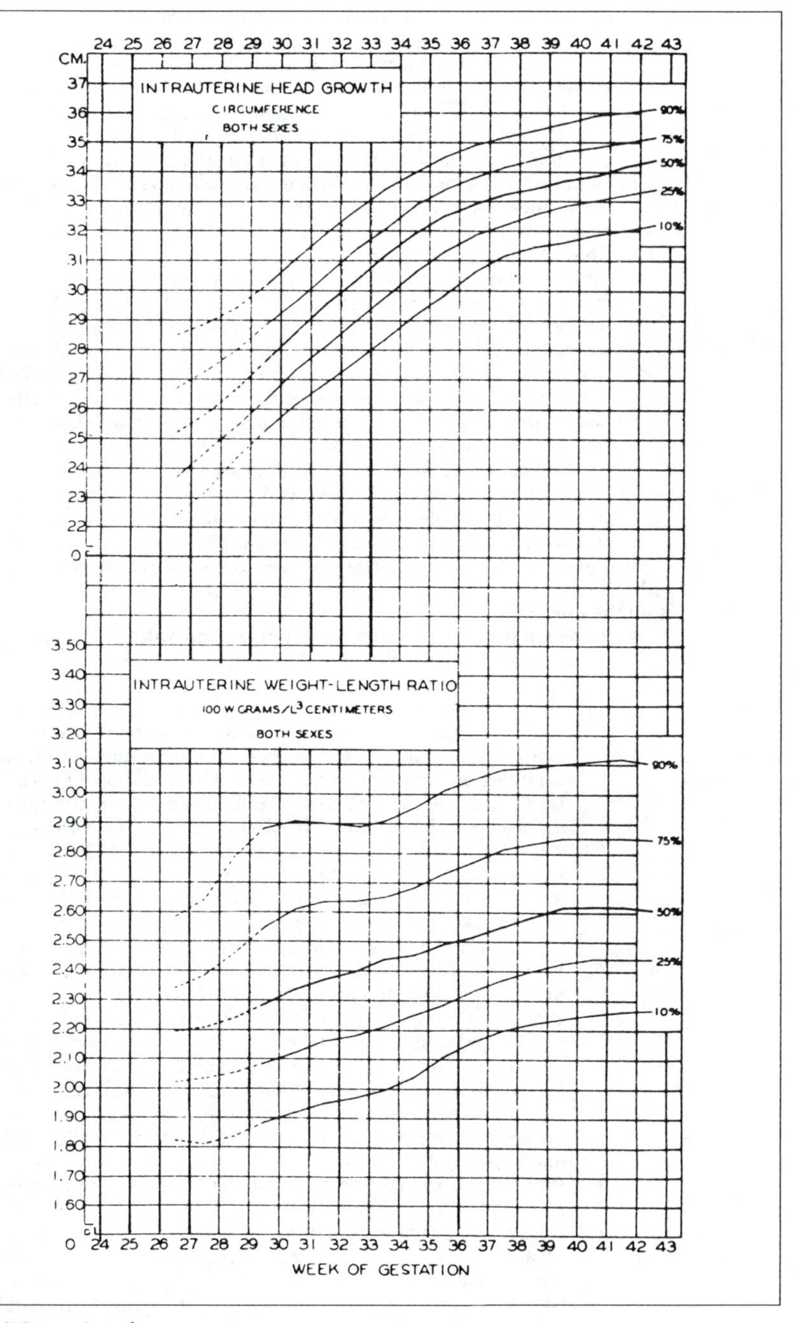

Fig. 9-5 (continued)

growth retardation (IUGR) is determined. Treatment should be initiated when available. The investigation includes a search for the factors included in subsection **IV.B** and usually includes a fetal ultrasound. An attempt should be made to assess the health of the fetus (see Chap. 3). Antepartum fetal monitoring, such as the nonstress test, the oxytocin challenge test, a biophysical profile, and serial ultrasound examinations, is often utilized. Doppler evaluation of placental flow is a more recent form of evaluation for uteroplacental insufficiency. Determination of the degree of pulmonary maturity should be considered if early delivery is being contemplated (see Chap. 13).

b. **Early delivery** is necessary if it is judged that the risk to the fetus staying in utero is greater than the risk of early delivery. Generally, indications are arrest of fetal growth, fetal distress, and pulmonary maturity near term, especially in a mother with hypertension. Acceleration of pulmonary maturity with steroids should be considered if amniotic fluid analyses suggest pulmonary immaturity. If there is poor placental blood flow, the fetus may not tolerate labor and may require delivery by cesarean section.

2. **During delivery.** Because very SGA infants are at risk for problems at the time of delivery and often require specialized care in the first few days of life, if at all possible, delivery should take place at a center with a high-risk nursery. The delivery team should be especially prepared to manage fetal distress, perinatal depression, meconium aspiration, hypoxia, and heat loss.

3. **In the nursery**

a. An **evaluation to determine the etiology of growth retardation** should be attempted, although in many cases the etiology will remain unclear.

(1) **Newborn examination.** The infant should be evaluated for any of the previously mentioned causes of poor fetal growth, especially chromosomal abnormalities, malformations, and congenital infection. Infants who have growth retardation due to factors that influence the last part of pregnancy (e.g., maternal renal disease, preeclampsia, or other factors interfering with placental circulation) will have a relatively normal head circumference, some reduction in length, but a more profound reduction in weight (see Figs. 9-1 and 9-2). Use of the ponderal index (weight in grams × 100/length in centimeters) or the weight-length ratio will quantify the loss of weight (see Fig. 9-5). The infant may have loss of subcutaneous tissue, peeling loose skin, a wasted appearance, and meconium staining.

When IUGR occurs in early pregnancy, head circumference, length, and weight may all be decreased in a proportionate way, and the ponderal index may be normal. As compared with infants whose IUGR begins in late pregnancy, these infants are more likely to have significant intrinsic fetal problems as a cause for growth retardation (chromosomal defects, malformations, and congenital infection).

(2) **Pathologic examination of the placenta** for congenital infection or infarction may be helpful.

(3) Generally, **serologic screening** for congenital infection is **not indicated** unless the history or examination suggests infection as a possible cause.

b. An **evaluation for complications related to growth retardation** should be undertaken. The following conditions occur more frequently in SGA than in AGA infants:

(1) Congenital anomalies

(2) Perinatal depression

(3) Meconium aspiration
(4) Pulmonary hemorrhage
(5) Persistent pulmonary hypertension
(6) Hypothermia
(7) Hypoglycemia
(8) Hypocalcemia
(9) Hyponatremia
(10) Polycythemia

Leukopenia, neutropenia, and thrombocytopenia may be seen in infants born to hypertensive mothers. The thrombocytopenia is often associated with maternal thrombocytopenia, but the neutropenia and leukopenia are not. The neutropenia is not associated with a shift to immature forms, as is seen in bacterial infections. There is an increased risk of nosocomial infection in these infants [7,31].

c. **Specific management considerations**

(1) **Feeding.** Start early feeding at 1 hour of age with glucose 5% and water, moving to milk feedings every 2 to 3 hours. If oral feedings are not tolerated, feed the infant by gavage or intravenously. If there was significant perinatal depression, the infant should be fed only intravenously for 1 to 2 days. Fluids should be limited, and the serum sodium concentration should be monitored (see Chap. 24). SGA infants require more calories per kilogram for growth than AGA infants.

(2) **Blood glucose level** should be monitored every 2 to 4 hours until it is stable.

(3) **Serum calcium level** may be depressed if the infant was asphyxiated or premature.

D. **Long-term problems of SGA infants.** It is difficult to determine the specific effects of IUGR, since several studies do not control well for parental height and socioeconomic status and because there are often overlapping effects from prematurity and asphyxia [37,64]. SGA infants are at risk for poor postnatal growth and neurologic and developmental handicaps [18,22]. These handicaps occur even in the absence of specific fetal disease (e.g., chromosomal abnormalities). This is especially true in infants who have IUGR in head circumference, height, and weight, suggesting early onset of IUGR [46], and in those who suffered perinatal asphyxia or hypoglycemia (or both) at birth [14,56,59]. For any weight group, the total proportion of infants who either die before 1 year of age or are handicapped at 1 year of age is similar for SGA and AGA infants. However, SGA infants have less risk of neonatal death compared with premature AGA infants of the same weight but a greater risk of morbidity at 1 year of age [52].

E. **Management of subsequent pregnancies** is important because recurrent IUGR is common. Specific recommendations include the following:

1. The mother should be cared for by personnel experienced in the care of high-risk pregnancies.
2. The health of the mother and the fetus should be assessed throughout the pregnancy by ultrasound and nonstress tests (see Chap. 3).
3. Early delivery should be considered if fetal growth is poor.

V. **Infants who are large for gestational age (LGA)** [4,37] (see Chap. 3)

A. **Definition.** The infant's weight is two standard deviations above the mean or above the ninetieth percentile (see Fig. 9-2).

B. **Etiology**

1. Constitutionally large infants (large parents)
2. Infants of diabetic mothers (class A, B, or C)
3. Some postterm infants
4. Transposition of the great vessels
5. Erythroblastosis fetalis
6. Beckwith-Wiedemann syndrome
7. Parabiotic syndrome (twins)

C. Management

1. The baby should be evaluated for problems listed in subsection **B**.
2. Observation should be made for evidence of birth trauma, including brachial plexus injury, and perinatal depression (see Chaps. 21 and 22).
3. The blood sugar level should be monitored. The infant should be fed early because some LGA infants may have hyperinsulinism and be prone to hypoglycemia (infants of diabetic mothers, infants with Beckwith's syndrome or erythroblastosis (see Chaps. 1 and 24).
4. The baby should be evaluated for polycythemia (see Chap. 18).

VI. Postmaturity [30,35]

A. Definition. The infant's gestation exceeds 42 weeks.

B. Etiology. The cause of prolonged pregnancy is not known in the majority of cases. The following are known associations:

1. **Anencephaly.** An intact fetal pituitary-adrenal axis is involved in the initiation of labor.
2. **Trisomy 16–18**
3. **Seckel's Syndrome** (bird-headed dwarfism)

C. Syndrome of postmaturity. These infants usually have normal length and head circumference. If they have the postmaturity syndrome, however, they will have lost weight. Infants with this syndrome are distinct from SGA infants in that they were doing well until they went beyond 42 weeks' gestation and became nutritionally deprived. SGA infants, of course, also may have these signs and symptoms. Postmature infants have been placed into three groups by Clifford [12,13]:

1. **Stage 1**
   a. Dry, cracked, peeling, loose, and wrinkled skin
   b. Malnourished appearance
   c. Decreased subcutaneous tissue
   d. Skin too big for baby
   e. Open-eyed and alert baby
2. **Stage 2**
   a. All features of stage 1
   b. Meconium staining
   c. Perinatal depression in some cases
3. **Stage 3**
   a. The findings in stages 1 and 2
   b. Meconium staining of cord and nails
   c. A higher risk of fetal, intrapartum, and neonatal deaths

D. Placenta. There is some correlation between low placental weights and increased mortality in postmaturity. One study [30] showed that the average placental weight in nonsurvivors was 452 gm, the average placental weight in survivors was 580 gm, and when the placental weight was over 700 gm, there were no deaths.

E. Risk. Figure 9-6 shows the pregnancy wastage associated with various gestational ages; mortality is increased with postmaturity. Kloosterman [30] showed that careful induction of labor or cesarean section after 42 weeks resulted in a decreased mortality compared with the results seen following conservative expectant therapy.

F. Management

1. **Prepartum management**
   a. Careful **estimation of true gestational age** using the date from the last menstrual period and techniques such as ultrasound
   b. Careful **monitoring of fetal well-being** using such studies as ultrasound, biophysical profiles, and nonstress tests
2. **Intrapartum management** involves preparation for perinatal depression and meconium aspiration and the use of fetal monitoring.
3. **Postpartum management**
   a. **An evaluation for complications related to postmaturity** should be

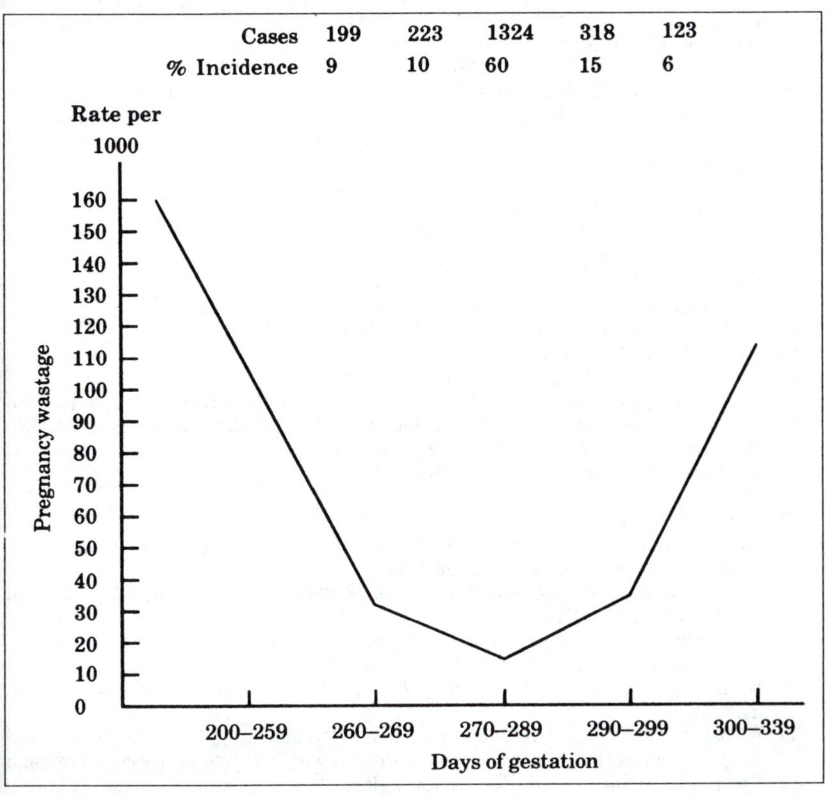

Fig. 9-6. Pregnancy wastage at various gestational ages in 2187 women with one and only one delivery between 1940 and 1950 at the Boston Hospital for Women. (From S. H. Clifford, Postmaturity with placental dysfunction: Clinical syndrome and pathologic findings. *J. Pediatr.* 44: 1, 1954.)

undertaken. The following conditions occur more frequently in postmature infants:

(1) Congenital anomalies
(2) Perinatal depression
(3) Meconium aspiration
(4) Persistent pulmonary hypertension
(5) Hypoglycemia
(6) Hypocalcemia
(7) Polycythemia

b. Early feeding

References

1. Allen, M. C. *Obstet. Gynecol.* 67: 427, 1986.
2. Ballard, J. L. *J. Pediatr.* 95: 769, 1979.
3. Ballard, J. *Pediatr. Res.* 11: 374, 1977.
4. Berk, M. *Pediatrics* 83: 1029, 1989.

5. Bernbaum, J. *Clin. Perinatol.* 11: 73, 1984.
6. Boyle, M. H. *N. Engl. J. Med.* 308: 1330, 1983.
7. Brazie, J. E. *J. Pediatr.* 100: 265, 1982.
8. Brazie, J. V., and Lubchenco, L. O. The Estimation of Gestational Age Chart. In C. H. Kempe, H. K. Silver, and D. O'Brien (Eds.), *Current Pediatric Diagnosis and Treatment,* 4th Ed. Los Altos, Calif.: Lange, 1976.
9. Campbell, S. *Obstet. Gynecol.* 65: 613, 1985.
10. Cashore, W. J. *Clin. Obstet. Gynecol.* 11: 391, 1984.
11. Chiswick, M. L. *Arch. Dis. Child.* 61: 708, 1986.
12. Clifford, S. H. *J. Pediatr.* 44: 1, 1954.
13. Clifford, S. H. *Am. J. Dis. Child.* 69: 327, 1945.
14. Commey, J. O. O. *J. Pediatr.* 94: 779, 1979.
15. Committee on Infectious Disease. *Pediatrics* 74: 303, 1984.
16. Drillien, C. M. *Clin. Perinatol.* 1: 197, 1974.
17. Dubowitz, L. M. *J. Pediatr.* 77: 1, 1970.
18. Fitzhandinge, P. M. *Pediatrics* 50: 50, 1972.
19. *Guidelines for Perinatal Care.* American Academy of Pediatrics and the American College of Obstetricians and Gynecologists, P.O. Box 1034, Evanston, Ill., 1983.
20. Hack, M. *J. Dev. Behav. Pediatr.* 4: 243, 1983.
21. Hack, M. *N. Engl. J. Med.* 321: 1642, 1989.
22. Harvey, D. *Pediatrics* 69: 296, 1982.
23. Herschel, N. *Obstet. Gynecol.* 60: 154, 1982.
24. Hittner, H. M. *J. Pediatr.* 91: 455, 1977.
25. Howie, P. W. *Br. Med. J.* 285: 156, 1982.
26. Institute of Medicine. *Preventing Low Birth Weight.* Washington, D.C.: National Academy Press, 1985.
27. Kauppila, O. *Acta Obstet. Gynecol. Scand.* [*Suppl.*] 39: 1, 1975.
28. Keirse, M. J. N. *Clin. Obstet. Gynecol.* 11: 415, 1984.
29. Klaus, M., and Fanaroff, A. *Care of the High-Risk Neonate.* Philadelphia: Saunders, 1973.
30. Kloosterman, G. J. The Obstetrician and Dysmaturity. In H. E. Leiden and K. N. V. Stenset (Eds.), *Aspects of Prematurity and Dysmaturity* (Second Nutricia Symposium). Springfield, Ill.: Thomas, 1968.
31. Koenig, J. M. *N. Engl. J. Med.* 321: 557, 1989.
32. Kramer, M. S. *J.A.M.A.* 260: 3306, 1988.
33. Levanthal, J. M. *Pediatrics* 68: 684, 1981.
34. Low, J. A. *Am. J. Obstet. Gynecol.* 142: 670, 1982.
35. Lubchenco, L. O. The Postterm Infant. In L. O. Lubchenco (Ed.), *Major Problems in Clinical Pediatrics,* Vol. 14: *The High Risk Infant.* Philadelphia: Saunders, 1976.
36. Lubchenco, L. O. The Estimation of Gestational Age. In L. O. Lubchenco (Ed.), *Major Problems in Clinical Pediatrics,* Vol. 14: *The High Risk Infant.* Philadelphia: Saunders, 1976.
37. Lubchenco, L. O. The Infant Who Is Large for Gestational Age. In: L. O. Lubchenco (Ed.), *Major Problems in Clinical Pediatrics,* Vol. 14: *The High Risk Infant.* Philadelphia: Saunders, 1976.
38. Lubchenco, L. O. The Infant Who Is Small for Gestational Age. In: L. O. Lubchenco (Ed.), *Major Problems in Clinical Pediatrics,* Vol. 14: *The High Risk Infant.* Philadelphia: Saunders, 1976.
39. Lubchenco, L. O. The Preterm Infant. In: L. O. Lubchenco (Ed.), *Major Problems in Clinical Pediatrics,* Vol. 14: *The High Risk Infant.* Philadelphia: Saunders, 1976.
40. Lubchenco, L. O. *Pediatrics* 37: 403, 1966.
41. Management of the high risk pregnancy: A symposium. *Clin. Perinatol.* 2: 1, 1974.
42. McCarthy, B. J. *Am. J. Obstet. Gynecol* 141: 252, 1981.
43. McCormick, M. C. *Pediatrics* 66: 991, 1980.
44. Naeye, R. *Pediatrics* 69: 724, 1983.

45. National Center for Health Statistics. Advanced Report of Final Natality Statistics, 1983. Monthly Vital Statistics Report Series 34, No. 6 (Suppl.), U.S. Dept. of Health and Human Services publication (PHS) 85-1120. Hyattsville, Md.: USDHHS, Sept. 20, 1985.
46. Parkenson, C. E. *Dev. Med. Child. Neurol.* 23: 411, 1981.
47. Persson, P.-H. *Acta Obstet. Gynecol. Scand.* 65: 481, 1986.
48. Primhah, R. A. *Clin. Pediatr.* 21: 417, 1982.
49. *Report of Committee on Infectious Disease: The Red Book.* Evanston, Ill.: Academy of Pediatrics, 1982. P. 20.
50. Selbing, A. *Acta. Obstet. Gynecol. Scand.* 64: 593, 1985.
51. The small-for-date infant. *Pediatr. Clin. North Am.* 17: 1, 1970.
52. Starfield, B. *J. Pediatr.* 101: 978, 1982.
53. Stein, Z. *Am. J. Public Health* 73: 1154, 1983.
54. Sweet, A. Y. Classification of the Low-Birth-Weight Infant. In M. H. Klaus and A. A. Fanaroff (Eds.), *Care of the High-Risk Neonate.* Philadelphia: Saunders, 1979.
55. Usher, R. J. *J. Pediatr.* 74: 910, 1969.
56. Vohr, B. R. *Am. J. Obstet. Gynecol.* 133: 425, 1979.
57. Westwood, M. *Pediatrics* 71: 376, 1983.
58. Williams, R. L. *Obstet. Gynecol.* 59: 624, 1982.
59. Winer, E. K. *Am. J. Obstet. Gynecol.* 143: 425, 1982.
60. Wise, P. H. *Pediatrics* 81: 542, 1988.

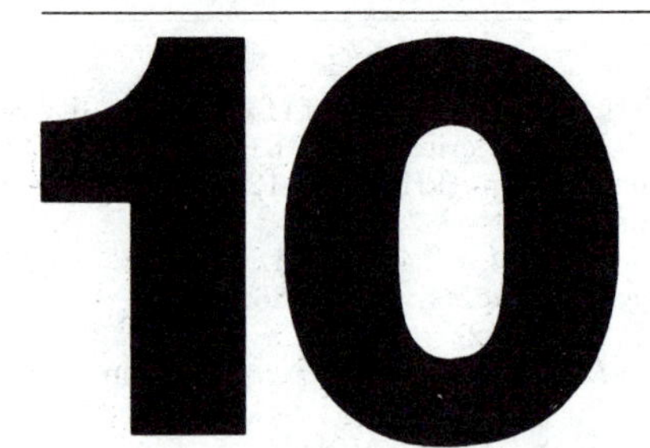

Multiple Gestation

DeWayne M. Pursley and
Ann R. Stark

Benirschke and Kim [4] have published an excellent review of multiple pregnancy.

I. **Incidence and types.** It is difficult to state the exact incidence of multiple gestation, since most epidemiologic studies do not account for the high rates of spontaneous abortions and stillborns that occur in these pregnancies. The rate of loss of a single fetus in twin gestations diagnosed by ultrasound in the first trimester has been reported to be as high as 63 percent [22]. In the United States, it is estimated that 12 per 1000 pregnancies result in a twin delivery.

   A. The rate of **monozygous (MZ)** or **identical twinning** is constant at 4 per 1000 pregnancies and results from a single ovulation with subsequent splitting of the developing egg within the first 15 to 16 days. Occasionally, a familial tendency for MZ twinning has been observed [8].

   B. **Dizygous (DZ)** or **fraternal twinning** results from double ovulation and fertilization and is probably determined by higher gonadotropin secretion rates. The rate of DZ twinning is variable and is influenced by heredity (transmitted autosomally but expressed only in the mother), race (high in some Nigerian tribes, low among Asians), maternal age (increased frequency with increased age), parity (increased rate with increased parity), nutrition (decreased rate with maternal malnutrition), "fertility" drugs (e.g., clomiphene, gonadotropins), and in vitro fertilization (resulting from multiple embryo implantation). Worldwide, the rate of DZ twinning ranges from 4 to 50 per 1000. In the United States, two-thirds of twins are dizygous, at the rate of 8 per 1000.

II. **Placentation.** There are basically two types of placentas in twins, monochorionic and dichorionic.

   A. **Monochorionic placentas** generally have two amnions, but occasionally have one. *Dichorionic placentas,* which always have two amnions, may be entirely separate or may be fused if implantation occurs side by side.

      1. Monochorionic placentas occur only in MZ twins, a useful finding for the determination of zygosity.

      2. Dichorionic placentas occur in all DZ twins but also occur in about 30 percent of MZ twins. This is related to the events of early development. In DZ twins, two blastocysts implant, each generating a separate placenta with chorion and amnion. Blood vessels of the two fetuses do not fuse [4].

   B. When MZ twinning occurs, the timing of the split of the single fertilized ovum determines the type of placentation.

      1. If twinning occurs soon after conception, before cells are set aside to make the chorion, two chorions will develop. Following that time, monochorionic placentation must occur, and the twins will generally be **monochorionic-diamnionic.**

      2. Similarly, once the amnion has formed, twinning at 15 to 16 days of development will result in a **monochorionic-monoamnionic** placenta, found in about 4 percent of MZ twins.

   C. To determine whether a placenta is monochorionic or dichorionic, identify the membrane that separates the two amniotic sacs [16]. In monochorionic twins, the two layers of amnion that form this membrane appear translucent when they are peeled apart and leave a single, fairly smooth chorionic surface on the placenta. In dichorionic twins, the two amnions and two chorions that form the dividing membrane are difficult to separate, and when peeled off, they disrupt the placental surface. These two-layer membranes are fairly opaque.

D. Antenatally, the chorionic type of a twin pregnancy can be accurately determined sonographically, and this information can be useful in the management of complicated multiple pregnancy [3].

III. Diagnosis of zygosity. Zygosity can be determined at birth in many twins on the basis of sex, examination of the placenta, and blood grouping.

A. Twins of unlike sex are dizygous. Monochorionic twins are monozygous. The remaining 45 percent are dichorionic, like-sexed twins. If blood grouping studies reveal differences, the twins are dizygous. If blood grouping fails to show differences, it is likely that the twins are monozygous.

B. If it becomes critical to prove monozygosity, e.g., for transplantation, immunologic studies can be performed. If it is not critical, adult twins classify themselves correctly on the basis of their similarities, with an error of 2 to 5 percent [9].

C. Of the 45 percent of twins who are dichorionic and like-sexed, 37 percent are DZ and 8 percent are MZ pairs [10].

D. Multiple pregnancies induced by fertility drugs are usually dizygous.

IV. Intrauterine growth

A. Through 29 weeks of gestation, the weight of each twin is nearly that of a singleton [15]. Subsequently, weight increments are not as great for twins as for singletons; after 33 weeks, twins weigh less than singletons. The average twin weight at term is approximately 2600 gm, compared with an average term singleton birth weight of 3200 gm. The peak of mean birth weight is reached at 37 to 38 weeks in twins rather than at 41 to 42 weeks, as is the case in singletons [6].

B. At most gestational ages, monochorionic twins weigh less than dichorionic twins. In addition, there can be a marked discordance in total-body weight and organ measurements within pairs of monochorionic twins affected by the transfusion syndrome (see sec. **VII.B**).

V. Diagnosis. Early diagnosis of multiple pregnancy is important because of the increased incidence of complications, including preeclampsia, polyhydramnios, gestational diabetes, anemia, fetal anomaly, fetal death, intrauterine growth retardation, and premature delivery.

A. Early diagnosis may be suggested by increased uterine size, polyhydramnios, or a family history of twins.

B. Diagnosis also may be suspected by palpation, auscultation of two heart beats, or increased maternal alpha-fetoprotein level and may be confirmed by ultrasonic studies.

VI. Perinatal mortality. Perinatal mortality among twins is greatly increased to 4 to 11 times that of singletons [13]. This increased mortality relates mostly to the increased frequency of premature delivery, since average twin delivery occurs at about 37 weeks. In fact, premature twins often have a birth weight–specific mortality that is equivalent to or even less than that for singletons. This might be explained in part by the fact that twins are more likely to be growth-retarded and thus more mature than singletons of an equivalent weight. On the other hand, more mature and larger twins appear to contribute disproportionately to perinatal mortality in twins, perhaps reflecting increasing uteroplacental insufficiency as they near term [6]. There are still other factors that influence mortality in twins.

A. Placentation is a major determinant of mortality in twins, with monochorionic twins experiencing greater mortality (26 percent) than dichorionic MZ or DZ twins (9 percent). This difference is largely related to vascular interconnections and the transfusion syndrome.

B. Studies disagree as to whether or not there is a difference in mortality between first and second twins.

1. The **second twin** is subjected to increased operative intervention, a longer period of hypoxia, and greater length of anesthesia.
2. Although optimal delivery time has been considered to be about 15 minutes after the first twin, with survival of the second twin progressively lower after a 30-minute interval, the use of continuous fetal monitoring may remove the need for a time restriction [17].
3. Although it is not the usual situation, some twin pregnancies are discordant in the development of pulmonary maturity. Indices of fetal lung maturation must be assessed individually in twins if premature delivery is planned [10]. The second twin is more likely to be malpresented, to be depressed at birth, and when premature, to have respiratory distress syndrome (RDS). Even after the second twin's greater risk for malpresentation (20 percent of first twins are nonvertex, while more than 40 percent of second twins are nonvertex [12]) and depression is accounted for, this twin, when vaginally delivered, is at an increased risk for RDS. Neither malpresentation nor depression is independently associated with RDS. The protective effects conveyed on the first twin may be related to greater benefits of labor. The second twin's increased risk for depression appears more closely associated with its greater likelihood of malpresentation [1].

C. **Rupture of the vasa previa** (leading to exsanguination of one of the twins) and **cord prolapse** are more common in twin deliveries than in single births. Monoamniotic twins, an infrequent occurrence, may have entangling of cords, associated with a 50 percent mortality.

D. Most studies have found a higher prevalence of anomalies at birth in twins as compared with singletons, and this contributes to their increased risk for mortality. The increased prevalence of anomalies in twins is, for the most part, confined to MZ twins [11].

VII. **Placental vascular shunts.** Vascular interconnections occur in almost all monochorionic twins and almost never in dichorionic placentas [18,21].

A. Usually these connections are **artery-to-artery** and are not of consequence. Rarely, they may cause acute problems during labor and delivery, with exsanguination of the second twin into the first. In addition, if this type of shunt occurs early in gestation, the arterial pressure of one twin can overpower that of the other. The lower part of the recipient twin's body is perfused more than the upper part, resulting in deterioration of existing tissues and malformation of developing tissues. This is referred to as the **twin reversed arterial perfusion (TRAP) sequence.** The degree of disruption is variable, including acephalic, acardiac, and amorphous twins.

B. **Artery-to-vein anastomoses** are of much greater importance and form the basis of the **transfusion syndrome.** The anastomoses are common; they usually go through a placental cotyledon, and their variable size, number, and direction determine their consequences. Clinically, the diagnosis of twin transfusion syndrome is made when twins exhibit a hemoglobin difference of more than 5 gm per 100 ml. It may be suspected when one twin appears plethoric and the other pale at birth.

1. In cases of chronic intrauterine transfer of blood, the **donor twin** will have severe growth retardation, with decreased cytoplasmic mass in all organs, anemia, hypovolemia, renal insufficiency, oligohydramnios, and amnion nodosum.
2. The **recipient twin** in chronic transfusion syndrome develops polycythemia (which may lead to jaundice or thrombosis postnatally), cardiac hypertrophy, hypervolemia, thickness of media of pulmonary and systemic arteries, and polyhydramnios. At times, the excessive volume load may lead to cardiac decompensation, secondary hepatic dysfunction, hypoalbuminemia, and edema and may even progress to hydrops.
3. These twins can differ in size by as much as 1000 gm. The transfusion syndrome explains how MZ twins can differ more at birth than DZ twins.
4. When the intrapair birth weight difference is small, the transfer of blood is thought to have occurred acutely.

C. Death of one monochorionic MZ twin may result in thromboplastic material entering the circulation of the surviving twin, causing **disseminated intravascular coagulation (DIC).** Alternatively, emboli from the dead twin could enter the cotwin's circulation. Either mechanism could result in destruction of tissue and in such defects as porencephalic cyst, hydranencephaly, limb amputation, aplasia cutis, gastroschisis, or intestinal atresia. Management of a pregnancy in which one twin dies involves consideration of risks to the mother and cotwin of prolonging the pregnancy as well as the risks of delivering a preterm infant [7,19]. Ultrasonic evaluation to see if the twins are dichorionic (with little risk of shared circulation) or monochorionic (with greater risk of shared circulation) should be done.

VIII. Anomalies. Congenital anomalies occur more frequently in twins compared with singletons [21]. The relative risk of anomalies for twins compared with singletons varies among different studies, and there are several possible epidemiologic and biologic explanations for this [11]. The increased frequency of early malformations in MZ twins might be the result of the same factor(s) that caused the twinning to occur. These defects include sacrococcygeal teratoma, sirenomelia sequence or less severe degrees of sirenomelia including the VATER association, anencephaly, holoprosencephaly malformation sequence, and extrophy of the cloaca malformation sequence. There is frequently discordance among MZ twins for anomalies, suggesting the importance of in utero environmental factors. Only 5 to 20 percent are concordant, and one twin may be less affected. When congenital heart disease occurs in one of the twins, it is concordant in 25 percent of MZ and in 5 percent of DZ pairs. Cleft lip and palate show a 40 percent concordance for MZ and an 8 percent concordance for DZ twins [4]. In cases of discordance of severe anomalies, early in utero recognition allows for the consideration of selective termination, hopefully allowing continuation of the pregnancy on behalf of the normal fetus. Conjoined twins are a rare event (1 in 33,000 to 165,000 live births) [5], and result from incomplete MZ twinning. The twins are most commonly joined at the thorax (thoracopagus), but they can be joined at the head, buttocks, or other sites, and other major anomalies occur frequently. Prenatal ultrasound is useful for diagnosis of the anatomy and site of the joining. Plans for treatment of thoracoabdominally conjoined twins depend on the anatomy of the cardiovascular systems. Prenatal echocardiography is a reliable method to diagnose the extent of the cardiovascular involvement [20]. After birth, ultrasound, x-ray, CT, MRI and angiography may be necessary to plan treatment.

IX. Follow-up data on 20 pairs of twins, of whom the smaller twin weighed less than 2000 gm (with the weight of the smaller twin at least 25 percent less than the weight of the larger twin), showed significant differences in height, weight, head circumference, and IQ; these differences were independent of birth order [2]. Overall, studies show that despite an initial postnatal period of rapid growth, the mean weights for twins remain below those for singletons for a given age. In addition, those with intrauterine growth retardation and born at low birth weight are at increased risk for developmental morbidity [14].

X. Pediatric management of twins

A. A pediatric team should attend the delivery; two teams should be present if problems are anticipated. It should be remembered that the second twin is at greater risk for asphyxia, bleeding, and intracranial hemorrhage.

B. The infants should be examined carefully for prematurity and growth retardation; these problems should be managed as usual. Mature, as well as growth-retarded, twins may be at increased risk for the consequences of placental insufficiency. Screening for polycythemia and hypoglycemia in growth-retarded twins should be considered.

C. The infants should be examined carefully for congenital anomalies. The survivor(s) of multiple gestation with intrauterine demise of one fetus must be carefully examined for disruptive structural defects and the consequences of embolic phenomena.

D. An attempt should be made to determine zygosity by sex, placenta, and blood types.

E. Blood pressure and hematocrit should be measured to determine whether or not twin transfusion syndrome is present. Both risks to the donor twin (hypovolemia, anemia, renal insufficiency, and IUGR) and to the recipient twin (CHF, hepatic dysfunction) need to be considered and treated in the usual manner.

F. Support should be arranged for the family, including home assistance and financial assistance.

G. If one twin dies, caregivers should encourage the grieving process to occur and not assume it will be minimized by the surviving twin [23].

References

1. Arnold, C. *N. Engl. J. Med.* 317: 1121, 1987.
2. Babson, S. G. *Pediatrics* 33: 327, 1964.
3. Barss, V. A. *Obstet. Gynecol.* 66: 779, 1985.
4. Benirschke, K. *N. Engl. J. Med.* 288: 1276, 1329, 1973.
5. Bergsman, D. *Birth Defects* 3: 1, 1967.
6. Ghai, V. *Clin. Perinatol.* 15: 123, 1988.
7. Hanna, J. H. *Obstet. Gynecol.* 63: 126, 1984.
8. Harvey, M. A. S. *J. Pediatr.* 90: 246, 1977.
9. Hrubec, Z. *N. Engl. J. Med.* 310: 435, 1984.
10. Leveno, K. J. *Am. J. Obstet. Gynecol.* 148: 405, 1984.
11. Little, J. *Semin. Perinatol.* 10: 50, 1986.
12. MacLennan, A. H. Multiple Gestation: Clinical Characteristics and Management. In R. K. Creasy and R. Resnik (Eds.), *Maternal-Fetal Medicine: Principles and Practices.* Philadelphia: Saunders, 1985. P. 527.
13. Marviate, M. *Clin. Obstet. Gynecol.* 9: 723, 1982.
14. McCulloch, K. *Clin. Perinatol.* 15: 141, 1988.
15. Naeye, R. E. *Pediatrics* 37: 409, 1966.
16. Purohit, D. M. *Pediatr. Clin. North Am.* 24: 481, 1977.
17. Rayburn, W. F. *Obstet. Gynecol.* 63: 502, 1984.
18. Robertson, E. G. *Am. J. Obstet. Gynecol.* 147: 170, 1983.
19. Romero, R. *N. Engl. J. Med.* 310: 772, 1984.
20. Sanders, S. P. *N. Engl. J. Med.* 313: 370, 1985.
21. Smith, D. W. (Ed.). *Recognizable Patterns of Human Malformation.* Philadelphia: Saunders, 1982. Pp. 504–516.
22. Wenstrom, K. D. *Clin. Perinatol.* 15: 1, 1988.
23. Wilson, A. L. *Pediatrics* 70: 587, 1982.

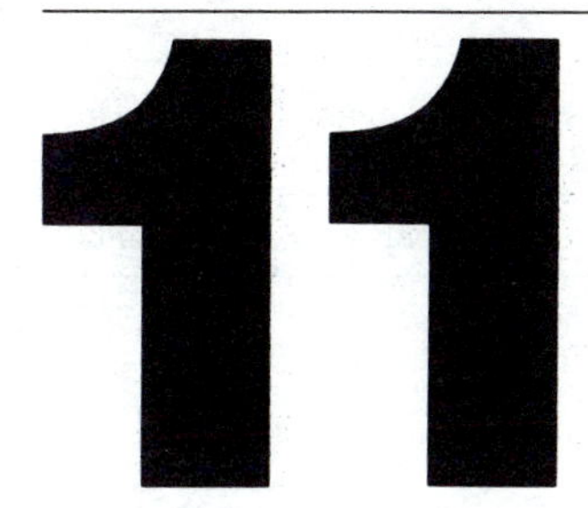

Genetic Issues Presenting in the Nursery

Diana W. Bianchi

I. **Introduction.** Although as many as 40 percent of pediatric hospital admissions have been shown to have a genetic basis [5], it is usually the infant with major malformations or an inborn error of metabolism who presents in the nursery setting. **Major malformations** are defined as those anomalies which are prenatal in origin and have cosmetic, medical, or surgical significance. The birth of an infant with major malformations, whether diagnosed antenatally or not, evokes an emotional parental response [14]. It is incumbent upon the medical staff to ensure that the affected infant has an expedient but thorough evaluation so that the appropriate diagnostic procedures and therapy may proceed.

II. **Incidence.** Major malformations occur in 2 to 3 percent of live births [9,13,17]. They have now surpassed prematurity as the leading cause of neonatal death.

III. **Etiology.** The etiology of congenital anomalies is shown in Table 11-1. Note that in the majority of cases, the cause is unknown. Only about 10 percent of cases are associated with a chromosome abnormality.

IV. **Approach to the Infant.**

A. **History**

1. **Prenatal.** If possible, the mother's obstetric chart should be reviewed, and the following points should be noted:
   a. History of chronic maternal illness such as diabetes, phenylketonuria, myasthenia gravis, myotonic dystrophy, or systemic lupus erythematosus (see Table 11-2).
   b. Drug and alcohol exposure during pregnancy. Table 11-2 includes the medications known to cause malformations in humans. For more details, see ref. 15.
   c. Abnormal uterine shape.
   d. Infections during pregnancy.
   e. Fetal growth patterns in utero (did the uterine size equal gestational age throughout pregnancy?)
   f. Results of antenatal ultrasound examinations (were anomalies, polyhydramnios, or oligohydramnios diagnosed?)
   g. Results of maternal serum alpha-fetoprotein (MSAFP) screening. A **low** value may be seen in trisomy 18 or 21 [4]. A **high** value may be indicative of impending fetal demise, open neural tube defect, abdominal wall defect, congenital nephrosis, epidermolysis bullosa, or Turner syndrome [2]. See Chap. 26.
   h. Quality and frequency of fetal movements in utero.
2. **Family history.** The parents and, if possible, the grandparents should be asked the following:
   a. Have there been any prior affected infants in the family?
   b. Is there a history of infertility, multiple miscarriages, neonatal death, or newborns with other malformations?
   c. What is their ethnic background?
   d. Is there a history of consanguinity?
3. **Perinatal events**
   a. Fetal position in utero
   b. Significant events during labor and type of delivery

Table 11-1. Etiology of congenital anomalies: Brigham and Women's Hospital Malformations Surveillance Data from 69,227 Newborns

	Number	Percent
Single gene (Mendelian inheritance)	48	4.1%
Chromosome Abnormality	157	10.1
Familial	225	14.4
Multifactorial	356	22.8
Teratogens	49	4.1
Uterine factors	39	2.5
Twinning	6	0.4
Unknown	669	43.1
TOTAL	1549	100%

Source: Data from Nelson, K., and Holmes, L. B. *N. Engl. J. Med.* 320: 19, 1989.

Table 11-2. Known human teratogens

Drugs
Aminopterin/amethopterin
Androgenic hormones
Busulfan
Chlorobiphenyls
Cyclophosphamide
Diethylstilbestrol
Heroin/methadone
Iodide
Isotretinoin (13-*cis*-retinoic acid)
Lithium
Phenytoin
Propylthiouracil
Tetracycline
Trimethadione
Valproic Acid
Warfarin

Heavy metals
Lead
Mercury

Radiation
Cancer therapy

Maternal conditions
Alcoholism
Insulin-dependent diabetes mellitus
Maternal phenylketonuria
Myasthenia gravis
Myotonic dystrophy
Smoking
Systemic lupus erythematosus

Intrauterine infections
Cytomegalovirus
Herpes simplex
Rubella
Syphilis
Toxoplasmosis
Varicella
Venezuelan equine encephalitis virus

Other exposures
Gasoline fumes
Heat
Hypoxia

   c. Length of umbilical cord (a positive association exists between fetal motor activity and cord length [12])
   d. Placental appearance
4. **Neonatal course**

B. **Physical examination.** A complete physical examination is **essential** to making an accurate diagnosis. Often, however, the critically ill neonate is partially hidden by monitoring equipment. Beware of making a diagnosis when (1) the midface is obscured by adhesive tape securing endotracheal and nasogastric tubes, (2) the extremities cannot be visualized because there are peripheral IV lines in place, and (3) the infant has received pancuronium bro-

Table 11-3. Physical findings in the three major live-born autosomal trisomies

	Trisomy 13	Trisomy 18	Trisomy 21
Birth weight:	Normal range	Growth retarded	Normal range
Skin:	Scalp defects		
CNS:	Major malformations: Holoprosencephaly Neural tube defects	Microcephaly	
Facies:	Abnormal midface Microphthalmia Cleft lip/palate	Micrognathia	Upslanting eyes Flattened facies Epicanthal folds Prominent tongue Small ears
Heart:	VSD, PDA, ASD Dextrocardia	VSD, ASD, PDA	AV canal VSD, PDA
Abdomen:	Polycystic kidneys	Omphalocele	
Extremities:	Polydactyly	Camptodactyly Overlapping fingers Abnormal dermatoglyphics Nail hypoplasia	Brachydactyly Simian crease in 45 percent Fifth finger clinodactyly Wide space between first and second toe
Neuro:		Hypertonic	Muscular hypotonia Weak Moro reflex

mide. Edema resulting from muscular paralysis can cause considerable distortion of facial features.

1. **Anthropometrics.** Specific physical parameters that should be measured in the affected neonate include length, head circumference, outer and inner canthal distance, palpebral fissure length, interpupillary distance, ear length, philtrum length, internipple distance, chest circumference, upper-lower segment ratio, and hand and foot length. Normal standards exist for all these measurements in infants of 27 to 41 weeks gestation [11].
2. Aspects of the physical examination not emphasized in a "routine" neonatal examination include a thorough inspection of the skin, the position of the hair whorls, head shape and facial feature characteristics, dermatoglyphics, and a description of the extremities. The dermatoglyphic pattern of low-arch dermal ridges is particularly useful in the bedside diagnosis of trisomy 18 (see Table 11-3).

C. Laboratory and other studies

1. **Placental pathology** should be obtained if possible.
2. **Chromosome studies.** Peripheral blood and skin are the most available sources of cells for a banded chromosome analysis. Generally, only 1 ml of peripheral blood is collected in a green-top tube (verify that sodium heparin is the anticoagulant). The sample should be kept at room temperature. It does not matter if the infant has been transfused. Stat results are usually available within 48 hours. Although 0.6 percent of newborns have abnormal chromosomes [9], only a third of these will have serious

Table 11-4. DNA mutations presenting as serious neonatal illness

Hemophilia
Ornithine transcarbamylase deficiency
Autosomal dominant polycystic kidney disease
Alpha-1-antitrypsin deficiency
Chronic granulomatous disease
21-OH deficiency (congenital adrenal hyperplasia)
Cystic fibrosis
Phenylketonuria
Myotonic dystrophy
Osteogenesis imperfecta

malformations. A summary of the physical findings in the three major live-born autosomal trisomies is shown in Table 11-3.

3. **DNA-based diagnosis and/or banking.** An increasing number of diseases presenting in the nursery have been cloned and result from single gene mutations [3]. Many of these disorders are potentially lethal. Obtaining blood or skin fibroblasts for DNA studies on an affected infant may facilitate genetic counseling and prenatal diagnosis in future pregnancies. A list of the relevant disorders is shown in Table 11-4. DNA studies are also useful in the determination of twin zygosity [7] and paternity [6].
4. **Radiographic studies** are important in the overall assessment of the infant.
   a. **Ultrasound examinations**—to detect cranial malformations, the presence of congenital heart disease, or liver and renal anomalies
   b. **Radiographs**—to define bony malformations or diagnose skeletal dysplasias (see ref. 16)
5. **Ophthalmologic examination** is indicated if there is a clinical suspicion of congenital infection or there are central nervous system or craniofacial anomalies.
6. **TORCH titers** need only be obtained if the physical findings are suggestive of congenital infection. [see Chap. 12]
7. **Urinary organic acids** are useful to diagnose metabolic disease in the dysmorphic newborn with metabolic acidosis. [see Chap. 24]

V. **Diagnosis.** Once the results of the history, physical examination, and laboratory studies are known, a diagnosis may become possible. Helpful references are refs. 1, 8, and 10. In many cases it is not possible to make a diagnosis in the nursery. Owing to the major changes in facial features that occur over the first year of life, certain diagnoses may become apparent later. Hence careful **follow-up** is important.

VI. **Counseling.** If a diagnosis is made, genetic counseling should be offered to discuss prognosis and potential therapy. A future counseling session should be scheduled to provide a **recurrence risk** as well as the **availability of prenatal diagnosis** for the condition.

VII. **Special issues for the perinatal death of an infant with malformations**

A. A complete **autopsy,** including radiographs and photographs, should be obtained.

B. Sterile **skin biopsy** for tissue culture. Cultured fibroblasts may serve as a source of chromosomes, enzymes, or DNA (see Chap. 24).

C. Arrangements should be made for a follow-up meeting with the family to summarize the results of the preceding studies.

References

1. Baraitser, M., and Winter, R. M. *A Colour Atlas of Clinical Genetics.* London: Wolfe Medical Publications, 1983.
2. Bergstrand, C. G. *Acta. Paediatr. Scand.* 75: 1, 1986.
3. Cooper, D. N., and Schmidtke, J. *Hum. Genet.* 73: 1, 1986.
4. Doran, T. A., Cadesky, K., Wong, P. Y., et al. *Am. J. Obstet. Gynecol.* 154: 277, 1986.
5. Hall, J. G., Powers, E. K., McIlvaine, R. T., et al. *Am. J. Med. Genet.* 1: 417, 1978.
6. Helminen, P., Ehnholm, C., Lokki, M. L., et al. *Lancet* 1: 574, 1988.
7. Hill, A. V. S., and Jeffreys, A. J. *Lancet* 2: 1394, 1985.
8. Jones, K. L. *Smith's Recognizable Patterns of Human Malformation,* 4th Ed. Philadelphia: Saunders, 1988.
9. Kalter, H., and Warkany, J. *N. Engl. J. Med.* 308: 424, 308: 491, 1983.
10. McKusick, V. A. *Mendelian Inheritance in Man,* 8th Ed. Baltimore: Johns Hopkins University Press, 1988.
11. Merlob, P., Sivan, Y., and Reisner, S. H. *Birth Defects* 20: 1, 1984.
12. Moessinger, A. C. *Pediatr. Res.* 16: 109, 1982.
13. Nelson, K., and Holmes, L. B. *N. Engl. J. Med.* 320: 19, 1989.
14. Nolan, T., and Pless, I. B. *J. Pediatr.* 109: 201, 1986.
15. Shephard, T. H. *Catalog of Teratogenic Agents,* 5th Ed. Baltimore: Johns Hopkins University Press, 1986.
16. Taybi, H. *Radiology of Syndromes and Metabolic Disorders,* 2d Ed. Chicago: Year Book Medical Publishers, 1985.
17. Van Regemorter, N., Dodion, J., Druart, C., et al. *J. Pediatr.* 104: 386, 1984.

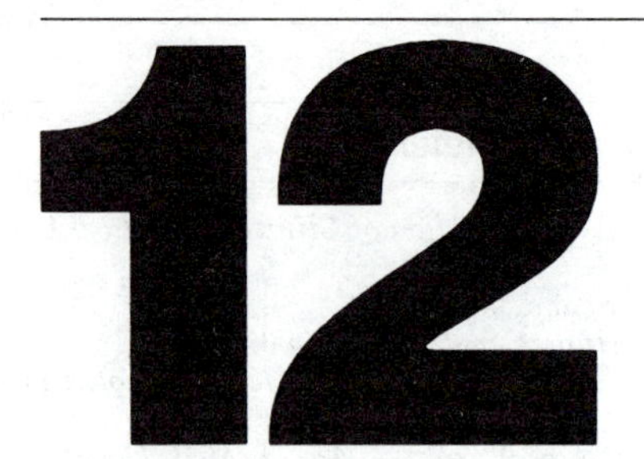

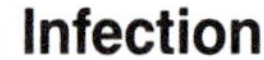

12 Infection

Viral Infections in the Newborn

Nicholas G. Guerina

Viral infections of the fetus and newborn can generally be divided into two major categories. The first is congenital infections and consists of viral infections that are transmitted to the fetus in utero. The second is perinatal infections and consists of viral infections that are acquired intrapartum or in the immediate postpartum period. It must be emphasized that many, if not all, of these agents can cause both congenital and perinatal infections and may be acquired outside the newborn period. However, classifying these viruses into congenital and perinatal categories emphasizes unique aspects of their pathogenesis in the fetus and newborn infant.

Classically, the congenital infections have been thought of by the acronym **TORCH** (**T** = **t**oxoplasma, **O** = **o**ther, **R** = **r**ubella, **C** = **c**ytomegalovirus, **H** = **h**erpes simplex virus) [81]. The recognition of other important agents causing congenital infections makes this term archaic. Also, herpes simplex virus infection does not share many of the features common to the other agents. In what follows, the concept of TORCH has been avoided given the preceding constraints. When congenital or perinatal infections are suspected, the diagnosis of each of the possible infectious agents should be considered separately. Useless information is often obtained when the diagnosis is attempted by drawing a single serum sample to be sent for TORCH titers.

I. Congenital infections

A. Cytomegalovirus. Cytomegaloviruses (CMV) are members of the herpesvirus family and derive their name from the cytopathology of infected cells, which is characterized by cellular enlargement with intranuclear and cytoplasmic inclusions. Human CMV is species-specific with no known vector for transmission in nature. Infection occurs as a result of intimate personal contact or exposure to infected breast milk, blood, or blood products. This virus is ubiquitous, and it is believed that nearly all individuals are infected at some time in their life [26]. Fortunately, asymptomatic infection occurs in most cases, but significant or life-threatening infection occurs in the immunocompromised or immunosuppressed patient. The fetus is particularly susceptible to severe disseminated CMV disease. Infection can occur at any time in gestation or in the perinatal period.

1. Intrauterine infection. Congenital CMV occurs in 1 percent of all live births in the United States, but only approximately 10 percent of these infections result in clinical symptoms [26]. Clinically apparent newborn disease is almost always associated with primary maternal infection in pregnancy [28]. It is estimated that the rate of intrauterine transmission is 30 to 40 percent with primary maternal infection, but less than 15 percent of newborns develop significant disease [26]. Recurrent maternal infection or viral reactivation can occur in pregnancy, and in these cases, transmission to the fetus can occur. However, the fetus and newborn rarely show clinical symptoms [43]. The risk of transmission to the fetus as a function of gestational age is uncertain. Infection in early gestation may carry a greater risk of severe fetal disease, but this has not been rigorously demonstrated [27].

Symptomatic CMV infection of the fetus presents with multiple organ involvement. The most common findings in the first 2 weeks following delivery in 34 infected newborn infants were petechiae (79 percent), hepatosplenomegaly (74 percent), and jaundice (63 percent) [26]. Microcephaly was found in 50 percent of infants, and 41 percent were small for gestational age. Twelve percent of infants had chorioretinitis. Other problems include prematurity (<38 weeks; 34 percent) and inguinal hernia in males (26 percent). Dental defects characterized by abnormal enamel production can be seen in later infancy [29]. Approximately a third of newborn infants with symptomatic disseminated CMV infection die. Infants surviving symptomatic CMV infection are at high risk for developing significant developmental abnormalities and neurologic dysfunction [30–33]. These include mental retardation, hearing deficits, language and learning disabilities, motor abnormalities, and visual disturbances. Hearing loss is very common with symptomatic congenital CMV infection, occurring in 60 to 70 percent of infants. In contrast to symptomatic newborn infants, those with asymptomatic infection have virtually no mortality, but 5 to 15 percent may have developmental abnormalities [26]. These include hearing loss, mental retardation, motor spasticity, and microcephaly [26,27,34,35].

Laboratory abnormalities in symptomatic CMV infections include intracranial calcifications, elevated hepatic transaminase levels, elevated bilirubin levels, anemia, and thrombocytopenia. The intracranial calcifications may occur anywhere in the brain. Bilirubin levels may be elevated at birth or rise over the first postnatal weeks. There is usually an elevated direct component that may increase to as high as 50 percent of the total bilirubin. Hyperbilirubinemia usually persists beyond the period of physiologic jaundice [26].

2. **Perinatal infection.** Perinatally acquired CMV may occur from (1) intrapartum exposure to the virus within the maternal genital tract, (2) postnatal exposure to infected breast milk [36], or (3) exposure to infected blood or blood products [37,38]. The incubation period varies from 4 to 12 weeks [26]. Almost all term infants who acquire infection perinatally from infected mothers remain asymptomatic. The majority of these infections arise from mothers with reactivated viral excretion. In these cases, long-term developmental and neurologic abnormalities are not seen. However, symptomatic perinatally acquired infections may occur at a higher frequency in preterm infants [39,40].
   a. **CMV pneumonitis.** CMV has been associated with pneumonitis occurring in infants less than 4 months of age [41,42]. Of 104 infants with pneumonitis, 21 (21 percent) had CMV compared with 3 of 97 (3 percent) hospitalized controls [42]. Twelve of the 104 infants with pneumonitis (12 percent) had CMV as the only infectious agent identified. Symptoms and radiographic findings in CMV pneumonitis are similar to those seen in afebrile pneumonia of other causes in neonates and young infants, including *Chlamydia trachomatis,* respiratory viruses, and *Ureaplasma urealyticum* [26]. In general, there is tachypnea, cough, coryza, and nasal congestion. Intercostal retractions and hypoxemia may be present, and apnea may occur. Radiographically, there is hyperinflation, diffuse increased pulmonary markings, thickened bronchial walls, and focal atelectasis. A small number of infants may have symptoms that are severe enough to require mechanical ventilation, and death may occur in approximately 3 percent of in-

fants [44]. Laboratory findings in CMV pneumonitis are nonspecific. The serum IgG level may be elevated in approximately two-thirds of patients, and a leukocytosis with an absolute eosinophilia may be present [26]. Long-term sequelae include recurrent pulmonary problems, including wheezing, and, in some cases, repeated hospitalizations for respiratory distress [44].

b. **Transfusion-acquired CMV infection.** Significant morbidity and mortality can occur in newborn infants receiving CMV-infected blood or blood products. Those most severely affected are preterm, low-birth-weight infants born to CMV-seronegative women [38,45–47]. Symptoms typically develop 4 to 12 weeks after transfusion, last for 2 to 3 weeks, and consist of respiratory distress, pallor, and hepatosplenomegaly [48]. Hematologic abnormalities are also seen and include hemolysis, thrombocytopenia, and atypical lymphocytosis. Mortality is estimated to be 20 percent in very low birth weight infants [48]. Disease can be prevented by the use of blood from donors who are seronegative for CMV [38]. Thus it is recommended that all blood and blood products for infants in the special care nursery be obtained from seronegative donors or that blood be prepared so as to virtually eliminate the risk of CMV transmission [49] (see Chap. 20).

3. **Diagnosis.** Congenital CMV infection should be suspected in any infant having typical symptoms of infection or if there is a maternal history of seroconversion or a mononucleosis-like illness in pregnancy [26]. The diagnosis of congenital CMV infection is made by the identification of virus in clinical specimens taken from infected newborn infants within the first 2 weeks of delivery. Virus may be isolated from urine or saliva, but urine has the greatest sensitivity because CMV is concentrated there in high titers. Specimens should be maintained at 4°C (ice or refrigerator) for transport and storage to optimize viral recovery. The identification of CMV in tissue culture may take from 2 days to 2 weeks. For this reason, various techniques for the rapid identification of CMV in clinical specimens have been developed. Of particular interest are assays incorporating specific antibodies that recognize CMV antigens present early in viral cultures [50–52]. These assays do not require unusual equipment for standard diagnostic virology laboratories, and virus can be detected with high sensitivity and specificity within 24 hours of inoculation. To differentiate perinatal from congenital CMV infection, the absence of viral excretion during the first 2 postnatal weeks should be documented.

   The determination of serum antibody titers to CMV has limited usefulness for the neonate, although negative IgG titers on both maternal and infant sera are sufficient to exclude congenital CMV infection. Unfortunately, the interpretation of a positive IgG titer in the newborn is almost always complicated by the presence of transplacentally derived maternal IgG. Uninfected infants usually show a decline in IgG within 1 month and have no detectable titer by 4 to 9 months [26]. Infected infants maintain their IgG titers throughout the same time period. Tests for CMV-specific IgM have limitations and are not widely available for routine clinical use at this time.

4. **Treatment.** There is no effective antiviral therapy currently available for the treatment of congenital or perinatal CMV infection in newborn infants. Clinical trials with several agents have been carried out, but the results have been disappointing or difficult to interpret [26]. Toxicity with these agents is a major limiting factor. The most promising antiviral drug is ganciclovir (9–13-dihydroxypropoxymethyl guanine). This agent has been shown to be effective in the treatment of chorioretinitis and pneumonitis in immunosuppressed transplant patients [53]. The drug is under investigation for use in newborn infants with CNS involvement associated with congenital CMV infection. It remains to be shown whether it is

safe and efficacious in altering the outcome of symptomatic CMV infection in the neonate.

Passive immunization with hyperimmune anti-CMV immunoglobulin and active immunization with a live attenuated CMV vaccine represent attractive therapies for prophylaxis against congenital CMV infections. However, data from clinical trials are lacking. The most likely use of immune globulin would be to provide prophylaxis of susceptible women against primary CMV infection in pregnancy. Two live attenuated CMV vaccines have been developed [54,55], but their efficacy has not been clearly established. The possibility of reactivation of vaccine-strain CMV in pregnancy with subsequent infection of the fetus must be carefully considered before adequate field trials can be completed in women of child-bearing age [26].

5. **Prevention.** Currently, it is difficult to identify the fetus at risk for symptomatic CMV infection. Approximately 2 percent of women acquire acute primary CMV infection in pregnancy. In general, these women are asymptomatic, and given the low overall risk for significant fetal disease, universal screening for CMV in pregnancy is not recommended [56–58]. Furthermore, isolation of virus from the cervix or urine of pregnant women has a poor predictive value for fetal infection [59]. There simply is not enough information known about fetal transmission to provide guidelines for obstetrical management. At this time, no recommendations for therapeutic abortion can be made, even if primary maternal CMV infection is documented.

   Although breast milk is a common source for perinatal CMV infection in the newborn infant, symptomatic infection is rare, especially in term infants. In this setting, protection against disseminated disease may be provided by transplacentally derived maternal IgG. However, there may be insufficient transplacental IgG to provide adequate protection in preterm infants. In this setting, the use of breast milk from CMV-negative mothers should be encouraged. At present there is no recommended method of minimizing the risk of exposure to CMV in infected breast milk; freezing milk at $-20°C$ will reduce the titer of CMV but will not eliminate active virus [60].

   Day care centers and hospitals are potential high-risk environments for acquiring CMV infection. Not surprisingly, a number of studies have confirmed an increased risk for infection in day care workers [62]. However, there does not appear to be an increased risk for infection in hospital personnel [63–66]. These studies demonstrate that good handwashing and infection-control measures practiced in hospital settings may be sufficient to control the spread of CMV to workers. Unfortunately, such control may be difficult to achieve in day care centers. Good handwashing should be suggested to pregnant women with children in day care. The determination of the CMV susceptibility of these women by serology may be useful for counseling.

   The risk of transfusion-acquired CMV infection in the neonate should be minimized by the use of blood and blood products obtained from CMV-negative donors [38]. For packed red blood cell transfusions, deglycerolized frozen cells provide a safe alternative [49]. It is particularly important to use blood from one of these sources in preterm, low-birth-weight infants [61] (see Chap. 20).

B. **Rubella.** This human-specific RNA virus is a member of the togavirus family. It causes a mild self-limiting infection in susceptible children and adults, but its effects on the fetus can be devastating. Prior to widespread immunization beginning in 1969, rubella was a common childhood illness, with 85 percent of the population being immune by late adolescence and nearly 100 percent of the population being immune by age 35 to 40 years [69]. Epidemics occurred every 6 to 9 years, with pandemics arising with a greater and more variable cycle [70]. During pandemics, susceptible women were at significant risk of exposure to rubella, resulting in a high number of fetal infections. In the mid-1960s, rubella accounted for an estimated 11,000 fetal deaths and 20,000 cases of congenital rubella syndrome [71]. Childhood immunization has dramatically reduced the number of cases of rubella in the United States. However, 12 to 24 percent of postpubertal individuals are susceptible, and outbreaks of rubella have occurred in several large urban areas over the past 10 years [67,71,72].

1. **Congenital rubella syndrome (CRS).** Fetal infection can occur at any time in pregnancy, but early gestation infection may result in multiple organ anomalies. Classically, congenital rubella syndrome (CRS) is characterized by the constellation of cataracts, sensorineural hearing loss, and congenital heart disease. The most common cardiac defects are patent ductus arteriosus and pulmonary artery stenosis. Other common features of CRS are intrauterine growth retardation, retinopathy, microphthalmia, meningoencephalitis, electroencephalographic abnormalities, mental retardation, behavioral disorders, hypotonia, dermatoglyphic abnormalities, hepatosplenomegaly, thrombocytopenic purpura, radiographic bone lucencies, and diabetes mellitus [67]. Some of the abnormalities of CRS may occur with a delayed onset of months to years. Many additional rare complications have been described, including myocarditis, glaucoma, microcephaly, chronic progressive panencephalitis, hepatitis, anemia, hypogammaglobulinemia, thymic hypoplasia, thyroid abnormalities, cryptorchidism, and polycystic kidney disease [67].

   The relative risk of fetal transmission and the development of CRS as a function of gestational age have been studied [23]. With maternal infection in the first 12 weeks of gestation, the rate of fetal infection was 81 percent. The rate dropped to 54 percent for weeks 13 to 16, 36 percent for weeks 17 to 22, and 30 percent for weeks 23 to 30. During the last 10 weeks of gestation, the rate of fetal infection again rose to 60 percent for weeks 31 to 36 and 100 percent for weeks 36 and beyond. When maternofetal transmission occurred during the first 10 weeks of gestation, 100 percent of the infected fetuses had cardiac defects and deafness. Deafness was found in one-third of fetuses infected at 13 to 16 weeks, but no abnormalities were found when fetal infection occurred beyond the sixteenth week of gestation.

2. **Diagnosis of maternal infection.** The diagnosis of acute rubella in pregnancy requires serologic testing. This is necessary because the clinical symptoms of rubella are nonspecific and can be seen with infection by other viral agents (e.g., enteroviruses, measles, human parvovirus) [67,68]. Furthermore, a large number of individuals may have subclinical infection. Several sensitive and specific assays exist for the detection of rubella-specific antibody [67,68]. Viral isolation from the nose, throat, and/or urine is possible, but this is costly and not practical in most instances.

   a. **Symptomatic maternal infection.** Symptoms typically begin 2 to 3 weeks after exposure and include malaise, low-grade fever, headache, mild coryza, and conjunctivitis occurring 1 to 5 days prior to the onset of rash [67]. The rash is a salmon-pink macular or maculopapular exanthem that begins on the face and behind the ears and spreads downward over 1 to 2 days. The rash disappears within 5 to 7 days from onset, and posterior cervical lymphadenopathy is common. Approximately one-third of women may have arthralgias without arthritis [67].

      In women suspected of having acute rubella infection, confirmation can be made by demonstrating a fourfold or greater rise in serum IgG titers when measured at the time of symptoms and approximately 2 weeks later [67]. The results of some assays may not directly correlate with a fourfold rise in titer, so other criteria for significant antibody increase may be required. When there is uncertainty about the interpretation of assay results, advice should be obtained from the laboratory running the test and an infectious diseases consultation. It is very important to have the acute serum titer determined again, in tandem with the convalescent titer. In some cases, the relative increase in titer within the first 2 weeks of symptoms may be less obvious because serum IgG has already begun to rise at the time of clinical symptoms. In this situation, repeated serum titers may be required. Obviously, a prior knowledge of a woman's immune status can be very useful. Also, a single, high-positive rubella-specific IgM titer may be diagnostic, but problems with the specificity of these assays and the persistence of IgM for many weeks make the interpretation of low-positive values difficult [68].

b. Recognized or suspected maternal exposure. Any individual known to have been immunized with rubella vaccine after their first birthday is generally considered immune [73]. However, it is best to determine immunity by measuring rubella-specific IgG, which has become a standard of practice in obstetrical care. If a woman exposed to rubella is known to be seropositive, she is immune and the fetus is considered not to be at risk for infection. Rarely, reinfections in previously immune women have been documented, but the risk of fetal damage appears to be very small [74]. If the exposed woman is known to be seronegative, a serum titer should be sent 3 to 4 weeks after exposure. A negative titer indicates that no infection has occurred, whereas a positive titer indicates infection. Women with an uncertain immune status and a known exposure to rubella should have titers sent as soon as possible after exposure. If this is done within 7 to 10 days of exposure, and the titer is positive, the patient is rubella immune and no further testing is required [68]. If the first titer is negative or was determined on serum taken more than 7 to 10 days after exposure, repeated testing (approximately 3 weeks later) and careful clinical follow-up are necessary. When both the immune status and time of exposure are uncertain, titers should be obtained 3 weeks apart. If both titers are negative, no infection has occurred. Alternatively, infection is confirmed if seroconversion or a fourfold increase in titer is observed. Further testing and close clinical follow-up are required if titers are inconclusive. In this situation, specific IgM determination may be helpful. Again, it should be emphasized that all serum samples should be tested simultaneously by the same laboratory when determining changes in titers with time. This can be accomplished by saving a portion of each serum sample prior to sending it for titer determination. The saved portion can be frozen until convalescent serum samples have been obtained.

3. Diagnosis of congenital rubella infection

a. Antenatal diagnosis. The risk of severe fetal anomalies is highest with acute maternal rubella infection during the first 16 weeks of gestation. However, not all early gestation infections result in adverse pregnancy outcomes. Approximately 20 percent of fetuses may not be infected when maternal rubella occurs in the first 12 weeks of gestation, and as many as 45 percent of fetuses may not be infected when maternal rubella occurs closer to 16 weeks of gestation. Unfortunately, there is no foolproof method of determining infected from uninfected fetuses early in pregnancy, but in utero diagnosis is being investigated. One method that has been used with some success is the determination of specific IgM in fetal blood obtained by percutaneous umbilical blood sampling (PUBS) [75,76] (see Chap. 3). Direct detection of rubella antigen and RNA in a chorionic villous biopsy specimen also has been used successfully [77]. Although these techniques offer promise, their use may be limited by sensitivity and specificity or the lack of widespread availability at this time.

b. Postnatal diagnosis. Guidelines for the establishment of congenital rubella infection or congenital rubella syndrome (CRS) in neonates have been summarized by the Centers for Disease Control [72]. The diagnosis of congenital infection is made when an infant has no congenital defects but has laboratory confirmation of infection based on one of the following:

(1) Isolation of rubella virus (oropharynx, urine)

(2) Detection of rubella-specific IgM in cord or neonatal blood

(3) Persistent rubella-specific titers over time (i.e., no decline in titer as expected for transplacentally derived maternal IgG). If, in addition, there are congenital defects present, the diagnosis of CRS is made.

4. Treatment. There is no specific therapy for either maternal or congenital rubella infection. Maternal disease is almost always mild and self-limiting. If primary maternal infection occurs during the first 5 months of pregnancy, therapeutic abortion should be considered [67].

Over one-half of newborn infants with congenital rubella may be asymptomatic at birth. If infection is known to have occurred beyond the sixteenth week of gestation, it is unlikely that any abnormalities will develop, and parents should be reassured. Nevertheless, repeated hearing evaluations should be carried out through childhood. Closer follow-up is required if early gestation infection is suspected or the timing of infection is unknown. This is true for asymptomatic infants as well as those with obvious CRS. The principal reason for close follow-up is to identify delayed-onset abnormalities or progressive disorders. In some cases, early interventions may be critical, such as therapy for glaucoma. Unfortunately, there is no specific therapy to halt the progression of most of the complications of CRS.

5. Prevention. The primary means of prevention of CRS is by immunization of all susceptible persons. Indeed, immunization is recommended for all nonimmune individuals 12 months of age or older. Documentation of maternal immunity is an important aspect of good obstetrical management. When a susceptible woman is identified, she should be reassured of the low risk of contracting rubella, but she should also be counseled to avoid contact with anyone known to have acute or recent rubella infection. Individuals with postnatal infection typically shed virus for 1 week before and 1 week after the onset of rash. On the other hand, infants with congenital infection may shed virus for many months, and contact should be avoided during the first year [67]. Unfortunately, once exposure has occurred, little can be done to alter the chances of maternal and subsequently fetal disease. Hyperimmune globulin does not diminish the risk of maternal rubella following exposure or the rate of fetal transmission [67]. Nevertheless, hyperimmune globulin should be given in large doses to any woman who is exposed to rubella and who does not wish to interrupt her pregnancy under any circumstances [68]. The lack of proven efficacy must be emphasized in these cases.

Susceptible women who do not become infected should be immunized soon after pregnancy [78]. There have been reports of acute arthritis occurring in women immunized in the immediate postpartum period, and a small percentage of these women have developed chronic joint or neurologic abnormalities or viremia [67,79]. Vaccine-strain virus also may be shed in breast milk and transmitted to breast-fed infants, some of whom may develop chronic viremia [67,79]. Thus it may be best to avoid breast-feeding in women receiving rubella vaccine. Conception also should be avoided for 3 months following immunization [68]. Immunization during pregnancy is not recommended because of the theoretical risk to the fetus.

Inadvertent immunizations in pregnancy have occurred, and fetal infection has been documented in a small percentage of these cases. However, no cases of CRS have been identified [80]. In fact, the rubella registry at the Centers for Disease Control has been closed with the following conclusions: The number of cases of inadvertent immunization in pregnancy is too small to be able to state with certainty that no adverse pregnancy outcomes will occur, but these would appear to be very uncommon. Thus it is still recommended that immunization not be carried out in pregnancy, but when this has occurred, reassurance of little risk to the fetus can be given.

C. Human immunodeficiency virus. Human immunodeficiency virus (HIV) has been firmly implicated as the causative agent of the acquired immunodeficiency syndrome (AIDS) [82–85]. The first reported cases of AIDS in the United States were in homosexual men, and although the majority of cases continue to occur in this population, a rising segment of the heterosexual population is also afflicted. As of May 1, 1990, approximately 130,000 cases of AIDS have been reported in the United States, with an estimate of between 650,000 and 1.4 million individuals currently infected with HIV [86–89]. Although a relatively small percentage of all cases of AIDS have been reported in the pediatric population, the number of cases occurring in infants and children less than 13 years of age is rapidly rising. As of the end of June 1989, there were 1681 cases of pediatric AIDS in the United States, and recent studies have shown that the number of infants at risk for HIV infection has risen by an alarming rate [90]. In Massachusetts, anonymous newborn screening revealed an overall seropositivity of 2.0 to 2.5 per 1000 [91]. This meant that approximately 0.2 percent of women giving birth were HIV-infected. In inner-city areas, the rate increased to 8.0 per 1000. Even more alarming are reports of seropositivity as high as 3 to 4 percent in some major metropolitan areas of the United States [90]. Considering these numbers, along with the epidemiology of adult HIV infections and estimates of the number of women engaged in high-risk behavior, the number of cases of pediatric AIDS in the United States has been projected to be from 6000 to 20,000 over the next several years [90]. The problem is considerably greater in other parts of the world. For example, from 5 to 10 percent of women of childbearing age in central and eastern Africa are seropositive for HIV [92]. Thus HIV poses a serious and challenging problem for obstetricians and pediatricians.

1. **The virus.** Human immunodeficiency virus (HIV) is a cytopathic retrovirus (lentivirus) formerly designated as lymphadenopathy-associated virus (LAV), human T-cell lymphotrophic virus III (HTLV-III), or AIDS-related virus (ARV). Two closely related types of HIV have been identified: HIV-1, which is found throughout the world and is the principal cause of HIV infection in the United States, and HIV-2, which was originally described in western Africa but now is found in other countries as well. HIV contains genomic RNA within a core that is surrounded by an inner protein shell and an outer lipid envelope. The genome consists of the three genes found in all retroviruses (*gag, pol, env*) along with at least six additional genes [82]. Multiple proteins are encoded for including group-specific antigen proteins (core structural proteins coded by *gag*); reverse transcriptase, which is required for DNA production from viral RNA (coded by *pol*); and the glycosylated peptide precursor gp160 (coded by *env*). gp160 is processed into the surface glycoprotein gp120, which is necessary for the binding of virus to target cells, and the associated transmembrane glycoprotein gp41, which is located in the viral lipid envelope. Other proteins readily identified are p24, which is the major core protein (function unknown), and p18, which is found in the inner shell (function unknown). The lipid envelope is derived from the host cell membrane as the virus buds from the infected cell surface.
2. **Pathogenesis.** The pathogenesis of HIV infection [82–85] begins with the binding of the virus to CD4 containing cells. These include T-helper/in-

ducer lymphocytes, monocytes, and macrophages. The virus then enters the cell, where genomic RNA is transcribed by reverse transcriptase, leading to the production of circularized proviral DNA, some of which becomes integrated into host chromosomal DNA. Once integration occurs, a latent (inactive) period follows, but under certain conditions of cellular activation, the proviral DNA is transcribed into viral genomic RNA and mRNA. Ultimately, viral regulatory and structural proteins are produced, resulting in the production of new virions that bud from the cell surface. The precise mechanisms of HIV-mediated cell death remain uncertain, but $CD4^+$ T-cell depletion is the hallmark of infection. However, the timing of the depletion is quite variable, possibly due to the ability of HIV to cause latent infection for months to years. It is also unclear if depletion results from cytolysis [83]. In addition to a decrease in cell number, altered T-cell function occurs. In particular, $CD4^+$ T-cell responsiveness to antigens is reduced, usually before cell depletion is observed. The other $CD4^+$ cells that may play a prominant role in HIV infection are monocytes and macrophages. These cells are relatively resistant to the cytopathic effects of HIV and thus may act as major viral reservoirs. They also may be important in the transport of HIV to other parts of the body, including the central nervous system (CNS).

The consequences of $CD4^+$ T-cell depletion is a cascade of immune deficiencies. Cell-mediated immunity is suppressed, and there is decreased production of lymphokines, including IL-2, IFN-γ, macrophage chemotactic factor, hematopoietic growth factors, and B-cell growth and differentiation factors [83]. Polyclonal B-cell activation resulting in hypergammaglobulinemia often occurs, but at the same time there is reduced antibody responses to new antigens. Such B-cell dysfunctions probably result from a combination of loss of T-helper cells, stimulation by polyclonal activators (e.g., other viruses such as CMV and EBV), and the direct action of HIV or HIV components on B cells. Finally, monocyte and macrophage functions are affected, as demonstrated by decreased chemotaxis and HLA class II antigen expression.

HIV-associated immune deficiencies can account for many of the clinical outcomes observed for infected individuals. These include susceptibility to opportunistic pathogens, neoplasms, and certain pyogenic infections. However, some of the clinical manifestations are not clearly linked to abnormal immunity. For example, severe CNS abnormalities [93,94], such as acute aseptic meningitis, subacute encephalitis, mild cognitive impairment, dementia, and progressive leukoencephalopathy, are common occurrences with HIV infection. A vacuolar myelopathy and peripheral neuropathy also have been described. Some of these abnormalities may result from toxic immunologic mediators released by macrophages entering the CNS, but there is evidence suggesting a direct effect of HIV on neuronal tissue [83–85]. Furthermore, HIV has been shown to infect CNS endothelial and glial cells. HIV infection of fibroblasts and bowel mucosal cells also has been demonstrated. Like monocytes and macrophages, infected fibroblasts could be an important reservoir for HIV in multiple tissues. HIV-infected individuals may develop a malabsorption syndrome, which may arise from the effects of macrophage-derived cytokines, but also could be related to the direct effects of virus on mucosal cells [85].

3. **Transmission.** There are three principal routes for HIV transmission: sexual contact, parenteral inoculation, and maternal-fetal or maternal-newborn infant transfer.
   a. **Sexual contact.** This remains the principal mode of transmission of HIV worldwide. In the United States, this has predominantly affected the homosexual population, but the rate of heterosexual transmission has increased considerably. Male-to-female transmission has been best documented, with viral exposure possibly arising from infected leukocytes present in semen [83]. It follows that the principal risk

factors for acquiring HIV in women of childbearing age are intravenous drug use (see **3.b**) and sexual contact with an infected male partner.

b. Parenteral transmission. Parenteral transmission of HIV results from the direct inoculation of infected blood or blood products. Not surprisingly, the major groups affected have been intravenous (IV) drug users (shared contaminated needles) and patients receiving transfusions. The largest group is the IV drug users, and transmission within this group is intimately linked to heterosexual transmission in the United States. Important among the transfusion group are hemophiliacs by nature of requiring factor VIII concentrates obtained from multiple donors. Careful screening of blood donors for risk factors for infection, universal HIV antibody testing of donated blood, and the special preparation of clotting factor to eliminate the risk of viral contamination have greatly reduced the incidence of transfusion-acquired HIV. However, donor screening is not 100 percent sensitive, and transfusion-acquired infection still occurs, although rarely. The most likely reason for false-negative HIV serology is the seronegative window that occurs between initial infection and the production of antiviral antibody. The odds of transfusion-acquired HIV infection from the transfusion of a single unit of tested blood have been estimated to be from 1:250,000 to 1:150,000 [83,95] (see Chap. 20).

c. Congenital and perinatal transmission. In utero and intrapartum transmissions from infected mothers constitute the principal modes of HIV infection in the pediatric population. Approximately 80 percent of pediatric AIDS cases have resulted from maternal transmission [90]. Most of the other 20 percent of cases are transfusion-related. With the reduction in transfusion-associated HIV infections, congenital and perinatal transmission will likely account for nearly 100 percent of pediatric AIDS in the future. The principal risk factors for maternal infection are IV drug use (52 percent) or sexual contact with IV drug-abusing partners (21 percent) [90]. Given the relatively high prevalence of IV drug abuse in inner-city areas, it is not surprising that most cases of pediatric AIDS have occurred in racial minority groups. Thus approximately 48 percent of infected children are black and 22 percent are Hispanic [90].

The risk of transmission of HIV from infected mothers to their fetuses and newborn infants has been estimated to be between 20 and 50 percent [96]. Initial studies suggested a rate in the 50 percent or greater range, but these studies focused on women who had already had infected children [96,97]. Subsequent prospective studies with variable follow-up indicate that the overall risk for transmission may be closer to 30 percent [96,98]. The fetuses of HIV-positive mothers may be adversely affected even in the absence of HIV transmission [92]. The timing of transmission remains uncertain. HIV has been isolated from cord blood specimens, and fetal infections as early as 14 to 20 weeks' gestation have been demonstrated [99]. The possibility of an HIV embryopathy also supports early gestation infection of the fetus [100]. Nevertheless, the risk of HIV transmission as a function of gestational age is not known, and transmission is also likely to occur by intrapartum exposure to mother's blood. It is possible that infants who become symptomatic in a relatively short time after birth represent those who were infected in utero as opposed to those infected perinatally. The mechanism of transplacental transfer of HIV is not known, but HIV can infect trophoblast cell lines [90]. It is interesting to note that infection has been documented to occur in only one infant of monozygotic twins [101].

Postnatal transmission of HIV from infected mothers to infants by means of breast milk appears to be well documented [102]. The risk for postnatal infection is small, but it is currently recommended that HIV-positive mothers in developed countries do not breast-feed.

4. **Natural history of HIV infection.** The initial response to HIV infection is the production of specific antibodies against the virus. Most often this occurs within 2 months, but seroconversion can take as little as 3 weeks or as long as 4 to 5 months [83]. Approximately 30 to 50 percent of patients may develop an acute illness [103] characterized by sore throat, myalgias, fever, and rash. This mononucleosis-like illness may be accompanied by aseptic meningitis and an atypical lymphocytosis. Whether or not this acute illness occurs, nearly all HIV-infected individuals develop persistent generalized lymphadenopathy. However, the development of further clinical symptoms has a considerably variable time course, and the time from seroconversion to the diagnosis of AIDS may take from 2 to 8 years [104]. Indeed, it is not even certain that all HIV-infected individuals will eventually develop AIDS [83]. At present, approximately 25 to 35 percent of patients will progress from the early stages of infection to AIDS within 5 to 7 years [83]. Those patients who have progressive HIV disease often develop a constellation of symptoms that has been referred to as the **AIDS-related complex (ARC).** Symptoms include prolonged fever, weight loss, and diarrhea. Coincident with the evolution of these symptoms is the development of abnormal T-cell mitogen responses followed by the reduction in $CD4^+$ T-cell numbers, a reversal of the $CD4^+$ to $CD8^+$ T-cell ratio, and other hematologic abnormalities.

   By the original CDC case definition, the diagnosis of AIDS essentially required the occurrence of one or more specified diseases resulting as a consequence of the underlying immunodeficiency. Recognizing the requirement for HIV infection and the spectrum of disease encountered, the CDC now suggests that patients be classified into one of three categories: group 1—HIV infection plus one or more specified infections or malignancies; group 2—HIV infection plus specified manifestations without a secondary infection or neoplasm found in group 1; and group 3—HIV infection without the specified manifestations required for groups 1 and 2 [105]. Patients formerly diagnosed with AIDS are included in group 1, whereas those formerly diagnosed with ARC are in group 2.

   a. **HIV in pregnancy.** At this time, the natural history of HIV infection in pregnancy is unknown (perinatal). Previous studies have been limited by selection bias, since HIV-positive women were identified through the recognition of HIV disease in their children or because they had symptomatic HIV infection. Information about the natural history of HIV infection in nonpregnant women is also lacking. Since pregnancy may itself lead to altered immunity, the need for pregnant seronegative controls in prospective studies may be important. Currently, prospective studies on HIV in pregnancy are underway. One such study is the Women and Infants Transmission Study (WITS), which is a multicenter NIH-sponsored investigation. Understanding more about the effect of pregnancy on HIV infection and the transmission of HIV to the fetus will be important in the obstetrical management and use of possible therapeutic modalities during pregnancy.

   b. **Pediatric HIV infection.** There are a number of features about pediatric HIV infection that set it apart from adult HIV disease. First of all, the majority of cases occur in infants and young children, reflecting the preponderance of congenital and perinatally acquired infections. Fifty percent of pediatric AIDS cases occur in the first year of life, and approximately 80 percent of cases occur by 3 years of age [106]. In these patients, the incubation period is most often only about 4 to 6 months, with HIV-related symptoms occurring in more than 80 percent of cases in the first year of life (median age of onset of symptoms is 9 months) [90,98,99,107]. It is estimated that 20 percent of infants with congenital/perinatal HIV infection will die within the first year of life, and 60 percent will have severe symptomatic disease by 18 months of age [98]. Conversely, a few perinatally infected children have gone as long as 7 to 10 years with latent (asymptomatic) infection [90]. The time to onset of HIV-related symptoms also appears to be shorter for transfusion-acquired HIV in children compared with adults [108] and in infants compared with older children [112]. Children also differ in their clinical presentation compared with adults [90,99,109,110]. As in adults, 90 percent of children develop diffuse, persistent lymphadenopathy. Hepatomegaly and splenomegaly are also common. Approximately 60 percent of infected infants and children develop failure to thrive. Fifty to 90 percent of HIV-infected children have CNS involvement characterized by an encephalopathy that can often be clinically devastating [90]. Although the clinical presentation may vary, developmental delay or loss of developmental milestones and diminished cognitive function are common features.

Of particular uniqueness to pediatric AIDS is the high frequency with which a chronic interstitial lung disease referred to as **lymphoid interstitial pneumonitis (LIP)** occurs. LIP is characterized by a diffuse lymphocytic and plasma-cell infiltrate. The clinical course of LIP is quite variable but may be progressive, resulting in marked respiratory distress (tachypnea, retractions, wheezing, hypoxemia). There is an association with Epstein-Barr virus infection, but the significance of this is uncertain. Overall, the prognosis appears to be more favorable for symptomatic HIV infections in children when the major symptom is LIP [90]. In addition to LIP, recurrent bacterial infections are a frequent feature of pediatric AIDS, owing in part to the early occurrence of B-cell dysfunction with dysfunctional hypergammaglobulinemia. Both focal and disseminated infections are encountered, with sepsis being most common. The organisms usually isolated from the bloodstream have been *Streptococcus pneumoniae, Haemophilus influenzae,* and *Salmonella* [99], but a variety of other bacteria have been recovered, especially from hospitalized patients. Other manifestations of HIV infection that may be more common in children are parotitis and cardiac dysfunction. Given the unique aspects of pediatric HIV infection, a separate classification scheme has been proposed [114].

The HIV-infected newborn infant is often asymptomatic, but symptoms may develop within the first month. These include persistent thrush, lymphadenopathy, and hepatosplenomegaly. In addition, opportunistic infections have been reported in HIV-infected neonates [111]. However, factors unrelated to HIV infection may complicate the clinical assessment of the newborn infant. These include intrauterine growth retardation and CNS abnormalities secondary to intrauterine exposure to illicit drugs. Some infants are believed to display a number of consistent dysmorphic features that constitute an AIDS embryopathy [100]. The features include growth failure (75 percent), microcephaly (70 percent), prominent (boxlike) forehead (75 percent), flat nasal bridge (70 percent), short nose with flattened columella (75 percent), triangular philtrum (75 percent), mild obliquity of the eyes (65 percent), long palpebral fissures with blue sclerae (60 percent), ocular hypertelorism (50 percent), patulous lips (60 percent), and a prominent upper vermilion border. It should be noted that the proposed embryopathy has not been widely accepted to date. Confirmation will likely require controls consisting of appropriately matched infants taking into account racial, socioeconomic, and demographic factors, in addition to confounding problems such as alcohol and IV drug abuse in pregnancy. A better understanding of the spectrum of HIV disease in the newborn infant will require carefully designed prospective studies such as the Women and Infants Transmission Study (WITS).

5. **Diagnosis.** The diagnosis of HIV infection in adults is made by the detection of specific antibody by an enzyme-linked immunosorbent assay (ELISA) with confirmation by Western blot analysis [113]. Testing should be offered to anyone at risk for HIV. Currently, testing requires informed consent.

   Unfortunately, serology is of limited value in diagnosing congenital HIV infection in infants less than 15 months old [90]. The reason for this is that maternal IgG crosses the placenta and can persist in infants throughout the first year or more of life. In the presence of symptomatology and/or specific laboratory findings strongly indicative of HIV [114], the diagnosis of HIV may still be made. However, the picture is less clear in infants with minimal or no symptomatology. Thus alternative tests have been employed to identify the presence of HIV in infants born to HIV-positive mothers. These include the following:

   a. In vitro tissue culture
   b. P24 antigen detection in peripheral blood [115]
   c. Polymerase chain reaction (PCR) to detect viral nucleic acid in peripheral blood [116]
   d. Enzyme-linked immunosorbent assay (ELISA) for the detection of specific IgM and IgA [117,118]
   e. In vitro stimulation of peripheral blood leukocytes to produce specific antibody [121]
   f. In situ hybridization to detect HIV-specific DNA in infected cells

   Of these, tissue culture and the p24 antigen assay are approved tests for the diagnosis of HIV infection. Culture is expensive, technically difficult, may require weeks to obtain results, and is not readily available. The p24 antigen assay suffers from a lack of sensitivity, particularly in infants [90,115]. More recently, PCR has been successfully used to identify HIV infections in neonates and infants [115,119,120], but its usefulness in the neonate may be limited to the identification of infants at greatest risk for developing fulminant HIV disease [90]. The importance of developing a rapid, sensitive, and specific test for the diagnosis of HIV in the neonate and asymptomatic infant is that early therapeutic interventions (e.g., zidovudine) may be available in the near future (see below).

6. **Treatment and prevention.** A major part of the management of HIV infection is symptomatic treatment. At present, there is no cure for HIV infection. Optimization of nutrition, prophylaxis against opportunistic infections (most notably *Pneumocystis carinii* pneumonia), and the prompt recognition and treatment of HIV-related complications (e.g., opportunistic infections, cardiac dysfunction, etc.) are paramount to the improvement in longevity and the quality of life for HIV-infected patients. In the newborn infant, special attention should be given to the possibility of congenitally and perinatally transmitted pathogens, such as *Mycobacteria, Toxoplasma,* and venereal agents, which may have a relatively high prevalence in HIV-infected adults.

   There are intense efforts to develop methods to treat and prevent HIV infections. Possibilities being investigated include vaccines to actively immunize against HIV and use of the following specific antiretroviral therapies [122]:

   a. Drugs that inhibit the action of viral proteins, especially reverse transcriptase
   b. Agents that block the binding of HIV to target cells
   c. Immunotherapy with interferon (IFN-α) or neutralizing monoclonal antibodies

   The greatest clinical experience has been with dideoxynucleoside analogues that interfere with viral reverse transcriptase [125–127,129,130]. Of these, zidovudine (3′-azido-2′,3′-dideoxythymidine, formerly known as

AZT) has been shown to be of benefit in at least transiently improving or slowing the development of some of the symptoms related to HIV infection in adults [125–127]. The drug has been approved by the FDA for use in HIV-infected adults. Zidovudine contains an N_3 group in place of a 3′-OH group. It is taken up by cells, where it is phosphorylated into a 5′-triphosphate form. In this form, zidovudine binds to the nucleotide recognition site on reverse transcriptase (competitive inhibition). Zidovudine is also incorporated into the growing DNA chain, but since it lacks a 3′-OH group, chain elongation is terminated [122].

Although there is less experience with the use of zidovudine in children, preliminary data are encouraging, at least for therapy in symptomatic infections. Pizzo et al. [123] reported the use of continuous intravenous infusion zidovudine in children with symptomatic HIV disease. Significant improvement, particularly in CNS abnormalities, was demonstrated: Thirteen of 13 children with encephalopathy and neurodevelopmental abnormalities improved based on a variety of controlled testing of psychomotor and cognitive functioning. An additional 5 of 8 patients showed neurodevelopmental improvement, even though they had unrecognized encephalopathy before treatment. Most patients showed an increase in appetite and weight, decreased lymphadenopathy and hepatosplenomegaly, decreased immunoglobulin levels (i.e., reduction in hypergammaglobulinemia), and an increase in $CD4^+$ cells. Larger clinical trials of orally dosed zidovudine have been conducted in symptomatic HIV-infected children, but the analyses of these studies are still underway. Preliminary results confirm some degree of efficacy with acceptable toxicity, and based on these results, zidovudine has been approved by the FDA for the treatment of symptomatic HIV infection in children over 3 months old. Additional studies are needed to determine the benefit of zidovudine in asymptomatic HIV infection and to establish the minimal effective dose to be administered. No data are available on the use of zidovudine in pregnancy, but the prospects for reducing the risk of fetal transmission are intriguing.

Intravenous gammaglobulin therapy has been used in children with HIV infections [124]. The most apparent use for this therapy is to provide functional IgG, since antibody responses to new antigens are frequently reduced in HIV-infected children. This may lead to a reduction in the frequency and severity of bacterial infections. Other benefits have been described in case reports, but no controlled studies have been completed. An interesting finding recently reported is the correlation between the absence of high-affinity/avidity maternal antibodies to the gp120 molecule of HIV and the risk of fetal transmission [128]. This raises the possibility of the use of specific maternal antibody as a marker for the relative risk of fetal infection, as well as suggesting a potential therapy to prevent fetal transmission. Similarly, one experimental therapy under clinical investigation is the infusion of soluble (recombinant) CD4 preparations. The goal of this therapy is to competitively block the binding of HIV to cells and thus prevent infection. The potential for this agent to prevent transplacental transfer of HIV is exciting [90].

Since HIV may be transmitted at the time of delivery, there has been speculation as to whether the risk of fetal infection may be reduced by cesarean section. There are no data to support this notion. Fetal transmission in early pregnancy has been documented, as has transmission in infants born by cesarean section [90]. No recommendations concerning mode of delivery can be made at this time.

Education plays an important role in the prevention of the spread of HIV infection. The aim here is to counsel the public about high-risk behavior. The hazards of IV drug use and measures to minimize the spread of HIV through sexual contact should be emphasized to all women in adolescent and gynecologic counseling. Eliminating unwarranted fears about casual contact with HIV-infected individuals is also a major goal of public education.

7. **HIV and the health care worker.** The transmission of HIV from patients to health care providers appears to be very uncommon. The precise risk is unknown and is the subject of considerable controversy. The greatest risk for transmission is from parenteral inoculation of infected blood by inadvertent needle sticks or cuts with contaminated sharp instruments. To minimize the risk of transmission of HIV to health care personnel, universal precautions have been recommended for all hospital environments [131]. Particular emphasis in perinatal/neonatal medicine should be placed on the avoidance of blood and bloody secretions in the delivery room by the wearing of gowns, gloves, and eye protection (preferably goggles with side shields). Meconium and gastric aspirates should never be suctioned by mouth; special meconium suction adapters and catheters are generally available that may be attached to wall suction (see Chap. 13). Of special concern in the nursery is the recapping of needles when drawing blood from umbilical lines. If recapping is required, it is best to use cap-holding devices to avoid needle sticks. Also, syringes should not be tapped or "flicked" to remove air when obtaining arterial blood gas samples. Specific guidelines have been suggested for the recognition and management of occupational exposures to HIV [132]. Types of exposures include percutaneous injury (needle sticks, cuts with a sharp instruments), mucous membrane contact, and skin contact (particularly with cuts, abrasions, dermatitis, or for prolonged time or over a large area) with potentially infectious tissues or body fluids. The guidelines recommend procedures for serologic testing in the worker and the patient contact. The use of zidovudine for postexposure prophylaxis is also discussed. Review of these guidelines is recommended for all individuals at risk for occupational exposure to HIV. The risk average of contracting HIV per episode of percutaneous exposure to HIV-infected blood is estimated to be approximately 0.4 percent [132]. It is unknown if postexposure zidovudine will further reduce this risk.

D. **Parvovirus.** Parvoviruses are small, unenveloped viruses that range in size from 18 to 26 mm and contain single-stranded DNA. Human infections are primarily due to strain B19, which is responsible for several clinical syndromes [133,134]. Although parvovirus B19 has genotypic variation, no antigenic variation between isolates has been demonstrated. Parvoviruses tend to infect rapidly dividing cells and can be transmitted across the placenta, posing a potential threat to the fetus.

1. **Epidemiology.** The seroprevalence of parvovirus B19 IgG reflects the age-related incidence of clinical disease [133,134]. Approximately 2 to 9 percent of children less than 5 years of age have detectable B19 IgG, compared with 15 to 35 percent for ages 5 years to less than 18 years. Studies in adults have varied, with seropositivity for B19 IgG ranging from 30 to 60 percent. Based on studies of household contacts, the incubation period for parvovirus B19 infection appears to be 4 to 14 days, with an attack rate of 50 to 60 percent for all ages. Of infected contacts (IgM positive), approximately 20 percent may be asymptomatic and 50 percent may not have a rash. Peak occurrence is from around midwinter through spring, with a cyclic peak activity every 5 to 7 years. The virus is probably spread by means of respiratory secretions, which clear in patients with typical erythema infectiosum at or shortly after the onset of rash.

2. **Common clinical presentations of parvovirus B19 infection**

   a. **Disease in children.** Parvovirus B19 has been associated with a variety of rashes, including the typical "slapped cheek" rash of erythema infectiosum (fifth disease) [135,136]. In approximately 60 percent of school-aged children with erythema infectiosum, fever occurs 1 to 4 days before the facial rash appears [133]. Associated symptoms include myalgias, upper respiratory or gastrointestinal symptoms, and malaise, but these symptoms generally resolve with the appearance of the rash. The rash is usually macular, progresses to the extremities and trunk, and may involve the palms and soles. The rash may be pruritic and may recur.

b. Disease in adults. The typical school-aged presentation of erythema infectiosum can occur in adults, but arthralgias and arthritis are more common [133,137,138]. As many as 60 percent of adults with parvovirus B19 infections may have acute joint swelling, most commonly involving peripheral joints (symmetrically). Arthritis may persist for years and may be associated with the development of rheumatoid arthritis.

3. Less common manifestations of parvovirus B19 infections

a. Infection in patients with hemolytic anemia or immunosuppression. Parvovirus B19 has been clearly identified as a cause of red blood cell aplasia. In particular, parvovirus B19 is the principal cause of aplastic crisis in individuals with chronic hemolytic anemia, including acquired diseases [135,139]. Severe anemia has been described in individuals with hemoglobin abnormalities (sickle-cell disease, hemoglobin SC disease, thalassemia), hereditary spherocytosis, and cellular enzyme deficits, such as pyruvate kinase deficiency. A viral prodrome usually occurs within 1 week of anemia. A rash also may occur but is less common. Parvovirus B19 also has been associated with acute and chronic red blood cell aplasia in immunosuppressed patients [140,141].

b. Fetal infection. Based primarily on the demonstration of viral DNA in fetal tissue samples, parvovirus B19 has been firmly linked to fetal nonimmune hydrops [142–145]. The presumed pathogenic sequence is as follows [146]:

Transplacental transfer of B19 virus → Infection of red cell precursors → Arrested red cell production → Severe anemia → Congestive heart failure → Edema

A study estimating the risk of fetal hydrops following maternal infection with parvovirus B19 showed that up to 15 percent of fetuses may be affected with maternal infection during the first 18 weeks of gestation [133]. However, in this study, B19 DNA was demonstrated in approximately one-third of the fetuses, suggesting that the attack rate for severe fetal disease was approximately 5 percent for maternal infection during the first 18 weeks of gestation. No adverse outcomes were noted for maternal infection occurring beyond 18 weeks, but more recent reports indicate that anemia may result from third-trimester infections.

B19 may infect cells other than those of the hematopoietic system. The finding of an ocular anomaly in one fetus infected with B19 suggests this possibility [144]. Furthermore, B19 DNA has been detected in cardiac tissues from aborted fetuses. It has been suggested that B19 may cause fetal myocarditis and that this may contribute to the development of hydrops. There is one report of B19-associated fetal hydrops dramatically responding to in utero digitalization. Despite this improvement, the fetus died and on postmortem examination was found to have intranuclear viral particles consistent with B19 present in cardiac tissue [147]. Finally, fetal hepatitis with severe liver disease has been documented [154].

The possibility of parvovirus B19-induced fetal anomalies has been questioned given the propensity for the virus to infect rapidly growing cells. Although there is one case report implicating B19 as a cause of an ocular anomaly [144], a study of 130 newborn infants to mothers with documented infection during pregnancy did not show any fetal anomalies [133].

4. **Diagnosis.** Parvovirus B19 is difficult to grow in vitro and will not grow in standard tissue cultures. Viral antigens may be directly detected in tissues either by radioimmunoassay [148], enzyme-linked immunosorbent assay (ELISA) [149], immunofluorescence, in situ nucleic acid hybridization [150], or polymerase chain reaction (PCR) [151]. While these techniques may be valuable for certain clinical settings, such as examining tissues from fetuses with nonimmune hydrops, determination of serum IgG and IgM levels may be more practical. Serum B19 IgG is absent in susceptible hosts, and IgM appears by day 3 of an acute infection. Serum IgM may be detected in up to 90 percent of patients with acute B19 infection, and serum levels begin to fall by the second to third month after infection. Serum IgG appears a few days after IgM and may persist for years.
5. **Treatment.** Treatment is generally supportive, but immunotherapy has been suggested under certain conditions. Specifically, intravenous gammaglobulin (IVIG) has been used with reported success in a limited number of cases of severe hematologic disorders related to persistent parvovirus infection [140,152]. The rationale for this therapy stems from the observations that (1) the primary immune response to B19 infection is the production of specific IgM and IgG, (2) the appearance of systemic antibody coincides with the resolution of clinical symptoms, and (3) specific antibody prevents infection. However, no controlled studies have been undertaken to establish the efficacy of IVIG prophylaxis or therapy for B19 infections.

   Given the potential for severe disease in immunocompromised patients exposed to parvovirus B19, IVIG prophylaxis is a reasonable consideration. Even more compelling is the use of IVIG to treat patients with symptomatic anemia and parvoviremia. IVIG is not currently recommended for prophylaxis in pregnancy.

   Intrauterine blood transfusions have been used with success in a few cases of fetal hydrops [153], but the institution of such therapy must take into account the severity of fetal disease and the risk to the fetus and mother of the procedure. Attempts to identify other causes of fetal hydrops are obviously important. The possible contribution of cardiac dysfunction that may not respond to blood transfusions also should be considered.
6. **Management of pregnant women at risk for parvovirus exposure.** Three groups of pregnant women of interest when considering the potential risk of fetal parvovirus disease are pregnant women exposed to an infected household contact, pregnant school teachers, and pregnant health care providers. In each case, the measurement of serum IgG and IgM levels may be useful to determine the women at risk or acutely infected after B19 exposure. The tests can be arranged through state departments of public health or the Centers for Disease Control, Atlanta, Georgia. In general, requests for these tests should be limited to pregnant women clearly at increased risk for acute parvovirus B19 exposure during the first 18 weeks of gestation. Consultation with your infectious disease service or state department of public health is recommended.
   a. **The pregnant woman exposed to an infected household contact.** Studies suggest that the risk of fetal B19 disease is very small for asymptomatic pregnant women in communities where outbreaks of erythema infectiosum occur [133,155]. In this setting, no special diagnostic tests or precautions may be indicated. However, household contacts with erythema infectiosum place the pregnant women at increased risk for acute B19 infection. It is estimated that the risk of B19 infection in a susceptible adult with a household contact is approximately 50 percent [135]. Considering an estimated risk of 5 percent for severe fetal disease with acute maternal B19 infection, the

risk of hydrops fetalis is approximately 2.5 percent for susceptible pregnant women exposed to an infected household contact during the first 18 weeks of gestation. Management of these women may include the following:

(1) Determination of susceptibility or acute infection by serum IgG and IgM determinations

(2) For susceptible or acutely infected women, serial fetal ultrasounds to monitor fetal growth and the possible evolution of hydrops

(3) Serial determinations of maternal serum AFP (AFP may rise up to 4 weeks before ultrasound evidence of fetal hydrops [146])

(4) Determination of fetal IgM by percutaneous umbilical blood sampling. The utility of this is questionable given the relatively high risk-benefit ratio at present, especially since it is unclear that obstetrical management will be altered by results. It may be useful to confirm B19 etiology when hydrops fetalis is present [153]

(5) Intrauterine fetal PRBC transfusions when B19 associated hydrops fetalis is present

b. The pregnant school teacher and health care provider. The epidemiology of community outbreaks of erythema infectiosum suggests that the risk of infection to susceptible school teachers is approximately 15 percent (compared with 50 percent for household contacts). This would lower the risk of B19 fetal disease in pregnant school teachers at less than 1 percent. It is not obvious that special precautions are necessary in this setting. In fact, there is likely to be widespread inapparent infection in both adults and children, providing a constant background exposure rate that cannot be altered. Considering the high prevalence of B19, the low risk of severe fetal disease, and the fact that attempts to avoid potential high-risk settings only reduce but do not eliminate exposure, exclusion of pregnant school teachers from the workplace is not recommended [156,157].

A similar approach may be taken for pregnant health care providers where the principal exposure will be from infected children presenting to the emergency room or physician's office. However, in many cases, the typical rash of erythema infectiosum may already be present, at which time transmission to contacts may be low. Furthermore, precautions directed at minimizing exposure to respiratory secretions may be taken to decrease the risk of transmission. Particular care should be exercised on pediatric wards where there are immunocompromised patients or patients with hemolytic anemias in whom B19 disease is suspected. These patients may shed virus well beyond the period of initial clinical symptoms, particularly when presenting with aplastic crisis. In this setting, there may be a significant risk for the spread of B19 to susceptible health care workers or other patients at risk for B19-induced aplastic crisis [158,159]. To minimize this risk, patients with aplastic crises from B19 infections should be maintained on contact precautions, masks should be worn for close contact, and pregnant health care providers should not be permitted to care for these patients [156,157].

II. Perinatal infections

A. Herpes simplex virus

1. Pathogenesis and epidemiology. There are two virologically distinct types of herpes simplex virus (HSV types 1 and 2). HSV-2 is the predominant cause of neonatal disease, but both types produce clinically indistinguishable syndromes. Infection in the newborn occurs as a result of direct exposure, most commonly in the perinatal period from maternal genital disease. The virus can cause localized disease of the skin, eye, or mouth or may disseminate by cell-to-cell contiguous spread or viremia.

After adsorption and penetration into host cells, viral replication proceeds, resulting in cellular swelling, hemorrhagic necrosis, formation of intranuclear inclusions, cytolysis, and cell death [1].
Seroprevalence studies indicate HSV to be highest in the lower socioeconomic groups. Recent studies using type-specific antigen showed the seroprevalence of HSV type 2 to be 35 percent in a middle-class population [2]. The overall occurrence of genital HSV is estimated to be 1 percent in pregnant women, and the majority of cases are recurrent infections [1]. It is estimated that 0.01 to 0.39 percent of women excrete virus at delivery [3]. The incidence of newborn infection with HSV is estimated to be 1:2000 to 1:5000 per year [3].

a. **Intrapartum transmission.** This is the most common cause of neonatal HSV and is primarily associated with active shedding of virus from the cervix at the time of delivery. Up to 90 percent of newborn infections occur as a result of intrapartum transmission. At least four factors have been identified that relate to intrapartum transmission. First, the amount and duration of maternal virus shedding is likely to be a major determinate of fetal transmission. These are greatest with primary maternal infections. Maternal antibody to HSV is also important and is associated with a decreased risk of fetal transmission. The exact mechanism of action of maternal antibody in preventing perinatal infection is not known, but transplacentally acquired antibody has been shown to reduce the risk of severe newborn disease following postnatal HSV exposure [4,5]. The risk of intrapartum infection increases with ruptured membranes, especially when greater than 6 hours [3]. Finally, direct methods for fetal monitoring, such as scalp electrodes, increase the risk of fetal transmission in the setting of active shedding. Thus it is best to avoid these techniques in women with a history of recurrent infection or suspected of primary HSV disease.

b. **Antenatal transmission.** In utero infection has been documented but is uncommon [1]. Spontaneous abortion has been described with primary maternal infection prior to 20 weeks' gestation, but the true risk to the fetus of early trimester primary infection is not known. Fetal infections may occur by either transplacental or ascending routes and have been documented in the setting of both primary and recurrent maternal disease. There may be a wide range of clinical manifestations from localized skin or eye involvement to multiorgan disease and congenital malformations [6,7]. Chorioretinitis, microcephaly, and hydranencephaly may be found in a small number of cases.

c. **Postnatal transmission.** There is increasing evidence that a significant percentage of neonatal HSV infections result from postnatal exposure. Potential sources include symptomatic and asymptomatic oropharyngeal shedding by either parent, hospital personnel, or other contacts; maternal breast lesions; and nosocomial spread [8–14]. Measures to minimize exposure from these sources are discussed below.

2. **Clinical manifestations.** Data from the NIAID Collaborative Antiviral Study Group indicate that morbidity and mortality of neonatal HSV best correlates with three categories of disease [1]. These are infection localized to the skin, eye, and/or mouth; encephalitis with or without localized mucocutaneous disease; and disseminated infection with multiple organ involvement. Some of the findings of the NIAID Collaborative Antiviral Study Group have recently been summarized for 291 HSV-infected infants [1]. The greatest mortality was seen in infants having disseminated disease; hemorrhagic shock and pneumonitis were the principal causes of death. Of the survivors for whom follow-up was available, significant neurologic sequelae were seen in a high percentage of the infants with encephalitis and disseminated disease. However, neurologic impairment

also occurred in 11 percent of infants with localized mucocutaneous disease despite the absence of clinical CNS disease.

a. **Skin, eye, and mouth infection.** With disease localized to the skin, vesicles typically appear in the second week of neonatal life. Often a cluster of vesicles may develop on the presenting part of the body, where extended direct contact with virus may occur. Vesicles occur in 90 percent of infants with localized mucocutaneous infection, and recurrent disease is common. Furthermore, significant morbidity has been described in these infants despite the absence of signs of disseminated disease at the time of diagnosis; up to 30 percent of infants may show later development of neurologic impairment [15–17], and infants with keratoconjunctivitis may develop chorioretinitis, cataracts, and retinopathy. Ophthalmologic and neurologic follow-up is important in all infants with mucocutaneous HSV.

b. **CNS infection.** Approximately one-third of neonates with HSV present with encephalitis in the absence of disseminated disease, and from 40 to 60 percent of these infants do not have mucocutaneous vesicles [16,18–20]. In the setting of disseminated disease, HSV is thought to invade the CNS from hematogenous spread. However, CNS infection in the absence of disseminated disease probably results from retrograde axonal spread. The latter condition most often occurs in infants having transplacentally derived viral neurtalizing antibodies, which may protect against widespread dissemination but not influence intraneuronal viral replication. Mortality is high without treatment, and approximately 50 percent of surviving infants develop neurodevelopmental impairment. Long-term sequelae from acute HSV encephalitis include microcephaly, hydranencephaly, porencephalic cysts, spasticity, blindness, chorioretinitis, and learning disabilities [1].

c. **Disseminated infection.** This is the most severe form of neonatal HSV. Symptoms usually begin within the first week of neonatal life. The liver, adrenals, and multiple other visceral organs are usually involved. Approximately two-thirds of infants have encephalitis. Clinical findings include seizures, shock respiratory distress, DIC, and pneumonitis. A typical vesicular rash may be absent in up to 20 percent of infants [16,18].

3. **Diagnosis.** HSV should be considered in the differential diagnosis of the ill neonates in a variety of clinical presentations. These include CNS abnormalities, fever, shock, DIC, and/or hepatitis. HSV also should be considered in infants with respiratory distress without an obvious bacterial etiology or clinical course and findings consistent with immature lung disease. The possibility of concomitant HSV infection with other commonly encountered problems of the preterm infant should be considered. Viral isolation in the appropriate clinical setting remains critical to the diagnosis. Serology is of little value, since specific IgM may not be detected for up to 3 weeks. However, the number of different viral antigen-specific antibodies produced seems to correlate with the extent of disseminated disease [21], and the presence of certain antigen-specific antibodies may have long-term prognostic value [22]. With mucocutaneous lesions, scrapings should be made of vesicles, placed in the appropriate viral transport medium and promptly processed for culture by a diagnostic virology laboratory. Virus also may be isolated from the oropharynx and nasopharynx, conjunctivae, stool, and urine. In the absence of a vesicular rash, viral isolation from these sites may aid in the diagnosis of disseminated HSV or HSV encephalitis. With encephalitis, an elevated CSF protein level and pleocytosis are often seen, but initial values may be within normal limits. Thus serial CSF examinations may be very important. Electroencephalography and CT scan are also useful in

the diagnosis of HSV encephalitis. Viral isolation from CSF has been reported to be successful in up to 40 percent of cases [1]. Laboratory abnormalities seen with disseminated disease include elevated hepatic transaminase levels, direct hyperbilirubinemia, neutropenia, thrombocytopenia, and coagulopathy. A diffuse interstitial pattern is usually observed on x-ray with HSV pneumonitis.

4. **Treatment.** Effective antiviral therapy exists for HSV, but the timing of therapy is critical. Treatment is indicated for all forms of HSV disease. Two currently used drugs are the nucleoside analogues vidarabine and acyclovir. The most extensive studies have been carried out with vidarabine, which has been shown to reduce the morbidity and mortality for all forms of neonatal HSV. Unfortunately, with disseminated disease, very high mortality occurs despite therapy. In a collaborative study examining the efficacy of vidarabine in the treatment of neonatal HSV [23], therapy reduced the mortality from disseminated disease from 90 to 70 percent. The mortality with encephalitis was reduced from 50 to 15 percent. The optimal dose is 30 mg/kg per day administered IV over 12 hours for a total of 14 days. Preliminary results from the NIAID Collaborative Antiviral Study Group indicate that acyclovir may be as efficacious as vidarabine for the treatment of neonatal HSV. Furthermore, acyclovir is a selective inhibitor of viral replication with minimal side effects on the host. It can be administered in relatively small volumes over short infusion times. Thus acyclovir has become favored in the treatment of neonatal HSV. The frequently used dose is 10 mg/kg every 8 hours.

5. **Management of the newborn at risk for HSV.** The principal problem in developing strategies for the prevention of HSV transmission is the inability to identify maternal excretion of virus at the time of delivery. Viral identification requires isolation in tissue culture, so any attempt to identify women who may be shedding HSV at delivery would require antenatal cervical cultures. Unfortunately, such screening cultures taken prior to labor fail to predict active excretion at delivery [24].

   Until more rapid techniques are made available for the identification of HSV, the only clear recommendation that can be made is to deliver infants by cesarean section if genital lesions are present at the start of labor. The efficacy of this approach may diminish when membranes are ruptured beyond 4 hours. Nevertheless, it is generally recommended that cesarean section be considered even with longer durations of membrane rupture, although data showing efficacy beyond 4 hours are lacking. The upper time limit for membrane rupture has been suggested to be 12 hours [25] to 24 hours [1]. For women with a history of prior genital herpes, careful examination should be performed to determine if lesions are present when labor commences. If lesions are observed, cesarean section should be carried out. If no lesions are identified vaginal delivery is appropriate, but cervical cultures should be obtained. At this time there are no data to support the prophylactic use of antiviral agents or immunoglobulin to prevent transmission to the newborn infant.

   Infants inadvertently delivered vaginally in the setting of cervical lesions should be isolated from other infants in the nursery, and cultures should be obtained from the oropharynx/nasopharynx and conjunctivae. The optimal time for culturing is 24 hours; cultures taken at earlier times may simply reflect transient contamination. Cultures should be repeated in another 48 to 72 hours and, if possible, several additional times over the next 2 weeks. Parents should be instructed to consult their pediatrician with the development of a rash or other clinical changes (lethargy, tachypnea, poor feeding, etc.), and weekly pediatric follow-up during the first month is recommended. Infants with a positive culture from any site or the evolution of clinical symptomatology should immediately have cultures repeated and antiviral therapy initiated. These infants should be evaluated for possible disseminated and CNS infection as well.

Currently, there is no indication for isolation of newborn infants from mothers with genital and/or recurrent mucocutaneous HSV. Careful hand washing and preventing the infant from having direct contact with lesions should be emphasized. Breast-feeding should be avoided if there are breast lesions [10–12].

Hospital personnel with orolabial HSV represent a low risk to the newborn, although the use of face masks can be recommended if active lesions are present. Of course, hand washing should again be emphasized. The exception to these guidelines is nursery personnel with herpetic whitlows. These individuals should not care for newborn infants because they have a high risk of viral shedding, and transmission can occur despite the use of gloves [1].

B. **Varicella-zoster virus.** The causative agent of varicella (chickenpox) is a member of the herpesvirus family. The same agent is believed to be responsible for herpes zoster (shingles). Hence this virus is now referred to as **varicella-zoster virus (V-Z virus)** [160]. Chickenpox results from primary V-Z virus infection, following which the virus may remain latent in sensory nerve ganglia. Zoster results from reactivation of latent virus later in life.

There are approximately 3 million cases of varicella yearly in the United States, primarily occurring in school-age children [160]. The majority of adults have antibodies to V-Z virus, indicating prior infection, even when there is thought to be no prior history of chickenpox. It follows that varicella is an uncommon occurrence in pregnancy. The precise incidence of gestational varicella is uncertain but has been estimated to be 0.8 to 5 per 10,000 [160]. Alternatively, zoster is primarily a disease of adults. The incidence of zoster in pregnancy is also unknown, but the disease is likely to be uncommon as well.

1. **Transmission.** It appears that the primary mode of transmission of V-Z virus is through respiratory droplets from patients with chickenpox. Spread through contact with vesicular lesions also may occur. Typically, individuals with chickenpox are contagious from 1 to 2 days before and 5 days after the onset of rash. Conventionally, a patient is no longer considered contagious when all vesicular lesions have dryed and crusted over. The incubation period for primary disease extends from 10 to 21 days, with most infections occurring between 13 and 17 days. Transplacental transfer of V-Z virus may take place in pregnancy, presumably secondary to maternal viremia, but the frequency of this event is unknown. Interestingly, maternal zoster in pregnancy also may result in fetal infection, although this is likely to be an uncommon event.

2. **Perinatal varicella.** Varicella may occur in approximately 25 percent of newborn infants whose mothers developed varicella within the peripartum period. The onset of disease usually occurs 13 to 15 days after the onset of maternal rash. Rarely neonatal disease has been observed to occur within 3 days of maternal rash, and the maximum incubation period has been 16 days (mean incubation of 11 days) [161]. When the newborn develops rash within 10 days, it is presumed to result from in utero transmission. The greatest risk for severe disease is seen when maternal varicella occurs within 4 days of delivery [161]. In these cases there is insufficient time for the acquisition by the fetus of transplacentally derived V-Z virus-specific antibodies. Symptoms generally begin 5 to 10 days after delivery, and the expected mortality is approximately 30 percent.

3. **Congenital varicella.** When in utero transmission of V-Z virus occurs prior to the peripartum period, there is no obvious clinical impact on the fetus in the majority of cases. However, three possible conditions related to congenital varicella deserve comment.

   a. **Varicella-associated chromosomal abnormalities.** It appears that chromosomal abnormalities may be common in varicella [162]. Although these are thought to be transient without adverse effects on the host, the possibility of more permanent abnormalities following in utero fetal infection has been suggested. Possible consequences include a higher incidence of childhood leukemia [163], but it must be emphasized that there are insufficient data to indicate the incidence of persistent chromosomal abnormalities or to confirm an increase in related disorders later in life.

b. **Congenital malformations.** Despite retrospective and prospective studies, it is unclear that there is an increased risk of congenital malformations with maternal V-Z virus infection in pregnancy [160,164]. Nevertheless, there is a strong association between gestational varicella and a spectrum of congenital defects comprising a unique syndrome [165,166]. Characteristic findings include cicatricial skin lesions, ocular defects, CNS abnormalities, intrauterine growth retardation, and early death. The syndrome most commonly occurs with maternal V-Z virus infection in weeks 7 to 20 of gestation [160]. It is primarily seen with gestational varicella but also can occur with maternal zoster.

3. **Zoster.** Zoster is uncommon in young infants but may occur as a consequence of in utero fetal infection with V-Z virus [167]. Similarly, children who develop zoster but have no prior history of varicella most likely acquired V-Z virus in utero. Zoster in childhood is usually self-limiting, with only symptomatic therapy indicated in otherwise healthy children.
4. **Postnatal varicella.** Varicella acquired in the newborn period as a result of postnatal exposure is generally a mild disease [160]. Rarely, severe disseminated disease may occur in newborn infants exposed shortly after birth. In these instances, treatment with acyclovir may be beneficial (see below).
5. **Diagnosis.** Infants with congenital varicella resulting from in utero infection occurring before the peripartum period do not shed virus, and the determination of V-Z virus-specific antibodies is often confusing. Thus the diagnosis is made on the basis of clinical findings and maternal history. With neonatal disease, the presence of a typical vesicular rash and a maternal history of peripartum varicella or postpartum exposure are all that is required to make the diagnosis. Laboratory confirmation can be made by (1) culture of vesicular fluid, although the sensitivity of this method is not optimal because the virus is quite labile, (2) demonstration of a four-fold rise in V-Z virus antibody titer by the FAMA (fluorescent antibody to membrane antigen) assay or by an enzyme-linked immunosorbent assay (ELISA). Antigen also may be detected in vesicular fluid by countercurrent immunoelectrophoresis, which is very sensitive and specific. Alternatively, indirect immunofluorescence may be used for rapid detection of virus from vesicular material.
6. **Treatment.** Infants with congenital infection, resulting from in utero transmission before the peripartum period, are unlikely to have active viral disease, so antiviral therapy is not indicated. However, infants with perinatal varicella acquired from maternal infection near the time of delivery are at risk for severe disease. In this setting, therapy with acyclovir is generally recommended. Data are not available on the most efficacious and safe dose of acyclovir for the treatment of neonatal varicella, but minimal toxicity has been shown with the administration of 30 mg/kg per day (divided q8h) for the treatment of neonatal herpes simplex virus. This dose given over 7 days may be efficacious for uncomplicated varicella, but a higher dose of 1500 mg/m^2 over a longer duration may be more appropriate for severe (disseminated) disease.

   At the present time, there is no established immunotherapy for the treatment of V-Z virus infections, but varicella-zoster immune globulin (VZIG) may be of prophylactic value. VZIG has been shown to be effective in preventing or attenuating V-Z virus infection when administered within 72 hours of exposure [168]. The dose for newborn infants is 125 U IM (see **7.b(2)**).

7. **Management of varicella in the nursery.** The risk of horizontal spread of varicella following exposure in the nursery appears to be low, possibly due to a combination of factors [160]. These include (1) passive protection due to transplacentally derived antibody in infants born to varicella-immune mothers and (2) brief exposure in most cases with a lack of intimate contact. Nevertheless, nursery outbreaks do occur, so steps should be taken to minimize the risk of nosocomial spread. The infected infant should be isolated in a separate room, and visitors and caretakers should be limited to individuals with a prior history of varicella. A new gown should be worn upon entering the room, and good hand washing should be used. Bedding and other materials should be bagged and sterilized. VZIG may be given to all other exposed neonates, but this may be withheld in full-term infants whose mothers have a prior history of varicella. Exposed personnel without a history of prior varicella should be tested for V-Z virus antibodies, and patient care by these individuals should be restricted as outlined in **7.a** below.

   In the regular nursery, all exposed infants will ordinarily be discharged home before they could become infectious. Occasionally, an exposed infant needs to remain in the nursery for more than 8 days, and in this circumstance, isolation may be required. In the special care nursery, exposed neonates are generally cohorted and isolated from new admissions within 8 days after exposure.

   Several situations of varicella exposure arise from time to time in the nursery for which the following guidelines may be useful [160]:

   a. **Antepartum exposure in mothers without a prior history of varicella.** The concern here is for women exposed within 21 days prior to admission to the hospital.
      (1) Mother and infant should be discharged as soon as possible from the hospital. If the exposure was from a household contact with current disease, VZIG should be administered to both mother and infant prior to discharge. Alternatively, arrangements to isolate the infectious household contact from the mother and infant may be done prior to discharge.
      (2) If exposure occurred 6 days or less prior to admission and the mother is discharged within 48 hours, no further action is required. Otherwise, mothers hospitalized between 8 to 21 days after exposure should be kept isolated from the nursery and other patients.
      (3) Personnel without a prior history of varicella should be kept from contact with a potentially infectious mother. If such an individual is inadvertently exposed, serologic testing (FAMA or ELISA) should be performed to determine susceptibility, and further contact should be avoided until immunity is proven. If the mother at risk for infection has not developed varicella for 48 hours after the staff member was exposed, no further action is required. Alternatively, if a susceptible staff member is exposed to any individual with active varicella lesions or in whom a varicella rash erupts within 48 hours of the exposure, contact with any patients should be restricted for that staff member from day 8 through day 21 after exposure.

   b. **Maternal varicella.** Of concern are mothers with active disease while in the hospital or in whom varicella has occurred within 21 days prior to delivery.
      (1) Resolution of the infectious stage prior to hospitalization
         (a) Maternal isolation is not required.
         (b) Isolate the newborn infant from other infants (room in with mother).
      (2) Active varicella lesions on admission to the hospital
         (a) Isolate mother.

(b) Administer VZIG (125 U IM) to newborn infant if maternal disease began less than 5 days before delivery or within 2 days postpartum [169,170]. (not 100% effective) [198,199]

(c) Isolate infant from mother until she is no longer infectious.

(d) If other neonates were exposed, VZIG may be administered and these infants may require isolation if they are still hospitalized by day 8 after exposure.

C. **Hepatitis.** Acute viral hepatitis is defined by the following clinical criteria [178]: (1) symptoms consistent with viral hepatitis, (2) elevation of serum aminotransferase levels to >2.5 times the upper limit of normal, and (3) the absence of other causes of liver disease. At least five agents have been identified as causes of viral hepatitis. These are hepatitis A virus (HAV), hepatitis B virus (HBV), hepatitis D virus (HDV), posttransfusion non-A, non-B hepatitis virus (NANB), and epidemic non-A, non-B hepatitis (Ep-NANB) [171]. It now appears that the major cause of posttransfusion NANB hepatitis is a flavivirus-like agent called hepatitis C (HCV) [171–173]. HDV, also referred to as the **delta agent,** is a defective virus that may require coinfection or superinfection with HBV [171,173]. HDV is coated with hepatitis B surface antigen (HBsAG). Specific antibodies to HDV can be detected in infected individuals, but there is no known therapy to prevent infection in exposed HBsAG-positive patients. For the newborn infant, therapy directed at the prevention of HBV infection also should prevent HDV, since coinfection is required.

1. **HAV.** This virus is spread by the fecal-oral route and can be detected by the presence of hepatitis A antigen (HAAg) in stool or by the presence of anti-HAV antibody. Anti-HAV IgG is present very early in infection and may already be significantly elevated at the time of clinical diagnosis. Thus a fourfold rise in IgG, ordinarily diagnostic of acute infection, may be difficult to demonstrate. However, specific IgM can be determined [174]. The usual incubation period for HAV is approximately 4 weeks (range 15 to 50 days). Symptoms include fever, malaise, anorexia, nausea, abdominal discomfort, dark urine, and jaundice [173]. Infectivity typically diminishes rapidly. Prophylaxis against HAV is recommended primarily for travelers to developing countries or individuals at risk from personal contact with infected patients [173].

   Studies of acute hepatitis in pregnancy have failed to demonstrate fetal transmission of HAV [175,176], although an increase in preterm deliveries may occur [177]. Nevertheless, acute maternal HAV infection near the peripartum period poses a threat to the neonate. **It is recommended that infants born to a mother who developed acute HAV infection within 2 weeks of delivery receive an injection of 0.5 ml immune serum globulin IM** [171]. Measures also should be taken to minimize fecal-oral spread of virus from the infected mother to her newborn infant and within the nursery. Of particular importance here are the appropriate disposal of contaminated materials and good hand washing practices.

2. **HBV.** This virus is one of the most common causes of acute and chronic hepatitis worldwide. In endemic populations, the carrier state is high and perinatal transmission is a common event. The risk of chronic infection is inversely proportional to age, with a 90 percent carriage rate following infection in neonates. The overall incidence of HBV infections in the United States is relatively low but still substantial. There is estimated to be approximately 300,000 infections yearly, with 250 deaths from fulminate disease [173]. As many as 1 million individuals are chronic carriers, approximately 25 percent of whom develop chronic active hepatitis. Patients with chronic active hepatitis are at increased risk for developing cirrhosis and hepatocellular carcinoma, and approximately 5000 of these patients die each year from HBV-related hepatic complications (primarily cirrhosis) [173]. The incubation period for HBV infection is approximately 120 days (range 45 to 160 days). Transmission occurs by percutaneous or

permucosal routes from infected blood or body fluids. Symptoms include anorexia, malaise, nausea, vomiting, abdominal pain, and jaundice [173].

a. **High-risk groups** for HBV infection in the United States [173] include the following:
   (1) Persons born in endemic areas: Alaskan natives and Pacific Islanders and natives of China, Southeast Asia, most of Africa, parts of the Middle East, the Amazon Basin
   (2) Descendants of individuals from endemic areas
   (3) Persons with high-risk behavior: homosexual activity, intravenous drug abuse, and multiple sexual partners
   (4) Close contacts with HBV-infected persons (sexual partners, family members)
   (5) Selected patient populations, particularly those receiving multiple blood or blood product transfusions
   (6) Selected occupational groups, including health care providers
b. **Diagnosis.** The diagnosis is made by specific serology and by the detection of viral antigens. The specific tests are as follows:
   (1) Hepatitis B surface antigen (HBsAG) determination: usually found 1 to 2 months after exposure; lasts a variable period of time
   (2) Anti-HB surface antigen (anti-HBs): appears after resolution of infection; provides long-term immunity
   (3) Anti-HB core antigen (anti-HBc): present in all HBV infections; lasts for an indefinite period of time
   (4) Anti-HBc IgM: appears early in infection; detectable for 4 to 6 months after infection; good marker for acute or recent infection
   (5) HB e antigen (HBeAG): present in both acute and chronic infections; correlates with viral replication and **high** infectivity
   (6) Anti-HB e antigen (anti-HBe): develops with resolution of viral replication; correlates with reduction in infectivity
   Infectivity correlates best with HBeAG positivity, but any patient positive for HBsAG is potentially infectious. Acute infection can be diagnosed by the presence of clinical symptoms and a positive HBsAG or anti-HBc IgM. The **chronic carrier state** is defined as the presence of HBsAG on two occasions, 6 months apart, or the presence of HBsAG without anti-HBc IgM [173].
c. **Prevention of HBV infection in the neonate.** The transmission of HBV from infected mothers to their newborn infants is thought to result primarily from exposure to maternal blood at the time of delivery. Transplacental transfer appears to occur in Taiwan, but this has not been found in other parts of the world, including the United States [171]. In Taiwan there is a high chronic carrier rate that may be related to the transplacental transfer observed in that country. When acute maternal HBV infection occurs in the first and second trimesters of pregnancy, there generally is little risk to the newborn infants, since antigenemia is usually cleared by term and anti-HBs is present. Acute maternal HBV infection in late pregnancy or near the time of delivery, however, may result in 50 to 75 percent transmission [179,180].
   The principal strategy for the prevention of neonatal HBV disease has been to immunoprophylax newborn infants at high risk for infection. Vaccination of these infants is also an important part of perinatal prevention and safeguards against postnatal exposure as well. Immunization of infants has been shown to effectively reduce the risk of chronic HBV infection in Taiwan [181]. Ultimately, universal immunization of infants promises to be one of the best options for disease control in the United States [182]. Other methods of disease control have been considered and include delivery by cesarean section. In one study in Taiwan, cesarean section in conjunction with maternal immunization dramatically reduced the incidence of perinatally ac-

quired HBV from highly infective mothers [183]. These results are promising and may offer a potential adjunctive therapy for very high risk situations (e.g., HBsAG/HBe-positive women). Currently, no specific recommendations can be made regarding mode of delivery.

It is recommended that all women be screened for HBsAG in pregnancy [173]. Screening should be done early in gestation. If the test is negative, no further evaluation is recommended unless there is a potential exposure history. With any concern about a possible infectious contact, development of acute hepatitis, or high-risk behavior in a nonimmunized woman, repeated testing should be performed. **All infants born to mothers confirmed to be positive for HBsAG should receive hepatitis B immune globulin (HBIG) and hepatitis B vaccine. Vaccine should also be given to all infants born to women originating from endemic areas** (see **a.(1)**). For the latter population, HBIG also should be given unless the mother is found to be HBsAG-negative. The dose for both HBIG and vaccine is 0.5 ml IM. The best injection site is the anterolateral thigh muscle, with one injection per thigh. Immunization with vaccine should be repeated at 1 and 6 months. If the maternal HBsAG status is unknown at delivery, testing should be performed as soon as possible.

Postnatal transmission of HBV by the fecal-oral route probably occurs, but the risk appears to be small. Nevertheless, this possibility adds further support to the need for the immunization of infants born to HBsAG-positive women. Another potential route of infection is by means of breast milk. This mode of transmission appears to be very uncommon in developed countries; there has been no documented increase in the risk of HBV transmission by breast-feeding mothers who are HBsAG-positive [171,189]. This is true even though HBsAG can be detected in breast milk. Recommendations regarding breast-feeding in developed countries should be individualized depending on how strongly breast-feeding is desired by the mother. The risk is certain to be negligible in infants who have received HBIG and hepatitis vaccine.

d. **Prevention of nosocomial spread.** HBsAG-positive infants pose a definite risk for nosocomial spread in the nursery [171]. To minimize this risk, nursery personnel are advised to wear gloves and gowns when caring for infected infants. Of course, universal precautions should currently be in effect in all nurseries (see **I.C.7**), so the risk of exposure to blood and body secretions already should be minimized. Immunization of health care workers is also strongly recommended, but if exposure should occur in a nonimmunized person, hepatitis serology should be sent and HBIG administered as soon as possible unless the individual is known to be anti-HBs-positive [173,189]. This should apply to personnel having close contact without appropriate precautions as well as those suffering a parenteral exposure (e.g., from a contaminated needle stick).

3. **NANB hepatitis.** The diagnosis of NANB hepatitis is made by the clinical picture of viral hepatitis in patients without serologic evidence of HAV or HBV. At least two clinical types of infection are seen. These are posttransfusion NANB and epidemic NANB. Posttransfusion NANB hepatitis may actually be transmitted by means other than blood transfusions. High-risk groups include transfusion recipients, parenteral drug users, and dialysis patients [173]. NANB hepatitis accounts for 20 to 40 percent of viral hepatitis in the United States. The incubation period ranges from weeks to months. Clinically, there is often a less fulminate and chronic course compared with HBV. Serum aminotransferases may fluctuate or remain chronically elevated for up to 1 year. Approximately 20 percent of patients may develop cirrhosis. Recently, a cDNA clone of a blood-borne

NANB viral hepatitis genome has been isolated, and a polypeptide was produced and incorporated into an immunoassay [171,184–186]. It now appears that this NANB virus, referred to as **hepatitis C virus (HCV),** may account for as much as 85 percent of transfusion-associated NANB viral hepatitis [187]. We are currently screening all donor blood for anti-HCV antibody (see page 365).

Epidemic NANB viral hepatitis (Ep-NANB) is primarily spread by fecal-contaminated water supplies. Epidemics have been documented in parts of Asia, Africa, and Mexico [173,188]. The agent does not appear to be endemic to the United States, but shellfish have been implicated as sources of infection. The clinical picture in infected individuals is similar to that of HAV except that there is a high mortality in pregnancy.

The efficacy of immunoglobulin prophylaxis against either form of NANB hepatitis is unknown. Maternal-infant transmission probably does occur, so empirical prophylaxis appears reasonable [171]. **Infants born to women with acute NANB hepatitis in the third trimester or perinatal period should receive immune serum globulin 0.5 ml IM.**

D. Enteroviruses

1. **Viruses.** The enteroviruses are ribonucleic acid (RNA) viruses belonging the genus *Picornaviridae* [190,191]. They are classified into four major groups: coxsackieviruses group A, coxsackieviruses group B, echoviruses, and polioviruses. All four groups have been reported to cause disease in the neonate. Infections occur throughout the year, with a peak incidence between July and November. The viruses are shed from the upper respiratory and gastrointestinal tracts. In most children and adults, infections are asymptomatic or produce a nonspecific febrile illness.
2. **Perinatal infection.** Most infections in newborn infants are caused by coxsackieviruses B and echoviruses. The mode of transmission appears to be primarily transplacental, although this is less well understood for echoviruses. Clinical manifestations are most commonly seen with transmission in the perinatal period.

   Symptoms in the newborn infant often appear within the first week postpartum. Clinical presentations vary from a mild nonspecific febrile illness to severe life-threatening disease. Krajden and Middleton [192] reported three major clinical presentations in a group of neonates with enterovirus infections. Approximately 50 percent had meningoencephalitis, 25 percent had myocarditis, and 25 percent had a sepsis-like illness. The mortality was lowest for the group with meningoencephalitis (approximately 10 percent). Of the infants with myocarditis, a mortality of approximately 50 percent was noted, but the mortality from the sepsis-like illness was essentially 100 percent. Similar results were noted in more recent reviews, except that the incidence of myocarditis appears to much lower [190,193]. A recent study also showed that the majority (70 percent) of severe enteroviral infections in neonates were caused by echovirus 11 [194].
3. **Diagnosis.** The primary task in symptomatic enterovirus infections is differentiating between viral and bacterial sepsis and meningitis. In almost all cases, presumptive therapy for possible bacterial disease must be initiated. Obtaining a careful history of a recent maternal viral illness, especially during the summer and fall months, may be helpful. The principal diagnostic laboratory aid generally available at this time is viral culture. Cultures should be obtained from nose, throat, stool, blood, urine, and CSF. Usually, evidence of viral growth can be detected within 1 week, although a longer time is required in some cases.
4. **Treatment.** In general, treatment of symptomatic enteroviral disease in the newborn infant is supportive only. There are no specific antiviral agents known to be effective against enteroviruses. However, protection against severe neonatal disease appears to correlate with the presence of

specific transplacentally derived antibody [190,195]. Furthermore, the administration of hyperimmune serum globulin appears to be beneficial in patients with agammaglobulinemia suffering from chronic enteroviral infection [196]. Given these observations, **it has been recommended that high-dose immune serum globulin be given to infants with severe, life-threatening enterovirus infections** [190]. **It may also be beneficial to delay the time of delivery if acute maternal enteroviral infection is suspected, provided there are no maternal or fetal contraindications** [197]. The clinical presentation in infants with a sepsis-like syndrome frequently evolves into shock, fulminate hepatitis with hepatocellular necrosis, and disseminated intravascular coagulation. This expectation dictates close monitoring with early interventions for any signs of cardiovascular instability and coagulopathy. In the initial stages of treatment, broad-spectrum antibiotic therapy is indicated for possible bacterial sepsis. Later, with the recognition of progressive viral disease, some form of antibiotic prophylaxis to suppress intestinal flora may be helpful. Neomycin (25 mg/kg every 6 hours) has been recommended [190].

5. **Nosocomial spread.** Nursery outbreaks of enterovirus infections have been well documented [191]. Several approaches to controlling the spread of virus in the nursery have been proposed. These include the administration of immune serum globulin to all infants in the nursery and closing the nursery to new admissions. These extreme measures are controversial. It has been suggested that emphasizing good hand washing and cohorting of infected infants may be adequate [191].

References

1. Whitley, R. J. Herpes Simplex Virus Infections. In J. S. Remmington and J. O. Klein (Eds.), *Infectious Diseases of the Fetus and Newborn Infant,* 3d Ed. Philadelphia: Saunders, 1990. P. 282.
2. Nahmias, A. J., et al. Prevalence of Herpes Simplex Virus (HSV) Type-Specific Antibodies in a USA Prepaid Group Medical Practice Population. Sixth International Meeting of the International Society for STD Research, London, England (Abstract No. 112), 1985.
3. Nahmias, A. J., Keyserling, K. L., and Kerrick, C. M. Herpes Simplex. In J. S. Remington and J. O. Klein (Eds.), *Infectious Diseases of the Fetus and Newborn Infant.* Philadelphia: Saunders, 1983, P. 638.
4. Yeager, A. S., et al. *Infect. Immun.* 29: 532, 1980.
5. Prober, C. G. *N. Engl. J. Med.* 316: 240, 1987.
6. Hutto, C., et al. *J. Pediatr.* 110: 97, 1987.
7. Florman, A. L., et al. *JAMA* 225: 129, 1973.
8. Linnemann, C. C., et al. *Lancet* 1: 964, 1978.
9. Hammerberg, O., et al. *Pediatr. Infect. Dis.* 2: 290, 1983.
10. Sullivan-Bolyai, J. Z., et al. *Pediatrics* 71: 455, 1983.
11. Dunkle, L. M., et al. *Pediatrics* 63: 150, 1979.
12. Kibrick, S. *Pediatrics* 64: 390, 1979.
13. Yeager, A. S., et al. *J. Pediatr.* 103: 905, 1983.
14. Douglas, J. M., et al. *J. Pediatr.* 103: 908, 1983.
15. Grossman, J. H., et al. *Obstet. Gynecol.* 58: 1, 1981.
16. Whitley, R. J., et al. *J. Infect. Dis.* 158: 109, 1988.
17. Mizrahi, E. M., et al. *Neurology* 31: 164, 1981.
18. Arvin, A. M., et al. *J. Pediatr.* 100: 715, 1982.
19. Whitley, R. J., et al. *Pediatr. Rev.* 7: 119, 1985.
20. Yeager, A. S., et al. *Pediatrics* 73: 188, 1984.
21. Sullender, W. M., et al. *J. Infect. Dis.* 155: 28, 1987.
22. Kahlon, J., et al. *J. Infect. Dis.* 158: 925, 1988.

23. Whitley, R. J., et al. *Pediatrics* 66: 495, 1980.
24. Arvin, A. M., et al. *N. Engl. J. Med.* 315: 796, 1986.
25. Freij, B. J., et al. *Clinics in Perinatology,* 15: 203, 1989.
26. Stagno, S. Cytomegalovirus. In J. S. Remmington and J. O. Klein (Eds.), *Infectious Diseases of the Fetus and Newborn Infant,* 3d Ed. Philadelphia: Saunders, 1990. P. 241.
27. Congenital Cytomegalovirus. In J. B. Hanshaw, J. A. Dudgeon, and W. C. Marshall (Eds.), *Viral Diseases of the Fetus and Newborn,* 2d Ed. Philadelphia: Saunders, 1985. P. 92.
28. Stagno, S., et al. *JAMA* 256: 1904, 1986.
29. Stagno, S., et al. *Pediatrics* 69: 646, 1982.
30. McCracken, G. J., et al. *Am. J. Dis. Child.* 117: 522, 1969.
31. Pass, R. F., et al. *Pediatrics* 66: 758, 1980.
32. Williamson, W. D., et al. *Am. J. Dis. Child.* 136: 902, 1982.
33. Berenberg, W., et al. *Pediatrics* 37: 403, 1970.
34. Saigal, S., et al. *Am. J. Dis. Child.* 136: 896, 1982.
35. Pearl, K. N., et al. *Arch. Dis. Child.* 61: 232, 1986.
36. Stagno, S., et al. *N. Engl. J. Med.* 302: 1073, 1980.
37. Yeager, A. S. *Am. J. Dis. Child.* 128: 478, 1974.
38. Yeager, A. S., et al. *J. Pediatr.* 98: 281, 1981.
39. Yeager, A. S., et al. *Pediatrics* 102: 918, 1983.
40. Paryani, S. G., et al. *J. Pediatr.* 107: 451, 1985.
41. Whitley, R. J., et al. *J. Pediatr.* 89: 11, 1976.
42. Stagno, S., et al. *Pediatrics* 68: 322, 1981.
43. Rutter, D., et al. *Lancet* 2: 1182, 1985.
44. Brasfield, D. M., et al. *Pediatrics* 79: 76, 1987.
45. Adler, S. P. *Rev. Infect. Dis.* 5: 977, 1983.
46. Pass, M. A., et al. *J. Pediatr.* 89: 646, 1976.
47. Adler, S. P., et al. *Pediatr. Infect. Dis.* 2: 114, 1983.
48. Ballard, R. B., et al. *Am. J. Dis. Child.* 133: 482, 1979.
49. Brady, M. T., et al. *J. Infect. Dis.* 150: 334, 1984.
50. Shuster, E. A., et al. *Mayo Clin. Proc.* 60: 577, 1985.
51. Alpert, G., et al. *J. Infect. Dis.* 152: 631, 1985.
52. Stirk, P. R., et al. *J. Med. Virol.* 21: 329, 1987.
53. Collaborative DHPG Treatment Study Group. *N. Engl. J. Med.* 314: 801, 1986.
54. Elek, S. D., and Stern, H. *Lancet* 1: 1, 1974.
55. Plotkin, S. A. *Infect. Immun.* 12: 521, 1975.
56. Griffiths, P. D., and Baboonian, C. A. *Br. J. Obstet. Gynaecol.* 91: 307, 1984.
57. Peckham, C. S., et al. *Lancet* 1: 1352, 1983.
58. Hunter, K., et al. *J. Obstet. Gynecol.* 145: 269, 1983.
59. Reynolds, D. W., et al. *N. Engl. J. Med.* 289: 1, 1973.
60. Dworsky, M. E., et al. *J. Pediatr.* 101: 440, 1982.
61. Holland, P. V., and Schmitt, P. J. In *Standards for Blood Banks and Transfusion Services,* 12th Ed. Arlington, Va.: Committee on Standards, American Association of Blood Banks, 1987. Pp. 30–31.
62. Pass, R. F., et al. *N. Engl. J. Med.* 314: 1414, 1986.
63. Dworsky, M. E., et al. *N. Engl. J. Med.* 309: 950, 1983.
64. Adler, S. P., et al. *J. Pediatr.* 108: 117, 1986.
65. Friedman, H. M., et al. *Pediatr. Infect. Dis.* 3: 233, 1984.
66. Balfour, C. L., and Balfour, H. H. *JAMA* 256: 1909, 1986.
67. Freij, B. J., et al. *Clin. Perinatol.* 15: 247, 1989.
68. Preblud, S. R., and Alford, C. A. *Rubella.* In J. S. Remmington and J. O. Klein (Eds.), *Infectious Diseases of the Fetus and Newborn Infant,* 3d Ed. Philadelphia: Saunders, 1990. P. 196.
69. Horstmann, D. M. *Clin. Obstet. Gynecol.* 25: 585, 1982.
70. Alford, C. A., and Pass, R. F. *Clin. Perinatol.* 8: 397, 1981.
71. Bart, K. J., et al. *Rev. Infect. Dis.* 7: S177, 1985.
72. Centers for Disease Control. *MMWR* 35: 770, 1986.
73. Centers for Disease Control. *MMWR* 33: 301, 1984.

74. Grangeot-Keros, L., et al. *N. Engl. J. Med.* 313: 1547, 1985.
75. Daffos, F., et al. *Lancet* 2: 1, 1984.
76. Enders, G., and Jonatha, W. *Infection* 15: 162, 1987.
77. Terry, G. M., et al. *Br. Med. J. (Clin. Res.)* 292: 930, 1986.
78. Preblud, S. R., et al. *J. Infect. Dis.* 154: 367, 1986.
79. Tingle, A. J., et al. *J. Infect. Dis.* 152: 606, 1985.
80. Centers for Disease Control. *MMWR* 36: 457, 1987.
81. Nahmias, A. J. *Hosp. Pract.* 9: 65, 1974.
82. Wong-Staal, F. Human Immunodeficiency Viruses and Their Replication. In B. N. Fields and D. M. Knipe (Eds.), *Virology,* 2d Ed. New York: Raven Press, 1990. P. 1529.
83. In R. S. Cotran, V. Kumar, and S. L. Robbins (Eds.), Diseases of Immunity. *Pathological Basis of Disease,* 4th Ed. Philadelphia: Saunders, 1989. P. 224.
84. Ho, D. D., et al. *N. Engl. J. Med.* 317: 278, 1987.
85. Levy, J. A. *JAMA* 261: 2997, 1989.
86. Centers for Disease Control. *MMWR* 37: 51, 1989.
87. Centers for Disease Control. *MMWR* 39: 81, 1990.
88. Centers for Disease Control. *MMWR* 39: 289, 1990.
89. Centers for Disease Control. *MMWR* 39: 110, 1990.
90. Pizzo, P. A. *J. Infect. Dis.* 161: 316, 1990.
91. Hoff, R., et al. *N. Engl. J. Med.* 318: 525, 1988.
92. Ryder, R. W., et al. *N. Engl. J. Med.* 320: 1637, 1989.
93. Report from the American Academy of Neurology AIDS Task Force. *Neurology* 39: 119, 1989.
94. Epstein, L. G., et al. *Ann. Neurol.* 23: S19, 1988.
95. Cumming, P. D., et al. *N. Engl. J. Med.* 321: 941, 1989.
96. Feinkind, L., and Minkoff, H. L. *Clin. Perinatol.* 15: 189, 1988.
97. Scott, G. B., et al. *JAMA* 253: 363, 1985.
98. Blanche, S., et al. *N. Engl. J. Med.* 320: 1643, 1989.
99. Falloon, J., and Pizzo, P. A. Acquired Immunodeficiency Syndrome in the Infant. In J. S. Remmington and J. O. Klein (Eds.), *Infectious Diseases of the Fetus and Newborn Infant,* 3d Ed. Philadelphia: Saunders, 1990. P. 306.
100. Marion, R. W., et al. *J. Dis. Child.* 141: 429, 1987.
101. Menez-Bautista, R., et al. *Am. J. Dis. Child.* 140: 678, 1986.
102. Rubinstein, A., et al. *JAMA* 249: 2350, 1983.
103. Tindall, B., et al. *Arch. Intern. Med.* 148: 945, 1988.
104. Curran, J. W., et al. *Science* 239: 610, 1988.
105. Centers for Disease Control. *MMWR* 36 (Suppl. 7): 1, 1987.
106. Centers for Disease Control. *MMWR* 35: 595, 1986.
107. Scott, G. B., et al. *N. Engl. J. Med.* 321: 1791, 1989.
108. Levy, J. A., et al. *Lancet* 2: 586, 1985.
109. Falloon, J., et al. *J. Pediatr.* 114: 1, 1989.
110. Pahwa, S., et al. *JAMA* 255: 2299, 1986.
111. Rubinstein, A. *Curr. Probl. Pediatr.* 16: 361, 1986.
112. Krasinki, K., et al. *Pediatr. Infect. Dis. J.* 8: 216, 1989.
113. Centers for Disease Control. *MMWR* 38(S7): 1, 1989.
114. Centers for Disease Control. *MMWR* 36: 225, 1987.
115. Krivine, A., et al. *J. Pediatr.* 116: 372, 1990.
116. Eisenstein, B. I. *N. Engl. J. Med.* 322: 178, 1990.
117. Weiblen, B. J., et al. *J. Immunol. Methods* 126: 199, 1990.
118. Weiblen, B. J., et al. *Lancet* 335: 988, 1990.
119. Rogers, M. F., et al. *N. Engl. J. Med.* 320: 1649, 1989.
120. Chadwick, E. G., et al. *J. Infect. Dis.* 160: 954, 1989.
121. Amadori, A., et al. *Pediatr. Infect Dis. J.* 9: 26, 1990.
122. Yarchoan, R., et al. *N. Engl. J. Med.* 321: 726, 1989.
123. Pizźo, P. A., et al. *N. Engl. J. Med.* 319: 889, 1988.
124. Hague, R. A., et al. *Arch. Dis. Child.* 64: 1146, 1989.
125. Volberding, P. A., et al. *N. Engl. J. Med.* 322: 941, 1990.
126. Schmidt, F. A., et al. *N. Engl. J. Med.* 319: 1573, 1988.

127. Fischl, M. A., et al. *N. Engl. J. Med.* 317: 185, 1987.
128. Devash, Y., et al. *Proc. Natl. Acad. Sci. USA* 87: 3445, 1990.
129. Cooley, T. P., et al. *N. Engl. J. Med.* 322: 1340, 1990.
130. Lambert, J. S., et al. *N. Engl. J. Med.* 322: 1333, 1990.
131. Centers for Disease Control. *MMWR* 36(Suppl. 2S): S3, 1987.
132. Centers for Disease Control. *MMWR* 39(RR-1): 1, 1990.
133. Anderson, L. J., and Hurwitz, E. S. *Clin. Perinatol.* 15: 273, 1988.
134. Anderson, M. J., and Cherry, J. D. Parvoviruses. In R. D. Feigen and J. D. Cherry (Eds.), *Textbook of Pediatric Infectious Diseases,* 2d ed. Philadelphia: Saunders, 1987. P. 1646.
135. Chorba, T., Coccia, R., Holman, R. C., et al. *J. Infect. Dis.* 154: 383, 1986.
136. Report of the Fifth Disease Working Party. *Community Dis. Rep.* 84/7: 4, 1984.
137. Ager, E. A., et al. *N. Engl. J. Med.* 275: 1326, 1966.
138. Cohen, B. J., et al. *Ann. Rheum. Dis.* 45: 832, 1986.
139. Lefrere, J. J., Courouce, A. M., Bertrand, Y., et al. *Am. J. Hematol.* 23: 271, 1986.
140. Koch, W. C., et al. *J. Pediatr.* 116: 355, 1990.
141. Kurtzman, G. J., et al. *N. Engl. J. Med.* 317: 287, 1987.
142. Anand, A., Gray, E. S., Brown, T., Clewley, J. P., and Cohen, B. J. *N. Engl. J. Med.* 316: 183, 1987.
143. Weiland, H. T., Vermey-Keers, C., Salimans, M. M., et al. *Lancet* 1: 682, 1987.
144. Woernle, C. H., Anderson, L. J., Tattersall, P., and Davison, J. M. *J. Infect. Dis.* 156: 17, 1987.
145. PHLS Working Party on Fifth Disease. *Community Dis. Rep.* 87/20: 3, 1987.
146. Carrington, D., Gilmore, D. H., Whittle, M. J., et al. *Lancet.* 1: 433, 1987.
147. Naides, S. J., et al. *Prenat. Diagn.* 9: 105, 1989.
148. Cohen, B. J., et al. *J. Hyg. (Camb.)* 91: 113, 1983.
149. Anderson, L. J., et al. *J. Clin. Microbiol.* 24: 522, 1986.
150. Clewley, J. P., Cohen, B. J., and Field, A. N. *J. Med. Virol.* 23: 367, 1987.
151. Clewley, J. P. *J. Clin. Microbiol.* 27: 2647, 1989.
152. Kurtzman, G. L., et al. *N. Engl. J. Med.* 321: 519, 1989.
153. Peters, M. T., and Nicolaides, K. H. *Obstet. Gynecol.* 75: 501, 1990.
154. Metzman, R., et al. *J. Pediatr. Gastroenterol. Nutr.* 9: 112, 1989.
155. Kinney, J. S., et al. *J. Infect. Dis.* 157: 663, 1988.
156. Committee on Infectious Diseases. *Pediatrics* 85: 131, 1990.
157. Centers for Disease Control. *MMWR* 38: 81, 1989.
158. Bell, L. M., et al. *N. Engl. J. Med.* 321: 485, 1989.
159. Evans, J. P., et al. *Br. Med. J.* 288: 681, 1984.
160. Gershon, A. A. Chickenpox, Measles, and Mumps. In J. S. Remmington and J. O. Klein (Eds.), *Infectious Diseases of the Fetus and Newborn Infant,* 3d ed. Philadelphia: Saunders, 1990. P. 395.
161. Meyers, J. D. *J. Infect. Dis.* 129: 215, 1974.
162. Aula, P. *Lancet* 1: 720, 1964.
163. Adelstein, A. M., and Donovan, J. W. *Br. Med. J.* 2: 629, 1972.
164. Siegel, M. *JAMA* 226: 1521, 1973.
165. La Foret, E. G., and Lynch, C. L. *N. Engl. J. Med.* 236: 534, 1947.
166. Srabstein, J. C., et al. *J. Pediatr.* 84: 239, 1974.
167. Hope-Simpson, R. E. *Proc. R. Soc. Med.* 58: 9, 1965.
168. Brunell, P. A., et al. *N. Engl. J. Med.* 180: 1191, 1969.
169. Centers for Disease Control. *MMWR.* 33: 84, 1984.
170. *Report of the Committee on Infectious Diseases,* 20th Ed. Elk Grove, Ill.: American Academy of Pediatrics, 1986. P. 399.
171. Zeldis, J. B., and Crumpacker, C. S. Hepatitis. In J. S. Remmington and J. O. Klein (Eds.), *Infectious Diseases of the Fetus and Newborn Infant,* 3d Ed. Philadelphia: Saunders, 1990. P. 574.
172. Choo, Q. L., et al. *Science* 244: 359, 1989.
173. Centers for Disease Control. *MMWR* 39(RR-2): 1, 1990.
174. Kluge, I. *Acta Med. Scand.* 174: 469, 1963.
175. Stokes, J., Jr., and Neefe, J. R. *JAMA* 127: 144, 1945.
176. Mosley, J. W., et al. *Am. J. Epidemiol.* 87: 539, 1968.

177. Woodson, R. D., and Cahill, K. M. *JAMA* 219: 1191, 1971.
178. Centers for Disease Control. *MMWR* 37: 429, 1988.
179. Schweitzer, I. L., et al. *Am. J. Med.* 55: 762, 1973.
180. Cossart, Y. E. *Postgrad. Med. J.* 50: 334, 1974.
181. Hsu, H.-M., et al. *JAMA* 260: 2231, 1988.
182. West, D. J., et al. *Pediatr. Clin. North Am.* 37: 585, 1990.
183. Lee, S.-D., et al. *Lancet* 2: 833, 1988.
184. Kuo, G., et al. *Science* 244: 362, 1989.
185. Esteban, J. I., et al. *Lancet* 2: 294, 1989.
186. van der Poel, C. L., et al. *Lancet* 2: 297, 1989.
187. Alter, H. J., et al. *N. Engl. J. Med.* 321: 1494, 1990.
188. Velazquez, O., et al. *JAMA* 263: 3281, 1990.
189. *Report of the Committee on Infectious Diseases,* 21st Ed. Edmonston, Ill.: American Academy of Pediatrics, 1988. P. 214.
190. Cherry, J. D. Enteroviruses. In J. S. Remmington and J. O. Klein (Eds.), *Infectious Diseases of the Fetus and Newborn Infant,* 3d Ed. Philadelphia: Saunders, 1990. P. 325.
191. Modlin, J. F. *Clin. Perinatol.* 15: 233, 1988.
192. Krajden, S., and Middleton, P. J. *Clin. Pediatr.* 22: 87, 1983.
193. Morens, D. M. *J. Pediatr.* 92: 374, 1978.
194. Modlin, J. F. *Rev. Infect. Dis.* 8: 918, 1986.
195. Modlin, J. F., et al. *N. Engl. J. Med.* 205: 368, 1981.
196. McKinney, R. E., et al. *Rev. Infect. Dis.* 9: 334, 1987.
197. Modlin, J. F. *Pediatrics* 66: 775, 1980.
198. King S., et al. *Pediatric Inf. Dis.* 5:588, 1986.
199. Danitner, W. *Pediatric Inf. Dis.* 5:582, 1986.

Bacterial and Fungal Infections

Nicholas G. Guerina

I. Bacterial Sepsis and Meningitis [1,160]

A. Introduction. Bacterial sepsis and meningitis continue to be major causes of morbidity and mortality in the newborn infant. This is despite improvements in antimicrobial therapy, advances in neonatal life support measures, and the prompt recognition of perinatal risk factors for infection. Sepsis neonatorum is frequently devastating, with the majority of survivors having significant neurologic sequelae as a consequence of central nervous system involvement, septic shock, or hypoxemia secondary to severe parenchymal lung disease or persistent pulmonary hypertension.

B. Epidemiology. The overall incidence of neonatal sepsis varies between 1 and 8 cases per 1000 live births [1]. Approximately one-third of septic newborn infants develop meningitis. Multiple risk factors for perinatal infection have been identified. These factors can generally be divided between maternal (obstetrical) and neonatal observations.

1. Maternal risk factors. Obstetrical factors include premature onset of labor, premature rupture of membranes (PROM), and maternal peripartum infection. The extent to which these factors increase the likelihood of newborn disease is best illustrated by studies in pregnant women with cervical colonization with group B beta-hemolytic streptococci (GBS). The attack rate for perinatally acquired sepsis in newborn infants born to GBS-colonized women is 1 to 2 percent, but this rate increases to 15.2 percent with premature onset of labor (<37 weeks) [2], 10.7 percent for chorioamnionitis or PROM > 24 hours [2], and 9.7 percent for maternal postpartum bacteremia [3]. Overt chorioamnionitis and maternal sepsis are relatively uncommon, so the only maternal indicator of intrauterine infection, aside from preterm labor, may be intrapartum fever. Boyer et al. [4] studied attack rates as a function of peak intrapartum temperature and length of rupture of membranes for GBS disease in 32,384 newborn infants. Their findings are summarized in Table 12-1, along with the attack rates by infant birth weight. The diagnosis of chorioamnionitis is usually manifested by maternal fever. Other findings may be chills, uterine pain and tenderness, foul vaginal discharge, hypotension, maternal tachycardia, and fetal tachycardia. Laboratory evidence of chorioamnionitis may be an elevated maternal white count (>20,000) with the differential showing 90 percent polys and bands. An uncontaminated, unspun sample of amniotic fluid from a febrile labor patient that shows bacteria and polymorphonuclear leucocytes is consistent with the diagnosis of chorioamnionitis. Many times these findings will be present in asymptomatic women who do not have perinatal or postpartum infection. If an amniotic fluid sample from a febrile labor patient shows no bacteria or polys, the diagnosis of chorioamnionitis can usually be excluded. The exceptions to this are infections of the placenta from maternal sepsis or ascending infections that reach the placenta without infecting amniotic fluid. Culture of the amniotic fluid may be helpful. The most common bacteria found are anaerobic streptococci, *Escherichia coli,* aerobic streptococci, and *Bacteroides* species. If group A streptococcus, *Neisseria gonorrheae,* or *Staphylococcus aureus* are found, they are treated as pathogens. Rarely, *Clostridium* species are found. *Bacteroides* and *Clostridium* may be maternal and neonatal pathogens.

2. **Neonatal risk factors.** The single most important neonatal risk factor is low birth weight. In the study of Boyer et al. [4], the attack rate for sepsis was 26 times greater in infants weighing less than 1000 g compared with those weighing more than 2500 g (see Table 12-1). In other studies, the rate of sepsis was 8 times greater in infants weighing 1000 to 1500 g compared with those weighing 2000 to 2500 g [5], and meningitis occurred from 3 to 17 times more often in those weighing less than 2500 g com-

Table 12-1. Attack rates for perinatally acquired group B streptococcal infections in newborn infants

Risk factor	Attack rate (cases per 1000 live births)	Death rate (of those infected)
Birth Weight (g)		
<1000	26	90
1001–1500	8	25
1501–2000	9	29
2001–2500	4	33
>2500	1	3
Rupture of Membranes (h)		
<6	0.8	33
7–12	1.9	10
13–18	1.5	40
19–24	5.7	27
25–48	8.6	18
>48	10.8	33
Peak Intrapartum Temperature (°C)		
<37.5	1.5	29
>37.5	6.5	17

Source: From Boyer et al. [4]; data from 32,384 newborn infants.

pared with infants weighing more than 2500 g [6]. Considering low birth weight and maternal risk factors [4], an attack rate of 7.6 per 1000 and a mortality rate of 33 percent were observed for the combined risk factors of birth weight less than 2500 g, rupture of membranes (ROM) more than 18 h, and intrapartum maternal temperature greater than 37.5°C [4]. By comparison, infants without these risk factors had an attack rate of 0.6 per 1000 and a mortality rate of 6 percent. Other perinatal risk factors have been recognized (Table 12-2) but they have less certain association with perinatally acquired bacterial infections. An intriguing finding is a substantial increase in the incidence of neonatal GBS disease (35 percent) associated with twin pregnancies in GBS-colonized women [7].

C. **Microbiology and pathogenesis.** Although a variety of bacteria have been isolated from newborn infants with sepsis, the principal etiologic agents are group B beta-hemolytic streptococci (GBS) and ***Escherichia coli.*** In addition, ***Listeria monocytogenes*** and nontypable ***Haemophilus influenzae*** appear to be increasingly common pathogens in neonatal sepsis.

1. **Group B beta-hemolytic streptococci (GBS).** Group B beta-hemolytic streptococcus is the most common cause of neonatal sepsis and meningitis in the United States. Infection most commonly occurs during the first few days of life (early-onset disease), with a mean onset of 20 h [7]. This form of the disease has an incidence of 2 to 4 per 1000. An epidemiologically distinct form of the disease occurs after the first week of life (mean onset 24 days) [7]. This form, referred to as **late-onset disease,** has an incidence of 1 to 2 per 1000.

   a. **Microbiology.** Three major capsular serotypes of GBS have been identified (types I, II, and III). These serotypes may be further divided into subclasses based on serologically distinct polysaccharide and protein antigens isolated from capsular and cell-wall extracts. There is an equal distribution of all three serotypes among isolates from women colonized with GBS. However, the distribution of serotypes

Table 12-2. Major and minor perinatal risk factors for sepsis and meningitis in the asymptomatic newborn infant

Major Risk Factors
ROM > 24 h
Intrapartum maternal fever (>38.0°C [>100.4°F])
Chorioamnionitis
Sustained fetal heart rate > 160 beats/min
Minor Risk Factors
Intrapartum maternal fever (>37.5°C [>99.5°F])
Twin gestation
Prematurity (<37 weeks)
Maternal WBC > 15,000
ROM > 12 h
Tachypnea (<1 h)*
Maternal GBS colonization
Low APGAR (<5 at 1 min)
Low birth weight (<1500 g)
Foul lochia

*Infants with any degree of respiratory distress persisting for more than 1 hour are considered symptomatic, and further evaluation and treatment for R/O sepsis are considered on that basis alone.

isolated from infected neonates depends on the site of infection and age of onset of disease. Nearly equal distribution of serotypes occurs among newborn infants with early-onset sepsis, but 85 to 90 percent of strains isolated from infants with early-onset meningitis or late-onset disease have type III capsules [7].

b. Pathogenesis and host susceptibility. Early-onset disease requires exposure to GBS colonizing the cervix, either from infected amniotic fluid or swallowed inoculum during transit through the vaginal canal. Approximately 15 to 20 percent of women have cervical colonization with GBS in the United States. Alternatively, late-onset disease may occur from maternally or nosocomially acquired organisms. Many studies have been designed to elucidate both host and bacterial factors critical for infection. One of the most significant findings is the correlation between the level of maternally derived capsular antibody and susceptibility of the neonate to infection [8–10]. Although this finding is best demonstrated for disease caused by serotype III, it may also be important for other serotypes, particularly serotype II. Other factors that may contribute to host susceptibility include deficiencies in the alternate and classical complement pathways [11–14] and neutrophil dysfunction [15,16–19].

2. *Escherichia coli K1 (ECK1).* *ECK1* is the second most prevalent cause of neonatal sepsis and meningitis in the United States, but it may actually exceed the incidence of GBS disease in certain regions of the United States and Europe. The overall incidence of *E. coli* infections in the newborn infant is estimated to be 1 to 2 per 1000 live births, and the majority of these infections are caused by strains possessing the K1 polysaccharide capsule [20].

a. Pathogenicity and host susceptibility. As for GBS disease, attempts have been made to identify host and bacterial factors associated with *ECK1* infections. *ECK1* poorly activates the classical complement pathway, so protection depends on antibody-mediated activation of the alternate pathway. Unfortunately, the K1 capsule is a poor immunogen, so virtually no maternally derived antibody is available for the neonate. Other bacterial components may contribute to the virulence of *ECK1,* including the O antigen serotype, hemolysin production, presence of the ColV plasmid, and expression of different classes of filamentous protein structures known as **pili** [21–23].

3. *Listeria monocytogenes.* It is difficult to know the true incidence of listeriosis, but a recently published study of the disease in the United States between the years 1980 and 1982 suggests that the incidence of neonatal infections may be as high as 0.6 per 1000 [24]. The true incidence is difficult to determine because *Listeria* infections have not been reportable. *Listeria* also may be a significant cause of stillbirths and spontaneous abortions. Major epidemics occur, usually associated with contaminated food products [25]. Three major populations are affected in these epidemics: (1) immunosuppressed patients (renal transplant recipients), (2) pregnant women, and (3) neonates (plus fetuses). As in GBS infections, there is both an early-onset (mean age 1.3 days) and a late-onset (mean age 14.0 days) form of the disease [26].

a. Pathogenesis and host susceptibility. Several cellular components of *Listeria* have been isolated and characterized, and some of the effects of these structures on the host immune system have been elucidated in vitro and in experimental animal models [27]. Alternatively, immunocompromised or *Listeria*-sensitive hosts may have defects in their immune system that allow *Listeria* to grow in the host tissues unchecked. The specific immune defects or deficiencies critical to *Listeria* infections in pregnant women and neonates are not completely defined. Both cell-mediated and humoral immunity appear to play roles in resistance to listeriosis. In vitro and in vivo (animal models) studies suggest that cell-mediated immunity may be altered in pregnancy, and the newborn infant may have a defect in macrophate–T-cell interaction [27,28]. Another important aspect of infection in pregnancy relates to the remarkable tropism of *Listeria* for the placenta. Recent studies in an animal model have demonstrated that *Listeria* can grow to high density in the decidua basalis of the placenta and in the fetal chorioallantoic plate [29]. This uncontrolled growth can result in spontaneous abortion or stillbirths and newborn infections by direct spread of *Listeria* to the fetus.

4. **Other bacterial pathogens.** A variety of other bacteria have been isolated from neonates with sepsis. Of these, nontypeable ***Haemophilus influenzae*** has received increasing attention recently [30]. Infection with this organism usually occurs in utero or in the immediate postpartum period. Mortality is high; the overall mortality rate is 55 percent, and it can be as high as 90 percent for newborn infants of less than 30 weeks' gestation.

5. **Nosocomial infections.** Nosocomial bacterial infections are significant problems for the neonate requiring extended care in the special care nursery. This is particularly true for very low birth weight infants. The overall incidence of nosocomial infections in neonates has been reported to be less than 5 percent, but infection rates for individual nurseries have been much higher [31–33]. Beyond the first 1 to 2 weeks of life, the neonate who has remained in the special care nursery is likely to be colonized with perinatally (endogenous) and nosocomially acquired flora. This places the neonate at risk of infection due to coagulase-negative staphylococci, enterococci, *Staphylococcus aureus* (including methacillin-resistant strains), and gram-negative bacteria, including multiply resistant enteric strains. In addition, late-onset disease caused by GBS and *Listeria* must be considered. The most frequently identified factors contributing to nosocomial infections are postnatal age (length of stay in nursery), low birth weight, foreign bodies (intravascular catheters, chest tubes, endotracheal tubes, etc.), nursery crowding, surgery, and prolonged treatment with broad-spectrum antibiotics. Strict isolation procedures should be enforced for all infants colonized or infected with multiply resistant bacteria.

   a. **Coagulase-negative staphylococci.** This organism has been recognized as an important cause of nosocomial bacteremia in the neonate in recent years. It is unclear whether there has actually been an increase in the incidence of coagulase-negative staphylococcal bacteremia or the realization that positive blood cultures represent true infection, not culture contamination [83,84]. This may be influenced, in part, by the changing population of the NICU, with an increase in the proportion of very low birth weight (VLBW) infants. Coagulase-negative staphylococci account for more than 50 percent of bacteremia in the NICU. Generally, many strains (40 to 80 percent) are methacillin-resistant; appropriate therapy for uncomplicated bacteremia is vancomycin 18 mg/kg/dose q24h for prematures under 29 weeks, 15 mg/kg/dose q12h for prematures between 30 to 36 weeks, 10 mg/kg/dose q8h for infants between 37 to 44 weeks, and 10 mg/kg/dose q6h for infants over 44 weeks. Treatment is usually given for 7 to 10 days. Central venous lines and intralipid infusions are significant risk factors for coagulase-negative staphylococcal infections [84,85] (see Appendix A).

D. **Evaluation and treatment—antenatal.** Evaluation and treatment of neonatal sepsis commonly begins in utero, especially in the presence of established obstetrical risk factors for infection. It is clear that the fetus at very high risk for infection should be delivered. However, the true risk of perinatally acquired bacterial infection is often difficult to assess, and the risk of other intrapartum or postnatal complications to the preterm infant must be considered.

1. **Preterm labor.** Although there are many noninfectious causes of preterm labor, the possibility of evolving bacterial disease must always be considered. Fetal activity and status of the mother must be carefully assessed. In the absence of fetal distress, signs or symptoms of chorioamnionitis, or any other developing maternal condition, it is often preferred to arrest labor with tocolysis. This is particularly true in early third-trimester pregnancies, where the high morbidity and mortality of very low birth weight infants obviates against delivery. Alternatively, delivery may be the best option for older fetuses, especially if there are maternal complications (pregnancy-induced hypertension, toxemia, etc.) or an uncertain fetal status (decelerations, decreased fetal movement, etc.) (see Chap. 3).
   a. **Antenatal steroids.** One of the most controversial issues in the management of preterm labor is the use of steroids to induce fetal lung maturation. In the presence of intact membranes, steroids have been shown to decrease the incidence of respiratory distress syndrome (RDS) in preterm newborn infants [34]. One argument against the use of steroids is the possibility of masking intrauterine infections, but there are little data to support this concept in the setting of intact membranes. Amniocentesis, to obtain amniotic fluid for the determination of fetal pulmonary maturation indices, may aid the obstetrician in his or her decision to use tocolytics and/or steroids (see Chap. 13).
   b. **Chemoprophylaxis.** The attack rate for sepsis neonatorum is relatively high (approximately 15 percent) with maternal GBS colonization and preterm labor (under 37 weeks). Thus the prevention of intrapartum transmission of GBS to the fetus and newborn has received much attention. Boyer and Gotoff [35] studied the prevention of GBS disease in neonates by selective intrapartum and postpartum chemoprophylaxis. Their experimental design and results are shown in Table 12-3. Intrapartum ampicillin, followed by limited postpartum treatment of the newborn, effectively prevented early-onset GBS disease in colonized mothers presenting with either preterm labor or PROM > 12 h.
2. **Premature rupture of membranes (PROM).** Premature rupture of membranes frequently complicates preterm labor by increasing the risk for sepsis. All the issues discussed for preterm labor apply, only now the increased risk for infection may tip the scales toward early delivery. In the setting of PROM, the use of steroids to facilitate fetal lung maturation is even more controversial. The available data suggest that the incidence of RDS is significantly decreased with PROM > 24 h, and antenatal steroids do not appear to further decrease the incidence [34]. Furthermore, steroids may complicate the assessment of intrauterine infection and increase the risk of infection with PROM [34].
   a. **Intrapartum antibiotics.** The use of intrapartum antibiotics with PROM should be considered whenever there is evidence of fetal distress (e.g., fetal tachycardia or poor variability on fetal monitoring), maternal chorioamnionitis, or PROM > 12 h with maternal GBS colonization (see Table 12-2).

   A study from Finland used a latex agglutinatum test from maternal vaginal smears taken during labor to detect heavy maternal colonization with GBS. Mothers with heavy colonization with GBS were randomized to receive penicillin during labor (5 million units of penicillin G IV q6h, or if no delivery within 18 hours, 1 million units every 8 hours until delivery) or no therapy. Use of penicillin appeared to reduce the incidence of early-onset GBS disease in the newborns [162].

E. **Evaluation and treatment—postnatal.** The evaluation and treatment of the newborn infant at risk for bacterial disease varies with clinical presentation. Asymptomatic infants or infants with minimal distress (e.g., mild tachypnea without an oxygen requirement) may require only routine newborn care and

Table 12-3. Experimental design and results of selective intrapartum and postpartum antibiotic therapy for the prevention of neonatal GBS disease

Experimental Design

1. Maternal vaginal and rectal cultures were taken at 26 to 28 weeks' gestation.
2. Women with positive cultures for GBS were included in the study if they had premature labor (under 37 weeks) or premature rupture of the membranes (>12 hours).
3. These women were randomized into a group that received ampicillin 2 g IV followed by 1 g q4h until delivery and a second control group that received no ampicillin.
4. If intrapartum fever developed (>37.5°C), the mothers were dropped from the study and treated with ampicillin.
5. Some infants were included in the study but not randomized. Some of these women were treated at the request of their obstetricians.
6. Surface and blood cultures were taken from the infants.
7. Normal infants whose mothers received ampicillin received four doses of ampicillin (50 mg/kg IV q12h).
8. Asymptomatic infants born to untreated mothers were not treated unless they developed signs of sepsis.
9. All infants with asphyxia, respiratory distress, or signs of infection at birth were fully cultured (including CSF) and treated.
10. Randomized and nonrandomized groups were followed.
11. Symptomatic infants and septic infants were treated with ampicillin and kandmycin.

Results

	Rate of early-onset GBS disease	
Randomization	Ampicillin	Control
Yes	0/85	5/79
No	0/235	15/1426
TOTAL	0/320	20/1505*

*Attack rate: 13.4 per 1000 live births.
Source: From K. M. Boyer et al. *N. Engl. J Med.* 314: 1665, 1986.

careful evaluation for infection. At the opposite end of the spectrum of disease are the infants with severe respiratory distress, persistent pulmonary hypertension, and shock. These infants challenge the limits of neonatal life support.

1. **Clinical signs of infection.** Infection in the newborn infant may present with nonspecific, often subtle clinical findings. These include the following:
   a. **Respiratory distress.** This is the most common symptom, occurring in up to 90 percent of infants with sepsis. The clinical presentation may vary from apnea, mild tachypnea, or a slight increase in oxygen requirement to severe RDS requiring mechanical ventilation.
   b. **Hypotension**
   c. **Acidosis (metabolic)**
   d. **Temperature instability.** The normal neonatal isothermic temperature range is 97°F (36°C) to 99.6°F (37°C). In a prospective study, sustained rectal temperatures above or below this range were correlated with bacterial infections in up to 30 percent of newborn infants [74]. Another study found that 10 percent of newborn infants with fever had positive cultures for bacterial infection [75].
   e. **Gastrointestinal symptoms.** These include vomiting, diarrhea, abdominal distension, ileus, and poor feeding.
   f. **Diminished activity or lethargy**

g. **Seizures**
h. **Petichiae or purpura**

2. **Laboratory studies.** No single laboratory test has been found to have acceptable specificity and sensitivity for predicting infection. Therefore, the results of laboratory studies must be assessed in conjunction with the presence of risk factors and clinical signs of sepsis.
   a. **Total neutrophil count and immature-to-total neutrophil ratio.** A total WBC of less than 5000 mm^3, a total neutrophil count of less than 1000/μl, or an immature (band) to total neutrophil ratio of greater than 0.2 have all been correlated with an increased risk of bacterial infection [76–80]. Noninfectious causes of an abnormal neonatal WBC include maternal toxemia (neutropenia) [81] and antenatal glucocorticoids (leukocytosis) [82]. There is some dispute about whether antenatal steroids raise the neonatal white count [161].
   b. **Cultures.** Cultures are critical in the diagnosis and treatment of bacterial infections. Blood cultures should be obtained from a peripheral site thoroughly cleansed with an antiseptic agent. No less than 0.5 ml per bottle of blood should be cultured [119,120]. The first blood sample from a freshly cut umbilical cord obtained under sterile conditions also may be adequate for cultures [121]. CSF samples should be plated promptly to avoid loss of viability of organisms due to changes in fluid pH. Urine culture has little value in the immediate perinatal period, but it may be very important for late-onset neonatal sepsis [122].
   c. **Chest x-ray**
   d. **Erythrocyte sedimentation rate (ESR), C-reactive protein concentration (CRP), and haptoglobin determination.** The sensitivity and specificity of each of these tests do not justify their individual use in the newborn; however, they may be useful in conjunction with each other and the CBC. Philip and Hewitt [36] found that if each of five separate tests were negative, the probability was 99 percent that infection was not present. The tests examined were (1) total WBC less than 5000/mm^3, (2) band/neutrophil ratio greater than 0.2, (3) positive C-reactive protein (CRP), (4) elevated haptoglobin level, and (5) an erythrocyte sedimentation rate (ESR) of 15 mm/h. Of these tests, the band/neutrophil ratio was the most useful, with a negative predictive value comparable with the full battery of five tests.
   e. **Gastric aspirate Gram stain.** This assay has low positive predictive value. Generally, if there are more than 5 neutrophils per high-power field or a large number of bacteria, particularly gram-positive cocci in clumps and chains, the test is positive. The low specificity of the test is not surprising, since a positive aspirate reflects an infected intrauterine environment, not a fetal inflammatory response. Thus the gastric aspirate may add little to what is already known from clinical information. However, if a gastric aspirate contains only occasional neutrophils or organisms, bacterial disease is unlikely [37].
   f. **Antigen detection methods.** Latex agglutination assays are available for both GBS and *ECK1*. These tests may complement other laboratory tests, particularly in the setting of antenatal maternal treatment with antibiotics or parenchymal lung disease with negative blood cultures. The significance of a positive urine test in a culture-negative, asymptomatic infant is uncertain, but it may represent a false-positive result.

3. **Assessment of the SYMPTOMATIC newborn infant.** The clinical signs and symptoms of sepsis in the newborn can be very nonspecific, and infection must be considered in virtually all cases of neonatal distress. This is particularly true with respiratory distress. Meconium aspiration pneumonitis, RDS, birth asphyxia, persistent pulmonary hypertension (primary or secondary to meconium aspiration or asphyxia), and apnea may all be indistinguishable from sepsis. Accordingly, the symptomatic new-

born infant should have a blood culture drawn and antibiotic therapy initiated. Meningitis also must be considered, but the clinical status of the ill neonate often requires that a lumbar puncture be deferred. Recently it has been suggested that premature infants with negative blood cultures and a clear-cut clinical course consistent with immature lung disease may not require a lumbar puncture [40]. Latex agglutination tests may aid in the diagnosis of GBS and *ECK1* infections, especially if intrapartum antibiotics have been administered.

4. **Assessment of the ASYMPTOMATIC newborn infant.** Identification of the asymptomatic but bacteremic newborn infant is often a difficult task. Given the low incidence of infection in asymptomatic newborn infants at risk for sepsis, careful observation may be all that is required in the perinatal period. Alternatively, all infants with identifiable risk factors could be treated for 48 hours to rule out R/O sepsis, particularly if close observation is not practical. One approach to this problem, somewhat in between the preceding two extremes, is currently in practice at the special care nurseries of the Beth Israel, Children's, and Brigham and Women's Hospitals in Boston. Perinatal risk factors are divided into major and minor categories (see Table 12-2). The significances of some of these risk factors have not been rigorously tested by clinical studies. Their inclusion is based upon extensive anecdotal experience. If one major or two minor risk factors are present, a CBC and blood culture are drawn and a gastric aspirate Gram stain is examined. Note that prematurity and low birth weight are often considered major risk factors by themselves but are listed under minor risk in Table 12-2. Their entry under the minor category emphasizes that other factors are considered that may act in concert. Thus the low-birth-weight infant is also likely to be premature, so two minor criteria would be met and the infant would be evaluated for sepsis. Similarly, the combination of prematurity and maternal GBS colonization would result in a workup for sepsis. However, the well 34- to 37-week newborn infant who has no other identifiable risk factors for infection would not be subjected to venipuncture or other testing. If the gastric aspirate Gram stain and CBC are benign, the infant at risk for infection is observed off antibiotics. Acknowledging the limitations of the tests employed, it is hoped that this approach will identify a group of well newborn infants who, despite risk factors, have a very low probability of perinatally acquired infection. However, it must be emphasized that infants may be asymptomatic at birth and have normal laboratory values but still be infected. In patients in whom there is clinical concern but normal laboratory tests, vital signs (temperature, pulse, respirations) are monitored every 4 hours and the CBC is repeated at 12 hours. All infants who are asymptomatic but have abnormal laboratory values receive a 48-hour course of antibiotics for R/O sepsis. Prior to starting antibiotics for R/O sepsis, a lumbar puncture is usually performed. This is also somewhat controversial, especially for the asymptomatic term infant. The principal argument for examination of the cerebral spinal fluid (CSF) is based on a study in which 15 percent of a small group of newborn infants had positive CSF cultures with negative blood cultures [38]. However, it is difficult to apply these data to the well term infant, in whom the incidence of meningitis without bacteremia is certain to be lower. If doses of antibiotics appropriate to treat meningitis are used, the lumbar puncture could be deferred pending the blood culture results and clinical course, but the results may be difficult to interpret. The most useful CSF assays for determining the likelihood of meningitis are the cell count and culture. Cultures are unreliable if the infant has been receiving antibiotics, and interpretation of the cell count may be limited if the lumbar puncture is traumatic or there is a coexisting subarachnoid or intraventricular hemorrhage. Furthermore, a small percentage of infants may have meningitis with normal CSF cell counts and chemistries [39]. The anticipated

rate of sepsis and/or meningitis is approximately 1–2% for infants meeting the above R/O sepsis criteria. This has been observed in our nurseries.

5. **Antibiotic therapy for neonatal septicemia and meningitis.** Presumptive antibiotic therapy in the neonate is directed toward the treatment of the most commonly encountered pathogens for a given clinical setting. In the perinatal period, the pathogens of greatest concern are GBS, *ECK1,* and *Listeria.* These organisms remain as the principal pathogens throughout the first month of life for otherwise healthy infants living at home. Ampicillin and an aminoglycoside, usually gentamicin, are effective against these bacteria. This combination also provides broad coverage for many other gram-positive and gram-negative bacteria less commonly isolated from the septic newborn infant. Another important consideration is the in vivo and/or in vitro synergy demonstrated for penicillins with aminoglycosides, especially against GBS and *Listeria* [40,41]. Third-generation cephalosporins also have been shown to be effective against gram-negative infections, but they have limited activity against *Listeria,* and no study has clearly demonstrated improved morbidity or mortality with their use [42–44]. Cephalosporins also displace bilirubin from albumin binding sites, which may place the neonate at increased risk for kernicterus in the setting of hyperbilirubinemia [45,46]. Nevertheless, with documented gram-negative meningitis, third-generation cephalosporins are recommended on the theoretical basis of greater CSF killing power. Cefotaxime is generally recommended because this agent has been used most frequently with proven efficacy for the newborn. The CSF killing power (KP) of an antibiotic is defined as

$$\text{KP} = \frac{\text{Concentration of antibiotic in CSF}}{\text{MBC of antibiotic for infecting organism}}$$

It is the low minimal bactericidal concentration (MBC), not the high CSF penetration, that gives third-generation cephalosporins a high CSF killing power. Recommended antibiotic therapy for specific perinatal infections are listed in Table 12-4.

6. **Antibiotic therapy for neonates at risk for nosocomial infections.** Although ampicillin and gentamicin provide excellent broad coverage for perinatal pathogens, this combination may not be preferred for neonates at risk for nosocomial infections (usually more than 1 week in the SCN). Considering the predominance of coagulase-negative staphylococci as the principal cause of nosocomial sepsis, vancomycin has become the principal agent for presumptive gram-positive bacterial coverage. Presumptive gram-negative coverage is provided with an aminoglycoside. The aminoglycoside of choice is usually gentamicin, but resistant organisms may be prevalent in many nurseries. An alternative aminoglycoside is amikacin; resistance to this antibiotic has been reported to be low, despite long-term use in the nursery [47]. In symptomatic infants who are at risk for nosocomial infection, blood, CSF, and urine (bladder tap or catheterization) cultures should be obtained. If the initial evaluation indicates meningitis or a urinary tract infection, ampicillin and gentamicin may be a preferable initial antibiotic combination. Gram-negative infections of the CSF are treated as in **D.5** (cefotaxime). Coagulase-negative staphylococci are treated with vancomycin. Vancomycin is dosed at 15 mg/kg IV q12h (preterm) or q8h (term) with the dose adjusted based on serum levels. (See C 6A pg. 150.)

7. **Immunotherapy for neonatal septicemia.** The human neonate may be considered an immunocompromised host with incomplete development of multiple components of the immune system. This is not to say that the newborn infants cannot limit the spread of disease, but defense mechanisms may frequently be overcome, especially in low-birth-weight infants. Problems with the immune system of the newborn may relate to decreased quantities and/or functions of multiple cellular and humoral con-

Table 12-4. Recommended antibiotic regimens for neonatal sepsis and meningitis (see Appendix A)

Organism	Site of infection	Antibiotic therapy*	Duration of therapy
GBS	Blood	Penicillin 200,000 U/kg per day	10–14 days
	CNS	Penicillin 400,000 U/kg per day	Complete 14–21 days
ECK1	Blood	Cefotaxime 50–100 mg/kg per day or other third-generation drug	Complete 14 days
	CNS	Cefotaxime 100 mg/kg per day (? gentamicin† 5 mg/kg per day for 5 to 10 days for synergy)	Complete 21 days
Listeria	Blood	Ampicillin 100–200 mg/kg per day (? gentamicin† 5 mg/kg per day for up to 1 week for synergy	Complete 14 days
	CNS	Ampicillin 300 mg/kg per day (? gentamicin† 5 mg/kg per day for up to 1 week for synergy)	Complete 14–21 days

*In all cases, therapy with ampicillin (300 mg/kg per day) and gentamicin (5 mg/kg per day) is initiated until an organism has been identified and antibiotic sensitivities are determined. Doses are divided q12h for term newborn infants and should be adjusted for increased renal clearance beyond the first week of life.

†Gentamicin is always 2.5 mg/kg per dose, with the interval adjusted based on gestational age and serum levels. In general, the intervals are q24h for infants less than 1000 g, q18h for infants of less than 35 weeks' gestation, and q12h for infants more than 35 weeks.

Note: For recommendations on the use of antibiotics in neonates weighing less than 1200 g, see ref. 164.

stituents [48,49]. Based on theoretical considerations and, in some cases, experimental evidence, the administration of blood and tissue factors to bolster the neonatal immune system has been proposed. Immunity factors that may augment neonatal defenses against infections due to GBS, *ECK1,* and *Listeria* are shown in Table 12-5.

a. **Immunoglobulin therapy.** This has received much attention in recent years. Shigeoka, Hall and Hill [60] observed increased survival when neonates infected with GBS received an exchange transfusion with blood containing elevated levels of GBS capsular antibodies. Thus the septic newborn infant may benefit from the administration of **GBS-specific** immunoglobulin preparations or from an exchange transfusion using blood from donors with high levels of GBS capsular antibodies. Protection against experimental GBS infections also has been demonstrated in animals receiving high-titer capsular antibody preparations, provided the therapy was given within the first few hours of infection [61]. Unfortunately, there are no data currently available that directly confirm the efficacy of exogenous specific immunoglobulin therapy for acute neonatal sepsis. Also, GBS-specific antibody preparations are not currently available, and commercial immunoglobulin preparations may not contain significant GBS-specific antibodies. Recent studies have suggested that nonspecific high-dose immunoglobulin therapy may actually be detrimental when given during acute GBS sepsis in an experimental animal model [62,130]. Although the utility of immunoglobulin therapy for acute bacterial disease remains uncertain, it may have a role in the prevention of nosocomial infection, especially in very low birth weight infants. A significant reduction in neonatal nosocomial infections has been

Table 12-5. Immunity factors in perinatal infections

Organism	Immunity factors [ref.]
GBS	Capsular antibody [10,50,51] Fibronectin [48,52] Complement [7] Neutrophils [7,48]
ECK1	Capsular antibody [53] Pilus antibody [23,54] Complement [55] Neutrophils [48]
Listeria	Interferon [27,56] Interlukins [27,57] Tumor necrosis factor [58,59]

found in clinical trials of immunoglobulin therapy using commercially available preparations [63,64,131]. However, these studies have limitations, and it is not clear that immunoglobulin prophylaxis significantly reduces the morbidity and mortality due to nosocomial infections. Furthermore, the half-life of exogenous immunoglobulins is very short, and weekly infusion may be required to sustain adequate levels in most cases. The results of additional controlled clinical trials currently underway are needed before prophylactic immunoglobulin therapy can be recommended as standard nursery practice.

b. Granulocyte infusions (see Chap. 20). There is some evidence that granulocyte transfusions may significantly improve the survival of the septic newborn infant who is also neutropenic and who has insufficient bone marrow reserve to replenish the granulocyte deficit. Christensen et al. [65] demonstrated survival in seven of seven (100 percent) septic newborns who received granulocyte transfusions compared with one of nine (11 percent) infected infants receiving supportive care alone. The infants in this study had severe depletion of bone marrow neutrophil storage pools (NSP = total metamyelocytes, band, and segmented forms less than 7 percent of marrow cells). Although a one-to-one correspondence between NSP and the percentage of neutrophils in peripheral smears has not been found, Christensen and coworkers [66] suggest that neutropenia with an immature-to-total neutrophil ratio greater than 0.8 reflects severe NSP depletion. Results from several other studies [48] incorporating granulocyte infusions for neonatal sepsis support the findings of Christensen and coworkers with a single exception. Stork et al. [67] were unable to demonstrate improved survival in a randomized, prospective clinical trial of granulocyte infusions in 25 septic newborn infants with neutrophil storage pool depletion. It is also important to note that only a small number of medical centers are currently established in the preparation and administration of granulocytes and that infusions may have significant side effects in the neonate [48].

c. Double-volume exchange transfusions (see Chaps. 15 and 20). Double-volume exchange transfusions using fresh whole blood have been used in neonatal septicemia to attempt to (1) remove bacterial toxins and/or decrease the bacterial burden, (2) improve peripheral and pulmonary perfusion, and (3) bolster the immune system of infected newborn infants. Unfortunately, there has been no prospective, randomized controlled study for the use of exchange transfusions in neonatal sepsis. Reports have suggested that improvements in hemodynamic and possibly pulmonary parameters may result from fresh whole-blood exchange transfusions [68–70]. Furthermore, fresh whole-blood transfusions provide an alternative method of providing neutrophils to septic newborn infants with severe NSP depletion [70]. Clearly, further studies are needed to confirm the efficacy of fresh whole-blood double-volume exchange transfusions in the septic newborn infant. Based on current knowledge, combined with the potential complications of the procedure, exchange transfusions should only be considered in the critically ill neonate with profound neutropenia and severe NSP depletion.

d. **Immunoprophylaxis against neonatal sepsis.** Although neonatal septicemia is a relatively low-incidence disease, it is frequently devastating. This continues to be so, despite improvements in the care of the critically ill septic infant. Selective intrapartum antibiotic therapy appears to be effective in preventing disease in many newborn infants, but this approach is currently limited only to cases of identifiable increased risk for perinatal disease. Many newborn infants who develop sepsis do not have recognized risks for infection (e.g., one-fourth to one-third of early-onset GBS infections). Infection in these infants may go undetected until overwhelming sepsis occurs. The ultimate solution to neonatal septicemia may be a combination of maternal immunization and postpartum immunotherapy (e.g., intravenous immunoglobulin; see above). Passive immunization of neonatal rats with anticapsular antibodies has been shown to prevent invasive disease due to GBS [7] and *ECK1* [53]. Immunization of pregnant rats with purified *ECK1* pili also has been shown to prevent invasive *ECK1* disease in their offspring [54]. These results are promising and suggest that passive immunization of the fetus may be possible by transplacental transfer of specific antibodies from immunized mothers. Further studies are currently underway to develop vaccines using these antigens and to determine the antigenicity and safety of a GBS type III polysaccharide [71].

e. **Management of severe parenchymal lung disease and persistent pulmonary hypertension in neonatal septicemia.** In addition to antibiotic therapy, the septic newborn infant may require considerable cardiopulmonary support [72]. This is particularly true in the setting of severe parenchymal lung damage from pneumonia or persistent pulmonary hypertension (PPHN). The etiology of PPHN in neonatal sepsis may be multifactorial, but there is evidence suggesting that GBS may directly induce PPHN through elevation in thromboxane production. In an animal model, the experimental thromboxane synthetase inhibitor Dazmegrel has been shown to reverse GBS-induced PPHN [73]. These results are promising, but further studies are needed to confirm the significance of thromboxane-induced PPHN in the septic newborn infant and to identify a safe and effective thromboxane synthetase inhibitor (Dazmegrel is not approved for human use) (see Chap. 13).

II. Focal bacterial infections

A. Skin infections (see Chap. 29). The newborn infant may develop a variety of rashes associated with bacterial disease. Some of these are related to systemic infection, while others are the direct result of primary cutaneous disease. The most frequently encountered clinical manifestations of localized skin infections are pustules, vesicles, cellulitis, and abscesses. The common bacteria colonizing the skin of the newborn infant include coagulase-negative staphylococci, *Staphylococcus aureus,* streptococci (including GBS), gram-negative enterics (including *E. coli*), and diphtheroids [111]. The colonizing organisms will vary with the vaginal flora present at the time of delivery and the organisms present in the environment of the nursery.

1. **Pustules.** Pustules in the newborn infant are most commonly caused by *Staphylococcus aureus,* but they must be distinguished from similar-appearing lesions of erythema toxicum.

a. **Diagnosis.** A lesion can be carefully cleansed with betadine, unroofed, and a Gram stain performed on the contents. With true pustules, numerous polymorphonuclear lymphocytes and gram-positive cocci can be seen. Culture of the material confirms the suspected pathogen. Cells consistent with eosinophils without organisms are seen with erythema toxicum. The eosinophils may best be demonstrated with a Wright stain.

b. **Treatment.** Topical treatment with bacitracin or Bactiban and close observation may be all that is required for a small number of pustules occurring on an otherwise well infant. Oral therapy with a penicillinase-resistant penicillin or first-generation cephalosporin also may be appropriate. More extensive lesions or lesions occurring in an ill infant should be treated with parenteral antibiotic after obtaining systemic cultures.

2. **Cellulitis.** The causative agents are usually streptococci, and parenteral antibiotic therapy is required. *Staphylococcus aureus,* gram-negative enteric bacteria or anaerobes also may be present with cellulitis associated with disruption of the skin (abrasions, scalp electrodes).

a. **Omphalitis.** This is characterized by erythema and/or induration with purulent discharge from the umbilical stump. Both gram-negative and gram-positive organisms may be involved, and in the setting of poor maternal immunity and poor aseptic technique, Clostridia may be common [106,107,109]. Routine cord care is discussed in Chapter 8. Treatment of omphalitis requires a full septic workup and parenteral antibiotics (usually oxacillin and an aminoglycoside). The seriousness of the condition is emphasized by the complications seen with progressive disease. These are related to contiguous spread to adjacent soft tissues or umbilical blood vessels. Abdominal wall cellulitis, necrotizing fasciitis, peritonitis, and umbilical arteritis or phlebitis with hepatic vein thrombosis or hepatic abscess have all been described [108,110,111].

B. **Ophthalmia neonatorum.** This condition refers to inflammation of the conjunctiva within the first month of life. Causative agents include topical antimicrobial agents (chemical conjunctivitis), bacteria, and herpesvirus (see Congenital Infections). Bacterial conjunctivitis is caused by *Neisseria gonorrhoeae, Chlamydia,* staphylococci, pneumonocci, streptococci, *E. coli,* and other gram-negative bacteria.

1. **Chemical conjunctivitis.** This is predominantly seen with silver nitrate 1% used to prophylax against bacterial conjunctivitis.

a. **Application of silver nitrate.** This should be done using single-dose ampules within the first hour of life [120]. The usual method of application is as follows:

(1) Cleanse the eyelid and surrounding skin with sterile cotton moistened with sterile water.

(2) Gently open the infant's eyelids and instill 2 drops of silver nitrate on the conjunctival sac. Allow the silver nitrate to run across the whole conjunctival sac. Carefully manipulate the lids to ensure spread of the drops. Repeat in the other eye.

(3) After 1 minute, wipe the excess silver nitrate from the surrounding skin and eyelids with sterile cotton. **Do not irrigate the eyes after this procedure.** This may reduce the efficiency of prophylaxis without altering the incidence of chemical conjunctivitis [120,121].

b. **Treatment of conjunctival irritation.** Approximately 90 percent of infants develop conjunctival hyperemia, edema, and eye drainage within hours of exposure to 1% silver nitrate ophthalmic drops. In some cases, periorbital edema also occurs. The reaction is usually self-limiting and resolves within 36 to 48 hours. Gentle wiping of the eyes with sterile cotton moistened with sterile saline or water is all that is required. Infectious conjunctivitis also may occur within hours of delivery, especially in the setting of prolonged rupture of membranes. A Gram stain can help differentiate between chemical and infectious conjunctivitis. With the former, only polymorphonuclear lymphocytes without organisms are seen. If doubt still exists, the exudate should be cultured and presumptive antimicrobial therapy initiated. A broad-spectrum agent such as cefotaxime provides coverage for *Staphylococcus aureus, N. gonorrhoeae,* and most gram-negative organisms. *Chlamydia* rarely causes conjunctivitis within the first day of life. Herpesvirus should be considered (see Congenital Infections).

c. **Alternative prophylaxis.** Tetracycline 1% and erythromycin 0.5% ophthalmic ointments also have been shown to be effective agents for the prophylaxis of bacterial conjunctivitis. The results of comparison studies using the various antimicrobial ophthalmic preparations vary [120,122,123,129], but overall there may be an advantage to using the ointments for the prevention of *Chlamydia* conjunctivitis. Alternatively, the ointments may impair vision and are more difficult to apply over the entire conjunctiva. Silver nitrate is still the most widely used agent, and the one with the longest record for safe and effective prophylaxis against gonococcal conjunctivitis. It also has the least potential for allergic reaction or the development of antibiotic resistance.

2. ***Neisseria gonorrhoeae.*** Gonococcal ophthalmia neonatorum (GON) usually presents as conjunctivitis with chemosis, purulent exudate, and lid edema starting 1 to 4 days after birth. Clouding or perforation of the cornea or panophthalmitis also may be present. Rhinitis, scalp infections, anorectal infection, funistitis, sepsis, arthritis, and meningitis have all been described with gonococcal infections in the newborn. A review of the rate of gonococcal infection in women as a function of age over a 12-year period reveals the highest incidence to be in adolescents and young adults (1 to 2 percent) [134]. This rate can be as great as 10 percent in selected populations of pregnant women. Furthermore, the recurrence rate can be high: A prenatal clinic in North Carolina reported an infection rate of 7.5 percent, with a recurrence rate of 30 percent by delivery [135]. Risk factors for a high incidence of perinatal gonococcal infection are low socioeconomic group, prior history of venereal disease, unmarried state, and urban populations. There is an increased risk of GON with premature rupture of membranes (PROM) in infected women [134].

a. **Diagnosis.** A Gram stain should be performed on conjunctival scrapings from any infant suspected of having infectious conjunctivitis. Routine bacteriologic cultures and prompt plating of exudate on appropriate growth medium (e.g., Thayer-Martin) for the isolation of *Neisseria* are required. Intracellular gram-negative diplococci are characteristically seen, and if they are present, the infant should have a blood culture taken prior to the initiation of antibiotic therapy. Presumptive therapy should be initiated if the clinical presentation is most consistent with GON but the Gram stain is equivocal. Maternal cervical cultures also should be obtained. Conjunctivitis can be caused by nongonococcal *Neisseria,* indicating the need for careful confirmation of gonorrhea by appropriate microbiologic techniques [128,132].

b. **Treatment.** Conventional management of GON consists of IV aqueous crystalline penicillin G (100,000 U/kg per day divided q12h for 7 days) with frequent saline irrigations [120,124]. With an increasing percentage of penicillinase-producing isolates of gonococcus [125,126], Cefotaxime 100 mg/kg per day divided q8h (q12h for preterm infants) for 7 days may be the more appropriate therapy, especially until antibiotic sensitivities are obtained. Topical antibiotic ointments or drops are not necessary, although consideration should be given to the possibility of concurrent *Chlamydia trachomatis* [124]. Of course, mothers should be treated for their own sake and to prevent postnatal infection of the neonate. All sexual partners of infected mothers should be evaluated and treated. Any infant suspected of being exposed to gonococcal infection should have secretion precautions for 24 hours after initiation of ocular and parenteral antimicrobial prophylaxis or treatment.

c. **Prevention.** Effective prevention of GON begins with maternal screening during pregnancy. **All pregnant women should have endocervical cultures for gonococci** as part of prenatal care. Cultures should be repeated at delivery for high-risk women. Treatment of infected pregnant women is the best means of preventing disease in the newborn. Ocular prophylaxis should be provided for all newborn infants within 1 hour of birth, as described above. In addition, infants born to culture-positive mothers should receive a single dose of parenteral antibiotic. Aqueous crystalline penicillin G, IV or IM (50,000 U for term and 20,000 U for preterm infants), has been used successfully. Alternatively, single-dose ceftriaxone 125 mg (50 mg/kg for preterm infants), IV or IM, can be used and would provide coverage for penicillin resistant strains [123,124,127].

3. ***Chlamydia trachomatis***
   a. **Incidence.** This is the most common cause of infectious conjunctivitis in the newborn infant [133,143]. The highest prevalence of cervical infection occurs in adolescents and ranges from 8 to 37 percent [143], and *Chlamydia* is identified in approximately 50 percent of women with mucopurulent cervicitis [145,146]. The principal mode of transmission is to the newborn upon vaginal delivery [144], with the organism being transmitted at a rate of 50 to 75 percent [143]. Between 20 and 50 percent of infants born to infected mothers will develop conjunctivitis [143].
   b. **Symptoms.** Chlamydial conjunctivitis usually appears 5 to 14 days after birth. There may be minimum inflammation or severe conjunctival inflammation with a purulent yellow discharge and swelling of the eyelids. Conjunctival scarring is possible. The cornea is usually not involved, although corneal pannus formation has been described.
   c. **Diagnosis.** The diagnosis of chlamydial conjunctivitis can be made by the demonstration of basophilic intracytoplasmic inclusion bodies on Giesma stain of scrapings taken from the palpebral conjunctival surface. The bodies are not found in the cells of the purulent exudate. Both polymorphonuclear and mononuclear lymphocytes are found in the exudate. Two rapid antigen detection methods as well as tissue culture are also available for the diagnosis of *Chlamydia* infection. A direct fluorescent antibody test (MicroTrak) and an enzyme-linked immunosorbent assay (Chlamydiazyme) have been approved for *Chlamydia* testing and have been shown to be very sensitive and specific for the detection of *Chlamydia* from conjunctival material [143]. Tissue culture may not be readily available at all centers; it requires special handling and at least 3 to 5 days for growth and detection.
   d. **Treatment.** Chlamydial conjunctivitis in the newborn can best be treated by systemic therapy with erythromycin ethylsuccinate 40 mg/kg per day in four divided doses for 3 weeks. This therapy also may eradicate the organism from the upper respiratory tract. Topical therapy with sulfonamide drops 10% or tetracycline ointment 1% or drops q6h for 3 weeks is also used. Systemic treatment with erythromycin is indicated for chlamydial pneumonia. Both parents should be treated with tetracycline or erythromycin.
   e. **Prevention.** See **B.1.C.**
4. **Bacterial conjunctivitis for agents other than *N. gonorrhoeae*.** *Staphylococcus* is the most common cause of bacterial conjunctivitis. Gram-negative organisms may be involved.

a. **Diagnosis** is by Gram stain and culture.
b. **Treatment** consists of local saline irrigation and instillation of the appropriate topical antibiotic ointment. Polymyxin B sulfate–bacitracin zinc–neomycin sulfate (Neosporin ophthalmic ointment) applied q6h is usually adequate. Any evidence of local or systemic spread of infection requires blood cultures and systemic treatment with appropriate systemic antibiotics, usually oxacillin and gentamicin.

5. **Herpes simplex** (see also Perinatal Viral Infections). Herpes simplex may cause eye infection during the neonatal period. The manifestations include conjunctivitis, optic neuritis, and chorioretinitis. The conjunctivitis has its onset between 2 and 14 days after birth. If there is a maternal history of herpes or other systemic signs or herpes infection, this diagnosis should be considered. Conjunctivitis of uncertain etiology that is not responding to antibiotic therapy may be herpetic in etiology.
   a. **Diagnosis.** Staining the corneal surface with fluorescein and examination of the eyes under a slit lamp with blue light may show the epithelial dendrite. Conjunctival scraping should be stained by the Papanicolaou method for the presence of multinucleated giant cells. Herpesvirus can be cultured from the conjunctiva or demonstrated by electron microscopy or fluorescent antibody.
   b. **Treatment.** Treatment of herpetic keratoconjunctivitis consists of trifluorothymidine 1 drop q2h or adenine arabinoside ointment q3h. Systemic therapy with acyclovir is also indicated.

C. **Urinary tract infection (UTI)**

1. **Incidence.** This varies with birth weight, increasing from 1 percent in infants weighing more than 2500 g to 3 percent for infants weighing less than 2500 g [86]. Bacteriuria may signal generalized sepsis with hematogenous spread to the kidney [87]. Alternatively, a primary UTI may result in bloodstream infection. There is a greater incidence in male infants than in female infants. The most common organism is *E. coli,* but other gram-negative bacteria, especially *Klebsiella pneumoniae,* and enterococci are also causative agents.
2. **Diagnosis.** Culture of urine obtained by superpubic bladder tap or bladder catheterization is essential for the diagnosis of UTI and should be part of the workup for sepsis in all neonates. The newborn at risk for intrapartum sepsis is the only exception to this rule; UTI is uncommon in early-onset sepsis [87]. Gram stain of unspun urine may identify bacteria. Perinatal maternal UTI increases the risk for infection in the newborn [88].
3. **Treatment.** Presumptive therapy consists of ampicillin and an aminoglycoside until antibiotic sensitivities are obtained. A repeat urine culture should have no growth after 48 to 72 hours of therapy. Persistence of bacteriuria may indicate renal abscess, obstructive uropathy, or inappropriate therapy. The duration of therapy is 14 days. All infants with UTI should have ultrasonic examination of the urinary tract early in the course of treatment. A cystourethrogram is also performed on most infants. The recurrence rate following a primary UTI is 25 percent for the first year [1].

D. **Pneumonia.**

1. **Perinatal disease.** The diagnosis of pneumonia in the immediate postpartum period can be difficult because of the frequency of other causes of respiratory distress, including hyaline membrane disease [90], retained fetal lung fluid [77], amniotic fluid aspiration, and meconium aspiration (see Chap. 13). In each of these cases, the radiographic findings can be identical to those seen with bacterial pneumonia. The diagnosis is best made by determining the risk factors for infection versus the other conditions and observing the clinical course. For example, an infant with transient tachypnea after being delivered by cesarean section, with membranes intact and no other identified risk factors for infection, may not

require antibiotic therapy unless symptoms persist and the likely diagnosis of retained fetal lung fluid becomes less certain. With greater than mild respiratory distress or when symptoms are progressing or not improving, appropriate cultures should be obtained and antibiotic therapy considered. When doubt exists, it is best to initiate therapy and later discontinue antibiotics if the clinical course is most consistent with a noninfectious etiology, cultures are negative, and subsequent radiographs do not support pneumonia. The microbiology of perinatally acquired pneumonia parallels that of sepsis and meningitis, and the choice and doses of antibiotics are the same. Culture-negative pneumonia is generally treated with ampicillin and gentamicin for 7 days.

2. **Ureaplasma urealyticum.** This organism is frequently isolated from the vagina of pregnant women and has been shown to be associated with chorioamnionitis, premature delivery, spontaneous abortion and stillbirth, and sepsis, pneumonia, and meningitis in the newborn [91–98]. Despite a relatively high rate of colonization, there appears to be no clear increased risk of respiratory disease in full-term infants [104]. However, there appears to be an association between the development of chronic lung disease and *Ureaplasma urealyticum* in low-birth-weight infants [99–103]. There are little data available on the efficacy of antibiotic therapy for newborn infection. In a double-blind, randomized, controlled trial, infants born to mothers with *Ureaplasma urealyticum* had a higher birth weight when erythromycin was administered during the third trimester compared with the placebo group [105]. It remains to be shown if treatment of low-birth-weight infants decreases the incidence of chronic lung disease.

E. **Osteomyelitis.** This is an uncommon infection in the neonatal period. When present, it may result from sepsis, direct inoculation in association with heel sticks and scalp electrodes, extension from soft-tissue infections [112–114].

1. **Microbiology and diagnosis.** The most common organisms are *Staphylococcus aureus,* group B streptococcus (GBS), gram-negative bacteria, *Neisseria gonorrhoeae,* and *Candida.* There is a good correlation between the most common causes of bacteremia in the newborn and the frequency of bone infections caused by a particular organism. Any bone can be involved, but most frequently, infection occurs in the femur, humerus, tibia, radius, and maxilla. Osteomyelitis of the skull has been associated with the use of scalp electrodes. Multiple simultaneous foci of infection can occur. Symptoms supporting the diagnosis include apparent pain on motion, localized erythema and/or swelling, or an apparent paralysis. Cultures should be obtained from blood, urine, and CSF, and any soft-tissue lesions such as skin pustules or an abscess should be aspirated for Gram stain and culture. Plain-film radiographs and Gram stain and culture of material obtained from needle aspiration of the involved bone and soft tissues are valuable in establishing the diagnosis.

2. **Treatment.** Therapy is initiated with oxacillin and gentamicin until an organism is identified and antibiotic sensitivities are determined. The duration of therapy is 3 to 4 weeks after systemic and local signs have resolved. Any local purulent collection should be drained.

F. **Septic arthritis.** This may occur by direct seeding associated with bacteremia, extension of infection from adjacent bone, or following local trauma [114–116]. In general, the etiologic agents are similar to those seen with osteomyelitis, reflecting the association with bacteremia or spread from involved bone in the neonate [117,118]. Open surgical drainage is recommended for diagnosis and relief of pressure in some joints (e.g., hip, shoulder), but needle aspiration may be sufficient for others (e.g., knee, wrist). Antibiotic therapy is the same as for osteomyelitis. Immobilization of joints is recommended until local signs have resolved and physiotherapy can be initiated.

G. **Otitis media.** The incidence of otitis media in the neonate is not known, but several risk factors for neonatal disease have been identified. These include nasotracheal intubation for more than 7 days, cleft palates, and other risk factors for sepsis, including prematurity [89]. The most commonly identified agents are *Staphylococcus aureus* and gram-negative enteric bacteria [89,151]. Tympanocentesis may be indicated if a clinical response is not observed within 48 hours of therapy with broad-spectrum antibiotics.

H. Diarrhea. In the United States, most neonatal diarrhea is due to feeding intolerance. Bacterial agents involved with infectious diarrhea in the neonate include enteropathogenic *E. coli, Salmonella, Pseudomonas, Klebsiella, Enterobacter, Proteus, S. aureus, Campylobacter fetus,* and rarely, *Shigella.* Viral illness may cause neonatal diarrhea.

1. **Diagnosis** is made by stool culture; there is a fluorescent antibody test for enteropathogenic *E. coli.* A Gram stain of the stool will show bacteria and cells. Noninfectious causes of diarrhea should be considered and ruled out (e.g., cystic fibrosis, Hirschsprung's disease), especially in cases of chronic diarrhea.
2. Small premature infants and newborns with diarrhea are at great risk of dehydration and electrolyte imbalance. Prevention and treatment of dehydration and electrolyte imbalance are important. In infants who appear sick, the infecting organism or other gastrointestinal flora may have extended to tissues with secondary sepsis; extensive cultures must be done and treatment with systemic antibiotics carried out in such infants.
3. **Treatment.** Oral treatment of enteropathogenic *E. coli* infection is controversial. Oral neomycin 100 mg/kg per day or oral colistin sulfate 15 mg/kg per day has been used. Treatment is for 5 days. Sick infants require systemic therapy. *Salmonella* gastroenteritis in the newborn usually requires treatment with ampicillin or chloramphenicol. *Shigella* gastroenteritis in the newborn is treated with ampicillin or trimethoprim-sulfamethoxazole for 5 days. Other organisms are treated with specific antibiotics according to the results of sensitivity testing.

III. Fungal infections

A. Mucocutaneous candidiasis. Fungal infections in the well, immunocompetent term infant are generally limited to immunocutaneous disease. The offending organism is *Candida albicans.* Oral candidiasis (thrush) is usually responsive to nystatin oral suspension (100,000 U/ml). A 1-ml dose is delivered to each side of the mouth every 6 hours and is continued for several days after the mouth clears of lesions. Alternate therapy is gentian violet 1%, which may be very effective with as few as one or two applications, but it may also be safely used over longer periods for refractory lesions. *Candida* diaper dermatitis is treated with nystatin ointment or powder (100,000 U/g) applied with each diaper change. Although mucocutaneous candidiasis most commonly occurs postnatally, rare intrauterine infections have been reported [136]. Intrauterine infection occurs by means of the ascending route and can result in mucocutaneous or disseminated disease.

B. Disseminated candidiasis. Systemic candidiasis has emerged as a serious nosocomial infection occurring is very low birth weight (VLBW) infants. As many as 3 percent of VLBW infants develop systemic candidiasis [84]. Risk factors may include prolonged use of antibiotics, parenteral hyperalimentation and intravenous fat emulsions, assisted ventilation, and the use of contaminated monitoring equipment [137,138]. *Candida albicans* remains the most common pathogen, but other *Candida* species should be considered. When an infectious process is suspected but bacterial pathogens are not identified and there is no response to antibiotic therapy, fungal disease should be considered. *Candida* sepsis may result in meningitis, arthritis, endophthalmitis, endocarditis, and obstructive uropathy [139,141]. Blood cultures are important but may be negative. CSF cultures are also important, and urine cultures may be valuable in identifying the infant with candidemia [140,141]. Other aids include microscopic examination of urine and the buffy coat of blood, the determination of serum *Candida* antigen levels, ophthalmologic examination, and renal ultrasonography [139–142]. Treatment consists of intravenous amphotericin B. The addition of 5-fluorocytosine may be beneficial, particularly with CNS involvement.

C. *Malassezia furfur.* This organism has been recognized as a cause of neonatal sepsis in the intensive care setting. In the neonatal SCN, 33 to 66 precent of infants may be colonized with this organism [158,159]. Infections have been found to occur primarily in preterm infants receiving intravenous fat emulsions [152–157]. The most common clinical presentation is apnea and bradycardia, although fever, thrombocytopenia, leukocytosis, and pulmonary infiltrates can occur. Treatment primarily consists of removal of the catheter used for lipid infusions. The need for an antifungal agent is uncertain, since symptoms usually resolve after catheter removal. Amphotericin is active against *Malassezia furfur* and may be used if clinical symptoms persist or are severe. *Malassezia furfur* should be considered in preterm infants receiving intravenous lipids who develop signs of sepsis but cultures fail to identify an organism. Yeast forms may be identified by Gram stain of the buffy coat from peripheral blood, but special culture techniques may be required to isolate the organism.

IV. Anaerobic infections [124,165]

A. Anaerobic infections. Table 12-6 shows the clinically important anaerobic bacteria [77]. Anaerobes make up a significant portion of the vaginal flora and are a well-known cause of maternal infection (see **I.B.1**). Many anaerobes have low virulence and are spontaneously cleaned from the maternal and neonatal bloodstreams. Most episodes of clinically significant anaerobic bacteremia are associated with either in utero infection, gastrointestinal disease (bowel perforation, necrotizing enterocolitis (NEC) (Chap. 28), or cord or wound infection. Sometimes there are local infections from skin trauma (scalp

Table 12-6. Clinically important anaerobic bacteria

Type of bacteria	Genus	Fermentation products from glucose or other major characteristics
Bacilli (spore-forming)	*Clostridium*	
Bacilli (non-spore-forming):		
Gram-positive	*Propionibacterium*	Propionic and acetic acids
	Lactobacillus	Lactic acid
	Bifidobacterium	Acetic and lactic acids
	Eubacterium	Butyric or acetic and formic acids or no major acids
	Actinomyces	Acetic, lactic, and succinic acids
Gram-negative (Bacteroidacese)	*Fusobacterium*	Butyric acid without isobutyric and isovaleric acids
	Bacteroides	Mixture of acids, including succinic, acetic, formic, lactic, and propionic acids
	Leptotrichia	Lactic acid
Cocci:		
Gram-positive	*Peptococcus*	Characteristically in clumps
	Peptostreptococcus	Characteristically in chains
Gram-negative	*Veillonella*	Propionic and acetic acids
	Acidaminococcus	Butyric and acetic acids

Source: Modified from A. W. Chow et al. Significance of anaerobes in neonatal bacteremia: Analyses of 23 cases and review of the literature. *Pediatrics* 54: 736, 1974.

monitors, forceps abrasions). While it is uncommon to have significant neonatal anaerobic bacteremia (under 1 percent of cases of neonatal sepsis), when it is present in a sick infant, it is often associated with severe disease. The pathogens associated with significant neonatal anaerobic infection are *Bacteroides fragilis, Peptostreptococcus, Clostridium perfringens,* and occasionally, *Fusobacterium.* These infections are often complicated by other aerobic bacterial infection occurring at the same time. Infections with an anaerobic bacteria either from chorioamnionitis, congenital pneumonia, or bowel perforation during the first few days of life are often due to gram-positive, penicillin G–susceptible organisms. After this time, the clinical setting is usually neonatal gastrointestinal disease (NEC, bowel perforation), and the organisms are often gram-negative penicillin G–resistant organisms.

B. Treatment. Penicillin is effective for most anaerobic infections but is ineffective against *B. fragilis.* Third-generation cephalosporins and vancomycin will not be effective against *B. fragilis.* Clindamycin is usually effective against *B. fragilis.* It may not penetrate the CSF well, and some resistant strains exist. Chloramphenicol is effective against *B. fragilis* and penetrates the CSF well. We usually treat intestinal perforation with ampicillin, gentimicin, and clindamycin. In cases of congenital pneumonia, considerations of anaerobic infection would suggest the need to include agents for *B. fragilis* in the antibiotic coverage.

C. Other anaerobic infection. Tetanus caused by *Clostridium tetani* is among the most severe anaerobic neonatal infections [124,166]. It often arises from infection of the umbilical stump. Treatment of tetanus includes administration of antitoxin (tetanus immune globulin 3000 to 6000 U IM), immunization with tetanus toxoid, parenteral penicillin G (100,000 to 200,000 U/kg per day for 10 to 14 days), and surgical care of the cord or wound, if necessary. For general sedation, although multiple drugs have been used, barbiturates afford good sedation as well as decreasing muscle spasms. Phenothiazines also may be used, but tachyphylaxis may develop to this drug. In extreme cases, muscle relaxation with neuromuscular blocking agents may be necessary if ventilation is compromised. Finally, neonatal infection with tetanus does not provide long-term immunity. These infants should therefore not be omitted from active immunization programs. Immunization of pregnant women will prevent neonatal tetanus.

References

1. Klein, J. O., and Marcy, S. M. Bacterial Sepsis and Meningitis. In J. S. Remmington and J. O. Klein (Eds.), *Infectious Diseases of the Fetus and Newborn Infant.* Philadelphia: Saunders, 1983. Pp. 679–735.
2. Pass, M. A. *J. Pediatr.* 95: 437, 1979.
3. Faro, S. *Am. J. Obstet.* 139: 686, 1981.
4. Boyer, K. M. *J. Infect. Dis.* 148: 795, 1983.
5. Buetow, K. C., Klein, S. W., and Lane, R. B. *Am. J. Dis. Child.* 110: 29, 1965.
6. Groover, R. V. *N. Engl. J. Med.* 264: 1115, 1961.
7. Baker, C. J., and Edwards, M. S. Group B Streptococcal Infections. In J. S. Remmington and J. O. Klein (Eds.), *Infectious Diseases of the Fetus and Newborn Infant.* Philadelphia: Saunders, 1983. P. 820.
8. Baker, C. J. *N. Engl. J. Med.* 294: 753, 1976.
9. Hemming, V. G. *J. Clin. Invest.* 58: 1379, 1976.
10. Baker, C. J. *Pediatrics* 68: 544, 1981.
11. Adamkin, D. *J. Pediatr.* 93: 604, 1978.
12. Strunk, R. C. *Pediatr. Res.* 13: 641, 1979.
13. Davis, C. A. *Pediatr. Res.* 13: 1043, 1979.
14. Mills, E. L. *Pediatr. Res.* 13: 1341, 1979.
15. Shigeoka, A. O. *J. Pediatr.* 95: 454, 1981.
16. Baker, C. J. *J. Exp. Med.* 143: 258, 1976.
17. Baker, C. J. *JAMA* 230: 1158, 1974.

18. Milligan, T. W. *Infect. Immun.* 21: 738, 1978.
19. Mattingly, S. J. *J. Clin. Microbiol.* 12: 633, 1980.
20. Robbins, J. B. *N. Engl. J. Med.* 290: 1216, 1974.
21. Evans, D. J. *J. Clin. Microbiol.* 13: 171, 1981.
22. Smith, H. W. *J. Gen. Microbiol.* 121: 387, 1980.
23. Guerina, N. G. *J. Infect. Dis.* 148: 395, 1983.
24. Ciesielski, C. A. *Arch. Intern. Med.* 148: 1416, 1988.
25. Schlech, A. F. *N. Engl. J. Med.* 308: 203, 1983.
26. Albritton, W. L. *Clin. Lab. Invest. Med.* 7: 311, 1984.
27. Bortolussi, R. *Surv. Synth. Pathol. Res.* 3: 311, 1984.
28. Lu, C. Y. *Infect. Immun.* 36: 169, 1982.
29. Redline, S. *J. Immunol.* 140: 3947, 1988.
30. Friesen, C. A. *Rev. Infect. Dis.* 8: 777, 1986.
31. Jarvis, W. R. *Pediatr. Infect. Dis.* 6: 344, 1987.
32. Townsend, T. R. *Am. J. Epidemiol.* 114: 73, 1981.
33. Goldmann, D. A. *J. Infect. Dis.* 144: 449, 1981.
34. Coustan, D. R. Clinical Aspects of Antenatal Enhancement of Pulmonary Maturation. In L. Stern (Ed.), *Clinics in Perinatology: The Respiratory System in the Newborn.* Philadelphia: Saunders, 1987. P. 697.
35. Boyer, K. M. *N. Engl. J. Med.* 314: 1665, 1986.
36. Philip, A. G. S. *Pediatrics* 65: 1036, 1980.
37. Mims, L. C. *Am. J. Obstet. Gynecol.* 114: 232, 1972.
38. Visser, V. E. *J. Pediatr.* 96: 1063, 1980.
39. Polk, D. B. *Pediatr. Infect. Dis. J.* 6: 1040, 1987.
40. Swingle, H. M. *J. Infect. Dis.* 152: 515, 1985.
41. Scheld, W. M. *J. Infect. Dis.* 140: 287, 1979.
42. McCracken, G. H., Jr. *JAMA* 252: 1427, 1984.
43. Odio, C. M. *Pediatr. Infect. Dis. J.* 6: 371, 1987.
44. Feldstein, T. J. *Pediatr. Infect. Dis. J.* 6: 471, 1987.
45. Robertson, A. *J. Pediatr.* 112: 291, 1988.
46. Fink, S. *Pediatrics* 80: 873, 1987.
47. Powell, K. R. *Pediatr. Infect. Dis. J.* 6: 461, 1987.
48. Yoder, M. C., and Polin, R. A. Immunotherapy of Neonatal Sepsis. In R. A. Polin and W. W. Fox (Eds.), *The Pediatric Clinics of North America: The Newborn II.* Philadelphia: Saunders, 1986. P. 481.
49. Wilson, C. B. *J. Pediatr.* 108: 1, 1986.
50. Fisher, G. W. *Acta Pediatr. Scand.* 71: 639, 1982.
51. Christensen, K. K. *Pediatr. Infect. Dis. J.* 5: S189, 1986.
52. Jacobs, R. F. *J. Infect. Dis.* 152: 695, 1985.
53. Bortolussi, R. *Infect. Immun.* 28: 111, 1980.
54. Guerina, N. G. *Microecol. Therapy* 14: 183, 1984.
55. Horwitz, M. A. *J. Clin. Invest.* 65: 82, 1980.
56. Buchweier, N. A. *Proc. Natl. Acad. Sci. USA* 82: 7404, 1985.
57. Czuprynski, C. J. *J. Immunol.* 140: 962, 1988.
58. Leist, T. P. *J. Exp. Med.* 167: 1743, 1988.
59. Nakane, A. *Infect. Immun.* 56: 2563, 1988.
60. Shigeoka, A. O. *Lancet* 1: 636, 1978.
61. Santos, J. I. *J. Pediatr.* 99: 873, 1981.
62. Kim, K. S. *Pediatr. Res.* 23: 474A, 1988.
63. Chirico, G. *J. Pediatr.* 110: 437, 1987.
64. Haque, K. N. *Pediatr. Infect. Dis. J.* 5: 622, 1986.
65. Christensen, R. D. *Pediatrics* 70: 1. 1982.
66. Christensen, R. D. *J. Pediatr.* 98: 101, 1981.
67. Stork, E. *Pediatr. Res.* 19: 366A, 1985.
68. Vain, N. E. *Pediatrics* 66: 683, 1980.
69. Belohradsky, B. H. *Infection* 6: S139, 1978.
70. Christensen, R. D. *J. Clin. Apheresis* 2: 177, 1984.
71. Baker, C. J. *N. Engl. J. Med.* 319: 1180, 1988.
72. Short, B. L., et al. *Clin. Perinatal* 14: 737, 1987.
73. Troug, W. E. *Pediatr. Res.* 23: 352, 1988.

74. Craig, W. S. *Arch. Dis. Child* 38: 927, 1962.
75. Voora, S. *Pediatrics* 69: 40, 1982.
76. Akenzua, G. I. *Pediatrics* 54: 38, 1974.
77. Boyle, R. J. *Pediatrics* 62: 744, 1978.
78. Christensen, R. D. *Pediatrics* 70: 1, 1982.
79. Manroe, B. L. *J. Pediatr.* 95: 89, 1979.
80. Philip, A. G. S. *Pediatrics* 65: 1036, 1980.
81. Brazy, J. E. *J. Pediatr.* 100: 265, 1982.
82. Anday, E. K. *J. Pediatr.* 101: 614, 1982.
83. Sidebottom, D. G. *J. Clin. Microbiol.* 26: 713, 1988.
84. Goldmann, D. A. *Infect. Dis. Clin. North Am.* 3: 779, 1989.
85. Freeman, J., et al. *N. Engl. J. Med.* 323: 301, 1990.
86. Bergstrom, T. *J. Pediatr.* 80: 858, 1972.
87. Visser, V. E. *J. Pediatr.* 94: 635, 1979.
88. Ries, K. *Clin. Perinatol.* 1: 423, 1974.
89. Klein, J. O. Bacterial Infections of the Respiratory Tract. In J. S. Remmington and J. O. Klein (Eds.), *Infectious Diseases of the Fetus and Newborn Infant.* Philadelphia: Saunders, 1983. P. 744.
90. Ablow, R. C. *N. Engl. J. Med.* 294: 65, 1976.
91. Kundsin, R. B. *Obstet. Gynecol.* 74: 679, 1989.
92. Romero, R. *Obstet. Gynecol.* 73: 532, 1989.
93. Hillier, S. L. *N. Engl. J. Med.* 319: 972, 1988.
94. Leng, J. J. *Rev. Fr. Gynecol. Obstet.* 82: 107, 1987.
95. Cassell, G. H. *Sex. Transm. Dis.* 10(Suppl. 4): 294, 1983.
96. Garland, S. M. *Pediatr. Infect. Dis. J.* 6: 868, 1987.
97. Waites, K. B. *Pediatrics* 83: 79, 1989.
98. Waites, K. B. *Lancet* 1: 17, 1988.
99. Holtzman, R. B. *J. Pediatr.* 114: 1061, 1989.
100. Wang, E. E. *Pediatr. Infect. Dis. J.* 7: 547, 1988.
101. Sanchez, P. J. *Pediatr. Infect. Dis. J.* 7: 542, 1988.
102. Cassell, G. H. *Pediatr. Infect. Dis. J.* 7: 535, 1988.
103. Cassell, G. H. *Lancet* 2: 240, 1988.
104. Sanchez, P. J. *Pediatr. Infect. Dis. J.* 6: 825, 1987.
105. McCormack, W. M. *Obstet. Gynecol.* 69: 202, 1987.
106. Mason, W. H. *Pediatr. Infect. Dis. J.* 8: 521, 1989.
107. Cushing, A. H. *Pediatr. Infect. Dis.* 4: 282, 1985.
108. Stunden, R. J. *J. Pediatr. Surg.* 23: 130, 1988.
109. Stoll, B. J. *Pediatr. Clin. North Am.* 26: 415, 1979.
110. Lally, K. P. *Ann. Surg.* 199: 101, 1984.
111. Marcy, S. M., and Klein, J. O. Focal Bacterial Infections. In J. S. Remmington and J. O. Klein (Eds.), *Infectious Diseases of the Fetus and Newborn Infant.* Philadelphia: Saunders, 1983. Pp. 801–808.
112. Overturf, G. D. *Pediatrics* 89: 19, 1975.
113. Weissberg, E. D. *Pediatrics* 53: 505, 1974.
114. Morrissy, R. T. *Pediatr. Annu.* 18: 33, 1989.
115. Pittard, W. B. *J. Pediatr.* 88: 621, 1976.
116. Samilson, R. L. *Pediatrics* 21: 798, 1958.
117. Glaser, A. A. *Pediatrics* 58: 692, 1976.
118. Granoff, D. M. *Am. J. Dis. Child.* 129: 730, 1975.
119. Visser, V. E. *J. Pediatr.* 94: 635, 1979.
120. American Academy of Pediatric's Committee on Drugs, Committee on Fetus and Newborn, and Committee on Infectious Diseases. *Pediatrics* 65: 1047, 1980.
121. Nishida, H. *Pediatrics* 53: 368, 1975.
122. Hammerschlag, M. R. *N. Engl. J. Med.* 320: 769, 1989.
123. Fransen, L. *Int. Ophthalmol.* 11: 189, 1988.
124. American Academy of Pediatrics. *Report of the Committee on Infectious Diseases (Redbook).* Elk Grove Village, Ill.: AAP, 1988.
125. Centers for Disease Control. *MMWR* 36(Suppl 5): 1S, 1987.
126. Centers for Disease Control. *MMWR* 36: 107, 1987.
127. Laga, M. *N. Engl. J. Med.* 315: 1382, 1986.

128. Denison, M. R. *Pediatrics* 81: 877, 1988.
129. Laga, M. *N. Engl. J. Med.* 318: 653, 1988.
130. Clapp, D. W., et al. *J. Pediatr.* 115: 973, 1989.
131. Weisman, L. E. *J. Pediatr.* 115: 445, 1989.
132. Kenny, J. F. *Clin. Pediatr.* 26: 473, 1987.
133. Lisby, S. M. *Clin. Pharmacol.* 6: 25, 1987.
134. Wilfert, C., and Gutman, L. Sexually Transmitted Diseases: Gonorrhea. In R. D. Feigin and J. D. Cherry (Eds.), *Textbook of Pediatric Infectious Diseases.* Philadelphia: Saunders, 1987. P. 595.
135. Jones, D. E. D. *J. Am. Venereal Dis. Assoc.* 2: 30, 1976.
136. van der Harten, J. J. *Arch. Dis. Child.* 50: 662, 1975.
137. Solomon, S. L. *Pediatr. Infect. Dis. J.* 5: 680, 1986.
138. Weese-Mayer, D. E. *Pediatr. Infect. Dis. J.* 6: 190, 1987.
139. Baetz-Greenwalt, B. *Pediatrics* 81: 826, 1988.
140. Ho, N. K. *Aust. Paediatr. J.* 20: 127, 1984.
141. Kozinn, P. J. *Can. Med. Assoc. J.* 126: 1386, 1982.
142. Schreiber, J. R. *Pediatrics* 74: 838, 1984.
143. Hammerschlag, M. R. *J. Pediatr.*114: 727, 1989.
144. Alexander, E. R. *Rev. Infect. Dis.* 5: 713, 1983.
145. Burnham, R. C., et al. *N. Engl. J. Med.* 311: 1, 1984.
146. Eager, R. M., et al. *West. J. Med.* 143: 37, 1985.
147. Schachter, J., et al. *JAMA* 225: 3374, 1986.
148. Beem, M. O. *N. Engl. J. Med.* 296: 306, 1977.
149. Tipple, M. A., et al. *Pediatrics* 63: 192, 1979.
150. Marcy, S. M., and Guerrant, R. L. Microorganisms Responsible for Neonatal Diarrhea. In J. S. Remmington and J. O. Klein (Eds.), *Infectious Diseases of the Fetus and Newborn Infant.* Philadelphia: Saunders, 1983. Pp. 917–1013.
151. Berman, S. A. *Pediatrics* 62: 198, 1978.
152. Shek, Y. H., et al. *Am. J. Clin. Pathol.* 92: 595, 1989.
153. Surmont, I., et al. *Eur. J. Pediatr.* 148: 435, 1989.
154. Larocco, M., et al. *Pediatr. Infect. Dis. J.* 7: 398, 1988.
155. Dankner, W. M., et al. *Rev. Infect. Dis.* 9: 743, 1987.
156. Redline, R. W., et al. *Hum. Pathol.* 16: 815, 1985.
157. Powell, D. A., et al. *J. Pediatr.* 105: 987, 1984.
158. Powell, D. A., et al. *J. Pediatr.* 111: 217, 1987.
159. Bell, L. M., et al. *Infect. Control. Hosp. Epidemiol.* 9: 151, 1988.
160. Freis, B. J., and Sever, J. L. (Eds.). Infectious Complications in Pregnancy. *Clin. Perinatol.* 15: 2 (whole issue), 1988.
161. Zackman, R. D. *J. Perinatol.* 8: 111, 1988.
162. Tuppuraenen, N., et al. *Obstet. Gynecol.* 73: 583, 1989.
163. Sanchez, P. J., et al. *J. Pediatr.* 116: 601, 1990.
164. Prober, C. G. *Pediatr. Infect. Dis. J.* 9: 111, 1990.
165. Noel, G. J., et al. *Pediatr. Infect. Dis. J.* 7: 858, 1988.
166. Stoll, B. J. *Ped. Clin. North Am.* 26: 415, 1979.

Tuberculosis (TB) [1,5,11,15]

John P. Cloherty

I. **Tuberculosis (TB)** is somewhat uncommon in the United States. In 1988, 22,517 cases were reported (9.1 per 100,000 U.S. population) [8]. The rates of TB infection are four- to ninefold higher for racial/ethnic minorities [4] (non-Hispanic blacks, Hispanics, Asian/Pacific Islanders, American Indian/Alaskan natives) than for non-Hispanic whites. The rates of TB infection have been increasing for non-Hispanic blacks and Hispanics. Although still high, the rates have been decreasing for Asian/Pacific Islanders and American Indian/Alaskan natives [7,8]. The rates of TB infection have been increasing in the age group from 25 to 44 years. In the racial and ethnic minorities, the greatest number of cases was in the 25- to 44-year-old group. While in non-Hispanics, the greatest number of cases was in the over 65-year-old group [7,8]. There has always been an association between TB and crowded housing, poor nutrition, poverty, and poor living conditions. Human immunodeficiency virus (HIV) infection in persons already infected with TB is a risk factor for the development of reactivated disease [8]. TB should be considered in patients with the preceding risk factors. The highest risk group for mortality from TB is patients under age 5. Untreated TB in the newborn is almost always fatal.

II. Diagnosis

A. Maternal tuberculosis. As in nonpregnant adults, the tubercle bacilli is contracted by pregnant women by inhalation. Most cases are asymptomatic or have minimal disease. Symptomatic women may present with cough, weight loss, fever, malaise, fatigue, or hemoptysis. Other manifestations may be mastitis, miliary tuberculosis, tuberculosis meningitis, and the later manifestation of tuberculosis of the skin, joints, kidney, and bone. Lymphohematogenous spread and endometritis are important in the pathogenesis of infection in the fetus and newborn [11]. Finding a peritoneal fibrinous exudate at cesarean section or an infected placenta may lead to the diagnosis of tuberculosis in the mother and newborn. Since the use of antituberculosis chemotherapy, there is no increased risk to the pregnant mother from tuberculosis as compared with nonpregnant women. Pregnant women with tuberculosis in the United States usually have no symptoms or have minimal disease. Diagnosis involves history, including epidemiologic and social information, and determination of PPD (purified protein derivative) status. Pregnancy has no effect on the reaction to PPD [10]. Finding a positive PPD reaction in an asymptomatic woman is the most common method of diagnosing TB in pregnancy in the United States. If there is a conversion reaction to PPD in a pregnant woman, a careful history should be taken, questions about employment, contacts, etc. should be asked, and a chest x-ray (with shielding of the fetus) should be done. Sputum samples should be obtained for smear, culture, and sensitivity. There should be a search for extrapulmonary TB, and if indicated, biopsies should be taken for examination and culture. If the history and clinical symptoms suggest TB in the absence of a positive skin test, material (sputum, nodes, biopsy) should be taken to confirm the diagnosis and treatment should be considered. Untreated TB is a far greater risk to the pregnant woman and her fetus than the risks of treatment [12]. Tuberculosis during pregnancy is not an indication for a therapeutic abortion [2]. There is no significant increase in malformations in infants born to mothers who had tuberculosis and were treated for it [3].

B. Tuberculosis of the fetus or newborn. Congenital tuberculosis is rare. Women with only pulmonary infection usually do not infect their offspring until after birth. In utero infection may occur by various mechanisms.

1. Miliary tuberculosis in the mother may cause infection of the placenta and then spread to the fetal circulation by the umbilical vein. The primary complex is usually the liver. The infant may be sick at birth with respiratory distress, poor feeding, fever, hepatomegaly, skin papules, lymphadenopathy, or ear drainage. Some infants may not have symptoms until the second or third week of life. Most patients have an abnormal chest x-ray, but some will have a normal film.
2. In women with tuberculosis endometritis, the fetus may aspirate infected amniotic fluid. If the aspiration was weeks before delivery, the baby will be symptomatic at birth and usually have an abnormal chest x-ray.
3. If the infection is acquired by aspiration of infected secretions at the time of birth, the infant will be well initially but will develop poor feeding, failure to thrive, anemia, and gastrointestinal and respiratory distress at 4 to 8 weeks. A purified protein derivative (PPD) tuberculin skin test (5 units) should be performed on any infant suspected of having congenital or perinatally acquired tuberculosis. It may not be positive unless the infection has been present for 4 to 6 months. Acid-fast stains and cultures

should be performed on blood, urine, gastric fluid, tracheal aspirates, and CSF. Tissue from lymph nodes, liver, lung, bone marrow, and the placenta may reveal organisms on pathologic examination and culture. Skin lesions should be examined and cultured, but may not contain organisms. Drug sensitivities should be performed on any organism grown from these cultures. If the mother has had recent active tuberculosis or develops an active lesion in the postpartum period, there should be aggressive investigation of the history and epidemiology and physical and laboratory examinations of the infant. If all direct smears are negative and the infant is ill, antituberculosis therapy should be started until the diagnosis is ruled out.

III. Management [1,5]

A. Mother. The recommended maternal treatment of **active** tuberculosis in pregnancy is **isoniazid (INH)** and **rifampin (RIF) daily,** and ethambutal is added if there is a possibility of INH resistance. Pyridoxine should be given in a dose of 50 mg daily. Other regimens used are INH and RIF and ethambutol daily for 1 to 2 months, then INH and RIF 2 times a week for 9 months or INH and ethambutol for 18 months with RIF added if resistance is likely [15]. If the organism is sensitive to all drugs, treatment can then be given twice weekly. The duration of therapy is usually 9 months. INH, RIF, and ethambutal have not been shown to be teratogenic. Streptomycin has teratogenic effects, causing vestibular damage and deafness. There are no data on the effects of pyrazinamide in pregnancy. Cycloserine and ethanamide should be avoided in pregnancy. Mothers infected with organisms that are resistant to many drugs may need treatment with medications that are usually contraindicated in pregnancy or have unknown fetal effects. This will leave the mother and physician difficult choices about treatment and continuation of the pregnancy. If the mother has a positive skin test, has never been treated, and active disease is ruled out, she should be treated with INH starting in the second trimester if the skin test conversion occurred during the previous 2 years. If the skin test conversion occurred over 2 years before the pregnancy and the chest x-ray is normal, maternal treatment can wait until the postpartum period. If a mother has HIV infection, a PPD skin test with redness and induration of 5mm or greater is an indication for treatment of tuberculosis. This is true even if the mother has had BCG in the past [14]. Table 12-7 is an outline of the usual management of tuberculosis in pregnant women. INH is excreted in breast milk in amounts that would not cause toxicity yet in amounts inadequate for treatment or prophylaxis of the infant [1,5].

B. Congenital or neonatal TB. Any infant with symptoms mentioned in **II.B** should cause one to consider TB as the diagnosis. Congenital tuberculosis is a serious illness. The prognosis is worse in premature infants. Once a diagnosis of congenital or neonatal tuberculosis is made or probable and all studies, cultures, and sensitivities are done, treatment should be started. The usual medications are INH and RIF given daily. If there is a possibility of infection with drug-resistant tuberculosis, treatment should be started with three or four drugs. INH, RIF, streptomycin (SM), and pyrazinamide (PZA) are often used in a daily dose. Streptomycin used for more than 6 to 8 weeks may be associated with eighth nerve damage. Tuberculosis meningitis is usually treated with INH, RIF, and PZA. Ethambutal may cause retrobulbar neuritis. Once sensitivities are known, treatment can be changed to two bactericidal drugs given twice weekly. Treatment is usually for 9 months. If INH, RIF, and PZA are given daily for the first 2 months, a total of 6 months of treatment is adequate. Other regimens are INH, RIF and PZA for 2 months, then INH and RIF for 4 months more or INH and RIF for 9 months and PZA and ethambutal if resistant [15]. The usual dose of INH is 10 to 20 mg/kg once daily or 20 to 40 mg/kg twice weekly. The usual dose of RIF is 10 to 20 mg/kg once daily and 10 to 20 mg/kg twice weekly. See refs. 5 and 15 for other doses of antituberculosis drugs. Syrup preparation of INH and RIF are unstable. Tablets should be used.

Table 12-7. Diagnosis and treatment of tuberculosis in the pregnant woman

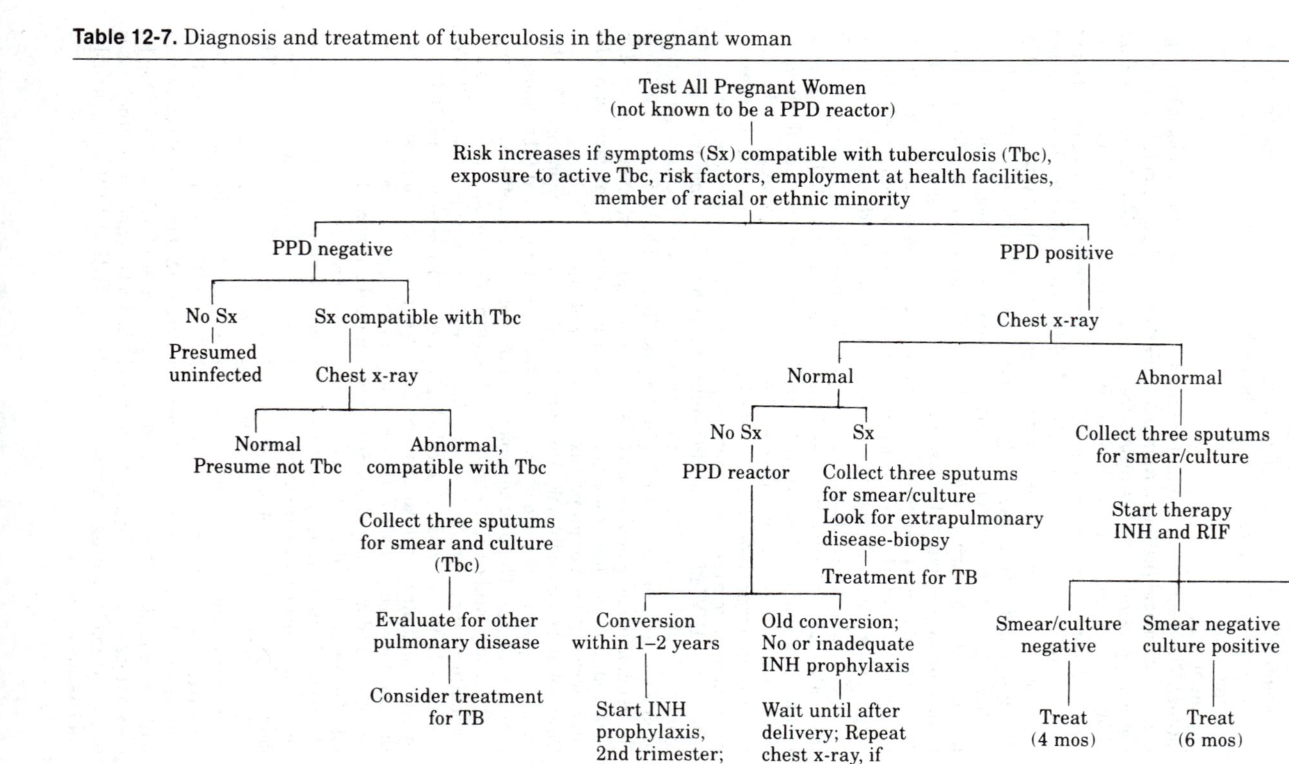

Source: Reprinted with permission, from Jacobs, R. F., and Abernathy, R. S. Management of tuberculosis in pregnancy and the newborn. *Clin. Perinatol.* 15: 310, 1988.

C. Other management of the infant of the mother with tuberculosis

1. Active infections in the mother

a. Hematogenous spread (miliary disease, bone disease, meningitis, endometrial disease, etc. in mother) or untreated pulmonary disease in mother. Do PPD, CXR, and culture on infant. If the baby appears to be infected, treat as in congenital TB (**III.B**). If there are no clinical or radiographic signs of infection in the infant, separate the infant from the mother until the mother is not contagious. The infant is given daily INH for at least 6 months. The PPD should be repeated at 4 to 6 weeks, 3 months, and 6 months of age. If it turns positive, INH should be given for 1 year. Other family members should be investigated for disease. Bacillus Calmette-Guerin (BCG) should be considered if compliance is a problem (see **V**)[15].

b. The mother has active disease, is on treatment, yet is suspected of being contagious. The baby is separated from the mother until the mother is felt to be noncontagious. This may take 6 to 12 weeks of culture negativity [15]. The baby is treated with INH and skin tested as in **a.** The household is carefully investigated. Bacillus Calmette-Guerin (BCG) vaccine should be considered for the infant if there is concern about compliance (see **V**).

c. The mother with newly diagnosed, untreated minimal disease or disease that has been treated for over 2 weeks and who is felt to be noncontagious. The infant should receive INH, providing the mother's organisms are susceptible to INH. The infant should have a chest x-ray at 4 to 6 weeks of age. A PPD should be done at 4 to 6 weeks of age, 3 months of age, and 6 months of age. If the PPD is negative at 6 months of age and there is no active disease in the family, INH can be discontinued in the infant. Separation of the infant from the mother is not necessary if compliance with the treatment plan is ensured. If there is concern about compliance, BCG vaccine for the infant should be considered.

2. No active infection in the mother

a. Mother with inactive infection, receiving treatment, with negative sputum and stable chest x-ray. The infant is at risk even if sputum is negative. The mother should have a chest x-ray at 3 and 6 months postpartum.

(1) In general, the infant is not separated from the mother.

(2) Specific therapy. The infant is treated with one of the following regimens:

(a) Isoniazid may be given (see **III.B**).

(b) BCG vaccine may be administered after ruling out active disease if there are compliance or follow-up problems.

b. Mother with history of adequate treatment. The mother should be observed with a chest film at 3 and 6 months postpartum, since there is some possibility that exacerbation may occur during pregnancy.

(1) The infant is not separated from the mother. PPD skin tests are performed on the baby every 3 months for 1 year; after that, tests are performed yearly.

(2) BCG vaccine and isoniazid are not given to the infant.

(3) The family is investigated for evidence of infection.

c. Mother with positive result on testing with PPD tuberculin only. The mother's sputum and chest x-ray are negative. There is some debate as to whether the mother should be treated during pregnancy or whether treatment should commence only after delivery, because there is an increased risk of hepatitis associated with isoniazid therapy during pregnancy. The current recommendation is to avoid isoniazid therapy in pregnant women if possible. Generally, the woman is treated if she is a known recent converter (within the previous 2 years), if she has an induration of 10 mm on testing with PPD tuberculin, or if there is any suggestion of immunosuppression. INH is started during the second trimester [1,5].

(1) The infant is not separated from the mother.

(2) Specific therapy for the infant.

(a) The infant is usually not given BCG vaccine, but it may be indicated if follow-up is poor.

(b) Isoniazid is usually not given. The baby is tested with PPD tuberculin every 3 months; if the result is positive, the baby should be treated for 1 year.

IV. Newborns exposed to tuberculosis in the nursery. The documented risk is low, but there is a possibility of spread from infected infants or personnel. If the exposure is considered to be significant, the infant should be tested with 5 units of PPD and, if negative, treated with isoniazid 10 mg/kg per day for 3 months. The skin test should then be repeated; if it still is negative, therapy can be stopped. Nursery personnel should be tested with PPD yearly.

V. Bacillis Calmette-Guerin (BCG) vaccine [1,5,6,9,13]. BCG vaccine is a live, attenuated strain of *Mycobacterium bovis*. These vaccines have been manufactured from many substrains of *M. bovis* that have been subcultured for years in many different laboratories. The last test of efficacy done in the United States was in 1955. There have been many culture passages done since then. Some recent trials show efficacy; some do not. It does appear to have some protective effect against the development of tuberculosis and may make the disease less serious in those who contract it. BCG vaccine should be considered (1) for individuals, especially infants, who are tuberculin skin test negative and who live in a household with exposure to untreated or ineffectively treated patients with contagious tuberculosis and (2) for groups in which an excessive rate of new infections occurs and the usual surveillance and treatment have failed or are not feasible. BCG is often given to infants in whom there is risk of exposure, preventive treatment might not be carried out, and there is uncertainty about the stability of the home situation. BCG may be given to infants from birth to 2 months of age. It is not necessary to skin test these infants. After 2 months, BCG is given only to individuals with negative skin tests. PPD should be repeated 2 to 3 months after vaccinations. If the PPD is negative, the vaccine should be readministered. The package insert should be read and the instructions for administration followed carefully. In normal individuals, BCG has rare side effects or complications. Complications reported are severe and include prolonged ulceration at the vaccination site, lymphadenitis, osteomyelitis, and lupoid reactions. In immunodeficient patients, disseminated BCG and death may occur. Patients with burns or generalized skin infection should not receive BCG. INH may decrease the effectiveness of BCG. INH has **documented efficacy** and should not be withheld in order to give BCG, which has doubtful efficacy.

Tuberculosis (TB)

1. American Academy of Pediatrics. *Report of the Committee on Infectious Diseases.* Elk Grove, Ill.: AAP, 1988. Pp. 429–447.
2. Bass, J. B. *Am. Rev. Respir. Dis.* 134: 355, 1986.
3. Bjerkedae, T., et al. *Scand. J. Respir. Dis.* 56: 245, 1975.
4. Hinmann, A. R. *Am. J. Epidemiol.* 103: 486, 1976.
5. Jacobs, R. F., and Abernathy, R. S. *Clin. Perinatol.* W.B. Saunders, Philadelphia, 15: 305, 1988.
6. Kendig, E. L. *N. Engl. J. Med.* 281: 520, 1969.
7. Centers for Disease Control. *JAMA* 257: 1290, 1987.
8. Centers for Disease Control. *MMWR* 39: 1, 1990.
9. Padungchan, S., et al. *Bull. WHO* 64: 247, 1986.
10. Present, P. A., et al. *Am. Rev. Respir. Dis.* 112: 413, 1975.
11. Smith, M. H. D., and Margues, J. R. Tuberculosis and Other Mycobacterial Infections. In R. D. Feign and J. D. Cherry (Eds.), *Textbook of Pediatrics Infectious Disease,* 2d Ed. Philadelphia: Saunders, 1987. P. 1342.
12. Snider, D. E., Jr., et al. *Am. Rev. Respir. Dis.* 122: 65, 1980.

13. Young, T. K. *Am. J. Public Health* 76: 783, 1986.
14. Centers for Disease Control. *MMWR* 38: 236, 1989.
15. Smith, M. H. D., and Teele, D. U. Tuberculosis. In J. S. Remmington and J. O. Klein (Eds.), *Infectious Diseases of the Fetus and Newborn Infant,* 3d ed., W. B. Saunders, Philadelphia, 1990.

Syphilis

John P. Cloherty

I. Epidemiology [10]. About 20,000 cases of primary or secondary syphilis are reported each year in the United States. It is estimated that only one-third of actual cases are reported. The incidence of congenital syphilis parallels the rate of primary and secondary syphilis in women 15 to 29 years of age. The incidence of syphilis in this group of women has been rising in the United States (4.2 per 100,000 population in 1977 to 8 per 100,000 population in 1986). The reported cases of congenital syphilis in the United States amounted to **168** in 1978 and **365** in 1986.

A. Congenital syphilis. In a review of 709 cases of congenital syphilis [6], the major factors contributing to the occurrence of congenital syphilis were as follows:

1. No prenatal care (46 percent of cases)
2. Prenatal care—negative serologic test for syphilis (STS) in first trimester, but test not repeated (15 percent)
3. No STS test performed (4 percent)
4. Negative maternal STS at delivery in a mother who had syphilis but had not yet converted her blood test (7 percent)
5. Laboratory error (0.3 percent)
6. Delay in treatment (8 percent)
7. Prenatal treatment failures (14 percent)
8. Insufficient data (7 percent)

B. High-risk factors. Epidemiologic factors suggesting high risk for exposure are as follows:

1. Inadequate prenatal care
2. Unwed mother
3. Teenaged mother
4. Drug abuse in mother or sexual partner
5. Sexual promiscuity
6. Sexual contact with someone known to have a sexually transmitted disease (STD)
7. Past history of a STD
8. Disadvantaged minority group
9. Poverty
10. HIV infection

The majority of congenital syphilis cases reported in Massachusetts between 1986 and 1989 were associated with late or no prenatal care. Many were associated with drug abuse [7].

II. Diagnosis of syphilis

A. Mother

1. **Clinical signs.** Maternal syphilis may be suspected because of the presence of a primary chancre in any area or because of signs of secondary syphilis, which include fever, sore throat, adenopathy, headache, and rash. The rash may involve the palms and soles. Condylomata lata may occur around moist areas. Signs of tertiary disease are gummas, neurosyphilis, and cardiovascular syphilis [4].
2. **Laboratory testing. All pregnant women should have serologic testing for syphilis (STS) at the first prenatal visit.** A second STS should be performed at about **28 weeks' gestation.** Women who are at high risk or if

the results of testing are unknown should have serologic screening at delivery. Infants should not be discharged from the hospital until negative maternal serologic status or adequate therapy has been documented [2,3,7]. In women at very high risk, consideration should be given to repeating serologic testing 1 month postpartum to capture the rare patient who had early primary infection at delivery and had not developed a positive blood test.

3. **Serologic testing.**
   a. **Nontreponemal tests** [6]
      (1) RPR (rapid plasma reagin)
      (2) VDRL (venereal disease research laboratory)

      These tests detect anticardiolipin antibody. These antibodies correlate with ongoing tissue damage. Seventy-five percent of symptomatic cases of primary syphilis, 100 percent of cases of secondary syphilis, and 75 percent of cases of latent and tertiary syphilis will have a positive RPR or VDRL. In secondary syphilis, the VDRL or RPR is usually positive in a titer greater than 1 to 16. If this is the first attack of primary syphilis, the RPR/VDRL will become nonreactive 1 year after treatment. Patients with secondary syphilis will usually become negative in 2 years. Those with early latent syphilis under 1 year's duration will usually become negative within 4 years. After the first attack of early latent syphilis of 1 to 2 years' duration, 75 percent of patients will become RPR/VDRL-negative in 5 years. Of those with late latent syphilis, 45 percent will become seronegative in 5 years. The rest will remain seropositive [4]. Nontreponemal antibody tests titers (VDRL/RPR) do correlate with disease activity, usually rising with each new infection and falling after treatment.

      One percent of the time, the positive RPR or VDRL is not caused by syphilis. This has been called a **biologic false-positive (BFP) reaction** and is probably related to tissue damage from various causes. **Acute BFP reactions** are those which resolve in 6 months and are usually associated with illnesses such as viral exanthems, vaccinations, hepatitis, mononucleosis, and *Mycoplasma* or *Protozoa* infections. These patients usually have low titers (1 to 8 or less) and normal treponemal tests. Rarely, BFP reactions are seen as a result of pregnancy. **Chronic BFP reactions** may be seen in chronic hepatitis, cirrhosis, tuberculosis, some very elderly patients, malignancy (if associated with excess gammaglobulin), or autoimmune disease. Many patients with systemic lupus erythematosus will have a positive RPR or VDRL. The titer is usually 1 to 8 or less. While most patients with BFP reactions have negative treponemal tests, some patients with systemic lupus erythematosus or rheumatoid arthritis and chronic BFP also may have positive treponemal tests. Another problem with the nontreponemal tests is the occasional negative reaction due to the **prozone phenomenon**; that is, a negative reaction may occur when undiluted serum is used. Negative reactions also may occur in late syphilis. Any positive nontreponemal test should be confirmed with one of the treponemal tests [6].

   b. **Treponemal antibody tests** [6]. These tests detect an interaction between surface antigens of *T. pallidum* and serum immunoglobulins. The test often used is the **fluorescent treponemal antibody absorption test (FTA-Abs).** This test is difficult to do and in many states has been replaced by the **microhemagglutination assay for antibody to *T. pallidum* (MHA-TP),** which gives similar results.

      Ninety percent of patients with a primary syphilitic chancre will have a positive FTA-Abs test. All patients with secondary and late syphilis will have a positive FTA-Abs test. Once these tests are positive, they will remain positive for life. They will tell if an infection ever occurred but not if an actual infection is present. Treponemal antibody titers do not correlate with disease activity and should be reported as positive or negative. In some cases, where an antibody to DNA is present, such as systemic lupus erythematosus, rheumatoid arthritis, polyarteritis, and other autoimmune diseases, a positive FTA-Abs will be present in the absence of any present or previous infection with syphilis. Rarely, pregnancy per se will cause a positive test. A negative test excludes previous or past infection except in very early primary infection or past infection that was treated before the FTA-Abs test turned positive.

B. Infant

1. **Infants should be evaluated for syphilis if they were born to a seropositive women who**
   - **a.** Were untreated or have poorly documented treatment
   - **b.** Were treated during pregnancy, especially in the last month
   - **c.** Were treated with a drug other than penicillin
   - **d.** Did not have the expected drop in nontreponemal titers after treatment
   - **e.** Were treated but did not have serologic evidence of cure
   - **f.** Have the risk factors listed in **I.B**
2. **Clinical signs.** Clinical signs in the infant may be a persistent rhinitis, snuffles, rash, hepatosplenomegaly, lymphadenopathy, anemia, hemorrhage, disseminated intravascular coagulation, jaundice, ascites, hydrops, nephrosis, chorioretinitis, meningitis, osteochondritis, or periostitis. Stillbirth, prematurity, intrauterine growth retardation, and a large placenta may be seen. There is a delayed effect in the nervous system, teeth, and eyes. Clinical signs of central nervous system (CNS) infection rarely appear in the newborn, even though one-third to one-half of infected infants will have CNS involvement. Some infants will have postnatal failure to thrive.
3. **Infant laboratory tests**
   - **a. Dark-field examination** of nasal discharge, spinal fluid, or scrapings from any cutaneous lesion
   - **b. X-rays** for evidence of periostitis or osteochondritis
   - **c. Cerebrospinal fluid (CSF) examination** may reveal an increased mononuclear count, elevated protein level, and positive serology (VDRL not RPR). If the VDRL is positive in the CSF, it is considered diagnostic of neurosyphilis. It may be negative in the presence of neurosyphilis and cannot be used to absolutely rule out neurosyphilis. The FTA-Abs test is less specific (more false-positive results) but is very sensitive. When the FTA-Abs test is negative in the CSF, it is good evidence against neurosyphilis.
   - **d. Pathologic examination** of the placenta
   - **e. Nontreponemal reagin serologic tests** (RPR) with titer, as in **A.3.**
   - **f. FTA-Abs test** with titer, as in **A.3.** Since the IgG portion of the antibody in the nontreponemal (RPR) and treponemal (FTA-Abs) tests is transported across the placenta, these tests will be positive even if the mother did not transmit the infection to her infant and whether she was adequately treated or not. Monthly determination of the nontreponemal tests with titer (RPR/VDRL with titer) will show a fall in titer to zero by 2 to 4 months if the antibody is passively acquired. If the baby was infected and made antibody, the titer will not fall or may rise. The tests may be negative at birth if the infection was acquired late in pregnancy. Repeating the test later will confirm the diagnosis.
   - **g. IgM–FTA-Abs test.** This test uses fluorescent-labeled antihuman IgM to detect fluorescent treponemal IgM antibodies in the newborn blood. Since IgM antibody is usually not transmitted across the placenta, a positive test should indicate congenital syphilis. However, clinical studies have shown false-negative results in 20 to 40 percent of cases and false-positive reactions possibly related to rheumatoid factor in 10 percent of cases [6]. The test cannot be recommended at this time.
   - **h. *T. pallidum* immobilization (TPI) test** is now performed in only a few

research laboratories for evaluation of other tests but is occasionally used to distinguish between patients with syphilis and those with BFP due to collagen-vascular disease.

III. Prevention of congenital syphilis by treatment of infected pregnant women [1,2,3,6,7,10]. Pregnant women should have serologic screening for syphilis as described in **II.**

A. Treatment protocol for pregnant women

1. Clinical disease in mother—treat.

2. No clinical disease in mother

a. Negative serologic test (RPR/VDRL)

(1) No disease—no treatment. Repeat test in late pregnancy, as in **II.**

(2) Early disease, symptomatic—treat.

(3) Exposure to a person with infectious syphilis in the past 90 days. It may be prudent to treat even if the exposure is before 90 days if tests are not available and follow-up is doubtful.

b. Known positive (VDRL/RPR)

(1) Previous adequate treatment—observe and follow titers.

(2) Untreated—treat.

(3) Previous inadequate treatment or questionable treatment—treat.

c. Possible false-positive reactions (VDRL/RPR)

(1) If positive FTA-Abs/MHA-TP, treat. See **II.**

(2) If negative FTA-Abs/MHA-TP, observe. See **II.**

d. Known biologic false-positive reaction—observe.

e. New positive

(1) Treat mother and infant.

(2) Previous adequate treatment—observe and follow titers.

(3) Previous inadequate treatment—treat.

(4) Untreated—treat.

f. Err on the side of treatment when the diagnosis of syphilis cannot be excluded with reasonable certainty. In pregnancy, nontreponemal test titers may rise for nonspecific reasons.

Patients who have adequate documentation of proper treatment for syphilis need not be retreated unless clinical, serologic, or epidemiologic evidence of reinfection exists, e.g., clinical lesions, a sustained (for ≥2 weeks) fourfold titer rise in a quantitative nontreponemal test, or a history of recent (within 90 days) sexual exposure to a person with early infectious syphilis. A person with recent venereal exposure to a person with syphilis has a 25 to 50 percent chance of acquiring syphilis and may have negative tests because she is in the early stage of infection. Some chancres may be difficult to see.

B. Specific recommendations for treatment of pregnant mothers who have syphilis. Penicillin is the drug of choice.

1. Syphilis under 1 year's duration. Benzathine penicillin G (Bicillin) in a total dose of 4.8 million units in two doses divided 1 week apart (2.4 million units IM weekly × 2) or procaine penicillin G 600,000 units IM daily for 15 days. If the patient is HIV-positive with either early or late syphilis, the dose is procaine penicillin G 1.2 million units IM daily for 15 days or 4.0 million units IV every 4 hours for 15 days. In HIV-positive patients, treatment may be extended for 3 weeks [6].

2. Syphilis over 1 year's duration. Benzathine penicillin G (Bicillin) in a total dose of 7.2 million units given as 2.4 million units IM weekly for 3 weeks (2.4 million units IM weekly × 3) or procaine penicillin G 600,000 units IM daily for 15 days.

3. Neurosyphilis is usually treated with 600,000 units of procaine penicillin G IM twice daily for 2 to 3 weeks. Some authorities recommended high-dose intravenous therapy 2.4 million units IV every 4 hours for 2 to 3 weeks [5,6]. Other recommendations for treatment of neurosyphilis in adults are as follows:

a. Aqueous penicillin G 2.4 million units every 4 hours IV for 10 days followed by benzathine penicillin G 2.4 million units IM weekly for 3 weeks.

b. Aqueous procaine penicillin G 2.4 million units IM divided in doses every 12 hours plus probenecid 500 mg orally four times a day for 10 days plus benzathine penicillin G 2.4 million units IM weekly for 3 weeks.

c. Benzathine penicillin G 2.4 million units IM weekly for 3 weeks.

None of these regimens has been well studied, and some have been associated with treatment failure in neurosyphilis [1,5]. The Jarisch-Herxheimer reaction may occur after treatment for syphilis. Febrile reactions with fetal distress, premature labor, or stillbirth are rare but possible. Therapy is necessary and must be given [3,10].

4. **If** the pregnant woman with syphilis is **allergic to penicillin,** she can still be treated with penicillin, and an attempt should be made to do this. The history of penicillin allergy should be reviewed, and the patient should be skin-tested against the major and minor determinants for penicillin allergy. If these tests are negative, penicillin can be given under medical supervision. If the tests are positive, the patient can be desensitized and then given penicillin. Desensitization should be done in consultation with an expert and in a facility where emergency treatment is available. The specific method of desensitization to penicillin is reviewed in refs. 3 and 9.

5. **Other drugs** have all been associated with problems and treatment failures and are only used when patients have documented penicillin allergy and are unable to be desensitized [5,6,7,9,10].

   a. **Erythromycin** is effective in syphilis but crosses the placenta in an unpredictable manner and has been associated with an **unacceptable rate of failure to adequately treat the fetus.** Its use in the treatment of pregnant women with syphilis is discouraged. Doses that have been used are as follows: early syphilis (<1 year's duration), 500 mg qid for 15 days orally, and latent syphilis (>1 year's duration), 500 mg qid for 30 days orally.

   b. **Tetracycline** is more effective than erythromycin but may cause liver damage in pregnant women and damage the teeth and bones of fetuses. Doses that have been used are as follows: early syphilis (<1 year's duration), 500 mg qid for 15 days orally, and latent syphilis (>1 year's duration), 500 mg qid for 30 days orally.

   c. **Doxycycline** is as effective as tetracycline and may have fewer fetal effects. Doses used are as follows: early syphilis (<1 year's duration), 100 mg PO q12h for 15 days, latent syphilis (>1 year's duration), 100 mg PO q12h for 30 days [4].

   d. **Chloramphenical** is effective, but its use is discouraged because of the immature renal function of the fetus and inability to monitor fetal levels. It also affects hepatic conjugating enzymes and has a potential to cause aplastic anemia.

   e. **Ceftriaxane** may be an acceptable alternative to penicillin therapy in pregnant women with syphilis. There have been small studies that suggest efficacy, but the optimal dose and duration of treatment are not clear [5,6]. Some patients who are allergic to penicillin are allergic to cephalosporins.

6. If a mother is treated for syphilis in pregnancy, monthly follow-up should be provided. The antibody response should be the same as for a nonpregnant patient. Retreatment is given if needed. All patients with syphilis should be evaluated for other sexually transmitted diseases, such as gonorrhea, chlamydia, herpes, and HIV infection.

IV. Treatment for the infant [1,2,3,6,10]

A. In untreated pregnant women, syphilis can be transmitted to the infant regardless of the duration of the maternal disease, but transmission is more common the first year after infection. The infection appears to be more easily transmitted after the fourth month of pregnancy but can occur any time in pregnancy. The organisms reach the fetus by way of the placenta and umbilical vein. The liver is the primary site of infection, with secondary spread to the skin, mucous membranes, bones, and CNS. Direct contact of the infant with infectious lesions at or after birth can result in infection. See **II.B** for diagnosis in the newborn. Remember that infection in late pregnancy or at delivery may be associated with negative infant serology at birth. Repeat clinical examination and testing are necessary for diagnosis.

1. **Negative serologic test**
   a. **No disease—no treatment.** If the mother is infected late in pregnancy, it is possible to have a serologic-negative mother and infant as well as an initially asymptomatic infant, since there is no primary infection stage in newborns who have in utero infection.
   b. **Early disease—treat.**
      (1) Symptomatic—treat.
2. **Positive serologic test**
   a. **Symptomatic** (e.g., snuffles, rash, hydrops, hepatomegaly, roentgenographic findings, abnormal cerebrospinal fluid)—treat.
   b. **Asymptomatic**
      (1) If the baby's titer is three or four times higher than the mother's, treat.
      (2) If FTA-Abs test is 3 to 4 +, treat.
      (3) If disease is poorly documented or the mother inadequately treated or untreated, treat.
      (4) If unreliable mother or doubtful follow-up, treat.
      (5) If the mother's infection was treated with any drug but penicillin, treat.
      (6) If the mother had a recent sexual exposure to an infected person, treat.
      (7) If the mother was treated in the last month of pregnancy, treat.
      (8) If the mother has HIV and was treated for syphillis with less than **neurosyphillis** regimen.
3. If the baby's VDRL/RPR, FTA-Abs, or both are positive and if history and clinical examination (including x-ray) make infection unlikely, it is safe to repeat titers on VDRL/RPR and FTA-Abs at monthly intervals. Any significant rise in titer or development of clinical signs requires treatment. If the serology is not negative by 6 months of age, treat.
4. If there are **only transferred antibodies,** the baby should have a falling titer and be negative by 4 months.
5. A **cerebrospinal fluid examination** should be performed on all infants to be treated for congenital syphilis.
6. Some would treat all newborns with a positive serologic test for syphilis because it may be difficult to document that the mother has had adequate treatment and falling serologic titers, a low titer may be present in latent maternal syphilis, infected newborns may have no clinical signs at birth, and follow-up/compliance may be difficult in the population at risk for congenital syphilis [6].

B. Specific therapy for the infant [3]

1. Infants who are felt to be infected but who have no evidence of CNS infection should be treated with **aqueous crystalline penicillin** G 100,000 to 150,000 units/kg per day IM or IV in two or three divided doses for 10 to 14 days or **aqueous procaine penicillin** G 50,000 units/kg per day IM once daily for 10 to 14 days.
2. Infants with CNS infection (CSF pleocytosis, elevated CSF protein, positive CSF serology) should be treated with **aqueous crystalline penicillin** 150,000 units/kg per day IV or IM divided into two or three doses for 2 to 3 weeks or **aqueous procaine penicillin** 50,000 units/kg per day IM for 3 weeks. Err on the side of higher doses and longer treatment.
3. If infants who have been evaluated appear to be at low risk for congenital syphilis but close follow-up is doubtful, then they should be given

benzathine penicillin G 50,000 units/kg per day IM as a one-time dose. It should be recognized that there will be treatment failures with this dosage.

4. Some cases of persistent hepatitis have been seen in infants treated for congenital syphilis [8].

V. Follow-up of infant

A. Infants treated for congenital syphilis should have follow-up serologic tests with titers at 2, 4, 6, and 12 months. Any rise in titer is an indication for retreatment. The nontreponemal tests will become negative in 90 percent of adequately treated infants. Patients with persistent titers, even though low, should be considered for retreatment. The FTA-Abs test may remain positive.

B. Infants with neurosyphilis should have follow-up serologic titers at monthly intervals for 3 months and then be followed as those with syphilis. Spinal fluid should be examined monthly for 3 months and then every 6 months for 3 years. If the infant is adequately treated, the cell count and protein will usually become normal in 2 to 3 months, and the nontreponemal titers will fall. The FTA-Abs test may remain positive. Any rise in titers or increase in cell count is an indication for retreatment. A positive nontreponemal RPR/VDRL in the CSF at 6 months is an indication for retreatment [1].

VI. Infection control. Nasal secretions and open syphilitic lesions are very infectious. Drainage secretions, blood, and bodily fluid precautions should be taken, and health care personnel should wear gloves when caring for the newborn at risk for congenital syphilis. The infant is not infectious 24 hours after penicillin therapy is begun. Those who had close contact with an infected infant or mother before precautions were taken should be examined and tested for infection. Treatment should be considered.

VII. Infants at risk for or with syphilis should be evaluated for the presence of other disease such as herpes, gonorrhea, chlamydia, and HIV.

VIII. Assistance and guidance is available from the Centers for Disease Control, Atlanta, Georgia, or state departments of health.

References

1. American Academy of Pediatrics. *Report of the Committee on Infectious Diseases (Redbook).* Elk Grove Village, Ill.: AAP, 1988. P. 400.
2. Centers for Disease Control. *MMWR* 37: S1, 1988.
3. Centers for Disease Control. *MMWR* 38(S8): 13, 1989.
4. Fiumara, N. J. *Pictoral Guide to Sexually Transmitted Diseases.* New York: Cahners, 1989.
5. Hook, E. W., III. *Rev. Infect. Dis.* 11(Suppl. 6): 1511, 1989.
6. Ingall, D., et al. Syphilis. In J. S. Remmington and J. O. Klein (Eds.), *Infectious Diseases in the Fetus and Newborn Infant.* Philadelphia: Saunders, 1990.
7. Massachusetts Department of Public Health. *Health Care Provider Update on Congenital Syphilis in Massachusetts.* January 1990.
8. Shah, M. C. *Pediatr. Infect. Dis. J.* 8: 891, 1989.
9. Wendel, G. D., Jr., et al. *N. Engl. J. Med.* 312: 1229, 1987.
10. Wendel, G. D. *Clin. Perinatol.* 15: 287, 1988.

Lyme Disease

Nicholas G. Guerina

I. *Borrelia burgdorferi* (Lyme disease). The discovery of Lyme disease began when two women from Lyme, Connecticut, noted a clustering of arthritis disease in family members and neighborhood children. Since then, Lyme disease has been reported in 32 U.S. states, and from 1983 to 1986, 5016 cases were reported to the Centers for Disease Control [1]. The causative agent is the spirochete *Borrelia burgdorferi,* which is carried by the ticks *Ixodes dammini.* Infection often causes a distinct rash (erythema chronicum migrans) and can produce a spectrum of disease from mild "flulike" symptoms to severe cardiac, CNS, and joint disease [7].

Fetal infection with *B. burgdorferi* has been documented with maternal infection in pregnancy, but the transmission appears to occur at a low frequency. However, data are insufficient to establish the true risk of fetal disease. Transmission has been documented in both early and late gestation, but the relative risk of transmission and severity of fetal disease as a function of gestational age has not been established. Schlesinger et al. [2] and Weber et al. [3] described newborn infants with multiple organ involvement with *B. burgdorferi*. The first infant died on day 2 from congenital heart disease and was found to have spirochetes in the spleen, kidney, and bone marrow. The second infant died on day 1 with respiratory failure and complications of CNS dysfunction, and spirochetes were identified in the liver and brain. In both cases, maternal infection was believed to have occurred in the first trimester. A third case report described the identification of spirochetes in a stillborn infant to a women with a history of clinical symptoms of Lyme disease [4].

The pregnancy outcomes of 19 women with Lyme disease in pregnancy have been reported [5]. Adverse fetal/newborn findings were present in 5 cases. Complications included prematurity, intrauterine fetal demise, cortical blindness, syndactyly, and rash. In one of the cases, erythema chronicum migrans and meningoencephalitis occurred in a woman at 37 weeks' gestation. The infant was delivered 7 days later and was asymptomatic in the immediate postpartum period. On day 5, the infant developed petechiae and a vesicular rash that resolved with IV penicillin G. Three of the cases with adverse outcomes occurred in women who received antibiotic therapy. In a second study, 17 women who developed Lyme disease in pregnancy were followed [6]. All these women received antibiotic therapy. There was one aborted fetus and syndactyly in a second infant who had no other abnormalities.

II. Diagnosis. Lyme disease may be diagnosed by the appearance of a typical rash (erythema chronicum migrans) in women living in or visiting an area where cases of Lyme disease have been previously reported. However, the spectrum of clinical symptoms may be quite variable [7]. At this time, there have been too few cases of neonatal disease to predict the likely clinical findings in newborn infants with active infection. Serology (IgG and IgM antibodies specific for *B. burgdorferi*) is an important aid in the diagnosis of Lyme disease and is currently available through the Centers for Disease Control. Cord blood specific IgM may be helpful for determining infected newborn infants.

III. Treatment. Treatment regimens for Lyme disease in pregnancy have been suggested [8,9]. For mild early symptoms, including rash, "flulike" illness, mild cardiac disease, and limited neurologic impairment (e.g., Bell's palsy), amoxicillin is recommended. With penicillin allergy, erythromycin is suggested. More severe symptoms or chronic disease requires intravenous therapy (penicillin G or ceftriaxone). Ceftriaxone may be preferable in late disease [9]. The relative risk of fetal transmission as a function of the severity of maternal disease, chronicity of maternal disease, or choice of antibiotic and route of administration is not known. Similarly, data are lacking on the optimal therapy for the newborn infant with symptoms of acute Lyme disease. In the study by Markowitz et al. [5], a 38-week infant born to a mother with acute Lyme disease 1 week prior to delivery developed petechiae and a vesicular rash that resolved with the intravenous administration of penicillin G for 10 days.

Lyme Disease

1. Ciesielski, C. A., et al. *Rev. Infect. Dis.* 2: S1435, 1989.
2. Schlesinger, P. A., et al. *Ann. Intern. Med.* 103: 67, 1985.
3. Weber, K., et al. *Pediatr. Infect. Dis. J.* 7: 286, 1988.
4. McDonald, A. B., et al. *N.Y. J. Med.* 87: 615, 1987.
5. Markowitz, L. E., et al. *JAMA* 255: 3394, 1986.

6. Ciesielski, C. A., et al. Prospective Study of Pregnancy Outcome in Women with Lyme Disease. Interscience Conference on Antimicrobial Agents and Chemotherapy, New York, 1987 (Abstract No. 39).
7. Stechenberg, B. *Pediatr. Infect. Dis. J.* 7: 402, 1988.
8. Treatment of Lyme disease. *Med. Lett. Drugs Ther.* 1989.
9. Luft, B. J., et al. *Rev. Infect. Dis.* 2: S1518, 1989.

Toxoplasmosis

Nicholas G. Guerina

I. ***Toxoplasma gondii*** is an obligate, intracellular protozoan parasite that is well recognized as an important human pathogen. This is particularly true for the fetus and newborn infant, as well as immunocompromised adults. Many animals may become infected, but the cat is the only definitive host. During an acute infection, the cat may shed up to 10 million oocysts in the stool per day for up to 2 weeks [1]. These oocysts may remain viable in soil for many months depending on climactic conditions. Susceptible farm animals may become infected by ingesting the oocysts, resulting in localization of viable organisms in muscle cysts. The primary mode of transmission to humans beyond the newborn period is by the ingestion of the cysts in undercooked meat or by the direct ingestion of oocysts. Transmission following the transfusion of whole blood or leukocytes may occur, but the risk is unknown. Normal children and adults are susceptible to acute infection if they lack specific antibody to the organism. Both humoral and cell-mediated immunity are important in the control of infection. Following an acute parasitemia, the organism invades tissues, where cysts are formed. The cysts persist in multiple organs, probably for life. Most often these are of little consequence to the normal host, but progressive, localized, or reactivated disease may occur in a subset of patients.

A. **Maternal infection.** The prevalence of *Toxoplasma* antibody varies with age and geographic location. In New York City, seroprevalence data indicate that approximately 16 percent of childbearing women aged 15 to 19 years are seropositive [2]. The seroprevalence steadily increases to approximately 50 percent for women 35 years of age or older. This survey indicates that over the period of investigation, 50 to 85 percent of women were at risk for primary acute *Toxoplasma* infection in pregnancy. Mass screening of newborn infants for the presence of *Toxoplasma* antibody was conducted over the past 4 to 5 years in Massachusetts [3]. The screening was carried out on filter-paper blood specimens routinely sent to the state laboratories for newborn screening of inborn errors of metabolism. Since maternal IgG readily crosses the placenta and is present in the term newborn at levels comparable with those in the mother, the prevalence of specific antibody in the newborn reflects the overall seroprevalence in childbearing women. It was found that 17 percent of newborn specimens had IgG to *Toxoplasma*. Thus 83 percent of mothers were at risk for acute infection.

   Many cases of acute *Toxoplasma* infection in pregnancy go undiagnosed, presumably because symptoms may be transient and nonspecific. Typical signs and symptoms are limited to generalized or localized lymphadenopathy and fatigue. In some cases, a mononucleosis-like syndrome with fever, malaise, sore throat, headache, myalgia, and an atypical lymphocytosis may be present. A single posterior cervical lymph node may be involved, and adenopathy may persist for months.

B. **Congenital infection.** Estimates of congenital *Toxoplasma* infection in the United States have varied from as little as 0.1 per 1000 to 1 to 2 per 1000 births. In a prospective screening study in New York City, a rate of 1.3 per 1000 births was reported in 1971 [4]. Based on the determination of cord blood IgM (followed by confirmatory titers in positive infants), a decreasing incidence (2 per 1000 to 0.1 per 1000) of congenital infection has been observed in Alabama [1,5]. In Massachusetts, the incidence of congenital infection based on IgM screening of filter-paper blood specimens (followed by confirmatory titers in the newborn) has been found to be around 0.1 to 0.13 per 1000 births.

The overall rate of fetal transmission during acute maternal *Toxoplasma* infection is approximately 40 percent, but the rate varies with gestational age [6]. Severe clinical disease is observed primarily with first-trimester infection, in which the rate of transmission is estimated to be approximately 15 percent. Conversely, the estimated rate of transmission in the third trimester is approximately 60 percent, but virtually all infected infants have mild or asymptomatic disease at birth. A major factor determining fetal transmission appears to be placental blood flow.

At least four forms of congenital infection have been recognized: (1) symptomatic neonatal disease, (2) symptomatic disease occurring in the first months of life, (3) sequelae or relapse in infancy or later childhood of previously undiagnosed infection, and (4) subclinical infection [1]. Severe neonatal disease invariably involves the CNS and also may include signs of generalized infection. Intracranial calcifications, abnormal CSF profiles, chorioretinitis, and convulsions are common findings in infants presenting with primarily neurologic disease [7]. Infants with signs and symptoms of generalized disease again frequently have chorioretinitis and abnormal CSF profiles, but they also have hepatosplenomegaly, lymphadenopathy, jaundice, and anemia [7]. Chorioretinal scars are the predominate feature of mild neonatal disease. Neurologic sequelae are common with severe neonatal disease, but it must be emphasized that the presence of neurologic abnormalities and/or hydrocephalus do not mean there has been extensive, irreversible CNS damage. These findings may occur as a result of active encephalitis, which may resolve with no sequelae after treatment [1].

The majority of infants with congenital *Toxoplasma* infection have subclinical disease [8,9], and several prospective studies have been conducted to determine the frequency of adverse outcomes in this group of infants [1,10–13,15]. These studies indicate that some degree of chorioretinal disease occurs in 20 to 85 percent of patients. The wide range may reflect differences due to (1) bias for the severity of infection, (2) the initiation of early treatment regimens, and (3) the length of follow-up. Nevertheless, it is clear that significant visual impairment, including bilateral blindness, may occur in congenitally infected individuals with inapparent disease at birth. Other sequelae occurring at lower frequencies include psychomotor retardation, seizures, hydrocephaly, microcephaly, reduced IQ, and sensorineural hearing loss.

II. Diagnosis. A number of methods may be employed in the diagnosis of congenital *Toxoplasma* infection [1]. These include isolation or histologic demonstration of the organism, detection of *Toxoplasma* antigens in tissues and body fluids, and serologic tests. Of these, serologic tests are the most frequently used at present. Several tests have been developed that determine specific IgG and/or IgM. Of particular interest are the Sabin-Feldman dye test and the indirect fluorescent antibody assay (IFA) for the detection of IgG and the IgM-IFA, IgM immunosorbent agglutination assay (IgM-ISAGA), and the double-sandwich IgM enzyme-linked immunosorbent assay (double-sandwich IgM-ELISA) [1].

III. Prevention and Treatment. The best way to prevent congenital *Toxoplasma* is by preventing acute maternal infection in pregnancy. At present, this requires the appropriate education of pregnant women about simple procedures that may minimize exposure [1]. These include the following:

A. Cats:

1. Keep indoors.
2. Empty litter every day (avoid if pregnant or wear gloves).
3. Feed only dry, canned, or cooked food.

B. Meat:

1. Avoid eating undercooked meat in pregnancy.

2. Wear gloves when handling meat, or wash hands thoroughly after handling.
3. Keep cutting boards and utensils thoroughly cleaned.

C. Vegetables:

1. Wear gloves when gardening.
2. Wash vegetables thoroughly before eating.
3. Wear gloves when handling vegetables, or wash hands thoroughly after handling.

A more definitive approach under development is the vaccination of cats and possibly intermediate hosts.

IV. Acute *Toxoplasma* in pregnancy. The diagnosis of acute *Toxoplasma* infection in pregnancy may be made by serologic testing with the possible results and interpretations as follows:

A. Initial serology performed at less than 2 months' gestation:

Negative dye test Negative IgM	Positive dye test Negative IgM	Positive dye test Positive IgM
↓	↓	↓
No infection	Infection before conception (no risk to fetus)*	Possible acute infection
		↓
		Repeat dye test in 3 weeks
		↓
		Stable or decreased titer
		↓
		Probable infection near or before conception (no risk to fetus)
		↓
		Increased dye titer
		↓
		Maternal acute infection (fetus at risk)

B. Initial serology performed later in gestation:

Negative dye titer (no infection)	Presence of two of the following: Clinical symptoms† High dye test titer‡ Positive IgM

C. Treatment of acute *Toxoplasma* in pregnancy with spiramycin has been shown to significantly reduce the rate of fetal transmission, but the severity of disease in infected infants may not be altered [6]. More recently, antenatal studies have been used to diagnose and treat congenital *Toxoplasma* infection in pregnancy [14]. Women were screened for susceptibility to *Toxoplasma* early in pregnancy in France. Women found to be susceptible were followed for seroconversion throughout pregnancy. Any women found to be acutely infected underwent percutaneous amniocentesis and umbilical blood sampling (PUBS), and serial ultrasound surveys were undertaken in an attempt to identify infected fetuses. The PUBS specimens were cultured for organisms, and specific IgM measurements were made along with a battery of other laboratory tests. All infected mothers were treated with spiramycin, and when fetal infection was suspected, pyrimethamine and a sulfa agent (sulfadoxine

*Seropositive immunocompromised patients (especially HIV-positive mothers) may be at risk for reactivation of *Toxoplasma* with subsequent fetal transmission.
†Lymphadenopathy consistent with acute *Toxoplasma* infection.
‡If clinical/IgM criteria are met but dye test shows titer low, repeat testing should demonstrate an increased titer.

or sulfadiazine) were added. The therapeutic regimen was pyrimethamine plus sulfonamide alternating every 3 weeks with spiramycin beginning at the twenty-fourth week of gestation. Folinic acid also was added to help prevent some of the potentially toxic side effects of pyrimethamine. Of 746 documented maternal infections, 42 cases of congenital infections were observed, 39 of which were identified by the antenatal screening tests. Twenty-four pregnancies were terminated. The remaining 15 pregnancies were carried to term; at 3 months follow-up, 13 of 15 infants remain asymptomatic. The other 2 infants were diagnosed with chorioretinitis. While these results are very exciting, they may not be easily applied to a relatively low incidence population.

In the French study population, the seroconversion rate is at least two to five times greater than that in the United States. It follows that the predictive value of the antenatal screening tests employed may be less in the U.S. population. Also, first-trimester screening was an important aspect of the study, but this is not always practical for many groups of patients in the United States. The expense of universal antibody screening in a low-incidence population is also a concern that has been raised.

Even if universal antibody screening in pregnancy is not feasible at this time, the results of the French study suggest that amniocentesis and PUBS may aid in the antenatal diagnosis of congenital infections. However, these procedures have definite risks to the fetus and mother that must measured against the uncertainty in predictive value in an unstudied population versus the risks of presumptive therapy with potentially toxic drugs. Nevertheless, it has been recommended that antenatal diagnosis of fetal infection be attempted in all women with confirmed acute *Toxoplasma* in pregnancy, provided testing can be done with minimal risks [1]. **In confirmed cases of fetal infection, or in cases where testing cannot be performed but acute maternal disease occurred in the second trimester, pyrimethamine (plus folinic acid)/sulfonamide alternating with spiramycin every 3 weeks beginning at 24 weeks' gestation is recommended** [1]. Long-term follow-up of infants treated in utero with this regimen is needed to better assess the impact of therapy on congenital *Toxoplasma* as well as the potential long-term effects of pyrimethamine exposure.

V. Infection in the newborn. Diagnosis of congenital *Toxoplasma* may be difficult because of the large number of asymptomatic presentations in the neonatal period. This is true even in symptomatic infants because of the wide spectrum of abnormalities and similarities with other congenital infections. Serology plays a key role, but in suspected cases, other laboratory tests, including placental pathology and cultures, as well as cultures of the infant's blood and CSF, may be helpful. The most useful serologic test is the determination of specific IgM by either the double-sandwich ELISA or IgM-ISAGA procedures [1]. In an attempt to diagnose most congenitally infected infants in Massachusetts, the New England Regional Screening Program was established in 1986. In this program, all newborn infants are screened for *Toxoplasma* antibodies, and for all infants with confirmed infection, antimicrobial therapy is recommended for 1 year. The protocol is as follows:

A. Serology performed on routine filter-paper specimens sent to the state laboratory for the screening of inborn errors of metabolism. Specific IgG and IgM (double-sandwich technique) are determined by ELISA.

B. The primary pediatrician is notified, and in conjunction with an infectious disease consult, the history, examination, and confirmatory serology are obtained (IgG/IgM ELISA on both mother and infant).

C. Treatment is initiated in confirmed or strongly suspected cases after a G6PD screen is performed (prior to initiating therapy with sulfa agents).

D. Initial and periodic follow-up tests are performed (the frequency of some tests varies as indicated for symptomatic infants).

1. Blood chemistries, weekly or biweekly CBCs to monitor toxic effects of pyrimethamine

2. CSF profiles, serology, and cultures (initial evaluation)
3. Ophthalmologic and neurologic evaluations
4. Head CTs
5. Audiometry and auditory brainstem responses if indicated

E. Two **treatment regimens** are employed depending on the severity of disease.
1. Treatment of moderate or severe disease (1-year therapy).
   a. Pyrimethamine 1 mg/kg per day for the first 3 days, followed by 1 mg/kg per day every other day
   b. Sulfadiazine 100 mg/kg per day divided bid
   c. Folinic acid (doses are increased with evidence of pyrimethamine toxicity):
      (1) 5 mg 3 times per week for <10 kg
      (2) 5 mg 3 times per week for 10 to 15 kg
      (3) 5 mg 4 times per week for 15 to 20 kg
2. Treatment of mild or asymptomatic infection (1-year therapy).
   a. First 6 months, as in **1** (moderate to severe disease)
   b. Final 6 months:
      (1) Sulfadiazine plus pyrimethamine for 1 month (doses as above) alternating with sulfadiazine alone for 1 month
      (2) Folinic acid while receiving pyrimethamine

   Variations on these regimens have been used, but there is general agreement that therapy should extend over 1 year from birth [1]. In addition, corticosteroids are recommended when there is evidence of acute inflammation, particularly chorioretinitis.

References

1. Remington, J. S., and Desmonts, G. Congenital Toxoplasmosis. In J. S. Remmington and J. O. Klein (Eds.), *Infectious Diseases of the Fetus and Newborn Infant,* 3d Ed. Philadelphia: Saunders, 1990. P. 89.
2. Desmonts, G., and Couvreur, J. *Bull. N.Y. Acad. Med.* 50: 146, 1974.
3. Weiblen, B., and Hoff, R. *Mass. Dept. Public Health* 5: 35, 1990.
4. Kimball, A. C., et al. *Am. J. Obstet. Gynecol.* 111: 211, 1971.
5. Hunter, K., et al. *Am. J. Obstet. Gynecol.* 145: 269, 1983.
6. Desmonts, G., and Couvreur, J. Toxoplasmosis. In O. Thalhammer, K. Baumgarten, and A. Pollak (Eds.), *Perinatal Medicine.* Stuttgart: Thieme, 1979. P. 51.
7. Eichenwald, H. In J. C. Siim (Ed.), *Human Toxoplasmosis.* Copenhagen: Munksgaard, 1960. P. 41.
8. Alford, C. A., Jr., et al. *Bull. N.Y. Acad. Med.* 50: 160, 1974.
9. Alford, C. A., Jr., et al. *J. Pediatr.* 75: 1167, 1969.
10. Couvreur, J., et al. *Ann. Pediatr. (Paris)* 31: 815, 1984.
11. Koppe, J. G., et al. *Eur. J. Obstet. Gynecol. Reprod. Biol.* 4: 101, 1974.
12. Wilson, C. B., et al. *Pediatrics* 66: 767, 1980.
13. Koppe, J. G., et al. *Lancet* 1: 254, 1986.
14. Daffos, F., et al. *N. Engl. J. Med.* 318: 271, 1988.
15. Sever, J. L., et al. *Pediatrics* 82: 181, 1988.

13 Respiratory Disorders

Introduction

This chapter presents those respiratory disorders most frequently seen in the newborn intensive care unit. A discussion of persistent pulmonary hypertension is also included. The following is a partial list of causes of respiratory distress in infants.

I. **Airway obstruction**
   A. **Nasal or nasopharyngeal**—choanal atresia, nasal edema, encephalocele
   B. **Oral cavity**—macroglossia, micrognathia
   C. **Neck**—congenital goiter, cystic hygroma
   D. **Larynx**—web, subglottic stenosis, hemangioma, cord paralysis, laryngomalacia
   E. **Trachea**—tracheomalacia, tracheoesophageal fistula, tracheal stenosis, tracheal agenesis, bronchial stenosis

II. **Lung parenchymal disease**
   A. **Aspiration syndromes**
   B. **Respiratory distress syndrome**
   C. **Atelectasis**
   D. **Air leak**—pneumothorax, pneumomediastinum, pneumopericardium, interstitial emphysema
   E. **Transient tachypnea** of the newborn
   F. **Pneumonia**
   G. **Pulmonary hemorrhage**
   H. **Bronchopulmonary dysplasia**
   I. **Wilson Mikity syndrome**
   J. **Chronic pulmonary insufficiency of prematurity**

III. **Thoracic malformations**
   A. **Pulmonary hypoplasia or agenesis**
   B. **Diaphragmatic hernia**
   C. **Intrathoracic cysts or tumors**
   D. **Congenital lobar emphysema**
   E. **Effusions, chylothorax**
   F. **Tracheosophageal fistula**

IV. **Nonpulmonary causes**
   A. **Congestive heart failure**
   B. **Metabolic causes**—acidosis, hypothermia, hypoglycemia
   C. **Persistent pulmonary hypertension**
   D. **Birth asphyxia**
   E. **Central nervous system lesions**

Respiratory Distress Syndrome/Hyaline Membrane Disease

Helen G. Liley and Ann R. Stark

The primary cause of respiratory distress syndrome (RDS) is inadequate pulmonary surfactant. The manifestations of the disease are caused by the consequent diffuse alveolar atelectasis, edema, and cell injury. During the past 30 years, significant advances have been made in the management of RDS [1,5,10,12]. These advances include the development of prenatal diagnosis to identify infants at risk, prevention of the disease by prenatal administration of glucocorticoids, improvements in perinatal care, advances in respiratory support, and surfactant replacement therapy. As a result, the mortality from RDS has decreased. However, the survival of increasing numbers of extremely immature infants has provided new challenges, and RDS remains a contributing cause of much neonatal mortality and morbidity.

I. Identification

A. Perinatal risk factors

1. **Factors that affect state of lung development at birth** include prematurity, maternal diabetes, and genetic factors (white race, history of RDS in siblings, male sex) [2,6].
2. **Factors that may acutely impair surfactant production, release, or function** include perinatal asphyxia in premature infants (e.g., secondary to antepartum hemorrhage or in some second-born twins) and cesarean section without labor. Infants delivered before labor commences do not benefit from adrenergic and steroid hormones released during labor, which increase surfactant production and release [8,15].

B. Prenatal prediction (see Tests for Pulmonary Surfactant below)

1. Prenatal prediction of lung maturity can be made by measurement of phospholipids in amniotic fluid. Prenatal prediction of risk for RDS is important because it will contribute to decisions regarding transfer of the mother to a perinatal center, administration of glucocorticoids to accelerate fetal lung maturation, and administration of artificial surfactant.
2. We recommend maternal glucocorticoid treatment if delivery of an infant with severe RDS seems imminent. In general, this applies to pregnancies shorter than 34 weeks or those in which lung immaturity is shown by amniotic fluid analysis and when delivery can be postponed for at least 24 hours to allow the glucocorticoid to take effect. Contraindications to glucocorticoid treatment include amnionitis or other indications for immediate delivery.

C. Postnatal diagnosis. The premature infant with RDS will have clinical signs shortly after birth. These include tachypnea, retractions, flaring of the nasal alae, grunting, and cyanosis. The classic radiographic appearance is of low-volume lungs with a reticulogranular pattern and air bronchograms. A **shake test** performed on swallowed amniotic fluid within 30 minutes may help confirm the diagnosis (see Tests for Pulmonary Surfactant, page 189).

II. Management. The key to management of infants with RDS are (1) to prevent hypoxia and acidosis (this allows normal tissue metabolism, optimizes surfactant production, and prevents right-to-left shunting), (2) to optimize fluid management (avoiding hypovolemia and shock on the one hand and edema, particularly pulmonary edema, on the other), (3) to reduce metabolic demands, (4) to prevent worsening atelectasis and pulmonary edema, and (5) to minimize barotrauma and hyperoxic lung damage.

A. Surfactant replacement therapy has been shown in numerous recent clinical trials to be successful in ameliorating RDS [12]. These trials have examined the effects of surfactant preparations delivered through the endotracheal tube either within minutes of birth (prevention studies) or after symptoms and signs of RDS are present (treatment or "rescue" studies). Research in animals suggests that preventive treatment of surfactant deficiency, before lung injury occurs, results in better distribution than supplementation once respiratory failure is severe. In human studies of such early treatment, study groups are inevitably "diluted," with infants whose lungs were mature, so it has not been established that preventive treatment is more successful. Surfactants of human, bovine, or porcine origin and two synthetic preparations have been studied. In general, they have shown short-term benefit in oxygenation and ventilation and, in many of the larger studies, decreased incidence of air leaks and death.

Surfactant treatment has not consistently reduced the incidence of such problems as intraventricular hemorrhage, necrotizing enterocolitis, and retinopathy of prematurity. It may be that although these disorders tend to be associated with severe RDS, they are primarily caused by immaturity of other organs. Likewise, single-dose treatment has had no consistent effect on the incidence of bronchopulmonary dysplasia. Studies using larger or more frequent doses may show an impact on these disorders [7]. Comparisons between surfactant preparations, causes of variability of response and the development of preparations containing human surfactant proteins produced by recombinant DNA technology are also the subjects of ongoing research. At the time of this writing, the synthetic preparation Exosurf Neonatal® is commercially available in the United States.

In general, we administer artificial surfactant as soon as the diagnosis of severe RDS is made, after adequate oxygenation, ventilation, perfusion and monitoring are established. The Exosurf dose is 67.5 mg phospholipid per kilogram and is administered gradually over 15–40 minutes, with changes in positioning of the infant to facilitate distribution. We use endotracheal tube adapters that permit administration without interruption of mechanical ventilation. Careful observation is necessary during treatment. Desaturation, bradycardia, and apnea are frequent adverse effects unless the dose is administered very slowly, and in synchrony with inspiration. Rate of infusion should be adjusted according to the infant's tolerance. Apnea is common at slow ventilator rates, so the rate should be at least 30/min during administration. In addition, some infants respond rapidly and need careful adjustment of ventilator settings to prevent pneumothorax secondary to sudden improvement in compliance. Others become transiently hypoxic during treatment and require additional oxygen. Pulmonary hemorrhage is an infrequent adverse effect of artificial surfactant therapy (according to a communication from the manufacturer). It most commonly occurs in extremely low birth weight infants, in males, and in those infants who have clinical evidence of patent ductus arteriosus. Risk is decreased by prenatal glucocorticoid therapy and by early postnatal treatment of PDA with indomethacin or ligation.

B. Oxygen

1. **Delivery of oxygen** should be sufficient to maintain arterial tensions at 50 to 80 mmHg. This range is generally sufficient to meet metabolic demands. Higher than necessary FIO_2 levels should be avoided because of danger of potentiating the development of lung injury and retinopathy of prematurity. The oxygen should be warmed and humidified and delivered through an air-oxygen blender that allows precise control over the oxygen concentration. For infants with acute RDS, oxygen should be ordered by concentration to be delivered to the infant's airway, not by flow, and oxygen concentration should be checked at least hourly. When ventilation with a bag and mask is required during suctioning of the airway, insertion of an endotracheal tube, or for an apneic spell, the oxygen concentration should be similar to that before bagging to avoid hyperoxia and should be adjusted in response to transcutaneous monitoring.
2. **Blood gas monitoring** (see Blood Gas Monitoring below). Frequent sampling is required to maintain arterial blood gases within appropriate

ranges. Arterial blood gases (PaO_2, $PaCO_2$, and pH) should be measured 15 to 20 minutes after changes in respiratory therapy, such as alteration in the FIO_2, ventilator pressures, or rate. We use either umbilical, radial, or posterior tibial arterial catheters for this purpose. To monitor trends in oxygenation continuously, we use pulse oximeters and transcutaneous PO_2 monitors. In more stable infants, capillary blood from warmed heels may be adequate for monitoring PCO_2 and pH.

C. Continuous positive airway pressure (CPAP)

1. **Indications.** We begin CPAP therapy in infants with RDS who have significant respiratory distress in the first 2 days and who require an FIO_2 of 0.3 to 0.5 to maintain a PaO_2 of 50 to 80 mmHg. Early CPAP therapy may reduce the need for mechanical ventilation and the incidence of long-term pulmonary morbidity [1]. In infants with RDS, CPAP probably helps to prevent atelectasis and may mitigate lung edema and preserve the functional properties of surfactant. PaO_2 therefore rises. $PaCO_2$ may fall if the CPAP enables the infant to inspire on a more compliant portion of his or her pressure-volume curve. However, minute ventilation may decrease on CPAP, particularly if the distending pressure is too great. We obtain a chest radiograph before or soon after starting CPAP to confirm the diagnosis of RDS and to exclude disorders in which this type of therapy should be approached with great caution, such as air leak. In infants who respond to CPAP, the risks and benefits of intubation and ventilation must be considered.
2. **Methods of administering CPAP.** CPAP can be applied by means of face mask, nasal prongs, nasopharyngeal tube, or endotracheal tube. Alternatively, distending pressure can be applied as continuous negative pressure in a negative-pressure respirator. In most infants we begin with CPAP by nasal prongs. CPAP is applied through a continuous flow respirator and is generally started at 5 to 7 cm H_2O pressure using a flow high enough to avoid rebreathing (5 to 10 L/min). The pressure is adjusted in increments of 1 to 2 cm H_2O, observing the baby's respiratory effort and monitoring the PaO_2. In infants in whom abdominal distension complicates nasal CPAP or who are being weaned from ventilator support, we also use CPAP by means of nasopharyngeal or endotracheal tube.
3. **Problems encountered with CPAP**
   a. CPAP may interfere with venous return to the heart and thus cardiac output. If administered by positive pressure, it may be transmitted to the pulmonary vascular bed, raising pulmonary vascular resistance and thereby promoting right-to-left shunting. The risk of these phenomena increases as lung compliance increases, for example, as RDS is resolving. In these circumstances, reduction of the CPAP may improve oxygenation.
   b. Hypercarbia may indicate that CPAP is too high and tidal volume is thereby reduced.
   c. Nasal prongs or nasopharyngeal tubes may be unsuccessful if crying or mouth opening prevents adequate transmission of pressure or if the infant's abdomen becomes distended. In these situations, endotracheal intubation is often necessary.
4. **Weaning.** As the infant improves, one should begin by reducing the FIO_2 in decrements of 0.05. Generally, when the FIO_2 is less than 0.40, CPAP can be reduced in decrements of 1 to 2 cm H_2O, checking blood gases after each adjustment. Physical examination will provide evidence of respiratory effort during weaning, and chest radiographs may help estimate lung volume. Lowering of the distending pressure should be attempted with caution if the lung volumes appear low and alveolar atelectasis persists. We generally discontinue CPAP at about 4 to 6 cm H_2O. The ambient oxygen is then adjusted appropriately.

D. Mechanical ventilation (see Mechanical Ventilation below)

1. **Indications** for starting respirator therapy are a $PaCO_2$ greater than 55

mmHg or rapidly rising, a PaO_2 less than 50 mmHg with a FIO_2 of 0.60 to 1.00, or severe apnea. The actual levels of PaO_2 and $PaCO_2$ necessitating intervention depend on the course of the disease. For example, a high $PaCO_2$ early in the course of severe RDS might indicate the need for a respirator, while the same $PaCO_2$ when the infant is recovering might be managed by observation and repeated sampling before any intervention is made.

2. **Respirators.** A continuous-flow, pressure-limited, time-cycled respirator is useful for ventilating newborns because pressure waveforms, inspiratory and expiratory duration, and pressure can be varied independently and because the flow of gas permits unobstructed spontaneous breathing.
   a. **Initial settings.** We generally start mechanical ventilation with a peak inspiratory pressure of 20 to 25 cm H_2O, positive end-expiratory pressure (PEEP) of 4 to 6 cm H_2O, frequency of 20 to 30 breaths per minute, inspiratory duration of 0.4 to 0.6 second, and the previously required FIO_2 (usually 0.50 to 1.00). It is useful to ventilate the infant first by hand, using an anesthesia bag and manometer to determine the actual pressures required. The infant should be observed for color, chest motion, and respiratory effort, and the examiner should listen for breath sounds. Adjustments in respirator settings may be required on the basis of these observations or arterial blood gas results.
   b. **Adjustments** (see **Mechanical Ventilation** below). $PaCO_2$ should be maintained in the range of 45 to 60 mmHg. It should be recognized that acidosis may exacerbate RDS, so if these $PaCO_2$ levels are accepted to minimize barotrauma, meticulous attention to control of any metabolic acidosis (e.g., by support of cardiac output) is necessary. Rapidly rising $PaCO_2$ levels may indicate the onset of complications of the disease, including atelectasis or air leak. Methods to decrease $PaCO_2$ will increase minute ventilation by affecting respiratory rate or tidal volume or both. Thus $PaCO_2$ is lowered by increasing peak inspiratory pressure, decreasing PEEP, increasing expiratory time, or increasing respiratory rate. Determining the appropriate maneuver requires some experience. PaO_2 usually rises in response to increases in FIO_2 or mean airway pressure (increases in peak inspiratory pressure, PEEP, or inspiratory time). Infants who remain hypoxemic despite these measures may improve when pancuronium (0.1 mg/kg per dose) is used for muscle relaxation. Occasional infants have pulmonary hypertension resulting in excessive right-to-left shunting through fetal pathways; in these infants, hyperventilation or alkalinization may improve oxygenation (see **Persistent Pulmonary Hypertension of the Newborn** below). More commonly, premature infants remain hypoxemic because of shunting through atelectatic lung and respond to measures that improve lung volumes.

4. **Care of the infant** receiving respirator therapy includes scrupulous attention to vital signs and clinical condition. FIO_2 and respirator settings must be checked frequently. Blood gas levels should be checked at least every 4 to 6 hours, or more frequently if the infant's condition is changing rapidly, and 15 to 20 minutes following any change in respirator settings. The effect of modest changes in FIO_2 can be assessed using a transcutaneous monitor. Airway secretions, if excessive, may require periodic suctioning and, occasionally, chest physiotherapy.

5. **Danger signs**
   a. If an infant receiving CPAP or mechanical ventilation deteriorates, the following should be suspected:
      (1) Blocked or dislodged endotracheal tube
      (2) Malfunctioning respirator
      (3) Pneumothorax
   b. **Remedial action.** The infant should be removed from the respirator and ventilated with an anesthesia bag. An appropriate suction cath-

eter is passed to determine patency of the tube, and its position is checked by laryngoscopy. If there is any doubt, the tube should be removed and the infant should be ventilated by bag and mask pending replacement of the tube. The ventilator should be checked to ensure that FIO_2 settings are appropriate. The baby's chest is auscultated and transilluminated to check for pneumothorax (see **Air Leak** below). If pneumothorax is suspected, chest radiographs should be obtained, but if the infant's condition is critical, immediate aspiration by needle is both diagnostic and therapeutic. Hypotension secondary to hemorrhage, capillary leak, or myocardial dysfunction also can complicate RDS and should be treated by blood volume expansion or pressors or both. An intraventricular hemorrhage also can cause a sudden deterioration. Immediate attention to treatable conditions is appropriate.

6. **Weaning.** As the infant shows signs of improvement, weaning from the ventilator should be attempted. The following steps are examples and should be varied depending on the infant's blood gases, physical examination, and responses.
   a. **Steps of weaning.**
      (1) Lower the inspiratory pressure to 30 cm H_2O by steps of 2 cm H_2O.
      (2) Reduce FIO_2 to 0.50 to 0.60, by decrements of 0.05.
      (3) Reduce inspiratory pressure to 20 cm H_2O and PEEP to 5 cm H_2O in decrements of 1 to 2 cm H_2O.
      (4) Decrease FIO_2 stepwise to 0.40.
      (5) Lower the respirator rate by 2 to 4 breaths per minute, usually to no less than 4 to 8 breaths per minute, as the infant's spontaneous breathing increases.
      (6) Settings at which mechanical ventilation can be successfully discontinued will vary with the size, condition, respiratory drive, and individual pulmonary mechanics of the infant. Larger infants often do well if changed to CPAP of 5 to 7 cm H_2O and then extubated if spontaneous breathing is well tolerated. Infants less than 2 kg are usually better weaned to respirator rates of 3 to 6 breaths per minute and then extubated if they are stable on FIO_2 less than 0.30 and peak inspiratory pressure less than 20 cm H_2O.
   b. **Failure to wean** may result from a number of causes, of which the following is a partial list (see **II.F**).
      (1) Recovery of the lung from RDS is not uniform, and segmental or lobar atelectasis, edema, or interstitial emphysema may delay weaning.
      (2) As the infant's lungs become more compliant, the inspiratory and expiratory times may have to be increased to allow optimal inflation and deflation of the lungs.
      (3) Pulmonary edema may develop secondary to patency of the ductus arteriosus.
      (4) Other reasons include onset of bronchopulmonary dysplasia and of apnea of prematurity. We frequently begin theophylline therapy in infants weighing less than 1250 gm to improve respiratory drive and prevent apnea (see also **Apnea** below). Glottic or subglottic edema resulting in obstruction may respond to inhaled racemic epinephrine or systemic glucocorticoids.

E. **Supportive therapy**
1. **Temperature** (see Chap. 32). Temperature control is crucial in all low-birth-weight infants, especially in those with respiratory disease. If the infant's temperature is too high or low, metabolic demands increase considerably. If oxygen uptake is limited by RDS, the increased demand cannot be met. An incubator or a radiant warmer must be used to maintain a neutral thermal environment for the infant.
2. **Fluids and nutrition** (see Chaps. 24 and 30).
   a. Most infants with RDS will initially require intravascular adminis-

tration of fluids. Generally we start fluid therapy at 60 to 70 ml/kg per day, using dextrose 10% in water. Very immature infants in whom poor glucose tolerance and massive transcutaneous losses are expected are usually started at 80 to 100 ml/kg per day; at higher fluid rates, the glucose concentration often must be lowered to 5%. We measure serum electrolytes early and frequently. Phototherapy, skin trauma, and radiant warmers increase insensible losses. Excessive fluid administration causes risk of pulmonary edema and may increase the risk for symptomatic patency of the ductus arteriosus. The key to fluid management is careful monitoring of serum electrolytes and body weight. Urine output and specific gravity also should be monitored but may not reliably reflect the state of hydration; fluid retention is common in infants with RDS. Conversely, extremely immature infants often lack renal concentration efficiency and have enormous evaporative losses.

b. By the second day, we usually add sodium (3 mEq/kg per day), potassium (2 mEq/kg per day), and calcium (100 to 200 mg/kg per day) to the fluids. Sodium acetate or bicarbonate can be used instead of sodium chloride if metabolic acidosis is present. Particularly in infants weighing less than 1000 gm, if it seems unlikely that adequate oral nutrition will be achieved within several days, we generally start adding an amino acid solution and intravenous fat solution by the second or third day.

c. In most infants with RDS, spontaneous diuresis occurs on the second to fourth day, preceding improvement in pulmonary function. Although furosemide may help stimulate water secretion, its use has been associated with increased incidence of symptomatic patent ductus arteriosus (PDA) [9,11]. If diuresis and improvement in lung disease do not occur by 1 to 2 weeks of age, this may signify the onset of bronchopulmonary dysplasia. In these infants, diuretics often improve pulmonary function.

3. **Circulation** is assessed by monitoring the heart rate, blood pressure, and peripheral perfusion. Judicious use of blood or volume expanders may be necessary, and pressors may be used to support the circulation. We often use dopamine (starting at 2.5 to 5 μg/kg per minute) to improve perfusion and urine output and to prevent metabolic acidosis. The volume of blood drawn should be monitored and generally should be replaced by packed red cell transfusion when it has reached 10 percent of the infant's blood volume or if the hematocrit falls below 40 to 45 percent.
4. **Possible infection.** Since pneumonia can duplicate the signs, symptoms, and radiographic appearance of RDS, we obtain cultures from all infants with RDS and treat with broad-spectrum antibiotics (ampicillin and gentamicin) for at least 48 hours.

F. Acute complications

1. **Air leak** (see **Air Leak** below). Pneumothorax, pneumomediastinum, pneumopericardium, or interstitial emphysema should be suspected when an infant with RDS deteriorates, typically with hypotension, apnea, bradycardia, or persistent acidosis.
2. **Infections** (see Chap. 12) may accompany RDS and may present in a variety of ways. Also, instrumentation, such as catheters or respiratory equipment, provides access for organisms to invade the immunologically immature preterm infant. Whenever there is suspicion of infection, cultures should be obtained and antibiotics administered promptly.
3. **Intracranial hemorrhage** (see Chap. 21). Infants with severe RDS are at increased risk for intracranial hemorrhage and should be monitored with cranial ultrasound examinations.
4. **Patent ductus arteriosus** (see Chap. 14) frequently complicates RDS. PDA typically presents as pulmonary vascular pressures begin to fall. If untreated, it may result in increasing left-to-right shunt and ultimately

congestive heart failure, manifested by respiratory relapse and cardiomegaly. Urine output decreases and jaundice worsens secondary to impaired renal and hepatic perfusion. We generally treat infants, especially those weighing less than 1500 g, with intravenous indomethacin if they develop signs of a PDA, such as a systolic or continuous murmur, hyperdynamic precordium, bounding pulses, and widened pulse pressure. We reserve surgical ligation for those infants in whom indomethacin is contraindicated (e.g., those with renal failure or necrotizing enterocolitis) or those in whom one or more courses of indomethacin have failed. In larger infants who are improving steadily despite PDA and who have no evidence of heart failure, mild fluid restriction and time may result in closure [4].

G. Long-term complications

1. **Bronchopulmonary dysplasia (BPD)** (see Chronic Lung Disease below). Chronic lung disease occurs in 5 to 30 percent of survivors of respirator therapy for RDS.
2. **Retinopathy of prematurity (ROP)** (see Chap. 38). Premature infants are at risk for ROP. Oxygen therapy should be monitored frequently, and all premature infants should have ophthalmologic examinations, the number and timing depending on gestational age at birth. In very premature infants, ROP may occur even if PaO_2 was never excessive.
3. **Neurologic impairment** is estimated to occur in 10 to 15 percent of the survivors of RDS. Contributing factors include circumstances of premature delivery, the immaturity of the infants at birth, and the accompanying risk for neurologic events such as intraventricular hemorrhage and periventricular leukomalacia. Prevention of perinatal asphyxia and careful attention to oxygenation, perfusion, nutrition, and metabolic demands may improve outcome.

References

1. Avery, M. E. *Pediatrics* 79: 26, 1987.
2. Bourbon, J. R. *Pediatr. Res.* 19: 253, 1985.
3. Carlo, W. A. *Pediatr. Clin. North Am.* 33: 221, 1986.
4. Clyman, R. I. *J. Pediatr.* 111: 718, 1987.
5. Crowley, P. *Br. J. Obstet. Gynecol.* 97: 11, 1990.
6. Farrell, P. M. *Am. Rev. Respir. Dis.* 3: 657, 1975.
7. Fujiwara, T. *Pediatrics* 86: 753, 1990.
8. Ghai, V. *Clin. Perinatol.* 15: 123, 1988.
9. Green, T. P. *J. Pediatr.* 103: 618, 1983.
10. Gregory, G. A. *N. Engl. J. Med.* 284: 1333, 1971.
11. Heaf, D. P. *J. Pediatr.* 101: 103, 1982.
12. Merritt, T. A. *Am. J. Dis. Child.* 142: 1333, 1988.
13. Stark, A. R. *J. Pediatr.* 94: 439, 1979.
14. Stark, A. R. *Pediatr. Clin. North Am.* 33: 533, 1986.
15. Wright, J. R. *Am. Rev. Respir. Dis.* 135: 426, 1987.

Tests for Pulmonary Surfactant

John S. Torday and
Douglas Richardson

I. Basis for the tests. Fluid formed in the fetal lung flows up the airways and into the amniotic fluid, carrying with it some of the pulmonary surfactant from the fetal lung. Surfactant is a complex mixture that lowers alveolar surface tension. It is composed of several phospholipids and at least three proteins. Infants with inadequate amounts commonly develop RDS. Tests are based on quantitation of surface-active phospholipids or on assessment of surfactant effects such as formation of stable foams [6].

Fluid obtained by amniocentesis or by removal from the vagina of a mother with rupture of membranes can be tested for the presence of pulmonary surfactant. The aspirated gastric fluid of a recently delivered newborn also can be assayed, although the interpretation is different (see **IV**).

II. L/S ratio. The lecithin-sphingomyelin (L/S) ratio, the most frequently used test, is performed by chromatography.

A. Clinical significance of specific results (see Table 13-1) Techniques such as centrifugation, acetone precipitation, and quantitation of chromatograms vary among laboratories and may affect results. Estimation of risk of RDS from the L/S ratio should therefore reflect the experience of the laboratory and clinical service [4]. At younger gestational ages, in which RDS occurs frequently, the risk of RDS, at any given L/S ratio, is somewhat higher than the averages noted in Table 13-1. Hence great care should be taken in interpreting L/S ratios in the transitional and borderline mature ranges. Conversely, at gestational ages close to term, in which RDS occurs infrequently, the actual risk of RDS is substantially lower for any given L/S ratio than those in the table [9].

B. Combination testing. The high rate of false prediction of RDS in the transitional zones has led to the use of test combinations, such as the lung profile [10,11]. The presence of phosphatidylglycerol (PG) [10] or the concentration of saturated phosphatidylcholine (SPC) [13] also has been used to improve the predictive value of the L/S ratio (Table 13-2). Preliminary reports suggest that assays of surfactant apoproteins may be another helpful adjunct [8].

C. Interpretation of contaminated samples. The effects of blood and meconium are due to the presence of lecithin and sphingomyelin in these substances. The L/S ratio in these contaminants has never been found to be higher than 2. Therefore, blood and meconium tend to elevate an immature L/S ratio (under 2) and depress a mature L/S ratio (over 2). Consequently, a contaminated specimen with an L/S ratio over 2 is probably mature, and one under 2 is probably immature. Amniotic fluid obtained vaginally by speculum examination is as reliable as that obtained transabdominally. Confirmation that such samples are amniotic fluid should be made with pH paper and Dextrostix®.

D. There are exceptions to the prediction of pulmonary maturity with an L/S ratio over 2:1 [2,6].

1. **Definite exceptions**
   a. Infants of diabetic mothers (IDM)
   b. Intrapartum asphyxia
   c. Erythroblastosis fetalis (EF)
2. **Possible exceptions**
   a. Intrauterine growth retardation (IUGR)
   b. Abruptio placentae
   c. Toxemia
   d. Hydrops fetalis

E. Predicting lung maturity in the IDM (see Chap. 1, **Maternal Diabetes**). Several cases of RDS have been documented in IDMs with L/S ratios over 2 or even 2.5. This is thought to be due to the poor surfactant activity for unknown reasons. Until the pathophysiology of RDS in the IDM is better understood, our experience has been that an L/S ratio between 2 and 3.5 is associated with a 7 to 10 percent risk of RDS, and an SPC concentration (see **B**) of 500 to 1000 μg/dl is also associated with a 7 to 10 percent risk of RDS. If the L/S ratio is greater than 3.5 and the SPC concentration is greater than 1000 μg/dl, the risk of RDS is very low (we have one probable case with this circumstance).

Table 13-1. Clinical significance of specific results

Ratio*	Clinical significance	Risk of RDS (%)
< 1.5	Immature lung	58
1.5–1.9	Transitional lung	17
2.0–2.5	Mature (caution)	11
> 2.5	Mature	0.5

*In samples uncontaminated by blood or meconium.
Source: Data from Hunink et al. [9].

Table 13-2. Use of lecithin sphingomyelin ratio and saturated phosphatidylcholine in predicting neonatal RDS alone and in combination*

	L/S ratio (number of infants)		
SPC (μg/dl)	Immature (<1.5)	Transitional (1.5 to 2.0)	Mature (>2.0)
500 or less			
Infants without RDS	22	22	17
Infants with RDS	36	19	13
More than 500			
Infants without RDS	3	35	600
Infants with RDS	2	5	11

*These values are from amniotic fluid samples analyzed regardless of sample contamination with blood, meconium, or complications of pregnancy, obtained within a 72-hour interval from tap to birth. Values were obtained at the Boston Hospital for Women, December 1976 to July 1983.
Key: SPC = saturated phosphatidylcholine; L/S ratio = lecithin-sphingomyelin ratio; RDS = respiratory distress syndrome.

The presence of phosphatidylglycerol in amniotic fluid may be particularly helpful in the IDM [7].

III. Other measures of surfactant. Numerous variations of the L/S ratio assay as well as other surfactant components have been developed (Table 13-3). Many of these tests have lower sensitivity and specificity; their principal use is as "stat" tests. Cautions in interpreting these tests are parallel to those for the L/S ratio but less well studied. Contamination may make the tests uninterpretable. Perinatal centers usually rely on more sensitive tests such as the L/S ratio, SPC concentration, or combinations such as the lung profile (see **II.B**). The SPC concentration is unaffected by contamination with blood or meconium [13].

IV. Shake test performed on gastric fluid [1,3]. A shake test performed on gastric fluid to predict RDS can be useful at referring hospitals to decide on the necessity for an infant's transfer to a neonatal intensive care unit. Its use in directing the administration of surfactant replacement therapy has yet to be clarified. The procedure described here is adapted from Evans [3]. This method also can be used on amniotic fluid.

A. Gastric aspirates should be obtained before the baby is 1 hour of age by passing a suction catheter with a mucus trap into the stomach. Specimens less than 1 ml in volume are inadequate.

B. Absolute alcohol, 0.5 ml, is added to 0.5 ml of gastric aspirate in a 4-ml glass test tube. The capped test tube is vigorously shaken for 15 seconds and allowed to stand for 15 minutes.

Table 13-3. Assessment of fetal pulmonary maturity

Test	Principle	Mature level
Primary Tests		
L/S ratio [6,7]	Surfactant lecithin compared with sphingomyelin by chromatography (TLC)	≥2.0
Lung profile [10,11]	Phosphatidylglycerol (PG) and phosphatidylinositol (PI) improve surfactant function by two-dimensional TLC	>50% acetone precipitated lecithin; 15 to 20% PI; 2 to 10% PG
Saturated lecithin [13]	Chromatography after oxidation with osmium tetroxide	≥500 mg/dl
Lecithin concentration	Direct measure of primary phospholipid in surfactant	≥3.5 mg/100 ml lecithin ≥0.1 mg/100 ml phosphorus
Adjunctive Tests		
Surfactant 35-kD protein (SP-A) [8]	Enzyme-linked immunosorbent assay (ELISA) using monoclonal antibodies	>3.0 μg/ml mature 0.6–3.0 μg/ml transitional
Stat Tests		
Microviscosimeter	Fluorescence depolarization used to estimate lamellar body concentration	$P < 0.310$ to 0.336
"Shake test" [1,3]	Generation of stable foam by pulmonary surfactant in presence of ethanol	Complete ring of bubbles 15 minutes after shaking at 1:2 dilution
Foam stability index (FSI)	Commercially produced quantitative shake test	≥0.48
Optical density	Evaluates turbidity changes dependent on total phospholipid concentration	At 650 nm, ≥0.15
Phosphatidylglycerol agglutination (Amniostat) [5]	Antibody-conjugated latex agglutination of PG	Present (trace to 1+)
TDx-FLM [12]	Automated fluorescence polarization using albumin as ratio	Surfactant/albumin 50 to 70 mg/g

Source: Adapted from Gabbe [4].

C. Result and interpretation:

Immature = no bubbles: high risk of RDS (60 percent)
1+ = Very small bubbles in meniscus extending one-third or less of distance around test tube (a magnifying glass is usually required to determine that these are bubbles, as opposed to particles): intermediate risk of RDS (20 percent)
2+ = Single rim of bubbles extending one-third to all the way around the test tube:
3+ = A rim of bubbles all the way around the test tube, with a double row in some areas: low risk of RDS (less than 1 percent)
4+ = A double row or more of bubbles all the way around the test tube: fully mature

References

1. Clements, J. A. *N. Engl. J. Med.* 286: 1077, 1972.
2. Cox, M. A. *Pediatr. Res.* 17: 310A, 1983.
3. Evans, J. J. *N. Engl. J. Med.* 292: 1113, 1975.
4. Gabbe, S. G. *J. Reprod. Med.* 23: 227, 1979.
5. Garite, T. J. *Am. J. Obstet. Gynecol.* 147: 681, 1983.
6. Gluck, L., and Kulovich, M. V. The Evaluation of Functional Maturity in the Human Fetus. In L. Gluck (Ed.), *Modern Perinatal Medicine.* Chicago: Year Book Medical Publishers, 1974.
7. Gluck, L. *Am. J. Obstet. Gynecol.* 120: 142, 1974.
8. Hallman, M. B. *Am. J. Obstet. Gynecol.* 158: 531, 1988.
9. Hunink, M. G. M. *Med. Decision Making* 10: 201, 1990.
10. Kulovich, M. V. *Am. J. Obstet. Gynecol.* 135: 57, 1979.
11. Kulovich, M. V. *Am. J. Obstet. Gynecol.* 135: 64, 1979.
12. Russell, J. C. *Clin. Chem.* 35: 1005, 1989.
13. Torday, J. S. *N. Engl. J. Med.* 301: 1013, 1979.

Mechanical Ventilation

Douglas Richardson

I. General principles. Mechanical ventilation is an invasive life-support procedure with multiple effects on the cardiopulmonary system. The goal is to optimize both gas exchange and clinical status. Use of any ventilatory strategy requires an understanding of how ventilator changes affect arterial blood gases (ABGs), a knowledge of the pathophysiology of common neonatal pulmonary disorders, and a collaborative approach among physicians, nurses, and respiratory therapists.

II. Indications for respiratory support. See Chapter 39 for intubation procedures and proper selection of endotracheal tube sizes.

A. Indications for continuous positive airway pressure (CPAP) in the preterm infant with RDS include

1. $FIO_2 > 0.40$ to 0.50 by hood with clinical distress
2. $FIO_2 > 0.60$ by hood
3. Clinically significant retractions after recent extubation
4. Frequent apnea with documented hypoxemia

B. Relative indications for mechanical ventilation in any infant include

1. Frequent intermittent apnea unresponsive to drug therapy
2. Early treatment when use of mechanical ventilation is anticipated because of deteriorating gas exchange
3. Relieving "work of breathing" in an infant with signs of respiratory difficulty

C. Absolute indications for mechanical ventilation

1. Prolonged apnea

2. PaO_2 < 50 mmHg on FIO_2 of > 0.80. This indication may not apply to the infant with cyanotic congenital heart disease.
3. $PaCO_2$ > 60 mmHg with persistent acidemia
4. Failure of optimal CPAP at FIO_2 > 0.60 to 0.70 in preterm infant with RDS
5. General anesthesia

III. Types of ventilatory support

A. Continuous positive airway pressure (CPAP)

1. **CPAP** can be administered by all neonatal ventilators or by homemade or commercial devices.
2. **General characteristics.** CPAP plays a central role in treating infants with RDS. A continuous flow of heated, humidified gas is circulated past the infant's airway at a set pressure of 3 to 8 cm H_2O while the infant breathes spontaneously. The air-oxygen mixture and airway pressure can be adjusted. CPAP can be delivered by means of nasal prongs, nasopharyngeal tube, or endotracheal tube. Positive-pressure hoods and continuous mask CPAP are not recommended.
3. **Advantages**
   a. CPAP is less invasive and causes less barotrauma than mechanical ventilation.
   b. It helps prevent alveolar and airway collapse, which might result in deterioration of PaO_2.
   c. CPAP decreases the frequency of apneic spells in some infants.
4. **Disadvantages**
   a. CPAP does not improve ventilation and may worsen it.
   b. It is inadequate in the face of severe changes in pulmonary compliance and resistance.
   c. It may be technically difficult to maintain nasal CPAP in large, active infants.
   d. Low levels of endotracheal CPAP (2 to 3 cm H_2O) may present a stressful resistive load to very small infants.
   e. Swallowed air can elevate the diaphragm and must be removed by a gastric tube.
5. **Indications**
   a. Early treatment of RDS
   b. Moderately frequent apneic spells
   c. After recent extubation
   d. Weaning chronic ventilator-dependent infants

B. Pressure-limited, time-cycled, continuous-flow ventilators are used most frequently in newborn intensive care units.

1. **General characteristics.** A continuous flow of heated and humidified gas is circulated past the infant's airway; the gas is a selected mixture of air with oxygen. Maximum inspiratory pressure (PI) and positive end-expiratory pressure (PEEP) are selected. Respiratory timing (rate and duration of inspiration and expiration) is selected.
2. **Advantages**
   a. The continuous flow of fresh gas allows the infant to make spontaneous respiratory efforts between ventilator breaths (intermittent mandatory ventilation, IMV).
   b. Good control is maintained over respiratory pressures.
   c. Inspiratory and expiratory time can be independently controlled.
   d. The system is relatively simple and inexpensive.
3. **Disadvantages**
   a. Tidal volume is poorly controlled.
   b. The system does not respond to changes in respiratory system compliance.
   c. Spontaneously breathing infants who breathe out of phase with too many IMV breaths ("bucking" or "fighting" the ventilator) may receive inadequate ventilation.

4. **Indications.** Useful in any form of lung disease in infants weighing less than 10 kg.

C. **Volume-cycled ventilators** are rarely used in newborn infants.

1. **Characteristics.** Similar to pressure-limited ventilators except that the volume delivered is selected. Numerous options are available.
2. **Advantages.** The pressure automatically varies with respiratory system compliance.
3. **Disadvantages**
   a. The system is complicated and requires more skill to operate.
   b. Because tidal volumes in infants are small, most of the tidal volume selected is lost in the ventilator circuit or from air leaks around uncuffed endotracheal tubes. A separate in-line tidal volume monitor is extremely helpful.
   c. It is more expensive than a pressure-limited device.
4. **Indications.** May be useful if there is rapidly changing compliance.

D. **High-frequency ventilators (HFVs)** may be used under special circumstances. There are three types of high-frequency ventilators used in newborns: oscillators (HFO), flow interrupters (HFFI), and jets (HFJ). Although some are still used under investigational protocols, most of these ventilators are now in clinical use [1,10].

1. **Characteristics.** These machines deliver extremely rapid rates (300 to 1500 breaths per minute, 50 to 250 Hz). Tidal volume is often smaller than dead space. The physiology is not well characterized. There are two major subgroups, those with active expiration (e.g., oscillators or HFO-A) and those with passive expiration (e.g., jets, or HFJ-P) [10]. Some are hybrids [e.g., an interrupter with active expiration (HFFI-A)].
2. **Advantages.** Achieves adequate ventilation at lower mean airway pressure (MAP). Because of this, it is most useful in pulmonary air leak syndromes (pulmonary interstitial emphysema, pneumothorax) [7,9]. It also may be useful during bronchoscopy.
3. **Disadvantages.** No advantage of this method has been demonstrated over more conventional ventilators for routine uses. These ventilators are more complex and expensive, and there is less long-term clinical experience. There may be an increased risk of significant intraventricular hemorrhage [14]. Early prototype HFJ ventilators were associated with tracheal damage. The relative advantages among oscillators, flow interrupters, and jets are not clear.
4. **Indications.** Currently, HFVs are used as a rescue therapy for infants failing conventional ventilation, particularly for air leak syndrome.

E. **Negative pressure.** These infant versions of the adult "iron lung" are rarely used because nursing access is limited by the negative-pressure cylinder and because the neck seal makes them feasible only for large babies. Their use is restricted to older infants with neuromuscular problems who can thus be ventilated without an endotracheal tube.

IV. **How ventilator changes affect blood gases.** This topic is reviewed well by Harris [11], Carlo [5], and Krauss [15].

A. **Oxygenation** (Table 13-4)

1. **F_{IO_2}.** The goal is to maintain adequate tissue oxygen delivery. Generally, this can be accomplished by achieving a PaO_2 of 50 to 80 mmHg. This results in a hemoglobin saturation of 89 to 95 percent [see Fig. 13-1 (oxyhemoglobin curve)]. Increasing inspired oxygen is the simplest and most direct means of improving oxygenation. In premature infants, the risk of retinopathy and pulmonary oxygen toxicity argue for miminizing PaO_2. For infants with other conditions, the optimum PaO_2 may be higher. Direct pulmonary oxygen toxicity begins to occur at F_{IO_2} values greater than 0.60 to 0.70.
2. **Mean airway pressure (MAP)** [2,3,6,11,18,20]
   a. **MAP** is the average area under the curve of the pressure waveform. Many ventilators now display MAP or can be equipped with a device

Table 13-4. Ventilator manipulations to increase oxygenation

Parameter	Advantage	Disadvantage
↑ F_{IO_2}	Minimizes barotrauma Easily administered	Fails to affect $\dot{V}/\dot{Q}$ matching Direct toxicity, especially >0.60
↑ PI	Critical openinng pressure Improves $\dot{V}/\dot{Q}$	Barotrauma: air leak, BPD
↑ PEEP	Maintains FRC/prevents collapse Splints obstructed airways Regularizes respiration	Shifts to stiffer compliance curve Obstructs venous return Increases expiratory work and CO_2 Increases dead space
↑ TI	Increases MAP without increasing PI "Critical opening time"	Necessitates slower rates, higher PI Lower minute ventilation for given PI-PEEP combination
↑ Flow	Square wave—maximizes MAP	Greater shear force, more barotrauma Greater resistance at greater flows
↑ Rate	Increases MAP while using lower PI	Inadvertent PEEP with high rates or long-time constants

Note: All manipulations (except F_{IO_2}) result in higher mean airway pressure (MAP).

to do so. MAP is increased by increases in PEEP, inspiratory pressure (PI), inspiratory time (TI), rate, and flow rate. All these changes lead to higher PaO_2, but each has different effects on $PaCO_2$. For a given rise in MAP, increasing PEEP gives the greatest improvement in PaO_2. Other ways of raising MAP are by increasing PI and by prolonging TI.

b. Optimum MAP results from a balance between optimizing PaO_2, minimizing direct oxygen toxicity, minimizing barotrauma, and achieving adequate ventilation. Barotrauma is probably most closely related to peak-to-peak swings in PI, although airway velocity and MAP are also implicated.

c. MAP as low as 5 cm H_2O may be sufficient in infants with normal lungs, whereas 20 cm H_2O or more may be necessary in severe RDS. Excessive MAP may impede venous return and adversely affect cardiac output.

3. Ventilation (Table 13-5)

a. CO_2 elimination depends on **minute ventilation.** Since minute ventilation is the product of respiratory rate and tidal volume, increases in ventilator rate will lower $PaCO_2$. Increases in tidal volume can be achieved by increasing the PI on pressure-cycled ventilators or by increasing volume on volume-limited machines. Because tidal volume is a function of the difference between PI and PEEP, a reduction in PEEP also improves ventilation. At very low tidal volumes, the volume of dead space becomes important and may lead to CO_2 retention.

b. Optimal $PaCO_2$ varies according to disease state. For very immature infants or infants with air leak, a $PaCO_2$ of 50 to 60 mmHg may be tolerated to minimize barotrauma, provided pH is greater than 7.25. When hyperventilation is used to reduce pulmonary vascular resistance, a $PaCO_2$ as low as 25 to 30 mmHg is occasionally required.

IV. Disease states

A. Effects of diseases. Respiratory failure can result from numerous illnesses through a variety of pathophysiologic mechanisms. Optimal ventilatory strategy must take into account the pathophysiology, expected time course, and particular vulnerabilities of the patient.

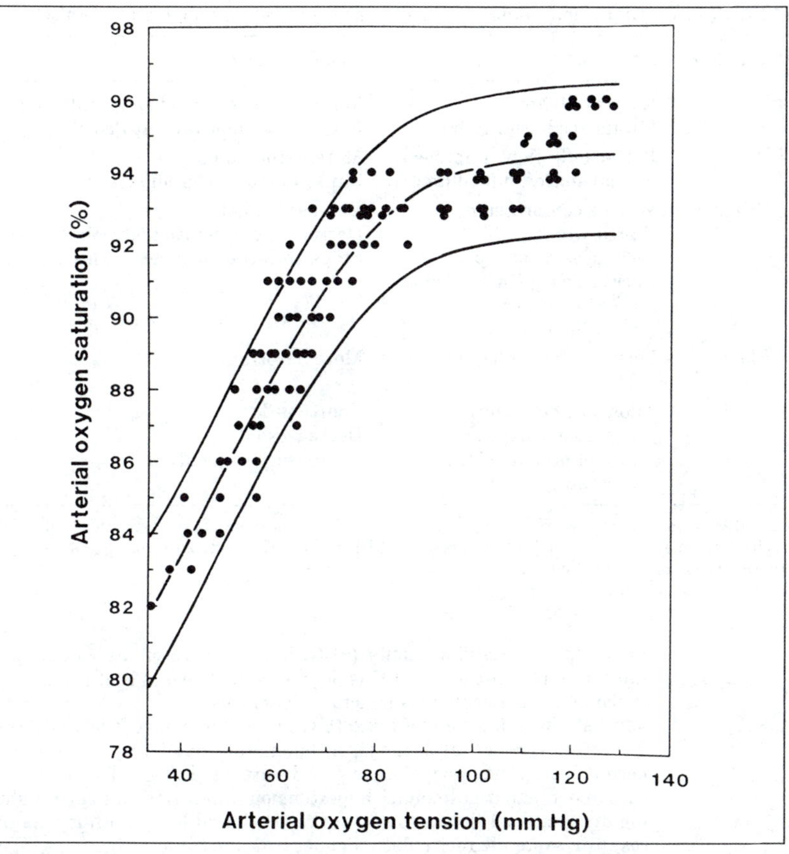

Fig. 13-1. Comparison of paired measurements of oxygen saturation by pulse oximetry and of oxygen tension by indwelling umbilical artery oxygen electrode. The lines represent ± 2 SD. (Modified, from A. Wasunna, A. G. Whitelaw. Pulse oximenry in preterm infants. *Arch. Dis. Child.* 62: 957, 1987.)

B. **Pulmonary mechanics** influence the ventilator strategy selected.

1. **Compliance** is the stiffness or distensibility of the lung and chest wall, i.e., the change in volume (ΔV) produced by a change in pressure (ΔP), or $\Delta V/\Delta P$. It is decreased with surfactant deficiency, excess lung water, and lung fibrosis. It is also decreased when the lungs are hyperexpanded.
2. **Resistance** is the impediment to airflow due to airway obstruction, turbulence, and viscous friction. Almost half of airway resistance is in the upper airways, including the endotracheal tube when in use. Resistance is high in airway diseases such as aspiration and bronchopulmonary dysplasia (BPD). Resistance can change rapidly if, for example, secretions partially occlude the endotracheal tube.
3. **Time constant** is the product of compliance and resistance. This is a measure of the time it takes to equibrate pressure between the proximal airway and the alveoli. Expiratory time constants are somewhat longer than inspiratory ones. When time constants are long, as in meconium aspiration, care must be taken to set inspiratory times and rates that permit adequate inspiration to deliver the required tidal volume and adequate expiration to avoid inadvertent PEEP.

Table 13-5. Ventilator manipulations to increase ventilation and decrease $PaCO_2$

Parameter	Advantage	Disadvantage
↑ Rate	Easy to titrate Minimizes barotrauma	Maintains same dead space/tidal volume May lead to inadvertent PEEP
↑ PI	Better bulk flow (improved dead space/tidal volume)	More barotrauma Shifts to stiffer compliance curve
↓ PEEP	Widens compression pressure Decreases dead space Decreases expiratory load Shifts to steeper compliance curve	Decreases MAP Decreases oxygenation/alveolar collapse Stops splinting obstructed/closed airways
↑ Flow	Permits shorter TI, longer TE	More barotrauma
↑ TE	Allows longer expiration for passive expiration in face of prolonged time constant	Shortens TI Decreases MAP Decreases oxygenation

Key: MAP = mean airway pressure; ↑ = increase; ↓ = decrease; TI = inspiratory time; TE = expiratory time; PI = peak inspiratory pressure; PEEP = positive end-expiratory pressure; FIO_2 = fraction of oxygen in inspired gas.

4. **Functional residual capacity (FRC)** is a measure of the volume of the lungs at end-expiration. FRC is decreased in diseases that permit alveolar collapse, particularly surfactant deficiency.
5. **Ventilation-perfusion matching ($\dot{V}/\dot{Q}$).** Diseases that reduce alveolar surface area (through atelectasis, inflammatory exudates, or obstruction) permit intrapulmonary shunting of desaturated blood. The opposite occurs in persistent pulmonary hypertension, when extrapulmonary shunting diverts blood flow away from the ventilated lung. Both mechanisms result in systemic recirculation of desaturated blood.
6. **Work of breathing** is especially important in the smallest infants and those with chronic lung diseases, whose high airway resistance, decreased lung compliance, compliant chest wall, and weak musculature may overwhelm their metabolic energy requirements and impede growth.

C. **Specific disease states.** Several of the more common neonatal disease processes are described below and are presented in Table 13-6 along with the optimal ventilatory strategies. Before initiating ventilatory support, however, clinicians must evaluate for mechanical causes of distress, including pneumothorax or airway obstruction.

1. **Respiratory Distress Syndrome (RDS)** (see Respiratory Distress Syndrome/Hyaline Membrane Disease above)
   a. **Pathophysiology.** RDS is caused by surfactant deficiency, which results in a severe decrease in compliance (stiff lung). This causes diffuse alveolar collapse with severe $\dot{V}/\dot{Q}$ mismatching and increased work of breathing.
   b. **Ventilatory strategy.** Early application of CPAP is used to prevent further atelectasis. CPAP is initiated at 5 to 6 cm H_2O and is escalated rapidly in increments of 2 cm H_2O up to a maximum of 9 to 10 cm H_2O. CPAP is titrated by clinical assessment of retractions and observation of transcutaneous PO_2 or O_2 saturation. Mechanical ventilation is used when $\dot{V}/\dot{Q}$ mismatching is severe enough that increased FIO_2 and CPAP are inadequate or in infants who tire from the increased work of breathing. Two basic conventional approaches used are slow and

Table 13-6. Neonatal pulmonary physiology by disease state

Disease	Compliance ml/cmH_2O	Resistance ml/cmH_2O/s	Time Constant (s)	FRC (ml/kg)	$\dot{V}/\dot{Q}$ Matching	Work
Normal term	4–6	20–40	0.25	30 ml/kg	–	–
RDS	↓ ↓	–	↓ ↓	↓	↓/↓ ↓	↑
Meconium aspiration	–/↓	↑/↑ ↑	↑	↑/↑ ↑	↓ ↓	↑
BPD	↑/↓	↑ ↑	↑	↑ ↑	↓ ↓/↓	↑ ↑
Air leak	↓ ↓	–/↑	–/↑	↑ ↑	↓/↓ ↓	↑ ↑
VLBW apnea	↓	–	↓ ↓	–/↓	↓/–	–/↑

Key: ↑ = increase; ↓ = decrease; – = little or no change; / = either/or.

rapid rate. A third approach is high-frequency ventilation. Controversy exists over the preferred method [17,21]. In all methods, PEEP should be escalated and weaned approximately in proportion to the FIO_2 (4 cm H_2O at 0.40, 5 cm H_2O at 0.50, etc). Our preferred approach is a modification of the low-rate technique in which TI does not exceed 1.0 second.

(1) The low-rate technique [18] achieves a high MAP with a long TI (0.5 to 1.0 second) but requires a moderate PI. TI should never exceed 1.5 seconds. Adequate PI, applied to recruit alveoli, is initially estimated by good chest excursion and is usually 20 to 25 cm H_2O. Rates are generally 20 to 40 breaths per minute. PEEP is set at 4 to 5 cm H_2O and may go up to 8 to 9 cm H_2O. Higher PEEP provides no benefit and may interfere with cardiac output. Flow rates of 10 to 15 liters per second are needed to provide a relatively square pressure waveform. When the patient becomes stable, FIO_2 and PI are weaned first, alternating with rate, as tolerated. This approach maximizes alveolar recruitment.

(2) Rapid rate, low pressure [12] relies on high rates to maintain MAP while reducing PI to minimize barotrauma. Rates of 60 to 80 breaths per minute are used, with TI as low as 0.2 to 0.3 second. Inadvertent PEEP is not encountered because the time constant in RDS may be as short as 0.05 second. PI is set as low as 12 to 18 cm H_2O, with PEEP of 4 to 5 cm H_2O. Initial settings are based on auscultation of good breath sounds and are increased as needed. In general, pressure is weaned first, while rate remains high, or by 10 percent drops in rate alternating with pressure, as tolerated.

(3) High-frequency ventilation may be initiated after conventional ventilation fails to maintain adequate gas exchange. Strategies differ depending on whether HFJ, HFO, or HFFI is used [5]. For HFJ, the frequency is set at 250 to 350 breaths per minute. Peak pressures are set 20 to 25 percent lower than those on conventional ventilation. PI and FIO_2 are adjusted as needed to maintain oxygenation. PEEP is maintained the same. Inspiratory-to-expiratory times are set at a 1:3 ratio. For HFO and HFFI-A, frequencies of 600 to 900 breaths per minute are selected, and PEEP is maintained. Stroke volume and FIO_2 are adjusted to provide a MAP similar to that on conventional ventilation and achieve adequate oxygenation. Inspiratory and expiratory ratios are fixed at 1:1. The ventilator manipulations in Table 13-4 also apply in general to high-frequency ventilators, although some parameters (e.g., TI/TE ratio in HFO) cannot be adjusted. In both HFJ and HFO, alveolar recruitment procedures may be important, both initially and as sighs delivered by conventional ventilators [4,10]. In both HFJ and HFO, weaning has usually been accomplished after transfer back to conventional ventilation.

Because RDS has such a distinctive time course of escalation, plateau, and weaning, ventilatory strategy should anticipate the increased risk of pneumothorax as compliance increases and time constants lengthen. In all approaches, a $PaCO_2$ value higher than physiologic is acceptable to minimize barotrauma. Extubation should be accomplished when ventilator rates are 3 to 10 breaths per minute. Aminophylline may be used to facilitate spontaneous breathing prior to extubation.

2. **Meconium aspiration syndrome (MAS)** (see Meconium Aspiration below)
   a. **Pathophysiology.** MAS results when a fetus or infant aspirates meconium-stained amniotic fluid. The severity of the syndrome is related to the associated asphyxial insult and the amount aspirated. The aspirated meconium causes acute airway obstruction, marked airway resistance, scattered atelectasis with $\dot{V}/\dot{Q}$ mismatching, and

hyperexpansion due to obstructive ball-valve effects. The obstructive phase is followed by an inflammatory phase 12 to 24 hours later that results in further alveolar involvement. Other aspiration syndromes (such as blood or amniotic fluid) have similar but milder effects.

b. **Ventilatory strategy.** Because of the ball-valve effects, application of positive pressure frequently results in pneumothorax or another air leak, so initiating mechanical ventilation requires careful consideration of the risks and benefits. Low levels of PEEP (4 to 5 cm H_2O) are helpful in splinting open partially obstructed airways and equalizing $\dot{V}/\dot{Q}$ matching. Higher levels only lead to hyperinflation. If airway resistance is high and compliance is normal, a slow-rate, moderate-pressure strategy [see **1.b(1)**] is needed. If pneumonitis is more prominent, more rapid rates can be used. Rapid rates may be required in the hyperventilation strategy employed for persistent pulmonary hypertension of the newborn (PPHN) that may be associated with MAS, but care must be taken to avoid inadvertent PEEP. Pancuronium is often used to minimize risks of air leak in severe MAS because of the high transpulmonary pressures these large infants can generate when "fighting" the ventilator and the ball-valve hyperexpansion caused by their disease. Weaning may be rapid if the illness is predominantly obstruction or very prolonged if complicated by barotrauma and severe inflammation.

3. **Bronchopulmonary dysplasia (BPD)** (see Chronic Lung Disease below)

a. **Pathophysiology.** BPD results from injury to the alveoli and airways. Bleb formation may lead to poor recoil. Fibrosis and excess lung water may cause stiffer compliance. Airways may be narrowed and fibrotic or hyperreactive. Upper airways may be overdistended and conduct airflow poorly. BPD is marked by shifting focal atelectasis, hyperinflation with $\dot{V}/\dot{Q}$ mismatching, chronic and acute increases in airway resistance, and a significant increase in the work of breathing.

b. **Ventilator strategy.** Optimal strategy is to wean infants off the ventilator as soon as possible to prevent further barotrauma and oxygen toxicity. If this is not feasible, ventilator settings should be minimized to permit tissue repair and long-term growth. Low rates (5 to 15 breaths per minute) and longer T_I (0.5 to 0.8 second) are used to maintain FRC. Higher pressures are often required (20 to 30 cm H_2O) because of the stiff lungs, although the high resistance prevents transfer of most of this to the alveoli. Acute decompensations can result from bronchospasm and interstitial fluid accumulation. These must be treated with adequately high P_I, bronchodilators and diuretics. Good oxygenation should be maintained (saturations of 90 to 92 percent), but higher $PaCO_2$ values can be permitted (55 to 65 mmHg), provided pH is normal. Weaning is a slow and difficult process, decreasing rate by 1 to 2 breaths per minute every day when tolerated. Occasional chronically ventilator-dependent infants require tracheostomy.

4. **Air leak** [11] (See Air Leak below)

a. **Pathophysiology.** Pneumothorax and pulmonary interstitial emphysema (PIE) are the two most common air leak syndromes. Pneumothorax results when air ruptures into the pleural space. In PIE, the interstitial air seriously reduces tissue compliance as well as recoil. In addition, peribronchial and perivascular air may compress the airways and vascular supply causing "air block."

b. **Ventilator strategy.** Since air is driven into the interstitium throughout the ventilatory cycle, the primary goal is to reduce MAP through any of its components (P_I, T_I, PEEP) and to rely on increased FiO_2 to provide oxygenation. This strategy holds for all air leak syndromes. If dropping the MAP is not tolerated, other techniques may be tried. Because the time constants for interstitial air are much longer than those for the alveoli, we sometimes use very rapid conventional rates

(80 to 120 breaths per minute), which may preferentially ventilate alveoli. High-frequency ventilation is emerging as an important alternative for severe airleak [9].

5. **Apnea** (See Apnea below.)
   a. **Pathophysiology.** Occasionally, apnea is severe enough to warrant ventilatory support, even in the absence of pulmonary disease. This may result from apnea of prematurity, during or following general anesthesia, or neuromuscular paralysis.
   b. **Ventilator strategy.** For infants completely dependent on the ventilator, the goal should be to provide "physiologic" respiration using moderate PEEP (3 to 4 cm H_2O), lower gas flow, and normal rates (30 to 40 breaths per minute), with PI adjusted to prevent hyperventilation (10 to 18 cm H_2O). Prolonged TI is unnecessary. For infants requiring a ventilator because of intermittent but prolonged apnea, low rates (3 to 10 breaths per minute) may be sufficient.

VI. **Adjuncts to mechanical ventilation**

A. **Sedation** can be used when agitation or distress are associated with excessive lability of oxygenation and hypoxemia. Although this problem is more common in the chronically ventilated neonate, acutely ill newborns may occasionally benefit from sedation. Morphine (0.1 to 0.2 mg/kg) or fentanyl (1–3 μg/kg/minute) can be used but may cause neurologic depression. Prolonged use may lead to dependence. Lorazepam (.05 to 0.1 mg/kg per dose given every 4 to 6 hours) has been used in more chronic situations because of its long duration of action.

B. **Muscle relaxation** with pancuronium bromide (0.1 mg/kg per dose repeated as needed) may be indicated in some infants who continue to breathe out of phase with the ventilator after attempts at finding appropriate settings and sedation have failed. High FIO_2 requirement (>0.75) or peak inspiratory pressure (>30 cm H_2O) are also relative indications for muscle relaxation. Although unequivocal data are not available, gas exchange may be improved in some infants following muscle relaxation, and the occurrence of chronic lung disease may be reduced [16,19]. Prolonged muscle relaxation leads to fluid retention and may result in deterioration in compliance. Sedation is routinely administered to infants receiving muscle relaxants.

C. **Blood gas monitoring** (see Blood Gas Monitoring below). All infants receiving mechanical ventilation require continuous monitoring and intermittent blood gas measurements.

D. **Pulmonary function testing (PFT)** of newborns has recently been adapted for clinical use. Systems are available to measure tidal volume, airflow, and transpulmonary pressure and then calculate and display dynamic compliance, pulmonary resistance, and work of breathing [8]. Although PFT may prove to be a valuable clinical tool, further studies documenting improved outcomes are needed.

VII. **Complications and sequelae.** As a complex and invasive technology, mechanical ventilation can result in numerous adverse outcomes, both iatrogenic and unavoidable.

A. **Barotrauma and oxygen toxicity**
   1. **Bronchopulmonary dysplasia (BPD)** is related to increased airway pressure, although oxygen toxicity, anatomic and physiologic immaturity, and individual susceptibility also contribute.
   2. **Air leak** is directly related to increased airway pressure, occurring frequently at MAPs in excess of 14 cm H_2O.

B. **Mechanical**
   1. **Obstruction** of endotracheal tubes may result in asphyxia.
   2. **Equipment malfunction,** particularly disconnection, is not uncommon and requires functioning alarm systems and vigilance.

C. **Complications of invasive monitoring**
   1. **Peripheral arterial occlusion with infarction**
   2. **Aortic thrombosis** from umbilical arterial catheters, occasionally leading to renal impairment and hypertension.

3. **Emboli** from flushed catheters, particularly to the lower extremities, splanchnic bed, or even brain.

D. **Anatomic**
1. **Subglottic stenosis**
2. **Palatal grooves** from prolonged orotracheal intubation
3. **Vocal cord damage**

References

1. Bancalari, E. *Clin. Perinatol.* 14: 581, 1987.
2. Boros, S. J. *J. Pediatr.* 91: 794, 1977.
3. Boros, S. J. *J. Pediatr.* 94: 114, 1979.
4. Boynton, B. R. *J. Pediatr.* 105: 297, 1984.
5. Carlo, W. A. *Pediatr. Clin. North Am.* 33: 221, 1986.
6. Chatburn, R. L. *Respir. Care* 28: 1579, 1983.
7. Clark, R. H. *Crit. Care Med.* 14: 926, 1986.
8. Cunningham, M. D. Monitoring Pulmonary Function. In J. P. Goldsmith and E. H. Karotkin (Eds.), *Assisted Ventilation in the Neonate,* 2d ed. Philadelphia: Saunders, 1988. Pp. 233–244.
9. Frantz, I. *Pediatrics* 71: 483, 1983.
10. Froese, A. B. *Am. Rev. Respir. Dis.* 135: 1363, 1987.
11. Harris, T. R. Physiological Principles. In J. P. Goldsmith and E. H. Karotkin (Eds.), *Assisted Ventilation of the Neonate,* 2d Ed. Philadelphia: Saunders, 1981. Pp. 22–67.
12. Heicher, D. A. *J. Pediatr.* 98: 957, 1981.
13. Herman, S. *Arch. Dis. Child.* 48: 612, 1973.
14. HiFi Study Group. *N. Engl. J. Med.* 320: 88, 1989.
15. Krauss, A. N. *Clin. Perinatol.* 7: 61, 1980.
16. Pollitzer, M. J. *Lancet* 1: 346, 1981.
17. Ramsden, C. A. *Arch. Dis. Child.* 62: 529, 1987.
18. Reynolds, E. O. R. *Arch. Dis. Child.* 46: 152, 1971.
19. Stark, A. R. *J. Pediatr.* 94: 439, 1979.
20. Stewart, A. R. *Pediatrics* 67: 474, 1981.
21. Tarnow-Mordi, W. *Br. Med. J.* 292: 575, 1986.

Blood Gas Monitoring

Douglas Richardson and
Ann R. Stark

I. **General principles.** The purpose of blood gas monitoring is to ensure adequate gas exchange while avoiding the risks of hypoxia or hyperoxia and excessive or inadequate ventilation. All sick infants with cardiopulmonary disorders should be monitored. The two major modes of monitoring are invasive blood gas analysis and noninvasive monitoring. Clinical circumstances, including severity and anticipated duration of lung disease, degree of instability, and availability of arterial access, will determine the appropriate combination of monitoring.

II. **Blood gas analysis.** Arterial blood gases (ABGs) are the gold standard for assessing the adequacy of oxygen delivery, ventilation, and pH. All noninvasive methods should be correlated with ABGs.

A. **Sampling.** Blood samples are usually obtained from indwelling arterial catheters. ABGs should be obtained every 1 to 6 hours when acute respiratory support is required and less frequently with stable chronic respiratory illness. Percutaneous arterial puncture is preferred when sampling is infrequent or course is expected to be short. Noxious stimuli, including arterial puncture, cause variable drops in measured PaO_2, especially in chronically ill infants with little pulmonary reserve, and this may influence interpretation. Sampling from venous catheters provides useful information on PCO_2 and pH only. Venous blood pH values are usually 0.02 to 0.04 lower and PCO_2 is usually 6 to 10 mmHg higher than paired arterial samples, but they vary depending on cardiac output and metabolic demands. Warmed capillary samples (CBGs) can be used to assess PCO_2 and pH. Capillary samples are unreliable in assessing oxygenation and may not always accurately reflect $PaCO_2$.

B. Measurements. Blood gas analyzers make direct readings of PO_2, PCO_2, and pH. The bicarbonate and oxygen saturation are generally calculated from standard nomograms. Direct measurement of oxygen saturation is possible but requires 0.5 ml more blood and a co-oximeter.

C. Interpretation. Extreme hypothermia or hyperthermia may lead to over- or underestimates (respectively) of arterial oxygenation. Since heparin solutions equilibrate with room air, excessive heparinization of sample syringes may have the same effect as air bubbles, raising PO_2 and lowering PCO_2.

III. Noninvasive monitoring [2,6]. Although ABGs are the gold standard, they have several drawbacks: (1) they require invasive catheters or painful and technically difficult arterial punctures, (2) they are not continuous, and (3) they are expensive both in terms of the cost of sample analyses and the clinical costs of iatrogenic anemia and transfusions. The continuous nature of noninvasive monitoring has made evident the inaccuracies of samples obtained by skin puncture. Continuous monitoring is especially useful in evaluating the clinical significance of apnea and acute changes such as pneumothorax and provides immediate feedback after changes in ventilator settings. It can be done at little risk to the patient. The long-term benefits of such monitoring are presumed but remain unproven.

IV. Noninvasive oxygen monitoring. The two technologies for monitoring oxygenation are transcutaneous ($PtcO_2$) and pulse oximetry ($StcO_2$).

A. Transcutaneous oxygenation ($PtcO_2$).

1. General characteristics. $PtcO_2$ monitoring uses a Clark-type sensor that is applied to the skin on an occlusive contact medium (usually distilled water or saline) and held in place by an adhesive ring. The sensor is heated to 43 to 44°C to produce localized hyperemia, which maximizes capillary blood flow under the sensor. Tissue oxygen then diffuses across the epidermis and sensor membrane, where it is chemically reduced, producing a current proportional to the PaO_2. A 10- to 15-minute equilibration time after sensor application is needed before the readings become reliable.

a. Calibration and maintenance. $PtcO_2$ sensors need to be calibrated before use at the temperature at which they will be used. This is usually 44°C for larger infants with a well-cornified epithelium and 43°C for small premature infants. To avoid the risk of thermal injury, sensors must be relocated every 4 to 6 hours and may need to be moved more frequently in hypoperfusion states. The sensors also require maintenance every week to replace the membrane and are recalibrated daily.

b. Limits and interpretations. Excessively high measurements may result from sensor dislodgment. Other errors may result from improper calibration. The accuracy of $PtcO_2$ measurements depends on diffusion of oxygen from tissues across the skin. Any factor that either affects local blood supply and oxygen delivery or creates a diffusion barrier will lead to underestimates of actual PaO_2 and must be interpreted with caution [11].

(1) Shock
(2) Severe acidosis, pH less than 7.06
(3) Hypothermia
(4) Severe anemia
(5) Tolazoline administration
(6) Marked skin edema or hydrops
(7) Hyperoxemia, PaO_2 greater than 160 mmHg

2. **Advantages**
   a. Under optimal steady-state conditions, correlations with ABGs are 0.90 to 0.95.
   b. Generally available in most NICUs.
   c. Provides estimates of hyperoxic status. This is useful for performing noninvasive hyperoxia tests to rule out cyanotic heart disease.
   d. Simultaneous pre- and postductal monitoring is possible to evaluate shunting in persistent pulmonary hypertension in the newborn.
3. **Disadvantages**
   a. Thermal injury, especially in extremely low birth weight infants or those with edema and poor perfusion
   b. Long equilibration time and sensor dislodgments may leave prolonged periods without monitoring.
   c. Not accurate in cases of shock or edema [11]
   d. Marked anemia will provide poor tissue oxygenation and result in discrepant $PtcO_2$.
   e. Less accurate in older infants with thicker epidermis
   f. High costs of fragile sensor and of technician time for frequent placements and maintenance

B. **Pulse oximetry** [10,12]
   1. **General characteristics.** Oximeters depend on the fact that reduced hemoglobin absorbs more red than infrared light and oxygenated hemoglobin absorbs more infrared than red. The oximeter probe consists of a light-emitting diode and a photodetector placed on opposite sides of a narrow part of the body. The diode emits equal intensities of red and infrared light into the tissue, and the photodetector senses the ratio of red to infrared light. The proportion of oxygenated and reduced hemoglobin, i.e., the percent saturated hemoglobin, is calculated and displayed. Since a ratio rather than an absolute value is measured, no calibration is required. The instrument is programmed to look only at pulsatile increases in oxygenated hemoglobin and thus depends on detection of a reasonable pulse. The correlations between transcutaneous estimates ($StcO_2$) and measured arterial saturations (SaO_2) are 0.90 to 0.95. The PaO_2 at any given SaO_2 is a function of the oxyhemoglobin dissociation curve (Fig. 13-1). Because SaO_2 increases little as the PaO_2 increases at the flat upper end of the curve, oximetry poorly distinguishes high normal oxygen tensions (80 to 100 mmHg) from dangerously hyperoxic ones (200 to 400 mmHg). This poor discrimination at the upper end of the curve is accentuated by any shifts in the curve itself [3,12]. Both higher concentrations of adult hemoglobin and acidosis shift the dissociation curve to the right [13]. A shift to the right means less saturation at a given PaO_2. Increases in $PaCO_2$, temperature, and concentration of 2,3-diphosphoglycerate (2,3-DPG) also shift the dissociation curve to the right.
      a. **Calibration and maintenance.** The photosensors do not need calibration. However, comparison of PaO_2 by ABG with transcutaneous saturation ($StcO_2$) allows the O_2 dissociation curve to be estimated for the individual infant. Interference by bright lights can be helped by shielding, but excessive motion artifacts can be a problem in active infants.
      b. **Limits and interpretation.** Because of the unpredictable location of the upper end of the O_2 dissociation curve, a measured $StcO_2$ of 97 percent might correspond to a PaO_2 ranging from 90 to 135 mmHg, given the ± 2 percent limits of accuracy of an oximeter. In preterm infants with predominantly fetal hemoglobin, saturations of 86 to 92 percent correspond to PaO_2 values of 37 to 97 mmHg. Thus, for a premature baby receiving oxygen or ventilatory support, PaO_2 should be monitored when the $StcO_2$ is greater than 90 percent. At the lower end of the curve, the effects of shifts in the curve are more evident in saturation

than in PaO_2. For example, at a PaO_2 of 45 mmHg, saturation may decrease from about 88 percent at pH 7.4 (which is satisfactory) to about 80 percent at pH 7.25 (which may be inadequate for tissue oxygenation). In general, saturation above 85 percent is adequate and below 80 percent is inadequate. $StcO_2$ between 80 and 85 percent may be adequate if the PaO_2 is greater than 45 mmHg. These values assume normal cardiac output and hemoglobin concentration. Although monitoring saturation is useful at lower levels, it must be remembered that partial pressure determines the rate of oxygen transferred to the tissues and also muscle tone in the wall of the ductus arteriosus and pulmonary arterioles.

2. **Advantages**
   a. Saturation is the basic physiologic determinant of tissue oxygen delivery.
   b. No warm-up or equilibration time
   c. Immediate readouts permit spot monitoring and shared equipment.
   d. Pulse-by-pulse detection of rapid or transient changes in saturation (e.g., apneic spells)
   e. Substantially lower maintenance and technician costs
3. **Disadvantages**
   a. Risk of hyperoxia at saturations between 90 and 100 percent
   b. Variability in hemoglobin saturation curve during first weeks makes estimates of PaO_2 unpredictable. This variability is affected by pH and relative amounts of adult and fetal hemoglobin.
   c. Motion and light artifacts disrupt monitoring.
   d. Not usable in cases of severe hypotension or marked edema
   e. Does not take clinical impact of anemia into account
   f. May provoke evaluation of transient, clinically insignificant desaturations
   g. Supplementary O_2 lowered too slowly because high PaO_2 not recognized

V. **Noninvasive PCO_2 monitoring.** The role of noninvasive PCO_2 monitoring is less well established. This is so because hyper- and hypocapnea are usually associated with acute changes in oxygenation. Noninvasive PCO_2 monitoring is useful to follow trends when unexpected changes in baseline PCO_2 may occur. Such clinical situations include rapid weaning in RDS, hyperventilation for persistent pulmonary hypertension, decompensation in established BPD, transition to high-frequency ventilation, and possibly in infants at high risk of pneumothorax. Two technologies available are transcutaneous PCO_2 ($PtcCO_2$) and capnography to estimate end-tidal PCO_2 ($PetCO_2$).

A. **Transcutaneous PCO_2 ($PtcCO_2$)** [2,6,8,9]

1. **General characteristics.** $PtcCO_2$ monitors use a Stow-Severinghaus pH-sensitive glass electrode. When applied occlusively to the skin, the heated sensor causes vasodilation of the underlying capillary bed. Tissue CO_2 equilibrates across the epidermis and membrane, where it combines with the internal electrolyte buffer. An electric current between the glass and reference electrodes is generated by the change in pH and is proportional to $PaCO_2$. Combined O_2/CO_2 sensors are available.
   a. **Maintenance and calibration.** The heated sensor causes more dissolved CO_2 to come out of solution and also raises the local tissue metabolic rate. Both effects result in a higher PCO_2 reading. At 44°C, the increase is a factor of 1.37 times. It is proportionally lower at lower temperatures, but accuracy and response time are worse. Most monitors have an electronic means of reducing the displayed $PtcCO_2$ by this factor. Reported correlations are 0.90 to 0.93, agreeing with $PaCO_2$ ± 4 mmHg. Sensors require 10 to 15 minutes of equilibration before providing stable readings. Before use, they must be calibrated against a standard CO_2 gas mixture, and they tend to drift during use.

Electrodes are costly and fragile, and replacement membranes are needed periodically. Sensor sites must be rotated every 2 to 6 hours to avoid burns.

b. **Interpretation and limits.** The $PtcCO_2$ sensor is conceptually similar to the more familiar $PtcO_2$ electrode. Both are dependent on adequate tissue blood flow and are adversely affected by hypotension and tissue edema, although the $PtcCO_2$ is less affected [1]. Rising $PtcCO_2$ and falling $PtcO_2$ should raise concerns about perfusion. Both sensors have relatively slow response times in vivo (30 to 90 seconds). Both require 5 to 15 minutes' equibration. Both are less accurate in older infants with thicker skin.

2. **Advantages.** $PtcCO_2$ can be used in any situation where continuous monitoring is indicated, including nonintubated infants. It may be particularly useful when initiating and adjusting high-frequency ventilation or for close monitoring after extubation.

3. **Disadvantages.** $PtcCO_2$ monitoring often fails to provide additional information beyond that readily available from intermittent blood gas analysis, and it is expensive and labor-intensive. Its slow response time makes it less useful for detecting acute rises in $PaCO_2$. It is not useful for intermittent monitoring of chronic BPD because of unpredictable variations in baseline.

B. **Capnography (end-tidal CO_2; $PetCO_2$)** [4,5]

1. **General characteristics.** Capnographs use infrared spectroscopy or mass spectrometry readings of expired gas to analyze CO_2 content. This technique depends on achieving an end-tidal CO_2 plateau from which to estimate alveolar CO_2. It is therefore rate- and flow-dependent. In adults, CO_2 waveform analysis is used qualitatively to assess ventilatory mechanics. In newborns, the relatively high rates and low tidal volumes (relative to the bias flow of fresh gas) and marked ventilation-perfusion mismatching mean that a stable $PetCO_2$ is often not achieved, resulting in inconsistent underestimates of $PaCO_2$, especially in sicker infants. Correlation coefficients with $PaCO_2$ are 0.69 to 0.92. Newer systems with lower dead space and mainstream sensors may make this method practical for use in neonates.

2. **Advantages.** $PetCO_2$ may provide intermittent trend monitoring for larger intubated infants with chronic lung disease. It can also be used qualitatively at the nostrils of nonintubated infants to detect airflow obstruction and apnea.

3. **Disadvantages.** The additional dead space introduced by the airway adapter can cause CO_2 retention of as much as 6 to 10 mmHg. $PetCO_2$ cannot be employed during high-frequency ventilation.

VI. **Other devices.** The noninvasive technologies have been employed invasively in arterial catheters: **oxygen electrode catheters** [7] and **oximetric catheters** [14]. Both techniques share all the advantages and disadvantages. They provide accurate direct arterial readings with rapid response times. Both require invasive monitoring. In both there is a significant rate of catheter tip occlusion. Such occlusions seem more frequent than with conventional catheters, presumably owing to the smaller lumen. Catheters are very expensive, cannot be reused, and require in vivo calibration.

VII. **Clinical applications.** The selection and appropriate use of blood gas monitoring technologies are complex and difficult. Clinical application requires careful clinical evaluation on an individual basis coupled with a thorough understanding of the advantages and limitations of the individual technologies. In order to assist clinicians in selecting the appropriate technology, four common clinical situations in which monitoring is necessary are sketched out in Table 13-7. Inevitably, patients do not fit neatly into these categories, and even when they do, they may change over time. Thus these guidelines cannot supplant thoughtful clinical judgment.

Table 13-7. Guidelines for use of blood gas monitoring

Clinical situation	Preferred technology	Supplemental monitoring	Rationale
Acutely ill premature infant Desired PaO_2 : 50–80 mmHg	Pulse oximetry $StcO_2$ 87–92 optimal	ABG via arterial line $PtcO_2$ if $StcO_2 > 95$ percent	Major concern is hypoxemia. Pulse oximetry minimizes invasiveness and cost, but risks hyperoxia; supplemental monitoring is therefore essential.
Chronically ill premature infant with BPD Desired PaO_2 : 60–80 mmHg	Pulse oximetry $StcO_2$ 90–92 optimal 90–95 acceptable	Periodic ABGs by arterial puncture to correlate. CBGs if only PCO_2 is of concern	Major concern is hypoxemia. Hyperoxia is less worrisome if ROP risk is low, but chronic excessive oxygen must be avoided. $PtcO_2$ shown to be less accurate in older infants
Premature infant with normal lung function on room air (e.g., apnea) Desired PaO_2 : > 50 mmHg	Pulse oximetry $StcO_2 \geqslant 87$	ABG or CBG to correlate and to check PCO_2	Hyperoxia risk is negligible. Pulse oximetry to monitor for hypoxemia; periodic blood gases to evaluate PCO_2
Acutely ill term infants with pneumonia/aspiration Desired PaO_2 : 60–80 mmHg	Transcutaneous $PtcO_2$ 60–80 Pulse oximetry $StcO_2$ 87–92	Pre- and postductal $PtcO_2$ if concern about pulmonary hypertension ABGs by arterial line to correlate and monitor PCO_2 $PtcCO_2$ may be helpful if hyperventilating	Higher PaO_2 goals used in treating pulmonary hypertension makes $PtcO_2$ preferable; dual pre- and postductal monitoring informative of shunt.

References

1. Brunstler, I., et al. *J. Pediatr.* 100: 454, 1982.
2. Cassady, G. *J. Pediatr.* 103: 837, 1983.
3. Dear, P. R. F. *Arch. Dis. Child.* 62: 879, 1987.
4. Epstein, M. F. *J. Pediatr.* 106: 282, 1985.
5. Meny, R. G. *Crit. Care Med.* 13: 1064, 1985.
6. Peabody, J. L. *Clin. Perinatol.* 12: 147, 1985.
7. Pollitzer, M. J. *Pediatrics* 66: 31, 1980.
8. Severinghaus, J. W. *Acta Anaesthesia. Scand. Suppl.* 68: 118, 1978.
9. Severinghaus, J. W. *Respir. Care* 27: 152, 1982.
10. Tremper, K. K. *Anesthesiology* 70: 98, 1989.
11. Versmold, H. T. *Birth Defects* 15: 285, 1979.
12. Wasunna, A. *Arch. Dis. Child.* 62: 957, 1987.
13. Wilkinson, A. R. *Am. Rev. Respir. Dis.* 122: 629, 1980.
14. Wilkinson, A. R. *Pediatrics* 93: 1016, 1978.

Air Leak: Pneumothorax, Pulmonary Interstitial Emphysema, Pneumomediastinum, Pneumopericardium

Rogers G. Howell, II

I. Background

A. Incidence. Air leak is a common respiratory complication in newborns. In 1987, 8 percent of 1615 infants admitted to Brigham and Women's Hospital or Children's Hospital NICUs developed air leak (Table 13-8). Multiple air leaks occurred in 15 percent. Twenty-five percent of infants treated with mechanical ventilation for RDS had air leak compared with 17 percent of infants ventilated with meconium aspiration syndrome (MAS). No infants with RDS treated with oxygen therapy alone developed air leak, although air leak developed in 21 percent of infants with MAS given similar therapy. In infants with lung disease, PIE occurred more often in preterm compared with term infants, 38 percent (28 of 74) versus 9 percent (3 of 34). Spontaneous pneumothorax requiring NICU care occurred in 0.07 percent (10 of ~15,000) of inborn infants 35 weeks' gestation and older without lung disease, a frequency similar to previous experience.

B. Mechanisms for development of air leak. Air leak may develop from prolonged tearing tension across alveolar walls due to excessive or uneven ventilation. This results in alveolar rupture either directly into the pleural space creating a pneumothorax or into the pulmonary interstitium. Pulmonary interstitial air also may result from disruption of overdistended distal airways, since during the early stages of RDS, the noncartilaginous, terminal airways are more compliant than the alveolar saccules [1]. Pulmonary interstitial air may become trapped and create pulmonary interstitial emphysema (PIE), track centrally by means of the lymphatics or perivascular tissue planes, and rupture into the mediastinal space causing a pneumomediastinum or disrupt the pleura and form a pneumothorax. Extrapulmonary air also may decompress into the fascial planes of the neck and result in subcutaneous emphysema, track through the esophageal hiatus and rupture through the retroperitoneum causing pneumoperitonium, dissect along perivascular sheaths of the great vessels or rupture through mediastinal connective tissue close to the pleural-pericardial connection into the pericardial sac and create pneumopericardium, or disrupt the pulmonary venous system and produce a systemic air embolus [5]. Trauma from endotracheal tube or suction catheter

Table 13-8. Number (percent) of patients with air leak

Number of patients	All types	Pneumothorax	PIE	Pneumomediastinum	Pneumopericardium
RDS					
327	68 (21%)	50 (15%)	26 (8%)	2 (<1%)	2 (<1%)
MAS					
81	15 (19%)	12 (15%)	1 (1%)	4 (5%)	1 (1%)
TTN					
107	7 (7%)	7 (7%)			

Key: PIE = pulmonary interstitial emphysema; RDS = respiratory distress syndrome; MAS = meconium aspiration syndrome; TTN = transient tachypnea of the newborn.

causing bronchial laceration or esophageal perforation also may result in pneumothorax [2,11].

II. Types of air leaks

A. Pneumothorax.
A. Pneumothorax. Risk factors include history of aspiration of blood, mucous, or meconium; difficult delivery; fetal distress; endotracheal intubation; resuscitation; positive-pressure ventilation; or pneumonia. Mechanically ventilated preterm infants who make expiratory efforts against ventilator breaths are prone to develop pneumothoraces and may benefit from pharmacologic muscle relaxation [8]. Mechanical ventilation using a long inspiratory time (1.0 versus 0.5 second) may result in more frequent pneumothoraces [9]. When pneumothorax occurs unexpectedly, ultrasound examination to detect possible renal malformations should be considered [3].

1. Diagnosis

a. Physical examination signs include the following:

(1) Respiratory distress, often tachypnea or retractions (or both)

(2) Cyanosis

(3) Chest asymmetry

(4) Apnea and bradycardia

(5) Shift of the cardiac point of maximum impulse

(6) Change in breath sounds

(7) Gradual deterioration of vital signs may precede the event, such as increased systolic blood pressure, pulse pressure, or heart rate or hypotension and bradycardia.

(8) Sudden deterioration may occur from elevated intrathoracic pressure collapsing the lung and restricting venous return, resulting in severe hypotension, bradycardia, apnea, hypoxia, and hypercapnia.

b. Chest radiograph is diagnostic. Anteroposterior (AP) and cross-table lateral views are useful. The lateral decubitus view, with the side of suspected pneumothorax up, will often show even a small pneumothorax.

c. Transillumination with a high-intensity, fiberoptic light source may demonstrate a pneumothorax for immediate treatment. Caution should be used interpreting results in infants with chest-wall edema or severe PIE or in extremely small infants. Baseline transillumination in these infants may be helpful in decreasing false-positive results.

d. Direct needle aspiration in the critically ill infant with clinical signs of pneumothorax may be diagnostic and therapeutic (see **2.b**).

2. Treatment

a. Conservative therapy may be adequate for infants who have no underlying lung disease or complicating therapy (such as mechanical ventilation), are in no distress, and have no continuous air leak. This therapy involves close observation for signs of deterioration, efforts to minimize crying, and following serial chest radiographs. The extrapulmonary air will usually resolve in 24 to 48 hours. Because of the danger of retinopathy of prematurity (ROP) and possible oxygen toxicity to the lungs, we do not use 100% oxygen, although this may speed up resorption of the pneumothorax.

b. Needle aspiration is useful as a therapeutic and diagnostic procedure in the critically ill infant with respiratory or hemodynamic compromise or both due to pneumothorax or in the occasional infant without intrinsic lung disease or continuing air leak but who is in distress from a pneumothorax. The procedure is as follows:

(1) Attach a 23- or 25-gauge "butterfly" needle to a large syringe through a three-way stopcock.

(2) Prepare the skin with antibacterial solution, and then insert the needle into the second intercostal space. With the infant lying supine, the needle should enter in the midclavicular line.

(3) Insert the needle until it touches the rib. Then slide it over the top of the rib to minimize the chance of bleeding from the intercostal artery. Apply continuous suction with the syringe as the needle is inserted. A rapid flow of air will occur when the pneumothorax is entered. Minimize needle penetration into the pleural space to reduce the risk of puncturing the lung while the free air is evacuated. Minimal penetration is likely when small drops of serous fluid are aspirated from the parietal pleura along with the air.

(4) Once airflow ceases, remove the needle, since, with the lung reexpanded, the visceral pleura may now appose the needle tip and be lacerated.

(5) If the air leak is continuous and the infant is compromised, the "butterfly" tubing, with the needle left in place, may be placed under sterile water and allowed to bubble while a chest tube is inserted (see **c**).

c. Chest tube insertion is necessary in infants with continuing air leak, in those with underlying pulmonary disease causing ongoing respiratory distress, and in those receiving positive-pressure ventilatory support. Chest tube insertion should be performed or supervised by experienced nursery personnel.

(1) Insertion of a chest tube

(a) Select a chest tube of the appropriate size. No. 10 and no. 12 French are most frequently used.

(b) Prepare the area with an antibacterial solution and infiltrate lidocaine 1% into the subcutaneous tissues overlying the sixth rib in the anterior axillary line. We generally administer a narcotic or neuroleptic to the patient if vital signs are stable.

(c) Make a small incision (1.0 to 1.5 cm) through the skin parallel to the sixth rib in the anterior axillary line.

(d) Bluntly dissect the tissues overlying the rib using a small curved hemostat. Then make a subcutaneous track to the third or fourth interspace. Care should be taken to avoid the nipple area and not to pierce the pectoralis muscle or lacerate the axillary artery.

(e) Enter the pleural space with the closed hemostat. Guide the tip over the top of the rib to avoid trauma to the intercostal artery, and push through the intercostal muscles and parietal pleura. Spread the tips to widen the opening and withdraw the hemostat with the tips spread to avoid pinching the lung. Confirm the location of the pleural opening with the closed hemostat. We rarely use trochars to enter the pleural cavity because of the risk of lung perforation.

(f) Hold the end of the chest tube with the curved hemostat. Advance the hemostat and chest tube through the skin incision into the pleural opening previously made. When the pleural space is entered, advance the chest tube after releasing the hemostat. A chest tube may be directed anteriorly by rotating the hemostat so that the curve points anteriorly and advancing the chest tube after releasing the hemostat.

(g) Note the chest tube to "steam up" once in the pleural space.

(h) Direct the chest tube to the location of the pleural air. The anterior pleural space is generally most effective.

(i) Palpate the chest wall around the entry site of the chest tube into the pleural space to confirm that placement is within the chest and not the subcutaneous tissues.

(j) Close the incision by placing either a purse-string suture around the tube or a single interrupted suture on each side of the tube with 3-0 or 4-0 silk. Secure the chest tube by firmly wrapping and tying the skin suture tails around the tube tight enough to crimp it. A loop may be made in the remaining silk to allow another tight tie around the chest tube 2 to 4 cm from the skin surface.

(k) Cover the incision site with petrolatum gauze and a small dressing or a clear plastic adhesive surgical dressing. We avoid extensive taping or large dressings because they interfere with chest examination and may delay discovery of a displaced chest tube.

(l) Place the chest tube to suction or water seal immediately after entering the pleural space. We generally apply suction at -10 to -20 cm H_2O. In large air leaks, -25 cm H_2O may be necessary.

(m) AP and lateral chest radiographs are taken to confirm tube position and to ascertain drainage of the pleural air.

(n) Radiographs frequently reveal chest tubes that are ineffective in evacuating extrapulmonary air. The most common cause of failure is tube placement in the posterior pleural cavity, away from the air. Other causes for ineffective drainage are tubes that perforate the lung, diaphragm, or mediastinum or are in subcutaneous tissue. Extrapulmonary air not in the pleural space, such as a pneumomediastinum or subpleural pulmonary pseudocyst, will not be drained by a chest tube. Complications of chest tube insertion include hemorrhage, lung infarction, and phrenic nerve injury.

(2) Removal of a chest tube. When the infant's lung disease has improved, the chest tube has drained no air for 24 to 48 hours, and the pneumothorax demonstrated by radiograph has been resolved for 24 to 48 hours, we discontinue suction and place the tube under water seal. If x-ray examination shows no reaccumulation of extrapulmonary air in 12 to 24 hours, we remove the chest tube. To reduce the chance of introducing air into the pleural space during chest tube removal, cover the chest wound with a small occlusive dressing while pulling the tube out. Also, remove the chest tube during expiration in spontaneously breathing infants and during inspiration in infants ventilated with positive pressure.

d. Persistent pneumothorax may require multiple chest tubes, needle aspirations, or rarely, innovative therapy such as briefly collapsing the affected lung by selective intubation or obstruction [14] (see **B.2**).

3. Complications of pneumothorax include the following:

a. Profound **ventilatory and circulatory compromise** may occur and, if uncorrected, result in death.

b. Intraventricular hemorrhage may result, possibly secondary to a combination of fluctuating cerebrovascular pressures, hypercapnia, hypoxia, and acidosis.

c. Inappropriate antidiuretic hormone secretion may occur by an unknown mechanism.

B. Pulmonary interstitial emphysema (PIE) develops most frequently in premature infants with RDS treated with mechanical ventilation and significantly increases mortality. Air tends to become trapped in the pulmonary interstitium because of increased pulmonary interstitial fluid and extensive intrapulmonary connective tissue. Pulmonary blood flow may be compromised by interstitial air impinging on the pulmonary vasculature. The two forms of PIE on pathologic examination are interstitial pulmonary emphysema in which air dissects through lymphatics near the pulmonary arteries and pulmonary pseudocysts formed by rupture of distal airways into large, air-filled spaces [1].

1. **Diagnosis**
   a. PIE most often develops in the first 2 postnatal days, appearing before or simultaneously with other air leaks.
   b. PIE may be accompanied by hypotension and bradycardia and may cause decreased chest excursion.
   c. PIE has two radiographic patterns: cystlike or linear, with the lucencies radiating out from the lung hilum.
2. **Treatment**
   a. Conservative management may be effective. Decrease the ventilator inspiratory time and pressures while maintaining adequate oxygenation and ventilation. High ventilator rates are often required.
   b. Unilateral PIE may improve if the infant is positioned with the affected lung dependent and chest physiotherapy and endotracheal suction are minimized [19]. Severe, localized PIE that has failed to improve with conservative management may improve with collapse of the affected lung by selective bronchial intubation or occlusion [4,13] or, rarely, by surgical resection [18].
   c. Infants with severe, diffuse PIE unresponsive to conventional therapy may respond to high-frequency ventilation or extracorporeal membrane oxygenation.
3. **Complications**
   a. PIE may result in air block, an extreme state of altered ventilation, oxygenation, and circulation.
   b. Other air leaks may be associated.

C. **Pneumomediastinum** develops when extraventilatory air dissects to the mediastinal pleura and ruptures into the mediastinal space.

1. **Diagnosis**
   a. **Physical examination** may detect distant heart sounds.
   b. **Positive transillumination** of a pneumomediastinum may be confused with a pneumothorax or pneumopericardium.
   c. **Lateral chest radiograph,** the most reliable method of diagnosis, will show air in the mediastinal space. An AP radiogram may have a "sail sign" caused by air outlining the thymus.
2. **Treatment**
   a. If possible, decrease ventilator inspiratory time and pressures while maintaining adequate oxygenation and ventilation.
   b. Observe closely for other air leaks.
   c. No specific drainage procedure is usually necessary. On rare occasions, tension pneumomediastium refractory to medical management may require mediastinostomy drainage [15].
3. **Complications**
   a. Pneumomediastinum is generally not clinically important. Rarely, cardiorespiratory compromise may develop if the air is under tension and does not decompress into the pleural space, the retroperitoneum, or soft tissues of the neck [15].
   b. Other air leaks may be associated with pneumomediastinum.
   c. Because adults with pneumomediastinum frequently report pain, we often provide mild analgesia or sedation to infants with pneumomediastinum who are extremely irritable.

D. **Pneumopericardium** is less common than other forms of air leak and is often accompanied by cardiovascular collapse. Occasionally, pneumopericardium may be asymptomatic and appear as an incidental finding on chest radiograph. It generally occurs in preterm infants with RDS during the first 3 days of ventilator support [7,12]. Mortality directly from pneumopericardium and its treatment is about 25 percent, but the overall mortality of infants with pneumopericardium is about 75 percent [7].

1. **Diagnosis** of symptomatic pneumopericardium is usually not difficult but must be made rapidly and accurately to institute appropriate therapy.

a. **Physical examination** will often reveal acute onset of a triad of hypotension, cyanosis, and bradycardia, although some infants have tachycardia and decreased pulse pressure. Heart sounds are muffled or distant.

b. **Transillumination** is sometimes useful to quickly establish the diagnosis in a moribund patient, but pneumopericardium may be confused with pneumothorax or pneumomediastinum.

c. **Chest radiographs** confirm the diagnosis, showing air outlining the cardiac silhouette in anterior and lateral views. Air under the inferior surface of the heart is diagnostic. The volume of pericardial air seen on radiograph may not correlate with the severity of circulatory compromise.

d. **Needle aspiration** in the severely compromised infant may be diagnostic as well as therapeutic and is appropriate in some situations on the basis of clinical signs alone (see **2.b**).

2. **Treatment**

a. Conservative therapy is appropriate if signs of impaired cardiac output are absent. If possible, decrease ventilator inspiratory time and pressures, monitor blood pressure closely (especially for narrowed pulse pressure), and observe for other air leaks.

b. Needle aspiration is indicated if tamponade or impaired cardiac output is present.

(1) Prepare the subxiphoid area with antibacterial solution.

(2) Use an 18- to 22-gauge intravenous catheter with inner needle attached by means of IV extension tubing and three-way stopcock to a syringe. Insert the needle subxiphoid at a 30- to 45-degree angle, aiming at the left shoulder, and aspirate with the syringe as the needle is advanced. Once air is aspirated, stop advancing the needle. Remove the needle while advancing the plastic catheter into the pericardial space, evacuate the remaining air, and then withdraw the catheter. If the air leak is persistent, continue to aspirate gently while preparing for pericardial tube placement. If blood is aspirated, immediately withdraw the catheter to avoid lacerating the ventricular wall.

c. If the air leak is persistent, a pericardial tube should be placed by experienced personnel. We manage the pericardial tube like a chest tube, although less negative pressure (-5 to -10 cm H_2O) is applied for suction. Observe the infant closely for signs of myocardial irritation or infection.

3. **Complications** of pneumopericardium result from hemodynamic compromise and may cause death.

E. **Other air leaks**

1. **Pneumoperitoneum** may result from intrathoracic extrapulmonary air decompressing into the abdominal space. If very large, pneumoperitoneum can compromise respiration by limiting diaphragmatic excursion. Usually the pneumoperitoneum is of little clinical importance, but it must be differentiated from abdominal air due to a ruptured viscus. In the sick newborn, radiographic examination of the bowel with an isotonic contrast agent, such as metrizamide, may help rule out the diagnosis of bowel perforation [6].

2. **Subcutaneous emphysema** is characterized by crepitus on physical examination and has little clinical importance, although it predisposes the affected skin to infection. Subcutaneous emphysema resolves once the positive pressure sustaining the air leak is removed.

3. **Systemic air embolism** is a rare but serious air leak that usually is fatal [16]. Air may enter the vasculature either by disruption of the pulmonary venous system or inadvertent injection through an intravascular catheter [5,16].

References

1. Ackerman, N. B. *Crit. Care Med.* 12: 512, 1984.
2. Anderson, K. D. *J. Pediatr. Surg.* 11: 687, 1976.
3. Bashour, B. N. *Pediatrics* 59: 1048, 1977.
4. Brooks, J. G. *J. Pediatr.* 91: 648, 1977.
5. Brown, Z. A. *Am. J. Dis. Child.* 131: 984, 1977.
6. Cohen, M. D. *Pediatrics* 69: 587, 1982.
7. Emery, R. W. *Ann. Thorac. Surg.* 37: 128, 1984.
8. Greenough, A. *Lancet* 1: 1, 1984.
9. Heicher, D. A. *J. Pediatr.* 98: 957, 1981.
10. Hill, A. *Pediatrics* 69: 144, 1982.
11. Krasna, I. H. *J. Pediatr. Surg.* 22: 784, 1987.
12. Lawson, E. E. *J. Pediatr. Surg.* 15: 181, 1980.
13. Lewis, S. *Arch. Dis. Child.* 63: 313, 1988.
14. Mathew, O. P. *J. Pediatr.* 103: 117, 1983.
15. Moore, J. T. *Am. J. Surg.* 154: 688, 1987.
16. Oppermann, H. C. *Pediatr. Radiol.* 8: 139, 1979.
17. Paxson, C. L. *J. Pediatr.* 91: 459, 1977.
18. Schneider, J. R. *J. Thorac. Cardiovasc. Surg.* 89: 332, 1985.
19. Swingle, H. M. *Pediatrics* 74: 354, 1984.

Apnea

Ann R. Stark

I. Background

A. Definition. An **apneic spell** can be defined as cessation of respiration accompanied by bradycardia (heart rate < 100 beats per minute) or cyanosis. Bradycardia and cyanosis are usually present after 20 seconds of apnea, although they may occur more rapidly in the small premature infant. After 30 to 45 seconds, pallor and hypotonia are seen, and infants may be unresponsive to tactile stimulation.

B. Incidence. Apneic spells occur frequently in premature infants. The incidence of apnea increases with decreasing gestational age. As many as 25 percent of all premature infants who weigh less than 1800 gm (about 34 weeks' gestational age) will have at least one apneic episode, while the majority of very small premature infants (under 30 weeks' gestational age) will have occasional apneic spells. These spells generally begin at 1 or 2 days of age; if they do not occur during the first 7 days, they are unlikely to occur later. Apneic spells persist for variable periods postnatally and generally cease by 37 weeks' postconceptional age [8]. Apneic spells occurring in infants at or near term are always abnormal and are nearly always associated with serious, identifiable causes, including birth asphyxia, intracranial hemorrhage, seizures, or depression from medication. Failure to breathe at birth in the absence of drug depression or asphyxia is generally caused by irreversible structural abnormalities of the central nervous system [3].

II. Pathogenesis. A number of mechanisms have been proposed to explain apnea in premature infants. Many clinical conditions also have been associated with apneic spells, and some may be causative. A full discussion of these conditions is found in ref. 13.

A. Developmental immaturity is a likely contributing factor, since apneic spells occur more frequently in immature infants.

1. The occurrence of apnea may correlate with **brainstem neural function.** The frequency of apnea decreases over a period in which brainstem conduction time of the auditory-evoked response shortens as postconceptional age increases [9].

2. Regularly occurring **oscillatory cycles** of waxing and waning ventilation occur in sleeping preterm infants. Apneic episodes are associated with the minimum phases of these cycles, which may be expressions of the instability of the respiratory control system [21].
3. Breathing in infants is strongly influenced by **sleep state.** Active or rapid-eye-movement (REM) sleep is marked by irregularity of tidal volume and respiratory frequency. REM sleep predominates in preterm infants, and apneic spells occur more frequently in this state than in quiet sleep.

B. Chemoreceptor response

1. In preterm infants, **hypoxia** results in transient hyperventilation, followed by hypoventilation and sometimes apnea, in contrast to the response in adults [16]. In addition, hypoxia makes the premature infant less responsive to increased levels of carbon dioxide [17]. Thus hypoxemia may be involved in the pathogenesis of some but not all [10] apneic spells. Clinical conditions in which both hypoxemia and apnea may occur include pneumonia, RDS (especially during weaning from ventilatory assistance), symptomatic patent ductus arteriosus, anemia, and hypovolemia.
2. The ventilatory response to increased **carbon dioxide** is decreased in preterm infants with apnea compared with a matched group without apnea [6], suggesting that abnormal respiratory control likely contributes to the pathogenesis of apnea.

C. Reflexes. Active reflexes invoked by stimulation of the posterior pharynx, lung inflation, fluid in the larynx, or chest-wall distortion can precipitate apnea in infants. These reflexes may be involved in the apnea sometimes associated, for example, with vigorous use of suction catheters in the pharynx or with the presence of fluid in the upper airway during feeding.

D. Respiratory muscles. Ineffective ventilation may result from impaired coordination of the inspiratory muscles (diaphragm and intercostal muscles) and the muscles of the upper airway (larynx and pharynx).

1. Although many infants have **central apnea,** in which inspiratory efforts and airflow cease simultaneously, a frequently observed type of apnea is **mixed apnea,** in which a central pause is either preceded or followed by airway obstruction [20]. Purely **obstructive apnea,** defined as absent airflow in the presence of inspiratory efforts, occurs less frequently. The site of this obstruction is probably in the upper pharynx.
2. Passive neck flexion, pressure on the lower rim of a face mask, and submental pressure (all encountered during nursery procedures) can obstruct the airway in infants and may lead to apnea, especially in a small premature infant. Spontaneously occurring airway obstruction is seen more frequently when preterm infants assume a position of neck flexion.

III. Monitoring and evaluation. All infants of less than 34 weeks' gestational age should be monitored for apneic spells for at least the first week of life because of the substantial risk of apneic spells in this group. Since impedance apnea monitors may not distinguish respiratory efforts during airway obstruction from normal breaths, heart rate should be monitored in addition to or instead of respiration. Even with careful monitoring, some prolonged spells of apnea and bradycardia may not be recognized [18].

A. When a monitor alarm sounds, one should remember to respond to the infant, not the monitor, checking for bradycardia, cyanosis, and airway obstruction.

B. Most apneic spells in premature infants respond to tactile stimulation. Infants who fail to respond to stimulation should be ventilated during the spell with bag and mask, generally with an FIO_2 of under 0.40 or equal to the FIO_2 prior to the spell to avoid marked elevations in arterial PO_2.

C. After the first apneic spell, the infant should be evaluated for a possible underlying cause (Table 13-9); if a cause is identified, specific treatment can then be initiated. One should be particularly alert to the possibility of a precipitating cause in infants who are more than 34 weeks' gestational age. Evaluation should include a history and physical examination, arterial blood gas

Table 13-9. Evaluation of an infant with apnea

Potential cause	Associated history or signs	Evaluation
Infection	Feeding intolerance, lethargy, temperature instability	Complete blood count, cultures if appropriate
Impaired oxygenation	Cyanosis, tachypnea, respiratory distress	Continuous oxygen monitoring, arterial blood gas measurement, chest x-ray examination
Metabolic disorders	Jitteriness, poor feeding, lethargy, CNS depression, irritability	Glucose, calcium, electrolytes
Drugs	CNS depression, hypotonia, maternal history	Magnesium, screen for toxic substances in urine
Temperature instability	Lethargy	Monitor temperature of patient and environment
Intracranial pathology	Abnormal neurologic examination, seizures	Cranial ultrasound examination
Gastroesophageal reflux	Difficulty with feeds	Specific observation, barium swallow

measurement with continuous transcutaneous oxygen monitoring, complete blood count, and measurement of blood sugar, calcium, and electrolyte levels.

IV. Treatment. When spells of apnea are repeated and prolonged (i.e., more than two to three times per hour) or when they require frequent bag and mask ventilation, treatment should be initiated in order of increasing invasiveness and risk.

A. Specific therapy should be directed at an underlying cause, if one is identified. If intermittent hypoxemia is identified by transcutaneous oxygen monitoring, supplemental oxygen is provided to maintain transcutaneous oxygen tension in the range of 60 to 80 mmHg or oxygen saturation about 90 percent.

B. Care should be taken to avoid reflexes that may trigger apnea. Suctioning of the pharynx should be done carefully, and oral feedings should be avoided. In addition, positions of extreme flexion or extension of the neck should be avoided to reduce the likelihood of airway obstruction.

C. Decreasing the environmental temperature to the low end of the neutral thermal environment range may lessen the number of spells. The placement of a heat shield around a small premature infant may decrease swings in temperature and may prevent apnea.

D. Oscillating water beds have no effect on reducing residual apnea in infants receiving theophylline and are probably of limited value.

E. Despite the absence of significant anemia, blood transfusion to elevate the hematocrit slightly (e.g., to above 40 percent) also seems to reduce the frequency of apneic spells in some infants [5] although this is controversial [12].

F. Nasal CPAP at low pressures (3 to 4 cm H_2O) has been shown to reduce mixed and obstructive apneic spells [14]. The additional airway care required and the difficulty with feeding often associated with use of nasal CPAP limit its usefulness.

G. Drug therapy with methylxanthines can markedly reduce the number of apneic spells.

1. Oral **theophylline** or intravenous **aminophylline** is given in a dose of 1.5 to 2.0 mg/kg q6h. A postdose serum level obtained after the fourth dose (0.5 to 1 hour after an intravenous dose, 1 to 2 hours after an oral dose)

will be approximately 50 percent of the steady-state blood concentration. The steady-state level should be measured on the fourth day [1]. If apneic spells are severe and more rapid onset of action is desired, a loading dose of 5 to 7 mg/kg aminophylline or theophylline will rapidly achieve the steady-state concentration. The loading dose is followed by the same maintenance dose as above.

a. There is no agreement on the appropriate serum level of theophylline, since efficacy for therapy of apnea does not necessarily correlate with the level achieved. We generally maintain levels at 7 to 12 μg/ml, although lower levels (3 to 4 μg/ml) achieved with lower doses of theophylline (2 mg/kg per day) may be effective [15].

b. Dose adjustments are made if therapeutic effect is not achieved or toxicity is observed.

(1) If the level is too low, an additional dose of 1 mg/kg of aminophylline is given to raise the serum level by 1 to 2 μg/ml; the maintenance dose is increased by 10 to 25 percent, and the level is rechecked.

(2) If level is too high, the next dose is withheld and the maintenance dose is decreased by 10 to 25 percent.

c. Theophylline is generally discontinued at 35 to 37 weeks' postconceptional age if no apneic spells have occurred for 1 week.

d. Mechanisms by which theophylline may decrease apnea include (1) respiratory center stimulation, (2) antagonism of adenosine, a neurotransmitter that can cause respiratory depression, and (3) improvement of diaphragmatic contractility.

e. **Toxicity of theophylline** is related to serum level. Clinical manifestations of toxicity usually begin with tachycardia, followed by jitteriness and irritability and signs of gastrointestinal dysfunction, including abdominal distension, feeding intolerance, or vomiting. Seizures may occur at extremely high drug levels. Metabolic changes, including increased glucose and insulin levels, occur following a theophylline loading dose in some infants [19]. Because some theophylline may be converted to caffeine in premature infants, the level of theophylline alone may not reflect the total xanthine load [2]. Despite theoretical risks related to decreased cerebral blood flow, retarded neuronal growth, and inhibition of constriction of the ductus arteriosus, no long-term sequelae have been demonstrated in infants following xanthine treatment.

2. **Caffeine citrate** also can be used to decrease the frequency of apneic spells. A suggested dosage schedule involves a loading dose of 20 mg/kg caffeine citrate (10 mg caffeine base) orally or intravenously, followed by maintenance doses of 2.5 to 5 mg/kg daily (caffeine base) in 1 dose beginning 24 hours after the loading dose.

a. Caffeine serum levels are maintained at 5 to 20 μg/ml, and should be monitored every 3 to 4 days.

b. Caffeine may be less toxic than theophylline, since side effects are not generally seen until blood levels are much higher than therapeutic levels. There may be no change in heart rate in infants treated with caffeine, in contrast to the tachycardia often associated with theophylline therapy.

3. If theophylline therapy fails to reduce the frequency of apneic spells, a trial of the respiratory stimulant **doxapram** may be considered [7]. Doxapram is administered only as a continuous infusion, initially at a rate of 1.0 to 1.5 mg/kg per hour. Once control is obtained, the infusion is decreased. Although increased doses up to 2.5 mg/kg per hour may be effective in infants who continue to have apnea at lower doses, the risk of toxicity is considerably increased. Toxicity includes hyperactivity, jitteriness, seizures, hyperglycemia, mild liver dysfunction, and hypertension.

Although these abnormalities resolve following discontinuation of the drug, toxicity and the need for continuous parenteral administration limit its widespread use.

H. If all the previously mentioned interventions fail, **mechanical ventilation** may be required.

V. Persistent apnea. In occasional infants, apneic spells may persist at 37 to 40 weeks' postconceptional age, when the infant may be otherwise ready for discharge home from the nursery. There is at this time no consensus on the appropriate management of these infants, but efforts are directed at reducing the risk of apneic spells so that the child can be cared for at home. A discussion of sudden infant death syndrome (SIDS) is found in ref. 11.

A. Recordings of impedance pneumography and ECGs for 12 to 24 hours ("pneumograms") can be used to document the occurrence of apnea and bradycardia during that time period, but they do not predict the risk of SIDS [18].

B. The infant should be reevaluated to detect an etiology for the apnea. Attention should be paid to possible neurologic problems and to feeding problems such as reflux. Possible anatomic causes of airway obstruction should be investigated.

C. Continued use of theophylline may be helpful in infants whose spells recur when the drug is discontinued. Attempts to withdraw the drug can be made at approximately 2-month intervals while the child is closely monitored.

D. Some infants are cared for with cardiorespiratory monitoring at home, although little data are available on its effectiveness [4].

E. Extensive psychosocial support must be provided for the family, who should be skilled in CPR and in the use of a monitor, if one is provided.

References

1. Aranda, J. V., et al. *N. Engl. J. Med.* 295: 413, 1976.
2. Bory, C. B. *J. Pediatr.* 94: 988, 1979.
3. Brazy, J. E., et al. *J. Pediatr.* 111: 163, 1987.
4. Consensus statement: National Institutes of Health Consensus Development Conference on Infantile Apnea and Home Monitoring, Sept. 29 to Oct. 1, 1986. *Pediatrics* 79: 292, 1987.
5. DeMaio, J. G. *J. Pediatr.* 114: 1039, 1989.
6. Gerhardt, T., et al. *Pediatrics* 74: 58, 1984.
7. Hayakawa, F. *J. Pediatr.* 109: 138, 1986.
8. Henderson-Smart, D. J. *Aust. Paediatr. J.* 17: 273, 1981.
9. Henderson-Smart, D. J., et al. *N. Engl. J. Med.* 308: 353, 1983.
10. Hiatt, I. M. *J. Pediatr.* 98: 288, 1981.
11. Hunt, C. E. *J. Pediatr.* 110: 669, 1987.
12. Keyes, W. G. *Pediatrics* 84: 412, 1989.
13. Martin, R. J. et al. *J. Pediatr.* 109: 733, 1986.
14. Miller, M. J., et al. *J. Pediatr.* 106: 91, 1985.
15. Muttitt, S. C., et al. *J. Pediatr.* 112: 115, 1988.
16. Rigatto, H., et al. *Pediatrics* 55: 604, 1975.
17. Rigatto, H., et al. *J. Appl. Physiol.* 39: 896, 1975.
18. Southall, D. P., et al. *Pediatrics* 70: 844, 1982.
19. Srinivasan, G., et al. *J. Pediatr.* 98: 815, 1981.
20. Thach, B. T., et al. *J. Pediatr.* 94: 275, 1979.
21. Waggener, T. B., et al. *J. Appl. Physiol.* 57: 536, 1984.

Persistent Pulmonary Hypertension of the Newborn

Linda J. Van Marter

I. **Definition. Persistent pulmonary hypertension of the newborn (PPHN),** also called **persistent fetal circulation (PFC),** is caused by a sustained elevation in **pulmonary vascular resistance (PVR)** after birth, preventing the transition to the normal extrauterine circulatory pattern. The disorder is most common in full-term or postterm infants. In 1985, 1 to 2 cases per 1000 live births occurred at Brigham and Women's Hospital. Until recently, PPHN has been associated with a mortality rate approaching 50 percent [11] and morbidities in survivors that include chronic pulmonary disease [22], neurodevelopmental disabilities [28,52], and intracranial hemorrhage or infarction [30].

The normal transitional circulation is characterized by a rapid fall in PVR with the first breath and a rapid rise in **systemic vascular resistance (SVR)** with the clamping of umbilical arterial flow to the placenta. These hemodynamic changes cause functional closure of the foramen ovale. The associated rise in arterial oxygen content results in constriction of the ductus arteriosus. These changes bring about the separation of the pulmonary and systemic circulations from parallel to series circuits. When PVR exceeds SVR, as a result of abnormal neonatal transition or other causes, right-to-left shunting occurs through the foramen ovale or ductus arteriosus, often resulting in severe hypoxemia. The sustained elevation in PVR may be idiopathic or secondary to identifiable pathophysiologic events.

II. **Epidemiologic associations.** The determinants of PPHN are not completely understood. Antenatal risk factors associated with PPHN include meconium-stained amniotic fluid and maternal conditions such as fever, anemia, and pulmonary disease [46]. Neonatal conditions linked with PPHN include the following:

A. **Intrauterine or perinatal asphyxia** is the diagnosis most commonly associated with PPHN. Prolonged fetal stress may result in remodeling and abnormal muscularization of the smallest pulmonary arteries [26,41]. Furthermore, acute asphyxia at birth may induce persistent pulmonary vasospasm [1,48]. Chronic hypoxemia may be associated with intrauterine growth retardation and more complex neonatal pathophysiology [55].

B. **Pulmonary parenchymal disease,** including RDS, pneumonia, and aspiration syndromes, especially meconium aspiration, may cause hypoxic pulmonary vasospasm or may be associated with anatomic pulmonary vascular abnormalities characteristic of PPHN [15,42]. The pulmonary vascular response to hypoxemia, asphyxia, or sepsis appears to be more prominent in more mature infants.

C. **Abnormalities of pulmonary development,** including vascular malalignment [9] and parenchymal hypoplasia, may be associated with PPHN.

D. **Myocardial dysfunction** has been associated with perinatal asphyxia, myocarditis, metabolic problems (such as hypoglycemia and hypocalcemia), and hyperviscosity. Intrauterine closure of the ductus arteriosus may result in increased PVR and right ventricular failure.

E. **Congenital heart disease,** both left- and right-sided, may be associated with right-to-left shunting with or without elevated pulmonary vascular resistance.

F. **Pneumonia and/or sepsis** of viral or bacterial origin may precede PPHN. The underlying mechanism may be endotoxin-mediated myocardial depression or pulmonary vasospasm associated with high levels of thromboxanes [3,19,54] and leukotrienes. In addition to more common etiologic agents, unusual organisms, including *Ureaplasma* [65] and echovirus 11 [61], have been linked with pulmonary hypertension.

III. **Pathology and pathophysiology**

A. **Pulmonary vascular remodeling** has been seen in autopsy studies of infants who died with idiopathic PPHN and in some cases of PPHN associated with meconium aspiration [26,40,41]. Abnormal muscularization of the normally nonmuscular intraacinar arteries, with increased medial thickness of the larger muscular arteries, results in a decreased cross-sectional area of the pulmonary vascular bed and elevated PVR. The cause of the vascular abnormalities usually is not known but may be mediated by chronic intrauterine hypoxemia [17,20,27]. Vascular changes also may occur following fetal exposure to nonsteroidal anti-inflammatory agents (prostaglandin synthetase inhibitors), which presumably cause constriction of the fetal ductus arteriosus and secondary pulmonary hypertension due to accumulation of vasoconstricting metabolites. Finally, humoral growth factors released by hypoxia-damaged endothelial cells may promote vasoconstriction and muscular overgrowth [25,34]. Whether the abnormal muscle in these cases causes irreversible vascular obstruction or increases the vasoreactivity is not known.

B. **Pulmonary hypoplasia** usually affects both alveolar and pulmonary arterial development. It may be seen as an isolated anomaly or in cases of congenital diaphragmatic hernia (see Chap. 27), oligohydramnios syndrome, severe renal anomalies, or abnormalities associated with decreased fetal breathing.

C. **Pulmonary vasospasm** is suspected in those infants with reversible PPHN. In addition to the underlying disease process, both the stage of the disease and the maturity of the host [21] seem to play a role in determining the mediators and response. The most potent pulmonary vasoconstricting influence is hypoxemia, a response exaggerated by acidemia. Neural and humoral vasoactive substances may contribute to the pathogenesis of PPHN, the response to hypoxemia, or both. These include factors associated with platelet activation, and the arachadonic acid metabolites. Thromboxanes (A_2 and its metabolite, B_2) [19,23] and leukotrienes (C_4 and D_4) [50,60] have been of interest, especially as mediators of increased PVR seen with sepsis and hypoxemia, respectively.

D. **Myocardial dysfunction with elevated PVR**

1. **Right ventricular (RV) dysfunction** may be caused by intrauterine closure of the ductus arteriosus, which results in altered fetal hemodynamics, postnatal pulmonary hypertension, RV failure, and a right-to-left shunt at the atrial level. RV failure resulting in altered diastolic compliance can cause right-to-left atrial shunting even in the absence of elevated PVR.
2. **Left ventricular (LV) dysfunction** causes pulmonary venous hypertension and reflex pulmonary arterial hypertension, often to suprasystemic levels. Right-to-left shunting by means of the ductus arteriosus may subsequently occur. This problem must be differentiated from the other causes of PPHN, since the treatment must be aimed at improving the LV function rather than at lowering elevated PVR.

E. **Mechanical factors** that can influence PVR include cardiac output and blood viscosity. Low cardiac output recruits fewer arteriolar channels and may raise PVR by this mechanism as well as its primary effect of lowering mixed venous oxygen content. Hyperviscosity, often associated with polycythemia, may lead to sludging in the pulmonary microvasculature. Pulmonary microthrombi have been seen at autopsy in some cases of intractable PPHN with [35] and without [2] thrombocytopenia.

IV. **Diagnosis.** PPHN must be suspected in any profoundly cyanotic newborn.

A. **Differential diagnoses** that are most common include uncomplicated pulmonary disease, sepsis, and congenital heart disease.

B. **The physical examination** is generally less remarkable for PPHN than for signs of the associated diagnoses. The precordial impulse may be quite prominent. The second heart sound is usually single or narrowly split and accentuated. In cases of perinatal asphyxia, a systolic murmur consistent with tricuspid regurgitation may be heard at the right or left lower sternal border.

C. A difference between simultaneous **pre- and postductal arterial blood gases (ABGs)** or transcutaneous oxygen monitors can be used to document a ductal right-to-left shunt. A gradient in **oxygen saturation** of at least 10 percent in the absence of structural heart disease indicates PPHN. If cutaneous monitors are used, the preductal electrode should be placed in the right upper quadrant of the infant's chest. Absence of a significant ductal shunt does not exclude pulmonary hypertension associated with isolated right-to-left atrial shunting.

D. Peckham and Fox [45] advocated as a provocative test of pulmonary hypertension the use of a **hyperventilation test** using 100% oxygen with manual or mechanical ventilation to achieve $PaCO_2$ in the 25 to 30 mmHg range. Infants with PPHN should respond by decreasing PVR and improved oxygenation. Because of the risk of barotrauma and pulmonary air leak, we advise caution in performing this test.

E. The **chest x-ray** is usually normal or shows associated pulmonary parenchymal disease or air leak. The cardiothymic silhouette is normal or borderline enlarged; pulmonary blood flow is normal or may appear reduced.

F. The **ECG** may show right ventricular predominance and be normal for age, or it may show signs of myocardial ischemia or infarction. It may be helpful in suggesting structural heart disease.

G. A **two-dimensional (2D) echocardiographic study** should be performed in all cases of unexplained cyanosis in order to exclude structural heart defects. Observation of bubbles produced by saline injection or color Doppler examination can confirm the presence of intracardiac shunting. Determination of right and left ventricular systolic time intervals allows estimation of ventricular function and the relative resistances of the pulmonary and systemic circuits, but this method has largely been replaced by Doppler studies. Additional echocardiographic markers of pulmonary hypertension can sometimes be identified [68].

H. **Cardiac catheterization** is virtually never needed now that 2D and Doppler echocardiography are available. If cardiac catheterization is performed, it should be performed in a catheterization laboratory or similar facility under fluoroscopic guidance.

I. **Diagnostic pitfalls** are not uncommon in the evaluation of patients with PPHN. The following diagnoses must be carefully considered:
   1. **Structural cardiovascular abnormalities** that may be associated with right-to-left ductal or atrial shunting are [38]
      a. **Obstruction to pulmonary venous return**—infradiaphragmatic total anomalous pulmonary venous return, hypoplastic left heart, cor triatriatum, congenital mitral stenosis
      b. **Myopathic LV disease**—endocardial fibroelastosis, Pompe's disease
      c. **Obstructions to LV outflow**—critical aortic stenosis, supravalvar aortic stenosis, interrupted aortic arch, coarctation of the aorta
      d. **Obligatory left-to-right shunts**—endocardial cushion defect, arteriovenous malformation, hemitruncus, coronary A–V fistula
      e. **Miscellaneous disorders**—Ebstein's anomaly, transposition of the great arteries.
   2. Left or right **ventricular dysfunction** may be associated with right-to-left shunting. **LV dysfunction,** due to ischemia or obstruction caused by myopathic LV disease or obstruction to LV outflow, may present with a right-to-left ductal shunt. **RV dysfunction** may be associated with right-to-left atrial shunting as a result of decreased diastolic compliance and elevated end-diastolic pressure. These diagnoses must be differentiated from PPHN caused by pulmonary vascular abnormalities.

J. **Signs favoring primary cardiac disease** over PPHN include cardiomegaly, weak pulses, pulse differential between upper and lower extremities, pulmonary edema, grade 3+ murmur and persistent PaO_2 at or less than 40 mmHg.

V. **Management. The cyanotic newborn must be considered a medical emergency.** Immediate, appropriate intervention is critical in reversing the rapid downhill spiral often seen with PPHN. Correction of hypoxemia and acidosis is especially important. Key principles for management include (1) rapid response to clinical decompensation and (2) conservative weaning of therapeutic measures that have proved effective; weaning should be done in small steps and only after a substantial period of stability (12 to 48 hours).

A. 100% oxygen should be administered by hood to any near- or full-term cyanotic newborn. Since hypoxemia is one of the most powerful stimuli to pulmonary vasoconstriction, oxygen therapy may greatly reduce elevated PVR. The generous use of oxygen is warranted in term infants who are at very low risk for retinopathy of prematurity in contrast to preterm infants, in whom oxygen must be more cautiously administered. After 10 minutes, the effects of oxygen therapy should be evaluated with a postductal ABG. If the postductal PaO_2 or transcutaneous oxygen monitor is less than 100 mmHg in 100% oxygen, simultaneous pre- and postductal ABGs should be obtained to assess transductal shunting. Transcutaneous monitoring is useful to follow rapid changes in oxygenation. Placement of two electrodes, one on the upper right thorax, and the other on the abdomen, can be used to monitor the effect of therapy on the gradient caused by a transductal shunt.

B. Intubation and mechanical ventilation should be instituted when hypoxemia is persistent despite maximal hood oxygen or when PaO_2 is borderline after prolonged supplementation with 100% oxygen. Contrasting approaches to mechanical ventilation have been used (see **VI**). Our practice is to maintain mild hyperoxia and moderate hyperventilation by attempting to keep the PaO_2 greater than 100 mmHg and the $PaCO_2$ equal to 25 to 35 mmHg and to take pathophysiologic mechanisms into account.

1. In the absence of alveolar disease, elevated intrapulmonary pressure associated with mechanical ventilation may impede cardiac output and raise PVR. We therefore use a strategy of rapid, low-pressure, short-inspiratory-time mechanical ventilation designed to minimize mean airway pressure. Typical ventilator settings are rate, 60 to 120 breaths per minute; PIP, 20 to 30 cm H_2O; PEEP, 2 to 3 cm H_2O; and inspiratory duration, 0.2 to 0.4 per second. High gas flow (20 to 30 liters per minute) may be required, and large-diameter ventilator tubing is used to maintain PEEP at low levels in the presence of high flow rates.
2. When PPHN complicates pulmonary disease such as RDS, pneumonia, or aspiration syndromes, mechanical ventilation must be modified accordingly. Slower rates, longer inspiratory times, and the use of PEEP may be required to adequately ventilate and oxygenate the baby who has parenchymal lung disease.
3. Because infants with PPHN are often large infants that vigorously resist mechanical ventilation, and because catecholamine release stimulates pulmonary alpha-adrenergic receptors, thereby raising PVR, we sometimes use **neuromuscular blockade with pancuronium** (0.1 mg/kg) and medication with **narcotic analgesics** to achieve muscle relaxation and sedation during positive-pressure ventilation. As an alternate to morphine, we frequently use fentanyl (Sublimaze) (3 to 5 μg/kg per hour), a potent, short-acting narcotic that reduces the extreme variability in oxygenation due to vasospasm by blunting sympathetic output from the central nervous system. Chest-wall rigidity that may inhibit ventilation, an occasional complication of fentanyl, is prevented by the simultaneous use of pancuronium [39].

C. After adequate oxygenation, **correction of acidosis** is the most important aspect of the treatment of PPHN. Alkalosis can be achieved by hyperventilation, metabolic therapy with sodium bicarbonate, or both and may result in a marked reduction in PVR. The pH should be maintained in the range of 7.45 to 7.60.

D. Maintenance of good cardiac output is necessary to maximize mixed venous oxygen concentration. Cardiotonic agents may be necessary to achieve adequate cardiac output in some infants with PPHN.

E. Other metabolic abnormalities can contribute to right-to-left shunting on the basis of poor cardiac output. Maintenance of a **neutral thermal environment** reduces the infant's energy demands. Correction of **hypoglycemia** and **hypo-**

calcemia [5] are important to provide adequate substrates for myocardial function.

F. **Polycythemia,** associated with hyperviscosity, mechanically increases PVR and may lead to release of vasoactive substances by platelet activation. On the other hand, a sufficient red blood cell mass is necessary for adequate oxygen-carrying capacity. Therefore, partial exchange transfusion is recommended to reduce the hematocrit to 45 to 55 percent in the infant with PPHN whose central hematocrit exceeds 70 percent.

G. **Intravascular volume** support with colloids such as albumin (5%), fresh-frozen plasma, or packed red blood cells may be necessary in the infant with pathophysiologic conditions associated with intravascular volume depletion (i.e., hemorrhage, hydrops, capillary leak) or decreased SVR (i.e., septic shock) or in whom SVR has been lowered by pharmacologic agents (i.e., sedative narcotics).

H. **Pharmacologic therapy** is directed at the simultaneous goals of optimizing cardiac output, enhancing systemic blood pressure, and reducing PVR. Since no selective pulmonary vasodilator has been identified, the relative effects of the available agents on the different subdivisions of the cardiovascular system must be considered in choosing the most appropriate agent (Table 13-10). Pharmacologic intervention should be reserved for those infants in whom hyperoxia and alkalosis have been attempted and for whom continuous monitoring of oxygenation and systemic arterial pressure is possible. Consideration of associated and differential diagnoses and the known or hypothetical pathogenesis of the right-to-left shunt may prove helpful in selecting the best agent or combination of agents for a particular infant.

1. **Dopamine (Intropin)** is often used in moderate (4 to 7 μg/kg per minute) to high (7 to 20 μg/kg per minute) doses for support of systemic blood pressure and improved cardiac output by means of alpha- and beta-adrenergic receptor stimulation. Dopamine in low dose (1 to 3 μg/kg per minute) also has a salutary effect of increasing renal blood flow. **Dobutamine,** a synthetic catecholamine with a structure similar to isoproterenol, has an inotropic more than a chronotropic effect on the heart through beta-1-adrenergic stimulation. Both drugs have potentially adverse effects on the PVR, especially at higher infusion rates (greater than 10 μg/kg per minute). If possible, we avoid high infusion rates of dopamine and dobutamine in newborns with PPHN.

2. **Isoproterenol (Isuprel)** is a beta-adrenergic agonist that relaxes the pulmonary circulation by means of vascular beta-receptor stimulation. SVR is also decreased but may be compensated by improved cardiac output through augmented inotropy and chronotropy. This agent may be useful in some cases of suspected or proven myocardial dysfunction in which dobutamine is insufficient and tachycardia is not present. Studies in animal models suggest that the hypoxic pulmonary circulation may be especially sensitive to beta-adrenergic stimulation [37]. A trial of isoproterenol should be initiated in very low doses (0.02 to 0.03 μg/kg per minute), and the infusion rate should be doubled every 10 minutes until oxygenation improves or maximal heart rate (180 to 185 beats per minute) is achieved. Moderate-dose dopamine is often useful, in conjunction with isoproterenol, to provide SVR support. The usefulness of isoproterenol is limited by its marked chronotropic effect, and it should not be used in an infant whose baseline heart rate exceeds 170 beats per minute.

3. **Tolazoline (Priscoline),** a drug described as an alpha-adrenergic antagonist, histaminic agonist, and direct vasodilator, has been used to treat PPHN with mixed results. In some cases, tolazoline has been credited with dramatic improvements in oxygenation, while other series [10] report a 50:50 response rate with a subgroup of patients who develop clinical deterioration. In order to avoid toxic levels and acute systemic hypotension, we recommend a conservative dose of tolazoline [66]. Tolazoline infusion is started at a dose of 1 to 2 mg/kg over 30 minutes. If a favorable

Table 13-10. Pharmacologic agents used in cardiovascular treatment of PPHN

	Receptor activator			Physiologic effects					
	Dopaminergic	Alpha-adrenergic	Beta-adrenergic	Cardiac output	PVR	SVR	SBP	Bronchodilation	Renal and GI perfusion
Dopamine [10,13,29,43,53]									
1 to 3 μg/kg/minute	+ + +	+	NE/+	NE/↑	NE	↑/↓	NE	NE	↑
4+ μg/kg/minute	+ + +	+ +/ + + +	+ +	↑/↑ ↑	NE/↑	↑ ↑	↑/↑ ↑	NE	NE/↑/↓
Dobutamine [58]	NE	+	+ +*	↑ ↑	NE/↓	NE/↓	↑	NE	NE
Isoproterenol [37]	NE	NE	+ + +	↑ ↑	↓ ↓	↓/↓ ↓	NE/↓ ↓	↑ ↑†	NE/↑
Tolazoline‡ [6,11,37,63]	NE	− −‡	NE	NE	↓ ↓	↓ ↓	↓/↓ ↓	NE	↓

*B_1 primarily.
†Effect may be diminished in the neonate.
‡Histamine-like and direct vasodilator properties, in addition to alpha-adrenergic antagonism.
Key: NE = no effect; PVR = pulmonary vascular resistance; SVR = systemic vascular resistance; SBP = systolic blood pressure.

response is achieved, a tolazoline infusion is maintained at 0.16 mg/kg per hour for each 1 mg/kg loading dose. Tolazoline is excreted by the kidney. Therefore, if urine flow is less than one ml/kg per hour, the infusion rate should be halved to 0.08 mg/kg per hour for each 1 mg/kg loading dose [66].

a. Therapeutic response to tolazoline is marked by a cutaneous flush, followed by an increased PaO_2. A fall in systemic arterial pressure may accompany the flush. Blood, plasma, or other colloid should be available for rapid infusion when necessary to prevent shock. Alternately, dopamine may be useful in supporting systemic blood pressure when tolazoline is used.

b. A successful response to tolazoline usually results in a rapid improvement in oxygenation, allowing reduction in the FIO_2. Lung compliance also may improve, and ventilator pressures may be cautiously lowered. When the PaO_2 can be maintained at 70 mmHg or higher with an FIO_2 of 0.50, tolazoline may be discontinued. We recommend gradual weaning, reducing the dose of tolazoline by halving the infusion rate at 15-minute intervals.

4. **Prostaglandins E_1 (PGE_1), I_2 (PGI_2), and D_2 (PGD_2)** have been used in a few therapeutic trials in PPHN. Known to possess potent vasodilator properties, PGE_1 has **not** been shown to be beneficial in human studies of PPHN [42]. Similarly, a trial of PGD_2 in newborn infants with PPHN met with mixed results [57]. PGI_2 (prostacyclin), one of the most potent vasodilators known, has had variable results in clinical trials. It is not now available for use.

H. **Use of other vasoactive pharmacologic agents,** including leukotriene inhibitors, amrinone, and calcium-channel blockers, in treatment of infants with PPHN requires further study.

VI. **Controversies in therapy** of PPHN focus on both old and new treatment strategies.

A. **Mechanical ventilation.** Hyperventilation and hyperoxia have been considered conventional therapy for PPHN since improvement in oxygenation, decline in PVR, or both often follow achievement of respiratory alkalosis [10,45]. More recently, the $pH/PaCO_2$-related decrease in PVR has been linked with alkalosis rather than hypocarbia [49]. In an uncontrolled study, Wung reported 100 percent survival in a group of infants with PPHN who were not hyperventilated [67]. His approach is to accomplish alkalosis with bicarbonate infusion and minimize barotrauma by permitting normocarbia or hypercarbia. Subsequent investigators have reported successful treatment of infants with PPHN without hyperventilation [12]. Still others report equal or better success using high-frequency oscillatory [31] or jet ventilation for PPHN [8,59].

Weighing the relative risks of barotrauma, oxygen toxicity, and sodium overload ($NaHCO_3$), our practice incorporates moderate conventional hyperventilation and augmentation of the respiratory alkalosis with metabolic support using sodium bicarbonate. As soon as some stability is achieved, usually at 36 to 72 hours, we accept lower levels of oxygenation and higher levels of carbon dioxide to avoid barotrauma.

B. **Extracorporeal membrane oxygenation (ECMO)** has been used as a lifesaving therapy for infants with PPHN who fail conventional management. [6] A larger, randomized trial conducted at our institution showed survival of 28 of 29 ECMO-treated critically ill infants with PPHN. Four of 10 similarly ill infants died with conventional maximal medical therapy [42a]. Improved survival notwithstanding, ECMO should be reserved for the most severely ill newborns with PPHN, since the long-term implications of the use of this technology are not yet known and significant morbidities have been reported, including thromboemboli, aluminum emboli [64], ocular vascular changes [44], and intracranial hemorrhage or other brain injuries [51,62].

C. Exchange transfusion for PPHN associated with sepsis. Exchange transfusion has been advocated in neonatal sepsis to provide antibodies, replete neutrophils, and decrease the endotoxin and humoral toxic burdens. If these factors contribute to pulmonary vasoconstriction, exchange transfusion may help to decrease PVR by diminishing these stimuli. However, no data clearly support exchange transfusion for this purpose, and the theoretical benefits must be weighed against the risks.

References

1. Abman, S. *Am. J. Physiol.* 253: H941, 1987.
2. Arnold, J. *J. Pediatr.* 106: 806, 1985.
3. Barefield, E. *Pediatr. Res.* 25: 237A, 1989.
4. Bartlett, R. *Pediatrics* 76: 479, 1985.
5. Bifano, E. *Pediatr. Res.* 25: 262, 1989.
6. Bloss, R. *J. Pediatr.* 97: 984, 1980.
7. Caplan, M. *Pediatr. Res.* 25: 305A, 1989.
8. Carlo, W. *Am. J. Dis. Child.* 143: 233, 1989.
9. Cater, G. *J. Pediatr.* 114: 293, 1989.
10. Drummond, W. *J. Pediatr.* 98: 603, 1981.
11. Drummond, W. *Clin. Pediatr.* 16: 335, 1977.
12. Dworetz, A. *Pediatrics* 84: 1, 1989.
13. Fiddler, G. *Arch. Dis. Child.* 55: 194, 1980.
14. Fox, W. *J. Pediatr.* 103: 505, 1983.
15. Fox, W. *Pediatrics* 59: 205, 1977.
16. Fuhrman, B. *J. Appl. Physiol.* 60: 114, 1986.
17. Geggel, R. *J. Pediatr.* 108: 756, 1986.
18. Gersony, W. *Circulation* 39: 87, 1969.
19. Gibson, R. *Pediatr. Res.* 23: 553, 1988.
20. Goldberg, S. *Pediatrics* 48: 528, 1971.
21. Gordon, J. *Pediatr. Res.* 23: 580, 1988.
22. Hageman, J. *Am. J. Dis. Child.* 142: 293, 1988.
23. Hammerman, C. *Am. J. Dis. Child.* 142: 319, 1988.
24. Hammerman, C. *J. Pediatr.* 110: 470, 1987.
25. Harker, L. *Pediatr. Res.* 15: 147, 1981.
26. Haworth, S. *J. Pediatr.* 88: 614, 1976.
27. Haworth, S. *Chest* 93: 133S, 1988.
28. Hendricks-Munoz, K. *Pediatrics* 81: 650, 1988.
29. Holloway, E. *Br. Heart J.* 37: 482, 1975.
30. Klesh, K. *Am. J. Dis. Child.* 141: 852, 1987.
31. Kohelet, D. *Crit. Care Med.* 16: 510, 1988.
32. Konduri, G. *Pediatr. Res.* 25: 317A, 1989.
33. Levin, D. *J. Pediatr.* 92: 265, 1978.
34. Levin, D. *Circulation* 60: 360, 1979.
35. Levin, D. *J. Pediatr.* 102: 299, 1983.
36. Lock, J. *J. Pediatr.* 95: 600, 1979.
37. Lock, J. *Am. J. Physiol.* 240: H697, 1981.
38. Long, W. *Clin. Perinatol.* 11: 601, 1984.
39. Marty, J. *Acta Anaesthesiol. Scand.* 25: 293, 1981.
40. Murphy, J. *J. Pediatr.* 104: 758, 1984.
41. Murphy, J. *J. Pediatr.* 98: 962, 1981.
42. Murphy, J. *Pediatr. Res.* 14: 606, 1980.

42a. O'Rourke, P. *Pediatrics* 84: 957, 1989.

43. Padbury, J. *J. Pediatr.* 110: 293, 1986.
44. Patrias, M. *Pediatrics* 82: 560, 1988.
45. Peckham, G. *J. Pediatr.* 93: 1005, 1978.
46. Reece, E. *Obstet. Gynecol.* 70: 696, 1987.
47. Rich, S. *Ann. Internal. Med.* 108: 425, 1988.
48. Rowe, R. *Pediatrics* 59: 573, 1979.

49. Schreiber, M. *Pediatr. Res.* 20: 113, 1986.
50. Schreiber, M. *Pediatr. Res.* 21: 176, 1987.
51. Schumacher, R. *Pediatrics* 82: 155, 1988.
52. Sell, E. *Am. J. Dis. Child.* 139: 25, 1985.
53. Seri, I. *Eur. J. Pediatr.* 142: 3, 1984.
54. Shook, L. *Pediatr. Res.* 25: 326A, 1989.
55. Siassi, B. *Semin. Perinatol.* 12: 80, 1988.
56. Sidi, D. *Pediatr. Res.* 23: 229, 1988.
57. Soifer, S. *J. Pediatr.* 112: 774, 1988.
58. Sonnenblick, E. *N. Engl. J. Med.* 300: 17, 1979.
59. Spitzer, A. *Clin. Perinatol.* 15: 389, 1988.
60. Stenmark, K. *N. Engl. J. Med.* 309: 77, 1983.
61. Toce, S. *Pediatr. Infect. Dis. J.* 7: 360, 1988.
62. Towne, B. *J. Pediatr. Surg.* 20: 410, 1985.
63. Truog, W. *J. Pediatr.* 100: 284, 1982.
64. Vogler, C. *N. Engl. J. Med.* 319: 75, 1988.
65. Waites, K. *Pediatrics* 83: 79, 1989.
66. Ward, R. *Pediatrics* 77: 307, 1986.
67. Wung, J. *Pediatrics* 76: 488, 1985.
68. Zellers, T. *J. Pediatr.* 114: 735, 1989.

Transient Tachypnea of the Newborn

Ann R. Stark and John M. North

I. **Definition.** Transient tachypnea of the newborn (TTN) is a mild, self-limited respiratory disorder characterized by an increased respiratory rate, usually without retractions, and mild cyanosis, usually with an F_{IO_2} requirement of less than 0.40 [1]. TTN is thought to be related to delayed resorption of fetal lung fluid, but TTN with profound hypoxemia may be related to myocardial failure [2,4]. Infants with TTN are generally born at or near term and frequently are born by cesarean section or under circumstances requiring large amounts of maternal IV fluids [5,6]. The chest x-ray examination shows prominent vascular markings, and fluid may be present in the interlobar fissures, although it should be noted that one series revealed that 17 percent of autopsy-proven pneumonia cases had premortem x-rays consistent with TTN [3]. Clearing of the lungs (as demonstrated by x-ray studies) and clinical improvement usually occur by 24 hours.

II. **Diagnosis and management.** It is important to remember that TTN is a diagnosis of exclusion. Other causes of respiratory distress, especially those related to infection, must be excluded. If an infant is at risk for pneumonia (e.g., if there has been prolonged rupture of membranes, polymorphonuclear leukocytes are present in the gastric aspirate, or a CBC is abnormal; see Chap. 12), or if respiratory symptoms do not improve in 4 to 6 hours, it is our policy to take appropriate cultures and treat the infant with broad-spectrum antibiotics. Oxygen is provided to maintain the Pa_{O_2} in the range of 60 to 80 mmHg; parenteral fluids are provided, since the tachypnea usually precludes enteral feedings. One controlled study has shown furosemide not to be effective in TTN [7].

References

1. Avery, M. E. *Am. J. Dis. Child.* 111: 380, 1966.
2. Halliday, H. L. *Arch. Dis. Child.* 56: 322, 1981.
3. Haney, P. J. *AJR* 143: 23, 1984.
4. Heinonen, K. *Acta. Paediatr. Scand.* 72: 111, 1983.
5. Rawlings, J. S. *Am. J. Dis. Child.* 138: 869, 1984.
6. Singhi, S. *Br. J. Obstet. Gynaecol.* 92: 356, 1985.
7. Wiswell, T. *Pediatrics* 75: 908, 1985.

Pulmonary Hemorrhage

John M. North

I. **Definition and association.** Pulmonary hemorrhage of any amount is a common finding on neonatal autopsies but is of unclear clinical significance [9,10,12]. **Massive pulmonary hemorrhage (MPH)** is defined on autopsy as confluent hemorrhage of two lobes or more that may be intraalveolar, interstitial, or both. With its appearance as the sole finding on some autopsies and case reports correlating with outcome, its clinical significance appears better established. Numerous retrospective autopsy surveys have been published indicating that the diagnosis of MPH is found on 4 to 17.8 percent of all neonatal autopsies, and when compared with concurrent live birth rates it has an incidence of 0.8 to 3.8 per 1000 live births [9–13]. When stratified by birth weight or gestational age, the incidence is considerably higher for premature and LBW births (as high as 50 per 1000 live births) [9,10,13,27]. The type of hemorrhage appears to be important, with interstitial hemorrhage most common in those dying at less than 48 hours of age and alveolar hemorrhage most common in those dying later [9]. The majority of deaths occur before the fourth day [9–11]. Since many of the studies are prior to mechanical ventilation, the mortality rates and timing of deaths are most likely different today. Since the interstitial hemorrhage is less likely to have frank blood per trachea, the incidence is most likely underestimated, with respiratory deterioration attributed to some other cause [13]. Statistical correlations have been made with prematurity, low birth weight, twin gestation, severe IUGR, fetal distress, hypothermia, breech delivery, male sex, and in one large British survey, smoking and extremes of maternal age [2,6,9,10,20]. Linkage of MPH with oxygen exposure is not firm [2,11,24]. Case reports have made possible associations with DIC, aspiration of maternal blood, coxsackie B viral infection, injection of hyperosmolar solutions, erythroblastosis fetalis, neonatal tetanus, rupture of an intercostal artery during chest tube placement, congenital hyperammonemia from urea cycle disorders, intrathoracic gastrogenic cysts, and neonatal anesthesia [4,7,8,14,16,18,21,23,25,26]. The pathogenesis of MPH remains open to speculation, with several theories being brought forward to attempt to explain a breakdown in the epithelial/endothelial barrier in the alveolus coupled with changes in the forces governing liquid flow across these membranes [3,5,17,22]. Factors tending to increase flow from the capillary space to the alveolar space are increased capillary fluid pressure (acute LV failure from asphyxia and/or congenital heart disease), decreased plasma oncotic pressure (hydrops fetalis, liver failure, prematurity), and abnormal coagulation in the face of endothelial damage. Hypothetically, increased surface tension will increase efflux to the alveolar space, as in RDS, ARDS, and possibly MAS [22]. To allow whole RBC efflux, damage to the tissues may be induced by ischemia, oxygen toxicity, inflammation/infection, and mechanical ventilation. From these postulates, autopsies, and case reports, the two highest-risk groups appear to be full-term asphyxiated infants and preterm infants with severe IUGR. MPH is seen infrequently after artificial surfactant therapy.

II. **Diagnosis.** The clinical picture is a sudden deterioration in respiratory status marked by cyanosis and bradycardia, often accompanied by blood per trachea, possibly an acute change in the chest x-ray with opacification of one or both lungs, a drop in the hematocrit, and in a few instances, clinical and/or hematologic evidence of a bleeding diathesis [1,10,22]. Coexisting IVH is not unusual.

III. **Treatment.** Loss of volume or blood or both is corrected. Mechanical ventilation with the use of PEEP is used to decrease fluid/blood efflux into the alveolar space. Inotropic/chronotropic support of cardiac dysfunction is instituted where appropriate. Correction of coagulopathy is essential. Anticipation of this disorder as a complication of mechanical ventilation with efforts to reduce predisposing factors should reduce its incidence.

References

1. Bomsel, F. *Ann. Radiol. (Paris)* 18: 419, 1975.
2. Boothby, C. *Arch. Dis. Child.* 48: 21, 1973.
3. Castile, R. *Mayo Clin. Proc.* 51: 155, 1976.
4. Ceballos, R. *J. Pediatr.* 72: 390, 1968.
5. Cole, V. *Pediatrics* 51: 174, 1973.
6. DeSa, D. *J. Obstet. Gynaecol. Br. Comm.* 77: 158, 1970.
7. Easa, D. *J. Pediatr.* 92: 989, 1978.
8. Ellis, M. *Q. J. Med.* 48: 211, 1979.
9. Esterly, J. *J. Pediatr.* 69: 3, 1966.
10. Fedrick, J. *Biol. Neonate* 18: 243, 1971.
11. Fekete, M. *Acta Paediatr. Hung.* 18: 53, 1977.
12. Fekete, M. *Acta Paediatr. Hung.* 9: 85, 1968.
13. Fekete, M. *Acta Paediatr. Hung.* 26: 65, 1985.
14. Fenton, A. *Anaesthesia* 43: 156, 1988.
15. Hurley, R. *Br. Med. J.* 3: 636, 1969.
16. Jung, A. *Clin. Pediatr.* 19: 624, 1980.
17. Kotas, R. *Pediatr. Res.* 9: 161, 1975.
18. MacPherson, R. *J. Can. Assoc. Radiol.* 24: 362, 1973.
19. Markestad, T. *Acta Paediatr. Scand.* 69: 425, 1980.
20. Parker, J. *Mayo Clin. Proc.* 43: 465, 1968.
21. Roberts, J. *J. Clin. Pathol.* 19: 334, 1966.
22. Rowe, S., and Avery, M. E. *J. Pediatr.* 69: 12, 1966.
23. Salimpour, R. *Arch. Dis. Child.* 52: 587, 1977.
24. Shanklin, D. *N. Engl. J. Med.* 277: 833, 1967.
25. Sheffield, L. *J. Pediatr.* 88: 450, 1976.
26. Simmons, M. *Am. J. Dis. Child.* 132: 208, 1978.
27. Sly, P. *Aust. Paediatr. J.* 17: 32, 1981.
28. Trompeter, R. *Arch. Dis. Child.* 50: 123, 1975.

Chronic Lung Disease

Richard B. Parad

I. **Definition.** Infants are considered to have **chronic lung disease (CLD)** if they continue to require supplemental oxygen to maintain adequate oxygenation after 28 days of life and have abnormal appearance of lung parenchyma on chest radiograph (CXR). This description includes the following categories:
   A. Preterm infants who develop bronchopulmonary dysplasia (BPD) after RDS
   B. VLBW infants who are initially well but develop chronic pulmonary insufficiency of prematurity (CPIP)
   C. Infants with or without mild initial respiratory distress who develop Mikity-Wilson (M-W) syndrome
   D. Term or preterm infants who require long-term O_2 supplementation after a prolonged course of mechanical ventilation for conditions including pneumonia, meconium aspiration syndrome, persistent pulmonary hypertension of the newborn, pulmonary hypoplasia, and surgical repair of major cardiothoracic and gastrointestinal congenital anomalies.

   The above definition predicts outcome only if gestational age at birth is beyond 30 weeks [41]. For infants weighing less than 1500 gm, the need for O_2 beyond 36 weeks' corrected age has a 63 percent positive predictive value for development of long-term pulmonary problems.

II. **Epidemiology.** LBW infants are most susceptible to developing CLD (Table 13-11). Differences in populations, clinical practices, and definitions account for wide variations in CLD incidence (7 to 35 percent) among centers [6]. Decreased

Table 13-11. Distribution by birth weight, birth weight specific survival, and incidence of RDS and CLD, and survival in inborn infants admitted to the NICU at Brigham and Women's Hospital, 1987 (total births 10,122)

Birth weight (g)	No. of infants	Survival (%)	RDS (%)	CLD (%)	RDS to CLD* (%)
501–750	40	50	63	40	64
751–1000	62	77	56	38	51
1001–1250	69	96	41	18	25
1251–1500	68	93	32	3	3
<1500	239	85	46	22	39
>1500	684	98	9	0.3	2

*Indicates percent of infants with RDS who develop CLD.
Key: CLD = chronic lung disease; RDS = respiratory distress syndrome.

risk for CLD is noted for blacks, females, and infants born to mothers who received antenatal glucocorticoid therapy [48].

III. **Pathogenesis** [3,17]

A. **Acute lung injury** is caused by prolonged hyperoxic exposure and barotrauma from mechanical ventilation. Cellular and interstitial injury results in release of mediators that cause secondary changes in alveolar permeability and recruit inflammatory cells into alveolar and interstitial spaces, which in turn causes leakage of water and protein. Airway and vascular tone may be altered. Proteolytic and oxidant injury may interfere with alveolar development and cause emphysematous changes. Sloughed cells and accumulated secretions not cleared adequately by the damaged mucocilliary transport system cause inhomogeneous peripheral airway obstruction that leads to alternating areas of collapse and hyperinflation and proximal airway dilatation.

B. In the **chronic phase** of lung injury, the interstitium may be altered by fibrosis and cellular hyperplasia that has resulted from excessive release of growth factors and mediators. Interstitial fluid clearance is disrupted resulting in pulmonary fluid retention. Airways develop increased muscularization and hyperreactivity. The physiologic effects are decreased lung compliance, increased airway resistance, and impaired gas exchange with resulting ventilation-perfusion mismatching and air trapping.

C. **Factors that may contribute to development of CLD** include the following:

1. Inadequate antioxidant enzyme activity (superoxide dismutase, catalase, glutathione peroxidase) or deficiency of free-radical sinks (vitamin E, glutathione, ceruloplasmin) or both may predispose a lung to oxygen toxicity. Similarly, inadequate antiprotease protection may predispose to lung injury from the unchecked proteases released by recruited inflammatory cells.
2. Excessive early intravenous fluid administration [49] and persistent left-to-right shunt through the PDA
3. Increase in vasopressin and decrease in atrial natriuretic peptide release may alter pulmonary and systemic fluid balance in the setting of obstructive lung disease [25,38].
4. Familial airway hyperreactivity
5. Increased inositol clearance, leading to diminished plasma inositol levels and decreased surfactant synthesis or impaired surfactant metabolism [24].
6. In utero or perinatal acquisition of organisms, including *Chlamydia trachomatis, Ureaplasma urealyticum,* and CMV (see Chap. 12) [11]

IV. **Diagnosis** [47]

A. **Physical examination** may reveal tachypnea, retractions, and irritability in an infant who is failing to thrive.

B. **Arterial blood gases (ABGs)** show hypoxemia and hypercarbia with eventual metabolic compensation.

C. **Chest x-ray (CXR)** changes as the disease progresses. **Stage I** has the same appearance as RDS, **stage II** shows diffuse haziness with increased density and normal to low lung volumes, **stage III** shows streaky densities with bubbly lucencies and early hyperinflation, and **stage IV** shows hyperinflation with larger hyperlucent areas interspersed with thicker, streaky densities. CXR abnormalities often persist into childhood.

D. **Cardiac evaluation. ECG** can show persistent or progressive RVH as cor pulmonale develops. LVH may develop with systemic hypertension. Nonpulmonary etiologies of respiratory failure should be excluded. **2D echocardiogram** may be useful in excluding left-to-right shunts (see Chap. 14).

E. **Pulmonary function testing (PFT)** can be used to evaluate pulmonary status. Increased respiratory tract resistance (Rrs) [20], dynamic compliance (Crs) [23], and presence and severity of airway reactivity predict risk for CLD development in ventilated infants [35].

F. **Pathologic changes** are detectable by the first few days of life, including upper airway mucosal and ciliary epithelial injury. By day 6, necrotizing bronchiolitis, obstruction of small airway lumens by debris and edema, and areas of peribronchial and interstitial fibrosis are present [14]. Emphysematous changes result in diminished surface area for gas exchange. Pulmonary vascular changes associated with pulmonary hypertension are seen early.

V. Inpatient treatment. Treatment goals are to minimize toxic exposures, maximize nutrition, and diminish oxygen consumption through lessening energy expenditures to direct energy toward growth and repair [51].

A. Mechanical ventilation. Acute phase: Ventilator adjustments are made to minimize airway pressures while providing adequate gas exchange (see Mechanical Ventilation above). In most circumstances, we avoid hyperventilation (keeping $PaCO_2$ at 45 to 65 mmHg, with pH > 7.25) and maintain SaO_2 at 90 to 95 percent (PaO_2 60–80 mmHg) [30]. **Chronic phase:** Once baseline ventilator settings are established with a $PaCO_2$ not higher than 65 mmHg, we delay decreasing ventilator rate until a pattern of steady weight gain is established.

B. Supplemental oxygen is supplied to maintain the PaO_2 above 55 mmHg and the $StcO_2$ above 90 percent. Although a PaO_2 less than 55 mmHg may allow adequate tissue O_2 delivery, pulmonary vasoconstriction can occur. When less than 30 percent O_2 by hood is required, we supply O_2 by nasal cannula if saturation can be maintained on less than 1 liter per minute flow. If the flowmeter is accurate at low rates, flow of 100% O_2 is gradually decreased to maintain $StcO_2$. Otherwise, the flow is decreased to ¼ liter per minute as tolerated and then O_2 concentration is decreased. $StcO_2$ should remain above 90 percent during sleep, feeds, and active periods before supplemental O_2 is discontinued.

C. Monitoring (see Blood Gas Monitoring above)

1. **Arterial blood gases (ABGs)** are used to monitor gas exchange and confirm noninvasive monitoring values. Because PO_2 may fall during arterial puncture, local anesthesia (1% lidocaine) prior to puncture may ensure more reliable values.
2. **Transcutaneous PO_2 ($PtcO_2$).** Decreased accuracy of $PtcO_2$ monitors in older babies limits their use in CLD [39]. $PtcO_2$ monitoring is less reliable for absolute values, but trends may be useful for ventilator adjustments.
3. We use **pulse oximetry** for long-term monitoring of infants with CLD, maintaining $StcO_2$ at 90 to 92 percent (PaO_2 60–80 mmHg).
4. **Capillary blood gases (CBGs)** are useful to monitor pH and PCO_2. Since pH and PCO_2 sometimes vary from central values, comparison with ABGs is prudent. If CBGs are similar to ABGs, we monitor stable, ventilator-dependent infants with pulse oximetry and one to two CBGs per day; less frequent CBGs are obtained in patients on O_2 by nasal cannula.
5. **Pulmonary function testing** can document functional responses to trials of bronchodilators, diuretics, and steroids (see **V.E.1–4**).

D. Fluid management [49]. Fluid intake is limited to the minimum required. Initially, we provide intake adequate to maintain urine output at least 1 cc/kg per hour and serum sodium of 140 to 145 mEq/L. Subsequently, we provide 130 to 150 cc/kg per day to supply sufficient calories for growth. We try to increase fluid intake when respiratory status is stable. We recalculate fluid intake each week to adjust for weight gain.

E. Drugs. When the infant remains ventilator-dependent on restricted fluid intake in the absence of PDA or intercurrent infection, additional pharmacotherapy is considered [10].

1. Pulmonary fluid retention is treated with **diuretics** [4,13]. Diuretics indirectly attenuate symptoms of respiratory distress and result in decreased Rrs and increased Crs; gas exchange is variably affected. An acute clinical response may be seen within 1 hour, although maximal effect may not be achieved until 1 week of therapy. The clinical improvement is likely due to decreased lung water content, with decreased interstitial and peribronchial fluid resulting in less resistance and better

compliance. The mechanisms of action may be due either to diuresis or nondiuretic effects.

a. **Furosemide** is used initially at doses of 0.5 to 1.0 mg/kg per dose IV one to two times daily. The dose may be given at time of blood transfusions if these have been associated with increased pulmonary fluid and respiratory distress. Immature infants are at increased risk of toxicity from larger or more frequent doses due to prolonged drug half-life [34]. Side effects include hypercalcuria, ototoxicity, electrolyte imbalance, and cholelithiasis. We use lower doses or combine furosemide with other diuretics rather than provide electrolyte supplementation (see **E.6**). When oral administration can be tolerated, the dose is converted to twice the current IV dose.

b. **Chlorothiazide and spironolactone.** If respiratory status improves with oral furosemide and deteriorates with its withdrawal, we substitute or add **chlorothiazide** (20 to 40 mg/kg per day PO divided bid) and **spironolactone** (2.5 mg PO qd). Chlorothiazide decreases calcium excretion and, in combination with furosemide, may minimize calcium loss and reverse nephrocalcinosis due to furosemide. The combination also allows use of a lower, less toxic furosemide dose. Spironolactone may be added for potassium sparing. This effect takes several days to develop and may last for days after the last dose. Use should be discontinued if potassium levels increase.

2. **Bronchodilators.** Acute obstructive episodes or chronically increased resistance may be related to increased airway tone or bronchospasm and may respond to bronchodilator therapy.

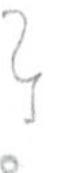

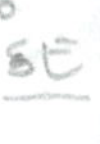

a. Administration of nebulized **beta-adrenergic agonists (BAA)** results in decreased Rrs and increased Crs [21,50]. Tachycardia is the major limiting side effect. Newer agents have increased beta-2 specificity with less beta-1 toxicity. Although isoproterenol (Isuprel®) has a short-term effect, inhalation of nebulized isoetharine (Bronkosol), metaproterenol (Alupent), and albuterol (Proventil® or Ventolin®) is associated with diminishing tachycardia and increasing duration of effect in that order. We use **albuterol** 0.5% solution (5 mg/ml) 0.02 to 0.04 cc/kg (up to 0.1 cc total) nebulized in 2 cc normal saline q6–8h. In ventilated infants, the nebulizer is placed in line with the ventilator near the endotracheal tube. In infants receiving both theophylline and BAA, we may stagger doses to avoid acute tachycardia. The combination of oral and aerosolized albuterol may decrease airway reactivity better than aerosol alone. Albuterol syrup (0.3 mg/kg per day PO/PG divided tid) given between aerosols can be tried in refractory infants.

b. **Muscarinic agents.** Nebulized **atropine** (50 μg/kg per dose) or ipratropium bromide (25 μg/kg per dose) [50] increase Crs and decrease Rrs and may have an additive effect with BAA. BAA and muscarinic agents can be concurrently nebulized.

c. **Theophylline** [28]. In addition to bronchodilation, infants with CLD may benefit from multiple actions of this drug, including diuresis, improved diaphragm contractility, inotropy, respiratory drive stimulation, and increased surfactant production. Improvements in mechanics have been demonstrated with low serum levels (5 to 10 μg/ml); however, increased levels used to treat reactive airway disease (RAD) (12 to 18 μg/ml) may be needed for maximal response. We use a loading dose of 7 mg/kg IV over 20 minutes and maintain a dose of 15 to 17 mg/kg per day IV divided q4–6h or by constant infusion, monitoring serum levels frequently. For enteral administration, the IV preparation given enterally may induce fewer GI side effects than syrup. Theophylline combined with diuretics produces a better response than either alone. Side effects include tachycardia, irritability, feeding intolerance, gastroesophageal reflux (GER), tremors, and lowered seizure threshold.

3. **Cromolyn** acts on both airway and pulmonary vascular tone. Therapeutic and prophylactic treatment of reactive airways has been demonstrated with nebulized cromolyn (10 to 20 mg q6–8h). We add this drug in infants who respond to bronchodilator therapy but remain symptomatic.
4. **Steroids.** Treatment with glucocorticoids in infants who remain ventilator-dependent for 2 to 3 weeks results in increased Crs and decreased Rrs and lowering of oxygen and ventilator requirements [12]. Mechanism of action may be related to diminished inflammation and fibrosis or increased functional surfactant. **Dexamethasone** (0.5 mg/kg per day IV divided q12h for 3 to 7 days, followed by slow taper over 5 to 6 weeks) may be indicated in infants with CXR evolving toward CLD who have failed ventilator weaning on conventional therapy by 2 to 3 weeks of age. Doses may be given orally. Acute complications include infection, systemic hypertension, and glucose intolerance. Adrenal suppression is transient. Growth, development, and bone age do not appear affected [32]. Postextubation airway edema, with stridorous obstruction (see **VI.A**) leading to respiratory failure, may be attenuated with dexamethasone 0.3 mg/kg per dose q12h starting 8 to 12 hours before the next extubation. Edema also may be acutely diminished with nebulized racemic epinephrine.
5. **Sedatives.** Sedation and, when necessary, analgesia are used for physical or autonomic signs of pain or discomfort. These responses may interfere with the ability to ventilate and oxygenate. Chloral hydrate, phenobarbital, short-acting benzodiazepines, or morphine sulfate are used.
6. **Electrolyte supplements.** Hyponatremia, hypokalemia, and hypochloremia with secondary hypercarbia are common side effects of chronic diuretic therapy that are corrected by lowering the diuretic dose or adding NaCl and KCl supplements. Adequate sodium intake should be provided. Serum sodium level can fall to the low 130's before intervention is required. Although hypochloremia may occur in compensated respiratory acidosis, low serum chloride from diuretic-induced loss and inadequate intake can cause metabolic alkalosis and $PaCO_2$ elevation. Chloride deficit is corrected with KCl.

F. **Chest physiotherapy (CPT) and suctioning** may diminish expiratory resistance. Damaged mucociliary clearance mechanisms and inability to cough during intubation result in obstruction of airways by secretions and debris. Vibration and percussion loosen peripheral plugs and secretions and move them centrally for clearance by suctioning. Normal saline distributed by positive-pressure ventilation may loosen this material for easier removal.

G. **Nutrition**

1. In CLD, metabolic rate and energy expenditure are elevated in the face of poor caloric intake [31,51]. To optimize growth, wasteful energy expenditure must be minimized and caloric intake maximized. Prolonged parenteral nutrition is often required. As enteral feeding is started, we feed by orogastric or nasogastric tube and limit oral feeding to avoid tiring the infant.
2. **Vitamin, trace element, and other dietary supplementation.** Vitamin E and antioxidant enzymes diminish oxidant toxicity, although vitamin E supplementation does not prevent CLD [10]. Vitamin A may promote epithelial repair and minimize fibrosis. Selenium, zinc, and copper are trace elements vital to antioxidant enzyme function, and inadequate intake may interfere with protection [26]. Vitamin A (retinyl palmitate, 2000 IU IM qod for 28 days) may reduce respiratory support and CLD incidence [40]. Inositol (120 to 160 mg/kg per day divided q4h IV or PG) may augment surfactant synthesis, diminish respiratory support, and decrease risk of CLD in infants with RDS [24].

H. **Blood transfusions.** We generally maintain hematocrit above 40 percent (Hb 14 gm/dl) during oxygen dependence. Improved O_2 utilization may allow better reserves for growth in the face of increased metabolic demands [5].

I. Behavioral factors. As with all sick infants, care is best provided with individualized attention to behavioral and environmental factors (see Chap. 35). The ideal environment is quiet. Interventions are coordinated at times appropriate for the baby. Regular times are designated for play, exercise, and sleep.

VI. Associated complications

A. Upper airway obstruction. Trauma to the nasal septum, larynx, trachea, and bronchi are common after prolonged or repeated intubation and suctioning. At postextubation bronchoscopy, 44 percent of chronically intubated infants had abnormalities (8 percent severe), including laryngotracheobronchomalacia, obstructive adenoids, granulomas, vocal cord paresis, edema, ulceration with pseudomembranes, subglottic stenosis, and congenital structural anomalies [15]. Stridor may develop when postextubation edema is superimposed on underlying stenosis. Abnormalities are not excluded by the absence of stridor and may be asymptomatic, becoming symptomatic at the time of a viral URI. Flexible fiberoptic bronchoscopy may be used to evaluate stridor, hoarseness, persistent wheezing, or repeated extubation failure.

B. Cor pulmonale. Chronic hypoxemia leads to hypoxic vasoconstriction, pulmonary hypertension, and eventual right ventricular hypertrophy and failure. Left ventricular function also can be affected. The ECG should be followed. Pulmonary hypertension may have reversible and fixed components. Supplemental O_2 is used to maintain the PaO_2 above 55 mmHg. Cardiac catheterization may be required to define the dysfunction and evaluate therapy. Pulmonary vasodilators including hydralazine and nifedipine have variable efficacy and should only be tried during pulmonary artery pressure and PaO_2 monitoring [22]. Echocardiographic studies can exclude structural heart disease and assess LV function but are less reliable to assess RV function and pulmonary hypertension.

C. Systemic hypertension, sometimes with LVH, developed in 43 percent of CLD infants on home O_2 therapy [2].

D. Systemic-to-pulmonary shunting. Left-to-right shunt through collateral vessels (e.g., bronchial arteries) can occur in CLD [22]. Risk factors include chest tube placement, thoracic surgery, and pleural inflammation. When left-to-right shunt is suspected and echocardiography fails to show intracardiac or PDA shunting, collaterals may be demonstrated by angiography. Occlusion of large vessels has been associated with clinical improvement.

E. Metabolic imbalance secondary to diuretics (see **V.E.1,6**)

F. Infection. Because these chronically ill, malnourished, and catheterized infants are at increased risk, episodes of pulmonary and systemic decompensation should be evaluated for infection. Monitoring of tracheal aspirate Gram stains may help distinguish endotracheal tube colonization from pneumonia. Viral and fungal infections should be considered when fevers or pneumonia develop. In infants who are not doing well, we frequently culture for possible infection with *Ureaplasma* and *Mycoplasma hominis* and treat if these organisms are identified [11].

G. CNS dysfunction. A neurologic syndrome presenting with extrapyramidal signs has been described in infants with CLD [37].

H. Hearing loss. Ototoxic drugs (furosemide, gentamicin) and ischemic or hypoxemic CNS injury increase the risk for sensorineural hearing loss. Screening with auditory brainstem responses is recommended at discharge (see Chap. 38).

I. Retinopathy of prematurity (ROP) (see Chap. 38). VLBW infants with CLD are at highest risk for developing ROP due to retinal immaturity and prolonged hyperoxic exposure. In one large multicenter cohort, 14 percent with RDS and 35 percent with BPD developed ROP.

J. Nephrocalcinosis is frequently documented on ultrasound examination [27]. Passage of stones and hematuria may occur. Most infants are asymptomatic with eventual spontaneous resolution, but renal function should be followed (see **V.E.1**).

K. Prematurity, inadequate calcium and phosphorous retention, and prolonged immobilization may lead to **osteoporosis.** Calcium loss due to furosemide and corticosteroids also may contribute. Supplementation with vitamin D, calcium, and phosphorous should be optimized.

L. Gastroesophageal reflux (GER). GER and some degree of aspiration occur in most premature infants. We try to document and treat GER when reflux or aspiration may contribute to pulmonary decompensation, apnea, or feeding intolerance with poor growth. Therapy includes upright or prone positioning, small frequent feeds, formula thickened with cereal, nasojejunal feeding, and metachlopromide with or without antacids. If these fail, fundoplication with gastrostomy [42] (in older infants), or gastrostomy alone with jejunal tube feeding may improve pulmonary status and growth.

M. Incidence of **inguinal hernia** is increased by the patent processus vaginalis in VLBW infants, particularly those with CLD. If reducible, surgical correction should be delayed until respiratory status is improved. Spinal rather than general anesthesia avoids reintubation and post-operative apnea.

N. Early **growth failure** may result from inadequate intake and excessive energy expenditure and may persist after clinical resolution of pulmonary disease [31] (see **VIII.B**). Premature withdrawal of supplemental O_2 may contribute to slowing of growth.

VII. Discharge planning. Timing of discharge depends on availability of home care support systems and parental readiness.

A. Weight gain/O_2 therapy. Supplemental O_2 should be weaned when the $StcO_2$ is maintained at 92 percent or greater, good weight gain has been established, and respiratory status is stable (see **V.B.** and **VI.N.**). We prefer to delay discharge until O_2 is discontinued. However, if long-term O_2 supplementation seems likely in an infant who is stable, growing, and has capable caretakers, we offer the option of home O_2 therapy.

B. Teaching. Involvement of parents in caregiving is vital to the smooth transition from hospital to home care. Parents should be taught CPR and early signs of decompensation. Teaching of equipment use, medication administration, and nutritional guidelines should begin when discharge planning is initiated.

C. Baseline values. Baseline values of vital signs, daily weight gain, discharge weight and head circumference, blood gases, $StcO_2$, hematocrit, electrolytes, CXR, and ECG must be documented at discharge. This information is useful to evaluate subsequent changes in clinical status. An eye examination and hearing screen should be performed prior to discharge.

VIII. Outpatient therapy. Several recent publications review outpatient therapy and follow-up [29,44,45].

A. Oxygen. Supplementary O_2 can be delivered by tanks or oxygen concentrator. Portable tanks allow mobility. Weaning is based on periodic assessment of $StcO_2$.

B. Home ventilation. Stable tracheostomized infants may qualify for home ventilator support if a suitable program is available.

C. Medications. Infants receiving diuretics require monitoring of electrolytes. When the infant is stable, we allow the infant to outgrow the diuretic dose by 50 percent before discontinuing the drug. Bronchodilators are tapered when respiratory status is stable in room air. Nebulized medications are tapered last. Discontinued medications should remain available for early use when symptoms recur.

D. Nutrition. Weight gain is a sensitive indicator of well-being and should be closely followed. Caloric supplementation is often required to maintain good growth after discharge.

E. Passive smoke exposure. Because smoking in the home increases respiratory tract illness in children [46], parents of CLD infants should be discouraged from smoking and should minimize the child's exposure to smoke containing environments.

IX. Natural history

A. Mortality. Mortality is estimated at 10 to 20 percent during the first year of life. Risk increases with duration of O_2 exposure and mechanical ventilation. Ventilation beyond 6 months is associated with 30 to 50 percent mortality [19]. Death is frequently caused by infection. Risk of unexpected death may be increased and may be related to abnormalities in control of breathing [1].

B. Long-term morbidity

1. **Pulmonary** [17]. Tachypnea, retractions, dyspnea, cough, and wheezing can be seen from months to years in seriously affected children. Although complete clinical recovery can occur, underlying PFT, gas exchange, and CXR abnormalities may persist to adolescence [7,9,18,36a]. The impact of persistent minor abnormalities of function and growth on long-term morbidity and mortality is not known. Reactive airway disease occurs more frequently, and infants with CLD are at increased risk for bronchiolitis and pneumonia.
2. **Neurodevelopmental delay/neurologic deficits.** Outcome in CLD is related to effects of low birth weight, but early behavioral differences exist between infants with CLD and VLBW and RDS controls. Later outcome varies widely; one-third to two-thirds of such infants are normal by 2 years [33], and subsequent improvement may occur. Our experience suggests specific motor coordination delays and visual-perceptual impairment rather than overall lower IQ, with resulting mean Bayley scores 1 SD below the normal mean by ages 4 to 6 years. Neurologic deficits occur in one-third of such children.
3. **Growth failure.** Degree of long-term growth delay is inversely proportional to birth weight and probably is influenced by CLD severity and duration. Weight is most affected, and head circumference is least affected. Delayed growth occurs in one-third to two-thirds of these infants at 2 years [33,45]. One-third of our school-age population is 3 SD below the mean for height and weight. Several recent reviews have been published on CLD [8,10,16,17,33,36,43].

References

1. Abman, S. H., et al. *Am. J. Dis. Child.* 143: 815, 1989.
2. Abman, S. H., et al. *J. Pediatr.* 104: 929, 1984.
3. Abman, S., et al. *Pediatr. Pulmonol.* 3: 185, 1987.
4. Albersheim, S. G., et al. *J. Pediatr.* 115: 615, 1989.
5. Alverson, D. C., et al. *J. Pediatr.* 113: 722, 1988.
6. Avery, M. E., et al. *Pediatrics* 79: 26, 1987.
7. Bader, D., et al. *J. Pediatr.* 110: 693, 1987.
8. Bancalari, E., et al. *Pediatr. Clin. North Am.* 33: 1, 1986.
9. Berman, W., Jr., et al. *J. Pediatr.* 109: 45, 1986.
10. Blanchard, P. W., et al. *Clin. Perinatol.* 14: 881, 1987.
11. Cassell, G. H. *Lancet* 2: 240, 1988.
12. Cummings, J. J., et al. *N. Engl. J. Med.* 320: 1505, 1989.
13. Engelhardt, B., et al. *J. Pediatr.* 114: 619, 1989.
14. Erickson, A. E., et al. *Am. J. Pathol.* 127: 474, 1987.
15. Fan, L. L., et al. *Crit. Care Med.* 10: 453, 1982.
16. Farrell, P. M. *Pediatr. Pulmonol.* 2: 44, 1986.
17. Farrell, P. M., and Taussig, L. M. *Bronchopulmonary Dysplasia and Related Chronic Respiratory Disorders.* Columbus, Ohio: Ross Laboratories, 1986. Pp. 1–149.
18. Gerhardt, T., et al. *J. Pediatr.* 110: 448, 1987.
19. Gibson, R. L., et al. *Am. J. Dis. Child.* 142: 721, 1988.
20. Goldman, S. L., et al. *J. Pediatr.* 102: 613, 1983.
21. Gomez-Del, Rio M., et al. *Pediatr. Pulmonol.* 2: 287, 1986.
22. Goodman, G., et al. *J. Pediatr.* 112: 67, 1988.

23. Graff, M. A., et al. *Pediatr. Pulmonol.* 2: 332, 1986.
24. Hallman, M., et al. *J. Pediatr.* 110: 604, 1987.
25. Hazinski, T. A., et al. *Pediatr. Res.* 23: 86, 1988.
26. Huston, R. K., et al. *J. Parenter. Enter. Nutr.* 11: 163, 1987.
27. Jacinto, J. S., et al. *Pediatrics* 81: 31, 1988.
28. Kao, L. C., et al. *J. Pediatr.* 111: 439, 1987.
29. Koops, B. L., et al. *Clin. Perinatol.* 11: 101, 1984.
30. Kraybill, E. N., et al. *J. Pediatr.* 115: 115, 1989.
31. Maisels, J. *Pediatrics* 77: 345, 1986.
32. Mammel, M. C., et al. *Dev. Pharmacol. Ther.* 10: 1, 1987.
33. Merritt, T. A., et al. *Bronchopulmonary Dysplasia.* Boston: Blackwell Scientific, 1988.
34. Mirochnick, M. H., et al. *J. Pediatr.* 112: 653, 1988.
35. Motoyama, E. K., et al. *Am. Rev. Respir. Dis.* 136: 50, 1987.
36. O'Brodovich, H., et al. *Am. Rev. Respir. Dis.* 132: 694, 1985.
36a. Northway, W. H. et al. *N. Engl. J. Med.* 323: 1793, 1990.
37. Perlman, J. M., et al. *Pediatrics* 84: 215, 1989.
38. Rao, M., et al. *Am. J. Dis. Child.* 140: 825, 1989.
39. Rome, E. S., et al. *Pediatrics* 74: 217, 1984.
40. Shenai, J. P., et al. *J. Pediatr.* 111: 269, 1987.
41. Shennan, A. T., et al. *Pediatrics* 82: 527, 1988.
42. Sindel, B. D., et al. *Am. J. Dis. Child.* 143: 1103, 1989.
43. Sinkin, R. A., et al. *Clin. Perinatol.* 14: 599, 1987.
44. Swanson, J. A., et al. *Mayo Clin. Proc.* 62: 613, 1987.
45. Taeusch, H. W., and Yogman, M. W. *Follow-Up Management of the High-Risk Infant.* Boston: Little, Brown, 1987. Pp. 1–353.
46. Tager, I. B., et al. *N. Engl. J. Med.* 309: 699, 1983.
47. Toce, S. S., et al. *Am. J. Dis. Child.* 138: 581, 1984.
48. VanMarter, L. J., et al. *Pediatrics* 86: 331, 1990.
49. VanMarter, L. J. *J. Pediatr.* 116: 942, 1990.
50. Wilkie, R. A., et al. *J. Pediatr.* 111: 278, 1987.
51. Yeh, T. F., et al. *J. Pediatr.* 114: 448, 1989.

Meconium Aspiration

Eric C. Eichenwald

I. Background

A. Cause. Acute or chronic hypoxia may result in the passage of meconium in utero. Gasping by the fetus or newly born infant can then cause aspiration of amniotic fluid contaminated by meconium. Meconium aspiration before or during birth can obstruct airways, interfere with gas exchange, and cause severe respiratory distress (Fig. 13-2).

B. The **incidence** of meconium-stained amniotic fluid is 8.8 percent of 1000 live births in Gregory's [7] series. Infants born with meconium-stained amniotic fluid frequently are postmature or have suffered antepartum or intrapartum asphyxia. In the same series [7], 46 percent of these infants had 1-minute Apgar scores less than 6 and 19 percent had Apgar scores less than 6 at 5 minutes. The timing of the insult can sometimes be suggested by the color of the fluid; yellow meconium is usually old, while green meconium suggests a more recent insult.

C. If the amniotic fluid is meconium-stained, about half the infants will have meconium in their tracheas on direct suction (Fig. 13-3). Meconium can be present in the trachea without any evidence of meconium in the mouth or larynx. The amount and thickness of meconium appear to be directly related to the severity of the respiratory symptoms and signs. Suctioning of the mouth and oropharynx before delivery of the shoulders, and direct suctioning of meconium from the trachea favorably affects the clinical course. Two-thirds

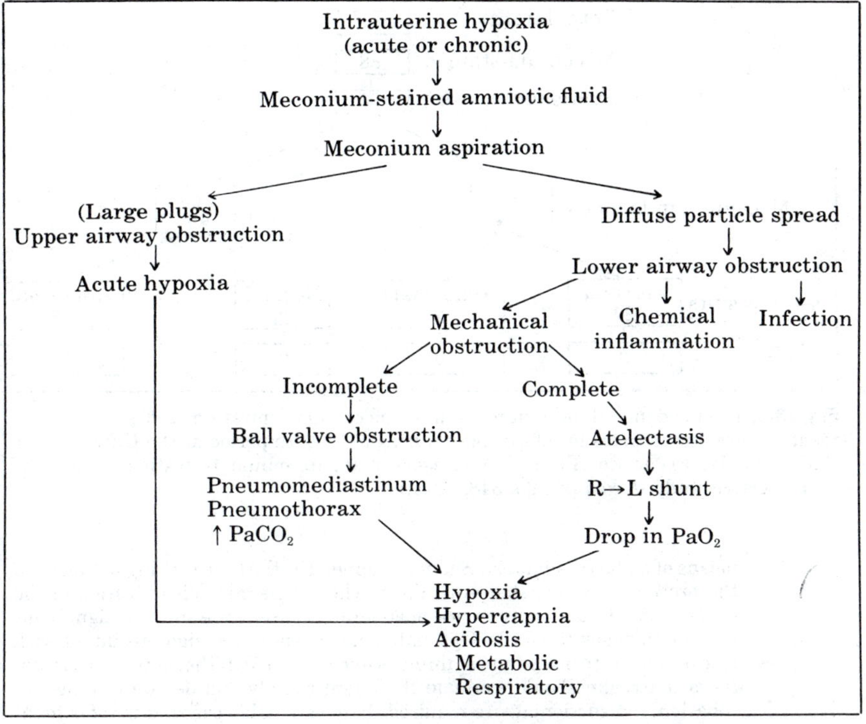

Fig. 13-2. Schema of the pathophysiology of meconium aspiration (From D. Vidyasagar et al., Assisted ventilation in infants with meconium aspiration syndrome. *Pediatrics* 56: 208, 1975. Copyright American Academy of Pediatrics, 1975.)

of Gregory's patients from whom meconium was suctioned had no respiratory difficulties, although half had abnormal results on chest x-ray examinations. In Ting's series [11], symptomatic meconium aspiration pneumonia was more common in meconium-stained infants who did not have tracheal suctioning performed. Adequate airway management, however, cannot prevent meconium aspiration altogether, since meconium may be aspirated by the fetus prior to delivery. [3,4] (see Chap. 5).

II. Prevention of passage of meconium in utero. Mothers who are at risk for uteroplacental insufficiency include those with toxemia or increased blood pressure, heavy smokers, those with chronic respiratory or cardiovascular disease, those with poor uterine growth, and those who are beyond their estimated day of confinement. These women should be carefully monitored during pregnancy, and they should have fetal heart rate monitoring during labor with fetal scalp blood samples for pH when indicated.

III. Prevention of meconium aspiration

A. When thick, particulate, "pea soup" meconium is present, the obstetrician should attempt to clear the nose and oropharynx before the chest is delivered. This can be done with a bulb syringe followed by a De Lee suction catheter passed through the nose to the oropharynx [2].

B. The infant should then be handed to the anesthesiologist or pediatrician, who intubates the trachea under direct laryngoscopy before inspiratory efforts have been initiated. A 3.0 or 3.5 I.D. endotracheal tube is used in term infants. After intubation, the tube is attached to wall suction of 80 to 90 mmHg by

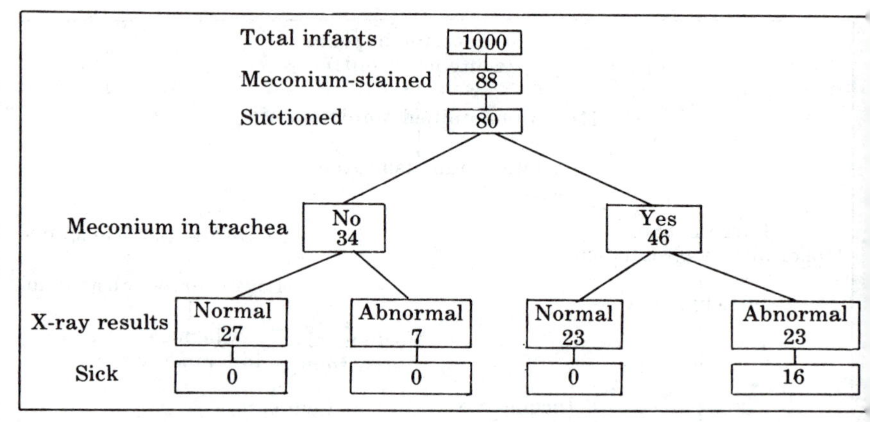

Fig. 13-3. The incidence of meconium staining, meconium aspiration, and roentgenographic changes in infants born during a 6-month period at the University of California, San Francisco. (From G. A. Gregory et al., Meconium aspiration in infants: A prospective study. *J. Pediatr.* 85: 848, 1974.)

means of a plastic adapter.* Suction is applied as the tube is being withdrawn; the procedure is repeated until the trachea is cleared. Visualization of the cords without suctioning is **not** adequate because there may be significant meconium below the cords. Optimal management of the vigorous infant with thin or moderate meconium staining is unclear [9,15]. If the meconium is thin, the pediatrician should **evaluate** the infant rapidly and **decide** whether intubation and suctioning are required. In questionable cases, it is safer to intubate and suction.

C. The child's general condition must not be ignored in compulsive attempts to clear the trachea. This procedure should be accomplished rapidly, and ventilation with oxygen should be initiated before significant bradycardia occurs. Since a few inspiratory efforts by the infant will move the meconium from the trachea to the smaller airways, exhaustive attempts to remove it are unwise [7,8].

D. No positive pressure should be used until after the trachea is suctioned. Direct tracheal suctioning also should be done in infants born through thin meconium who have Apgar scores of 6 or less at 1 minute.

IV. Management of meconium aspiration. Infants who are depressed at birth and have had meconium suctioned from the trachea are at risk for meconium aspiration pneumonia and thus should be observed closely for respiratory distress. Chest x-ray examination may help determine which infants are most likely to develop respiratory distress, although a significant number of infants without respiratory distress will have an abnormal chest film. Chest physiotherapy and suctioning of the oropharynx should be done during the period of observation—every 30 minutes for the first 2 hours and then continued if respiratory symptoms develop. Transcutaneous monitoring of PO_2 or oxygen saturation during this period aids assessment of the severity of the infant's condition and allows for prevention of hypoxemia during chest physiotherapy. Infants frequently require supplemental oxygen during physiotherapy.

A. Drug therapy. Meconium promotes the growth of bacteria [1], and differentiating between bacterial pneumonia and meconium aspiration may be diffi-

*Touch-Trol. Manufactured by Argyle, Division of Sherwood Medical, St. Louis, MO 63103.

cult. Thus the use of broad-spectrum antibiotics (e.g., ampicillin and gentamicin) is usually indicated in infants when an infiltrate is seen on chest x-ray studies. Appropriate cultures should be taken to identify bacterial disease, if present. There is no evidence that steroids are beneficial [6,17].

B. **Routine care.** The thermal environment of all infants at risk for meconium aspiration pneumonia should be watched closely. Blood glucose and calcium levels should be assessed and corrected if necessary. In addition, these infants may have acute asphyxia and a severe metabolic acidosis that should be corrected with bicarbonate. Asphyxiated infants may require specific therapy for hypotension, which can be aided by monitoring of central venous pressure. Hypotension and poor cardiac output may require temporary support with colloid infusion or cardiotonic medications such as dopamine. Fluids should be restricted as much as possible to prevent cerebral and pulmonary edema. Renal function should be continuously monitored (see Perinatal Asphyxia in Chap. 21).

C. **Obstruction.** In infants with significant meconium aspiration, mechanical obstruction of both large and small airways can occur, as well as a chemical pneumonitis (see Fig. 13-2). This results in severe arterial hypoxemia, partly secondary to right-to-left shunting through atelectatic lung and partly due to the inflammatory change.

D. **Management** of hypoxemia should be accomplished by increasing the inspired oxygen concentration and by monitoring of blood gases and pH. Usually an indwelling arterial catheter is required for blood sampling and infusion. It is crucial to provide sufficient oxygen, because repeated hypoxic insults may contribute to pulmonary artery hypertension. If FiO_2 requirements exceed 0.40, a trial of CPAP may be considered. CPAP is often helpful, and the appropriate pressures must be individualized for each infant [5,13]. In some instances, CPAP may aggravate air trapping and should be instituted with caution if hyperinflation is apparent clinically or radiographically [12,16].

E. **Mechanical ventilation.** Hypercapnia may become a problem in infants with very severe disease. For severe carbon dioxide retention ($PaCO_2 > 60$ mmHg) or for persistent hypoxemia ($PaO_2 < 50$ mmHg), mechanical ventilation is indicated [14]. In these infants, higher inspiratory pressures (about 30 to 35 cm H_2O) are more often required than in infants with RDS; the PEEP (usually 2 to 6 cm H_2O) selected should depend on the individual's response. Adequate expiratory time should be permitted to prevent air trapping behind partly obstructed airways. Useful starting points are inspiratory time of 0.50 to 0.75 second at a rate of 20 to 25 breaths per minute. Some infants may respond better to rapid-rate ventilation with rates of 60 to 150 breaths per minute and inspiratory times as short as 0.2 second (see Mechanical Ventilation above).

F. **Air leak.** There is a 10 to 20 percent incidence of pneumothorax or pneumomediastinum associated with meconium aspiration [7,8], which may increase when mechanical ventilation is required; thus a high index of suspicion for air leak is required. Equipment should be available to evacuate a pneumothorax promptly (see Air Leak above).

G. **Pulmonary hypertension** often accompanies meconium aspiration, and specific measures should be taken to ascertain the degree to which this is contributing to the infant's hypoxemia [10] (see Persistent Pulmonary Hypertension of the Newborn above).

References

1. Bryan, C. S. *Johns Hopkins Med. J.* 121: 9, 1967.
2. Carson, B. S. *Am. J. Obstet. Gynecol.* 126: 712, 1976.
3. Davis, R. O. *Am. J. Obstet. Gynecol.* 151: 731, 1985.
4. Falciglia, H. S. *Obstet. Gynecol.* 71: 349, 1988.
5. Fox, W. *Pediatrics* 56: 214, 1975.

6. Frantz, I. D. *J. Pediatr.* 86: 438, 1975.
7. Gregory, G. A. *J. Pediatr.* 85: 848, 1974.
8. Klaus, M. *J. Pediatr.* 85: 853, 1974.
9. Linder, N. *J. Pediatr.* 112: 613, 1988.
10. Murphy, J. D. *J. Pediatr.* 104: 758, 1984.
11. Ting, P. *Am. J. Obstet. Gynecol.* 122: 767, 1975.
12. Tran, N. *Pediatr. Res.* 14: 34, 1980.
13. Truog, W. E. *J. Pediatr.* 100: 284, 1982.
14. Vidyasagar, D. *Pediatrics* 56: 208, 1975.
15. Wiswell, T. *Pediatrics* 85: 715, 1990.
16. Yeh, T. F. *Crit. Care Med.* 10: 588, 1982.
17. Yeh, T. F. *J. Pediatr.* 90: 140, 1977.

14 Congenital Heart Disease

Alan M. Fujii and James E. Lock

I. Recent advances in pediatric cardiology, cardiac surgery, and neonatology have greatly improved our capacity to manage neonates with congenital heart disease. Two-dimensional echocardiography with color-flow Doppler now provide reliable anatomic and physiologic information to aid in the medical and surgical management of neonates with congenital heart disease (CHD). Fetal echocardiography has become very important in the obstetric management of fetal arrhythmias, hydrops, and patients at risk for structural heart disease. Pharmacologic maintenance of the ductus arteriosus in certain types of cyanotic congenital heart disease [30,38,47] and closure of the ductus in premature infants with respiratory distress syndrome [16,26,27] are now routine. Advances in pediatric cardiac catheterization techniques and angiography have made precise physiologic and anatomic diagnoses with very low complication rates possible [20]. Therapeutic cardiac catheterizations are now being investigated and are routinely performed for selected lesions [59]. Advances in surgical management of infants with congenital heart disease have made primary repair rather than staged repair the treatment of choice for many lesions [33,57]. The overall mortality for infants with congenital heart disease is improving [22,25].

Advances in pediatric cardiology, neonatology, and other pediatric subspecialties have made it important for pediatricians and neonatologists to be able to rapidly evaluate and participate in the initial medical management of neonates with congenital heart disease. A multidisciplinary approach involving several subspecialty services is sometimes required, especially since one-fifth of patients with severe congenital heart disease weigh less than 2500 gm at birth [25] and have a higher mortality than term infants [23]. This chapter is intended as a practical guide for the initial evaluation and management, by pediatricians and neonatologists, of infants suspected of having congenital heart disease. For a more detailed discussion of the individual lesions, the clinician should consult current textbooks of pediatric cardiology [1,35,40,52].

II. **Incidence and mortality.** The incidence of structural heart disease is about 8 per 1000 live births [42]. Data from the New England Regional Infant Cardiac Program (NERICP) show that approximately 3 per 1000 live births have heart disease that results in death or requires cardiac catheterization or surgery during the first year of life [25]. Half these infants presented before the second week of life [24]. Of these infants, 19 percent have birth weights less than 2500 gm. Patent ductus arteriosus (PDA), coarctation of the aorta, and ventricular septal defects are common among infants with low birth weights, while transposition of the great vessels is usually associated with normal birth weights. The most common congenital heart lesions presenting in the first week of life are transposition of the great arteries and hypoplastic left heart syndrome (Table 14-1). The mortality 1 year after diagnosis for an infant hospitalized in the first 28 days of life with symptomatic cardiac disease is shown in Table 14-2. These mortality statistics continue to improve, as can be seen from the table [25].

III. **Diagnosis and approach.** Congenital heart disease (CHD) most commonly presents as a heart murmur, heart failure, cyanosis, arrhythmia, or some combination of these clinical signs. Recently, many infants with congenital heart disease have been diagnosed by fetal echocardiography.

Table 14-1. Top five diagnoses presenting at different ages

Diagnosis	%
Age on Admission: 0–6 Days (*n* = 1603)	
D-TGA	15%
HLH	12%
TOF	8%
Coarctation	7%
VSD	6%
Other	52%
Age on Admission: 7–13 Days (*n* = 311)	
Coarctation	20%
VSD	14%
HLH	9%
D-TGA	8%
TOF	7%
Other	42%
Age on Admission: 14–28 Days (*n* = 306)	
VSD	18%
TOF	17%
Coarctation	12%
D-TGA	10%
PDA	5%
Other	38%

Key: D-TGA = D-transposition of the great arteries; HLH = hypoplastic left heart syndrome; TOF = tetralogy of Fallot; VSD = ventricular septal defect; PDA = patent ductus arteriosus.
Source: D. C. Fyler and P. Lang, Neonatal Heart Disease. In G. B. Avery (ed.), *Neonatology: Pathophysiology and Management of the Newborn.* Philadelphia: Lippincott, 1981.

A. Fetal echocardiography. Preliminary diagnosis by fetal echocardiography has assumed greater importance as experience has increased. Two-dimensional echocardiography of in utero fetal cardiac structure is most accurate between 18 and 24 weeks' gestational age [55]. Indications for fetal echocardiography may include the following:

1. **Fetal factors**
    a. Extracardiac fetal anomalies on fetal ultrasound
    b. Fetal cardiac anomalies on fetal ultrasound
    c. Fetal arrhythmia
    d. Hydrops fetalis [37]
2. **Maternal factors**
    a. Maternal CHD
    b. Polyhdramnios
    c. Poorly controlled diabetes mellitus
    d. Collagen-vascular disease
    e. Exposure to environmental teratogens (Table 14-3)
3. **Familial factors**
    a. Family history of CHD
    b. Family history of inherited syndromes (Table 14-4)
    c. Abnormal fetal genetic screen (see Table 14-3)

    Most severe forms of CHD can be accurately diagnosed by fetal echocardiography. Coarctation of the aorta and ventricular and atrial septal defects are exceptions that are frequently missed [54].

B. Heart murmur in an acyanotic infant. Initial evaluation of neonates suspected of having congenital heart disease should include a complete physical examination (including a careful search for other anomalies; see Tables 14-3 and 14-4), blood pressures in all four extremities, electrocardiogram (ECG), chest x-ray, and evaluation of oxygenation in 100% oxygen. Demonstration of a

Table 14-2. Mortality (percent) to first birthday by diagnosis over various time periods (52 months)

Diagnosis	July 1968 to November 1972		November 1972 to March 1977		March 1977 to June 1981	
	No. of cases	Percent (mortality)	No. of cases	Percent (mortality)	No. of cases	Percent (mortality)
VSD	265	12	290	12	328	13
D-TGA	185	43	129	38	172	27
TOF	152	30	166	30	181	15
PDA	112	6	91	13	100	6
HLH	141	92	101	97	116	90
COARCT	133	53	136	31	170	31
ECD	85	47	88	34	128	28
HETRO	67	55	69	52	70	53
PS	55	18	49	16	71	7
SV	50	48	47	47	37	32
PA & IVS	56	79	50	68	41	68
TAPVR	42	81	43	51	31	32
AS	26	50	37	49	25	40
Truncus	27	63	21	76	36	64
ASD	44	14	64	5	40	0.8
Myocard	49	33	28	50	35	34
TA	49	43	32	41	32	47
DORV	27	37	20	45	28	50
L-TGA	15	40	11	55	14	21
Other	84	46	84	31	132	25
TOTAL	1664	41	1556	37	1787	29

Key: VSD = ventricular septal defect; D-TGA = D-transposition of the great arteries; TOF = tetralogy of Fallot; PDA = patent ductus arteriosus; HLH = hypoplastic left heart syndrome; COARCT = coarctation of the aorta; ECD = endocardial cushion defect; Hetero = heterotaxia; PS = pulmonary stenosis; SV = single ventricle; PA & IVS = pulmonary atresia & intact ventricular septum; TAPVR = total anomalous pulmonary venous return; AS = aortic stenosis; Truncus = truncus arteriosus; ASD = atrial septal defect; Myocard = myocardial disease; TA = tricuspid atresia; DORV = double outlet right ventricle; L-TGA = L "corrected" transposition of the great arteries.

Source: D. C. Fyler, L. P. Buckley, J. Cartier, M. Breibart, and A. S. Nadas, The regionalization of infant cardiac care in New England. *Rev. Lat. Card. Inf.* 2: 10, 1986.

Table 14-3. Syndromes with cardiac defects

Syndrome	Incidence of congenital heart disease (5%)	Characteristic cardiac defect
Chromosomal Anomalies		
Trisomy 21 (Down's syndrome)	40–50	AVC, VSD
Trisomy D (Patau's syndrome)	80–90	VSD, PDA
Trisomy E (Edward's syndrome)	95	VSD, PDA
4P (Wolf's syndrome)	40	ASD, VSD
5P (Cri-du-chat syndrome)	20–30	Variable
XO (Turner's syndrome)	30	Coarctation, AS
Environmental Teratogens		
Rubella syndrome	50	PDA, peripheral PS
Thalidomide	19	TOF, truncus
Fetal alcohol syndrome	30–40	VSD, ASD, TOF
Fetal hydantoin syndrome	10	Variable
Fetal trimethadione syndrome	50	VSD, TOF
Maternal lupus	?	Congenital heart block

Key: AVC = atrioventricularis communis; VSD = ventricular septal defect; PDA = patent ductus arteriosus; ASD = atrial septal defect; AS = aortic stenosis; PS = pulmonary stenosis; TOF = tetralogy of Fallot.
Source: Modified from J. A. Noonan, Association of congenital heart disease with syndromes or other defects. *Pediatr. Clin. North Am.* 25: 797, 1978.

Table 14-4. Syndromes of genetic or unknown etiology with cardiac defects

Syndrome	Etiology	Characteristic cardiac defect
Skeletal Defects Predominant		
Ellis van Creveld	R	Single atrium
Laurence-Moon-Biedl	R	TOF, VSD
Carpenter	R	PDA, VSD
Holt-Oram	D	ASD, VSD
Fanconi	R	PDA, VSD
Thrombocytopenia absent radius	R	ASD, TOF
Rubinstein-Taybi	?	PDA
VATER	?	Variable
Diabetic embropathy	Maternal diabetes	Variable
Characteristic Facies		
Noonan	?D	PS (dysplastic PV), ASD
DiGeorge	?	TOF, RAA
Smith-Lemli-Opitz	R	VSD, PDA
Facial dysmorphism	D	PDA
de Lange	?	TOF, VSD
Goldenhar	?	TOF, variable
Williams elfin facies	?	Supravalvular AS, peripheral PS
Asymmetric crying facies	?	Variable

Table 14-4 (continued)

Syndrome	Etiology	Characteristic cardiac defect
Skin Lesions Prominent		
Forney (deafness, freckles)	D	Mitral insufficiency
Leopard (deafness, lentigines)	D	PS
Neurofibromatosis (hamartoma)	D	PS, renal artery stenosis
Tuberous sclerosis (adenoma sebaceum)	D	Rhabdomyoma
Situs Inversus		
Kartagener (bronchiectasis)	R	Dextrocardia
Ivemark asplenia or polysplenia	?	Complex
Connective-Tissue Disorders		
Marfan	D	Aortic aneurysm, MVP, cystic medial necrosis
Ehlers Danlos	D	Dissecting aneurysm, arterial rupture
Cutis laxa	R	Peripheral PS
Osteogenesis	D,R	MVP, aortic insufficiency
Pseudoxanthoma elasticum	R	Coronary artery disease
Metabolic Disorders		
Glycogen storage II (Pompe)	R	Massive glycogen deposition
Homocystinuria	R	Thromboses of medium-sized arteries
Mucopolysaccharidoses:		
Type I Hurler	R	Pseudoatherosclerosis AI, MI
Type II Hurler	X-linked	AI
Type IV, V, VI	R	AI
Neuromuscular Disorders		
Friedreich's ataxia	R	Cardiomyopathy
Myotonic dystrophy	D	MVP, cardiomyopathy
Muscular dystrophy	X-linked	Cardiomyopathy
Arrhythmia		
Jervell Lange Nielson (deafness)	R	Prolonged Q–T, VF
Romano Ward (no deafness)	D	Prolonged Q–T, VF
Refsum's (polyneuritis)	R	Arrhythmia, heart block
Familial periodic paralysis	D	Hypokalemia, SVT

Key: R = recessive; TOF = tetralogy of Fallot; VSD = ventricular septal defect; PDA = patent ductus arteriosus; D = dominant; ASD = atrial septal defect; ? = unknown; PS = pulmonary stenosis; PV = pulmonary valve; RAA = right aortic arch; MVP = mitral valve prolapse; AI = aortic insufficiency; MI = mitral insufficiency; SVT = supraventricular tachycardia.

Source: From J. A. Noonan, Associate of congenital heart disease with syndromes or other defects. *Pediatr. Clin. North Am.* 25: 797, 1978.

rapid rise in PO_2 by transcutaneous monitor or arterial blood gas analysis to greater than 200 mmHg in 100% oxygen (hyperoxia test) largely eliminates cyanotic congenital heart disease from the differential diagnosis. If only a soft systolic murmur (the murmur being no louder than the heart sounds) is found in an acyanotic infant ($PO_2 > 60$ mmHg in room air and/or $PO_2 > 200$ mmHg in 100% oxygen), elective referral to a pediatric cardiologist or careful follow-up by the pediatrician 2 to 4 weeks after discharge from the hospital may be arranged.

Hemodynamically "benign" heart murmurs may be heard in 60 percent and transient murmurs of a patent ductus arteriosus are heard in 14 percent of healthy term infants [8]. Murmurs consistent with trivial ventricular septal defects that later resolve spontaneously may be heard in 4 percent of term infants after 16 hours of age [8,19]. Murmurs from transient mitral or tricuspid regurgitation following perinatal asphyxia are noted in the early perinatal period [17].

Pathologic murmurs tend to appear at characteristic ages. Stenotic (systolic ejection murmurs) and artrioventricular valvar insufficiency (systolic regurgitant) murmurs tend to be noted shortly after birth. In contrast, left-to-right shunt murmurs (systolic regurgitant VSD murmur or continuous PDA murmur) may not be heard until the second to fourth week of life, when the pulmonary vascular resistance has decreased. Conversely, a characteristic continuous PDA murmur heard on the first day of life may represent a closing ductus arteriosus in a patient with ductal-dependent pulmonary blood flow, e.g., tetralogy of Fallot and pulmonary atresia. Thus the age of the patient when the murmur was first noted and the character of the murmur provide important clues to the nature of the malformation (Table 14-5).

C. **Congestive heart failure.** The neonate in congestive heart failure may present with tachypnea, tachycardia, hepatomegaly, diaphoresis, poor perfusion, feeding intolerance, edema, growth failure, or cardiovascular collapse. The age when congestive heart failure develops depends on the type and hemodynamics of the lesion responsible. For congestive heart failure to develop in the first weeks of life, there is usually either a severe pressure or volume overload lesion or primary myocardial dysfunction. Table 14-5 lists some acyanotic lesions that may cause congestive heart failure in the neonatal period.

1. **Aortic stenosis (AS)** is usually valvar and rarely is severe enough to produce symptoms in infancy [36]. Two-dimensional echocardiography will establish the diagnosis and assess the severity of the lesion. Critical AS presenting in infancy may be associated with hypoplasia of the left ventricle and other left-sided obstructive lesions (e.g., coarctation of the aorta). The initial medical management of symptomatic infants with critical AS includes inotropic support, diuretics, oxygen, and positive-pressure ventilation. Prostaglandin E_1 infusion to maintain patency of the ductus arteriosus may be beneficial. Cardiac catheterization should be performed as soon as possible to confirm the diagnosis, assess the left ventricular size (an end-diastolic volume ≥ 20 ml/m^2 is needed to support systemic circulation), and perform balloon valvotomy [32,58]. Alternatively, surgical valvotomy may be performed. Patients do poorly if the valvotomy induces severe aortic regurgitation. Asymptomatic AS requires long-term evaluation because the stenosis will frequently increase with time.
2. **Coarctation of the aorta (COARCT)** occurs in nearly 10 percent of newborns with severe congenital heart disease, is usually preductal, and is more common in males and premature infants. Eighty to 90 percent of infants with symptomatic coarctation have associated cardiac malformations (**complex coarctation**). The infant with severe coarctation may present with absent femoral pulses, differential (lower extremity) cyanosis, or congestive heart failure. Poor lower extremity perfusion and/or heart failure also may be observed in patients with interrupted aortic arch and

in patients with a large aortic thrombus. Clinical deterioration may occur as the ductus arteriosus constricts and lower body perfusion is compromised. Two-dimensional echocardiography will usually establish the diagnosis. Initial therapy is with anticongestive measures. Prostaglandin E_1 infusion to maintain patency of the ductus arteriosus [30,47] may be used in severe cases as preparations are made for cardiac catheterization and/or surgical repair. In infants with symptomatic coarctation and VSD, the coarctation is usually repaired through a left thoracotomy incision, and the patient is observed to determine whether further intervention is necessary. We have not routinely performed balloon dilatation in infants with coarctation because of the high incidence of restenosis and aneurysms.

3. **Interrupted aortic arch (IAA)** is a rare lesion in which there is discontinuity of the aortic arch, and it is usually associated with other cardiovascular malformations and with DiGeorge syndrome. It may present with clinical manifestations that are similar to severe coarctation of the aorta. Fetal echocardiograms have recently detected IAA and severe coarctation in utero. The initial management includes medical palliation with prostaglandin E_1 and management of heart failure and metabolic abnormalities. Surgical reconstruction should be performed as soon as possible, since the mean age of death in unoperated cases is 10 days.
4. **Ventricular septal defect (VSD)** is the most common cause of congestive heart failure after the second week of life, although only 10 percent of all VSDs ever become hemodynamically significant. Moderate to large VSDs become hemodynamically significant as the pulmonary vascular resistance decreases and pulmonary blood flow increases. Premature infants, who have a lower initial pulmonary vascular resistance, tend to develop heart failure earlier than term infants. Two-dimensional echocardiography usually establishes the diagnosis of a VSD. Medical management of congestive heart failure includes digoxin, diuretics, low-sodium formula, and caloric supplementation. Cardiac catheterization and surgery should be performed in infants with persistent evidence of heart failure or pulmonary hypertension. Our surgeons prefer the infant to be more than 2000 gm prior to undertaking primary operative repair of premature infants with a VSD.
5. **Endocardial cushion defect (ECD), ostium primum,** and **common atrioventricular canal defects (CAVC)** account for only 5.5 percent of newborns with severe congenital heart disease. The ECG has a characteristic superior axis with a counterclockwise frontal vector loop. Patients with ostium primum atrial septal defects (ASD) do not usually develop congestive heart failure in infancy unless there is severe mitral insufficiency. Patients with a CAVC (atrial and ventricular septal defects) tend to develop congestive heart failure after the second week of life and may develop irreversible pulmonary vascular obstructive disease in the first year of life. When congestive heart failure can be medically controlled, cardiac catheterization and surgical repair are usually performed electively between 6 and 12 months of age [50]. Patients with Down syndrome are frequently found to have CAVC defects (up to 50 percent have congenital heart disease), so that an ECG is warranted in all patients in whom the diagnosis of Down syndrome is made.
6. **Patent ductus arteriosus (PDA)** occurs in only 5.6 percent of term newborns with congenital heart disease and is associated with coarctation of the aorta and VSD and is a component of vascular rings. Premature infants, mechanically ventilated for respiratory distress syndrome (RDS), commonly show evidence of a PDA as early as the second or third day of life [9]. The earliest manifestation is frequently a harsh systolic ejection murmur heard over the entire precordium, but loudest at the left upper sternal border and left infraclavicular areas. If the PDA persists and as

Table 14-5. Acyanotic cardiac lesions that may result in congestive heart failure

Diagnosis	Physical findings	Onset of heart murmur	Onset of CHF	ECG findings	CXR findings	Associated pathology
Severe AS	SEM and SEC	Birth onward	3 days onward	Usually LVH; RVH if hypoplastic LV	CE with PV congestion	EFE, MS, or MR
Severe coarctation	Decreased femoral pulses; differential cyanosis	Variable	First month	Usually RVH	CE with PV congestion	Bicuspid AoV, VSD, AS, AR
IAA	Decreased femoral pulses; differential cyanosis	Variable	4 days onward	Usually RVH	CE with PV congestion	VSD, PDA, complex CHD, DiGeorge's syndrome
VSD	SRM; MDR	2–3 days onward	Usually 3–6 weeks	RVH or BVH	CE with ↑ PBF	Prematurity; chromosomal anomalies
CAVC	SRM	Birth onward	Usually 3–6 weeks	Superior axis with CCWL, RVH, or BVH	CE with ↑ PBF	Down syndrome; heterotaxy

PDA	Continuous murmur; bounding pulses; hyperdynamic precordium	2–3 days onward	First week onward	RVH normal for age	CE with ↑ PBF	Prematurity
Transient myocardial ischemia	Transient SRM; quiet precordium	Birth	Birth	NSSTTWA	CE with PV congestion	Perinatal asphyxia
Myocarditis	Other signs of infection (e.g., seizures)	Variable	Birth onward	NSSTTWA; arrhythmia (20%)	CE with PV congestion	Perinatal infection
EFE	Muffled heart sounds; gallop rhythm	Variable	Usually in first 6 months	RVH in newborns; LVH in infants	CE with PV congestion	
Pompe's disease (acid maltase deficiency)	Hypotonia and weak cry; protruding tongue	Variable	Usually within 2 months	LAD with LVH; deep q waves; PR < 0.09 second	CE	

Key: CHF = congestive heart failure; ECG = electrocardiogram; CXR = chest x-ray; AS = aortic stenosis; SEM = systolic ejection murmur; SEC = systolic ejection click; LVH = left ventricular hypertrophy; RVH = right ventricular hypertrophy; LV = left ventricle; CE = cardiac enlargement; PV = pulmonary venous; EFE = endocardial fibroelastosis; MS = mitral stenosis; MR = mitral regurgitation; AoV = aortic valve; VSD = ventricular septal defect; AR = aortic regurgitation; IAA = interrupted aortic arch; PDA = patent ductus arteriosus; CHD = congenital heart disease; SRM = systolic regurgitant murmur; MDR = middiastolic murmur; BVH = biventricular hypertrophy; PBF = pulmonary blood flow; CAVC = common atrioventricular canal defect; CCWL = counterclockwise vector loop; NSSTTWA = nonspecific ST-T wave abnormalities; LAD = left axis deviation.

the pulmonary vascular resistance (PVR) decreases over the next few days, the intensity of the murmur increases and later becomes continuou (i.e., extends through the second heart sound), the peripheral pulses in crease in amplitude (increased pulse pressure greater than 25 mmHg bounding pulses), the precordial impulse becomes hyperdynamic, and th patient's respiratory status deteriorates (manifesting as tachypnea or ap nea, carbon dioxide retention, and an increasing mechanical ventilatio requirement). As the patient develops CHF from a hemodynamically sig nificant PDA, the liver enlarges and extends more than 3 cm below th right costal margin, while serial chest x-rays show an increase in hear size and the lungs may appear more radiopaque. This typical progressio of clinical signs does not occur in every patient with a hemodynamicall significant PDA. Conversely, other lesions may produce bounding pulses a hyperdynamic precordium, and cardiac enlargement (e.g., an arterio venous fistula or an aorticopulmonary window). Generally, however, th clinical assessment of a premature infant with the typical findings of a hemodynamically significant PDA are adequate to guide therapeutic de cisions. If the diagnosis is in doubt, a two-dimensional echocardiogram will usually clarify the anatomic diagnosis.

In a collaborative study [26] that involved 13 centers and enrolled 355 low-birth-weight infants (between 500 and 1750 gm), 21 percent had a hemodynamically significant PDA. Based on this study, indomethacin is now the treatment of choice for medical treatment of PDA. In this study 79 percent of significant PDAs closed with indomethacin. Those that di not respond at all underwent surgical ligation. Birth weight did not affec the efficacy of indomethacin, and there was no increase in complication associated with surgery after unsuccessful indomethacin therapy.

Prophylactic administration of indomethacin does not appear beneficia [31,41]. Owing to the low risk of indomethacin therapy, we recommenc treatment of *mechanically ventilated infants* with indomethacin when a PDA first becomes apparent. Up to three doses of intravenous indometh acin (Table 14-6) may be administered. We recommend that asymptom atic premature infants less than 34 weeks' postconceptional age who *do not require mechanical ventilation* or supplemental oxygen be treatec with indomethacin only after cardiovascular or respiratory signs of a he modynamically significant PDA develop [16]. Some infants who fail to respond to the first course of treatment with indomethacin may responc to a second course. Contraindications to use of indomethacin are listed ir Table 14-7. Early closure of PDA by either indomethacin or surgical li gation may decrease the duration of mechanical ventilation and incidence of bronchopulmonary dysplasia. Two-dimensional echocardiography to confirm diagnosis should be performed prior to surgical ligation of a he modynamically significant PDA.

7. **Transient myocardial ischemia** with myocardial dysfunction should be suspected in any neonate with a history of perinatal asphyxia. A tricuspid or mitral regurgitant murmur may be heard. A serum creatine kinase MB fraction greater than 5 to 10 percent may be helpful in determining the

Table 14-6. Dose of intravenous indomethacin in premature infants with PDA

	Dose (12–18 hour intervals)	
Age	Initial	Second and third
<48 hours	0.2 mg/kg	0.1 mg/kg
2–7 days	0.2 mg/kg	0.2 mg/kg
>7 days	0.2 mg/kg	0.25 mg/kg

Table 14-7. Contraindications for indomethacin in infants with PDA

BUN $\geq$ 30 mg/dl
Serum creatinine $\geq$ 1.8 mg/dl
Total urine output $\leq$ 0.6 ml/kg/per hour over preceding 8 hours
Platelet count < 60,000/mm^3
Stool hematest > 3+ (or moderate to large)
Evidence of bleeding diathesis
Clinical or radiographic evidence of necrotizing enterocolitis
Evidence of enlarging intraventricular hemorrhage

Key: PDA = patent ductus arteriosus; BUN = blood urea nitrogen.
Source: Adapted from W. M. Gersony et al., Effects of indomethacin in premature infants with patent ductus arteriosus: Results of national collaborative study. *J. Pediatr.* 102; 895, 1983.

presence of myocardial damage [44]. Treatment is dictated by the severity of the myocardial dysfunction. Care must be taken with volume administration [11] because this may actually worsen the patient's condition. (See Chapter 21.)

8. **Myocarditis** is usually the result of a viral infection acquired by the infant perinatally. Enterovirus [12], rubella, varicella, and other viruses have been shown to cause myocarditis and myocardial necrosis. Severe bacterial infections also may cause a myocarditis. Myocardial dysfunction may be associated with maternal autoimmune disease such as systemic lupus erythematosus (SLE). Careful initiation of anticongestive therapy, digoxin and diuretics, may be helpful.
9. Cardiomyopathies such as Pompe's disease, the cardiomyopathy associated with maternal diabetes, primary myocarditis, and idiopathic hypertrophic subaortic stenosis may be rare causes of myocardial dysfunction.

D. **Cyanosis.** Differentiation of cardiac from respiratory causes of cyanosis in the neonatal intensive care unit is a common problem. After an initial clinical assessment and stabilization of the infant, an arterial blood gas should be obtained in 100% oxygen. A chest x-ray, ECG, and hematocrit should be examined. If an obvious pulmonary etiology is not apparent from the client chest x-ray and hypoxemia (PO_2 < 100 mmHg) persists, then simultaneous pre- and postductal arterial blood gases should be obtained to determine whether there is right-to-left shunting through the ductus arteriosus (persistent pulmonary hypertension, critical coarctation, or interrupted aortic arch). Early use of the hyperoxia test in an infant with progressive pulmonary disease may be helpful in assessing the neonate suspected of having cyanotic congenital heart disease. If the arterial PO_2 is greater than 200 mmHg in 100% oxygen, then cyanotic congenital heart disease may generally be excluded from the differential diagnosis.

1. **Cyanotic CHD** (PO_2 < 50 mmHg in 100% oxygen). Infants with profound cyanosis and a normal to low PCO_2 should be evaluated for cyanotic congenital heart disease. A scheme for the initial clinical evaluation is outlined in Table 14-8 [21].
   a. **D-Transposition of the great arteries (D-TGA)** is the most common form of cyanotic congenital heart disease presenting in the neonatal period. In D-TGA the aorta arises from the right ventricle and the pulmonary artery from the left ventricle. Associated cardiac anomalies such as ventricular septal defects, patent ductus arteriosus, coarctation of the aorta, and hypoplastic right ventricle are common. In D-TGA with an **intact ventricular septum (IVS),** the pulmonary and systemic circuits are in parallel instead of in series. Survival of the

Table 14-8. Cyanotic congenital heart disease presenting with PaO_2 less than 50 mmHg

Diagnosis	Heart murmur	ECG findings	CXR findings
D-TGA with IVS	None	RVH normal for age	No CE with ↑ PBF
TAPVR with PV obstruction	None	RVH	PV congestion
Ebstein's anomaly	± TR murmur	RAE, RBBB, WPW	Massive CE; normal or ↓ PBF
Tricuspid atresia with PS or PA	± PS murmur	Superior axis, LVH	No CE with ↓ PBF
PA with IVS	± TR murmur, ± continuous murmur	LVH, QRS axis 0–90 degrees	± CE with ↓ PBF
Severe PS	PS murmur	RVH, QRS axis 0–90 degrees	± CE with ↓ PBF
Severe TOF	PS murmur	RVH	No CE with ↓ PBF
TOF with PA	± Continuous murmur	RVH	No CE with ↓ PBF

Key: ECG = electrocardiogram; CXR = chest x-ray; D-TGA = D-transposition of the great arteries; IVS = intact ventricular septum; RVH = right ventricular hypertrophy; CE = cardiac enlargement; PBF = pulmonary blood flow; TAPVR = total anomalous pulmonary venous return; PV = pulmonary venous; TR = tricuspid regurgitation; LVH = left ventricular hypertrophy; RAE = right atrial enlargement; RBBB = right bundle branch block; WPW = Wolff-Parkinson-White syndrome; PS = pulmonary stenosis; PA = pulmonary atresia; LVH = left ventricular hypertrophy; TOF = tetralogy of Fallot; ↑ = increased; ↓ = decreased; ± = present or absent.
Source: Adapted from M. D. Freed, Congenital Cardiac Malformations. In M. E. Avery and H. W. Taeusch (eds.), *Schaffer's Diseases of the Newborn,* 5th Ed. Philadelphia: Saunders, 1984.

infant depends on mixing of systemic and pulmonary venous blood at some level, usually through a restrictive patent foramen ovale. The diagnosis of D-TGA with IVS should be suspected in any term neonate with profound cyanosis, clear lung fields with increased to normal pulmonary blood flow on chest x-ray, and a normal ECG. Two-dimensional echocardiography will usually confirm the diagnosis. Cardiac catheterization with balloon atrial septostomy should be performed to improve intraatrial mixing of blood and systemic oxygenation. Prostaglandin E_1 infusion may temporarily improve the oxygenation if there is adequate decompression of the left atrium. Surgical atrial septal defect creation or early "repair" (great artery switch, Senning or Mustard procedure) may be performed if adequate palliation by balloon atrial septostomy to maintain an arterial saturation greater than 55 to 60 percent is not achieved. We prefer to perform a primary great artery switch procedure during the first 2 weeks of life, with reimplantation of the coronary arteries into the neoaortic root. A great artery switch procedure performed after 2 weeks requires preparatory banding of the pulmonary artery to prepare the left ventricle for the systemic pressure load.

b. Total anomalous pulmonary venous return (TAPVR) is an uncommon lesion that is surgically correctable, but it is often initially misdiagnosed as pulmonary disease. In TAPVR, the pulmonary venous return is to the systemic venous system. The time and severity of presentation depend on the presence or absence of pulmonary venous obstruction. Infants with TAPVR without pulmonary venous obstruction usually present after the neonatal period with mild cyanosis and congestive heart failure. Infants with TAPVR and pulmonary venous obstruction may present in the first week of life with profound cyanosis, pulmonary venous congestion, and poor perfusion. The chest x-ray may show pulmonary venous congestion with a "ground glass" opacification of the lungs fields. Two-dimensional echocardiography will usually establish the diagnosis [13]. Surgical repair should be performed as soon as possible and may be performed without cardiac catheterization. Prostaglandin E_1 infusion is generally not helpful in patients with TAPVR with pulmonary venous obstruction and may precipitate pulmonary edema.

c. **Ebstein's anomaly** is an uncommon lesion in which there is "downward" displacement of the tricuspid valve and "atrialization" of a portion of the right ventricle. In severe Ebstein's anomaly there is marked cardiac enlargement on chest x-ray owing to massive right atrial enlargement. Tricuspid stenosis and/or regurgitation may cause marked right-to-left atrial shunting. Two-dimensional echocardiography provides the best means of confirming the clinical diagnosis. Prostaglandin E_1 infusion may be used in the profoundly cyanotic infant to augment pulmonary blood flow until regression of the pulmonary vascular resistance occurs. Ebstein's anomaly is often associated with Wolff-Parkinson-White syndrome and supraventricular tachycardia. The prognosis is guarded for infants with Ebstein's anomaly who present with profound cyanosis in the neonatal period.

d. **Tricuspid atresia** consists of complete absence of the right atrioventricular connection and absence to severe hypoplasia of the right ventricle. The ECG shows a superior axis with a counterclockwise frontal vector loop and left ventricular hypertrophy in over 80 percent of patients. Most infants with tricuspid atresia have an associated VSD, allowing blood to pass from the left ventricle to the right ventricular outflow and pulmonary arteries. Thus a neonate with profound cyanosis and tricuspid atresia usually has associated pulmonary stenosis or atresia limiting pulmonary blood flow. Prostaglandin E_1 infusion may be used to augment pulmonary blood flow in severely cyanotic infants with tricuspid atresia until surgery can be performed.

e. **Pulmonary atresia with intact ventricular septum (PA with IVS)** consists of pulmonary valvar or infundibular atresia and varying degrees of right ventricular and tricuspid valve hypoplasia. Associated cardiovascular lesions include coronary artery–myocardial sinusoidal communications, a lesion that markedly compromises long-term survival. Tricuspid regurgitation is usually present. There is an obligatory right-to-left shunt at the atrial level, and pulmonary blood flow is dependent on a PDA. Prostaglandin E_1 infusion will improve oxygenation until surgery can be performed.

f. **Severe pulmonary stenosis (PS)** is usually valvar and associated with muscular hyperplasia of the right ventricle. There may be marked right-to-left atrial shunting. Severe PS in the neonate may show one of two ECG patterns: (1) left or biventricular hypertrophy with a QRS axis of -10 to 100 degrees or (2) right ventricular hypertrophy with right-axis deviation. Prostaglandin E_1 infusion may be needed to palliate the infant until cardiac catheterization and pulmonary valvotomy can be performed. Transcatheter balloon valvotomy has become the treatment of choice for this lesion at our institution [59].

g. **Severe tetralogy of Fallot (TOF)** consists of infundibular PS or PA, malalignment-type VSD, "overriding" aorta, and right ventricular hypertrophy. TOF may be associated with an absent pulmonary valve,

PDA, ASD, absence of the ductus arteriosus, right aortic arch (19 percent), origin of the left anterior descending coronary artery from the right coronary artery (5 to 7 percent), tracheoesophageal fistula, Down syndrome, Noonan's syndrome, rubella syndrome, and multiple congenital anomalies. There is right-to-left shunting at the ventricular level; the degree of cyanosis depends on the severity of the PS. Pulmonary blood flow may be dependent on a PDA or pulmonary collateral vessels. Absence of a pulmonary stenosis murmur suggests PA. Prostaglandin E_1 infusion may palliate the infant until cardiac catheterization and/or surgery can be performed. Failure to respond to prostaglandin E_1 infusion may be due to absence of the ductus arteriosus [9].

2. **Cyanosis with congestive heart failure** ($PO_2 < 150$ mmHg in 100% oxygen). Clinical differentiation of these lesions with arterial hypoxemia and congestive heart failure in the first month of life is difficult. There is usually increased pulmonary blood flow, cardiac enlargement, and an obligatory mixing of pulmonary and systemic venous blood within the heart. The differential diagnosis includes hypoplastic left heart syndrome, truncus arteriosus, single ventricle, TAPVR without significant obstruction, D-TGA with a VSD, and tricuspid atresia with increased pulmonary blood flow.
   a. **Hypoplastic left heart syndrome (HLH)** accounts for 6.6 percent of infants with severe congenital heart disease and is one of the most common lesions presenting in the first week of life. The syndrome includes malformations producing similar hemodynamic manifestations: aortic atresia, mitral atresia, premature closure of the foramen ovale, hypoplastic left ventricle with critical mitral stenosis or AS, or aortic atresia. These lesions reduce or eliminate blood flow through the left side of the heart, cause an obligatory left-to-right shunt at the atrial level, and a right-to-left shunt at the ductal level. Constriction of the ductus arteriosus may rapidly result in hypotension and shock. Prostaglandin E_1 infusion may palliate the infant until the diagnosis is established. In the past, no surgical treatment was available. Recently, experimental surgery [46] has met with increasing success, with 3-year survival approaching 50 percent [33].
   b. **Truncus arteriosus** consists of a single arterial vessel arising from the base of the heart from which arises the coronary, systemic, and pulmonary arteries. Associated cardiovascular anomalies include truncal valve stenosis or regurgitation, right aortic arch (34 percent), coarctation or IAA, PS, and inconsistent coronary artery anatomy [10]. There is a frequent association with DiGeorge syndrome. Pulmonary blood flow is usually excessive, and the infants tend to develop congestive heart failure in the second week of life. Medical anticongestive therapy and supplemental nutritional support may be helpful. Palliative or reparative surgery is usually required in the first year of life because of intractable congestive heart failure and to avoid the development of pulmonary vascular obstructive disease.
3. **Pulmonary disorders responsible for cyanosis** (see Chap. 13).
   a. **Primary lung disease** causing alveolar hypoventilation, decreased lung compliance, ventilation-perfusion inequality, intrapulmonary right-to-left shunts, or increased diffusion distance may produce varying degrees of cyanosis in the neonate. The patient is usually in respiratory distress, and carbon dioxide retention is characteristic. The patient will usually increase the arterial PO_2 to more than 150 to 200 mmHg in 100% oxygen with adequate ventilation, has a normal ECG for age, and has evidence of lung disease on chest x-ray. The differential diagnosis includes the following:
      (1) Transient tachypnea of the newborn.
      (2) Aspiration syndromes (e.g., meconium and blood)

(3) RDS
(4) Pneumonia
(5) Pulmonary hemorrhage
(6) BPD
(7) Atelectasis
(8) Pulmonary lymphangiectasia
(9) Wilson-Mikity syndrome
(10) Cystic adenomatoid malformation
(11) Pulmonary hypoplasia or aplasia

b. **Airway obstruction** causes mechanical interference with ventilation and results in alveolar hypoventilation. The patient is usually in obvious respiratory distress, and stridor may be present. Physical examination may reveal the source of the airway obstruction. The chest x-ray may show a right aortic arch or anterior mediastinal calcifications. The ECG is usually normal for age. The patient's PO_2 will usually increase above 150 mmHg in 100% oxygen with adequate ventilation (e.g., an oral airway or endotracheal intubation). The differential diagnosis includes the following:
(1) Choanal stenosis or atresia
(2) Pierre-Robin syndrome
(3) Macroglossia
(4) Thyroid goiter
(5) Cystic hygroma
(6) Vocal cord paralysis
(7) Laryngomalacia
(8) Laryngeal web
(9) Subglottic hemangioma, stenosis, or hematoma
(10) Vascular ring or pulmonary sling
(11) Tracheomalacia
(12) Tracheoesophageal fistula
(13) Tracheal or bronchial stenosis
(14) Mucus plug
(15) Mediastinal masses (e.g., thymoma or teratoma)

c. **Extrinsic compression of the lungs** may cause mechanical interference with ventilation. The patient is usually in respiratory distress. The ECG is usually normal for age, and the chest x-ray is often diagnostic. The PO_2 generally improves markedly following treatment of the underlying disorder. The differential diagnosis includes the following:
(1) Pneumothorax
(2) Pulmonary interstitial or lobar emphysema
(3) Chylothorax or other pleural effusion
(4) Congenital diaphragmatic hernia (CDH)
(5) Thoracic dystrophies or dysplasia

d. **Central nervous system (CNS) or neuromuscular diseases** (See Chapter 21) may cause alveolar hypoventilation. The patient's respiratory efforts are slow, diminished, or absent. Other signs of nervous system dysfunction may be apparent. The patient's PO_2 will generally increase above 150 mmHg in 100% oxygen with adequate ventilation. The chest x-ray and ECG are generally normal, but secondary atelectasis or pneumonia may occur. The differential diagnosis includes the following:
(1) Drug-induced depression of respiratory drive
(2) Postasphyxial cerebral dysfunction
(3) Intraventricular hemorrhage
(4) Subarachnoid hemorrhage
(5) Subdural hematoma
(6) Meningitis
(7) Sepsis and shock

(8) Encephalitis
(9) Seizure
(10) Intracranial malformations
(11) Phrenic nerve paralysis
(12) Neuromuscular disorders (e.g., neonatal myasthenia gravis)
(13) Hypoglycemia

4. **Cyanosis with normal PO_2**

a. **Methemoglobinemia** causes reduced blood oxygen-carrying capacity owing to an abnormal hemoglobin or to enzyme abnormalities. The patient is cyanotic without respiratory or cardiac signs and has a normal arterial pO_2 even with the existing cyanosis. In addition, the blood does not become bright red when exposed to air (e.g., when a drop of blood is allowed to dry on a piece of filter paper). Neonates with cyanosis due to methemoglobinemia should be treated with methylene blue (1.0 mg/kg as a 1% solution in normal saline). A rapid decrease in cyanosis over 1 to 2 hours suggests a toxic etiology or an autosomal-recessive nicotinamide adenine dinucleotide (NADH)–methemoglobin reductase deficiency. Failure to respond to methylene blue implies an associated glucose-6-phosphate dehydrogenase (G-6-PD) deficiency or the autosomal-dominant hemoglobin M. Toxic causes of methemoglobinemia in neonates include the following:

(1) Nitrate or nitrite ingestion from well water or certain vegetables (e.g., carrots)
(2) Aniline dyes
(3) Prilocaine

b. **Polycythemia** may produce an apparent cyanosis despite a normal oxygen saturation if increased viscosity and capillary stasis occurs. The patient may be an infant of a diabetic mother, is usually plethoric and asymptomatic, but may manifest respiratory distress, convulsions, CHF, persistent pulmonary hypertension (PPH), priapism, or renal vein thrombosis. The chest x-ray, ECG, and arterial blood gases are usually normal (see Chapter 18.)

c. **Altered capillary blood flow** due to exposure to cold

IV. **Medical management of patients with congenital heart disease (CHD).** The medical management of these neonates may be separated into the management of patients with a ductal-dependent circulation or the management of congestive heart failure and its sequelae.

A. **Prostaglandin E_1.** (See Appendix A) Among newborns with cyanotic CHD resulting in decreased pulmonary blood flow, the patency of the ductus arteriosus may be important to their survival until they receive definitive medical or surgical therapy. Infants with poor mixing (D-TGA) and left-sided obstructive lesions also may benefit from therapy to keep the ductus open. The use of prostaglandin E_1 (PGE_1) infusion in these neonates improves oxygenation, perfusion, and acid-base balance. PGE_1 infusions have been used in coarctation of the aorta, Ebstein's anomaly, hypoplastic left heart syndrome, IAA, pulmonary atresia or stenosis (with or without a VSD), severe TOF, D-TGA, tricuspid atresia, and tricuspid insufficiency. Since PGE_1 infusions may make some conditions worse (e.g., TAPVR with pulmonary venous obstruction), its use in transport should be limited to those infants in whom poor perfusion, acidosis, or profound cyanosis ($PO_2 < 25$ mmHg, arterial hemoglobin saturation < 60 percent) precludes a safe transport or a clearly established diagnosis at the referring hospital indicates the need for PGE_1 therapy. All such patients should be intubated prior to leaving the referring hospital, since 10 to 12 percent of infants treated with PGE_1 will develop apnea. A separate intravenous line should be started for volume administration, since 4 percent of these infants develop hypotension with PGE_1 administration. Our usual starting dose of PGE_1 is 0.05 μg/kg per minute. Our pharmacy dispenses PGE_1, 20 μg/ml, in a 10-ml vial to be prepared prior to use as follows:

PGE_1 (Prostin VR Pediatric R) 10 ml of 20 μg/ml + 30 ml 5% D/W = 40 ml (5 μg/ml) infused at 0.6 ml/kg per hour = 0.05 μg/kg per minute. The dose may be increased to 0.1 μg/kg/minute (see pages 295, 625). If mixed from the standard vial (500 μg/ml), 1 ml of 500 μg/ml + 100 ml of 5% D/W = 5 μg/ml.

Once an effect has been achieved, the effect may often be maintained by an infusion rate of 0.01 μg/ng/minute. The dose is titrated to the response of the infant. Reconstituted PGE_1 expires within 24 hours. The response to PGE_1 is often immediate if patency of the ductus arteriosus is important to the infant. Failure to respond to PGE_1 may mean that the initial diagnosis was incorrect, the ductus was unresponsive to PGE_1 (e.g., in an older infant), or the ductus is absent. The infusion site has no significant effect on the ductal response to PGE_1 infusion. Other adverse reactions to PGE_1 include fever (14 percent), seizures (4 percent), cutaneous flushing (10 percent), bradycardia (7 percent), tachycardia (3 percent), cardiac arrest (1 percent), and edema (1 percent).

B. Treatment of CHF should not only improve inadequate cardiac output and tissue perfusion caused by a hemodynamically significant cardiovascular lesion, but also reduce pulmonary congestion. This may be achieved by increasing myocardial contractility, decreasing preload, or decreasing myocardial afterload. Digoxin remains the mainstay of chronic anticongestive therapy. Sympathomimetic amines may be used for acute management of CHF. Diuretics, caloric supplementation, and fluid (120 to 150 ml/kg per day) and sodium restriction (e.g., breast milk or a low sodium formula) may be sequentially added (see Chapter 30). Other measures include reducing the infant's energy expenditure (maintaining the infant in a thermoneutral environment and gavage feedings) and improving tissue oxygenation (supplemental oxygen to maintain an arterial PO_2 at 60 to 80 mmHg and maintaining a hematocrit above 40 percent). Supplemental oxygen also may decrease myocardial workload by decreasing the pulmonary vascular resistance. Although afterload-reduction therapy is commonly used in older children and adults, it is uncommonly used in neonatal intensive care units.

1. **Digoxin** (See Appendix A) remains the cornerstone in the treatment of CHF in the neonate, although it may be of little benefit to the premature infant with PDA [6]. Term infants can usually be safely treated with a total dose of 30 μg/kg; premature infants can usually be effectively digitalized with a total dose of 20 μg/kg [6,48,56]. One-half of this **total digitalizing dose (TDD)** may be given IV, IM, or PO, followed by one-fourth of the TDD every eight to twelve hours for the remaining two doses. An initial maintenance dose of one-fourth to one-third of the TDD (range 5 to 10 μg/kg per day) may then be adjusted according to the patient's clinical response and tolerance for the drug (Table 14-9). When oral digoxin is used, we prefer the pediatric Lanoxin preparation (50 μ/ml). When converting from an established oral to parenteral dose, 75 percent of the oral dose should be used. Lead II ECGs should be obtained prior to each dose for the first few days of digoxin therapy, and the digoxin should be withheld for signs of toxicity (PR interval greater than 0.14 seconds or arrhythmias, including sinus bradycardia < 100 beats per minute). Serum electrolytes and calcium should be monitored, especially when digoxin is administered with a diuretic. Infants with mild CHF or primary myocardial disease, who may have increased sensitivity to digoxin toxicity, may

Table 14-9. Digoxin dosage

	TDD	Maintenance
Premature infants	20 μg/kg	5 μg/kg/per day
Term infants	30 μg/kg	8–10 ug/kg/per day

be digitalized using only the maintenance dose (omitting the loading dose). Digoxin therapy may be used in conjunction with a low-sodium formula, caloric supplementation, diuretics and fluid restriction.

Infants suspected of having digoxin toxicity should have a digoxin level drawn (a level less than 2.0 μg/ml virtually excludes toxicity). Digoxin toxicity in neonates is usually manageable by withholding further doses until the signs of toxicity resolve and by correcting the predisposing factors such as hypokalemia. Severe ventricular arrhythmias associated with digoxin toxicity may be managed with phenytoin, 2 to 4 mg/kg over 5 minutes, or lidocaine, 1 mg/kg loading dose, followed by an infusion at 1 to 2 mg/kg per hour. Atrioventricular block may be treated with atrophine (0.01 mg/kg IV, repeated as needed). Severe dysrhythmias (including severe bradycardia in the presence of a high digoxin level) may be refractory to these therapies and require temporary cardiac pacing or the use of digoxin antibody preparation (Digibind).

2. **Diuretics** (see Appendix A) should be used in patients with CHF that is refractory to digoxin therapy alone. Oral or intravenous potassium supplementation (3 to 4 mEq/kg per day) or an aldosterone antagonist should accompany the use of thiazide or "loop" diuretics. Diuretics most commonly used in the nursery are

   Chlorothiazide (Diuril), 5 to 40 mg/kg per day, PO divided bid
   Furosemide (Lasix), 1 to 2 mg/kg per dose, IV or PO q24 h in a premature q12h in a term infant
   Spironolactone (Aldactone), 2 to 3 mg/kg per day, PO in a single daily dose

   Intravenous furosemide, 1 to 2 mg/kg per dose, usually results in a brisk diuresis within an hour of administration. If no response is noted in an hour, a second dose (double the first dose) may be given. Chronic use of furosemide may produce urinary tract stones as a result of its calciuric effects. Nephrocalcinosis may be monitored radiographically or by ultrasound. A more potent diuretic effect may be achieved using a combination of a thiazide and a "loop" diuretic. Combination diuretic therapy may be complicated by hyponatremia and hypokalemia. When changing from an effective parenteral to oral dose of furosemide, the dose should be increased by 50 to 80 percent. Furosemide may increase the nephro- and ototoxicity of concurrently used aminoglycoside antibiotics.

3. **Sympathomimetic amine infusions** (see Chapter 6) are used to improve myocardial performance and are indicated for the treatment of shock (hypoperfusion syndrome), especially when accompanied by hypotension and severe CHF requiring parenteral support. Patients should be closely monitored, usually with an electrocardiographic monitor and an arterial catheter. When appropriate, the intravascular volume should be repleted, with care being given not to fluid overload the already precariously balanced cardiovascular system. **Dopamine** (Intropin) is a precursor of norepinephrine and stimulates beta-1, dopaminergic, and alpha-adrenergic receptors in a dose-specific manner. Dopamine can be expected to increase mean arterial pressure, improve ventricular function, and improve urine output with a low incidence of side effects at doses less than 10 μg/kg per minute. A combination of low-dose dopamine ($\leq$5 μg/kg per minute) and **dobutamine** (Dobutrex) or **isoproterenol** (Isuprel) may be used to minimize the potential peripheral vasoconstriction induced by high doses of dopamine while maximizing the dopaminergic effects on the renal circulation. Dobutamine is an analogue of dopamine, with predominantly beta-1 effects and relatively weak beta-2 and alpha-receptor stimulating activity. Dobutamine, in comparison with dopamine, lacks the direct renal vasodilating properties, has less chronotropic effect in adult patients, and does not depend on norepinephrine release from peripheral nerves for its effect. There are little published data available concerning

the use of dobutamine in neonates, although clinical experience has been favorable. **Isoproterenol,** a beta-adrenergic receptor agonist, improves ventricular function, increases heart rate, and induces peripheral vasodilation. Isoproterenol alone should probably not be used in the treatment of hypotensive cardiogenic shock because of its peripheral vasodilator properties. **Epinephrine** is a potent alpha- and beta-adrenergic receptor agonist that is commonly used in cardiopulmonary resuscitation (0.1 ml/kg of 1:10,000 solution), IV, endotracheally, or rarely, by intracardiac injection. Although epinephrine is rarely the inotropic drug of choice, it may be useful in situations of overwhelming disease in which maximal doses of the more commonly used inotropic agents have failed to produce the desired effect. Epinephrine may be started at 0.05 μg/kg per minute and increased up to 1.0 μg/kg per minute. The epinephrine infusion should be combined with a peripheral vasodilator. Convenient initial infusions of the commonly used inotropic agents are shown below and in Tables 14-10 and 14-11.

Dopamine, 2 to 25 μg/kg per minute (inactivated by alkaline solution), 0.75 ml of 40 mg/ml solution + 100 ml 5% D/W = 30 mg/dl (See Table 14–10.)
Dobutamine, 2 to 15 μg/kg per minute, 2.5 ml of 12 mg/ml solution + 100 ml 5% D/W = 30 mg/dl (See Table 14–10.)
Isoproterenol, 0.05 to 0.5 μg/kg per minute (titrated to keep the heart rate less than 200 beats/min), 3.0 ml of 0.2 mg/ml solution + 100 ml 5% D/W = 0.6 mg/dl (See Table 14–10.)

These infusions may be modified to meet the individual requirements of the patient. A quick check of the dosage may be obtained using the following formula:

$$\text{Dose } (\mu\text{g/kg}) \text{ per minute} = \frac{\text{concentration (mg/dl)} \times \text{rate (ml/hour)}}{6 \times \text{weight (kg)}}$$

Table 14-10. Dopamine and dobutamine infusion rates and dosages

Rate (ml/kg per hour) of above dopamine and dobutamine solutions	Dose (ug/kg per minute)
0.5	2.5
1.0	5
2.0	10
3.0	15
4.0	20

Table 14-11. Isoproterenol infusion rates and dosages

Rate (ml/kg per hour) of above isoproterenol solutions	Dose(ug/kg/per minute)
0.5	0..05
1.0	0.10
2.0	0.20
3.0	0.30
4.0	0.40

4. **Vasodilators** (see Chapter 6) act to improved cardiac output and pulmonary congestion by decreasing ventricular afterload and preload. Vasodilators may be especially useful in infants with congestive cardiomyopathies [3], in whom conduction disturbances may occur with low doses of digoxin. Additional benefit may be achieved with a combination of inotropic and vasodilator therapy. While there is very little published experience using vasodilators in premature neonates [4], vasodilators are potentially beneficial. These drugs should be used in cooperation with a pediatric cardiologist. Patients should initially be closely monitored, with an ECG monitor and arterial and central venous catheters. **Sodium nitroprusside** (Nipride) is a direct arteriolar and venodilator that has been used extensively in adults and children with myocardial dysfunction. Nitroprusside has a short half-life of 1 to 2 minutes, is given by continuous infusion, with the dose (0.5 to 6.0 μg/kg per minute) adjusted to improve cardiac output, tissue perfusion, and urine output without causing hypotension. Its effect dissipates within minutes of discontinuation. The intravascular volume should be repleted using the central venous pressure as a guide. Cyanide levels should be checked within 48 hours of starting nitroprusside infusion, since nitroprusside is metabolized to thiocyanate, which is renally excreted. **Captopril** (0.05 to 0.5 mg/kg per dose, po q6–24h) is an angiotensin-converting enzyme inhibitor effective for chronic afterload reduction. **Hydralazine** (0.1 to 1 mg/kg per dose q4–6h) is a direct arteriolar vasodilator that may be used to specifically reduce afterload. It is seldom used as the initial vasodilator because it has a long half-life and chronic use may produce a lupus-like syndrome. **Amrinone** (5 to 10 μg/kg per minute) is a relatively new bipyridine compound that is a phosphodiesterase inhibitor, inducing increases in cAMP [2]. Amrinone increases inward flux of calcium, enhancing myocardial contractility, and causes a peripheral vasodilation. Amrinone may have a pronounced negative inotropic effect in some newborn animals [7,51], and thus it is not widely used in the newborn.

V. **Electrocardiography.** The ECG records electrical depolarizations of the myocardium and in the neonate reflects the chamber relationships that existed in utero. When interpreting an ECG, the following determinations should be made (1) rate and rhythm; (2) axis: P, QRS, and T (a quick assessment of the frontal plane axes may be obtained by examining orthogonal leads I and aV_F); (3) intervals: PR, QRS, QT, and QTc = $QT\sqrt{R\text{-}R}$; (4) ventricular loop (*q* waves in the left lateral precordial leads may not be apparent until V_{6-8}) or L loop (*q* waves in the right precordial leads); (5) evidence for chamber enlargement or hypertrophy; (6) evidence for pericardial disease, ischemia, infarction, metabolic abnormalities, and drug effect; (7) confirmation of lead placement (complexes in leads I and V_6 usually have a similar morphology if the limb leads have been properly placed); and (8) how the ECG pattern fits with the clinical picture. The criteria for interpretation are based on normal values, which are shown in Figures 14-1 to 14-21 [14]. The ECG of the "normal" premature infant is somewhat different from that of the term infant [39,43]. The differences are discussed in **V.A.**

A. **ECG in premature infants**

1. **The ECG rhythm** is primarily a sinus rhythm with marked sinus bradycardia as low as 50 beats per minute, including nodal escape beats during sleep and with defecation. Atrial dysrhythmias are common and typically decrease in frequency with maturation.
2. **QRS complex**
   a. The QRS axis is directed more leftward, and there is a wider range of QRS axes than in the term infant.
   b. The QRS amplitude is generally lower in premature infants, presumably because of the small ventricular mass.
   c. The precordial leads show less right ventricular dominance than in term infants, and with growth, the QRS pattern changes toward an "adult-type" pattern more rapidly than in term infants.

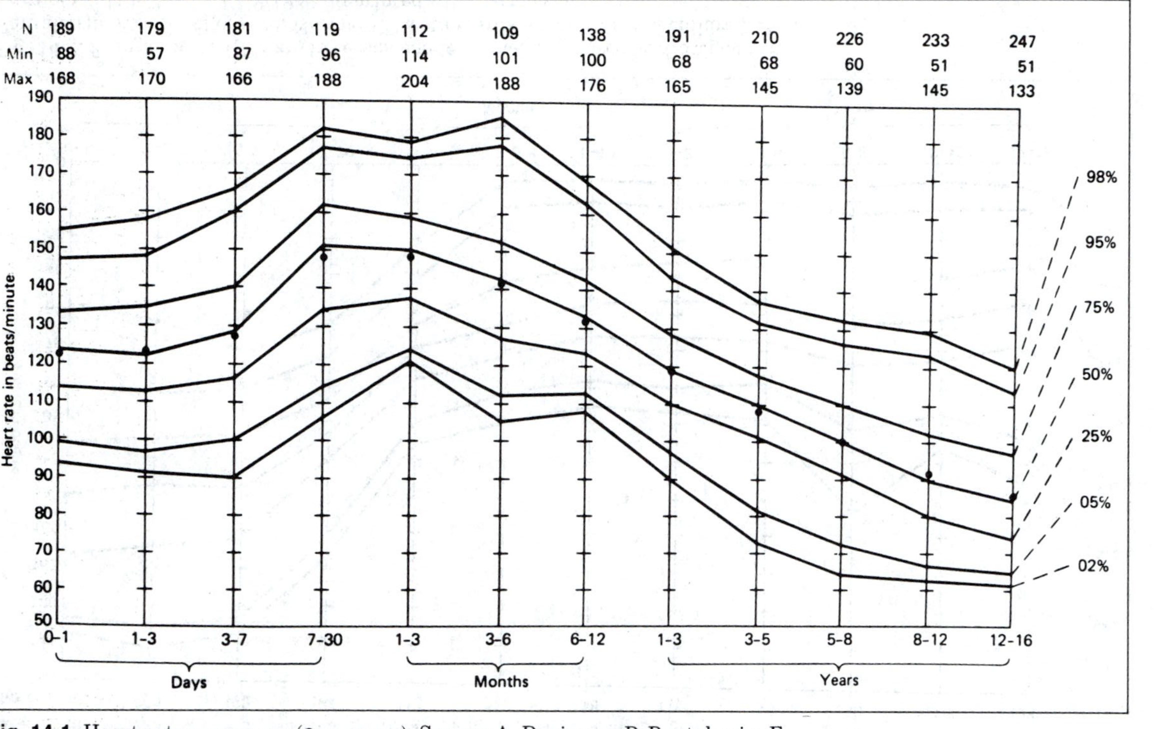

Fig. 14-1. Heart rate versus age (● = mean). Source: A. Davignon, P. Rautaharju, E. Boisselle, et al. Normal ECG standards for infants and children, *Ped. Cardiology* 1: 123–131, 1979/1980. Reprinted with permission.

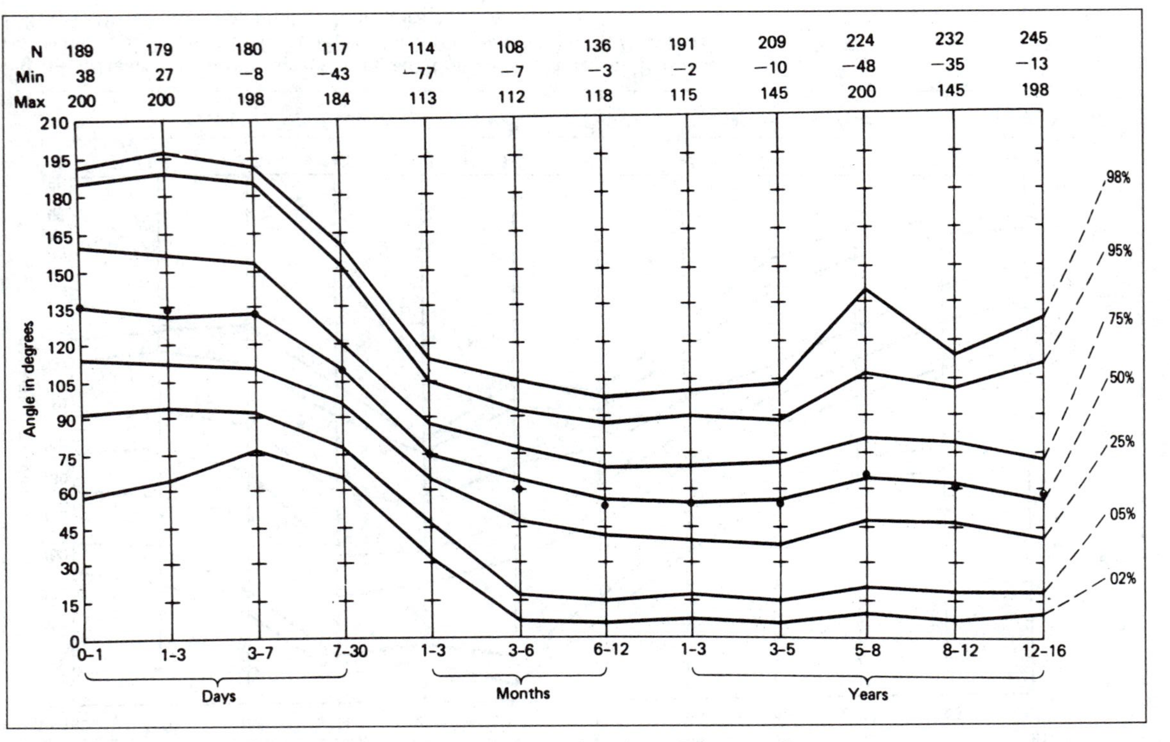

Fig. 14-2. Frontal plane QRS angle versus age (● = mean). Source: A. Davignon, P. Rautaharju, E. Boisselle, et al. Normal ECG standards for infants and children, *Ped. Cardiology* 1: 123–131, 1979/1980. Reprinted with permission.

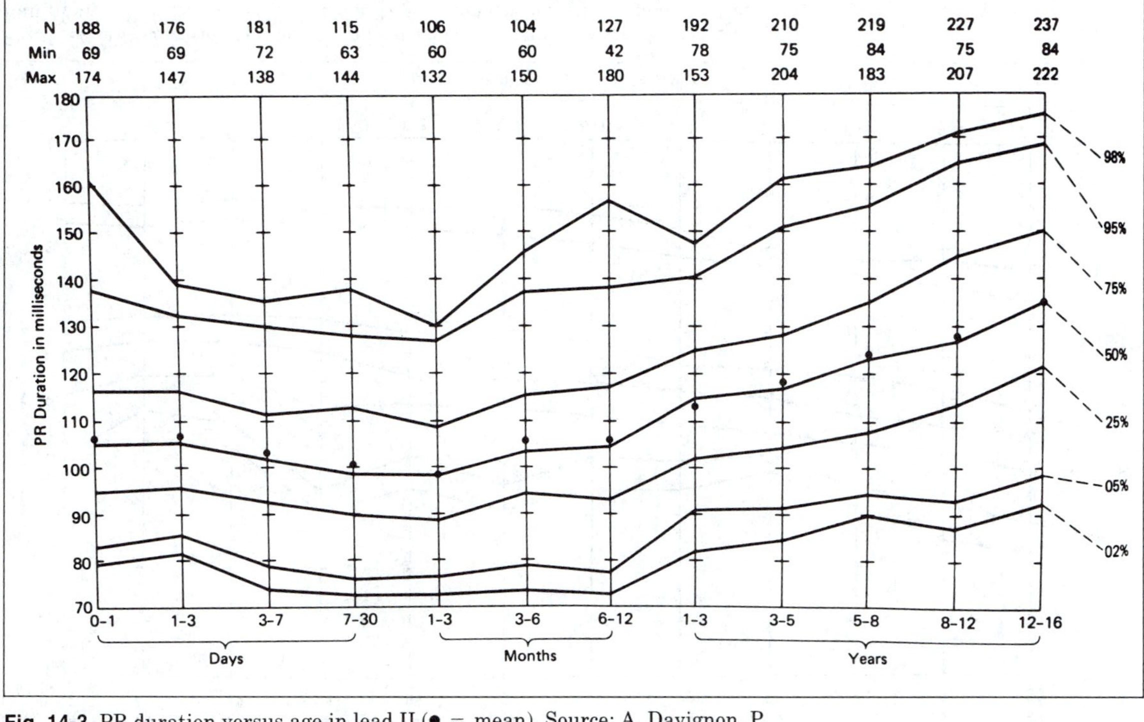

Fig. 14-3. PR duration versus age in lead II (● = mean). Source: A. Davignon, P. Rautaharju, E. Boisselle, et al. Normal ECG standards for infants and children, *Ped. Cardiology* 1: 123–131, 1979/1980. Reprinted with permission.

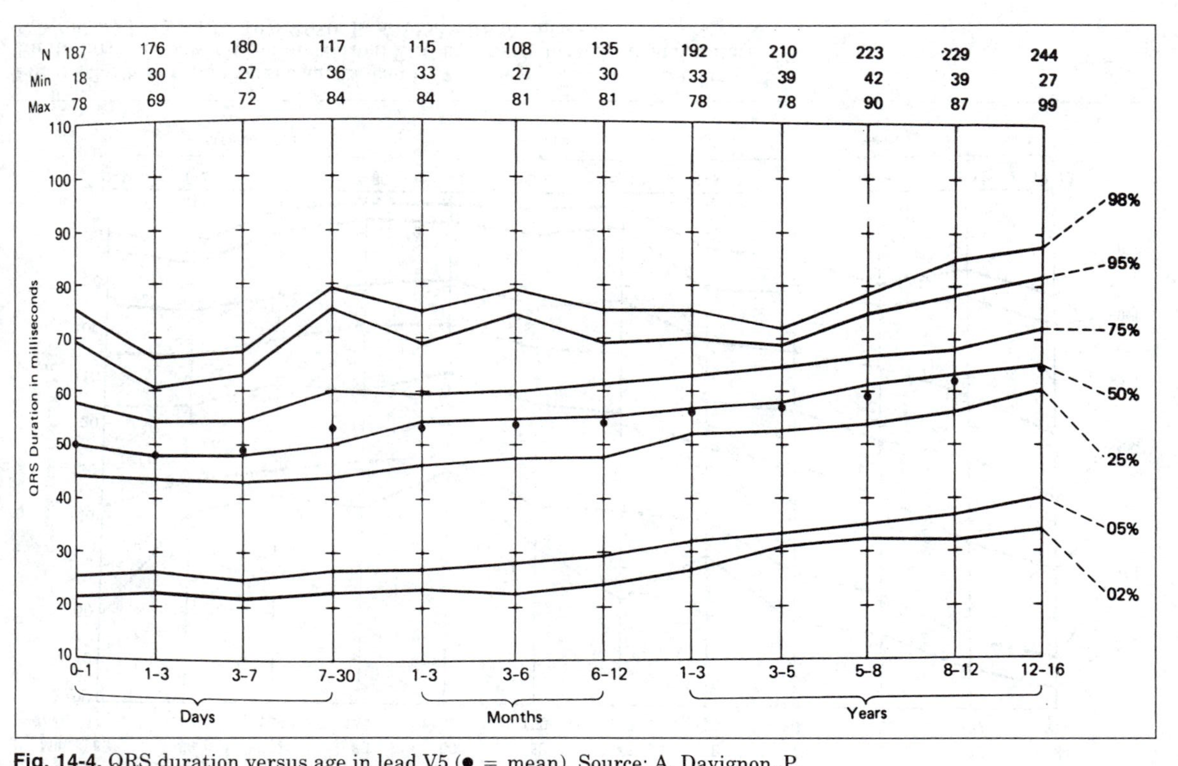

Fig. 14-4. QRS duration versus age in lead V5 (● = mean). Source: A. Davignon, P. Rautaharju, E. Boisselle, et al. Normal ECG standards for infants and children, *Ped. Cardiology* 1: 123–131, 1979/1980. Reprinted with permission.

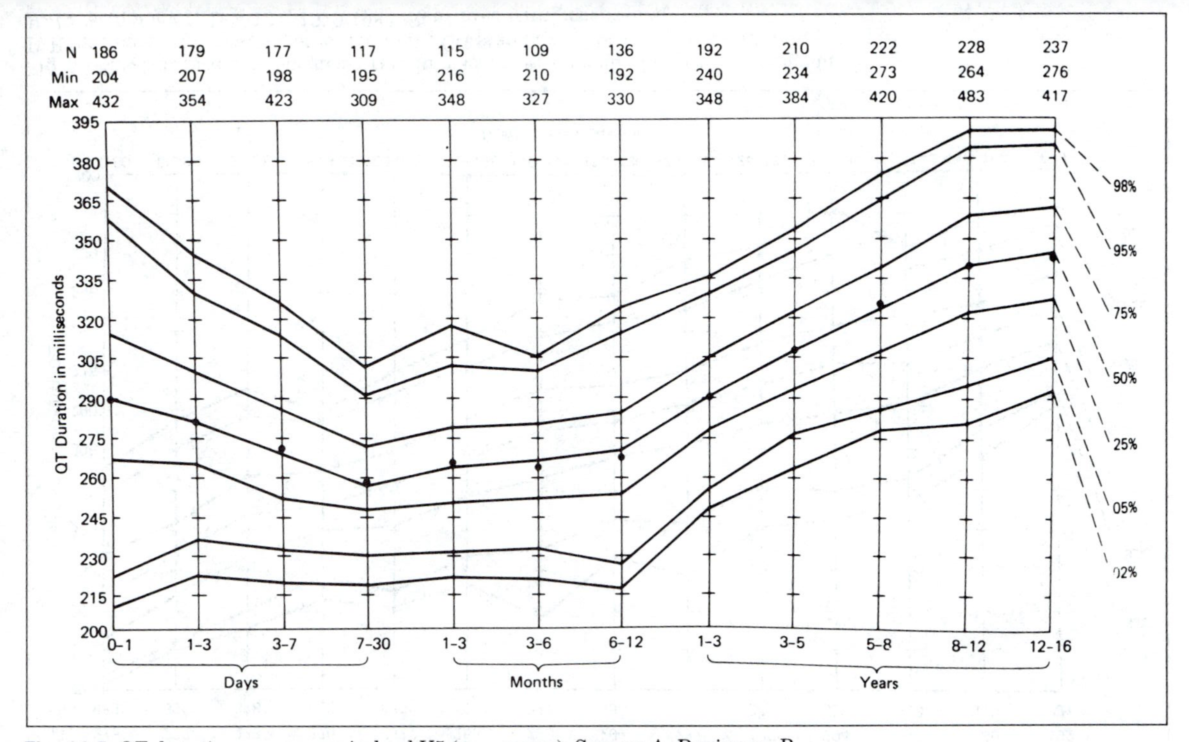

Fig. 14-5. QT duration versus age in lead V5 (● = mean). Source: A. Davignon, P. Rautaharju, E. Boisselle, et al. Normal ECG standards for infants and children, *Ped. Cardiology* 1: 123–131, 1979/1980. Reprinted with permission.

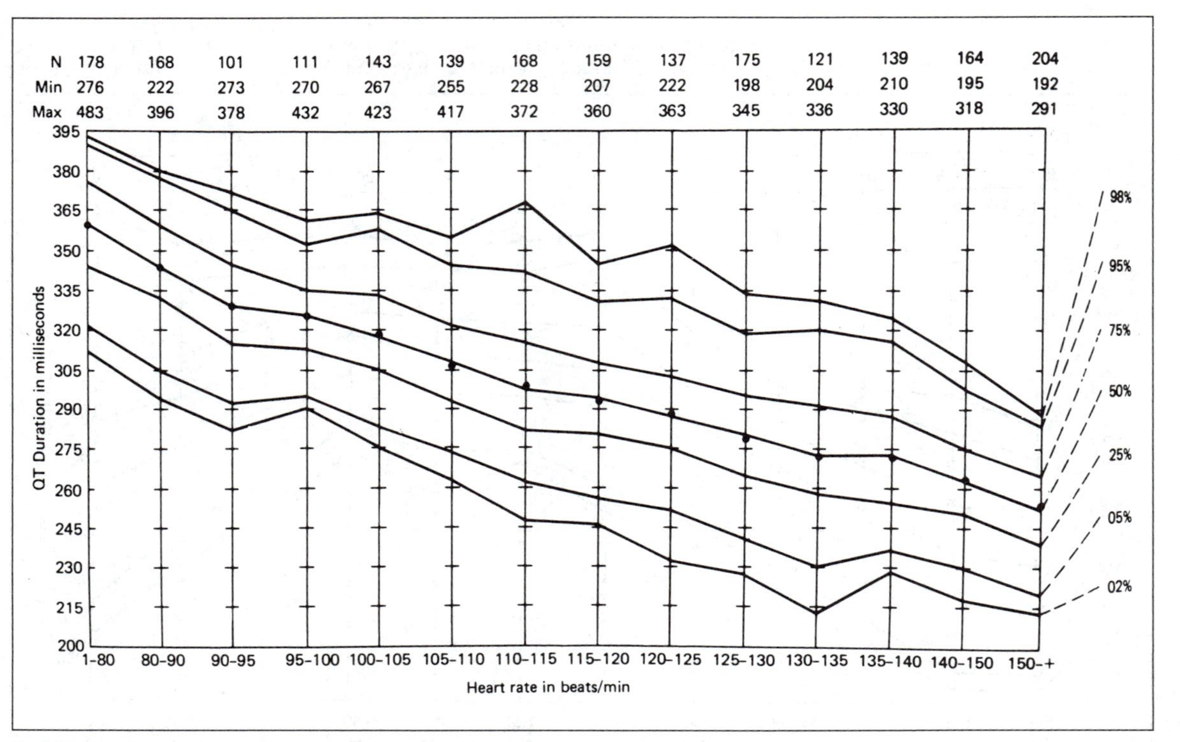

Fig. 14-6. QT duration versus heart rate in lead V5 (● = mean). Source: A. Davignon, P. Rautaharju, E. Boisselle, et al. Normal ECG standards for infants and children, *Ped. Cardiology* 1: 123–131, 1979/1980. Reprinted with permission.

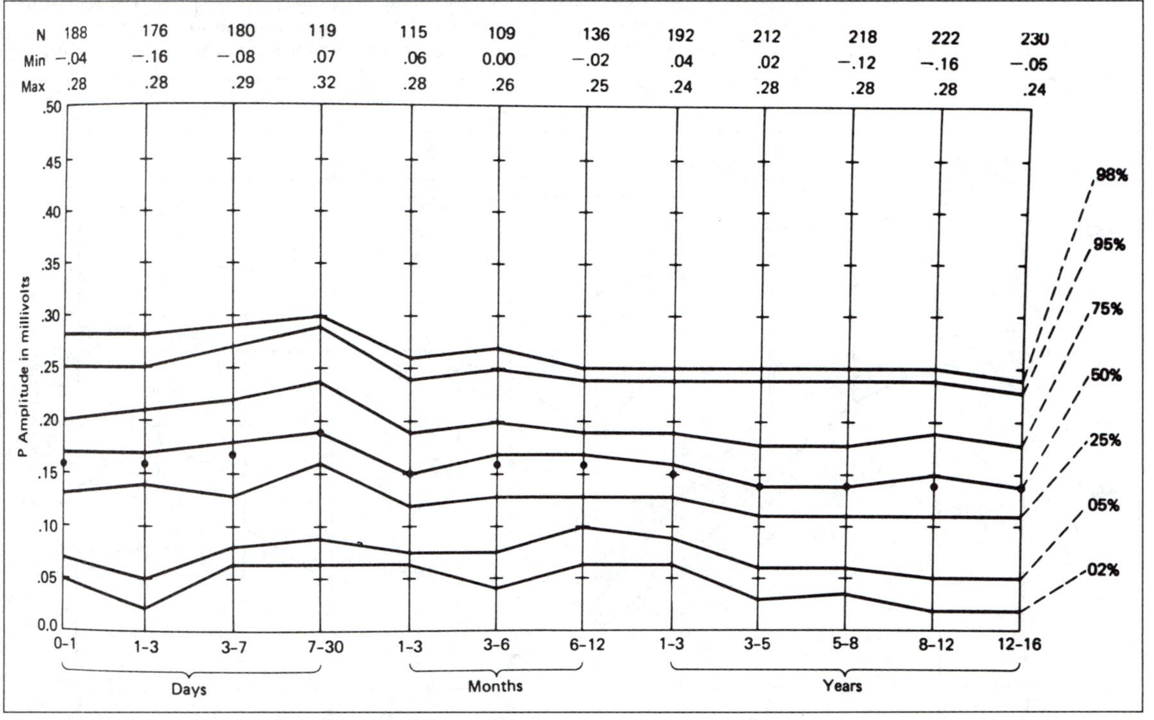

Fig. 14-7. P amplitude versus age in lead II (● = mean). Source: A. Davignon, P. Rautaharju, E. Boisselle, et al. Normal ECG standards for infants and children, *Ped. Cardiology* 1: 123–131, 1979/1980. Reprinted with permission.

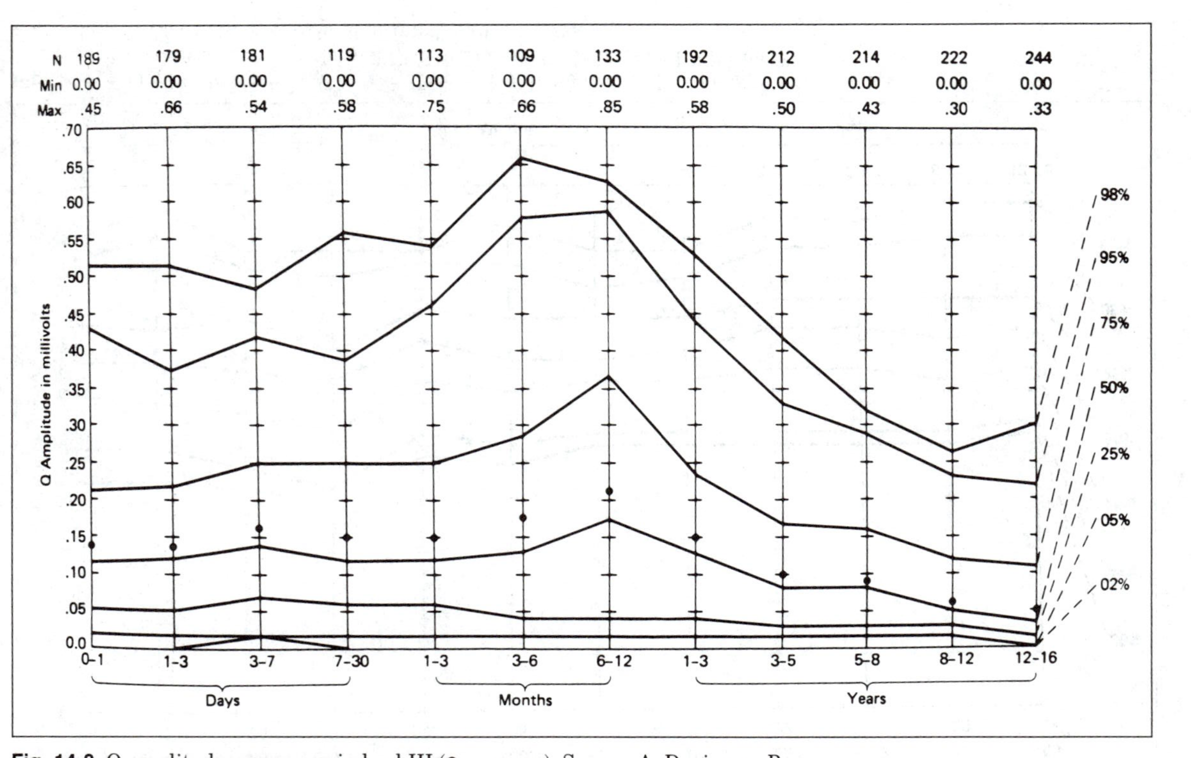

Fig. 14-8. Q amplitude versus age in lead III (● = mean). Source: A. Davignon, P. Rautaharju, E. Boisselle, et al. Normal ECG standards for infants and children, *Ped. Cardiology* 1: 123–131, 1979/1980. Reprinted with permission.

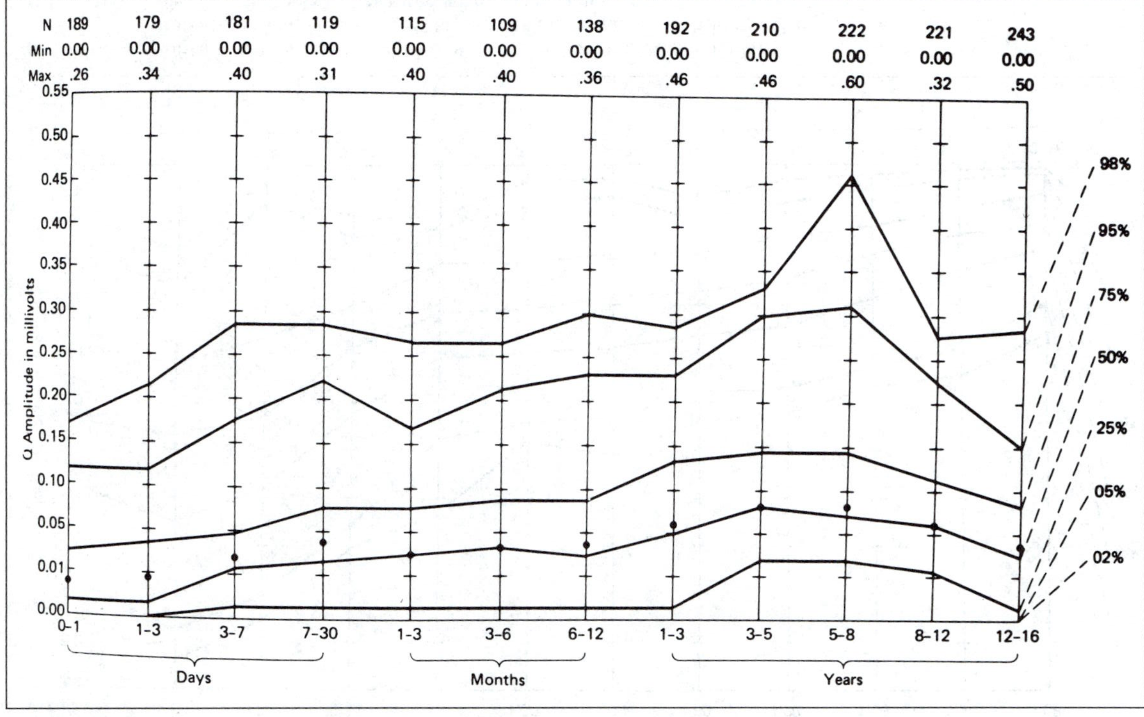

Fig. 14-9. Q amplitude versus age in lead V6 (● = mean). Source: A. Davignon, P. Rautaharju, E. Boisselle, et al. Normal ECG standards for infants and children, *Ped. Cardiology* 1: 123–131, 1979/1980. Reprinted with permission.

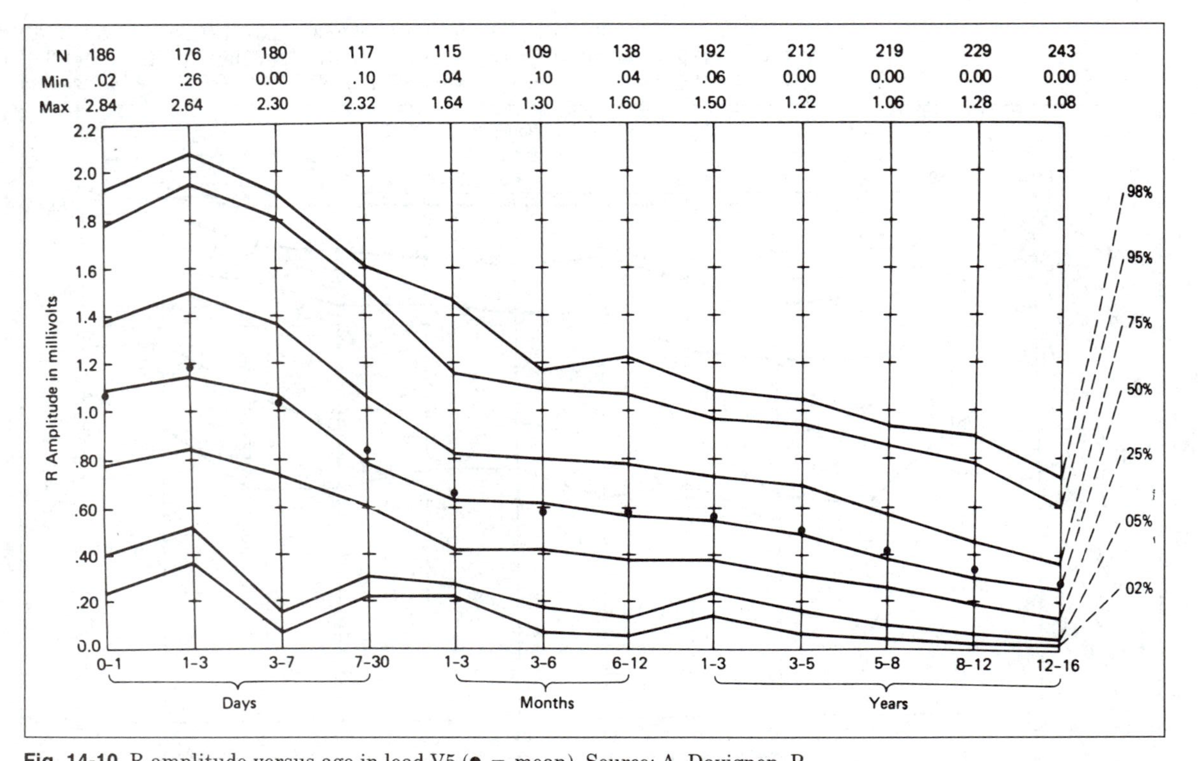

Fig. 14-10. R amplitude versus age in lead V5 (● = mean). Source: A. Davignon, P. Rautaharju, E. Boisselle, et al. Normal ECG standards for infants and children, *Ped. Cardiology* 1: 123–131, 1979/1980. Reprinted with permission.

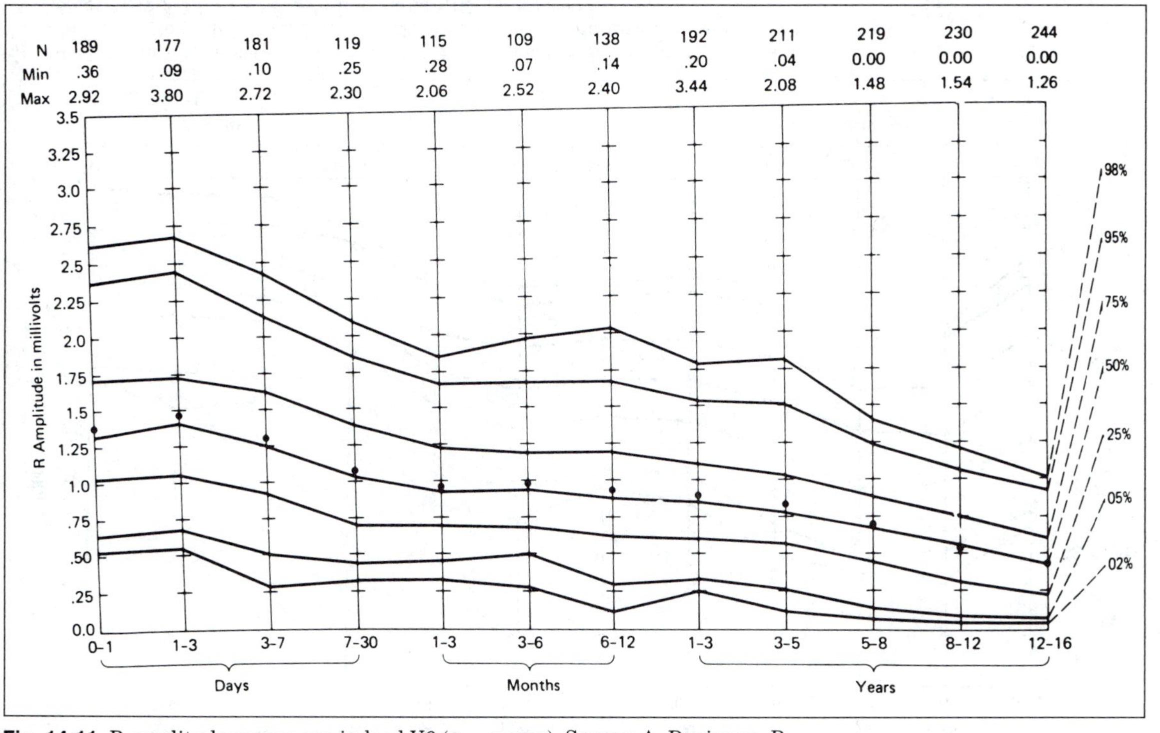

Fig. 14-11. R amplitude versus age in lead V6 (● = mean). Source: A. Davignon, P. Rautaharju, E. Boisselle, et al. Normal ECG standards for infants and children, *Ped. Cardiology* 1: 123–131, 1979/1980. Reprinted with permission.

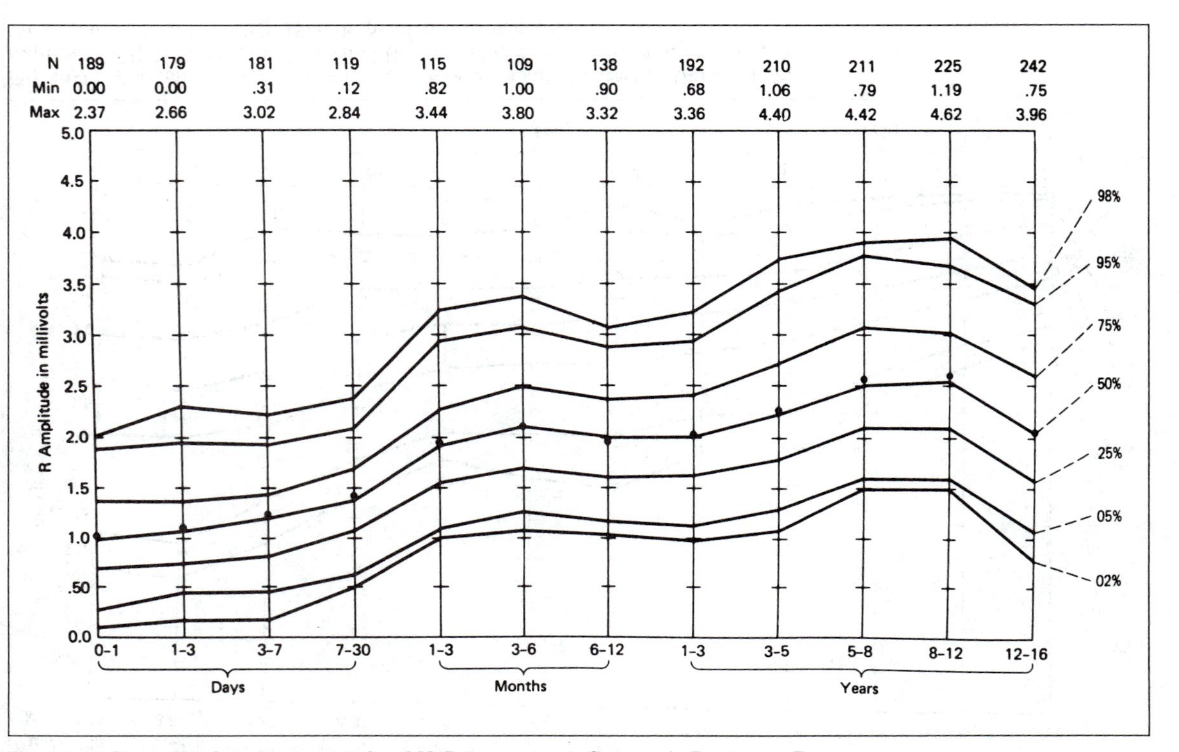

Fig. 14-12. R amplitude versus age in level V3R (● = mean). Source: A. Davignon, P. Rautaharju, E. Boisselle, et al. Normal ECG standards for infants and children, *Ped. Cardiology* 1: 123–131, 1979/1980. Reprinted with permission.

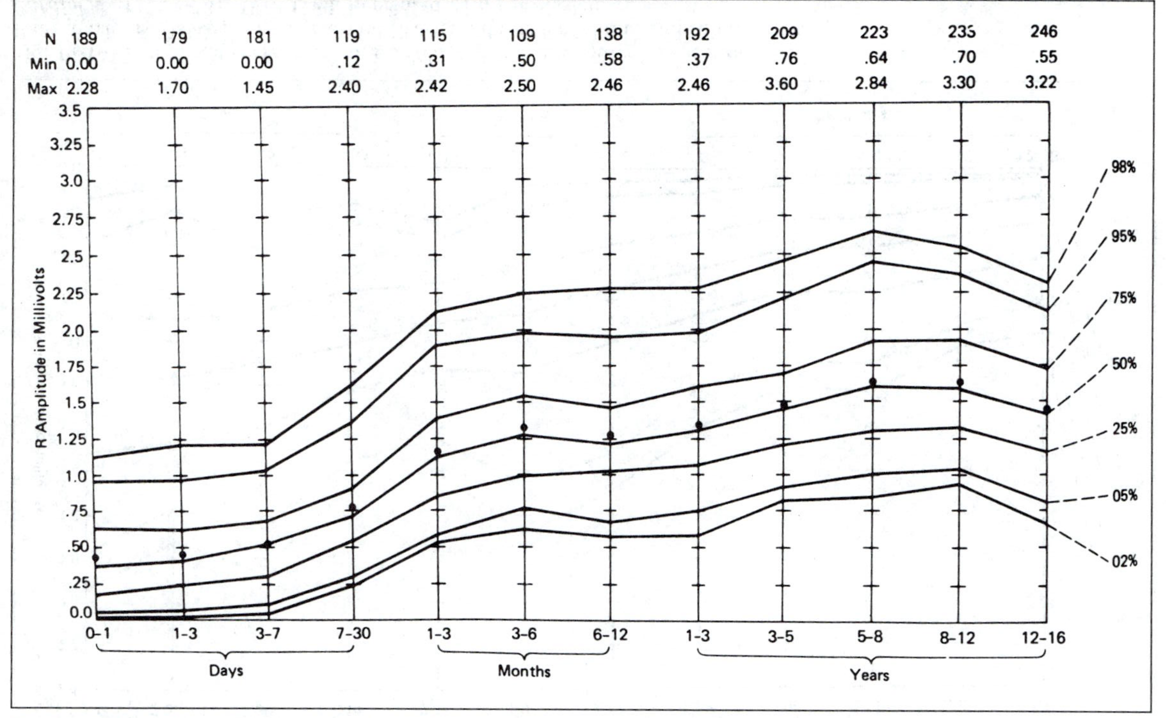

Fig. 14-13. R amplitude versus age in lead V1 (● = mean). Source: A. Davignon, P. Rautaharju, E. Boisselle, et al. Normal ECG standards for infants and children, *Ped. Cardiology* 1: 123–131, 1979/1980. Reprinted with permission.

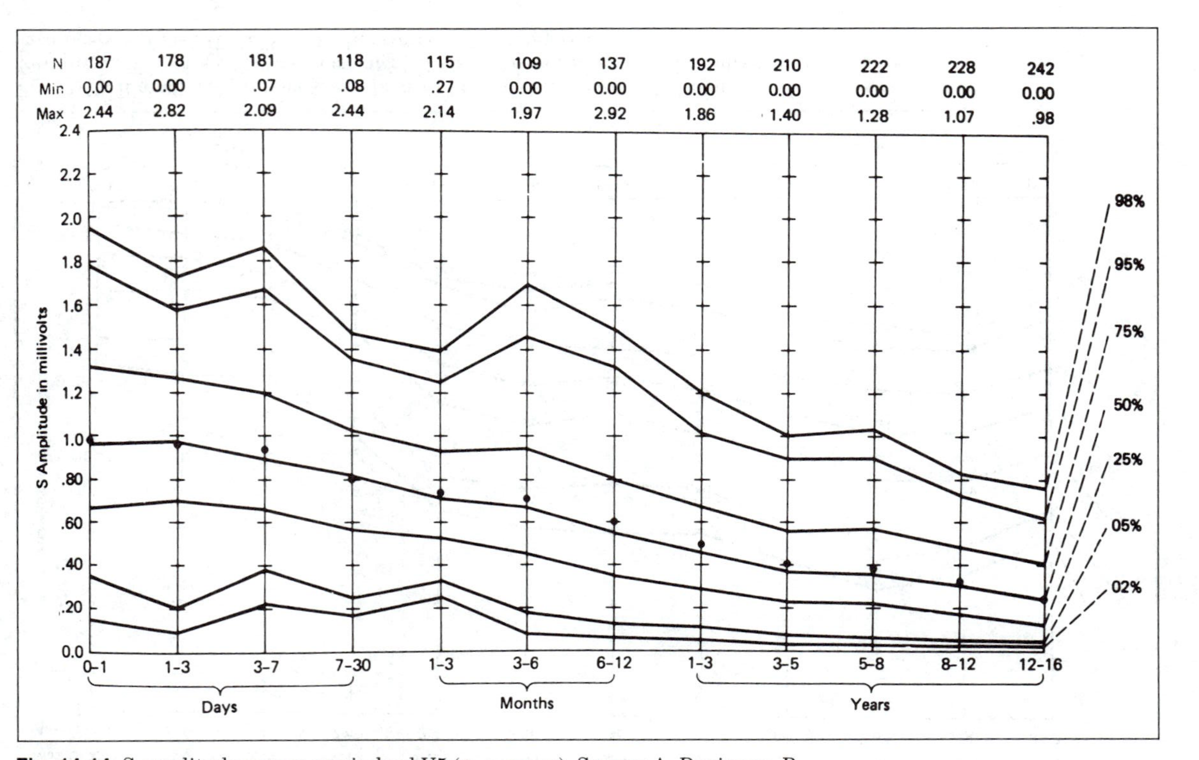

Fig. 14-14. S amplitude versus age in lead V5 (● = mean). Source: A. Davignon, P. Rautaharju, E. Boisselle, et al. Normal ECG standards for infants and children, *Ped. Cardiology* 1: 123–131, 1979/1980. Reprinted with permission.

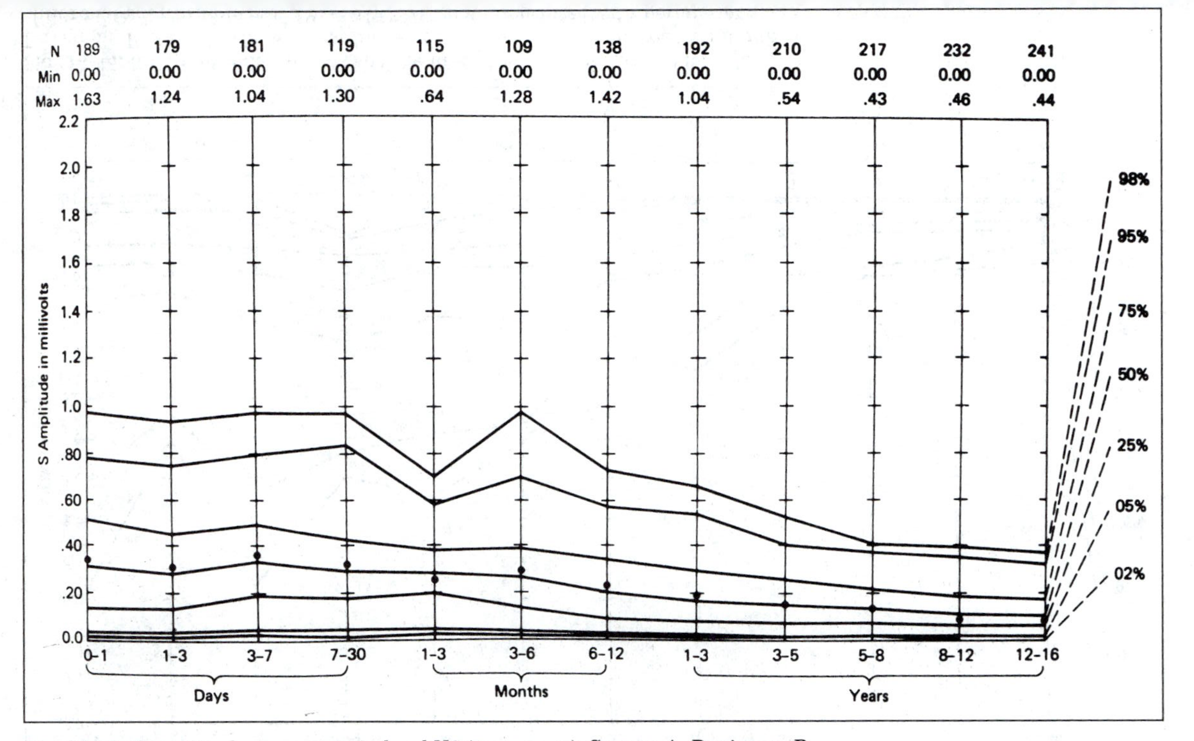

Fig. 14-15. S amplitude versus age in level V6 (● = mean). Source: A. Davignon, P. Rautaharju, E. Boisselle, et al. Normal ECG standards for infants and children, *Ped. Cardiology* 1: 123–131, 1979/1980. Reprinted with permission.

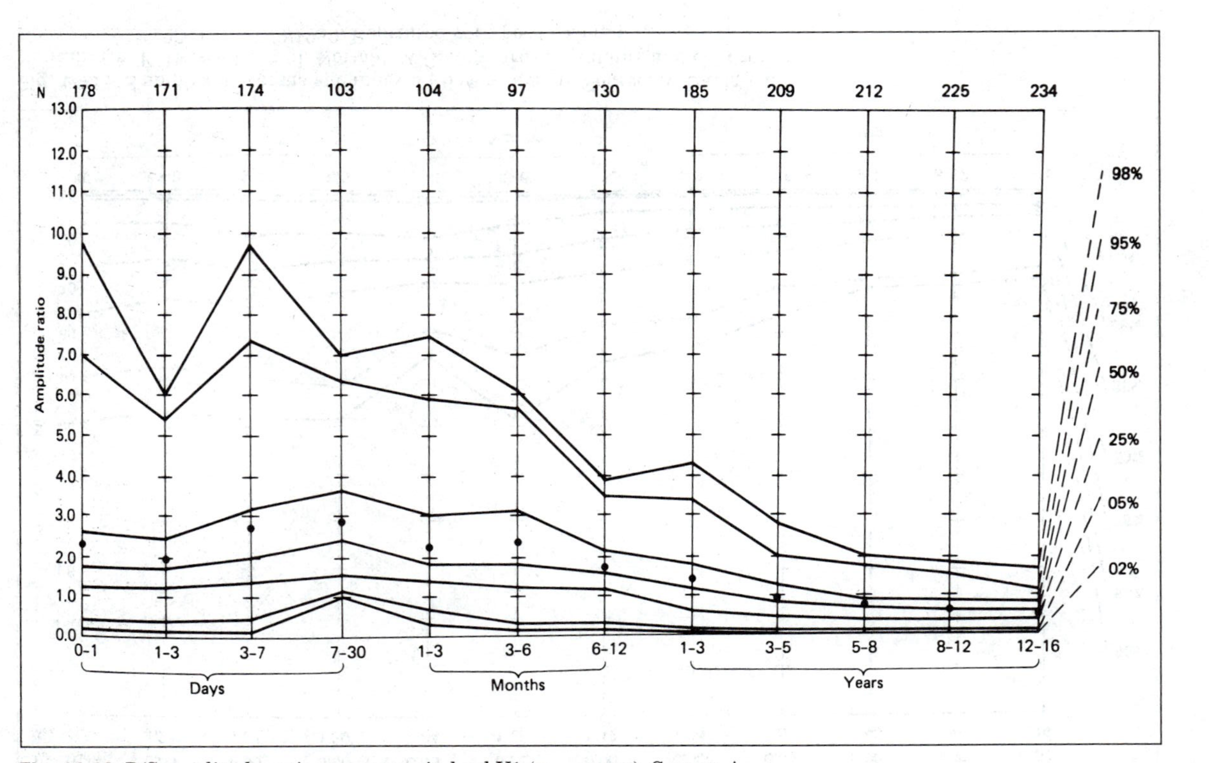

Fig. 14-16. R/S amplitude ratio versus age in lead V1 (● = mean). Source: A. Davignon, P. Rautaharju, E. Boisselle, et al. Normal ECG standards for infants and children, *Ped. Cardiology* 1: 123–131, 1979/1980. Reprinted with permission.

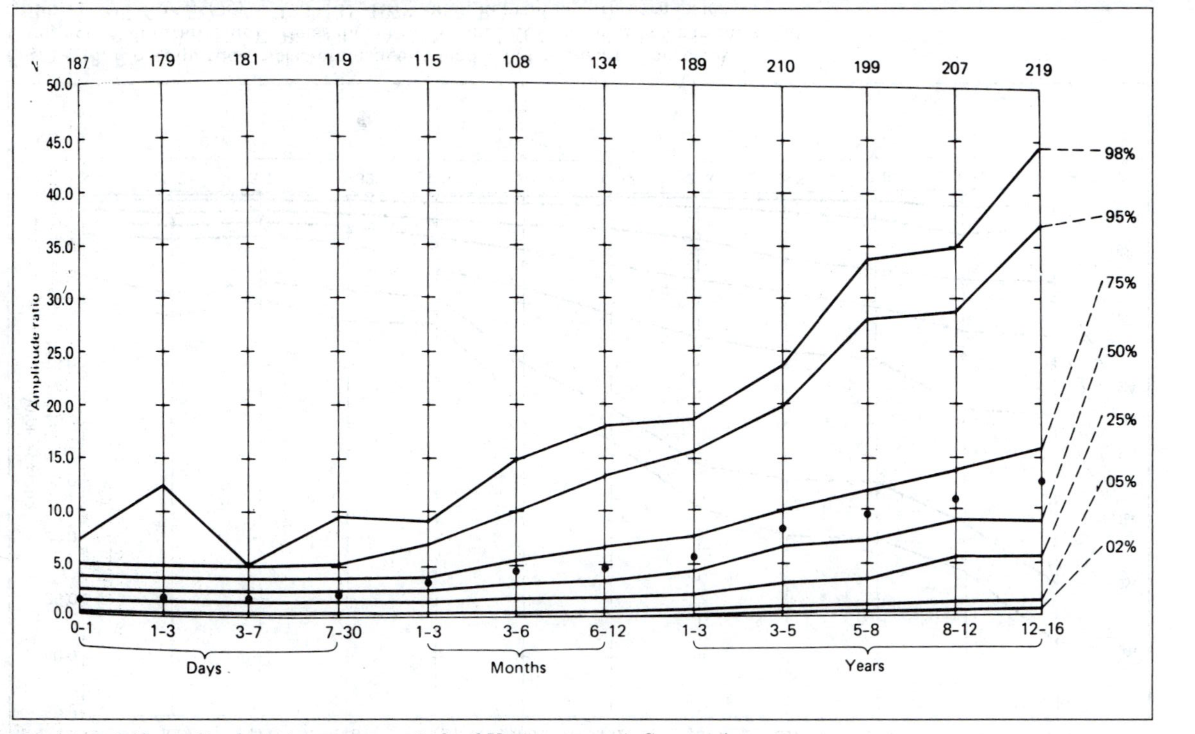

Fig. 14-17. R/S amplitude ratio versus age in lead V5 (● = mean). Source: A. Davignon, P. Rautaharju, E. Boisselle, et al. Normal ECG standards for infants and children, *Ped. Cardiology* 1: 123–131, 1979/1980. Reprinted with permission.

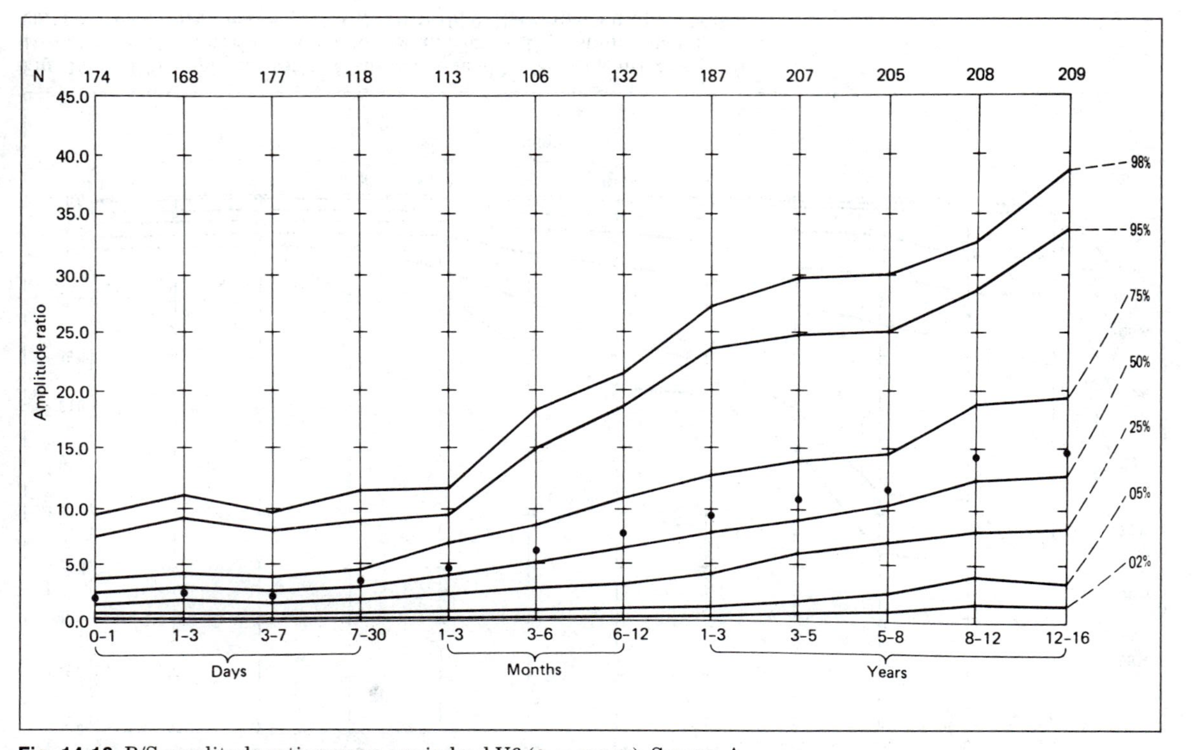

Fig. 14-18. R/S amplitude ratio versus age in lead V6 (● = mean). Source: A. Davignon, P. Rautaharju, E. Boisselle, et al. Normal ECG standards for infants and children, *Ped. Cardiology* 1: 123–131, 1979/1980. Reprinted with permission.

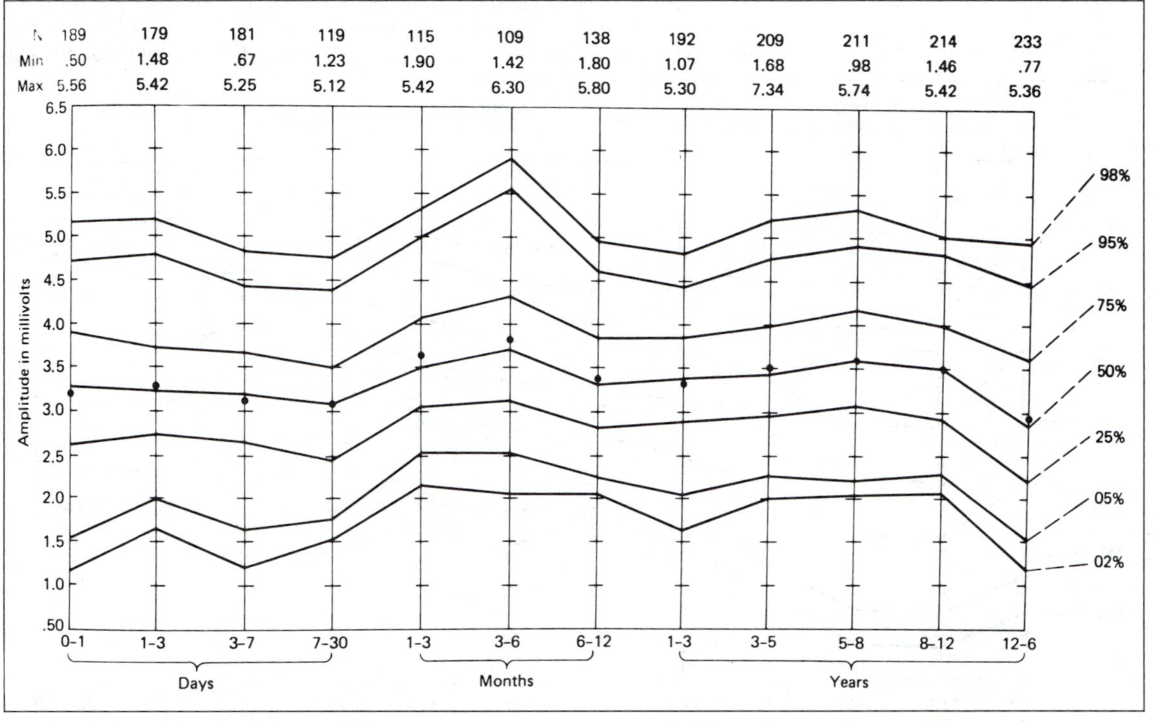

Fig. 14-19. R + S amplitude versus age in lead V4 (● = mean). Source: A. Davignon, P. Rautaharju, E. Boisselle, et al. Normal ECG standards for infants and children, *Ped. Cardiology* 1: 123–131, 1979/1980. Reprinted with permission.

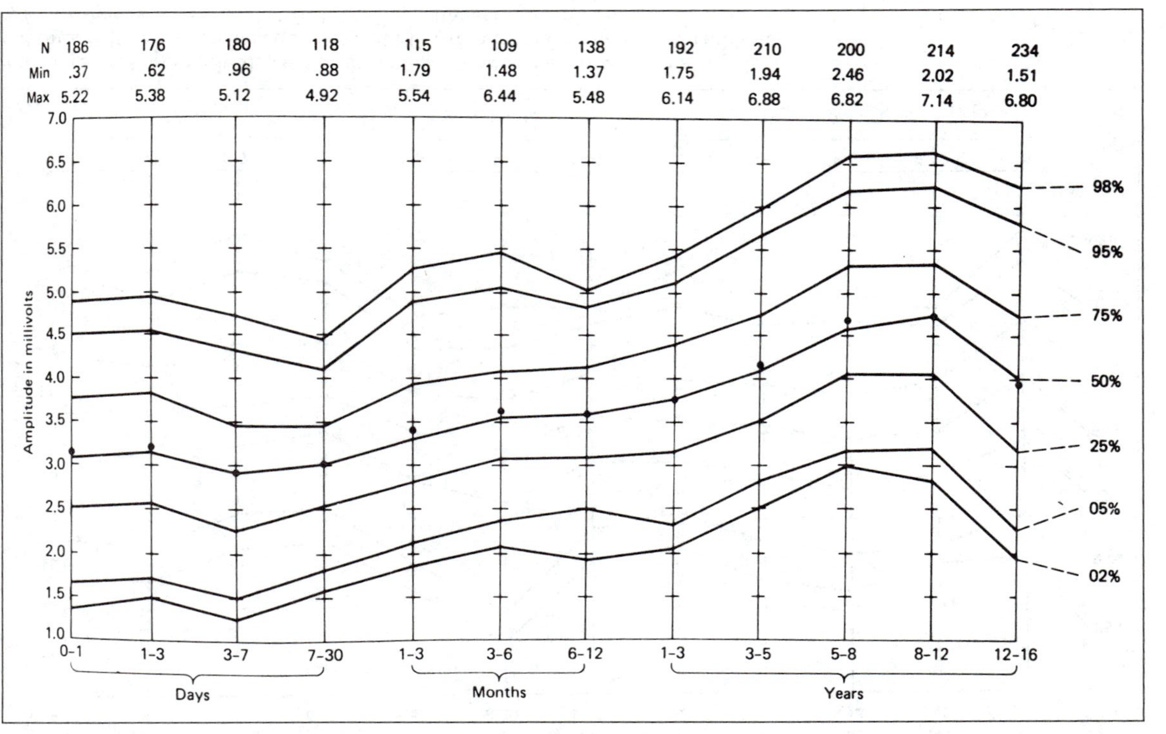

Fig. 14-20. Amplitude R in lead V2 versus age (● = mean). Source: A. Davignon, P. Rautaharju, E. Boisselle, et al. Normal ECG standards for infants and children, *Ped. Cardiology* 1: 123–131, 1979/1980. Reprinted with permission.

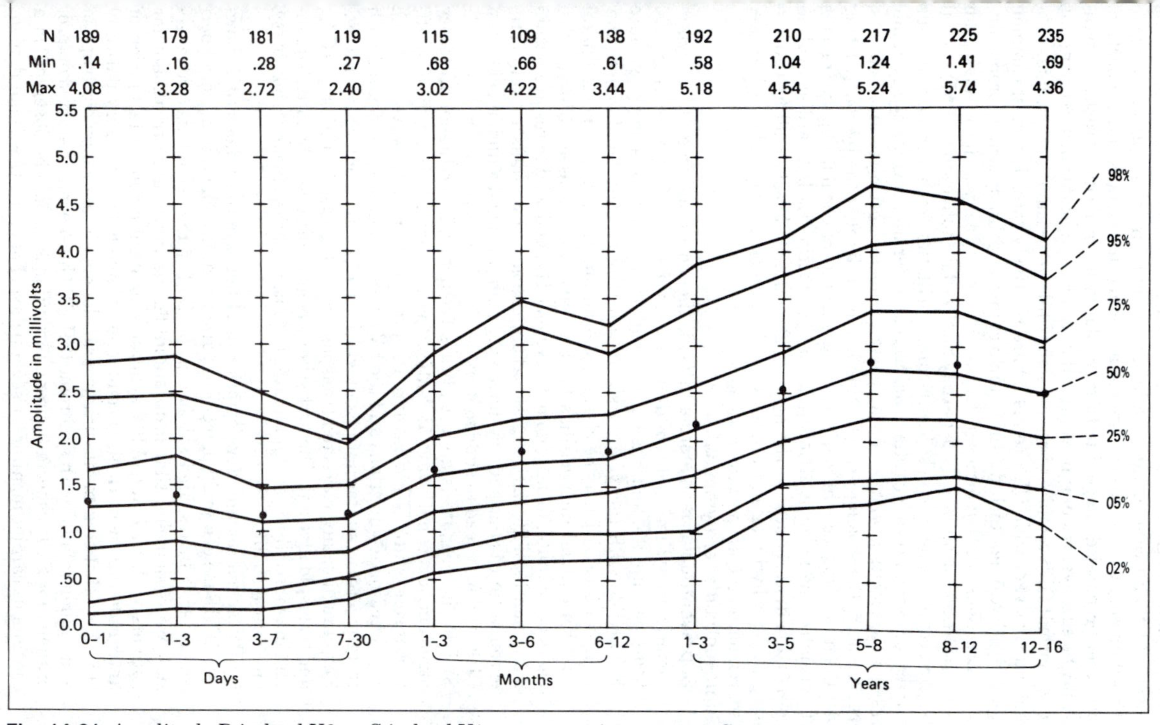

Fig. 14-21. Amplitude R in lead V6 + S in lead V1 versus age (● = mean). Source: A. Davignon, P. Rautaharju, E. Boisselle, et al. Normal ECG standards for infants and children, *Ped. Cardiology* 1: 123–131, 1979/1980. Reprinted with permission.

d. At birth, the R/S ratio in V_1 may be less than 1.0, and with age, the R/S ratio increases until at least 6 weeks of age rather than decreases.
e. Premature infants often have a tall R wave in lead V_6.
f. ST segment abnormalities are commonly present in the premature infant and include "scooped out" and depressed ST segments in the right precordial leads and ST elevation in the standard leads.
g. The QT interval is 0.24 to 0.30 second and decreases with age. The QTc interval early in premature infants is about 0.44 second, longer than for term infants.

VI. **Rhythm disturbances.** Symptomatic dysrhythmias are being recognized with increasing frequency in the neonate and fetus as neonatal and obstetric monitoring improves [29]. Significant sustained fetal arrhythmias are most commonly due to congenital anomalies, e.g., an extranodal accessory atrioventricular connection, tumors, and prenatal damage due to transplacental antibodies. Tachyarrhythmias may be supraventricular or ventricular. Supraventricular tachyarrythmias (narrow, normal QRS complex) are common, while ventricular arrhythmias (abnormal, but not very wide QRS complex) are relatively rare. The most common neonatal dysrhythmias include sinus tachycardia and bradycardia, premature atrial contractions (PACs), atrioventricular reentrant tachycardia involving an accessory connection often called **paroxysmal atrial tachycardia (PAT),** atrial flutter, and complete heart block. Ventricular fibrillation, tachycardia, and sinus node arrest or extreme bradycardia usually occur as terminal events of a systemic illness or in association with severe hypoxia, acidosis, electrolyte disturbances, or drug toxicity. Diagnosing arrhythmias is most reliably done by constructing "ladder diagrams" to trace the sequence of atrial and ventricular depolarizations and to visualize the mode of atrioventricular conduction [28]. A cardiac evaluation of rhythm disturbances in the neonate should include a 12-lead ECG documenting the dysrhythmia and in sinus rhythm, a chest x-ray, echocardiogram, and search for metabolic and toxic etiologies.

A. **Supraventricular arrhythmias**

1. **Supraventricular tachycardia (SVT)** is the most common group of symptomatic arrhythmias in children, usually has a rate greater than 200 beats per minute, and has normal ventricular complexes on the surface ECG (wide QRS tachycardia should initially be considered ventricular tachycardia). SVT may be classified as automatic or reentrant. Neonatal automatic atrial tachycardias tend to have rates between 170 and 210 beats per minute, usually do not develop CHF, and tend to resolve within a few months of life [29]. Junctional automatic tachycardias are very rare, except after cardiac surgery, have very high rates and a high incidence of CHF, and may lead to sudden death.

   SVT in the neonate is almost always reentrant, involving an accessory atrioventricular pathway [5]. Half of these patients will manifest Wolff-Parkinson-White (WPW) syndrome, preexcitation delta wave, on ECG. The accessory connections and the SVT they produce are associated with certain cardiac malformations in which there is atrial enlargement [e.g., Ebstein's anomaly, corrected transposition of the great arteries (L-TGA), and tricuspid atresia]. The arrhythmia begins and ends abruptly. The infant may initially be asymptomatic, but later may become irritable, fussy, and refuse feedings.

   CHF does not usually develop prior to 24 hours of continuous SVT; however, CHF is seen in 20 percent of patients after 36 hours and in 50 percent after 48 hours. Medical therapy for SVT in the neonate is controversial. We recommend that **propranolol** be the initial drug treatment for patients with SVT and WPW syndrome to avoid potential faciliation of antegrade (atrioventricular) conduction through the accessory pathway [15]. Note that treatment with propranolol may be associated with apnea and sudden infant death syndrome (SIDS). Thus neonates started on propranolol for SVT, especially premature infants, should be observed on a continuous cardiac monitor for several days. For patients without demonstrable WPW syndrome, **digoxin** should be the initial therapy in the treatment of SVT in patients without CHF. Parenteral digitalization is described in **IV.B.1.** During digitalization, vagal maneuvers (facial/malar ice wrapped in a towel to elicit the "diving reflex") may be tried in stable neonates. This may be performed with caution in sick infants. Parenteral digitalization usually abolishes the arrhythmia within 10 hours. If digoxin successfully maintains the patient in sinus rhythm, it should be continued for 6 to 12 months. The addition or substitution of other antiarrhythmic drugs such as propranolol, flecainide, quinidine, or amiodarone alone or in combination [28] may be necessary. Esophageal electrode overdrive pacing has become the initial treatment of choice for sustained SVT. Synchronized direct current (dc) cardioversion (starting at 1 to 2 Watt-seconds/kg) may be necessary in infants with refractory arrhythmias and in very ill infants. Resuscitation equipment must be available when either esophageal pacing or DC cardioversion is used. *Oral* verapamil, 3 to 5 mg/kg per day divided tid, is safe and efficacious for the treatment of SVT [49] and does not lead to cardiovascular collapse, as does the intravenous form [29]. Verapamil is contraindicated in patients who have received prior beta-adrenergic blockade, since pretreatment with propranolol is associated with the development of complete heart block.

In utero SVT may be suspected when a very rapid fetal heart rate is noted by fetoscopy. The diagnosis may be confirmed by in utero fetal echocardiography. At that time, an initial search for CHD and fetal hydrops may be made. In utero treatment of the immature fetus with SVT may be accomplished by treatment of the mother with antiarrhythmic drugs that cross the placenta. Use of digoxin, propranolol, procainamide, quinidine, and verapamil has been reported. Failure to control the fetal SVT in the presence of fetal hydrops is an indication for delivery. Cesarean delivery of an infant in persistent SVT may be necessary because the fetal heart rate is not a reliable indicator of fetal distress.

2. **Atrial flutter** is a less common form of SVT that may be idiopathic or associated with the same cardiac lesions seen with SVT. CHF is rare because some degree of atrioventricular block is almost always present. The atrial rate may be 200 to 380 beats per minute. Flutter waves are best seen in leads II and V_1. Digoxin is the initial drug of choice and will increase the degree of atrioventricular block even if it does not induce medical cardioversion. Synchronized DC cardioversion (starting at 1 to 2 Watt-seconds/kg) is sometimes necessary. Maintenance therapy with digoxin should probably be continued for 1 year. The addition of propranolol or other drugs such as amiodarone [28] may be necessary. Quinidine should probably not be used, especially in the absence of digoxin, owing to the risk of 1:1 atrioventricular conduction and the risk of ventricular fibrillation [53].
3. **Atrial fibrillation** is an uncommon atrial arrhythmia that may be associated with cardiac lesions that produce atrial enlargement. The ventricular response is irregularly irregular, distinct P waves are not identifiable, and the ventricular rate may be slowed with digoxin. Those with chronic atrial fibrillation may develop atrial thrombi and should be anticoagulated before cardioversion to prevent systemic embolization. Medical cardioversion of the digitalized patient may be achieved with quinidine. Synchronized DC cardioversion (starting at 1 to 2 Watt-seconds/kg) or esophageal pacing is often necessary. Maintenance therapy with digoxin should probably be continued for 1 year.
4. **Multifocal atrial tachycardia** in the neonate is very rare and is not always associated with pulmonary disease, as is often true in adults. It consists of a chaotic, irregular supraventricular tachycardia (SVT) with P waves of varying morphology. This arrhythmia is well tolerated unless the ventricular response is excessively rapid. Digoxin may be used to slow the

ventricular rate. Propranolol or quinidine may be used to suppress the ectopic atrial activity, but DC cardioversion is probably not beneficial.

5. **PACs** are common in normal neonates, are usually benign, and do not require specific therapy. Blocked PACs may occur if the PAC occurs when the atrioventricular conduction pathway is refractory. The pause after a blocked PAC often gives the appearance of marked sinus bradycardia. If the PAC occurs after the atrioventricular pathway is only partially repolarized, an aberrantly conducted ventricular depolarization pattern may be observed on the surface ECG.
6. **Sinus tachycardia** in the neonate at rates greater than 2 standard deviations above the mean for age is common and occurs in response to stress, fever, hypovolemia, and xanthine toxicity. Medical management consists of identifying and treating the underlying cause.
7. **Sinus bradycardia** in the neonate at rates less than 2 standard deviations below the mean for age is also common. If the blood pressure is normal, it is not of major concern. Transient sinus bradycardia may occur with hypoxemia, acidosis, and elevated intracranial pressure. A stable sinus bradycardia may occur with digoxin toxicity, hypothyroidism, and sinus node dysfunction (usually a complication of cardiac surgery).

B. Ventricular arrhythmias

1. **Ventricular tachycardia** in the neonate is relatively rare and is often associated with hypoxemia, shock, electrolyte disturbances, digoxin toxicity, catecholamine toxicity, prolonged QT syndrome, and cardiac tumors. The finding of rapid, wide QRS complexes, three or more consecutive PVCs in the absence of P waves, is diagnostic (this ECG pattern may be simulated by SVT in patients with WPW syndrome, in whom there is antegrade conduction through the anomalous pathway). Ventricular tachycardia may be a hemodynamically unstable rhythm. The underlying cause should be rapidly sought and treated. The patient should be treated with a lidocaine bolus, 1 to 2 mg/kg, followed by a lidocaine infusion, 1 to 2 mg/kg per hour. DC cardioversion (starting dose to 1 to 2 Watt-seconds/kg or 5 to 10 Watt-seconds) will usually induce cardioversion if the patient is hemodynamically compromised. Phenytoin, 2 to 4 mg/kg, may be effective if the arrhythmia is due to digoxin toxicity (see **IV.B.1**).
2. **Ventricular fibrillation** in the neonate is usually an agonal arrhythmia in a patient dying from another cause. There is a coarse irregular pattern on ECG with no identifiable QRS complexes. There are no peripheral pulses or heart sounds on physical examination. If the underlying problem is correctable, cardiopulmonary resuscitation (CPR) should be instituted and DC cardioversion (starting dose 1 to 2 Watt-seconds/kg or 5 to 10 Watt-seconds) performed as soon as possible. A bolus of lidocaine, 1 mg/kg, followed by a lidocaine infusion, 1 mg/kg per hour, should be started. When the infant is hemodynamically stable, the underlying problems should be corrected and the patient observed for signs of organ ischemia.
3. **Premature ventricular contractions (PVCs)** are occasionally seen in the normal neonate and do not generally require treatment. When PVCs are due to digoxin toxicity, hypoxemia, electrolyte disturbances, or catecholamine or xanthine toxicity, the underlying problem should be corrected. If the PVCs are of several forms or in couplets, they may require treatment with lidocaine.

C. Conduction disturbances

1. **Congenital complete heart block (CHB)** has a slow, regular ventricular rate that is independent of the atrial rate. It is frequently detected in utero as a fetal bradycardia. About half the infants with CHB have an associated cardiovascular malformation (corrected L-TGA, VSD, or ASD). An association with myocarditis and with maternal systemic lupus erythematosus and other collagen-vascular diseases has been reported. The presence of symptoms is usually related to the severity of the associated

cardiac malformation and the degree of bradycardia. Infants with isolated congenital CHB usually have a heart rate greater than 50 beats per minute, are asymptomatic, and grow normally [18]. Infants with slower heart rates may require an epicardial pacemaker. We have paced an infant as small 900 gm with temporary epicardial electrodes in our institution. A soft systolic ejection murmur and apical diastolic rumble are common in patients with isolated CHB. Stokes-Adams episodes and CHF are indications for an artificial pacemaker. Isoproterenol may sometimes temporarily increase the ventricular rate and cardiac output in an infant who develops CHF. A transvenous pacemaker is a helpful temporary measure in acute situations and in preparation for placement of permanent epicardial pacemaker leads.

2. **First-degree atrioventricular block** (PR interval > 0.15 second) in the neonate may be a digitalis effect, a nonspecific conduction disturbance, or associated with certain types of CHD (e.g., CAVC). No specific treatment is generally indicated.
3. **Second-degree atrioventricular block** may occur with SVT, digitalis toxicity, and a nonspecific conduction disturbance. No specific treatment is usually necessary other than treatment of the underlying cause. Two forms of second-degree atrioventricular block are recognized: (1) Mobitz I (Wenkebach phenomenon) and (2) Mobitz II (intermittent failure to conduct P waves, with a constant PR interval).

VII. Transport of the neonate with symptomatic CHD (see Chapter 33). Transport of an infant suspected of having severe CHD to a tertiary medical center can be an intimidating experience. The assessment of the neonate at the referring hospital, based on history, physical examination, chest x-ray, ECG, and an arterial blood gas analysis, should provide a reasonable working cardiac diagnosis. The process may be facilitated by requesting that these tests be obtained by the referring hospital prior to the arrival of the transport team. Having made an initial assessment of the infant, routine stabilization, as indicated by the clinical status of the infant, is provided. Since only limited diagnostic and therapeutic resources are available to the transport team, a rapid, safe transport to the receiving hospital is the best strategy.

Use of PGE_1 (see **IV.A**) in transport should be limited to those infants in whom poor perfusion, acidosis, or profound cyanosis ($PO_2 < 25$ mmHg, arterial hemoglobin saturation < 60 percent) preclude a safe transport or a clearly established diagnosis at the referring hospital indicates the need for PGE_1 therapy. All such patients should be intubated prior to leaving the referring hospital, since 10 to 12 percent of infants treated with PGE_1 will develop apnea. A separate intravenous line should be started for volume administration, since 4 percent of the infants develop hypotension with PGE_1 administration. If the patient deteriorates acutely after starting PGE_1, stop the infusion, since the patient may have TAPVR with pulmonary venus obstruction (see page 625).

In infants with cyanotic CHD, an inspired oxygen concentration greater than 50% is usually of no significant benefit and may cause excessive pulmonary vasodilation and pulmonary blood flow. A call to the receiving cardiologist or neonatologist and a visit to the parents of the child prior to departure from the referring hospital are imperative.

References

1. Adams, F. H. et al. *Moss's Heart Disease in Infants, Children and Adolescents*, 3d Ed. Baltimore, Williams & Wilkins, 1983.
2. Alousi, A. A., et al. *Circulation* 73: 10, 1986.
3. Beekman, R. H., et al. *Pediatrics* 73: 43, 1984.
4. Benitz, W. E., et al. *J. Pediatr.* 106: 102, 1985.
5. Benson, D. W., et al. *Am. J. Cardiol.* 52: 1002, 1983.
6. Berman, W., et al. *J. Pediatr.* 93: 652, 1978.

7. Binah, O., et al. *Circ. Res.* 52: 747, 1983.
8. Braudo, M., et al. *Am. J. Dis. Child.* 101: 575, 1961.
9. Braunlin, E., et al. *Pediatr. Cardiol.* 1: 231, 1981.
10. Calder, L., et al. *Am. Heart J.* 92: 23, 1976.
11. Cassady, G. The Pathophysiologic Picture of the Postasphyxiated Infant. In G. J. Peckham and M. A. Heymann (Eds.), *Cardiovascular Sequelae of Asphyxia in the Newborn: Report of the Eighty-Third Ross Conference on Pediatric Research.* Columbus, Ohio: Ross Laboratories, 1982. Pp. 66–70.
12. Cherry, J. D. Enteroviruses. In J. S. Remington and J. O. Klein (Eds.), *Infectious Diseases of the Fetus and Newborn Infant.* Philadelphia: Saunders, 1976. Pp. 366–413.
13. Chin, A. J., et al. *Am. Heart J.* 113: 1153, 1987.
14. Davignon, A., et al. *Pediatr. Cardiol.* 1: 123, 1979/80.
15. Deal, B. J., et al. *J. Am. Coll. Cardiol.* 5: 130, 1985.
16. Ellison, R. C., et al. *Pediatrics* 71: 364, 1983.
17. Emmanouilides, G. C., et al. *Curr. Probl. Pediatr.* 9: 1, 1979.
18. Esscher, E., et al. *Acta Paediatr. Scand.* 70: 131, 1981.
19. Evans, J. R., et al. *Circulation* 22: 1044, 1960.
20. Fellows, K. E., et al. *Circulation* 56: 485, 1977.
21. Freed, M. D. Congenital Cardiac Malformations. In M. E. Avery and H. W. Taeusch (Eds.), *Schaffer's Diseases of the Newborn,* 5th Ed. Philadelphia: Saunders, 1987. Pp. 243–290.
22. Fyler, D. C. Non-Pump Cardiac Surgery in the New England Regional Infant Cardiac Program. In B. L. Tucker and G. G. Lindesmith (Eds.), *Proceedings of the First Clinical Conference on Congenital Heart Disease.* San Francisco: Grune and Stratton, 1979. Pp. 295–306.
23. Fyler, D. C., Rothman, K. J., Buckley, L. P., Cohen, H. E., Hellenbrand, W. E., and Castaneda, A. The Determinants of Five Year Survival of Infants with Critical Congenital Heart Disease. In A. N. Brest (Ed.), *Pediatric Cardiovascular Disease.* San Francisco: Davis, 1980.
24. Fyler, D. C., and Lang, P. Neonatal Heart Disease. In G. B. Avery (Ed.), *Neonatology: Pathophysiology and Management of the Newborn.* Philadelphia: Lippincott, 1981. Pp. 438–470.
25. Fyler, D. C., et al. *Rev. Lat. Cardiol. Infant.* 2: 10, 1986.
26. Gersony, W. M., et al. *J. Pediatr.* 102: 895, 1983.
27. Gersony, W. H., et al. *Pediatr. Clin. North Am.* 33: 545, 1986.
28. Gillette, P. C., and Garson, A. *Pediatric Cardiac Dysrhythmias.* New York: Grune and Stratton, 1981.
29. Gillette, P. C., et al. *Clin. Perinatal.* 15: 699, 1988.
30. Graham, T. P., et al. *South Med. J.* 71: 1238, 1980.
31. Hammerman, C., et al. *Dev. Pharmacol. Ther.* 10: 393, 1987.
32. Helgason, H., et al. *J. Am. Coll. Cardiol.* 9: 816, 1987.
33. Jonas, R. A., et al. *J. Thorac. Cardiovasc. Surg.* 92: 6, 1986.
34. Jonas, R. A., et al. *Aust. N.Z. J. Surg.* 55: 39, 1985.
35. Keith, J. D., Rowe, R. D., and Vlad, P. *Heart Disease in Infancy and Childhood,* 3d Ed. New York: Macmillian, 1978.
36. Keane, J. F., et al. *Circulation* 52: 1138, 1975.
37. Kleinman, C. S., et al. *N. Engl. J. Med.* 306: 568, 1982.
38. Lang, P., et al. *J. Pediatr.* 91: 805, 1977.
39. Liebman, J., Plonsey, R., and Gillette, P. C. *Pediatric Electrocardiography.* Baltimore: Williams & Wilkins, 1982.
40. Lock, J. E. *Diagnostic and Interventional Catheterization in Congenital Heart Disease.* Boston: Nijhoff, Kluwer Academic, 1986.
41. Mahony, L., et al. *J. Pediatr.* 106: 801, 1985.
42. Mitchell, S. C., et al. *Circulation* 43: 323, 1971.
43. Moller, J. H., and Neal, W. A. *Heart Disease in Infancy.* Norwalk, Conn.: Appleton-Century-Crofts, 1981.
44. Nelson, R. M., et al. *N. Engl. J. Med.* 298: 146, 1978.
45. Noonan, J. A., et al. *Pediatr. Clin. North Am.* 25: 797, 1978.

46. Norwood, W. I., et al. *N. Engl. J. Med.* 308: 23, 1983.
47. Olley, P. M.,, et al. *Circulation* 53: 728, 1976.
48. Pinsky, W. W., et al. *J. Pediatr.* 94: 639, 1979.
49. Porter, C. J., et al. *Am. J. Cardiol.* 48: 487, 1981.
50. Rastelli, G. C. *Atrioventricular Canal Defects.* Philadelphia: Saunders, 1976.
51. Ross-Ascuitto, N., et al. *Circ. Res.* 61: 847, 1987.
52. Rowe, R. D., et al. *The Neonate with Congenital Heart Disease,* 2d Ed. Philadelphia: Saunders, 1981.
53. Rowland, T. W., et al. *Pediatrics* 61: 52, 1978.
54. Silverman, N. H., et al. *J. Am. Coll. Cardiol.* 5: 20S, 1985.
55. Snider, A. R., et al. *Clin. Perinatol.* 15: 523, 1988.
56. Spangler, J. G., et al. *J. Pediatr.* 95: 1087, 1979.
57. Turley, K., et al. *Circulation* 66: 214, 1982.
58. Zeevi, B., et al. *Clin. Perinatol.* 15: 633, 1988a.
59. Zeevi, B., et al. *J. Am. Coll. Cardiol.* 11: 821, 1988b.

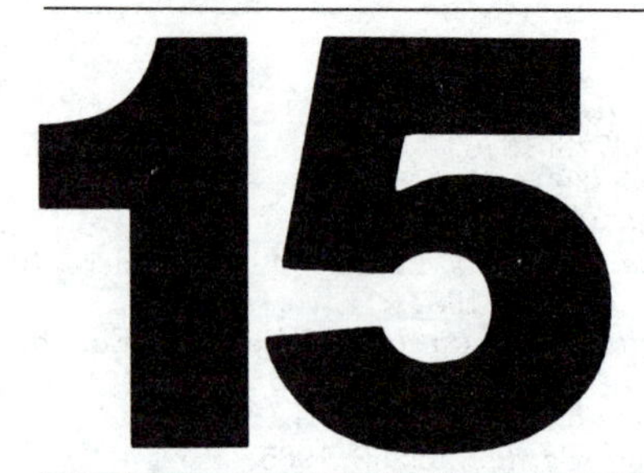

Neonatal Hyperbilirubinemia

John P. Cloherty

I. Background [56B,67]. The normal adult serum bilirubin level is less than 1 mg/dl. Adults appear jaundiced when the serum bilirubin level is greater than 2 mg/dl, and newborns appear jaundiced when the serum bilirubin level is greater than 7 mg/dl. Between 25 and 50 percent of all term newborns and a higher percentage of premature newborns develop clinical jaundice. Also, 6.1 percent of well term newborns will have a maximal serum bilirubin level over 12.9 mg/dl. A serum bilirubin level over 15 mg/dl is found in 3 percent of normal term babies [52].

A. Source of bilirubin. Bilirubin is produced from the breakdown of heme-containing proteins.

1. The major heme-containing protein is **red cell hemoglobin,** which is the source of 75 percent of bilirubin production. Red cell hemolysis makes this protein available for catabolism. Heme **protoporphyrin** is oxidized to **biliverdin,** and biliverdin is reduced to bilirubin with the production of **carbon monoxide (CO)** (which is excreted from the lung) and **iron** (which is reutilized). This reaction is catalyzed by microsomal heme oxygenase. Catabolism of 1 gm hemoglobin produces 34 mg bilirubin. Measurement of carbon dioxide production rate has been used in the study of hyperbilirubinemia and hemolysis [85]. Bilirubin is then reduced to bilirubin IXα (naturally occurring isomer in humans) by the enzyme bilirubin reductase.
2. The other 25 percent of bilirubin is called **early-labeled hemoglobin** and comes from
   - a. The breakdown of free heme, heme proteins, myoglobin, and heme-containing enzymes in the liver
   - b. Ineffective erythropoiesis with destruction of nonsenescent red cell precursors in the bone marrow
3. The normal newborn produces 6 to 10 mg of bilirubin per kilogram per day, as opposed to the production of 3 to 4 mg/kg per day in the adult. The newborn has a greater red cell mass per kilogram than the adult, has red cells with a life span of 80 to 90 days (as opposed to 120 days for the adult), and has greater production of bilirubin from sources others than senescent erythrocytes.
4. Bilirubin IXa, the usual unconjugated bilirubin, is a weakly polar weak acid with low solubility in water at neutral pH. It is not very soluble in fat but is somewhat soluble in weakly polar solvents.

B. Bilirubin metabolism [53,111]

1. **Transport.** Bilirubin IXα is bound to albumin for transport in the blood to the liver. The tightness of the albumin-bilirubin bond is of importance in bilirubin toxicity. Bilirubin bound to albumin does not usually enter the central nervous system (CNS) and is nontoxic.
2. **Uptake.** Bilirubin, but not albumin is transported into the liver cell, probably by a bilirubin-binding protein on the surface of the liver cell. Once within the liver cell, bilirubin is bound to ligandin (Y protein, glutathione S-transferase B), Z protein, and other glutathione S-transferases for transport to the smooth endoplasmic reticulum for conjugation [48]. Phenobarbital increases the concentration of ligandin.

3. **Conjugation.** Unconjugated (indirect) bilirubin (UCB), which is lipid-soluble, is converted to a water-soluble (direct) bilirubin by conjugation in the liver cell.
   a. **Bilirubin uridine diphosphate glucuronyl transferase (UDPG-T)** is inducible by phenobarbital and catalyzes the formation of bilirubin monoglucuronide in the endoplasmic reticulum.
   b. The **bilirubin monoglucuronide** may be excreted as is, stored, or converted to bilirubin diglucuronide in the plasma membrane of the liver cell. This reaction is catalyzed by a transferase enzyme.
4. **Excretion.** After conjugation, bilirubin is excreted into the bile through the canalicular membrane. In the presence of bacteria, particularly *Clostridium perfringens* and *Escherichia coli,* most of the conjugated bilirubin (CB) is reduced to **stercobilin** and not resorbed. Because the gut is sterile in the newborn, this reduction does not occur. The newborn gut contains **beta-glucuronidase,** which hydrolizes bilirubin glucuronide, producing UCB that may be resorbed (enterohepatic circulation) [73].
5. **Fetal bilirubin metabolism**
   a. Most UCB formed by the fetus is cleared by the placenta into the maternal circulation.
   b. **Conjugation** of bilirubin is limited in the fetus because of decreased fetal hepatic blood flow, decreased hepatic ligandin, and decreased UDPG-T activity. CB is excreted into the fetal gut and is usually hydrolyzed and resorbed. Infants with hemolytic disease may have increased levels of CB at birth.
   c. Bilirubin is normally found in amniotic fluid by 12 weeks' gestation and is usually gone by 37 weeks' gestation. Increased amniotic fluid bilirubin is found in hemolytic disease of the newborn and in fetal intestinal obstruction below the bile ducts.

II. **Physiologic hyperbilirubinemia** (Figure 15-1). Most newborn infants develop a serum UCB level over 2 mg/dl in the first week of life. This level usually rises in full-term infants to a peak of 6 to 8 mg/dl by 3 days of age and then falls. A rise to 12 mg/dl is in the physiologic range. In premature infants, the peak may be 10 to 12 mg/dl on the fifth day of life, possibly rising over 15 mg/dl without any specific abnormality of bilirubin metabolism. Levels under 2 mg/dl may not be seen until 1 month of age in both full-term and premature infants. This "normal jaundice" is called **physiologic hyperbilirubinemia.** It is caused by an increased bilirubin load presented to the liver cells, by difficulty clearing the bilirubin from the plasma, and by impaired conjugation and excretion of the bilirubin. All these problems are transient in physiologic hyperbilirubinemia; however, there are certain conditions in which bilirubin levels normally considered in the physiologic range might be pathologic (e.g., sick infants, premature infants). Physiologic jaundice is attributed to the following mechanisms:

A. An increased bilirubin load on the hepatic cell ($>$8.5 mg/kg per day) due to
   1. Increased red blood cell (RBC) volume per kilogram in infants as compared with adults
   2. Decreased survival of fetal RBC: 90-day survival as compared with 120-day survival of adult RBC
   3. Increased early-labeled bilirubin
   4. Increased resorption of bilirubin from intestine (enterohepatic circulation) [73]
      a. Beta-glucuronidase converts conjugated bilirubin to UCB in the intestine. This UCB is then resorbed.
      b. **Early feeding** reduces serum bilirubin levels, possibly by decreasing the bilirubin resorption through the following mechanisms:
         (1) The increased gut motility caused by the feedings
         (2) The introduction of bacteria into the gut; the bacteria convert CB to urobilin, which cannot be resorbed [53]

B. Defective uptake of bilirubin from plasma [48] as a result of
   1. Decreased ligandin (Y protein)

2. Binding of Y and Z proteins by other anions
3. Decreased caloric intake in the first 24 to 72 hours (this mechanism is considered possible, but it is not certain)

C. Defective conjugation due to
1. Decreased UDP G-T activity
2. Decreased UDP glucose dehydrogenase activity

D. Decreased excretion of bilirubin

Healthy term infants usually do not need their bilirubin levels measured unless jaundice occurs in the first 2 days of life or it appears that the bilirubin level may rise into the 20s. There is no evidence that healthy term infants without a pathologic cause of jaundice are at risk of brain damage with bilirubin levels in the 20–24 mg/dl range (26, 56A, 56B). Most of our healthy term infants are sent home by 48 hours of age, and many are leaving at 24 hours of age. If they return at day 4 of life with a bilirubin level of 15–17 mg/dl, they can be safely followed without phototherapy. If the age of the baby, the level of the bilirubin, and rate of rise suggest that the bilirubin will rise into the 20s, treatment may be indicated (see **V.E**).

III. **Nonphysiologic hyperbilirubinemia** (Figs. 15-1 and 15-2 and Table 15-1) [11]. Nonphysiologic hyperbilirubinemia may not be easy to distinguish from physiologic hyperbilirubinemia. In small, sick, premature infants, even a bilirubin concentration in the "physiologic range" may cause kernicterus. The following situations suggest nonphysiologic hyperbilirubinemia and require investigation.

A. **General conditions**
1. Clinical jaundice prior to 36 hours of age
2. Serum bilirubin concentrations increasing by more than 5 mg/dl per day
3. Total serum bilirubin level greater than 15 mg/dl in a formula-fed term infant
4. Total serum bilirubin level greater than 17 mg/dl in a breast-fed term infant
5. Clinical jaundice persisting after 8 days in a term infant or after 14 days in a premature infant
6. Investigation for an elevated bilirubin may only require history taking and following the bilirubin levels. The common factors associated with elevated bilirubin levels without abnormality of bilirubin metabolism are

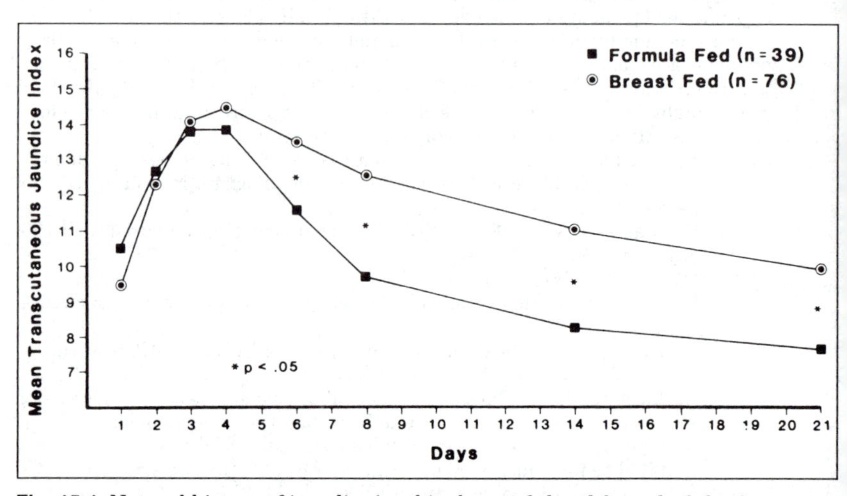

Fig. 15-1. Natural history of jaundice in white breast-fed and formula-fed infants. (From C. Kivlahan and E. J. P. James, The natural history of neonatal jaundice. *Pediatrics* 74: 368, 1984.)

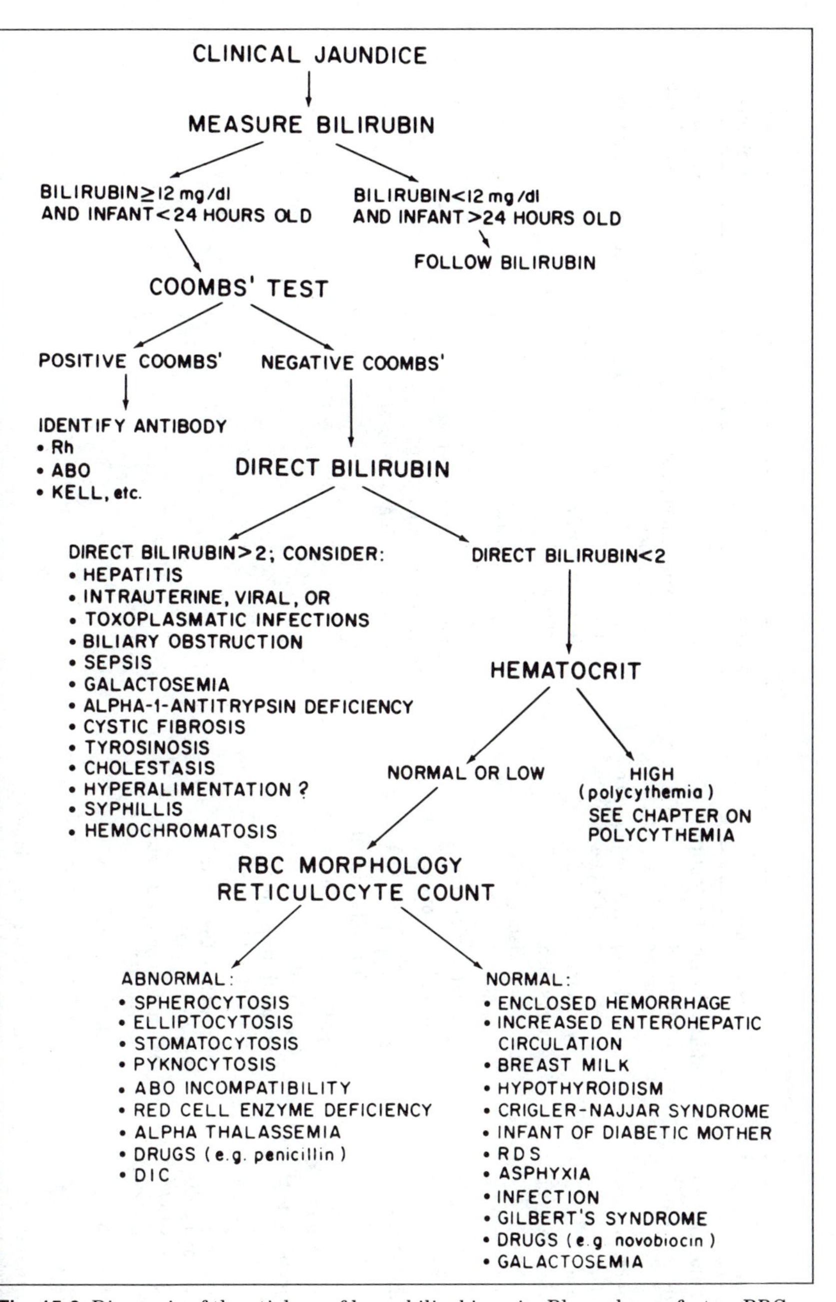

Fig. 15-2. Diagnosis of the etiology of hyperbilirubinemia. Rh = rhesus factor; RBC = red blood cell; DIC = disseminated intravascular coagulation; RDS = respiratory distress syndrome.

Table 15-1. Causes of neonatal hyperbilirubinemia

Overproduction	Undersecretion	Mixed	Uncertain mechanism
Fetomaternal blood group incompatibility (e.g., Rh, ABO	**Metabolic and Endocrine Conditions**	Sepsis	Chinese, Japanese, Korean, and American Indian infants
Hereditary spherocytosis (eliptocytosis, somatocytosis	Galactosemia	Intrauterine infections:	Breast-milk jaundice
Nonspherocytic hemolytic anemias	Familial nonhemolytic jaundice types 1 and 2 (Crigler-Najjar syndrome)	Toxoplasmosis	
G-6-PD deficiency and drug	Gilbert's disease	Rubella	
Pyruvate-kinase deficiency	Hypothyroidism	CID	
Other red-cell enzyme deficiencies	Tyrosinosis	Herpes simplex	
Alpha thalassemia	Hypermethioninemia	Syphilis	
Delta-beta thalassemia	Drugs and hormones:	Hepatitis	
Acquired hemolysis due to vitamin K_3, nitrofurantoin, sulfonamides, antimalarials, penicillin oxytocin?, bupivacaine, or infection	Novobiocin	Respiratory distress syndrome	
	Pregnanediol	Asphyxia	
	Lucey-Driscoll syndrome	Infant of diabetic mother	
	Infants of diabetic mothers	Severe erythroblastosis fetalis	
	Prematurity		
	Hypopituitarism and anencephaly		
Extravascular Blood	**Obstructive Disorders**		
Petechiae	Biliary atresia*		
Hematomas	Dubin-Johnson and Rotor's syndrome*		
Pulmonary, cerebral, or occult hemorrhage	Choledochal cyst*		
	Cystic fibrosis (inspissated bile)*		
	Tumor* or band* (extrinsic obstruction)		

Polycythemia	Alpha-1-antitrypsin deficiency*
Fetomaternal or fetofetal transfusion	Parenteral nutrition
Delayed clamping of the umbilical cord	
Increased Enterohepatic Circulation	
Pyloric stenosis*	
Intestinal atresia or stenosis including annular pancreas	
Hirschsprung's disease	
Meconium ileus and/or meconium plug syndrome	
Fasting or hypoperistalsis from other causes	
Drug-induced paralytic ileus (hexamethonium)	
Swallowed blood	

Key: G-6-PD = glucose-6-phosphate dehydrogenase; CID = cytomegalovirus inclusion disease, as in TORCH.
*Jaundice may not be seen in the neonatal period.
Source: Modified from G. B. Odell, R. L. Poland, and E. Nostrea, Jr., Neonatal Hyperbilirubinemia. In M. H. Klaus and A. Fanaroff (Eds.), *Care of the High Risk Neonate*. Philadelphia: Saunders, 1973. Chap. 11.

breast-feeding, maternal diabetes, Asian race, decreased gestational age, bruising, and possibly induction of labor with oxytocin. In these situations, since jaundice is not only expected but likely, especially when several factors are present, extensive laboratory investigations may not be indicated [55,56A,56B].

B. History. The history may suggest a nonphysiologic cause of jaundice.

1. A **family history of jaundice,** anemia, splenectomy, or early gallbladder disease suggests hereditary hemolytic anemia such as spherocytosis.
2. A **previous sibling with jaundice or anemia** may suggest blood group incompatibility.
3. A **previous sibling with jaundice** suggests breast-milk jaundice or jaundice associated with certain racial groups (e.g., Asian and American Indian).
4. A **history of liver disease in the family** or in a sibling may suggest galactosemia, alpha-1-antityrpsin deficiency, tyrosinosis, hypermethioninemia, Gilbert's disease, Crigler-Najjar syndrome types I and II, or cystic fibrosis [16,34].
5. **Maternal illness during pregnancy** may suggest congenital viral or toxoplasmosis infection. Infants of diabetic mothers tend to develop hyperbilirubinemia (see Chap. 1, **Maternal Diabetes**).
6. **Maternal drugs** such as sulfonamides, nitrofurantoin, and antimalarials can cause hemolysis in a G-6-PD–deficient infant.
7. **The labor and delivery history** may show **trauma** that may be associated with extravascular bleeding and hemolysis. The use of **oxytocin** in labor may be associated with neonatal hyperbilirubinemia, although this is controversial [41,55]. **Asphyxiated infants** may have elevated bilirubin levels due either to inability of the liver to process bilirubin or to intracranial hemorrhage. **Delayed cord clamping** may be associated with neonatal polycythemia and jaundice. **Prematurity** is associated with an exaggeration of physiologic hyperbilirubinemia.
8. The infant's history may show **poor caloric intake,** which decreases bowel motility and increases bilirubin resorption from the bowel. Poor caloric intake also may decrease bilirubin uptake by the liver. Vomiting may be associated with sepsis, pyloric stenosis, or galactosemia. Delayed or infrequent stooling may be caused by intestinal obstruction, and bilirubin resorption may be increased.
9. A history of **maternal intake of drugs** that may interfere with the binding of bilirubin to albumin (e.g., sulfonamides) should make one concerned about toxicity of bilirubin at relatively low levels.
10. **Breast-feeding.** A distinction must be made between **breast-milk jaundice,** in which breast milk is the primary factor causing significant jaundice, and **jaundice associated with breast-feeding,** in which the bilirubin level may be only slightly elevated compared with formula-fed babies [34].
    a. True **breast-milk jaundice** occurs in about 1 percent of breast-fed infants. The jaundice is of late onset. After the third day, instead of the usual fall in the serum bilirubin level, the bilirubin level continues to rise and may reach 20 to 30 mg/dl by 14 days of age. If breast-feeding is continued, the levels will stay elevated and then fall slowly at 2 weeks of age, returning to normal by 4 to 12 weeks of age. If breast-feeding is stopped, the bilirubin level will fall rapidly in 48 hours. If nursing is resumed, the bilirubin may rise 2 to 4 mg/ml, but usually will not reach the previous high level. These infants show good weight gain, have normal liver function tests, and show no evidence of hemolysis. The mechanism of true breast-milk jaundice syndrome is unknown. Factors suggested as causes include the following:
        (1) Some mothers with breast-milk jaundice have a hormone (3-alpha,20-beta-pregnanediol) in their breast milk that inhibits bil-

irubin conjugation in incubated liver slices. Some infants have the usual pattern of breast-milk jaundice without this hormone in their mother's milk. In the breast milk of some mothers, this hormone does not inhibit conjugation, and conjugation may be inhibited by breast milk that does not contain 3-alpha, 20-beta-pregnanediol.

(2) Mothers with breast-milk jaundice syndrome have higher lipoprotein lipase activity. This enzyme releases free fatty acids from triglycerides. Free fatty acids may interfere with the hepatic uptake or conjugation of bilirubin.

(3) Decreased excretion of bilirubin in the stool. Breast-fed infants have less stool and less bilirubin in the stool in the first 3 days of life [19].

(4) Increased resorption of bilirubin from the stool. This may be related to decreased passage of stool due to less stool volume and the increased B-glucuronidase activity in breast milk causing cleavage of B-bilirubin glucuronide and readsorption of the unconjugated bilirubin [30,37]. **Kernicterus** has not been reported in a case of pure breast-milk jaundice, but there have been no prospective studies of the effect of this condition on the neonate. There is no evidence that bilirubin is any less toxic in this situation, so it seems reasonable to discontinue breast-feeding for 48 hours in cases of significant indirect hyperbilirubinemia if it is possible that breast-feeding is the cause. Breast-feeding should be discontinued if it appears that the bilirubin will reach levels that may be toxic and also to prevent prolongation of hospitalization as well as the performance of many laboratory tests. In well term infants we usually do this at a level of 16 to 18 mg/dl depending on the age of the baby and the rate of rise in bilirubin level. Discontinuance of breast-feeding is useful to rule out other causes of prolonged unconjugated hyperbilirubinemia, such as hemolytic disease, hypothyroidism, and familial nonhemolytic jaundice (Crigler-Najjar syndrome). Mothers with infants who have breast-milk jaundice syndrome have a recurrence rate of 70 percent in future pregnancies. They can usually successfully nurse their infants if they pump their breasts and resume nursing in 48 hours. They will need much encouragement and support. As they get older, most infants will be able to handle whatever factors in breast milk caused the jaundice. This may be due to an increased ability of the liver to take up and conjugate bilirubin as well as decreased readsorption of bilirubin from the bowel because of increased stool volume and bacterial colonization. These infants may have a higher than average level of unconjugated bilirubin for many weeks. Phototherapy should be used for treatment if the bilirubin level is very high (approaching 20 mg/dl) in healthy term infants. Phototherapy should be used to prevent the bilirubin level from rising to 20 mg/dl in healthy term infants or to levels that may be considered hazardous in premature infants. This is suggested despite the lack of evidence of bilirubin toxicity in term breast-fed infants who have jaundice because of breast-feeding.

b. Jaundice associated with breast-feeding. Infants who are breast-fed have bilirubin levels slightly higher in the first 3 to 4 days of life than bottle-fed infants. The differences in the levels of bilirubin are not clinically significant [19,37,55] (see Fig. 15-1). The factors mentioned in true breast milk jaundice (**10.a.1–4**) may be operative here. Maternal smoking is associated with lower newborn bilirubin levels. In most reported series, breast-feeding mothers were much less likely to smoke than bottle-feeding mothers [54]. When carbon monoxide is used as a marker for bilirubin production, breast-feeding and caloric deprivation were not associated with increased bilirubin production [54]. We encourage breast-feeding mothers to feed their infants every 2 to 3 hours. If an infant has enough jaundice to require treatment or repeated laboratory tests, we may ask the mother to supplement feeding with formula or stop feeding temporarily in case breast-feeding is a factor causing the jaundice. We then resume the breast-feeding when the bilirubin level is under control. These situations require clinical judgment and good communication skills with the parents.

C. **The physical examination** may suggest the cause of nonphysiologic jaundice. The baby should be examined for the following:
  1. **Prematurity**
  2. Evidence of **small size for gestational age (SGA),** which may be associated with polycythemia and in utero infections
  3. **Microcephaly,** which may be associated with in utero infections
  4. **Extravascular blood**—bruising, cephalohematoma, or other enclosed hemorrhage
  5. **Pallor** associated with hemolytic anemia or extravascular blood loss
  6. **Petechiae** associated with congenital infection, sepsis, or erythroblastosis
  7. **Hepatosplenomegaly** associated with hemolytic anemia, congenital infection, or liver disease
  8. **Omphalitis**
  9. **Chorioretinitis** associated with congenital infection
  10. Evidence of **hypothyroidism** (see Chap. 1B)

D. **Clinical tests.** The following tests are indicated in the presence of nonphysiologic jaundice:
  1. Serum bilirubin (direct and indirect)
  2. Determination of blood type and Rh of the mother and infant. Infants of women who are Rh-negative should have a blood type, Rh, and Coombs' test performed at birth. All mothers should have had a blood type and an antibody screen done in pregnancy. This will pick up antibodies to fetal red cell antigens (see **IX**). It will not diagnose the presence of hemolytic anti-A and anti-B antibodies in maternal serum. The cost-effectiveness of routine typing and Coombs' testing of all infants born to O-positive mothers is controversial. It may be wise to perform these tests if skin pigmentation is such that clinical jaundice may be missed. Early hospital discharge makes this approach more desirable.
  3. Direct Coombs' test on the infant
  4. Identification of antibody (this test is performed if the Coombs' test is positive)
  5. Hematocrit
  6. Evaluation of peripheral smear for RBC morphology and reticulocyte count
  7. In prolonged jaundice, tests of liver function [serum glutamic oxaloacetic transaminase (SGOT), alkaline phosphatase), thyroid function [thyroxine (T_4)], as well as tests for viral or bacterial infection and tests of urine for galactosemia (see Chap. 24) may be indicated.
  8. Measurement of serum albumin level and pH may be useful in deciding the risk of toxicity from various levels of bilirubin.
  9. Many tests to measure the binding of bilirubin to albumin and to measure unbound bilirubin have been proposed. Some measurement of bilirubin binding to albumin may be useful, but no test can yet be recommended for routine clinical use [54,75].
  10. **Transcutaneous bilirubinometry** is a useful screening test for the identification of significant jaundice in term infants. It measures the yellowness of the skin and subcutaneous tissues. The instrument is expensive. Each hospital should correlate the instrument they are using with serum bilirubin measurements [54,86,105].

11. Use of the simple card **icterometer** to estimate the level of jaundice has been found by some to be helpful [4]. Transcutaneous **bilirubinometry** and the **icterometer,** although available, have not been felt by many of the clinicians in our hospitals to be superior to the naked eye [56B].

IV. Diagnosis of neonatal hyperbilirubinemia (see Table 15-1 and Fig. 15-2)

V. Bilirubin toxicity. The subject of CNS toxicity from bilirubin has become somewhat confused in recent years [50,72,98]. Jaundiced infants dying from erythroblastosis have a characteristic yellow staining of the brain known as **kernicterus.** The staining is most severe in the basal ganglia, globus pallidus, putamen, and caudate nuclei. The cerebral hemispheres and the bulbar and cerebellar nuclei also may be involved. There also may be necrosis, neuronal loss, and replacement of neurons by glial cells. Clinically, kernicterus [95] presents as follows:

A. **Stage 1:** Poor Moro reflex, decreased tone, lethargy, poor feeding, vomiting, and high-pitched cry
B. **Stage 2:** Opisthotonus, seizures, fever, rigidity, oculogyric crises, and paralysis of upward gaze. Many infants die in this phase.
C. **Stage 3:** Spasticity is decreased at about 1 week of age.
D. **Stage 4:** Late sequelae include spasticity, athetosis, partial or complete deafness, mild mental retardation, paralysis of upward gaze, and dental dysplasia.
E. Some bilirubin encephalopathy may be asymptomatic in the neonatal period but may present with neurologic or intellectual problems years later. There has been general agreement that there is a direct association between **classic, clinical, and pathologic kernicterus** and **marked elevation of UCB in hemolytic disease.** In a retrospective study of full-term infants with Rh disease, Hsia et al. [39] found that 18 percent of infants with bilirubin levels between 16 and 30 mg/dl and 50 percent of infants with bilirubin levels over 30 mg/dl developed kernicterus. Using a policy of keeping the bilirubin level below 20 mg/dl, they found no kernicterus in 200 consecutive cases of Rh disease. A British study [62] showed no kernicterus in infants whose bilirubin level was kept below 18 mg/dl and a 46 percent incidence if the bilirubin level was over 18 mg/dl. Some infants did not develop kernicterus with levels between 30 and 40 mg/dl [62]. Kernicterus has been described in infants who were jaundiced from ABO incompatibility [106]. Serial bilirubins were not obtained in these studies of full-term infants with hemolytic disease; therefore, a safe serum bilirubin level for these infants could not be established. Subsequent clinical experience has shown that in the full-term infant with **hemolytic disease,** if the UCB level is kept under 20 mg/dl, the occurrence of kernicterus is unlikely. This probably should apply to any other causes of hemolytic disease, such as hereditary spherocytosis, pyruvate kinase deficiency, or glucose-6-phosphate dehydrogenase (G-6-PD) deficiency. Some studies suggest that toxic effects of bilirubin (bilirubin encephalopathy) may be asymptomatic in the newborn period but show up later as mild neurologic or intellectual defects. These effects were seen in infants whose serum bilirubin level never reached 20 mg/dl [40,64,78]. Other studies showed no relationship between serum bilirubin level and neurodevelopmental outcome, although there was some relationship at the highest bilirubin levels [15,18,76]. **In well full-term infants without hemolytic disease, there are no data to show any ill effect from bilirubin values under 25 mg/ml** [26,56A]. Because of reports of the presence of "kernicterus" at autopsy in premature infants whose bilirubin level did not exceed 10 mg/dl, guidelines have been developed for treatment of elevated bilirubin levels. Despite these recommendations, studies of low-birth-weight infants have been unable to establish a relationship between bilirubin levels and neurologic damage if the bilirubin level was under 20 mg/dl [10,15,18,44,76]. Kernicterus may occur when UCB is free in the serum. Normally, 1 gm of albumin tightly binds 8.5 mg/dl of bilirubin. The ability of albumin to bind bilirubin tightly may vary from 4.0 to 8.5 mg/dl of bilirubin. Medications that may decrease the ability of albumin to bind bilirubin are

listed in Table 15-2. Infants who have hemolysis, respiratory distress, hypoxia, hypercarbia, acidosis, asphyxia, sepsis, hypothermia, or hypoglycemia may have less ability to bind bilirubin to albumin. Factors that may alter the blood-brain barrier making it more permeable to bilirubin are hyperosmolarity, seizures, hypercarbia, hypertension, vasculitis, and hypoxic ischemic injury [54,75]. Decisions on treatment must be based on the clinical status of the baby as well as the bilirubin level. In one prospective study [102], 100 preterm infants whose serum bilirubin levels exceeded 18 mg/dl were randomly assigned to receive an exchange transfusion or not. There was no difference in the rate of kernicterus or neurologic outcome at age 1 to 2 years if the peak bilirubin level was under 24 mg/dl. The incidence of abnormal neurologic outcome was the same in 87 matched control infants whose bilirubin levels stayed under 15 mg/dl. The one infant with kernicterus had a bilirubin level of 27.6 mg/dl [102]. Other studies compared infants with kernicterus at autopsy with a group matched for birth weight and gestational age who did not have kernicterus at autopsy. There was no difference in the groups in the incidence of sepsis, hypothermia, asphyxia, acidosis, hypercarbia, hypoxia, hypoglycemia, hypoalbuminemia, and serum bilirubin level [44]. Many of the previous studies relating asphyxia, hypoxia, acidosis, and hypernatremia to kernicterus in low-birth-weight infants were done before it was realized that almost half of low-birth-weight infants have intracranial bleeding. The elevated bilirubin levels may have been part of the picture of an intracranial bleed. One of the major problems in this matter is the lack of accuracy of bilirubin measurements at high concentrations [51,80]. The use of phototherapy also may confuse these studies, because during phototherapy bilirubin is photoisomerized into nontoxic isomers of bilirubin. Although these isomers are nontoxic, they cannot be distinguished from naturally occurring toxic bilirubin by the tests used to measure bilirubin [51,80]. The current hypothesis for the occurrence of kernicterus in low-birth-weight infants is that bilirubin must be **"free" or unbound to albumin** for it to cross the blood-brain barrier. Bilirubin is normally carried bound to albumin, and substances bound to albumin cannot usually cross the blood-brain barrier. An explanation for the lack of correlation between bilirubin levels and kernicterus is an alteration in the permeability of the blood-brain barrier [49]. It is possible that the blood-brain barrier may be altered by anoxia, asphyxia, hypertonic solutions, seizures, etc., thus allowing for the development of kernicterus at low levels of bilirubin. A recent study of premature infants showed no relationship between the presence of kernicterus at autopsy and the free or total bilirubin

Table 15-2. Drugs that cause significant displacement of bilirubin from albumin in vitro

Sulfonamides
Moxalactam
Fusidic acid
Radiographic contrast media for cholangiography (sodium iodipamide, sodium ipodate, iopanoic acid, meglumine ioglycamate)
Aspirin
Apazone
Tolbutamide
Rapid infusions of albumin preservatives (sodium caprylate and *N*-acetyltryptophan)
Rapid infusions of ampicillin
Long-chain free fatty acids (FFA) at high molar ratios of FFA:albumin

Source: From P. Roth, and R. A. Polin, Controversial topics in kernicterus. *Clin. Perinatol.* 15: 970, 1988.

level. The presence of kernicterus could not be predicted by the presence of low Apgar scores, hypothermia, hypoglycemia, sepsis, acidosis, hypoxia, or hypercapnia. Three infants with kernicterus did have prolonged acidosis, hypoxemia, or hypothermia in the 24 hours prior to death. The premature infants with kernicterus did not show staining of the basal ganglia (as is seen in term infants) but showed staining in the subthalamic, pontine, and cranial nerve nuclei [51,74]. The neuropathologic changes seen in preterm infants with kernicterus may be due to the prior nonspecific damage and not to the bilirubin [88]. It has been shown that when the blood-brain barrier is altered, albumin-bound bilirubin will enter the brain. These new data indicate that there is **no specific bilirubin level that is definitely "safe" or "toxic" for all infants.** There are no hard guidelines for exchange transfusions in low-birth-weight infants. The following statement from the *Guidelines for Perinatal Care* from the American Academy of Pediatrics and the American Academy of Obstetricians and Gynecologists [2] gives an idea of the current confusion in management of hyperbilirubin:

> Many physicians currently use published guidelines and are aggressive in their treatment of jaundice in low-birth-weight neonates, initiating phototherapy early and performing exchange transfusions in certain neonates with very low bilirubin levels (<10 mg/dl). Nevertheless, it must be recognized that this will not prevent kernicterus consistently. Some pediatricians may prefer to adopt a more conservative therapeutic stance and allow serum bilirubin levels to approach 15 to 20 mg/dl (257 to 342 μmol/liter), even in low-birth-weight neonates, before considering exchange transfusion. At present, both of these approaches to treatment must be considered acceptable. In either case, the finding of low bilirubin kernicterus at autopsy in certain low-birth-weight neonates cannot necessarily be interpreted as a therapeutic failure. Like retinopathy of prematurity, kernicterus is a condition **that cannot be prevented in certain neonates,** given the current state of knowledge. Although there is some evidence of an association between hyperbilirubinemia and neurodevelopmental handicap less severe than classical kernicterus, it has not been established that this represents a cause-and-effect relationship. Futhermore, there is no information presently available to suggest that treating mild jaundice will prevent such a handicap [2].

A recent study from the Netherlands suggests a causal relationship between maximal serum total bilirubin levels and neurodevelopmental outcome in infants under 32 weeks' gestation and/or under 1500 gm in weight [94]. There are problems with the study because all infants did not have ultrasound examination of the head, duration of the elevated bilirubin level was not measured, and bilirubin level was measured only when clinically indicated. This study causes concern and must be confirmed with other follow-up studies of low-birth-weight infants [66]. We are not certain of the best way to manage these low-birth-weight jaundiced infants, but until better data are available, we in the nursery have to do or not do something. These are the general guidelines that we follow:

1. **Infants under 1500 gm, phototherapy** if bilirubin level is over 5 mg/dl
2. **Infants between 1500 and 2000 gm, phototherapy** at bilirubin levels of 8 to 12 mg/dl
3. **Infants between 2.0 and 2.5 kg, phototherapy** at bilirubin levels of 13 to 15 mg/dl
4. **Term formula-fed healthy infants** Consider phototherapy when the bilirubin level is between 15–20 mg/dl
   The decision to use phototherapy will vary with the age of the baby and the judgment as to what the natural history of the rise and fall of the

bilirubin level will be. See **V.E**, the following paragraph, and reference 56A.

5. **Term breast fed healthy infant [see B10]**
   - **a.** Frequent nursing
   - **b.** If the bilirubin level is over 15 mg/dl, be certain that there is adequate fluid intake and stool output
   - **c.** If the bilirubin level is over 18 mg/dl, consider stopping nursing for 48 hours
   - **d.** If the bilirubin level is approaching 20 mg/dl, phototherapy

All these treatments are adjusted according to the age of the baby at the time of the specified bilirubin level. This level must be viewed within the background of the natural history of bilirubin conjugation in the newborn (see **II**). A well, term, formula-fed infant with a bilirubin level of 13 mg/dl at 48 hours of age will probably have a rise to above 15 mg/dl by 72 hours of age, while a similar term infant with a bilirubin level of 13 mg/dl at 96 hours of age would not merit attention [56A]. A premature infant may not start to effectively metabolize the bilirubin load until it is 5 to 6 days old. All the preceding guidelines assume that there is no pathologic cause of jaundice. Sick infants would have phototherapy started at lower levels. In **hemolytic disease** (except ABO incompatibility), phototherapy is started immediately. In **ABO hemolytic disease** we start phototherapy if the bilirubin level exceeds 10 mg/dl at 12 hours, 12 mg/dl at 18 hours, 14 mg/dl at 24 hours, or 15 mg/dl anytime. If the bilirubin reaches a level where kernicterus is likely to occur, an exchange transfusion is done. Some methods of using the serum bilirubin levels as a criteria for exchange transfusion are shown in Tables 15-3 and 15-4. It is generally agreed that exchange transfusions should be done in **full-term** infants with Rh sensitization to prevent the unconjugated bilirubin from rising above 20 mg/dl (Fig. 15-3). Some have chosen a level of 18 mg/dl. A reversible change in audio-evoked potentials has been seen in term isoimmunized infants with bilirubin levels of 15 mg/dl [71]. There is great controversy about the best management of hyperbilirubinemia in the term nonisoimmunized infant and in the premature infant. In well, term, nonisoimmunized infants there is much data to support withholding exchange transfusion if the level of bilirubin stays below 25 mg/dl [75]. In term infants with ABO incompatibility we try to keep the bilirubin level below 20 mg/dl. If there is brisk hemolysis from any cause, the infants are managed as in Rh isoimmunization. In premature infants a plan as in Tables 15-3 and 15-4 may be followed, but this will vary with the age of the baby, the trend of the bilirubin, and the clinical status of the baby. This approach may lead to many unnecessary exchange transfusions

Table 15-3. Serum bilirubin level (mg/dl) as a criterion for exchange transfusion*

	Birth weight (gm)				
	<1250	1250–1499	1500–1999	2000–2499	⩾2500
Standard risk	13	15	17	18	20
High risk†	10	13	15	17	18

*Both treated and untreated infants received an exchange transfusion if bilirubin levels exceeded these values in each weight category.

†High-risk criteria are met when one or more of the following apply: birth weight < 1000 gm, 5-minute Apgar score of 3, PaO_2 < 40 mmHg for >2 hours, pH < 7.15 for >1 hour, rectal temperature < 35°C for >4 hours, serum total protein value < 4 gm/dl × 2, serum albumin level < 2.5 gm/dl × 2, hemolysis, or clinical deterioration.

Source: From W. J. Keenan, K. K. Novak, J. M. Sutherland, D. A. Bryla, and K. L. Fetterly, Morbidity and mortalilty associated with exchange transfusion. *Pediatrics* 75(Suppl.): 417, 1985.

Table 15-4. Management of jaundice in low-birth-weight infants

	Indirect bilirubin concentrations					
Birth weight	5–6 mg/dl	7–9 mg/dl	10–12 mg/dl	12–15 mg/dl	15–20 mg/dl	>20 mg/dl
≤1000 gm	Phototherapy* →	→	Exchange transfusion† →	→	→	→
1000–1500 gm	Observe and repeat BR	Phototherapy →	→	Exchange transfusion →	→	→
1500–2000 gm	Observe and repeat BR →	→	Phototherapy →	→	Exchange transfusion →	→
>2000 gm	Observe	Observe and repeat BR	Phototherapy (<2500 gm)	Phototherapy (>2500 gm) →	→	Exchange transfusion

Key: BR = bilirubin determination.
*Perform binding tests (titration with bilirubin and Sephadex gel filtration) if an infant under phototherapy approaches the next treatment interval.
†Exchange if albumin binding is saturated or if serum indirect BR continues to rise.
Source: From W. J. Cashore and L. Stern, The management of hyperbilirubinemia. *Clin. Perinatol.* 11: 339, 1984.

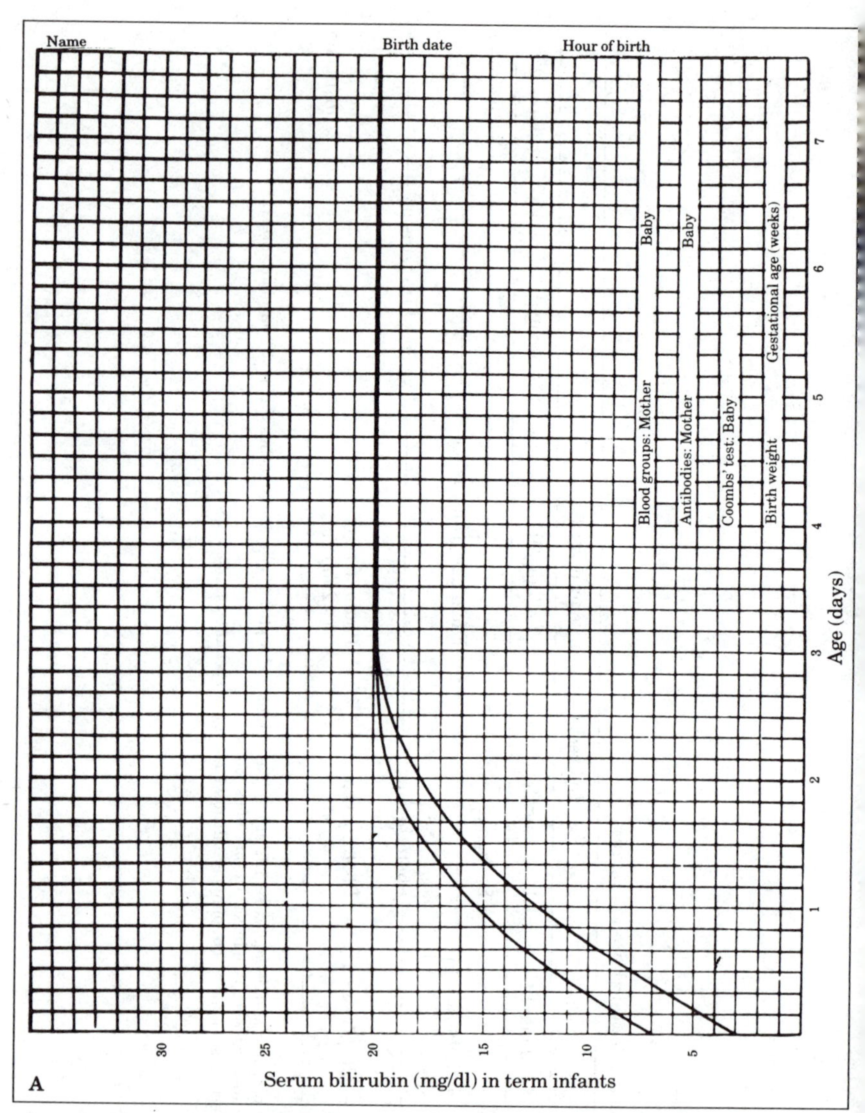

Fig. 15-3. Serum bilirubin levels plotted against age in term infants (**A**) and premature infants (**B**) with erythroblastosis. Levels above the top line are predictive of an ultimate bilirubin level that will be over 20 unless the natural course is altered by treatment. Levels below the bottom line predict that the level will not eventually reach 20. Between the lines is an intermediate zone, in which the ultimate level could be

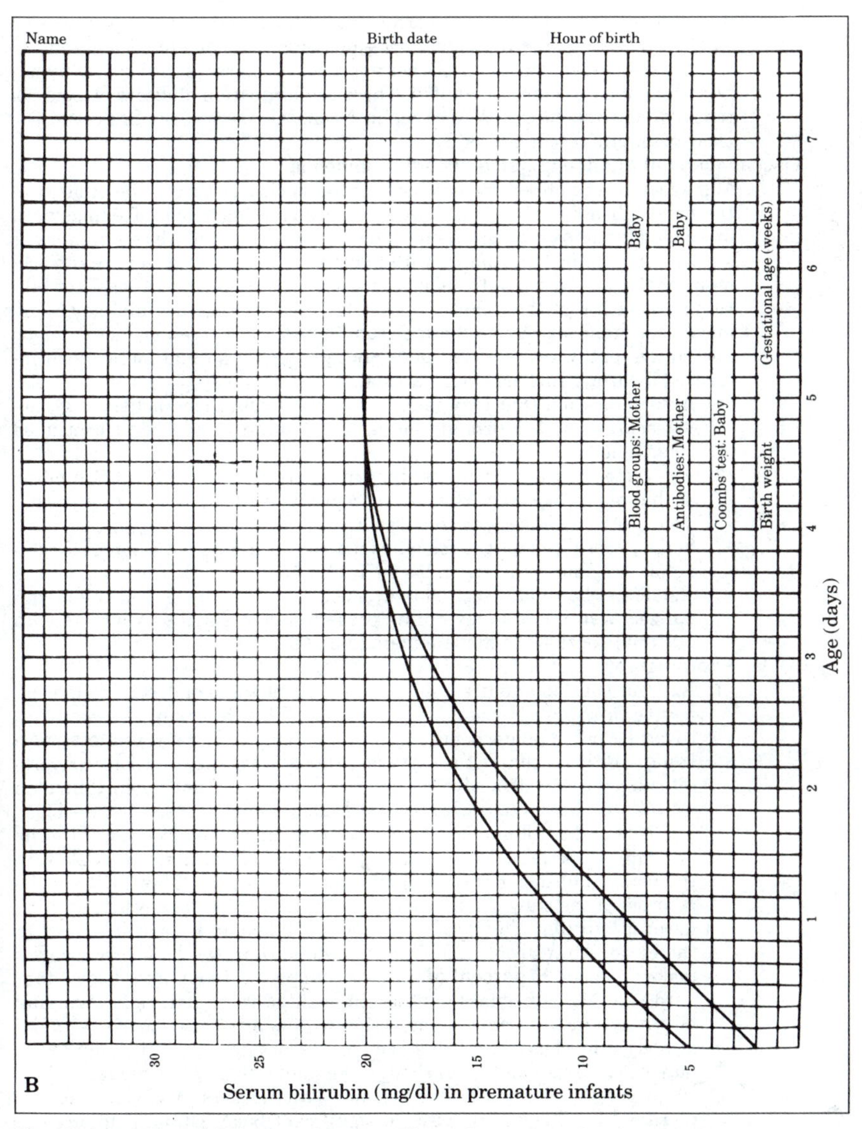

Fig. 15-3 (continued) below or above 20. These charts were developed before phototherapy was used in this country and before the discovery of many factors that might lead to kernicterus at low bilirubin levels; however, the charts still offer good guidelines to the natural progression of bilirubin leels in infants with Rh incompatibility. (From F. H. Allen, Jr., and L. K. Diamond, *Erythroblastosis Fetalis: Including Exchange Transfusion Technique*. Boston: Little, Brown, 1957. P. 57.)

and will not definitely prevent kernicterus. All these data must be reviewed by the caregivers, and individual decisions must be made in each case as to what is the best management. Other approaches to assess the risks of hyperbilirubinemia are being evaluated. These are brainstem auditory evoked potentials, analysis of cry, the Brazelton Neonatal Assessment Scale and nuclear magnetic resonance (56B).

VI. Management of unconjugated hyperbilirubinemia

A. Management of indirect hyperbilirubinemia is clearly tied to the etiology of the hyperbilirubinemia. Infants who are receiving inadequate feedings need **increased feedings** both in volume and in calories to reduce the enterohepatic circulation of bilirubin. Infants with hypothyroidism need adequate replacement of thyroid hormone to treat their hyperbilirubinemia. If levels of bilirubin are such that the infant is at risk for kernicterus, bilirubin may be removed mechanically by **exchange transfusion,** its excretion increased by alternative pathways by using **phototherapy,** or its normal metabolism increased by **drugs** such as phenobarbital.

1. Any medication that may interfere with bilirubin metabolism (e.g., novobiocin) or with bilirubin binding by albumin should be discontinued (see Table 15-2).
2. Any factor (drugs or acidosis) that may interfere with bilirubin binding or that may make the CNS more susceptible to bilirubin toxicity (hypoxia, ischemia) should be corrected (see **V**).
3. Some general guidelines for management of infants with hyperbilirubinemia are shown in section **V** and Tables 15-3A and B. These guidelines should not be rigidly applied to every infant. Therapy should be individualized. **Kernicterus may not be preventable in small sick infants with current programs of management** [2,51,66].

B. Phototherapy [8,52,56A,65,88]

1. Exposure of the jaundiced infant to blue, cool white or green lights is effective in reducing serum bilirubin level. When bilirubin absorbs light, several types of photochemical reactions occur. The first is **photoisomerization,** which occurs in the extravascular space of the skin. This converts bilirubin produced in vivo by the breakdown of hemoglobin (bilirubin 4Z,15Z) to a bilirubin isomer (4Z,15E). This isomer diffuses into the blood and is bound to albumin, transported to the liver, and excreted with the bile into the bowel. No conjugation is required. Excretion is very slow. In the bowel the isomer may be converted back to UCB. This UCB may be resorbed if the baby is not having stools [52]. During phototherapy, both natural bilirubin (UCB) (4Z,15Z) and the bilirubin isomer are found in the blood. After about 12 hours of phototherapy, the less toxic isomers make up about **20 percent of the bilirubin** pool in the infant's body. Standard tests for bilirubin do not distinguish **between** naturally occurring bilirubin and the isomer. Conversion to this less toxic isomer is rapid, although the clearance of this isomer is somewhat slow. Bilirubin levels may not change much even though the phototherapy has made the bilirubin present less toxic. Photoisomerization occurs at low-dose phototherapy (6 $\mu W/cm^2/nm$), with no significant benefit from doubling the irradiance. Another reaction occurring in phototherapy is the **intramolecular cyclization of bilirubin to lumirubin** [59]. Lumirubin makes up 2 to 6 percent of serum concentration of bilirubin during phototherapy. It is rapidly excreted in the bile and urine without conjugation. Since the conversion of bilirubin to lumirubin is an irreversible reaction it is not changed back to bilirubin for readsorption. It is the most important pathway for the lowering of serum bilirubin level [52]. There is a strong dose-effect relationship between the excretion of lumirubin and the dose of phototherapy in the range of 6 to 12 $\mu W/cm^2/nm$. Some bilirubin is converted to polar colorless products by **photo-oxidation**. These products are probably excreted in the urine and account for a small part of the drop in bilirubin level by phototherapy.

2. The amount of irradiance (measured in microwatts per square centimeter per nanometer) to which the skin is exposed determines the effectiveness of phototherapy. Since bilirubin adsorbs visible light in the 400- to 500-nm range, any light source with irradiance in this range will be effective. The most effective lights are those with high-energy output near the maximum adsorption peak of bilirubin (450 to 460 nm). Blue lamps with a peak output at 425 to 475 nm are the most efficient for phototherapy. Cool white lamps with a principal peak at 550 to 600 nm and a range of 380 to 700 nm are usually adequate for treatment; they do not overheat the baby, and they do not mask cyanosis. We have found that light banks with alternate blue and white lights are effective and do not make the baby appear cyanotic [33]. The irradiance can be measured at the skin by a radiometer and should exceed 5 $\mu W/cm^2$ at 425 to 475 nm. There is not much benefit in exceeding 9 $\mu W/cm^2/nm$. Other methods of checking irradiance are to change the bulbs after they have been used for an amount of time specified by the manufacturer [i.e., when the irradiance in the desired spectrum (425 to 475 nm) falls] (GE 20-W daylight lamps, 2000 hours). This requires keeping a log book for each unit. Our practice is to change all the bulbs every 3 months, because this approximates the correct number of hours of use and irradiance for our unit.
3. **Indications for phototherapy**
   a. Phototherapy should be used (1) when there is an abnormal rise in the bilirubin level (see Figs. 15-1 and 15-3) or (2) when a level of bilirubin exists that may be hazardous to the infant if it were to increase, even though it has not reached levels requiring exchange transfusion (see Tables 15-3A and B and Fig. 15-3).
   b. **Prophylactic phototherapy** may be indicated in special circumstances (i.e., tiny infants who are likely to develop dangerous levels of bilirubin, severely bruised premature infants). In hemolytic disease of the newborn, phototherapy is used while the rise in the serum bilirubin level is plotted (see Fig. 15-3) and while waiting for exchange transfusion.
   c. In hemolytic disease of the newborn, phototherapy is started immediately at birth.
   d. Before phototherapy is started, a diagnosis as to the probable cause of jaundice should be made. The minimum would be a history, physical examination, and a Coombs' test, as well as a hematocrit and blood smear.
   e. It is usually best that each hospital set general guidelines for an acceptable bilirubin level for infants of various gestational ages and clinical situations.
   f. A 4-day-old term infant who has no medical problems and has nonhemolytic jaundice with a bilirubin level of 15 mg/dl can usually be observed; however, a 2-day-old term infant with the same bilirubin level will usually need treatment with phototherapy because the bilirubin may continue to rise until the fourth or fifth day.
   g. In term babies who have no other medical problems and have nonhemolytic jaundice, we usually try to keep the bilirubin level below 20 mg/dl. If the bilirubin level is 16–17 mg/dl on day 4, we may treat with phototherapy. This depends on the rate of rise. If it was 13 mg/dl on day 4, we would not treat. We would evaluate fluid intake, urine and stool output, and state of hydration. We would then follow the bilirubin level.
   h. Parents of infants who are born at home or who leave the hospital less than 24 hours after birth should be informed about neonatal jaundice.
   i. The ideal management of premature infants to prevent bilirubin toxicity is unknown (see **V** and refs. 2, 51, 74, and 75). Until there is greater understanding of the mechanisms of bilirubin toxicity, the guidelines in Tables 15-3A and B are probably reasonable. It is best

to decide in each case what would be an acceptable bilirubin level and at what level an exchange transfusion should be performed. Phototherapy is usually started at a level of bilirubin that is one-half the "exchange level." Most infants under 1000 gm are started on phototherapy immediately after birth.

j. Phototherapy should not be used in infants with liver disease or obstructive jaundice. These infants might develop the "bronze baby" syndrome [47]. This is probably caused by retention of some product of phototherapy. Since most babies with obstructive jaundice do not have high indirect bilirubin levels, phototherapy is usually not indicated. If the indirect bilirubin level is high, exchange transfusion is probably safer than phototherapy because it is not known if the bronze pigment is toxic [34].

4. Technique of phototherapy [104]

a. The **light source** is usually four daylight and four special blue light fluorescent lamps 45 cm above the infant. Some currently used units are ineffective because the radiant energy is inadequate or because the units are placed too far away from the infant. We use the Airshield phototherapy unit (manufactured by Airshield, Inc., Hatboro, Pa. 19040). We also use 20-W Westinghouse special blue fluorescent lamps (F/20T12), alternating with Criticolor white fluorescent lamps (Vero-a-Ray, F/20TIC/cc) (available from North American Phillips Corp., Toledo, Ohio 43605). The irradiance should be at least 6 $\mu W/cm^2/nm$ in wavelengths of 400 to 500 nm at the infant's skin. The ideal is 8 to 9 $\mu W/cm^2/nm$. For infants on critical care open beds we use the Ohmeda Ohio infant warmer system with phototherapy light II, stock no. 6600-0055-900 (Ohmeda Columbia, Md. 21046-1801, Division of BOC Health Care). This is a spot phototherapy quartz halide white light with output in the blue spectrum. There is increased output in the center of the beam and decreased output at the edges of the beam. Another system we use for infants in critical care beds is the Airshield phototherapy system 2850. Green light is effective but has no advantage over blue light (56B). We have recently used a woven fiberoptic blanket which delivers light in the 425-475 nm range for phototherapy. The blanket remains cool. Bili-Blanket® stock # 6600-0104-900 OHMEDA, Columbia, Md, 21046-1801.

b. The lamps should be changed after 2000 hours of use (see **B.2**). The manufacturer provides data on the decay of lamps after various hours of use. These data should be used in planning a method of monitoring the energy output of the lamps. Monitoring the energy output in the 425- to 475-nm range will give more precise information on energy output.

c. All electrical outlets must be properly grounded.

d. A Plexiglas cover or shield is used to prevent harm to the infant in case of lamp breakage and to screen out wavelengths below 300 nm, protecting the infant from ultraviolet light. Infrared energy (wavelengths over 650 nm) is also screened out by Plexiglas.

e. Infants are kept naked except for eyepatches and a face mask used as a diaper.

f. Care should be taken to ensure that the eyepatches do not occlude the nares.

g. Large infants may be treated in an open crib; small infants may need a servocontrolled incubator for temperature control or a servocontrolled warmer bed.

h. If an incubator is used, there should be a 5- to 8-cm space between it and the lamp cover to prevent overheating.

i. The infants are turned every 2 hours.

j. If one wishes to treat a larger skin area and thus increase the efficiency of phototherapy, the infant can be placed in a clear plastic crib on a plastic air bubble mattress (Aircap, Sealed Air Corporation, 2030 Lower Homestead Avenue, Holyoke, Mass. 01040), and another bank of lights can be placed under the baby [87]. If clear plastic cribs are not available, an extra light can be placed beside the infant. Another method of increasing the amount of skin exposure to light with an organza hammock has been described [22].

k. Temperature is monitored every 2 hours using a control alarm if possible.

l. Infants should be weighed daily (small infants are weighed twice each day); extra fluid should be provided as necessary.

m. Between 10 and 20 percent extra fluid over usual requirements is given to compensate for the increased insensible water loss and to increase stooling to prevent the resorption of bilirubin from the bowel (see Chap. 24).

n. Skin color is not a guide to hyperbilirubinemia in infants undergoing phototherapy; consequently, bilirubin level should be monitored at least every 12 hours.

o. Infants are removed from phototherapy for feedings and to let the baby and mother enjoy visual and tactile contact.

p. Phototherapy is stopped when it is felt that the level is low enough to eliminate concern about toxic effects of bilirubin, when risk factors for toxic levels of bilirubin are gone, and when the baby is old enough to handle the bilirubin load (e.g., in nonhemolytic jaundice in a term infant, the infant is often 4 to 5 days of age and the bilirubin is 13 mg/dl). A bilirubin level is usually checked 12 hours after lights are stopped.

q. Home phototherapy is effective and is cheaper than hospital phototherapy. Most candidates for home phototherapy are breast-fed infants whose bilirubin problems can be resolved with a brief interruption of breast-feeding. Asphyxia and apnea from nasal obstruction from the eyepatches has been reported in hospital phototherapy. Constant supervision is required. All the other details of phototherapy, such as temperature control and fluid intake, are also required. The Academy of Pediatrics has issued guidelines for home phototherapy but has not endorsed its use [3]. Use of the Bili-Blanket® may make this treatment safer [B4a]. (Bili-Blanket®) stock #6600-0104-900 OHMEDA, Columbia, Maryland 21046-1801.

r. Telling mothers who have jaundiced babies to put them in sunlight at home may be **hazardous.** Severe hyperthermia may result from putting infants in direct sunlight.

5. Side effects of phototherapy [8,14,52]. Light has many biologic effects. Some side effects are the following:

a. Insensible water loss

(1) There is increased insensible water loss in infants undergoing phototherapy. In term infants this loss may increase by 40 percent, whereas in low-birth-weight infants it may increase by 80 to 200 percent. This is especially true in infants in open cribs and beds. Servocontrolled warmers and incubators will decrease this water loss. These infants must be given extra fluid to make up for these losses (see Fluid and Electrolyte Management of the Newborn in Chap. 24).

(2) Gastrointestinal effects. Phototherapy is associated with **watery diarrhea** and increased **fecal water loss.** The diarrhea may be caused by increased bile salts and unconjugated bilirubin in the bowel.

(3) Decreases in **serum calcium level** in preterm infants have been described with phototherapy.

(4) **Retinal damage** has been described in animals whose eyes have been exposed to phototherapy. **The eyes should be shielded with eyepatches.** Follow-up studies of infants whose eyes have been adequately shielded show normal clinical vision and normal electroretinography [52].

(5) **Skin.** The bilirubin in the skin is removed by phototherapy, so skin color can no longer be used as a guide to serum bilirubin levels. Phototherapy is effective in black infants. There may be some tanning of the skin of black infants under phototherapy owing to exposure to light in the 300- to 600-nm range. Exposure to wavelengths in the 360- to 400-nm range may cause erythemia and increased skin blood flow.

(6) "Bronze baby" syndrome (see **B.3.j**)

(7) **Cell damage** effects in tissue culture cells exposed to phototherapy have been seen. These include mutations, sister chromatid exchange, and DNA strand breaks. It may be wise to shield the scrotum during phototherapy.

(8) Tryptophan is reduced in amino acid solutions exposed to phototherapy. Methionine and histidine are also reduced in amino acid solutions if multivitamins are added and the solution is exposed to phototherapy. These solutions should probably be shielded from phototherapy by using aluminum foil on the lines and bottles.

(9) Effects of phototherapy on **growth and head circumference** have been described in some studies but not in others [52].

(10) Phototherapy upsets the usual maternal-infant interaction and should be used only with adequate thought and explanation.

(11) No significant long-term developmental differences have been found in infants treated with phototherapy as compared with controls [8,52,54,65].

C. Exchange transfusion is performed to correct anemia in infants severely affected with erythroblastosis and hydrops or to prevent or correct hyperbilirubinemia that might lead to neurologic sequelae. Double-volume exchange transfusion lowers the bilirubin level in the plasma to about one-half the preexchange level. Bilirubin is removed from the extravascular space because extravascular bilirubin will equilibrate and bind to the albumin in the exchanged blood. The infant's antibodies are washed out, and red cells that are partially hemolyzed or antibody coated are washed out. Exchange transfusion should be instituted if evaluation of bilirubin and albumin levels indicate any significant risk of bilirubin toxicity (see **V** and Fig. 15-3 and Tables 15-3A and B). Asphyxia, hypoalbuminemia, acidosis, hypoxia, or shock should be corrected prior to exchange transfusion. All these infants are in intense phototherapy while a decision to exchange is being made.

1. **Early exchange transfusion** is indicated in the presence of hydrops and is often indicated by a history of previously severely affected infants or a known sensitized infant [100].

   a. The objective of early exchange transfusion is to correct anemia, stop hemolysis, and prevent a rise in bilirubin level (see Fig. 15-3). In **hemolytic disease,** immediate exchange transfusion is usually indicated if

   (1) The cord bilirubin level is over 4.5 mg/dl and the cord hemoglobin level is under 11 gm/dl

   (2) The bilirubin level is rising over 1 mg/dl per hour despite phototherapy

   (3) The hemoglobin level is between 11 and 13 gm/dl and the bilirubin level is rising over 0.5 mg/dl per hour despite phototherapy

   (4) The bilirubin level is 20 mg/dl or it appears that it will reach 20 mg/dl at the rate it is rising (see Fig. 15-3)

(5) There is progression of anemia in the face of adequate control of bilirubin by other methods (e.g., phototherapy)

These guidelines are somewhat historical, and they do not take into account intensive phototherapy [23,52]. In hemolytic disease, we usually do an early exchange if there is significant anemia (Hbg level under 11 gm/dl) and we cannot control the bilirubin by phototherapy. Figure 15-3 shows the natural history of the bilirubin use in infants with Rh sensitization without phototherapy.

b. **Effects of early exchange.** Early exchange removes sensitized RBCs before hemolysis and removes bilirubin prior to extravascular space distribution.

c. When a hydropic infant is expected, as in the case of an infant who has received intrauterine transfusions, cooperation among the pediatrician, obstetrician, and blood bank is essential. In such cases, immediate partial exchange transfusion may be necessary to correct anemia, improve congestive heart failure (CHF), and remove sensitized red blood cells.

2. **Rebound of bilirubin levels after exchange**
   a. The exchange with fresh blood introduces unbound albumin.
   b. A two-volume exchange (see **5.24**) leaves 13 percent of the baby's RBCs. After the exchange, bilirubin level is often 45 percent of preexchange levels, and it rises to 60 percent of preexchange levels within half an hour; this demonstrates the rapid influx of bilirubin into the vascular space.
   c. A larger increase in bilirubin reflects newly formed bilirubin as a result of the following:
      (1) Previously sequestered (in bone marrow or spleen) sensitized RBCs
      (2) Early-labeled bilirubin
      (3) Hemolysis of transfused RBCs. The importance of this as a cause of later increases in bilirubin is demonstrated by the high frequency of repeat exchange transfusions required in nonhemolytic disease.

3. **Later exchange transfusions** are indicated at bilirubin levels that may be toxic or if the bilirubin level may be expected to reach such levels. Repeat exchanges are usually indicated when, after the early rebound, the bilirubin continues to rise over 1 mg/dl per hour or when there is a severe persistent hemolytic anemia. If the initial bilirubin level was over 25 mg/dl, there will usually be a high rebound, and the infant should usually be exchanged again within 8 to 12 hours.

4. **Blood used in exchange transfusion** should be whole blood collected in citrate-phosphate-dextrose (CPD). Blood should be as fresh as possible (<24 hours old for hydropic or sick neonates and <72 hours old for all others). Blood collected in acid-citrate-dextrose (ACD) is usually not used because of the high acid load. Blood prepared from components (packed red cells and fresh-frozen plasma) has ACD as the anticoagulant. Blood may be produced from components when fresh blood is not available and young red cells and active plasma factors are required. The blood can be made up to the desired hematocrit. Heparinized blood is usually not available in the United States. Preparation of blood for exchange transfusion is discussed in Chapter 20.
   a. Citrate binds ionic calcium and magnesium. The fall in magnesium level associated with exchange transfusion has not been associated with clinical problems. Hypocalcemia associated with exchange transfusion may produce cardiac and other effects (see Hypocalcemia in Chap. 24). The original recommendation for exchange transfusion was to give 1.0 ml of calcium gluconate 10% intravenously after every 100 ml of exchanged blood [1]. This has only a temporary effect on the

ionized calcium [56]. Sometimes if the calcium is given too fast, bradycardia is seen. If given, it should be given over 1 minute. We have performed exchange transfusions in infants with and without added calcium, and we see no real difference. Some recommend that no extra calcium be given unless the electrocardiogram (ECG) and clinical assessment suggest hypocalcemia.

b. The high glucose content of ACD or CPD blood (300 mg/dl) may stimulate insulin secretion from the hyperplastic islets of Langerhans present in infants with erythroblastosis. This hypoglycemia often occurs 1 to 2 hours after an exchange. Blood glucose level should be monitored for several hours after the exchange, and the infant should have a reliable glucose intake by bottle, gavage, or intravenous infusion. Blood made from components may have a low glucose level, causing hypoglycemia during the exchange. The glucose levels of the blood and the infant should be checked during the exchange, and intravenous glucose should be given as needed. It is often useful to have a reliable intravenous line with glucose 5% and water running during the exchange.

c. Acid-base balance. The pH of donor blood is low; however, citrate is metabolized to alkali by the liver. If the baby is very ill and unable to metabolize citrate, the citrate may produce significant acidosis. If the infant is well, buffer usually should not be added because citrate is converted to bicarbonate by the liver, eventually resulting in a late metabolic alkalosis. If the blood is over 24 hours old, measure the pH before using it.

d. CPD blood has less than one-half the acid load of ACD blood, and the pH usually remains above 7.0 after storage for 7 days. In contrast, the pH of ACD blood is about 6.7 by 2 to 3 days of storage. CPD blood is preferred in our nurseries over ACD blood for this reason. Blood made from components has fresh-frozen plasma, which has ACD as the anticoagulant. The pH of ACD plasma is 6.6.

e. In hydropic or critically ill neonates, it is probably wise to buffer the blood with tromethamine (THAM), 10 m*M* of 1.0 *M* THAM per unit of blood. If the blood is less than 48 hours old, this buffering is not necessary. We usually use fresh blood less than 24 hours old for all exchange transfusions in hydropic or ill neonates; therefore, buffering is not a concern.

f. Potassium levels may be elevated in blood over 24 hours old. Levels as high as 9 mg/L may occur in blood 24 hours old and as high as 20 mg/L in blood 48 hours old [4]. If packed red cells are washed before reconstitution, this excess potassium is removed. Washing by some methods (IBM cell washer) may cause hypokalemia. If blood or packed cells are over 24 hours old, it is best to check the potassium level before using it.

g. If the exchange is for nonimmune hyperbilirubinemia, blood is typed and cross-matched against the plasma and red cells of the infant. In Rh hemolytic disease of the newborn, if blood is prepared before delivery, it should be type O Rh-negative cross-matched against the mother. If the blood is obtained after delivery, it also may be cross-matched against the infant. In ABO incompatibility, the blood should be type O Rh-negative or Rh-compatible with the mother and infant, cross-matched against the mother and infant, and have a low titer of naturally occurring anti-A or anti-B antibodies. Sometimes O cells are used with AB plasma to be certain no anti-A or anti-B antibodies are present. In other isoimmune hemolytic disease, the blood should not contain the sensitizing antigen and should be cross-matched against the mother.

h. Subsequent transfusions should be done with blood that is compatible with that of the mother and the infant.

5. **Technique of exchange transfusion.** This technique is reviewed extensively elsewhere [6,24]; some details are listed below:
    1. Sick infants need attention to asphyxia, hypoglycemia, acidosis, and temperature control before exchange transfusion is performed.
    2. In all infants, exchange transfusion should be performed under a radiant heater that is servocontrolled to the infant.
    3. Infants should be restrained with binders on their arms and legs.
    4. A cardiac monitor should be in place as well as a cuff to monitor blood pressure.
    5. Suction, oxygen, and equipment for resuscitation should be available.
    6. Usually, a reliable intravenous line should be in place for administration of glucose and medication.
    7. An assistant should be assigned to the infant to record volumes of blood, to observe the infant, and to check vital signs. An assistant experienced in resuscitation should be available for the rare complications.
    8. The glucose concentration in the blood to be used should be measured before an exchange with reconstituted blood.
    9. The infant's blood glucose level should be measured during an exchange with reconstituted blood and after an exchange with citrated blood (see **4.b**).
    10. When blood is more than 24 hours old or reconstituted, measurement of potassium level and pH may be indicated.
    11. The blood should be warmed to 37°C. A controlled water bath (Hemokinetitherm Controlled Fluid Warmer, Dupaco, Inc., Arcadia, Calif. 91006, or Blood Warming Coil, Abbott Laboratories, North Chicago, Ill. 60064) is the safest means for warming the blood. The temperature of the bath should be monitored by the thermometer in the unit and by an extra external thermometer to guard against failure of the thermometer in the unit.
    12. Sterile techniques should be used.
    13. We do most exchanges by the push-pull technique through the umbilical vein. See Chapter 39 for insertion of an umbilical venous catheter. We use the Plasmaseal exchange transfusion tray (American Pharmaseal Laboratories, Glendale, Calif. 91209).
    14. When the umbilical cord is old and dried up, it is difficult to use for the exchange transfusion. The cord can be softened by soaking it for 30 to 60 minutes with saline; this makes it easy to insert the catheter into the vein.
    15. When an umbilical venous catheter is inserted, a loose tie should be placed around the skin of the cord.
    16. The catheter should be inserted only as far as required to permit free blood exchange. A catheter in the heart may cause arrhythmias.
    17. It is not usually helpful to check the position of the umbilical catheters by x-ray examination, because it is often necessary to move them around during the exchange. The position of central venous catheters should be checked by x-ray studies.
    18. The venous cathether should not be left open to air; the baby may cry and suck in air, causing air embolism.
    19. When the exchange transfusion is finished, a silk purse-string suture should be placed around the vein; the tails of the suture material should be left. This localization of the vein will facilitate the next exchange transfusion.
    20. When the catheter is removed, the tie around the cord should be tightened snugly for about 1 hour. It is important to remember to loosen the tie after 1 hour to avoid necrosis of the skin.
    21. When the venous catheter is removed, it should be pulled out quickly; otherwise, the blood will flow from the distal side hole out the

proximal side hole, which can cause panic in the inexperienced practitioner.

22. If it is not possible to insert the catheter in the umbilical vein, exchange transfusion is most safely accomplished through a **central venous pressure line** placed through the antecubital fossa. This line can be left in for future exchanges. Methods of exchange using peripheral arteries and veins have been described [9,36,83].
23. Isovolumetric exchange transfusion (taking blood out of the umbilical artery and putting new blood in the umbilical vein) may be tolerated better in small, sick, or hydropic infants. We usually do this by a pull out of the umbilical artery with a simultaneous push in the umbilical vein, but a method of doing it with a Holter pump has been described [17].
24. Exchange transfusion usually involves double the volume of the infant's blood; this is termed a **two-volume exchange.** The blood volume in an infant is usually 80 ml/kg; therefore, the exchange transfusion uses 160 ml/kg of blood. In the push-pull method, the blood is removed in aliquots that are tolerated by the infant. This usually is 5 ml for infants under 1500 gm, 10 ml for infants 1500 to 2500 gm, 15 ml for infants 2500 to 3500 gm, and 20 ml for infants over 3500 gm. If the aliquots are large, there will be a greater fall in serum bilirubin level and a greater rebound. If the aliquots are small, the postexchange bilirubin level will be higher but the rebound will be less. If at the end of 3 ml of each withdrawal the blood is pushed back into the baby and then the full aliquot is drawn, the exchange will be more efficient because of less catheter deadspace.
25. A single-volume exchange removes 63 percent of the infant's blood volume. A two-volume exchange removes 87 percent of the infant's blood volume.
26. Sick infants who are anemic (hematocrit < 35 percent) are best given a partial exchange transfusion with packed RBCs (25 to 80 ml/kg) to raise the hematocrit to 40 percent. After the infant has been stabilized, further exchanges can be performed for hyperbilirubinemia. The blood for these exchanges should be set up prior to delivery and packed with the plasma separated into an attached side bag; the components can be remixed if a packed-cell exchange is not necessary.
27. The rate of exchange has little effect on the amount of bilirubin removed [82] because bilirubin is in two compartments—intravascular and extravascular. Small aliquots and a slower rate, however, place less stress on the cardiovascular system. The recommended time for the exchange transfusion is 1 hour.
28. The blood should be shaken gently after every deciliter of exchange, because the RBCs will settle rapidly. Settling may lead to exchange with relatively anemic blood at the end of the exchange.
29. Albumin (in the form of 25 percent salt-poor albumin, 1 gm/kg, 1 to 2 hours prior to exchange) increases the amount of bilirubin removed by the exchange [99]. Some evidence shows that bilirubin is removed from the brain, and neurotoxicity may be alleviated by albumin [5,21] in experimental animals. Albumin is contraindicated in babies with CHF or severe anemia. There is some difference of opinion as to the efficacy of albumin in removing extra bilirubin [12].
30. After exchange transfusion, phototherapy is continued. Bilirubin level is measured every 4 hours. Glucose levels should be monitored.
31. We usually do not treat these infants with antibiotics unless an old, dirty cord was entered or there was some break in sterile technique. If so, the baby may be treated with oxacillin and gentamicin for 3 days.

6. **Complications of exchange transfusions**
    a. **Vascular**—embolization (with air or clots), vasospasm, thrombosis, and infarction
    b. **Cardiac**—arrhythmias, volume overload, and arrest
    c. **Electrolyte**—hyperkalemia, hypoglycemia, hypernatremia, hypocalcemia, hypercalcemia (rapid infusion of calcium), and acidosis
    d. **Bleeding**—thrombocytopenia, deficient clotting factors
    e. **Infections**—bacteremia, hepatitis, cytomegalic viral infection, acquired immune deficiency syndrome (AIDS), malaria (see Chap. 20)
    f. **Miscellaneous**—perforation of vessels, hypothermia, hyperthermia, and possibly necrotizing enterocolitis [89]
    g. Hemoglobinemia, hemoglobinuria, and hyperkalemia have been reported due to overheating of the blood, with resultant hemolysis [96].
    h. Massive hemolysis and intravascular sickling and death from the use of hemoglobin SC have been described. Donor blood with sickle-cell trait or disease should not be used for exchange transfusions in the newborn.
    i. Transient maculopapular rash with eosinophilia, lymphopenia and thrombocytopenia has been described in infants receiving multiple exchange transfusions, both intrauterine and extrauterine. This does not usually progress to **graft-versus-host disease,** as has been described in some neonates who had both intrauterine and extrauterine transfusions [70]. We use irradiated blood in newborns to prevent graft-versus-host disease (see Chap. 20). If the above-mentioned rash is transient and not associated with other signs of immunodeficiency, we do not investigate it [13].

D. **Phenobarbital,** 5 to 8 mg/kg every 24 hours, induces microsomal enzymes and increases bilirubin conjugation and excretion. It has been shown to be effective in lowering the serum bilirubin level and to reduce the need for exchange when given to the mother, the infant, or both.
1. **Side effects** include lethargy and slow feeding. Also, phenobarbital takes 3 to 7 days to become effective and may take much longer in premature infants.
2. There is no advantage in combining phenobarbital with phototherapy [93].
3. Phenobarbital is useful in treatment of Crigler-Najjar syndrome type II and may be useful for treatment of direct hyperbilirubinemia secondary to "inspissated bile" syndrome [92].
4. Phenobarbital may be used in the treatment of the direct hyperbilirubinemia associated with the use of parenteral hyperalimentation.
5. Phenobarbital has been given for 7 days prior to delivery to mothers who are known to have a fetus affected with hemolytic disease. The evidence for benefit is controversial [61,90].
6. Because of effects on neuronal developmental seen in laboratory animals, phenobarbital should not be used routinely for prevention or treatment of hyperbilirubinemia [27,92]. The benefit of phenobarbital in decreasing the need for exchange transfusion with its attendant complications must be balanced with any possible risk of using it (see Chap. 2).

E. **Other methods of management**
1. Full-term infants who are being breast-fed and have bilirubin levels of 18 to 20 mg/dl should be given formula feedings for 48 hours. If breast milk is the cause of the jaundice, the bilirubin level will fall by 2 to 6 mg/dl during this time. This will help rule out other causes and reassures the family. If breast-feeding is restarted, the bilirubin level may rise again and may take 4 to 12 weeks to fall below 2 mg/dl. Kernicterus has not been observed in this group of infants, and it is felt that these mothers should continue to breast-feed them once the bilirubin is at a safe level.

In premature infants who are at any special risk for kernicterus, this policy may have to be altered (see **III.B.10**).

2. Other agents such as agar and activated charcoal have been used to decrease the resorption of bilirubin by the enterohepatic circulation [58,73
3. TIN-protoporphyxin is an inhibitor of heme oxygenase, which is the enzyme necessary for conversion of heme to bilirubin. This is an area of promise for study [42,84].

VII. Direct or conjugated hyperbilirubinemia (CB) [28,35,56B,97] is due to failure to excrete CB from the hepatocyte into the duodenum. It is manifested by a CB level over 2.0 ml/dl or a CB level greater than 15 percent of the total bilirubin level. It may be associated with hepatomegaly, splenomegaly, pale stools, and dark urine. CB is found in the urine; UCB is not. The preferred term to describe it is **cholestasis,** which includes retention of conjugated bilirubin (CB), bile acids, and other components of bile.

A. The differential diagnosis of direct hyperbilirubinemia includes the following:
   1. **Liver cell injury (normal bile ducts)**
      a. **Toxic**—cholestatic jaundice related to the use of intravenous hyperalimentation in low-birth-weight infants. This is the major cause of elevated CB in the newborn intensive care unit. It appears to be unrelated to the parenteral use of lipid.
      b. **Infection—viral**—hepatitis (B, non-A, non-B, A?), **giant cell neonatal hepatitis,** rubella, cytomegalovirus, herpes, EBV, coxsackie, adenovirus; **bacterial**—syphilis, *E. coli,* GBS, *Listeria, Staphyloccus;* **parasitic**—toxoplasmosis
      c. **Metabolic (normal bile ducts)**—alpha-1-antitrypsin deficiency, cystic fibrosis, galactosemia, tyrosinemia, hypermethionemia, fructosemia, storage diseases (Gaucher's, Niemann-Pick, glycogenosis type IV, Wolman's), Roter syndrome, Dubin-Johnson syndrome, Byler disease, Zellweger's syndrome, idiopathic cirrhosis, Aagenaes syndrome (hereditary cholestasis with lymphedema), porphyria
   2. **Excessive bilirubin load (normal bile ducts) (inspissated bile syndrome)**—erythroblastosis fetalis (especially in infants who have been treated with intrauterine transfusion), any other severe red cell hemolytic disease
   3. **Bile flow obstruction (biliary atresia, extrahepatic or intrahepatic).** The extrahepatic type may be isolated or associated with a choledochal cyst, trisomy 13 or 18, or polysplenia. The intrahepatic type may be associated with the Alagille syndrome, coprostanic acidemia, **choledochal cyst, bile duct stenosis, rupture of bile duct, lymph node enlargement, hemangiomas, tumors,** pancreatic cyst, inspissated bile syndrome, and cystic fibrosis.
   4. In the newborn intensive care unit, the most common causes of elevated CB, in decreasing order of frequency, are hyperalimentation, idiopathic hepatitis, biliary atresia, alpha-1-antitrypsin deficiency, intrauterine infection, choledochal cyst, galactosemia, and increased bilirubin load from hemolytic disease.

B. **Diagnostic tests and management**
   1. Evaluate for hepatomegaly, splenomegaly, petechiae, chorioretinitis, and microcephaly.
   2. Evaluate liver damage and function by measurement of serum glutamic oxaloacetic transaminase (SGOT) level, serum glutamic pyruvic transaminase (SGPT) level, alkaline phosphatase level, prothrombin time (PT), partial thromboplastin time (PTT), and serum albumin level.
   3. Rule out known causes of conjugated hyperbilirubinemia (see **A.4**). This usually involves the following:
      a. Stopping parenteral hyperalimentation with amino acids. If this is the cause, the liver dysfunction will usually resolve.
      b. Tests for bacterial, viral, and intrauterine infections (TORCH) (see Chap. 12).

   c. Serum analysis for alpha-1-antitrypsin deficiency.
   d. Serum and urine amino acids determinations (see Chap. 24)
   e. Urinalysis for glucose and reducing substances (see Chap. 24)

4. If known causes are ruled out, the problem is to differentiate idiopathic neonatal hepatitis from bile duct abnormalities such as intrahepatic biliary atresia or hypoplasia, choledochal cyst, bile plug syndrome, extrahepatic biliary atresia, hypoplasia, or total biliary atresia.
   a. An abdominal ultrasound should be done to rule out a choledochal cyst or mass. An upper GI series also may help in this diagnosis.
   b. We use a hepatobiliary scan with technetium (**^{99m}Tc**) diisopropyliminodiacetic (**DISIDA**) as the next step to visualize the biliary tree [81].
   c. Iodine-131–rose bengal fecal excretion test may be useful if the ^{99m}Tc-DISIDA scan is not available.
   d. A nasoduodenal tube can be passed and fluid collected in 2-hour aliquots for 24 hours. If there is no bile, treat with phenobarbital, 5 mg/kg per day for 7 days, and repeat the duodenal fluid collection [38].
   e. If the duodenal fluid collections, scans, and ultrasound suggest no extrahepatic obstruction, a percutaneous needle liver biopsy is done. If the biopsy shows no features of extrahepatic obstruction, the child may be observed with careful follow-up. Sometimes features of both bile duct disease and hepatocellular disease are present, and the pathologist will be unable to give a definite diagnosis.
   f. If the ultrasound, scans, or fluid collections suggest extrahepatic obstruction disease, the baby will need an exploratory laparotomy, cholangiogram, and open liver biopsy to make a definite diagnosis.
   g. If the diagnosis of extrahepatic obstruction disease cannot be ruled out, the baby must have the studies outlined because surgical therapy for choledochal cyst is curative if done early and hepatoportoenterostomy has better results if done early.

VIII. Hydrops. *Hydrops* is a term used to describe generalized subcutaneous edema in the fetus or neonate. It is usually accompanied by ascites and often by pleural or pericardial effusions (or both).

A. Etiology [60,91]. Hydrops fetalis is discussed here because in the past hemolytic disease of the newborn was the major cause of both fetal and neonatal hydrops. Because of the decline in Rh sensitization, nonimmune conditions are now the major causes of hydrops. The elements involved in the pathogenesis of hydrops include anemia, cardiac failure, decreased colloid oncotic pressure (hypoalbuminemia), increased capillary permeability, asphyxia, and placental perfusion abnormalities. There is a general but no constant relationship between the degree of anemia, serum albumin level, and the presence of hydrops. There is no correlation between the severity of hydrops and the blood volume of the infant. Most hydropic infants have normal blood volume (80 mg/kg).

1. Hematologic (chronic in utero anemia) (10 percent of cases)—isoimmune hemolytic disease (e.g., Rh incompatibility), homozygous alpha thalassemia, homozygous G-6-PD deficiency, chronic fetomaternal transfusion, twin-to-twin transfusion, chronic fetomaternal transfusion, hemorrhage, thrombosis, bone marrow failure (chloramphenical, maternal papovirus infection), bone marrow replacement (Gaucher's disease)

2. Cardiovascular (failure or poor output) (20 percent of cases)
   a. Rhythm disturbances—heart block, paroxysmal auricular tachycardia, atrial flutter
   b. Major cardiac malformation (e.g., hypoplastic left heart, Epstein's disease)—myocarditis (coxsackievirus), endocardial fibroelastosis, cardiac neoplasm (rhabdomyoma), cardiac thrombosis, arteriovenous fistulas, premature closure of foramen ovale, generalized arterial calcification

3. Renal (5 percent of cases)—nephrosis, renal vein thrombosis, renal hypoplasia, urinary obstruction

4. **Infection** (8 percent of cases)—syphilis, rubella, cytomegalovirus, congenital hepatitis, toxoplasmosis, leptospirosis, Chagas' disease, parvovirus (see Chapter 12)
5. **Pulmonary** (5 percent of cases)—diaphragmatic hernia, pulmonary lymphangiectasia, cystic adenomatoid malformations, intrathoracic mass
6. **Placenta or cord** (rare cause)—chorangioma, umbilical vein thrombosis arteriovenous malformation, chorionic vein thrombosis, true knot in umbilical cord, cord compression, choriocarcinoma
7. **Maternal conditions** (5 percent of cases)—toxemia, diabetes
8. **Gastrointestinal** (5 percent of cases)—meconium peritonitis, in utero volulus, atresia
9. **Chromosomal** (10 percent of cases)—Turner syndrome, trisomy 13, 18 21, triploidy, aneuploidy
10. **Miscellaneous** (10 percent of cases)—cystic hygroma, Wilms' tumor, angioma, teratoma, neuroblastoma, CNS malformations, amniotic band syndrome, lysosomal storage disorders, congenital myotonic dystrophy skeletal abnormalities (osteogenesis imperfecta, achondrogenesis, hypophosphatasia, thanatophoric dwarf, arthroglyposis), Noonan syndrome acardia
11. **Unknown** (20 percent of cases)

B. Diagnosis. Pregnant women with polyhydramnios, severe anemia, toxemia and isoimmune disease should have an ultrasonic examination of the fetus. If the fetus is hydropic, a careful search by ultrasound and real-time fetal echocardiography may reveal the cause and may guide fetal treatment. The accumulation of pericardial or ascitic fluid may be the first sign of impending hydrops in a Rh-sensitized fetus. Investigations should be carried out for the causes of fetal hydrops mentioned in **A.** The usual investigation includes the following:

1. **Maternal**—blood type and Coombs' as well as red cell antibody titers, complete blood count and red blood cell indices, hemoglobin electrophoresis Kleihauser-Betke stain of maternal blood for fetal red cells, VDRL, studies for viral infection and toxoplasmosis (see Chap. 12), sedimentation rate, lupus tests
2. **Fetal**—ultrasound echocardiography for cardiac and other structural lesions as well as arrhythmia [45], fetal blood sampling for karyotype hemoglobin electrophoresis, hematocrit, albumin, cultures and titers for infection
3. **Amniocentesis**—karyotype, metabolic studies, fetoprotein, cultures
4. **Neonatal.** After birth many of the same studies may be carried out on the infant. A complete blood count, type and Coombs', ultrasound of the head heart, and abdomen, and a search for the etiologies listed in **A** should be done. Liver function tests, urinalysis, viral titers, chromosome studies placental examination, and x-rays may be indicated. If the infant is stillborn or dies, a detailed autopsy should be done [63].

C. Management

1. A hydropic fetus is at great risk for intrauterine death. A decision must be made about intrauterine treatment if possible, e.g., fetal transfusion in isoimmune hemolytic anemia (see Chap. 3) or maternal digitalis therapy for paroxysmal atrial tachycardia (see Chap. 14). If fetal treatment is not possible, the fetus must be evaluated for the relative possibility of intrauterine death versus the risks of premature delivery. If premature delivery is planned, pulmonary maturity should be induced with steroids if it is not present (see Chap. 13).
2. The infant delivered with hydrops will require the usual resuscitation and stabilization at birth (see Chap. 5).
3. Paracentesis may be required if ventilation is difficult. We usually use a 20-gauge angiocatheter for this.
4. If hydrothorax is present, thoracentesis or chest tubes may be required.

5. Intubation, ventilation with 100% oxygen, a constant distending airway pressure at 4 to 6 cm H_2O, and an inspiratory time of 0.6 to 1.0 second are usually required because of pulmonary edema.
6. Central arterial and venous lines are required to monitor arterial pressure, venous pressure, oxygenation, and acid-base balance.
7. If the hematocrit is under 30 percent, a partial exchange transfusion with 50 to 80 ml/kg packed red cells (hematocrit of 70 percent) should be performed to raise the hematocrit. If the problem is Rh isoimmunization, the blood should be type O Rh-negative. We often use O-negative cells and AB serum prepared before delivery cross-matched against the mother. We do an exchange out the umbilical artery and in the umbilical vein at a rate of 2 to 4 ml/kg per minute.
8. Since most hydropic infants are normovolemic, manipulation of the blood volume is usually not initially indicated. It may be indicated after measurement of arterial and venous pressures and after correction of acidosis and asphyxia.
9. If a low serum albumin level is contributing to hydrops, fresh-frozen plasma may help. Care must be taken not to volume-overload an already failing heart.
10. Dopamine at a rate of 2.5 to 5.0 μg/kg per minute may be required to improve cardiac output.
11. There should be careful measurement of intake, output, and central venous and arterial pressures.
12. Fluid intake is usually kept at 40 to 60 ml/kg per day as dextrose and water at a glucose infusion rate of 4 to 8 mg/kg per minute as 10% to 20% D/W.
13. Measure blood sugar, electrolytes, calcium, phosphorus, bilirubin, blood urea nitrogen (BUN), creatinine, albumin, liver function tests, CBC, blood smear, reticulocyte count, platelet count, chest x-ray, and ECG.
14. An echocardiogram may help evaluate cardiac structure and function.
15. Abdominal ultrasound may reveal renal or other masses.
16. Furosemide may help pulmonary edema.
17. Hyperbilirubinemia should be treated as in **VI.**
18. Many infants with hydrops will survive if aggressive neonatal care is provided.

IX. Isoimmune hemolytic disease of the newborn

A. Etiology. Isoimmune hemolytic disease of the newborn is caused by maternal immunoglobulin G (IgG) antibodies directed against fetal red cell antigens that are foreign to the mother [1,31,69]. The usual antigen involved prenatally is the Rh(D) antigen, and postnatally, the A and B antigens. Maternal antibodies to antigens other than Rh antigen have been associated with isoimmune hemolysis of the fetus or the newborn [77] (Tables 15-5 to 15-7). The finding of a positive Coombs' test in an infant born to an Rh(D)-positive mother should cause one to identify the antibody. The antibody may be anti-A or anti-B. If one of these antibodies is not found, the mother's serum should be tested against a panel of red cells and the father's cells. This may have implications for subsequent pregnancies. These "other" antigens make up 1 percent of cases of hemolytic disease of the newborn. As hemolytic disease from Rh antigen becomes less common as a result of treatment with Rhogam, these antigens assume more relative importance. The most commonly implicated "other" antigens are Kell, Duffy, E, C, and c.

B. Fetal management [31]. All pregnant women should have a blood type, Rh, and an antibody screening performed on their first prenatal visit. This will identify the Rh-negative mothers and identify any antibody due to Rh or any rare antigen sensitization that may be a result of a previous transfusion, abortion, or injection of blood. In a Caucasian population in the USA, 15 percent of people will lack the D antigen (*dd*). Of the remainder, 48 percent will be heterozygous (*dD*) and 35 percent will be homozygous (*DD*). Approximately

Table 15-5. Common antigens other than Rh implicated in hemolytic disease of the newborn

Antigen	Alternative symbol or name	Blood group system
Do^a		Dombrock
Fy^a		Duffy
Jk^a		Kidd
Jk^b		Kidd
K	K:1	Kell
Lu^a	Lu:1	Lutheran
M		MNSs
N		MNSs
S		MNSs
s		MNSs

Table 15-6. Other antigens involved in hemolytic diseases of the newborn

Antigen	Alternative symbol or name	Blood group system
Co^a		Colton
Di^b		Diego
Ge		Gerbich
Hy	Holley	
Jr		
Js^b	Matthews, K:7	Kell
k	Cellano, K:2	Kell
Kp^b	Rautenberg, K:4	Kell
Lan	Langereis	
Lu^b		Lutheran
LW	Landsteinder-Weiner	
P, P1, P^k	Tj^a	P
U		MNSs
Yt^a		Cartwright

15 percent of matings in this population will have a fetus with the D antigen and a mother without it. If the mother has antibodies that have been associated with severe immune hemolytic disease of the fetus, the antibody titer is repeated at 20 weeks and monthly thereafter. If the mother is Rh-positive and her antibody screening is negative, it may be advisable to repeat an antibody screening later in pregnancy, but this will have a low yield [2]. If the mother is Rh-negative and her serum is negative for antibodies, she should be retested at 28 and 35 weeks' gestation (see **D** for prenatal Rhogam). If the mother has an antibody, it should be identified, and consultation should be obtained with someone experienced in neonatal isoimmunization. If the titer is in the range of 1:16 by the indirect Coombs' test (each center should have its own standards for action on various titers), titers should be repeated more frequently in the last trimester. If the titer is over 1:16 or at a level at which the local center has had a fetal demise, amniocentesis should be performed to

Table 15-7. Infrequent antigens implicated in hemolytic diseases of the newborn

Antigen	Alternative symbol or name	Blood group system
Be^a	Berrens	Rh
Bi	Biles	
By	Batty	
C^w	Rh:8	Rh
C^x	Rh:9	Rh
Di^{*a}		Diego
Evans		Rh
E^w	Rh:11	Rh
Far	See Kam	
Ga	Gambino	
Go^a	Gonzales	Rh
Good		
Heibel		
Hil	Hill	MNSs Mi sub +
Ht^a	Hunt	
Hut	Hutchinson	MNSs Mi sub
Js^a	Sutter	Kell
Kam (Far)	Kamhuber	
Kp^a	Penney	Kell
Mit	Mitchell	
Mt^a	Martin	MNSs#
Mull	Lu:9	Lutheran
Mur	Murrell	MNSs Mi sub
Rd	Radin	
Re^a	Reid	
R^N	Rh:32	Rh
Vw(Gr)	Verweyst (Graydon)	MNSs Mi sub
Wi^a	Wright	
Zd		

measure the optical density at a wavelength of 450 nm and to classify the risk for fetal death from hydrops.

Amniocentesis can be performed starting at 22 weeks of pregnancy. The fetus also should be followed by ultrasound and tests of fetal well-being (see Chap. 3). Fetuses in the high-risk group may be treated by early delivery if the risk of fetal demise or intrauterine transfusion exceeds the risk of early delivery. In our institution, this is usually 30 weeks, but this requires careful fetal monitoring, induction of pulmonary maturity, and close cooperation between obstetrician and neonatologist. If the fetus is too immature to consider early delivery, intrauterine transfusion is indicated. The fetus is transfused every 10 to 14 days until judged capable of extrauterine survival. There is an association between fetal transfusion and sudden fetal demise. Careful ultrasound surveillance for fetal distress of the fetus with Rh hemolytic disease may allow one to hold off on intrauterine transfusion [32]. Percutaneous fetal umbilical vein sampling can give an exact fetal hematocrit (see Chap. 3). The fetus may be transfused by the usual intraperitional route or by transfusion directly into the umbilical vein (usually reserved for the hydropic fetus at this time). Some of these infants will be born with all adult O-negative red cells because all the fetal cells are destroyed. Although one should be prepared, not all infants will need postnatal exchange transfusion. These infants are at risk to develop a conjugated hyperbilirubinemia.

C. **Neonatal management.** About half the infants with a positive Coombs' test from Rh hemolytic disease will have minimum hemolysis and hyperbilirubinemia (cord bilirubin level < 4 mg/dl and hemoglobin level > 14 gm/dl). These infants may require no treatment or only phototherapy. They may develop an exaggerated physiologic anemia at 12 weeks of age. One-fourth of the infants with Rh hemolytic disease will present with anemia, hemoglobin level less than 14 gm/dl, and hyperbilirubinemia (cord bilirubin > 4 mg/dl). They will have increased nucleated red cells and reticulocytes on blood smear. These infants may have thrombocytopenia and a very elevated white blood cell count. They have an enlarged liver and spleen, and they require early exchange transfusion and phototherapy (see **VI.B–C**). Figure 15-3 and Tables 15-3A and B can be used to help decide what treatment to use. Hydropic fetuses have a high mortality and are managed during pregnancy as in the treatment of hydrops (see **VIII.C**).

D. **Prevention** [29,31]. Elimination of the exposure of women to foreign red cell antigens will prevent immune hemolytic disease of the newborn. Avoiding unnecessary transfusions and injection of blood will eliminate sensitization. Since anti-C antibodies are a cause of hemolytic disease of the newborn, if Rh-negative blood is to be given to an Rh-positive woman, her blood should be tested with anti-C serum before transfusion. If she is C-negative, C-negative blood should be used. Rh hemolytic disease is now being prevented by administration of Rho(D) immune globulin to unsensitized Rh-negative mothers. This is usually done at 28 weeks' gestation and within 72 hours of delivery. Other indications for Rho(D) immune globulin and for larger doses are given in ref. 101.

X. **ABO hemolytic disease of the newborn** [69]. Since the introduction of Rh immune globulin, ABO incompatibility is the most common cause of hemolytic disease of the newborn in the United States.

A. **Etiology.** It is caused by the reaction of maternal anti-A or anti-B antibodies to the A or B antigen on the red cells of the fetus or newborn. It is usually seen only in A or B infants born to type O mothers because these mothers make anti-A or anti-B antibodies of the IgG class, which cross the placenta, while mothers of type A or B usually make anti-A or anti-B antibodies of the IgM class, which do not cross the placenta. The combination of a type O mother and a type A or type B infant occurs in 15 percent of pregnancies in the United States. Only one-fifth of infants with this blood group setup (or 3 percent of all infants) will develop significant jaundice. Some bacterial vaccines such as tetanus toxoid and pneumococcal vaccine had A and B substance in the culture media and were associated with significant hemolysis in type A or type B neonates born to type O mothers who were given these vaccines. New preparations of the vaccine are said to be free of these A and B substances.

B. **Clinical presentation.** The situation is a type O mother with a type A or type B infant who becomes **jaundiced in the first 24 hours of life.** Approximately 50 percent of the cases occur in **first-born infants.** There is no predictable pattern of recurrence in subsequent infants. The majority of ABO-incompatible infants have anti-A or anti-B antibody on their red cells, yet only a small number have significant ABO hemolytic disease of the newborn. Infants may have a low concentration of antibody on their red cells; consequently, their antibody will not be demonstrated by elution techniques or by a positive direct antiglobulin test (Coombs' test). As the antibody concentration increases, the antibody can be demonstrated first by elution techniques and then by the Coombs' test. Although all ABO-incompatible infants have some degree of hemolysis, **significant hemolysis is usually associated only with a positive direct Coombs' test** on the infants red cells [20]. If there are other causes of neonatal jaundice, ABO incompatibility will add to the bilirubin production. In infants with significant ABO incompatibility, there will be many spherocytes on the blood smear and an elevated recticulocyte count. RBCs from infants with ABO incompatibility may have increased osmotic fragility and autohemolysis as in hereditary spherocytosis (HS). The autohemolysis is not corrected by glucose, as in HS. The family history and long-term course will usually help with the diagnosis of HS.

C. **Management.** If a type and Coombs' test are done on the cord blood of infants born to type O mothers, these infants can have bilirubin levels followed and therapy instituted early enough to prevent severe hyperbilirubinemia. If the results are not available within 24 hours after birth, this screening test will not be of much aid. Another (and less expensive) method is to do bilirubin levels at 12 hours of age on all infants born to type O mothers. In the absence of a routine test on all infants born to type O mothers, one must rely on clinical observation to notice the jaundiced infants. This will depend on the observation of the caretakers and may not be reliable in infants whose skin pigmentation makes the diagnosis of jaundice difficult.

Transcutaneous bilirubinometry may be useful in Caucasian infants. We are evaluating the cost-effectiveness of various ways to make an early diagnosis of the occasional infants with ABO incompatibility who will have severe hyperbilirubinemia. A bilirubin level at 12 hours of age or a cord blood type and Coombs' test on all black or Asian infants born to type O mothers may be a reasonable compromise. Infants born to type O mothers who are to have an early discharge (within 24 hours) should be evaluated for ABO incompatibility; the parents should be made aware of the possibility of jaundice. Only 10 percent of infants with a positive direct Coombs' test for ABO incompatibility will need phototherapy [68]. Many infants will have an initial rise in bilirubin that will quickly fall to normal levels. If the criteria for treatment suggested in Rh disease are used, many of these infants will undergo unnecessary treatment. A reasonable approach in term infants without medical problems is shown in Table 15-8.

Most infants with clinical jaundice from ABO incompatibility can be managed by phototherapy if it is started before bilirubin levels get too high. If the bilirubin level is approaching 20 mg/dl and is not controlled by phototherapy, an exchange transfusion should be done to keep the bilirubin under 20 mg/dl.

Table 15-8. Approach to term infants with ABO incompatibility and no medical problems

Age in hours	Total serum bilirubin level, mg/dl	Treatment
Under 12	Under 10	Observe
	Over 10	Phototherapy
Under 18	Under 12	Observe
	Over 12	Phototherapy
Under 24	Under 14	Observe
	Over 14	Phototherapy
Over 24	Over 15	Phototherapy

From L. M. Osborn, et al. *Pediatrics,* American Academy of Pediatrics, 4:371, 1984 [68].

Figure 15-3 may be used as a guide. Kernicterus has been reported in ABO incompatibility [106]. If exchange transfusion is necessary, it should be with type O blood that is of the same Rh type as the infant. Blood with a low titer of anti-A or anti-B antibody is best. We often use type O cells resuspended in type AB plasma. There is no need for prenatal diagnosis or treatment and no need for early delivery.

References

1. Allen, F. H., Jr., and Diamond, L. K. *Erythroblastosis Fetalis: Including Exchange Transfusion Technique.* Boston: Little, Brown, 1957. P. 57.
2. American Academy of Pediatrics and the American College of Obstetricians and Gynecologists. Hyperbilirubinemia. In F. P. Frigoletto and G. A. Little (Eds.), *Guidelines for Perinatal Care,* 2d Ed. Elk Grove Village, Ill.: American Academy of Pediatrics, 1988. P. 261.
3. American Academy of Pediatrics Committee on Fetus and Newborn. *Pediatrics* 76: 136, 1985.
4. Batton, D. G. *Transfusion* 23: 163, 1983.
5. Bowen, W. R. *Am. J. Dis. Child.* 98: 568, 1959.
6. Bowman, J. M. Hemolytic Disease of the Newborn. In S. S. Gellis and B. N. Kagen (Eds.), *Current Pediatric Therapy.* Philadelphia: Saunders, 1971. P. 262.
7. Brown, A. K., Kim, M. H., and Bryla, D. Report on the NIH Cooperative Study of Phototherapy: Efficacy of Phototherapy in Controlling Hyperbilirubinemia and Preventing Kernicterus. In R. L. Levine and M. J. Maisels (Eds.), *Hyperbilirubinemia in the Newborn: Report of the Eighty-Fifth Ross Conference on Pediatric Research.* Columbus, Ohio: Ross Laboratories, 1983. P. 55.
8. Brown, A. K. *Pediatrics (Suppl.)* 75: 393, 1985.
9. Campbell, N. *J. Pediatr.* 94: 820, 1979.
10. Cashore, W. J. *Clin. Perinatol.* 11: 339, 1984.
11. Cashore, W. J. Bilirubin Binding Tests. In R. L. Levine and M. J. Maisels (Eds.), *Hyperbilirubinemia in the Newborn: Report of the Eighty-Fifth Conference on Pediatric Research.* Columbus, Ohio: Ross Laboratories, 1983. P. 101.
12. Chan, G. *J. Pediatr.* 88: 609, 1976.
13. Chudwin, D. S. *Am. J. Dis. Child.* 136: 612, 1982.
14. Cohen, A. N. *Pediatrics* 65: 740, 1980.
15. Crichton, J. U. *Pediatrics* 49: 656, 1972.
16. Crigler, J. F., Jr. *Pediatrics* 10: 169, 1952.
17. Cropp, G. J. *J. Pediatr.* 77: 881, 1970.
18. Culley, P. *Br. Med. J.* 2: 383, 1970.
19. DeCarvaho, M. *J. Pediatr.* 107: 786, 1985.
20. Desjardins, L. *J. Pediatr.* 95: 447, 1979.
21. Diamond, I. *J. Clin. Invest.* 45: 678, 1966.
22. Ebbesen, F. *Eur. J. Pediatr.* 130: 279, 1979.
23. Ebbesen, F. *Eur. J. Pediatr.* 133: 37, 1980.
24. Edwards, M. C. Exchange Transfusions. In M. A. Fletcher, M. G. MacDonald, and G. B. Avery (Eds.), *Atlas of Procedures in Neonatology.* Philadelphia: Lippincott, 1983.
25. Epstein, M. F. *Pediatrics* 82: 350, 1988.
26. Fargusova, K. *Acta Paediatr. Scand.* 48: 590, 1959.
27. Fishman, R. H., et al. *Exp. Neurol.* 79: 212, 1983.
28. Fitzgerald, J. F. *Pediatr. Clin. North Am.* 35: 357, 1988.
29. Freda, V. J. *N. Engl. J. Med.* 292: 1014, 1975.
30. Freed, L. M. *Pediatr. Res.* 21: 267A, 1987.
31. Frigoletto, F. P. *Clin. Perinatol.* 1: 321, 1974.
32. Frigoletto, F. *N. Engl. J. Med.* 315: 430, 1986.
33. Furst, E. *J. Pediatr.* 93: 102, 1978.
34. Gartner, L. M. Breast Milk Jaundice. In R. L. Levine and M. J. Maisels (Eds.),

Hyperbilirubinemia in the Newborn: Eighty-Fifth Ross Conference on Pediatric Research. Columbus, Ohio: Ross Laboratories, 1983.
35. Gartner, L. M. *Pediatr. Rev.* 5: 163, 1983.
36. Goldman, S. L. *J. Pediatr.* 102: 115, 1983.
37. Gourley, G. R. *Lancet* 1: 644, 1986.
38. Green, H. L. *J. Pediatr.* 95: 412, 1979.
39. Hsia, D. Y. Y. *N. Engl. J. Med.* 247: 668, 1952.
40. Johnson, L., and Boggs, T. R. Bilirubin-Dependent Brain Damage: Incidence and Indications for Treatment. In G. B. Odell, R. Schaffer, and A. P. Simopoulos (Eds.), *Phototherapy in the Newborn: An Overview.* Washington: National Academy of Sciences, 1974. P. 122.
41. Johnson, J. D. *Am. J. Dis. Child.* 138: 1047, 1984.
42. Kappas, A. *Pediatrics* 81: 485, 1988.
43. Kim, M. H. *J. Pediatr.* 66: 502, 1980.
44. Kim, M. H. *Pediatrics* 66: 852, 1980.
45. Kleinman, C. S., et al. *N. Engl. J. Med.* 306: 568, 1982.
46. Kopelman, A. Editorial Comment. In F. A. Oski and J. A. Stockman (Eds.), *Yearbook of Pediatrics.* Chicago: Year Book Medical Publishers, 1984. P. 37.
47. Kopelman, A. *J. Pediatr.* 84: 473, 1972.
48. Levi, A. J. *J. Clin. Invest.* 48: 2156, 1969.
49. Levine, R. L. *Pediatrics* 69: 255, 1982.
50. Lucey, J. F. *Pediatrics* 69: 381, 1982.
51. Lucey, J. F. Editorial Comment. In F. A. Oski and J. A. Stockman (Eds.), *Yearbook of Pediatrics.* Chicago: Year Book Medical Publishers, 1983. P. 37.
52. Maisels, M. J. Neonatal Jaundice. In G. B. Avery (Ed.), *Neonatology.* Philadelphia: Lippincott, 1987.
53. Maisels, M. J. *Pediatr. Clin. North Am.* 19: 447, 1972.
54. Maisels, M. J. Clinical Studies of the Sequelae of Hyperbilirubinemia. In R. L. Leven and M. J. Maisels (Eds.), *Hyperbilirubinemia in the Newborn: Eighty-Fifth Ross Conference on Pediatric Research.* Columbus, Ohio: Ross Laboratories, 1983. P. 26.
55. Maisels, M. J., et al. *Pediatrics* 81: 505, 1988.
56A. Maisels, M. J. and Newman, T. B. Jaundice in the Healthy Term Infant: Time for Reevaluation. In *Yearbook of Neonatal and Perinatal Medicine,* Mosby Yearbook Inc., New York. 1990. P. xiii.
56B. Maisels M. J. Neonatal Jaundice Maisels M. J. (ed) Clinics in Perinatology 17:1, 1990.
57. Martin, J. R. *N.Z. Med. J.* 77: 167, 1973.
58. Maurer, H. M. *J. Pediatr.* 82: 73, 1973.
59. McDonagh, A. F. *Pediatrics* 75: 443, 1985.
60. McGillivroy, B. C. *Pediatr. Rev.* 9: 197, 1987.
61. McMullin, G. P. *Lancet* 2: 949, 1970.
62. Mollism, P. L. *Blood* 6: 777, 1951.
63. Mostoufl-Zadeh, M., et al. *Hum. Pathol.* 16: 785, 1985.
64. Naeye, R. L. *Pediatrics* 62: 497, 1978.
65. National Institute of Child Health and Development. *Pediatrics (Suppl.)* 72: 385, 1985.
66. Newman, T. B., et al. *Pediatrics* 83: 1064, 1989.
67. O'Dell, G. B. Bilirubin. In *Neonatal Hyperbilirubinemia.* New York: Grune and Stratton, 1982.
68. Osborn, L. *Pediatrics* 74: 371, 1984.
69. Oski, F. A., and Naimen, J. L. (Eds.) Erythroblastosis Fetalis. In *Hematologic Problems in the Newborn.* Philadelphia: Saunders, 1982. Chap. 10.
70. Parkman, R. P. *N. Engl. J. Med.* 290: 359, 1974.
71. Perlman, M. *Pediatrics* 72: 658, 1983.
72. Perlman, M. *Pediatrics* 81: 304, 1988.
73. Poland, R. D. *N. Engl. J. Med.* 284: 1, 1971.
74. Ritter, D. A. *Pediatrics* 69: 260, 1982.
75. Roth, P., et al. *Clin. Perinatol.* 15: 965, 1988.

76. Rubin, R. A. *J. Pediatr.* 94: 601, 1979.
77. Sabo, B. H. Antigens Implicated in Hemolytic Disease of the Newborn. In C. A. Bell (Ed.), *Seminar on Prenatal Blood Banking.* Arlington, Va.: American Association of Blood Banks, 1978.
78. Scheidt, P. C. *J. Pediatr.* 91: 292, 1977.
79. Schmacher, R. E. *Pediatrics* 76: 10, 1985.
80. Schreiner, F. L. *Pediatrics* 69: 277, 1982.
81. Spivak, W. *J. Pediatr.* 110: 855, 1987.
82. Sproul, A. *J. Pediatr.* 65: 12, 1964.
83. Srinivasan, G. *Crit. Care Med.* 8: 338, 1980.
84. Stevenson, D. K. *Am. J. Dis. Child.* 143: 353, 1989.
85. Stevenson, D. K. Estimation of Bilirubin Production. In R. L. Levine and M. J. Maisels (Eds.), *Hyperbilirubinemia in the Newborn: Report of the Eighty-Fifth Ross Conference of Pediatric Research.* Columbus, Ohio: Ross Laboratories, 1983. P. 64.
86. Strange, M., et al. *Clin. Perinatol.* 12: 51, 1985.
87. Tan, K. L. *Pediatrics* 56: 550, 1975.
88. Tan, K. L. *Pediatrics* 57: 836, 1976.
89. Thangarel, M. *Pediatrics* 69: 199, 1982.
90. Towers, S. H. *Arch. Dis. Child.* 52: 324, 1977.
91. Turkel, S. B. *Clin. Perinatol.* 9: 613, 1988.
92. Vaisman, S. L. *Clin. Perinatol.* 2: 37, 1975.
93. Valdes, O. S. *J. Pediatr.* 78: 1015, 1971.
94. Van de Bor, M. *Pediatrics* 83: 915, 1989.
95. Van Praagh, R. *Pediatrics* 28: 870, 1961.
96. Vaughn, R. L. *Am. J. Dis. Child.* 136: 646, 1988.
97. Wanek, E. A. *Pediatr. Rev.* 11: 57, 1989.
98. Watchko, J. F. *Pediatrics* 71: 680, 1983.
99. Waters, W. J. *J. Pediatr.* 33: 789, 1964.
100. Wennberg, R. P. *J. Pediatr.* 92: 789, 1978.
101. Wible-Hart, J. *Clin. Perinatol.* 10: 343, 1983.
102. Wishingrad, L. *Pediatrics* 36: 102, 1965.
103. Wood, B. *Arch. Dis. Child.* 54: 111, 1979.
104. Wu, P. K. *Perinatal-Neonatal Med.* 5: 49, 1981.
105. Yamanouchi, I. *Pediatrics* 65: 195, 1980.
106. Zuelzer, W. W. *Am. J. Dis. Child.* 88: 319, 1954.

Anemia

John P. Cloherty

I. Hematologic physiology of the newborn [1,2,4]. Significant changes occur in the red cell mass of an infant during the neonatal period and ensuing months. The evaluation of anemia must take into account this developmental process, as well as the infant's physiologic needs.

A. Normal development: The physiologic anemia of infancy

1. In utero, fetal aortic oxygen saturation is 45 percent; erythropoietin levels are high, red cell production is rapid, and reticulocyte counts are 3 to 7 percent.
2. After birth, oxygen saturation is 95 percent, and erythropoietin is undetectable. Red blood cell (RBC) production by day 7 is less than one-tenth the level in utero. Reticulocyte counts are low, and hemoglobin level falls (Table 16-1).
3. Despite dropping hemoglobin levels, the ratio of hemoglobin A to hemoglobin F increases, and the levels of 2,3-diphosphoglycerate (2,3-DPG) (which interacts with hemoglobin A to decrease its affinity for oxygen, thus enhancing oxygen release to the tissues) are high; as a result, oxygen delivery to the tissues actually increases. This physiologic "anemia" is not a functional anemia in that oxygen delivery to the tissues is adequate. Iron from degraded red blood cells is stored.
4. At 8 to 12 weeks, hemoglobin levels reach their nadir (Table 16-2), oxygen delivery to the tissues is impaired, erythropoietin production is stimulated, and RBC production increases.
5. Infants who have been transfused in the neonatal period have lower nadirs than normal, due to their higher percentage of hemoglobin A [11].
6. During this period of active erythropoiesis, iron stores are rapidly utilized. The reticuloendothelial system has adequate iron for 15 to 20 weeks in term infants. After this time, the hemoglobin level decreases if iron is not supplied.

B. Anemia of prematurity is an exaggeration of the normal physiologic anemia (see Tables 16-1 and 16-2).

1. RBC mass is decreased at birth, although the hemoglobin level is the same as in the term infant.
2. The hemoglobin nadir is reached earlier than in the term infant because
   a. RBC survival is decreased compared with the term infant.
   b. There is a relatively more rapid rate of growth in premature babies as compared with term infants.
   c. Vitamin E deficiency is common in small premature infants, unless the vitamin is supplied exogenously.
3. The hemoglobin nadir in premature babies is lower than in term infants because erythropoietin is produced by the term infant at a hemoglobin level of 10 to 11 gm/dl but is produced by the premature infant at a hemoglobin level of 7 to 9 gm/dl. This reflects the lower oxygen requirements in healthy preterm infants rather than a defect in erythropoietin production [6,11,12].
4. Iron administration before 10 to 14 weeks of age does not increase the

Table 16-1. Hemoglobin changes in babies in the first year of life

	Hemoglobin Level		
Week	Term babies	Premature babies (1200–2400 gm)	Small premature babies (<1200 gm)
0	17.8	17.0	15.6
1	18.8	15.3	14.8
3	15.9	13.2	12.0
5	12.7	9.6	8.2
10	11.4	9.8	8.1
20	12.0	9.8	9.0
50	12.0	11.0	11.0

Source: From B. Glader. Erythrocyte Disorders in Infancy. In A. J. Schaffer and M. E. Avery (eds.), *Diseases of the Newborn*. Philadelphia: Saunders, 1977.

Table 16-2. Hemoglobin nadir in babies in the first year of life

Maturity of baby at birth	Hemoglobin level at nadir	Time of nadir
Term babies	9.5–11.0	6–12 wk
Premature babies (1200–1400 gm)	8.0–10.0	5–10 wk
Small premature babies (<1200 gm)	6.5– 9.0	4– 8 wk

Source: From B. Glader. Erythrocyte Disorders in Infancy. In A. J. Schaffer and M. E. Avery (eds.), *Diseases of the Newborn*. Philadelphia: Saunders, 1977.

nadir of the hemoglobin level or diminish its rate of reduction. However, this iron is stored for later use.

5. Once the nadir is reached, RBC production is stimulated, and iron stores are rapidly depleted because there is less iron stored in the premature infant as compared with the term infant.

II. Etiology of anemia in the neonate

A. Blood loss is manifested by a decreased or normal hematocrit, increased or normal reticulocyte count, and a normal bilirubin level (unless the hemorrhage is retained) [7,8]. If blood loss is recent (e.g., at delivery), the hematocrit and reticulocyte count may be normal and the infant may be in shock. The hematocrit will fall later due to hemodilution. If the bleeding is chronic, the hematocrit will be low, the reticulocyte count up, and the baby normovolemic.

1. **Obstetric causes of blood loss,** including malformations of placenta and cord
   - a. Abruptio placentae
   - b. Placenta previa
   - c. Incision of placenta at cesarean section
   - d. Rupture of anomalous vessels (e.g., vasa previa, velamentous insertion of cord, or rupture of communicating vessels in a multilobed placenta)
   - e. Hematoma of cord caused by varices or aneurysm
   - f. Rupture of cord (more common in short cords and in dysmature cords)
2. **Occult blood loss**
   - a. **Fetomaternal bleeding** may be chronic or acute. It occurs in 8 percent of all pregnancies, and in 1 percent of pregnancies the volume may be

as large as 40 ml. The diagnosis of this problem is by Kleihauer-Betke stain of maternal smear for fetal cells [2]. Many conditions may predispose to this type of bleeding:

(1) Placental malformations—chorioangioma or choriocarcinoma
(2) Obstetric procedures—traumatic amniocentesis, external cephalic version, internal cephalic version, breech delivery
(3) Spontaneous

b. **Fetoplacental bleeding**
(1) Chorioangioma or choriocarcinoma with placental hematoma
(2) Cesarean section, with infant held above placenta
(3) Tight nuchal cord or occult cord prolapse

c. **Twin-to-twin transfusion**

3. **Bleeding in the neonatal period** may be due to the following causes:

a. **Intracranial bleeding** associated with
(1) Prematurity
(2) Second twin
(3) Breech delivery
(4) Rapid delivery
(5) Hypoxia

b. **Massive cephalohematoma,** subgaleal hemorrhage, or hemorrhagic caput succedaneum

c. **Retroperitoneal bleeding**

d. **Ruptured liver or spleen**

e. **Adrenyl or renal hemorrhage**

f. **Gastrointestinal bleeding**
(1) Peptic ulcer
(2) Enterocolitis
(3) Nasogastric catheter
(4) Maternal blood swallowed from delivery or breast should be ruled out by the Apt test (see Chap. 17)

g. **Bleeding from umbilicus**

4. **Iatrogenic causes.** Excessive blood loss may result from blood sampling with inadequate replacement.

B. **Hemolysis** is manifested by a decreased hematocrit, increased reticulocyte count, and an increased bilirubin level [7,8].

1. **Immune hemolysis** (see Chap. 15)

a. **Rh incompatibility**

b. **ABO incompatibility**

c. **Minor blood group incompatibility** (e.g., c, E, Kell, Duffy)

d. **Maternal disease** (e.g., lupus), autoimmune hemolytic disease, rheumatoid arthritis (positive direct Coombs' test in mother and newborn, no antibody to common red cell antigen Rh, AB, etc.), or drugs (e.g., penicillin antibodies in mother and child, child on penicillin [3]).

2. **Hereditary red cell disorders**

a. **RBC membrane defects** such as spherocytosis, elliptocytosis, stomatocytosis.

b. **Metabolic defects**—glucose 6-phosphate dehydrogenase (G6PD) deficiency (significant neonatal hemolysis due to G6PD deficiency is usually seen only in Mediterranean or Asian G6PD-deficient males; blacks in the United States have a 10 percent incidence of G6PD deficiency but rarely have significant neonatal problems unless an infection or drug is operative), pyruvate-kinase deficiency, 5′-nucleotidase deficiency, and glucose phosphate isomerase deficiency.

c. **Hemoglobinopathies**
(1) Alpha- and gamma-thalassemia syndromes
(2) Alpha- and gamma-chain structural abnormalities

3. **Acquired hemolysis**

a. **Infection**—bacterial or viral

b. **Disseminated intravascular coagulation**

c. **Vitamin E deficiency**
d. **Microangiopathic hemolytic anemia**—cavernous hemangioma, renal artery stenosis, severe coarctation of the aorta

C. **Diminished RBC production** is manifested by a decreased hematocrit, decreased reticulocyte count, and normal bilirubin level (see Chap. **Hydrops** 15).
1. **Diamond-Blackfan syndrome**
2. **Congenital leukemia** or other tumor
3. **Infections,** especially rubella and parvovirus
4. **Osteopetrosis,** leading to inadequate erythropoiesis
5. **Drug-induced red cell suppression**
6. **Physiologic anemia or anemia of prematurity** (see **I.A** and **B**)

III. **Diagnostic approach to anemia in the newborn** (Table 16-3)

A. The **family history** should include questions about anemia, jaundice, gallstones, and splenectomy.

B. The **obstetric history** should be evaluated.

C. The **physical examination** may reveal an associated abnormally and provide clues as to the **origin** of the anemia.
1. **Acute blood loss** leads to shock, with cyanosis, poor perfusion, and acidosis.
2. **Chronic blood loss** produces pallor, but the infant may exhibit only mild symptoms of respiratory distress or irritability.
3. **Chronic hemolysis** is associated with pallor, jaundice, and hepatosplenomegaly.

D. **Complete blood count.** Capillary blood samples are 3.7 ± 2.7 percent higher than venous hematocrits. Warming the foot reduced the difference from 3.9 to 1.9 percent [2].

E. **Reticulocyte count** (elevated in chronic blood loss and hemolysis, depressed in infection and production defect)

F. **Blood smear** (see Table 16-3)

G. **Coombs' tests and bilirubin level**

H. **Apt test** (see Chap. 17) on gastrointestinal blood of uncertain origin

I. **Kleihauer-Betke preparation** of the mother's blood. A 50-ml loss of fetal blood into the maternal circulation will show up as 1 percent fetal cells in the maternal circulation [2].

J. **Ultrasound of abdomen and head**

K. **Test on parents**—CBC, smear, red cell indices, red cell enzymes (G6PD, PK)

L. **Studies for infection** (TORCH infection; see Chap. 12)

M. **Bone marrow** (rarely used except in cases of bone marrow failure from hypoplasia or tumor)

IV. **Therapy**

A. **Transfusion** (see Chap. 20)
1. **Indications for transfusion.** The decision to transfuse must be made in consideration of the infant's condition and physiologic needs.
   a. Infants with respiratory disease should probably have their hematocrit maintained above 40 percent. Transfusion with adult red cells provides the added benefit of lowered oxygen affinity, which augments oxygen delivery to tissues. Blood should be fresh (<3 days old) to ensure adequate 2,3-DPG levels.
   b. Healthy, asymptomatic newborns will self-correct a mild anemia, provided that their iron intake is adequate.
   c. Infants with ABO incompatibility who do not have an exchange transfusion may have protracted hemolysis and may require a transfusion several weeks after birth. If they do not have enough hemolysis to require treatment with phototherapy, they will usually not become anemic enough to need a transfusion.
   d. Premature babies may be quite comfortable with hemoglobin levels of 6.5 to 7.0 mg/dl. The level itself is not an indication for transfusion. Sick infants (e.g., with sepsis, pneumonia, or bronchopulmonary dys-

Table 16-3. Classification of anemia in the newborn

Reticulocytes	Bilirubin	Coombs' test	RBC morphology	Diagnostic possibilities
Normal or ↓	Normal	Negative	Normal	Physiologic anemia of infancy or prematurity; congenital hypoplastic anemia; other causes of decreased production
Normal or ↑	Normal	Negative	Normal	Acute hemorrhage (fetomaternal, placental, umbilical cord, or internal hemorrhage)
			Hypochromic microcytes	Chronic fetomaternal hemorrhage
↑	↑	Positive	Spherocytes	Immune hemolysis (blood group incompatibility or maternal autoantibody)
Normal or ↑	↑	Negative	Spherocytes	Hereditary spherocytosis
			Elliptocytes	Hereditary elliptocytosis
			Hypochromic microcytes	Alpha- or gamma-thalassemia syndrome
			Spiculated RBCs	Pyruvate-kinase deficiency
			Schistocytes and RBC fragments	Disseminated intravascular coagulation; other microangiopathic processes
			Bite cells (Heinz bodies with supravital stain)	Glucose 6-phosphate dehydrogenase deficiency
			Normal	Infections; enclosed hemorrhage (cephalohematoma)

Key: RBC = red blood cell; ↓ = decreased; ↑ = increased.
Source: Adapted from the work of Dr. Bertil Glader, Director of Division of Hematology-Oncology, Children's Hospital at Stanford, CA.

plasia) may require increased oxygen-carrying capacities and therefore need transfusion. Growing premature infants also may manifest a need for transfusion by exhibiting poor weight gain, apnea, tachypnea, or poor feeding.

2. **Blood products and methods of transfusion** (see Chap. 20)
   a. **Packed RBCs.** The volume of transfusion may be calculated as follows:

$$\frac{\text{Weight} \times \text{blood volume per kilogram} \times (\text{hematocrit desired} - \text{hematocrit observed})}{\text{Hematocrit of blood to be given}}$$

   The average newborn blood volume is 80 ml/kg; the hematocrit of packed RBCs is 60 to 90 percent and should be checked prior to transfusion. The maximum transfusion should usually be 10 ml/kg.
   b. **Whole blood** is indicated when there is acute blood loss.
   c. **Exchange transfusion** with packed red cells may be required in severely anemic infants, when routine transfusion of the volume of packed RBCs necessary to correct the anemia would result in circulatory overload (see Chap. 15).
   d. **Irradiated** (5000 rads) [9] or **frozen RBCs** may be used if there is concern about the immunocompetence of the infant. Premature infants in particular may be unable to reject foreign lymphocytes in transfused blood. Frozen RBCs probably reduce the incidence of transfusion-related cytomegalovirus infection. We use blood from CMV-negative donors for all neonatal transfusions (see Chap. 20).

B. **Prophylaxis**
1. **Term infants** do not require iron supplementation until 2 months of age, when reticulocytosis resumes. These infants are usually sent home from the hospital on iron-fortified formula (2 mg/kg per day) if they are not breastfeeding.
2. **Premature infants** (preventing or ameliorating the anemia of prematurity). The following is a description of our usual nutritional management of premature infants from the point of view of providing RBC substrates and preventing additional destruction:
   a. **Vitamin E** (25 IU of water-soluble form) is given daily until the baby is 2 to 3 months of age (usually stopped at discharge from hospital).
   b. **Mother's milk** or formulas similar to mother's milk in that they are low in linoleic acid are used to maintain a low content of polyunsaturated fatty acids in the RBCs [4].
   c. **Iron** is **not used** for the first 2 months, since the therapeutic dose (6 mg/kg per day) enhances lipid peroxidation of RBC membranes. Iron in lower doses (i.e., in iron-fortified formula at a dose of 12 mg/L or 1.5 to 2.0 mg/kg per day when fed with a diet high in linoleic acid) was associated with hemolysis; however, a diet low in linoleic acid protected the red cells from this effect [4]. Since iron is not necessary in the first 2 months, it is not used even at the low dose, although this study suggests that it probably does no harm if used with the proper formula.
   d. After the baby is 8 weeks old, iron supplements (2 mg/kg per day as fortified formula or therapeutic iron) are used to prevent late anemia of prematurity, since premature babies have less total-body iron stores.
   e. These infants should be followed carefully, and additional iron supplementation may be required [10].
   f. Methods and hazards of transfusion are discussed in Chapter 20.

References

1. Blanchelte, V. S., and Ziplensky, A. *Clin. Perinatol.* 11: 489, 1984.
2. Blanchelte, V., and Ziplensky, A. Neonatal Haematology. In G. B. Avery (Ed.), *Neonatology,* 3d Ed. Philadelphia: Lippincott, 1987. Chap. 29.
3. Clayton, E. M. *Am. J. Clin. Pathol.* 52: 370, 1969.
4. Glader, B. Erythrocyte Disorders in Infancy. In M. E. Avery, and H. W. Taeusch (Eds.), *Diseases of the Newborn.* Philadelphia: Saunders, 1984.
5. Melhorn, D. K. *J. Pediatr.* 79: 281, 1971.
6. Mestyan, J. *Biol. Neonatal* 7: 11, 1964.
7. Nathan, D. G., and Oski, F. A. *Hematology of Infant and Childhood.* Philadelphia: Saunders, 1981.
8. Oski, F. A., and Naiman, J. L. *Hematologic Problems in the Newborn,* 3d Ed. Philadelphia: Saunders, 1982.
9. Parkman, R. *N. Engl. J. Med.* 290: 359, 1974.
10. Siimes, M. A. *J. Pediatr.* 101: 277, 1982.
11. Stockman, J. A., III. *Clin. Perinatol.* 4: 239, 1977.
12. Stockman, J. A. *N. Engl. J. Med.* 296: 647, 1977.

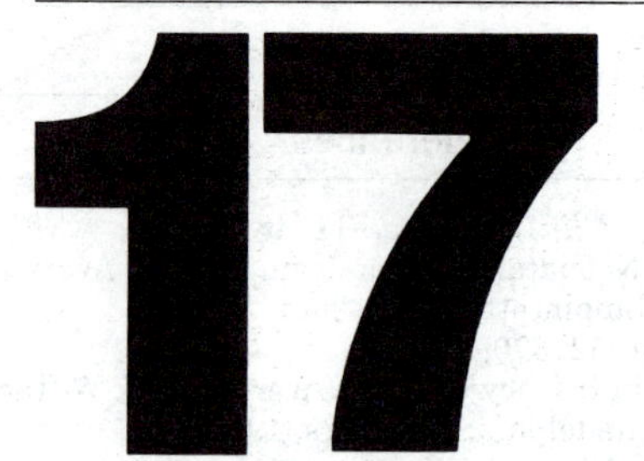

Bleeding

Allen M. Goorin and
John P. Cloherty

The neonatal hemostatic mechanism differs from that of the older child. In neonates there is decreased activity of certain clotting factors, impaired platelet function, and suboptimal defense against clot formation.

I. Etiology

A. Deficient clotting factors

1. **Transitory deficiencies** of the vitamin K–dependent factors II, VII, IX, and X and protein C [13] are characteristics of the newborn period and may be accentuated by the following:
   - **a.** The administration of total parenteral alimentation or antibiotics or the lack of administration of vitamin K to premature infants.
   - **b. Term infants** may develop vitamin K deficiency by day 2 or 3 if they are not supplemented with vitamin K parenterally, because of negligible stores and inadequate intake.
   - **c. The mother** may have received certain drugs during pregnancy that can cause bleeding in the first 24 hours of the infant's life.
     - **(1)** Phenytoin (Dilantin [6,8], phenobarbital, and salicylates [16] interfere with the vitamin K effect on synthesis of clotting factors (see Appendix B).
     - **(2)** Coumadin compounds given to the mother interfere with the synthesis of vitamin K–dependent clotting factors by the liver of both the mother and the fetus, and the bleeding may **not** be immediately reversed by administration of vitamin K (see Appendix B).
2. **Disturbances of clotting** may be related to associated diseases such as **disseminated intravascular coagulation (DIC)** due to infection, shock, anoxia, necrotizing enterocolitis, renal vein thrombosis, or the use of vascular catheters. Any significant liver disease may interfere with the production of clotting factors by the liver.
3. **Inherited abnormalities of clotting factors**
   - **a. Sex-linked recessive (expressed in males)**
     - **(1)** Factor VIII clotting activity and factor VIII procoagulant antigen are decreased in the fetus with classic hemophilia.
     - **(2)** Christmas disease is due to an inherited quantitative deficiency of **plasma thromboplastin component (PTC) (factor IX).**
   - **b. Autosomal dominant (expressed in males and females with one parent affected)**
     - **(1)** Von Willebrand's disease involves decreased levels of factor VIII and platelet dysfunction due to decreased platelet adhesiveness.
     - **(2)** Dysfibrinogenemia is due to fibrinogen (factor I) dysfunction.
     - **(3)** Factor XI [plasma thromboplastin antecedent (PTA)] deficiency (see **c.4**).
   - **c. Autosomal recessive (occurs in both males and females; the parents are carriers)**
     - **(1)** Deficiencies of factors V, VII, X, XII, and XIII. (Factor XIII deficiency appears to be inherited as an X-linked trait in some kindreds.)

(2) Prothrombin (factor II) or fibrinogen (factor I) deficiency
(3) Dysprothrombinemia due to an abnormal factor II
(4) Factor XI or PTA deficiency is incompletely recessive and is often classified as autosomal dominant, since heterozygotes will have some minor bleeding problems.
(5) Variants of von Willebrand's disease

B. Platelet problems (see Chap. 19)

1. **Qualitative disorders** include hereditary conditions [e.g., Glanzmann's disease (thromboasthenia)] and disorders that result from the mother's use of aspirin.
2. **Quantitative disorders**
   a. **Immune disorders** are seen in infants with isoimmune thrombocytopenia and erythroblastosis, infants of mothers with autoimmune diseases such as idiopathic thrombocytopenia purpura (ITP) and disseminated lupus erythematosus, and infants of mothers who received drugs such as quinine, quinidine, sulfonamides, and digitalis.
   b. **Infectious disorders** include bacterial infections, viral infections (e.g., cytomegalovirus and rubella), and protozoal infections.
   c. **Congenital megakaryocytic hypoplasia** may occur either as an isolated disorder or associated with pancytopenia or other congenital anomalies (e.g., Fanconi's syndrome).
   d. **Leukemia** (rare)
   e. **DIC** (common).
   f. **Inherited thrombocytopenia**
   g. **Giant hemangiomas** (Kasbach-Merritt) [2]
   h. **Hyperviscosity syndrome**
   i. **Renal vein thrombosis**
   j. **Necrotizing enterocolitis**

C. Other causes of bleeding

1. **Vascular problems**
   a. Central nervous system (CNS) or pulmonary hemorrhage may result from hypoxia, acidosis, obstetric trauma, or prematurity (see Chap. 21).
   b. Cephalohematoma (massive type)
2. **Miscellaneous problems**
   a. Rupture of spleen or liver associated with breech delivery (see Chap. 13 and 22)
   b. Retroperitoneal or intraperitoneal hemorrhage may present as scrotal ecchymosis [1].
   c. Alpha-1-antitrypsin deficiency [10]

II. Diagnostic workup of the bleeding infant

A. The **history** includes (1) family history of excessive bleeding, (2) information about illnesses during pregnancy and birth, (3) maternal medications (aspirin, phenytoin), and (4) maternal history of a previous birth of an infant with a bleeding disorder.

B. Examination. The crucial decision in diagnosing and managing the bleeding infant is determining whether the infant is sick or well [3,7,9,15] (Table 17-1).

1. **Sick infant.** Consider DIC, infection, or liver disease (vascular injury induced by hypoxia may lead to DIC).
2. **Well infant.** Consider vitamin K deficiency, isolated clotting factor deficiencies, or immune thrombocytopenia.
3. **Petechiae, small superficial ecchymosis, or mucosal bleeding** suggest a platelet problem.
4. **Large bruises** suggest deficiency of clotting factors, DIC, liver disease, or vitamin K deficiency.
5. **Enlarged spleen** suggests infection or erythroblastosis.
6. **Jaundice** suggests infection or liver disease.
7. **Abnormal retinal findings** suggest infection (TORCH; see Chap. 12).

Table 17-1. Differential diagnosis of bleeding in the neonate

Clinical evaluation	Laboratory studies			Likely diagnosis
	Platelets	PT	PTT	
"Sick"	D−	I+	I+	DIC
	D−	N	N	Platelet consumption (infection, necrotizing enterocolitis, renal vein thrombosis)
	N	I+	I+	Liver disease
	N	N	N	Compromised vascular integrity (associated with hypoxia, prematurity, acidosis, hyperosmolality)
"Healthy"	D−	N	N	Immune thrombocytopenia, occult infection, thrombosis, bone marrow hypoplasia (rare)
	N	I+	I+	Hemorrhagic disease of newborn (vitamin K deficiency)
	N	N	I+	Hereditary clotting factor deficiencies
	N	N	N	Bleeding due to local factors (trauma, anatomic abnormalities); qualitative platelet abnormalities (rare); factor XIII deficiency (rare)

Key: PT = prothrombin time; PTT = partial thromboplastin time; D− = decreased; I+ = increased; DIC = disseminated intravascular coagulation; N = normal.
Source: Modified from B. E. Glader, Bleeding Disorders in the Newborn Infant. In A. J. Schaffer and M. E. Avery (Eds.), *Diseases of the Newborn*. Philadelphia: Saunders, 1977. Chap. 64.

C. Laboratory tests (Table 17-2)

1. **The Apt test** is used to rule out maternal blood. If the child is well and only gastrointestinal bleeding is noted, an Apt test is performed on gastric aspirate or stool to rule out the presence of maternal blood swallowed during labor or delivery or from a bleeding breast (a breast pump can be used to collect milk to confirm the presence of blood in the milk or the infant's stomach can be aspirated before and after breast-feeding).
   a. **Procedure.** Mix 1 part stool or vomitus with 5 parts water; centrifuge it and separate the clear pink supernatant (hemolysate); add 1 ml of sodium hydroxide 1% to 4 ml of hemolysate.
   b. **Result.** Hemoglobin A (HbA) changes from pink to yellow brown (maternal blood); HbF stays pink (fetal blood).
2. **Blood smear** is used to determine the number, size and kind of platelets and the presence of fragmented red blood cells as seen in DIC. Large platelets are young platelets and imply an immune etiology for thrombocytopenia.
3. **Platelet count.** The platelet count from the smear equals the number of platelets from 10 oil-immersion fields times 1000. A platelet count also should be performed on the mother if the infant's count is decreased. Significant bleeding from thrombocytopenia is usually associated with platelet counts under 20,000 to 30,000/μl.
4. **Prothrombin time (PT)** is a test of (1) the extrinsic clotting system, (2) the activation of factor X by factor VII, and (3) factors VI, X, V, and II and fibrinogen.
5. **Partial thromboplastin time (PTT)** is a test of the intrinsic clotting system

Table 17-2. Normal values for laboratory screening tests in the neonate

Laboratory test	Premature infant having received vitamin K	Term infant having received vitamin K	Child over 1 to 2 months of age
Platelet count/μl	150,000–400,000	150,000–400,000	150,000–400,000
Platelets on peripheral blood smear	10–20/Platelets/oil-immersion field, including 1 or 2 small clumps	Same as premature infant	Same as premature infant
PT (sec.)*	14–22	13–20	12–14
PTT (sec.)*	35–55	30–45	25–35
Fibrinogen (mg/dl)	150–300	150–300	150–300

Key: PT = prothrombin time; PTT = partial thromboplastin time.
*Normal values may vary from laboratory to laboratory, depending on the particular reagent employed. In full-term infants who have received vitamin K, the PT and PTT values generally fall within the normal "adult" range by several days (PT) to several weeks (PTT) of age. Small premature infants (under 1500 gm) tend to have longer PT and PTT than larger babies. In infants with hematocrit levels greater than 60 percent, the ratio of blood of anticoagulant (sodium citrate 3.8 percent) in tubes should be 19:1 rather than the usual ratio of 9:1; otherwise, spurious results will be obtained, since the amount of anticoagulant solution is calculated for a specific volume of plasma. Blood drawn from heparinized catheters should not be used. The best results are obtained when blood from a clean venipuncture is allowed to drip directly into the tube from the needle or scalp vein set. Factor levels II, VII, IX, and X are decreased. Three-day-old full-term baby not receiving vitamin K has levels similar to a premature baby. Factor XI and XII levels are lower in premature infants than in term infants and account for prolonged PTT. Fibrinogen, factor V, and factor VIII are normal in premature and term infants. Factor XIII is variable.
Source: Data from normal laboratory values at the Hematology Laboratory, The Children's Hospital, Boston; J. B. Alpers and M. T. Lafonet (Eds.), *Laboratory Handbook*. Boston: The Children's Hospital, 1984.

and of the activation of factor X by factors XII, XI, IX, and VIII. PTT is also a test of the final coagulation pathway (factors V and II and fibrinogen).

6. **Fibrinogen** can be measured on the same sample used for PTT. Fibrinogen may be decreased in liver disease.
7. **Fibrin split products (FSP)** are degradation products of fibrin and fibrinogen found in the sera of patients with DIC and in patients with liver disease who have problems clearing FSP. Improper collection of blood will result in increased FSP in the sample.
8. **D-Dimer test.** This replaces the FSP in most laboratories. D-Dimers are formed from the action of plasmin on the fibrin clot, generating derivatives of cross-linked fibrin containing D-dimer. Normal levels are less than 0.5 μg/ml. Levels are higher in DIC, deep vein thrombosis, and pulmonary embolism [12].
9. **Bleeding time.** This test measures platelet quantity and quality, as well as vascular integrity. It is useful to diagnose von Willebrand's disease and functional platelet disorders. The template bleeding time is 3.4 ± 1.3 minutes for preterm infants [9].

III. **Treatment of neonates with abnormal bleeding parameters who have not had clinical bleeding.** In one study, preterm infants with respiratory distress syndrome (RDS) or term infants with asphyxia were treated for abnormal bleeding parameters (without DIC) to correct the hemostatic defect. Although the treatment was successful in correcting the defect, no change in mortality was seen when compared with controls [17].

In general, clinically ill infants or infants weighing less than 1500 gm are given the benefit of transfusion with fresh-frozen plasma (10 ml/kg) if the PT or PTT or both are greater than two times normal or with platelets (1 unit; see **IV.C**) if the platelet count is under 20,000/μl (see Chaps. 19 and 20).

IV. Treatment of bleeding

A. Vitamin K_1 oxide (Aquamephyton). An intravenous dose of 1 mg is administered in case the infant was not given vitamin K at birth. Infants on total parenteral nutrition and infants on antibiotics for more than 2 weeks should be given 0.5 mg of vitamin K_1 IM or IV weekly to prevent vitamin K depletion. Vitamin K should be given before transfusion therapy is begun, since it takes several hours to work and should not be forgotten.

B. Fresh-frozen plasma (see Chap. 20) (10 ml/kg) is given intravenously for active bleeding and is repeated every 8 to 12 hours as needed. This is used because it replaces the clotting factors immediately.

C. Platelets (see Chap. 19). If there is no increased platelet destruction (as a result of DIC, immune platelet problem, or sepsis), 1 unit of platelets given to a 3-kg infant will raise the platelet count to 50,000 to 100,000/μl. If no new platelets are made or transfused, the platelet count will drop slowly over 3 to 5 days. Platelets from the mother or from a known PLA_1-negative donor should be used if the infant has an isoimmume platelet disorder. The blood of the donor should be matched for Rh factor and type, since red cells will be mixed in the platelet concentrates.

D. Fresh whole blood (see Chap. 20). The baby is given 10 ml/kg; more is given as needed. Fresh blood should be used for exchange transfusion, since it removes antibodies and provides fresh platelets and clotting factors.

E. Clotting factor concentrates (see Chap. 20). When there is a known deficiency of factor VIII or IX, one needs to raise the plasma concentration to 20 percent of normal to stop serious bleeding; 10 ml/kg of fresh-frozen plasma will do this. If a higher plasma concentration is desired, factor concentrates or cryoprecipitate must be used to avoid volume overload.

F. Diagnosis and treatment should be aimed at the underlying cause (e.g., infection, liver rupture, catheter, or enterocolitis).

G. Treatment of specific disorders

1. DIC. The baby usually appears sick and may have petechiae, gastrointestinal hemorrhage, oozing from venipunctures, infection, asphyxia, or hypoxia. The platelet count is decreased, and PT and PTT are increased. Fragmented red blood cells (RBCs) are seen on the blood smear. Fibrinogen is decreased, and FSPs or D-dimers are increased. Treatment involves the following steps:

a. The underlying cause should be treated (e.g., sepsis, necrotizing enterocolitis).

b. Vitamin K_1, 1.0 mg IV, is given.

c. Platelets and fresh-frozen plasma are given as needed to keep the platelet count over 50,000/μl and to stop the bleeding.

d. If the bleeding persists, one of the following steps should be taken, depending on the availability of blood, platelets, or fresh-frozen plasma:

(1) Exchange transfusion with fresh citrated whole blood or packed cells mixed with fresh-frozen plasma

(2) Transfusion with platelets and fresh-frozen plasma

e. If DIC is associated with thrombosis of large vessels, heparin is given as a bolus of 25 to 35 units/kg, followed by 10-15 units/kg per hour as a continuous infusion. Platelets and plasma are continued after the heparin has been started. Platelet counts should be kept at or above 50,000/μl. The aim of heparin treatment is to keep the PTT at $1\frac{1}{2}$ to 2 times normal [15].

2. **Hemorrhagic disease of the newborn** occurs in 1 per 200 to 400 neonates not given vitamin K prophalaxis [4,13].
   a. In the healthy infant, hemorrhagic disease of the newborn may occur when the infant is not given vitamin K (the infant may have been born in a busy delivery room, at home, or transferred from elsewhere). Bleeding and bruising may occur after the infant is 48 hours of age. The platelet level is normal, and PT and PTT are prolonged. If there is active bleeding, 10 ml/kg of fresh-frozen plasma and an IV dose of 1 mg of vitamin K are given.
   b. If the mother has been treated with phenytoin (Dilantin), primidone (Mysoline), methsuximide (Celontin), or phenobarbital, the infant may be vitamin K deficient and bleed during the first 24 hours. The mother should be given vitamin K 24 hours prior to delivery (10 mg of vitamin K_1 IM) [6]. The newborn should have PT, PTT, and platelet counts monitored if any sings of bleeding occur. The usual dose of vitamin K_1 (1 mg) should be given to the baby postpartum and repeated in 24 hours. Repeated infusions of fresh-frozen plasma (FFP) are given if any bleeding occurs.
   c. **Delayed hemorrhagic disease** of the newborn can occur at 4 to 12 weeks of age. This can be seen in infants with malabsorption from diseases such as cystic fibrosis or in infants treated with prolonged broad-spectrum antibiotics.

References

1. Amoury, R. A. *South Med. J.* 75: 1471, 1978.
2. Bowles, L. J. *Clin. Pediatr. (Phila).* 20: 428, 1981.
3. Buchanan, G. R. Hemorrhagic Diseases. In D. G. Nathan and F. A. Oski (Eds.), *Hematology of Infancy and Childhood,* 3d Ed. Philadelphia: Saunders, 1987.
4. Caravella, S. J., et al. *Pediatrics* 80: 1, 1987.
5. Chaou, W. T. *J. Pediatr.* 105: 880, 1984.
6. Dalessio, D. J. *N. Engl. J. Med.* 312: 559, 1985.
7. Glader, B. E. Bleeding Disorders in the Newborn Infant. In M. E. Avery and H. W. Taeusch (Eds.), *Schaffer's Diseases of the Newborn,* 5th Ed. Philadelphia: Saunders, 1984.
8. Hall, J. G. *Am. J. Med.* 68: 122, 1980.
9. Hathaway, W. E. *Clin. Perinatol.* 2: 83, 1975.
10. Hope, P. L. *Arch. Dis. Child.* 57: 68, 1982.
11. Kisker, C. T. *Am. J. Pediatr. Hematol. Oncol.* 3: 193, 1981.
12. Alpers, J. B. (Ed.). *Laboratory Handbook.* Stow, Ohio: The Children's Hospital, Lexi-Comp, Inc., 1988.
13. Lane, P. A., et al. *J. Pediatr.* 106: 351, 1985.
14. O'Connor, M. E., et al. *J. Pediatr.* 108: 616, 1986.
15. Oski, F. A., and Naiman, J. L. *Hematologic Problems in the Newborn,* 3d Ed. Philadelphia: Saunders, 1982.
16. Stuart, M. J., et al. *N. Engl. J. Med.* 307: 909, 1982.
17. Turner, T. *Br. J. Haemtaol.* 47: 65, 1981.

Polycythemia

Allen M. Goorin

As the central hematocrit rises, there is increased viscosity and decreased blood flow; when the hematocrit increases to more than 60 percent, there is a fall in oxygen transport [5] (Fig. 18-1). Newborns have erythrocytes that are less deformable than the erythrocytes of adults. As viscosity increases, there is impairment of tissue oxygenation and decreased glucose in plasma, with a tendency to form microthrombi. If these events occur in the cerebral cortex, kidneys, or adrenal glands, significant damage may result. Hypoxia and acidosis increase viscosity and deformity further. Poor perfusion increases the possibility of thrombosis.

I. Definitions

- **A. Polycythemia**—venous hematocrit of over 65 percent [3,8], a venous hematocrit over 64 percent or more at 2 hours of age [19], or an umbilical venous hematocrit over 63 percent or more [18].
- **B. Hyperviscosity** is defined as greater than 14.6 centipoise at a shear rate of 11.5 sec^{-1} as measured by a viscometer [24]. The relationship of hematocrit and viscosity is nearly linear below a hematocrit of 60 percent, but viscosity increases exponentially at a hematocrit of 70 percent or greater.

II. Incidence. The incidence of polycythemia in newborns is increased in small for gestational age and postterm babies, but on average is 0.4 to 5 percent [16,17,28,29].

III. Causes of polycythemia

- **A. Placental red cell transfusion**
  1. **Delayed cord clamping** may occur either intentionally or in unattended deliveries.
     - a. When the cord is clamped within 1 minute after birth, the blood volume of the infant is 83.4 ml/kg.
     - b. When the cord is clamped 2 minutes after delivery, the blood volume of the infant is 93 ml/kg.
     - c. In newborns with polycythemia, blood volume per kilogram of body weight varies inversely in relation to birth weight [17] (Fig. 18-2).
  2. **Cord stripping** (thus pushing more blood into the infant)
  3. **Holding the baby below the mother** at delivery
  4. **Maternal-to-fetal transfusion** is diagnosed with the Kleihauer-Betke stain technique of acid elution to detect maternal cells in the newborn circulation [14] (see Chap. 16).
  5. **Twin-to-twin transfusion** [22]
- **B. Placental insufficiency (increased fetal erythropoiesis secondary to intrauterine hypoxia)**
  1. Small-for-gestational-age infants [11]
  2. Infants of toxemic mothers
  3. Postmature infants
  4. Infants born to mothers with Eisenmenger syndrome [15]
- **C. Other causes**
  1. Infants of diabetic mothers (increased erythropoiesis)
  2. Large for gestational age babies

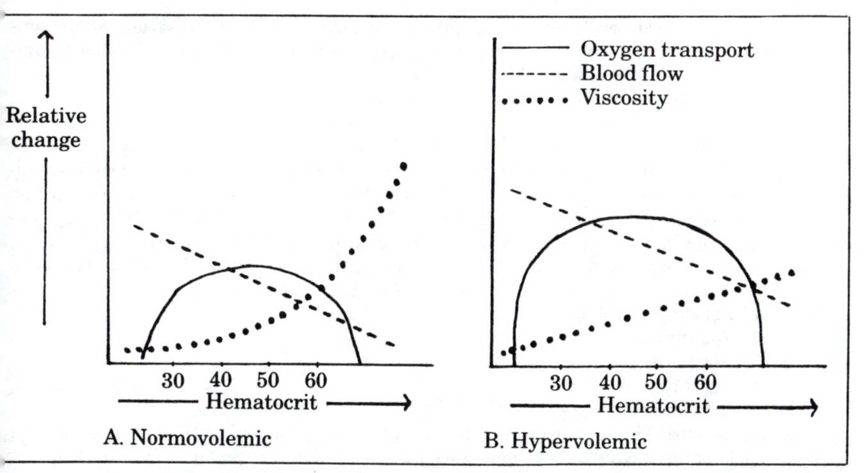

Fig. 18-1. Effect of hematocrit on viscosity, blood flow, and oxygen transport. (Adapted from B. Glader, Erythrocyte Disorders in Infancy. In A. J. Schaffer and M. E. Avery (Eds.), *Diseases of the Newborn.* Philadelphia: Saunders, 1977. P. 624.)

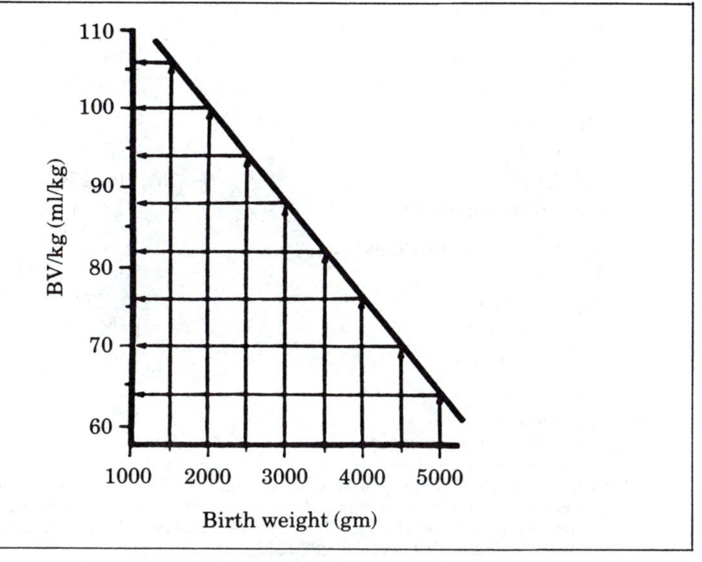

Fig. 18-2. Nomogram designed for clinical use, correlating blood volume per kilogram with birth weight in polycythemic neonates (BV = blood volume). (From J. S. Rawlings et al., Estimated blood volumes in polycythemic neonates as a function of birth weight. *J. Pediatr.* 101: 594, 1982.)

3. Infants with congenital adrenal hyperplasia, Beckwith-Wiedemann syndrome, Down syndrome, neonatal thyrotoxicosis, congenital hypothyroidism [27], trisomy 13, and trisomy 18
4. Drugs (maternal use of propranolol) [6]

IV. Symptoms. Case reports indicate that most infants with polycythemia are asymptomatic, but a large study of 987 polycythemic infants showed that over half had clinical symptoms [29]. Clinical findings include feeding problems; plethora; jitteriness; hypotonia; respiratory symptoms such as tachypnea; cardiac symptoms such as cyanosis, murmurs, or congestive heart failure; lethargy; hypoglycemia; poor suck; convulsions; renal vein thromboses; increased jaundice; cerebral infarcts; necrotizing enterocolitis; priapism; and testicular infarcts. The most consistent clinical findings (Table 18-1) include the following:

A. Feeding problems
B. Tachypnea
C. Plethora
D. Lethargy
E. Cyanosis [7,26,29]

V. Screening. The routine screening of all newborns for polycythemia/hyperviscosity is being advocated by some authors [8,29]. Timing and site of blood sampling alter the hematocrit value [19,24]. We do not routinely screen well term newborns for this syndrome, since there are little data showing that treatment of asymptomatic patients with partial exchange transfusion is beneficial in the long term [3].

Table 18-1. Neonatal hyperviscosity syndrome

Neonatal hyperviscosity	Incidence (percent)
Clinical Symptoms	
Feeding problems	21*
Cyanosis	7†, 12‡
Plethora	20*
Lethargy	14*
Jitteriness	7*
Hypotonia	7*
Tachypnea	6*, 10†, 15§
Necrotizing enterocolitis	1*, 2†, 4‡
Laboratory Abnormalities	
Hyperbilirubinemia	33*
Hypoglycemia	13*, 27†
Hypocalcemia	9*, 9‡
Hypomagnesemia	30‡
Thrombocytopenia	1*, 20¶
Prominent vascular markings or chest x-ray	85§

*Source: From T. E. Wiswell, J. D. Cornish, and R. S. Northam, Neonatal polycythemia: Frequency of clinical manifestations and other associated findings. *Pediatrics* 70: 26, 1986.
†Source: From B. D. Black et al., Developmental and neurologic sequelae of neonatal hyperviscosity syndrome. *Pediatrics* 4: 426, 1982.
‡Source: From J. R. Humbert, H. Abelson, W. E. Hathaway, and F. C. Batagglia, Polycythemia in small for gestational age infants. *J. Pediatr.* 75: 812, 1969.
§Source: From G. R. Gladstone, A. Horodof, and W. M. Gersoney, Propranolol administration during pregnancy: Effects on the fetus. *J. Pediatr.* 86: 962, 1975.
¶Source: From A. Host and M. Ulrich, Late prognosis in untreated neonatal polycythemia with minor or no symptoms. *Acta Paediatr. Scand.* 71: 629, 1982.

VI. Diagnosis. The capillary blood or peripheral venous hematocrit level should be determined in any baby who appears plethoric, who has any predisposing cause of polycythemia, who has any of the symptoms mentioned in **IV.**, or who is not well for any reason.

- **A.** Depending on local perfusion, the **capillary blood hematocrit** will be 5 to 20 percent higher than the central hematocrit. Warming the heel prior to drawing a capillary hematocrit will give a better correlation with the peripheral venous or central hematocrit. If the capillary blood hematocrit is above 65 percent, a peripheral venous hematocrit should be done.
- **B.** Any **venous hematocrit** more than 60 percent is of concern.
- **C.** Measurement of **blood viscosity** should be done if available, because some infants with hematocrits less than 65 percent will have hyperviscous blood [28].

VII. Management

- **A.** Any child with symptoms that could be due to hyperviscosity should have a partial exchange transfusion if the peripheral **venous hematocrit** is more than 65 percent.
- **B.** **Asymptomatic infants** with a peripheral venous hematocrit between 60 and 70 percent can usually be managed by pushing fluids.
- **C.** Most neonatologists perform an exchange transfusion when the peripheral venous hematocrit is more than 70 percent in the absence of symptoms, but this is controversial [1,3,7,16].
- **D.** The following formula can be used to calculate the exchange with albumin 5% on normal saline that will bring the hematocrit to 60 percent. In infants with polycythemia, the blood volume varies inversely with the birth weight [20] (see Fig. 18-2). We usually take the blood from the umbilical vein and replace it with albumin 5% or normal saline in a peripheral vein. There are many methods of exchange (see Chap. 15).

  Volume of exchange (in ml)

  $$= \frac{\text{blood volume} \times (\text{observed hematocrit} - \text{desired hematocrit})}{\text{observed hematocrit}}$$

  Example: A 3-kg infant, hematocrit 75 percent, blood volume 80 ml/kg—to bring hematocrit to 60 percent:

  $$\text{Volume of exchange (in ml)} = \frac{(80 \text{ ml} \times 3 \text{ kg}) \times (75 - 60)}{75}$$

  $$= \frac{240 \text{ ml} \times 15}{75}$$

  $$= 48\text{-ml exchange}$$

  Total usual volume is 10 to 20 ml/kg of body weight.

VIII. Outcome

- **A.** Infants with polycythemia and hyperviscosity who have decreased cerebral blood flow velocity and increased vascular resistance develop normal cerebral blood flow following partial exchange transfusion [16]. They also have improvement in systemic blood flow and oxygen transport [24].
- **B.** The long-term neurologic outcome of asymptomatic polycythemic/hyperviscostic infants treated or untreated remains controversial.
  1. One trial, randomizing treatment with small numbers of patients, has shown decreased IQ scores of school-aged children who had neonatal hyperviscosity syndrome whether or not the newborns were treated [2,3].
  2. Another retrospective study, with small numbers of patients, showed no difference in the neurologic outcome of patients with asymptomatic neonatal polycythemia whether they were treated or not [10].
  3. Some earlier preliminary prospective studies favored treatment [2,7].
  4. An increased incidence of necrotizing enterocolitis following partial exchange transfusions by umbilical vein has been reported [1,4,25]. Enter-

ocolitis was not seen in one retrospective analysis of 185 term polycythemic babies given partial exchange transfusions with removal of blood from the umbilical vein and reinfusion of a commercial plasma substitute through peripheral veins [9].

5. A large prospective, randomized clinical trial comparing partial exchange transfusion with symptomatic care (increased fluid intake, etc.) equally balanced for risk factors and the etiologies of the polycythemias is necessary to give guidelines for treatment of the asymptomatic newborn with polycythemia/hyperviscosity.

References

1. Black, V. D. *Pediatr. Clin. North Am.* 5: 1137, 1982.
2. Black, V. D. *Pediatrics* 69: 426, 1982.
3. Black, V. D. *Pediatrics* 83: 662, 1989.
4. Black, V. D. *Pediatrics* 76: 225, 1985.
5. Glader, B. Erythrocyte Disorders in Infancy. In A. J. Schaffer and M. E. Avery (Eds.), *Diseases of the Newborn.* Philadelphia: Saunders, 1977.
6. Gladstone, G. R. *J. Pediatr.* 86: 962, 1975.
7. Goldberg, K. *Pediatrics* 69: 419, 1982.
8. Hathaway, W. E. *Pediatrics* 72: 567, 1983.
9. Hein, H. A. *Pediatrics* 80: 75, 1987.
10. Host, A. *Acta Paediatr. Scand.* 71: 629, 1982.
11. Humbert, J. R. *J. Pediatr.* 75: 812, 1969.
12. Katz, J. *J. Pediatr.* 101: 99, 1982.
13. Malan, A. D. *Early Hum. Dev.* 4: 393, 1980.
14. Michael, A. F., Jr. *Pediatrics* 28: 604, 1959.
15. Mukhtar, A. I. *Obstet. Gynecol.* 5: 651, 1982.
16. Oski, F. A., and Naiman, J. L. *Hematologic Problems in the Newborn,* 3d Ed. Philadelphia: Saunders, 1982. Pp. 87–96.
17. Ramamurthy, R. S. *Perinatol. Neonatol.* Sept.–Oct.: 38, 1979.
18. Ramamurthy, R. S. *Pediatrics* 68: 168, 1981.
19. Ramamurthy, R. S. *J. Pediatr.* 110: 929, 1987.
20. Rawlings, J. S. *J. Pediatr.* 101: 594, 1982.
21. Rosenkrantz, T. S. *J. Pediatr.* 101: 94, 1982.
22. Sacks, M. O. *Pediatrics* 24: 604, 1961.
23. Shohat, M. *Pediatrics* 73: 7, 1984.
24. Swetnam, S. M. *J. Pediatr.* 110: 443, 1987.
25. Thilo, E. H. *Pediatrics* 73: 476, 1984.
26. Wesenberg, R. L. *Hosp. Pract.* 13: 137, 1978.
27. Weinblatt, M. E. *Am. J. Dis. Child.* 141: 1121, 1987.
28. Wirth, F. H. *J. Pediatr.* 63: 833, 1979.
29. Wiswell, T. E. *Pediatrics* 78: 26, 1986.

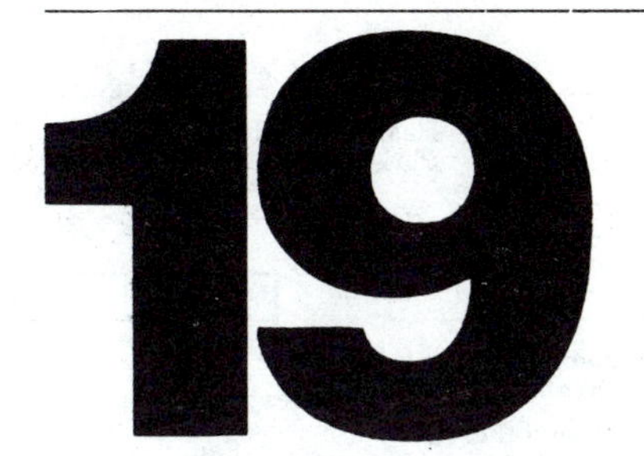

Thrombocytopenia

Allen M. Goorin

Thrombocytopenia is defined as a platelet count of less than 150,000/ml of blood in both term and premature infants. The expected life span of platelets in newborns is 8 to 9 days, as in older subjects. In one prospective study, thrombocytopenia developed in 22 percent of 807 consecutive infants admitted to a neonatal intensive care unit. The platelet count nadir usually occurred by day 4 and usually resolved by day 10. A potential etiology of increased platelet destruction, including immune-mediated platelet destruction, disseminated intravascular coagulation (DIC), and having had an exchange transfusion, was found in 80 percent of patients [9]. Furthermore, more severe grades of intraventricular hemorrhage and serious neurologic morbidity were noted in the small surviving thrombocytopenic infants.

I. **General approach to diagnosis of thrombocytopenia** (Fig. 19-1)
   A. **Maternal history.** There may be a history of thrombocytopenia, bleeding before or during pregnancy, having undergone a splenectomy, drug use, or infection.
   B. **Infant.** The baby may seem healthy or may appear sick. Petechiae or large bruises, hepatosplenomegaly, jaundice, and congenital anomalies may be seen.
   C. **Laboratory work**
      1. The **mother** needs to have a platelet count and platelet typing (if the maternal count is normal).
      2. The **baby** needs
         a. Complete blood count (CBC)
         b. Platelet count
         c. Prothrombin time (PT)
         d. Partial thromboplastin time (PTT)

II. **General approach to therapy for thrombocytopenia**
   A. **Platelet transfusion in the newborn**
      1. **Indication**—clinical bleeding or platelet count less than 20,000/ml.
      2. **Source.** A random donor is used, except in the infant with alloimmune thrombocytopenia, in which case either the mother's platelets or platelets from a platelet antigen–compatible donor are used.
      3. **Quantity.** One unit of platelets per 3 kg raises the platelet count by 50,000 to 100,000/μl, unless there is peripheral destruction of the platelets.
      4. **Frequency.** The normal half-life is 4 to 5 days; it is shorter if increased platelet consumption is present.
      5. **Route. Never give platelets through an arterial line or into the liver because thrombosis may occur.** Platelets are given intravenously through a peripheral vein.
      6. **All platelet transfusions** should be irradiated because of the white blood cells (WBCs) in platelet transfusions (see Chap. 20).
   B. **Steroid therapy** in bleeding infants. Prednisone 2 mg/kg per day may reduce bleeding by as yet undefined mechanisms.
   C. In an **emergency** situation, fresh whole blood is used for exchange transfusion.

III. **Thrombocytopenia with decreased platelet survival** [3,11]. Plasma **glycocalicin,** a fragment of the platelet membrane glycoprotein (Ib), was recently reported to

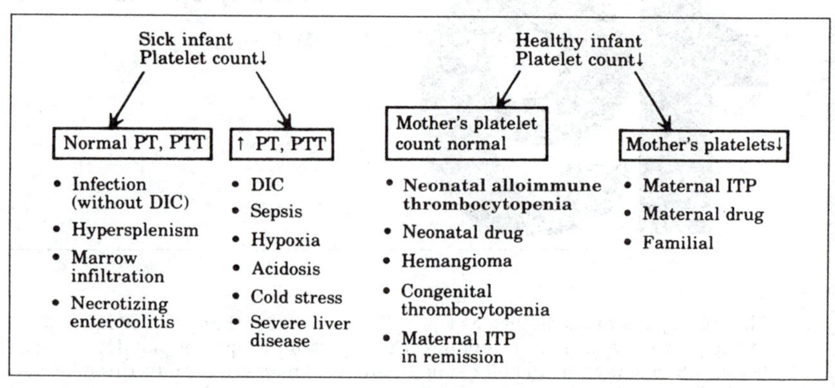

Fig. 19-1. Clinical status in neonatal thrombocytopenia with features that determine a quick differential diagnosis (PT = prothrombin time; PTT = partial thromboplastin time; DIC = disseminated intravascular coagulation; ITP = immune thrombocytopenic purpura; ↑ = increased; ↓ = decreased).

be decreased in patients with thrombocytopenia secondary to underproduction and normal or increased in patients with thrombocytopenia caused by a reduction in platelet life span [28].

A. **Immune thrombocytopenia.** In **autoimmune** thrombocytopenia, the antibody is formed against the antigen on the mother's platelets. In **alloimmune** thrombocytopenia, the antibody is formed against the antigen on the infant's platelets. Recent advances in direct and indirect antiplatelet antibodies have helped differentiate the two syndromes [22,25] (Table 19-1).

1. **Maternal immune thrombocytopenia purpura (ITP)**

a. **Clinical picture.** The baby appears healthy but has petechiae, bruises, bleeding, and a low platelet count. The mother has thrombocytopenia or a history of ITP in the past. Eight percent of 1357 normal women at delivery had mild thrombocytopenias, with platelet counts ranging from 97,000 to 150,000/μl, without discernible clinical effects on the mothers or infants [5].

b. **Pathophysiology.** The mother produces immunoglobulin G (IgG) antibody, which reacts against the "public antigen" found on all platelets (i.e., hers and the baby's). Some mothers have mild thrombocytopenia and platelet antibodies in the second half of pregnancy. If the mothers have never had any bleeding problem, are not on steroids, have an intact spleen, had a normal platelet count just before the pregnancy or in the first half of the pregnancy, and never had a platelet count under 80,000/ml, there appears to be little risk to the fetus. Additionally, if a mother is found to have thrombocytopenia and has no history of immune thrombocytopenia and has no circulatory platelet antibodies there is little risk to her offspring [26A]. This entity is called **pseudo-ITP** [6].

c. **Treatment**

(1) Even if the mother has true ITP, it appears that in utero fetal hemorrhage is very rare as compared with the small but definite risk of such hemorrhage in alloimmune thrombocytopenia [6]. One uncontrolled report [20] showed a 3.6-fold increase in neonatal platelet counts following **steroid** administration to mothers with ITP and positive antiplatelet antibodies. Prednisone 10 to 20 mg qd was given for 10 to 14 days prior to delivery. This study needs to be confirmed before steroid administration becomes rou-

Table 19-1. Interpretation of antiplatelet antibodies on the mother's platelets (direct) or in her serum (indirect)

Antiplatelet antibody test		
Direct	Indirect	Immune syndrome
+	+	Auto- and sometimes isoantibody
+	−	Autoantibody
−	+	Isoantibody

Key: + = positive; − = negative.

tine practice. Intravenous IgG given prenatally to the mother with ITP has not been clearly shown to affect the fetal platelet count.

(2) Percutaneous umbilical blood sampling (PUBS) is beginning to be used as a safe, accurate, and direct method of obtaining the fetal platelet counts. In experienced hands, the mortality from this procedure is less than 1 percent [6]. This 1 percent mortality still may be too great a risk for cases of maternal ITP (see Chap. 3).

(3) There may be little correlation between fetal and maternal platelet counts.

(4) **Antiplatelet antibodies.** The level of maternal circulating antiplatelet antibody (direct test; see Table 19-1) is reported to be correlated with both presence and extent of neonatal thrombocytopenia [11]. This needs to be confirmed by other investigators before decisions regarding cesarean section are based on the maternal level of circulating antiplatelet antibody.

(5) Mothers who have had recent platelet counts under 80,000/μl, are on steroids, or have had a splenectomy are at increased risk to have a child with significant thrombocytopenia.

(6) Since a **cesarean section** reduces trauma to the infant, it would decrease the risk of bleeding in the occasional infant who is severely thrombocytopenic. The issue of when to do cesarean section in mothers known to have ITP is controversial [6,11,17,21]. The maternal mortality from cesarean sections in some centers is the same as from vaginal deliveries [14]. Our usual management of these cases is to allow vaginal delivery to progress until a fetal scalp platelet count can be done. If the fetal scalp platelet count is over 50,000/μl and labor is progressing normally, the infant is delivered vaginally [27]. If these criteria are not met, then a cesarean section is done. One should remember that obstetricians would like a maternal platelet count of 50,000 to 100,000/μl before they are willing to operate and anesthesiologists are often unwilling to give epidural anesthesia to mothers with platelet counts under 100,000/μl [6].

(7) **Therapy for infants** severely affected includes intravenous **gammaglobulin** (IgG), **prednisone** (2 mg/kg per day), **platelet transfusion,** and possibly **exchange transfusion** (see **II**). **Gammaglobulin** (IgG) 0.4 gm/kg per day for 5 days or 1.0 gm/kg per day for 2 days with or without concomitant steroids given to 12 infants with platelet counts of 5000 to 54,000/μl raised the platelet count 75 percent of the time to over 50,000/μl and to at least twice the pretreatment value 48 hours after completion of the IgG. Additionally, 4 patients required repeated doses of IgG to maintain the platelet count in a safe range [4,10]. Both steroids and IV IgG appear to be helpful in a majority of babies with bleeding and/or low platelet counts secondary to maternal ITP.

(8) **Outcome.** Most reports regarding the outcome of infants born to mothers with ITP are retrospective analyses and may overstate the problem. Antenatal intracranial hemorrhage occurs but appears to be an extremely uncommon event [6]. A prospective study [21] reported 5 of 99 conceptions in 95 pregnancies died, but all deaths occurred in utero between 18 and 28 weeks of gestation. Of the liveborn infants, 51 percent had thrombocytopenia, but only 6 of 94 infants had serious bleeding.

2. **Drug-induced immune destruction** of platelets may be seen if the mother or the newborn receives quinine, quinidine, digoxin, chlorothiazide, sulfonamide derivatives, phenylbutazone, or *para*-aminosalicylic acid. The list of drugs causing this problem is growing [15]. The mechanism of drug-induced immune destruction is similar to autoimmune destruction.
3. **Neonatal thrombocytopenia** associated with systemic lupus in the mother is similar to autoimmune destruction.
4. **Alloimmune neonatal thrombocytopenia** involves antibodies against naturally occurring platelet antigens, usually $P1^{A1}$ antigen. Other platelet antigens that are mostly HLA-related make up about 20 percent of the cases [3].
   a. **Clinical picture.** The baby appears healthy but has petechiae, bruising, bleeding, and a low platelet count. The mother has a normal platelet count; it may be her first pregnancy, or she may have a history of a previously affected pregnancy. There may be a history of alloimmune thrombocytopenia in children born to the mother's sisters.
   b. **Pathophysiology.** In 50% of cases, the mother is $P1^{A1}$-negative and the fetus is $P1^{A1}$-positive; 98 percent of all individuals are $P1^{A1}$-antigen positive. The mother's IgG antibody, which is directed against a $P1^{A1}$ locus, coats the baby's platelets. Other platelet antigens make up the other cases by a similar mechanism. Coated platelets are destroyed in the infant's reticuloendothelial system. We have seen two fetal deaths with bleeding associated with fetal alloimmune thrombocytopenia.
   c. **Prenatal therapy**
      (1) **Gammaglobulin.** Intravenous gammaglobulin (IgG) with or without dexamethasone given once a week to seven pregnant women who had previously delivered infants with severe alloimmune thrombocytopenia was recently reported to significantly increase newborn platelet counts to over 30,000/ml. None of the infants had an intracranial hemorrhage [7].
      (2) **Platelet transfusion.** In utero repeated platelet transfusions to six fetuses with low platelet counts as measured by PUBS as early as 32 weeks' gestation was successful in raising fetal platelet counts to near or above normal levels (see Chap. 3). All neonates did well with no signs of bleeding at birth [19].
      (3) Close cooperation between the obstetrician, neonatologist, and hematologist is required to decide which fetuses would benefit from prenatal treatment. The infant with alloimmune thrombocytopenia is clearly at greater risk for in utero and perinatal bleeding than those born to mothers with ITP. Mothers who had a previous infant with significant in utero bleeding would certainly qualify for PUBS at 20 to 22 weeks' gestation. If the fetal platelet count is low, treatment of the mother with weekly intravenous gammaglobulin seems reasonable [7]. PUBS can be repeated in 4 weeks. We have no set policy in cases of prenatal alloimmune thrombocytopenia yet, but we consider PUBS, steroids, intravenous gam-

maglobulin, fetal scalp platelet counts, elective cesarean section, and vaginal delivery on a case-by-case basis.

d. **Therapy** at delivery and during the neonatal period

(1) **Delivery.** If the fetal platelet count is over 50,000/ml as measured by PUBS (see **III.A.4.C.(3)**) or fetal scalp platelet count, we allow **vaginal delivery** if presentation and labor are normal. If these criteria are not met, a **cesarean section** is done.

(2) **Transfusion.** The mother's platelets are collected 24 hours prior to delivery. If the baby has a platelet count of less than 20,000/μl, or if the baby shows any signs of bleeding or oozing, the mother's platelets ($P1^{A1}$-negative) are transfused into the baby. The mother's serum will have $P1^{A1}$-positive antibody, which potentially can react with the newborn's platelets for up to 6 weeks; using washed maternal platelets resuspended in plasma will avoid this complication. If there is an emergency secondary to bleeding in the newborn and the mother's platelets have not been previously collected, either the mother's whole blood or platelets from a previously typed $P1^{A1}$-negative platelet donor can be used. Random platelets should be used if there is serious bleeding and $P1^{A1}$-negative platelets are not available. To avoid the possibility of the infant developing **graft-versus-host (GVH) disease,** the blood products should be irradiated (see Chap. 20).

(3) **Gammaglobulin.** Successful postnatal use of intravenous IgG 0.4 gm/kg per day for 2 to 5 days has been reported [1].

(4) **Prednisone** 2 mg/kg per day is usually given to newborns with continued low platelet counts or continued bleeding.

(5) Sisters of $P1^{A1}$-negative mothers should have platelet typing done to anticipate problems. If they are $P1^{A1}$-negative and their husbands are $P1^{A1}$-positive, anticipatory planning is indicated.

(6) **Outcome.** We have seen two fetal deaths with bleeding associated with fetal alloimmune thrombocytopenia. In one report, 7 of 50 patients had intracranial hemorrhage and in 2 of the 7 patients the intracranial bleeding occurred prenatally [8]. We recommend obtaining a cranial ultrasound study after delivery to document any intracranial bleeding, since intracranial hemorrhages are sometimes clinically silent.

B. Peripheral consumption of platelets

1. **Disseminated intravascular coagulation (DIC)** (see Chap. 17)

a. **Clinical picture.** The infant appears sick and has thrombocytopenia, a prolonged PT, and a prolonged PTT. Fibrinogen is decreased, and split products or D-dimers are increased.

b. **Therapy**

(1) The underlying disorder (e.g., sepsis, acidosis, hypoxia, or hypothermia) should be treated. Vitamin K should be given, and clotting factors and platelets should be replaced.

(2) Exchange transfusion with fresh whole blood is performed for patients with active bleeding not responsive to repeated plasma and platelet transfusions.

2. **Giant hemangioma (Kasabach-Merritt syndrome)** [13]

a. **Clinical picture.** The baby appears healthy and has a large hemangioma and thrombocytopenia.

b. **Therapy** involves platelet transfusion, clotting factors, and prednisone. Most hemangiomas involute by 1 to 2 years of age, so medical management should be attempted. We have recently treated some of these hemangiomas with α Interferon and have had good results. Surgical approach to the hemangioma is sometimes necessary.

3. **Necrotizing enterocolitis** (see Chap. 28)

a. **Clinical picture**—thrombocytopenia with necrotizing enterocolitis

b. **Therapy.** The underlying disorder is treated, and platelet transfusions are given as necessary [18].

C. **Direct toxic injury to platelets**

1. **Sepsis** may be of bacterial or viral origin. Therapy involves treatment of the underlying disorder; platelet transfusion is necessary if there is bleeding.
   a. Thrombocytopenia as an early detection of sepsis in newborns is nonspecific [24,29].
   b. Thrombocytopenia as an indication of a high-risk factor associated with increased hemorrhage, morbidity, and mortality has been described [13].
   c. There is some evidence that an immune mechanism may be involved in the thrombocytopenia of neonatal sepsis [31].
2. **Drug injury.** Thiazides, tolbutamide, hydralazine, and aspirin have been implicated. Therapy involves the removal of the offending drug; platelet transfusion is necessary if there is bleeding.

   Maternal ingestion of aspirin during pregnancy should be avoided. If ingestion has occurred within 1 week of delivery, 90 percent of newborns will have bleeding tendencies [30]. Maternal use of aspirin has been associated with a reduced mean birth weight of the offspring, prolongation of gestation and labor, increased blood loss at delivery, and increased perinatal mortality [3].

D. **Hypersplenism**

1. **Clinical picture.** The baby has an enlarged spleen and thrombocytopenia; there may or may not be hemolytic anemia. The condition is associated with congenital hepatitis, congenital viral infection, and portal vein thrombosis.
2. **Therapy.** The underlying disorder is treated. Platelet transfusion is administered if there is bleeding. Splenectomy is performed only as a last resort for uncontrollable bleeding.

E. **Familial shortened platelet survival** results from intrinsic problems with platelets. Production also may be abnormal.

1. **Wiskott-Aldrich syndrome** is manifested by the presence of abnormal, small platelets.
2. **May-Hegglin anomaly.** The infant has giant, bizarre platelets with Doehle bodies, abnormal platelet survival, and impaired production of platelets.
3. **Bernard-Soulier syndrome.** There are large platelets with granules clumped to appear as a nucleus.

IV. **Thrombocytopenia with normal platelet survival and decreased platelet production**

A. **Toxic injury to megakaryoctyes**

1. **Bacterial or viral infections**
2. **Drug-induced injury**

B. **Congenital thrombocytopenias**

1. **Syndrome of thrombocytopenia with absent radii** [16]
2. **Familial thrombocytopenias**
3. **Fanconi's anemia**
4. **Marrow aplasia,** which may be isolated or general

C. **Marrow infiltration**

1. **Neonatal leukemia**
2. **Congenital neuroblastoma**
3. **Storage disease**

V. **Thrombocytopenia associated with erythroblastosis fetalis.** The mechanism may possibly involve platelet trapping in the liver and spleen, anoxia with secondary intravascular coagulation, or associated antiplatelet antibodies.

VI. **Thrombocytopenia after exchange or other transfusion.** Blood more than 24 hours old has few viable platelets.

References

1. Amato, M. *J. Pediatr.* 107: 650, 1988.
2. Androw, M., et al. *J. Pediatr.* 110: 457, 1987.
3. Buchanan, G. R. Hemorrhagic Diseases. In D. G. Nathan and F. A. Oski (Eds.), *Hematology of Infancy and Childhood,* 3d Ed. Philadelphia: Saunders, 1987.
4. Ballin, A., et al. *J. Pediatr.* 112: 789, 1988.
5. Burrows, R. F., et al. *N. Engl. J. Med.* 319: 142, 1988.
6. Bussel, J. B. *J. Pediatr.* 113: 497, 1988.
7. Bussel, J. B., et al. *N. Engl. J. Med.* 319: 1374, 1988.
8. Bussel, J. B. *Pediatr. Res.* 23: 337a, 1988.
9. Castle, V., et al. *J. Pediatr.* 108: 749, 1986.
10. Chirico, G., et al. *J. Pediatr.* 103: 654, 1983.
11. Cines, D. B. *N. Engl. J. Med.* 306: 826, 1982.
12. Collins, E. *Obstet. Gynecol.* 58: 575, 1981.
13. Esterly, N. B. *J. Am. Acad. Dermatol.* 8: 504, 1983.
14. Frigoletto, F. D. *Am. J. Obstet. Gynecol.* 139: 969, 1980.
15. Gill, F. A. *Pediatr. Ann.* 12: 71, 1974.
16. Hall, J. G. *Medicine* 48: 411, 1969.
17. Handen, R. I. *N. Engl. J. Med.* 305: 951, 1981.
18. Hutter, J. J. *J. Pediatr.* 88: 1026, 1976.
19. Kaplan, O. *Blood* 72: 340, 1988.
20. Karpatkin, M. *N. Engl. J. Med.* 305: 936, 1981.
21. Kelton, J. G. *Ann. Intern. Med.* 99: 796, 1983.
22. Kelton, J. G. *N. Engl. J. Med.* 302: 1401, 1980.
23. Mehta, P. *J. Pediatr.* 97: 791, 1980.
24. Modanlou, H. D. *Clin. Pediatr. (Phila.)* 20: 402, 1981.
25. Moore, S. B. *Mayo Clin. Proc.* 57: 778, 1982.
26. Oski, F. A., and Naiman, J. L. *Hematologic Problems in the Newborn,* 3d Ed. Philadelphia: Saunders, 1982.

26A. Samuels, P. *N. Engl. J. Med.* 323: 229, 1990.

27. Scott, J. R. *Am. J. Obstet. Gynecol.* 136: 495, 1980.
28. Steinberg, M. H., et al. *N. Engl. J. Med.* 317: 1037, 1987.
29. Storm, W. *Acta Paediatr. Acad. Sci. Hung.* 23: 349, 1982.
30. Stuart, M. J. *N. Engl. J. Med.* 307: 909, 1982.
31. Tate, D. Y. *J. Pediatr.* 98: 449, 1981.

Blood Products Used in the Newborn

Sherwin V. Kevy

I. Products and components

A. Whole blood. Three different anticoagulants are available. Citrate-phosphate-dextrose (CPD), CPD with adenine (CPD A-1), and CPD with a nutrient solution (one of which contains adenine and mannitol, the other adenine and additional glucose). Heparinized blood is no longer available.

1. **Contents of 1 unit of whole blood** [14,21]
   a. Total volume is 510 ml; red cell volume is 210 ml, and plasma volume is 300 ml.
   b. Sodium citrate, 1.66 gm; dextrose, 1.61 gm; citric acid, 206 mg; and sodium biphosphate, 140 mg per 500 ml (total volume).
   c. Sodium, 25 mEq; potassium, 15 mEq; and plasma acid, 80 mEq.
   d. Plasma pH and plasma potassium values are as follows:

	CPD				CPD A-1			
Day:	0	7	14	21	0	7	14	21
pH:	7.20	7.00	6.90	6.87	7.35	7.25	6.95	6.90
Plasma K^+ (mEq/L):	4	10	21	27	4	9	18	25

   e. Red cell contents
      (1) Hemoglobin A (HbA) only (we exclude donors with sickle-cell trait because of the potential for extreme hypoxia in neonates)
      (2) 2,3-Diphosphoglycerate (2,3-DPG) levels (in CPD blood):

Day:	0	7	14	21
μM/gm Hb:	13.2	14.1	9.8	3.2

      Units stored at room temperature for 6 hours in order to prepare components lose 25 percent of their 2,3-DPG content. Adenine-fortified anticoagulants reduce the 2,3-DPG content by 10 percent during storage [16].
   f. Storage longer than 24 hours ablates half the coagulation factor activity; otherwise, 20 ml/kg will provide enough plasma to restore a normal prothrombin time (PT) and partial thromboplastin time (PTT) in the absence of consumption or severe liver failure.
   g. Normal immunoglobulins
   h. Fresh, nonrefrigerated whole blood (used within 4 hours) contains clotting factors, active platelets, and a functional white blood count (WBC) of 6000 to 10,000/μl [9].
2. **Production from components of a whole-blood unit** for exchange transfusion
   a. May be used when fresh blood is not available, but the clinician requests very young red cells or active plasma factors.

b. Mix packed red cells and fresh-frozen plasma (FFP).
Example: Creation of a unit with a hematocrit (Hct) of 50 percent:

$$\text{Volume of packed cells} = \frac{\text{total exchange volume} \times 0.5 \text{ (desired Hct)}}{0.7 \text{ (Hct of packed cells)}}$$

$$\text{Volume of FFP} = \text{total exchange volume} - \text{packed cell volume}$$

c. Beware of increased acid load from FFP made with the anticoagulant [acid-citrate-dextrose (ACD) plasma pH = 6.6].

d. There is no platelet activity in old or reconstituted blood.

3. Indications for the neonate

a. Exchange for neonatal hyperbilirubinemia

(1) Uncomplicated term infant—up to 5-day-old whole blood

(2) Premature or sick newborn—as fresh as possible

b. Exchange for sepsis, respiratory distress syndrome (RDS), toxic substances—as fresh as possible (<4 hours old, nonrefrigerated for sepsis to preserve white cell function) [8,9]

c. When anemia is present with **a** or **b,** one may wish to elevate the hematocrit in the unit by removing plasma. To create a whole-blood unit with a hematocrit of 50 percent:

Plasma to be removed

$$= \text{total volume of the unit} - \frac{0.4 \times \text{total volume of the unit}}{0.5}$$

d. Treatment of acute blood loss and shock. (*Note:* Whole blood is not a useful product to increase hematocrit acutely; for this purpose, use packed red cells (see Chap. 16).

4. Amount of infusion

a. Shock or blood loss. Estimate amount of blood loss and infuse at maximum rate (usually 10 to 20 ml/kg per hour), monitoring vital signs and slowing infusion when vital signs begin to improve.

b. For **exchange transfusion** see Chapter 15.

5. Preparation of product

a. Whole blood is drawn into quad or quint packs so that the unit can be split to create several red cell or whole blood infusions.

b. Group, type, direct antiglobulin test, and two-cell antibody screening are performed on the mother and baby.

c. Type-specific red cell product is used unless

(1) Type-specific product is unavailable (use type O Rh-negative)

(2) ABO incompatibility is present (use type O RH-negative)

(3) Maternal or infant direct antiglobulin test or screening is positive (e.g., Rh sensitization; use compatible blood) (see Chap. 15)

(4) Special product is available (e.g., cytomegalovirus-negative) in all blood types except AB negative.

d. Major and minor cross-matching is performed against maternal or infant serum or both [22]. Cross-matching need not be repeated up to age 4 months, provided that the patient has not had exchange transfusion or multiple plasma infusions [21]. In neonates on chronic red cell and plasma infusions, weekly screening may be performed to search for antibody development [22].

e. Blood is drawn up through a 150-μm macroaggregate filter prior to infusion [6].

B. Fresh-frozen plasma (collected in ACD, CPD, CPD A-1)

1. Contents

a. Volume: 250 ml; smaller aliquots can be aseptically prepared with an SCD (sterile connection device, Dupont).

b. Electrolyte concentration: sodium, 160 to 170 mEq/L; potassium, 3.5 to 5.5 mEq/L; pH, 6.6 to 6.75
c. Clotting factors
d. Plasma proteins, including colloid (e.q., albumin) and antibodies
e. White cells, 30 to 50/μl

2. **Indications**
a. Replacement of clotting factors (see Chap. 17)
b. Volume expansion (see Chap. 6)
c. Use of hyperimmune plasma [e.g., as adjunctive treatment of group B streptococci sepsis (experimental); do not treat patients who have only been exposed]. The specific antibody concentration of different lots of intravenous gammaglobulin can be obtained from the manufacturer (see Chap. 12).

3. **Amount of infusion**
a. To replace clotting factors, 10 ml/kg will normalize the PT and PTT if chronic consumption [e.g., bleeding, disseminated intravascular coagulation (DIC)] is not going on. Active bleeding from clotting factor deficiency may require treatment every 8 or 12 hours [12].
b. **Volume expansion.** Usually use 5 to 10 ml/kg given over at least ½ hour (see Chap. 6).

4. **Preparation of product**
a. Use type-specific product or AB-negative.
b. No cross-matching is necessary.
c. Filter through a macroaggregate (150 μm) filter.

C. **Packed red blood cells (PRBC)**

1. **Contents of 1 unit of packed red cells**
a. Volume: 300 ml; red cell volume, 210 ml, and plasma volume, 90 ml. The unit can be aseptically subdivided using a multiple pack system or a sterile connection device.
b. Sodium, 15 mEq; potassium, 4 mEq; and plasma acid, 25 mEq.
c. White cells, 6000 to 10,000/μl
d. No immunoglobulin or clotting factors

2. **Indications**
a. **Replacement of phlebotomy losses**
b. **Improvement of oxygen-carrying capacity** in patients with pulmonary or cardiac disease
c. **Chronic anemia** when there is no expectation that therapy other than transfusion would increase red cell mass before life-threatening effects of anemia (e.g., congestive heart failure) supervene

3. **Amount of infusion**
a. Volume of packed cells to be infused is determined by the following equation:

$$\text{PRBC volume to be infused} = \frac{\text{Patient's blood volume} \times (\text{hematocrit desired} - \text{hematocrit observed})}{\text{hematocrit of packed cells (usually 0.7)}}$$

In most circumstances, this volume is about 10 ml/kg.
b. In patients without congestive heart failure, maximum rate of infusion is 10 ml/kg per hour.
c. In patients with impending heart failure, do not exceed 2 ml/kg per hour. Intravenous furosemide (0.25 to 0.50 mg/h may be given during the transfusion to prevent worsening heart failure. Careful attention must be paid to vital signs under either circumstance.
d. Patients in overt heart failure or with unstable vital signs may benefit from partial exchange transfusion with packed cells to increase the hematocrit but maintain isovolemia.

4. **Special red cell products**
   a. In general, these products are used for patients in whom low WBC levels and decreased plasma protein levels in blood will be valuable. Situations of concern for neonates are the following:
      (1) Nonhemolytic transfusion reactions (see **F.2**)
      (2) Prevention of cytomegalovirus infection (see **G**) (see Chap. 12).
   b. Washed packed red cells—70 percent hematocrit in normal saline; 92 percent reduction in WBCs and significant dilution of plasma proteins
   c. Filters are now available that will remove more than 98 percent of the white cells. They do retain a 37-cc volume of packed cells or whole blood in the filter.
   d. Frozen washed red cells—volume, 200 ml; hematocrit, 70 percent; sodium, 9 mEq; potassium, 1 to 2 mEq; pH, 6.8; 98 percent reduction in WBCs and no plasma proteins; most expensive of all
5. **Preparation of product** (see **A.5**)

D. **Platelets** (see Chap. 19)
1. **Contents of 1 unit of platelets**
   a. Total volume of concentrated unit is 20 ml (platelets, 5×10^{10}; plasma volume, 6 ml; pH, 6.35 to 6.85).
   b. CPD (see **A.1b**)
   c. White cells, $10^7/\mu l$
2. **Indications for the neonate**
   a. Absolute thrombocytopenia (platelet count $< 50{,}000/\mu l$) **with bleeding.** The aim should be to raise the platelet count to approximately $100{,}000/\mu l$.
   b. Absolute thrombocytopenia **without bleeding.** The use of prophylactic platelet transfusion is controversial. Since spontaneous bleeding can occur with a platelet count less than 20 to $30{,}000/\mu l$, we currently recommend transfusion at this point. Prophylactic platelet transfusion is indicated when the platelet count is under $50{,}000/\mu l$ in sepsis, DIC, or necrotizing enterocolitis [12].
   c. Thrombocytopenia secondary to massive transfusion or exchange transfusion
3. **Amount of infusion**
   a. If no ongoing consumption, 0.1 unit/kg raises the platelet count to $30{,}000/\mu l$ if the platelet unit is less than 3 days old.
   b. Failure to achieve this increment suggests consumption (sepsis, DIC, bleeding), maternal idiopathic thrombocytopenic purpura (ITP), neonatal isoimmune thrombocytopenia, splenomegaly, or injured platelets (prolonged storage, washed processed platelets).
4. **Preparation for patient**
   a. A single donor is used to produce 1 unit of platelets. The unit is concentrated to a volume of 15 to 20 ml. In the case of neonatal isoimmune thrombocytopenia, maternal platelets are concentrated and resuspended in appropriate plasma to reduce infusion of maternal antibody-laden plasma [12]. Compatible platelets from any source may be used (see Chap. 19).
   b. Patients should be given type-specific or group O platelets in plasma compatible with the patient.
   c. Washing and resuspending platelets may slightly decrease platelet function or survival or both.
   d. Platelets are drawn up through a macroaggregate filter and **must always be given** through a peripheral **venous** line to avoid serious embolic phenomena. (*Do not use arterial lines to infuse platelets.*)
   e. Platelets should be irradiated to 1500 to 5000 rads to avoid graft-versus-host (GVH) disease [3,7,11].

E. **Granulocyte transfusion**
1. **Contents of granulocyte transfusion** depends on collection technique. Continuous-flow centrifugation (most common) yields a 450-ml unit con-

taining approximately 2×10^{10} granulocytes per unit with a hematocrit of 20 percent and the equivalent of 4 units of platelets in CPD.

2. **Indications (controversial)**—severe neutropenia (600/μl absolute neutrophil count or the criteria of Manroe [15]) without expectation of rapid bone marrow recovery and with clinical evidence of sepsis [6] (see Chap. 12)
3. **Amount of infusion**
   a. If tolerated, 10 to 15 ml/kg infusions can be administered every 12 hours [9,11]. Beware of pulmonary symptoms with granulocyte concentrates.
   b. Between 20 and 30 ml/kg may be given by partial exchange transfusion, but beware of decreasing the child's hematocrit by dilution.
   c. Whole blood (nonrefrigerated) used within 4 hours of collection can be used for a two-volume exchange transfusion. This will significantly raise the neutrophil count as well as provide platelets, clotting factors, and immunoglobulins [8,9].
4. **Preparation of product for patient**
   a. In the event that type-specific products are unavailable, a product containing type O-negative red cells and compatible plasma may be used.
   b. Major cross-matching of baby and maternal sera against red cells in granulocyte unit; minor cross-matching of donor unit plasma against baby red cells
   c. Irradiate to 2500 to 5000 rads to prevent GVH disease [13].

F. Blood product transfusion reactions

1. **Acute hemolytic transfusion reactions (rare)**
   a. Caused by incompatibility, usually of donor red cells with patient's plasma
   b. In neonates one may observe changes in vital signs and red urine only, since there will be no report of chills or back pain. Sudden fall in hematocrit, documentation of hemoglobinemia, and demonstration of incompatibility in the blood bank confirm the diagnosis.
   c. **Treatment**
      (1) Restore hematocrit with compatible red cells.
      (2) Administer volume to maintain blood pressure.
      (3) If vital signs permit, a dose of furosemide (0.5 to 1.0 mg/kg) should be given to enhance urine flow and prevent renal failure.
      (4) If shock occurs, use dopamine at a dose of 5 to 10 μg/kg per minute.
      (5) In the presence of DIC or refractory shock, fresh whole blood exchange transfusion may be attempted.
2. **Nonhemolytic transfusion reactions**
   a. Caused by allergic or nonspecific response to protein antigens or white cell fragments
   b. Clinical diagnosis depends on small changes in vital signs, loss of temperature control, wheezing, rash, and demonstration of compatibility in the blood bank.
   c. Treatment consists of prevention of future reactions by using plasma and white cell–poor products (see Chap. **4**).
3. **Ancillary effects of transfusion**
   a. Hypothermia may occur if cool blood is infused into small babies. Blood should be placed through a blood warmer for very small babies or babies with temperature control problems.
   b. Overheating of blood in warmers can lead to a syndrome of hyperthermia and the effects of heat damage to red cells (hemoglobinuria, hemoglobinemia, hyperbilirubinemia, and anemia).
   c. Rapid infusion. Rapid infusion (<30 minutes) of blood products, especially FFP, has been associated with sudden deterioration of vital signs and should be reserved for urgent situations only.

   - **d.** Hypoglycemia. Babies receiving hyperalimentation may suffer hypoglycemia during a prolonged infusion (>30 minutes) without glucose; therefore, the baby's blood glucose level should be monitored carefully. If a drop in blood sugar occurs, either the transfusion can be interrupted intermittently for glucose infusion or a separate constant glucose drip can be given simultaneously.
   - **e.** Hypocalcemia is a well-known complication, because calcium is bound by citrate in blood. For treatment see Chapter 24.

4. **Graft-versus-host disease (GVH)** [7,13,17]
   - **a.** GVH disease can occur with any cellular blood product but is proportional to the number of white cells in the product.
   - **b.** GVH disease can probably occur in any neonate (even full-term neonates) receiving granulocytes or platelets.
   - **c.** GVH disease has been reported in babies undergoing intrauterine transfusion [17].
   - **d.** There is no evidence that GVH disease occurs in any normal full-term neonate from red cell products. This is theoretically possible for high-risk premature infants, and severely ill full-term infants. Since irradiation does not have a deleterious effect on red cells, these are routinely irradiated to 2500 rads prior to transfusion.
5. **Infection** (see Chap. 12)
   - **a.** Transmission of infection is the most frequent serious complication of blood transfusion.
   - **b.** Blood bank laboratory procedures currently screen for syphilis, hepatitis B surface antigen, surrogate testing for non-A, non-B hepatitis, hepatitis C, HIV antibody (AIDS) [5], and HTLV-I antibody by direct testing. The donor medical history includes questions relating to AIDS and other transmissible viral diseases. High-risk groups are eliminated by direct questioning and a confidential donor exclusion form. Donor room standards include rejection of donors with recent minor viral or bacterial infections as well as parasitic and endemic infections (e.g., malaria). In creating a neonatal donor program, one should be particularly careful to use only volunteers with carefully taken donor histories.

G. Cytomegalovirus (CMV) is a serious potential nosocomial infection in the neonate [2,3,4,18]. The risk of CMV acquisition is proportional to the dose of white cells in blood or blood product. Different approaches may be adopted to handle the threat of this disease in babies receiving transfusion:

1. Use of white cell–poor blood products exclusively, regardless of donor
2. Identification of a CMV antibody–negative units
3. Exposure of high-risk babies to as few units as possible by using quint packs.
4. Review of our transfused neonatal population indicates that more than 90 percent are very premature or acutely ill. We therefore have found it prudent and cost-effective to provide CMV antibody–negative blood products in all instances of neonatal transfusion.

H. Testing for **hepatitis B** surface antigen and elimination of paid donors resulted in a dramatic decline in hepatitis B cases. It became evident that more than 90 percent of posttransfusion hepatitis was caused by non-A, non-B (NANB) hepatitis. In a multicenter cooperative study, NANB hepatitis developed in 12 percent of multitransfused patients (three donor exposures). Current estimates following the adoption of surrogate testing indicate that 2.5 percent of transfusion survivors develop NANB posttransfusion hepatitis [1,18,19,23]. A recent test developed to screen blood for NANB hepatitis (hepatitis C) is now in use in our blood banks. Since commencing HIV antibody testing of blood donors, the risk of transfusion-associated AIDS is estimated to be 4 cases per 1 million units transfused. Units such as ours, which exclusively transfuse CMV-negative blood to neonates, have an additional protective effect since 94 to 100 percent of AIDS patients are positive for the CMV antibody. Present estimates indicate that the possibility of acquiring AIDS by transfusion is 1 in 300,000 for units of blood not tested for CMV [5,10,20].

References

1. Aach, R. D., et al. *N. Eng. J. Med.* 204: 989, 1981.
2. Adler, S. P. *Pediatr. Infect. Dis. J.* 2: 114, 1983.
3. Adler, S. P., et al. *J. Pediatr.* 108: 117, 1986.
4. Adler, S. P., and Lawrence, L. *Transfusion* 24: 333, 1984.
5. Berkman, S. A., and Groopman, J. E. *Trans. Med. Rev.* 2: 1, 1988.
6. Butch, S. *Transfusion Techniques in Hemotherapy of the Infant and Premature.* Arlington, Va.: American Association of Blood Banks, 1983.
7. Button, L. N. *Transfusion* 21: 643, 1981.
8. Christensen, R. D. *J. Pediatr.* 98: 101, 1981.
9. Christensen, R. D. Pediatrics 70: 1, 1982.
10. Drew, W. L., et al. *J. Infect. Dis.* 143: 188, 1981.
11. Fisher, M. C. *Pediatrics* 79: 157, 1987.
12. Kevy, S. V. *The Use of Platelets, Plasma, and Plasma Derivatives in the Newborn in Hemotherapy of the Infant and Premature.* Arlington, Va.: American Association of Blood Banks, 1983.
13. Leitman, S. F. *Posttransfusion Graft-Versus-Host Disease in Special Considerations in Transfusing the Immunocomprised Patient.* Arlington, Va.: American Association of Blood Banks, 1985.
14. Mollison, P. L., Engelfriet, B. L., and Contreras, M. *Blood Transfusion in Clinical Medicine.* Oxford: Blackwell Scientific, 1987.
15. Manroe, B. J. *J. Pediatr.* 95: 89, 1979.
16. Morrof, G., et al. *Transfusion* 28: 365, 1988.
17. Parkman, R. N. *N. Eng. J. Med.* 290: 359, 1974.
18. Stevens, C. E., et al. *Ann. Intern. Med.* 101: 733, 1984.
19. Tabor, E. *Lancet* 1: 743, 1985.
20. Ward, J. W., et al. *Ann. Intern. Med.* 106: 61, 1987.
21. Widmann, F. K. (Ed.). *Technical Manual.* Arlington, Va.: American Association of Blood Banks, 1985.
22. Wolfe, L. C. *Hum. Pathol.* 14: 256, 1983.

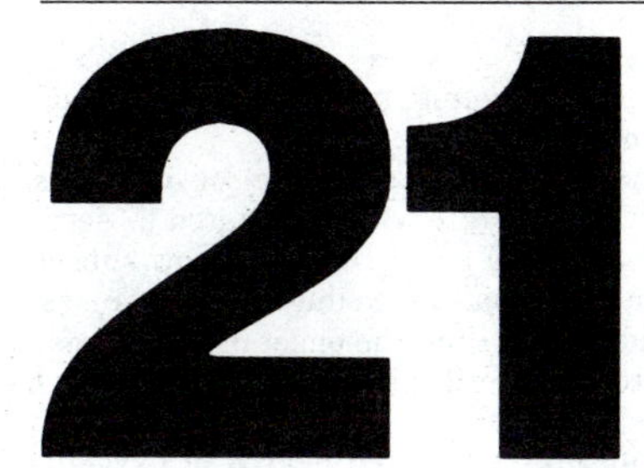

Neurology

Neonatal Seizures

Karl Kuban and James Filiano

I. **Clinical patterns.** The usual well-organized tonic-clonic seizure patterns seen in older infants are not seen in the newborn because of immaturity of the newborn brain [98]. The predominance of oral and buccal phenomena (such as chewing, lip smacking, and sucking), as well as gaze abnormalities and apnea, may relate to the advanced development of the limbic structures and their connections to the brainstem and diencephalon [98] in comparison with other forebrain structure.

A. **Seizure patterns**

1. **Focal clonic seizures.** In focal clonic seizures, the movements involve well-localized clonic jerking. These types of seizures are not associated with loss of consciousness. They are most often provoked by metabolic disturbances [80], but they may be associated with focal traumatic injury (i.e., cerebral contusion), subarachnoid hemorrhage (SAH) [98], or focal infarct [26]. The electroencephalogram (EEG) is most often unifocally abnormal. The prognosis is generally good [4].
2. **Multifocal clonic seizures.** These seizures are characterized by random clonic movements of limbs similar to those seen in normal infants under 34 weeks' gestation. The EEG most often is multifocally abnormal.
3. **Tonic seizures.** The movements are focal or generalized and may resemble decerebrate or decorticate posturing seen in older children; the movements are most often associated with eye deviation and occasionally with clonic movements or apnea. This condition is more often seen in premature babies and is most often associated with diffuse central nervous system (CNS) disease or intraventricular hemorrhage (IVH) [80]. The prognosis is mixed but is generally poor [4]. Most often, the EEG is multifocally abnormal, has a burst-suppression pattern, or has extremely attenuated amplitude [80,98]. When tonic seizures occur on the heels of an apneic or hypoxic episode, the prognosis is better.
4. **Myoclonic seizures.** Manifestations include synchronous single or multiple slow jerks of the upper or lower limbs (or both) and are associated with diffuse CNS pathology [51]; the prognosis is poor [4,51]. The EEG shows a burst-suppression pattern or focal sharp, transient waves and may evolve into hypsarrhythmia. Rapid multifocal polymyoclonus frequently is not associated with an epileptiform EEG [63].
5. **Subtle seizures** constitute 50 percent of seizures in newborns (both term and premature) and most often occur in infants who manifest other seizure types described above [24,51,98]. Subtle seizures may not be associated with an epileptiform or hypersynchronous EEG, may be subcortical in origin, and may not be ameliorated by anticonvulsant therapy [10,47,63]. Examples of subtle seizures include the following:
   a. Tonic horizontal deviation, usually with jerking of the eyes
   b. Repetitive blinking or fluttering of the eyelids

c. Oral and buccal movements—drooling, sucking, and yawning
d. Tonic posturing of a limb
e. Apnea (see Apnea in Chap. 13) due to seizure most often has either an accelerated or a normal heart rate when evaluated 20 seconds following its onset [23,100,101]; the heart rate may slow subsequently as a result of sustained hypoxemia. Apnea due to other causes is usually associated with bradycardia from the onset of the episode [102]. Apnea without associated epileptic movements is rarely the sole manifestation of seizure [84].
f. **Rhythmic fluctuations in vital signs** and degree of oxygenation in pharmacologically paralyzed infants. These observations, although suggestive, are not diagnostic of seizure, and establishment of the diagnosis requires an EEG [36].
g. Complex, purposeless movements, such as "swimming" or "bicycling" movements

B. **Jitteriness and clonus** may be associated with hypocalcemia, hypoglycemia, neonatal encephalopathy, and drug withdrawal; however, the problem is most commonly seen in infants, particularly premature infants, who have none of these problems [8,98]. Infants of diabetic mothers (IDMs) are frequently "jittery" with normal blood sugar and calcium levels. Jitteriness or clonus in infants may be confused with seizures. Characteristics of jitteriness and clonus that help to differentiate them from seizures [98,100] are as follows:
1. Absence of abnormal gaze or eye movements
2. Provocation by stimulation of the infant or by stretching a joint, in contrast to the usual spontaneous occurrence of seizures
3. Cessation of movements with passive flexion or gentle restraint [63]
4. Absence of fast and slow components characteristic of a clonic fit (tremor and clonus oscillate rhythmically)
5. Tremor and clonus have no associated EEG abnormality.
6. Repetitive jerks in seizures tend to be between 2 and 3 per second, whereas clonus tends to be faster (5 to 6 per second) [63].
7. Jitteriness and nonseizure clonus are not accompanied by increased blood pressure, bradycardia, or tachycardia.

C. **Use of EEG in diagnosis.** The EEG is an adjunct to the clinical determination of seizures. As a result of the immaturity of the CNS, ictal and interictal abnormalities can take many, often nonspecific forms. The EEG may have sharp or, more rarely, spike forms, but they also may have rhythmic activity in the delta, theta, or alpha frequency as the EEG correlate of seizures [4,49,104]. Focal and multifocal clonic seizures often, but not invariably have focal and multifocal EEG abnormalities; subtle, tonic, and myoclonic seizures usually have a greater range of EEG correlates to include most of the forms mentioned previously. There are at least two reasons that apparent clinical seizures may not be correlated with EEG discharges. First, many of the motor phenomena often thought to represent subtle seizures or complex motor patterns may reflect subcortical EEG-negative spells or behaviors that may be refractory to anticonvulsant therapy. Whether any or some of these clinical phenomena should be viewed as seizures is controversial. Second, neonates with severely damaged nervous systems may not be able to transmit electrical activity from deeper cerebral structures to the cortex, which is where surface EEG electrodes are most likely to pick up discharges. In such circumstances, the background EEG is usually blunted, flat, or shows a burst-suppression pattern. Conversely, epileptiform discharges seen on the EEG tracings do not necessarily guarantee the presence of clinical seizures. Nonetheless, we would advocate treating paralyzed neonates who have epileptiform discharges. In nonparalyzed babies, treatment should be administered to babies with clonic seizures. Although one cannot be certain that tonic, myoclonic, or subtle events are epileptic, if they occur in the absence of an acute metabolic disturbance, are associated with an epileptiform EEG, or interfere with the care of the neonate, we would advocate a trial of anticonvulsant treatment. A normal interictal EEG does not rule out seizures [30,50].

II. Etiology of seizures

A. Perinatal complications include neonatal encephalopathy, cerebral contusion, and intracranial hemorrhage (ICH). **Neonatal encephalopathy** is a term used to designate cerebral dysfunction in the neonate, including seizures, when the etiology is not known. We specifically avoid the term **hypoxic-ischemic encephalopathy** unless there is very clear and direct evidence of prenatal ischemia or postnatal hypoxia and/or ischemia. Hypoxic-ischemic encephalopathy should never be a diagnosis of exclusion. Furthermore, even clear or direct evidence of compromised oxygen delivery to the fetus or the neonate does not preclude the presence of an underlying neurologic disorder that may have predisposed the fetus or neonate to the subsequent hypoxic or ischemic disturbance. Criteria traditionally used to identify past hypoxic-ischemic events, including abnormal fetal heart rate patterns, low Apgar scores, jitteriness, lethargy, and seizures, simply are not specific for hypoxic-ischemic events. In fact, hypoxic-ischemic events are an infrequent cause of any of these signs, and the vast majority of babies with these signs do not have long-term repercussions [29,68,69,70,95]. Continued presumptive use of the term **hypoxic-ischemic encephalopathy** impedes further search for other or underlying etiologies and tends to implicate the perinatal period as the time frame for the insult with little or no firm substantiation. Neonatal encephalopathy, cerebral contusion, and intracranial hemorrhage account for greater than 40 percent of all neonatal seizures and a larger proportion in premature babies.

1. **Neonatal encephalopathy** includes babies with severe fetal distress who are apneic at birth and accounts for 24 to 40 percent of neonatal seizures [49,98]. Seizures usually occur on the first day of life, most often beginning in the first 12 hours [98].
   a. **Ictal manifestations** of neonatal encephalopathy include subtle seizures, tonic seizures, and multifocal seizures [50]. Seizures occur in 8 percent of infants with well-defined asphyxia [27,28]. Metabolic disorders that may be associated include hypoglycemia, hypocalcemia, inappropriate secretion of antidiuretic hormone (ADH) with hyponatremia, and diabetes insipidus [41,42,51,98].
   b. Early seizures associated with clear hypoxic or ischemic events are often difficult to control. Infants who require multiple medications have high morbidity and mortality [28,50,98] (see Perinatal Asphyxia, p. 393).
2. **ICH and CNS trauma** may result from breech delivery or difficult forceps extraction. Trauma in these circumstances may cause cerebral contusion or hemorrhage, subdural hematomas, or subarachnoid bleeding and may be manifest by focal seizures and lateralized neurologic signs often occurring after the first day of life. ICH is usually associated with prematurity and signs of neonatal encephalopathy (see Intracranial Hemorrhage below and Chap. 23).
   a. **Primary subarachnoid hemorrhage (SAH)** occurs in infants subjected to trauma but may occur without apparent trauma. It occurs more often in premature than in term infants. The majority of infants with SAH are asymptomatic. When seizures occur, however, they usually do so on the second day. The baby appears well between seizures, and 90 percent develop normally [24,51,80,98].
   b. **Periventricular hemorrhage (PVH)** usually occurs in premature infants. This problem is likely to occur within 3 days of birth and may present with tonic seizures [50]. The seizures may be associated with rapid deterioration, respiratory arrest, and death. Most babies with PVH do not have seizures.
   c. **Subdural hemorrhage (SDH)** results from a tear of the falx, tento-

rium, or superficial cortical veins. It is most likely to occur in large babies and in breech deliveries [12,46]. The seizures are associated with cerebral contusion or hemorrhage and may have focal features. The seizures occur on the first days of life [12,46]. When considering this diagnosis, one should consider bleeding below the tentorium, which may not be seen on ultrasound [5] and which may cause sudden, acute brainstem dysfunction.

d. **Choroid plexus hemorrhage** occurs in full-term infants and its triggers are unknown.

B. **Metabolic problems.** These seizures usually present as focal or multifocal clonic seizures (see Chap. 24).

1. **Hypoglycemia** is defined as a blood glucose level of less than 30 mg/dl (see Hypoglycemia and Hyperglycemia in Chap. 24). Most often, it occurs in IDMs, babies who are small for gestational age (SGA), premature babies, and infants in whom asphyxia or other stress occurs. Hypoglycemia is often associated with or is a complication of other causes of seizures, such as sepsis and meningitis. Neonatal hypoglycemia also occurs in hereditary fructose intolerance [31], Beckwith-Wiedemann syndrome, congenital glucagon deficiency, maternal oral hypoglycemic agent ingestion, the glycogenoses, and other metabolic disorders. Symptoms of hypoglycemia include hypotonia, apnea, stupor, jitteriness, and seizures [43]. Seizures occur in the minority of babies with hypoglycemia [43]. When they do occur, however, they usually imply longstanding hypoglycemia, and as a result, such infants often have poor outcome [43, 98].
2. **Hypocalcemia** [24] is defined as a calcium level less than 7 mg/dl with an albumin level of greater than 3.5 gm/dl (see Hypocalcemia, Hypercalcemia, and Hypermagnesemia in Chap. 24).
   a. Early hypocalcemia occurs in babies who are premature, babies in whom asphyxia or trauma has occurred, infants of mothers with hyperparathyroidism, and IDMs [24,98]. Hypocalcemia is often accompanied by other causes of seizures, such as hypoglycemia, and may occur as part of neonatal encephalopathy. As a result, treatment with calcium may not stop the seizures [51,98]. Prognosis reflects the prognosis of the underlying problem.
   b. Late hypocalcemia results from ingestion of formula with a suboptimal ratio of calcium to phosphorus, from abnormalities in vitamin D metabolism, or from renal disease. Symptoms include clonus, jitteriness, and hyperactive deep tendon reflexes. Seizures occur after the first week of life, are usually focal with a focally abnormal EEG, and respond to treatment with calcium [15,50,97]. The prognosis for normal outcome is excellent.
3. **Hypomagnesemia** is defined as a magnesium level of less than 1.2 mg/dl (see Hypocalcemia, Hypercalcemia, and Hypermagnesemia in Chap. 24); it is most often associated with hypocalcemia, but it may occur in isolation [15].
4. **Hyponatremia** may result from inappropriate ADH secretion, excessive renal salt loss, or excessive administration of hyponatremic fluids.
5. **Hypernatremia** may be caused by dehydration, renal disease, or diabetes insipidus [41], or it may be iatrogenic (see Fluid and Electrolyte Management in Chap. 24).
6. **Pyridoxine dependency** [52,74]
7. **Disorders of amino acid metabolism** may cause seizures after the second day of life (see Inborn Errors of Metabolism in Chap. 24). Diagnosis is made by serum, urine, and CSF amino acid determinations. Acidosis with an elevated anion gap is common. Dietary and metabolic interventions may be helpful for many of these disorders (e.g., "maple syrup" urine disease, isovaleric acidemia, urea cycle disorders, methylmalonic acidemia, proprionic acidemia, congenital lactic acidosis, and biotin responsive dis-

orders), and therefore, appropriate consultation is indicated. The more common disorders associated with seizures include the following:

a. **"Maple syrup" urine disease** [24]. Seizures occur after institution of feeding and are associated with alteration of consciousness, poor feeding, and hypotonia occasionally alternating with opisthotonus or decerebration.

b. **Phenylketonuria** [29] is more likely to occur in the third or fourth week of life or later.

c. **Hyperglycinemia** [56,86] occurs in ketotic and nonketotic forms.

d. **Isovaleric acidemia** presents with vomiting, anion gap acidosis, tremor, convulsions, coma, and a cheesy odor. Death occurs a few weeks after birth in half the patients.

e. **Urea cycle disorders** [24] are usually associated with hyperammonemia.

f. **Beta-alanine abnormalities** [73,88]. This class of disorders is composed of two related disorders: hyperbetaalaninemia and carnosinemia. They present with severe seizures early in neonatal life and have progressive neurologic deterioration. Diagnosis is made by the presence of elevated serum levels of either beta-alanine or carnosine. Beta-aminoaciduria and gamma-aminobutyric aciduria may be present in hyperbetaalaninemia.

8. **Organic acidemias.** Both methylmalonic acidemia and proprionic acidemia usually present with vomiting and stupor and are associated with acidosis, an elevated anion gap, hyperammonemia, and ketotic hyperglycinemia [2,99,105]. Diagnosis is made by urine and serum organic acid screen.

   a. **Methylmalonic acidemia** [2,99]. Some infants are vitamin B_{12} responsive.

   b. **Propionic acidemia** [99]. Biotinidase deficiency may be associated with multiple carboxylase deficiency.

   c. **Congenital lactic acidosis** is caused by a number of inborn errors of metabolism, some of which respond to dietary therapy or pharmacologic dosages of thiamine [1].

   d. **Glutaric aciduria type II** [77]. Hypoglycemia, hyperammonemia, a sweaty-feet odor, anemia, seizures, and death within 90 hours of life are common.

9. **Biotin-responsive disorders.** These disorders include deficiencies in either biotinidase, holocarboxylase synthetase, or the multiple carboxylase complex. Metabolic acidosis, alopecia totalis, scaly eruption, hypotonia, an odor of cat urine, and elevated glycine and organic acid levels are common but not universal features. Diagnosis is made by blood or cultured fibroblast assay of the enzymes. Patients with these disorders are usually very responsive to pharmacy-grade biotin 10 mg PO qd [16].

10. **Fructose intolerance.** Seizures and other symptoms occur only if fructose-containing foods are ingested [31,47].

11. **Peroxisomal disorders** [64,67] are a heterogeneous collection of disorders that includes Zellweger's cerebrohepatorenal syndrome and neonatal adrenoleukodystrophy. Diagnosis is made by elevations of one or more of the following serum metabolites: very long chain fatty acids, plasmalogens, phytanic acid, and pipecolic acid. X-linked dominant and recessive forms have been identified. Babies with Zellweger's disease frequently have prepatellar calcifications on x-ray.

12. **Mitochondrial disorders** are another heterogeneous collection of encephalopathies with multiorgan involvement caused by a variety of enzyme deficiencies involved in pyruvate metabolism and electron transport–respiratory chain metabolism. Some forms of Leigh's disease (subacute necrotizing encephalomyelopathy) [1,50] and Alper's disease may be so induced. Pyruvate, lactate, and alanine levels may be elevated in the serum and/or CSF.

13. **Storage diseases**—G_m1 and G_m3 gangliosidoses [24,50]
14. **Menkes' kinky hair disease** [1,19,35,60]. Menkes' disease in the newborn is characterized by seizures, pili torti (kinky hair), connective-tissue defects, and hypothermia. Diagnosis is made by demonstration of decreased serum levels of copper and ceruloplasmin and the characteristic gross and microscopic appearance of the hair. This is an X-linked disorder of cellular copper distribution that is not improved by copper supplementation. In the neonate, the hair may not appear kinky, although, if present, it has the characteristic sandy brown color.

C. **Infections may lead to seizures at any time** (see Chap. 12) and include [80,98] the following:
1. **Bacterial meningitis**, including brain abscess [79]
2. **Viral infections** (coxsackie and echovirus, rubella, cytomegalovirus, and herpesvirus). Sometimes, a characteristic EEG pattern may be present during herpes encephalitis [62].
3. **Toxoplasmosis**
4. **Syphilis**
5. Seizures in the neonate caused directly by the human immunodeficiency virus, without opportunistic infection, has not been established.

D. **Developmental problems**
1. **Cerebral dysgenesis** [49,80,98]. The absence of obvious morphologic disturbances on CT scan, head ultrasound, or MRI scan does not rule out microscopic forms of cerebral dysgenesis (heterotopias, neuronal disorganization, etc.).
2. The **phakomatoses** include Sturge-Weber anomaly, neurofibromatosis, tuberous sclerosis, incontinentia pigmenti, and the organoid nevus syndrome [14,24,50,98] (see Chap. 29).

E. **Drug-associated seizures**
1. Narcotic and sedative withdrawals are characterized by jitteriness, irritability, autonomic instability, and occasionally, seizures (see Chap. 2). Seizures occur within 2 days with heroin withdrawal but may be delayed for 1 to 2 weeks with methadone or barbiturate withdrawal. Methadone withdrawal will lead to seizures six times more often than heroin withdrawal [24,38,98]. Seizures and tremor have been associated with direct effects of cocaine and methamphetamine intoxication and cocaine withdrawal. Infarcts can be associated with maternal cocaine use in pregnancy [11,13,71].
2. **Inadvertent administration of local anesthetic** into the fetal circulation either directly by scalp injection or indirectly by transplacental transmission during labor and delivery can lead to seizures that are usually tonic. The clinical picture includes hypotonia, bradycardia, fixed and dilated pupils, and complete external ophthalmoplegia [91]. Such babies have an excellent prognosis if properly diagnosed and managed.
3. **Theophylline** at toxic blood levels can lead to seizures [32].
4. **Propylene glycol**, a diluent in IV nutrition formulations and several medications, has been associated with seizures and other disorders in premature infants [53].

F. **Polycythemia/hyperviscosity** (see Chap. 18). Lethargy and hypotonia are more common signs of this condition, although seizures can occur. Hypoglycemia is a possible complication as well.

G. **Focal infarcts** from arterial or venous occlusion [26,106]. These events may be provoked by deficiency in protein C or S, thrombocytosis, polycythemia, maternal lupus, maternal cocaine use, cardiac anomalies (including myomata seen in tuberous sclerosis), and paradoxical emboli. Most focal infarcts have no recognized antecedents and are presumed to be emboli seeded from the placenta.

H. **Familial neonatal seizures** occur as an autosomal-dominant inherited trait. These seizures occur late in the first week of life and generally do not continue after the perinatal period [78,96].

- **I. Hypertensive encephalopathy** was associated with seizures in one newborn with coarctation of the aorta [54].
- **J. Unknown causes** are involved in 3 to 25 percent of cases [4,8,24,30,75,98].

III. Treatment. Recurrent or continuous seizures may cause biochemical or physiologic effects that may lead to brain injury [58,59,84,99,100,101].

- **A.** Optimize ventilation, cardiac output, blood pressure, serum electrolytes, and pH.
- **B.** The underlying disease should be treated. Certain specific causes of seizures such as narcotic withdrawal (see Chap. 2), metabolic abnormalities (see Chap. 24), and meningitis (see Chap. 12) need specific therapy. Diuresis and, occasionally, gastric lavage are required to remove inadvertently administered local anesthetic from symptomatic infants [39]. Most of the therapy of neonatal seizures is symptomatic. To date, there is no evidence to confirm that high-dose phenobarbital is a useful therapy for the nonepileptic aspects of neonatal encephalopathy.
- **C. Intravenous therapy.** A reliable intravenous line should be established, using an umbilical vein if necessary.
- **D. Glucose** given prior to induced seizures in experimental animals appears to reduce mortality and brain damage; it also prevents the secondary fall in the blood glucose level seen in status epilepticus [101]. Excessive glucose, however, promotes accumulation of cerebral lactic acid, which also may be damaging to the brain [62,65,66]. Thus we advocate maintenance of the serum glucose level within physiologic bounds (70 to 120 mg/dl).
  1. If rapid screen with Dextrostix shows low blood glucose levels, this should be corrected, even if it is not the primary cause of the seizures. The patient is given 2 to 4 ml/kg of dextrose 25% in water (25% D/W) (0.5 to 1.0 gm/kg) over 3 minutes. The glucose dosage should be tapered slowly. Intravenous glucose is given at a rate of 0.25 to 0.50 gm/kg per hour to keep the blood serum level normal (70 to 120 mg/dl). For example, 10% D/W given at 100 ml/kg per day is equal to 0.4 gm/kg per hour (see Chap. 24).
  2. If the glucose levels remain low, treatment with glucagon or hydrocortisone should be considered even if signs are not present (see Chap. 24).
- **E. Pyridoxine dependency** is diagnosed by giving pyridoxine 50 mg IV as a therapeutic trial (under EEG control, if possible) [51,80,87,98]. Cessation of seizures will occur within minutes if pyridoxine dependency or deficiency is the cause of seizures. Maintenance therapy in dependency calls for a dose of 10 to 100 mg of pyridoxine PO qd. In deficiency, the dose is 5 mg PO qd, and the EEG does not always normalize immediately on cessation of seizures during pyridoxine infusion [74]. Rarely, pyridoxine therapy has been associated with hypotonia and apnea [45].
- **F. Anticonvulsants.** If hypoglycemia or metabolic problems are not the evident cause of seizures, anticonvulsant medications should be administered.
  1. **Phenobarbital**
     - **a. Ongoing seizures (acute administration).** Phenobarbital 15 to 20 mg/kg is given intravenously over several minutes in the presence of seizures [48,72]. If the seizures continue after 60 minutes, a second dose of phenobarbital (10 mg/kg) may be given, usually concomitantly with loading dosages of phenytoin [22] (see **2**). With continued seizures, another 10 mg/kg dose of IV phenobarbital may be administered 2 to 4 hours later, given over 15 minutes [22]. The maximum total phenobarbital loading dose is 30 to 40 mg/kg (serum values of 30 to 45 μg/ml). If phenobarbital is unsuccessful in controlling seizures, phenytoin should be administered (see **2**). Cumulative loading doses greater than 20 mg/kg of phenobarbital require careful monitoring of blood pressure and respiratory status for the possible development of hypotension and, more rarely, apnea. Hypotension, usually due to peripheral vasodilation, but occasionally due to myocardial depression in neonates with diseased hearts, may be treated with volume expansion. Rarely, dopamine may be necessary (see Chap. 6). Apnea occurs

frequently after serial intravenous administration of a benzodiazepine and phenobarbital.

b. **Interictal (acute administration).** If an infant had a seizure but is not currently having seizures, the administration of 15 to 20 mg/kg of phenobarbital given intravenously will lead to therapeutic plasma levels [48,72].

c. **Maintenance doses** range from 3.5 to 4.5 mg/kg per day of phenobarbital, given as a single dose or divided in two doses given q12h IV or PO. Serum phenobarbital levels tend to rise during the first 1 to 2 weeks with doses of 5 to 6 mg/kg per day [48,72,75]. Phenobarbital half-life diminishes subsequently [72].

d. Therapeutic plasma levels range from 15 to 45 μg/ml, measured at least 1 hour after an IV dose or 2 to 4 hours after a PO dose. The goal is to maintain the lowest therapeutic level that controls seizures; this level is usually in the range of 15 to 30 μg/ml. Phenobarbital can cause sedation and hypotonia in neonates. One study suggests that phenobarbital increases theophylline requirement in premature infants with apnea [107].

2. **Phenytoin (Dilantin)** 15 to 25 mg/kg is given intravenously, administered in normal saline at a rate not greater than 1 mg/kg per minute [72,103]. Phenytoin is generally given if there has been no response to phenobarbital or if there is a critical need to monitor the level of consciousness. A maintenance dose of 4 to 8 mg/kg per day, divided into two or three doses, can be given intravenously [7,72,103]. The therapeutic plasma level is 10 to 20 μg/ml, taken at least 1 hour after IV administration. Phenytoin is poorly absorbed from the gastrointestinal tract and/or the half-life is very short when administered in the newborn period [72].

3. **Diazepam (Valium)** is used only when immediate cessation of seizures is required (e.g., when seizures interfere with vital functions). Although diazepam has a rapid therapeutic onset, redistribution pharmacodynamics result in an anticonvulsant half-life measured in minutes [98]. Its sedative-effect half-life, in contrast, exceeds 24 hours.

   a. If diazepam is required, it should be administered after dilution of 0.2 ml (1 mg) of diazepam with 0.8 ml of normal saline [24,50,92]. Titration of dosage is otherwise difficult.

   b. The initial dose should be 0.1 to 0.3 mg/kg given slowly, IV, until the seizure stops.

   c. Diazepam acts synergistically with phenobarbital to increase the risk of provoking respiratory arrest [76,98]. Appropriate facilities for circulatory and ventilatory support should be available.

   d. Diazepam contains sodium benzoate, which may interfere with bilirubin binding to albumin [24,85,98].

4. **Lorazepam (Ativan)** is an effective anticonvulsant when administered acutely. However, experience with lorazepam is limited. Its anticonvulsant effect lasts longer than that of diazepam. The current recommended dose is 0.05 mg/kg per dose IV over 2 to 5 minutes [21]. The dose may be repeated. Complications are the same as with diazepam.

5. **Paraldehyde** is used as an adjunct only after maximum therapeutic levels of phenobarbital and phenytoin are attained and seizures are not controlled.

   a. It may be given rectally, 0.1 to 0.3 ml/kg diluted in a ratio of 1:1 or 2:1 with mineral oil [22,24,97]. It should be given no more frequently than three times daily.

   b. Excretion is predominantly hepatic, but 7 to 18 percent is excreted by the lung [22,34]. One of the important toxic effects provoked by paraldehyde is pulmonary hemorrhage [22].

   c. Paraldehyde also can provoke mucosal slough and circulatory collapse, particularly when old paraldehyde is used [6,22,24,90].

d. Intravenous paraldehyde can be used but is corrosive to blood vessels and is more apt to provoke circulatory instability. Some plastic bottles and tubing are dissolved by old paraldehyde [6,22,24,90]. Paraldehyde can be administered in burettes and tubing made of polyethylene or polypropylene but not polyvinyl. When used to terminate status epilepticus, the drug should be diluted into a 5% solution that is mixed with dextrose 5%. This solution is given at the rate of 50 to 150 mg/kg per hour. Paraldehyde may be tapered after cessation of seizures. Continuous infusion of paraldehyde should not be continued beyond 3 hours [34]. Therapeutic levels are 10 to 16 mg/dl [44, 47].

6. Other anticonvulsants with which there is limited experience in the newborn period include primidone (Mysoline), carbamazepine (5 to 10 mg/kg PO bid), pentobarbital, and rectal administration of valproic acid [3,27, 33,98].

7. Adequacy of therapy may be difficult to judge. Electrical seizures may be seen despite absence of clinical seizures. We attempt to stop all clinical evidence of seizures, including blood pressure and heart rate changes, in infants who are paralyzed. We use phenobarbital to attain levels of 40 μg/ml if necessary. Other drugs are used as indicated if clinical seizures continue. Do not attempt to stop all electrical epileptiform activity because of the side effects of doses required to do this [100].

G. Follow-up anticonvulsant medications. If possible, all medications except maintenance phenobarbital at 3.5 to 5 mg/kg per day should be discontinued before the infant is discharged [98]. The other medications, except phenobarbital, are often stopped when intravenous therapy is stopped. A normal examination, absence of recurrent seizures, and a nonepileptiform EEG are indications for discontinuation of all anticonvulsants. Occasionally, this may be done prior to discharge; more often, however, anticonvulsants are continued for the first 2 months of life [61,94,98]. Decisions to treat longer are based on the risk of recurrence of seizures. Factors entering into this risk are the original cause of the seizure, the neurologic examination, and the EEG [98,100]. Infants whose seizures were caused by a **transient metabolic disturbance** have little risk of recurrent seizures, infants whose seizures were caused by **hypoxic-ischemic encephalopathy** have a 30 to 50 percent risk of recurrent seizures, and infants whose seizures were caused by **malformations of the cerebral cortex** have a high incidence of recurrent seizures.

H. Other medications

1. Calcium. If hypocalcemia is the cause of the seizure, calcium gluconate 10%, 2 ml/kg (18 mg of elemental calcium per kilogram) mixed with an equal volume of water, is given intravenously over 3 minutes. The patient's condition is checked during the administration using an electrocardiogram (ECG) or cardiac monitor [15,51,98] (see Hypocalcemia, Hypercalcemia, and Hypermagnesemia in Chap. 24).

a. Calcium should not be mixed with sodium bicarbonate.

b. If the infusion is too rapid, bradycardia can result.

c. Calcium should not be given through the umbilical vein unless the catheter tip is in the inferior vena cava.

d. The peripheral veins should be observed directly when calcium is being rapidly infused to avoid tissue necrosis caused by extravasation.

e. If hypocalcemia is the cause of the seizures, they will stop immediately after the calcium level in the blood is returned to normal; maintenance calcium should be given (see Hypocalcemia, Hypercalcemia, and Hypermagnesemia in Chap. 24).

f. When the hypocalcemia is a secondary cause of seizures (as is most common), or when there is concurrent untreated hypomagnesemia, the seizures may continue after calcium administration.

2. **Magnesium.** Hypomagnesemia is treated with magnesium sulfate 50%, 0.2 ml/kg. Half of all hypocalcemic infants also have hypomagnesemia; failure to treat hypomagnesemia may cause a lack of clinical response to administration of calcium for hypocalcemia [15,51,98] (see Chap. 24).

IV. **Prognosis.** At the present time, the overall prognosis in neonatal seizures is **death in 15 percent, neurologic sequelae** such as mental retardation, motor deficits, and seizures **in 30 percent** of survivors, and **normal outcome in 56 percent** of survivors. Fifteen to 20 percent of survivors will develop a chronic seizure disorder [98]. In the individual case, prognosis is estimated by the level of maturity, underlying etiology of the seizures, EEG, neurologic examination, and imaging studies of the brain (ultrasound, CT, MRI, etc.).

A. **Prognosis by maturity.** Newborns with seizures have a prognosis that is related to maturity regardless of etiology or other clinical factors. Older literature generally has combined outcome data of full-term and premature neonates. Recent reports, however, have considered these two groups separately [4,17,24,47,81,89]. In one study, seizures developed in 22.7 percent of infants

Table 21-1. Prognosis of seizures by etiology*

Etiology	Normal outcome (percent)
Subarachnoid hemorrhage	90
Uncertain	75
Early hypocalcemia	50
Late hypocalcemia	100
Hypoglycemia	33–71
Neonatal encephalopathy	31–50
Intraventricular hemorrhage	10
Meningitis	11–65
Dysgenesis	0

*This means prognosis for the etiology when **seizures** are a manifestation of the etiology [4,20,57,98].
Sources: Data from I. Bergman et al., Outcome in neonates with convulsions treated in an intensive care unit. *Ann. Neurol.* 14: 642, 1983; J. Dennis, Neonatal convulsions: Aetiology, late neonatal status and long-term outcome. *Dev. Med. Child Neurol.* 20: 143, 1978; T. K. McInerny and W. K. Schubert, Prognosis of neonatal seizures. *Am. J. Dis. Child.* 117: 261, 1969; and J. J. Volpe, Neonatal Seizures. In *Neurology of the Newborn.* Philadelphia: Saunders, 1987, pp. 129–158.

Table 21-2. Prognosis of seizures by seizure pattern: Normal outcome (percent) by gestational age at birth

Seizure pattern	Full-term (percent)	Premature (percent)
Focal clonic	100*	33
Multifocal	33	33
Generalized	59	41
Tonic	50	36
Myoclonic	0	0
Subtle	57	44

*Probably not normal in cases of neonatal stroke [26,83,93].
Source: Data from I. Bergman et al., Outcome in neonates with convulsions treated in an intensive care unit. *Ann. Neurol.* 14: 542, 1983.

Table 21-3. Prognosis of seizures by ictal and interictal electroencephalogram patterns

Pattern	Normal (percent)*,†	Normal (percent)‡,§		
		≤ 31 weeks	32–36 weeks	≥ 37 weeks
Ictal				
Normal background (focal discharge)	57			
Abnormal background (multifocal discharge)	24			
Alpha, beta, theta, or delta discharge	20	38	67	83
Repeated sharp waves (abnormal background)	21			
No discharge	0			
Interictal				
Normal	89	20	50	77
Unifocal discharge		33		80
Multifocal discharge		52	41	62
Flat	0			
Low amplitude	11			
Burst suppression	8	17	33	18
Focal status				0
Generalized status				
Persistent dysmaturity for age	33			

*Data from J. Dennis, Neonatal convulsions: Aetiology, late neonatal status and long-term outcome. *Dev. Med. Child Neurol.* 20: 143, 1978.
†Premature and full-term infants were grouped together in this study.
‡Data from I. Bergman et al., Outcome in neonates with convulsions treated in an intensive care unit. *Ann. Neurol.* 14: 642, 1983.
§Infants in this study were grouped together according to gestational age.

with a gestational age of 31 weeks or less, in 1.6 percent of infants between 32 and 36 weeks' gestation, and in 0.16 percent of infants born at 37 weeks' gestation or more [4]. Neonatal mortality associated with seizures was 84 percent in infants with a gestational age of 31 weeks or less, 57 percent in infants between 32 and 36 weeks' gestation, and 17 percent in infants with a gestational age of 37 weeks or more [4]. Other studies show the same relationship among seizures, mortality associated with seizures, and gestational age [89].

B. **Prognosis by etiology.** Seizures represent signs and not a disease state [49]. Outcome, in general, reflects the seriousness of the disorder that provokes the seizures [4,20,43,57,83,84,89,98] (Table 21-1).

C. **Prognosis by seizure pattern** [4]. Certain patterns are associated with poor prognosis. This is summarized in Table 21-2.

D. **Prognosis by EEG.** Both ictal and interictal EEG patterns have prognostic value. Table 21-3 reviews outcome data by EEG pattern. Prognostication on the basis of either clinical or EEG findings should generally be made from assessments performed 5 to 10 days after the initial evaluation [46,82]. Abnormalities of background rhythm are more strongly associated with future clinical outcome than an epileptiform, maturationally delayed, or asymmetrical EEG [81]. A **normal background EEG** is associated with **under 10 percent** incidence of neurologic sequelae; **severe background abnormalities** such as burst-suppression pattern, electrical silence, or marked voltage suppression are associated with a **90 percent incidence** of neurologic sequelae; and **moderate background abnormalities** such as immaturity and voltage asymmetries are associated with a **50 percent incidence** of neurologic sequelae [50,51,81,98]. Caution must be used in predicting a bad prognosis in infants under 33 weeks' gestation who have a burst-suppression pattern on EEG because of the sometimes normal finding of this pattern in small premature infants [98]. High levels of phenobarbital and other anticonvulsant medications may cause abnormalities in the EEG background.

E. **Other prognostic features.** Results of the National Collaborative Perinatal Project found that in neonatal seizures, death, mental retardation, cerebral palsy, or epilepsy is related to the following factors [40]: (1) Apgar scores of less than or equal to 6 at 5 minutes, (2) the need for 5 minutes of positive-pressure ventilation following birth, (3) early onset of seizures, (4) seizures lasting longer than 30 minutes, (5) hypotonia at 5 minutes following birth, (6) 3 or more days with uncontrolled seizures, and (7) the presence of tonic or myoclonic seizures. Nonetheless, when evaluated at 7 years of age, 70 percent of surviving neonates with seizures had normal outcome [68,69,70,95]. Other reports suggest that 20 to 30 percent of neonates with seizures will develop epilepsy [83]. Bergman et al. [4] confirmed the prognostic importance of the duration of seizures and the presence of tonic seizure patterns. They were not able, however, to support the importance of low Apgar scores to development of early seizures. They further noted that poor outcome was associated with the need for more than one anticonvulsant, an observation also reported by Finer et al. [27]. Most studies, unfortunately, have limited long-term follow-up [83].

References

1. Adams, R. D., and Lyon, G. Early Infantile Progressive Metabolic Encephalopathies. In *Neurology of Hereditary Metabolic Diseases of Children.* New York: Hemisphere, 1982. Pp. 37–108.
2. Ampola, M. G. *N. Engl. J. Med.* 293: 313, 1975.
3. Andre, M. *J. Clin. Pharmacol.* 30: 585, 1986.
4. Bergman, I. *Ann. Neurol.* 14: 542, 1983.
5. Blank, N. K. *Arch. Neurol.* 35: 106, 1978.

6. Bostrom, B. *Am. J. Dis. Child.* 136: 414, 1982.
7. Bourgeois, B. F. D. *Neurology* 33: 173, 1983.
8. Brown, J. K. *Dev. Med. Child Neurol.* 15: 823, 1973.
9. Calciolari, G. *Clin. Pediatr.* 27: 119, 1988.
10. Camfield, P. R. *J. Child Neurol.* 2: 244, 1987.
11. Chaney, N. E. *J. Pediatr.* 112: 133, 1988.
12. Chaplin, E. R. *Pediatrics* 63: 812, 1979.
13. Chasnoff, I. J. *J. Pediatr.* 108: 456, 1986.
14. Clancy, R. R. *Arch. Neurol.* 42: 236, 1985.
15. Cockburn, F. *Arch. Dis. Child.* 48: 99, 1973.
16. Committee on Genetics, American Academy of Pediatrics. *Pediatrics* 83: 449, 1989.
17. Connell, J. *Arch. Dis. Child.* 64: 452, 1989.
18. Connell, J. *Arch. Dis. Child.* 64: 459, 1989.
19. Daish, P. *Arch. Dis. Child.* 53: 956, 1978.
20. Dennis, J. *Dev. Med. Child Neurol.* 20: 143, 1978.
21. Deshmukh, A. *Am. J. Dis. Child.* 140: 1042, 1986.
22. Dodson, W. E. *J. Pediatr.* 89: 527, 1976.
23. Fenichel, G. M. *Ann. Neurol.* 7: 577, 1980.
24. Fenichel, G. M. Convulsions. In *Neonatal Neurology.* New York: Churchill-Livingstone, 1980. Pp. 20–44.
25. Fenichel, G. M. *Yale J. Biol. Med.* 60: 139, 1987.
26. Filipek, P. A. *Pediatr. Neurol.* 3: 141, 1987.
27. Finer, N. N. *Am. J. Dis. Child.* 137: 21, 1983.
28. Finer, N. N. *J. Pediatr.* 98: 112, 1981.
29. Freeman, J. M. Neonatal Seizures. In K. F. Swaiman and F. S. Wright (Eds.), *The Practice of Pediatric Neurology,* 2d Ed. St. Louis: Mosby, 1982. Pp. 1064–1077.
30. Freeman, J. M. *J. Pediatr.* 77: 701, 1970.
31. Froesch, E. R. Essential Fructosuria. In J. B. Stanbury (Ed.), *Metabolic Basis of Inherited Disease,* 4th Ed. New York: McGraw-Hill, 1978.
32. Gal, P. *Pediatrics* 65: 547, 1980.
33. Gal, P. *Neurology* 38: 467, 1988.
34. Giacoia, F. P. *Pediatrics* 104: 291, 1984.
35. Goka, T. *Monogr. Hum. Genet.* 10: 148, 1978.
36. Goldberg, R. N. *Pediatrics* 69: 583, 1982.
37. Gross, G. J. *J. Pediatr.* 82: 1004, 1973.
38. Herzlinger, R. A. *J. Pediatr.* 91: 638, 1977.
39. Hillman, L. S. *J. Pediatr.* 95: 472, 1979.
40. Holden, K. R. *Pediatrics* 70: 165, 1982.
41. Kaplan, S. L. *J. Pediatr.* 92: 431, 1978.
42. Khare, S. K. *J. Pediatr.* 90: 628, 1977.
43. Koivisto, M. *Dev. Med. Child Neurol.* 14: 603, 1972.
44. Koren, G. *Neurology* 36: 108, 1986.
45. Kroll, J. S. *Dev. Med. Child Neurol.* 27: 377, 1985.
46. Leblanc, R. J. *Neurosurgery* 53: 642, 1980.
47. Legido, A. *Pediatr. Neurol.* 4: 79, 1988.
48. Lockman, L. A. *Neurology* 29: 1445, 1979.
49. Lombroso, C. T. *Adv. Neurol.* 34: 101, 1983.
50. Lombroso, C. T. Seizures in Newborns, Epilepsy and Electroencephalography Course Syllabus. Harvard Medical School, March 1983.
51. Lombroso, C. T. Seizures in the Newborn Period. In P. J. Vinken and G. W. Bruyn (Eds.), *Handbook of Clinical Neurology.* Amsterdam: North-Holland, 1973. Pp. 189–218.
52. Lott, I. T. *Neurology* 28: 47, 1978.
53. MacDonald, M. G. *Pediatrics* 79: 622, 1987.
54. Mace, S. *Am. J. Dis. Child.* 137: 32, 1983.
55. MacIntosh, D. *Developmental Pharmacology Therapy* 10: 100, 1987.
56. Markand, O. N. *Neurology* 32: 151, 1982.

57. McInerny, T. K. *Am. J. Dis. Child.* 117: 261, 1969.
58. Meldrum, B. S. *Arch. Neurol.* 28: 10, 1973.
59. Meldrum, B. S. *Arch. Neurol.* 29: 82, 1973.
60. Menkes, J. H. *Pediatrics* 29: 769, 1962.
61. Ment, L. R. *Neurology* 32: 169, 1982.
62. Mizrahi, E. M. *Neurology* 32: 1215, 1982.
63. Mizrahi, E. M. *Clev. Clin. J. Med.* 37: 1837, 1987.
64. Moser, H. W. *Neurology* 38: 1617, 1988.
65. Myers, R. E. Lactic Acid Accumulation as a Cause of Brain Edema and Cerebral Necrosis Resulting from Oxygen Deprivation. In C. Korobkin and C. Guilleminault (Eds.), *Advances in Perinatal Neurology,* Vol. 1. New York: Spectrum, 1979. Pp. 85–114.
66. Myers, R. E. *Arch. Neurol.* 34: 65, 1977.
67. Naidu, S. *Neurology* 38: 1100, 1988.
68. Nelson, K. B. *JAMA* 251: 1843, 1990.
69. Nelson, K. B. *Pediatrics* 68: 36, 1981.
70. Nelson, K. B. *JAMA* 25L: 1843, 1984.
71. Oro, A. S. *J. Pediatr.* 111: 571, 1987.
72. Painter, M. J. *Neurology* 31: 1107, 1981.
73. Perry, T. L. Carnosinemia. In W. L. Nyhan (Ed.), *Heritable Disorders of Amino Acid Metabolism.* New York: Wiley, 1974.
74. Pettit, R. E. *J. Child Neurol.* 2: 38, 1987.
75. Pitlick, W. *Clin. Pharmacol. Ther.* 23: 346, 1978.
76. Prensky, A. L. *N. Engl. J. Med.* 276: 779, 1967.
77. Przyrembel, H. *Clin. Chim. Acta* 66: 227, 1976.
78. Quattlebaum, T. G. *Pediatrics* 95: 257, 1979.
79. Renier, D. J. *Neurosurgery* 69: 877, 1988.
80. Rose, A. L. *Pediatrics* 45: 404, 1970.
81. Rowe, J. C. *Electroencephalogr. Clin. Neurophysiol.* 60: 183, 1985.
82. Sarnat, H. B. *Arch. Neurol.* 33: 696, 1976.
83. Scher, M. S. *Pediatr. Neurol.* 5: 17, 1989.
84. Scher, M. S. *Pediatr. Clin. North Am.* 36: 281, 1989.
85. Schiff, D. *Pediatrics* 48: 139, 1971.
86. Schiffman, R. *Ann. Neurol.* 25: 201, 1989.
87. Scriver, C. R. *Pediatrics* 25: 62, 1960.
88. Scriver, C. R. Hyper-beta-alanemia associated with beta-aminoacidemia and gamma-amino-butyric aciduria, somnolence, and seizures. *N. Engl. J. Med.* 274: 636, 1966.
89. Seay, A. R. *Arch. Neurol.* 34: 381, 1977.
90. Sinal, S. *Pediatrics* 57: 158, 1976.
91. Sinclair, J. C. *N. Engl. J. Med.* 273: 1173, 1965.
92. Smith, B. T. *Dev. Med. Child Neurol.* 13: 630, 1971.
93. Sran, S. K. *Am. J. Dis. Child.* 142: 1086, 1988.
94. Sun, S. *Pediatr. Res.* 15: 712, 1981.
95. Susser, M. Quantitative Estimates of Prenatal and Perinatal Risk Factors for Perinatal Mortality, Cerebral Palsy, Mental Retardation and Epilepsy. In J. M. Freeman (Ed.), *Prenatal and Perinatal Factors Associated with Brain Disorders* (NIH Publication 85-1149). Bethesda, Md.: NIH, 1985.
96. Tibbles, J. A. R. *Dev. Med. Child Neurol.* 22: 664, 1980.
97. Tibbles, J. A. R. *Pediatrics* 35: 778, 1965.
98. Volpe, J. J. Neonatal Seizures. In *Neurology of the Newborn,* 2d Ed. Philadelphia: Saunders, 1987. Pp. 129–158.
99. Volpe, J. J. Disorders of Organic Acid Metabolism. In *Neurology of the Newborn,* 2d Ed. Philadelphia: Saunders, 1987. Pp. 434–455.
100. Volpe, J. J. *Pediatrics* 84: 422, 1989.
101. Wasterlain, C. G. *Arch. Neurol.* 33: 821, 1976.
102. Watanabe, K. *Am. J. Dis. Child.* 136: 980, 1982.
103. Whelan, H. T. *Neurology* 33: 106, 1983.
104. Willis, J. *Dev. Med. Child Neurol.* 22: 214, 1980.

105. Wolf, B. *Pediatrics* 68: 113, 1981.
106. Wong, V. K. *Pediatr. Neurol.* 3: 235, 1987.
107. Yazdani, M. *Am. J. Dis. Child.* 141: 97, 1987.

Intracranial Hemorrhage

Karl Kuban

I. **Intracranial hemorrhage (ICH)** occurs in 20 to more than 40 percent of infants with birth weights less than 1500 gm but is less common among more mature newborns. Bleeding within the skull can occur extracerebrally (1) into epidural, subdural, or subarachnoid spaces, (2) into parenchyma of the cerebrum or cerebellum, or (3) into ventricles from the subependymal germinal matrix or choroid plexus. The incidence, pathogenesis, presentation, diagnosis, management, and prognosis of these hemorrhages vary according to location (Table 21-4); each type of hemorrhage will be considered separately.

A. **Subependymal hemorrhage–intraventricular hemorrhage (SEH-IVH)**

1. **Incidence.** Bleeding from the subependymal germinal matrix with or without subsequent rupture into a ventricle occurs in approximately 17 to 40 percent of infants born before 34 weeks' gestation [92]. The incidence appears to have diminished over the past 5 years so that most tertiary centers currently report an incidence of 17 to 25 percent [6,7,120]. Although IVH can occur in the full-term neonate, it is rare, and the source for bleeding is usually the choroid plexus [59].

2. **Pathogenesis.** Germinal matrix or subependymal tissue overlies the head of the caudate nucleus; after 26 weeks' gestation it is comprised of glial cells, which subsequently migrate into the adjacent cerebrum [25]. The supportive tissue of the germinal matrix then involutes and almost disappears by 34 weeks' gestation [27]. The maximum rate of involution occurs between 26 and 32 weeks, the period of greatest risk for development of SEH-IVH [28].

   The predisposing associations for development of SEH-IVH may be organized as intravascular inflow, intravascular outflow, and structural (both vascular and extravascular) factors (Table 21-5). The vasculature of the germinal matrix region lacks musculorum, is poorly supported by perivascular structures, and is an end bed to the only muscularized arterioles (striatal arteries) in the cerebrum before term [56,114]. Loss of vascular autoregulation in these arterioles, leading to a pressure-passive state, makes vessels just distal to them unusually vulnerable to rupture during surges in arterial blood flow. This is particularly true if there is resistance to egress of blood as occurs with increases in venous pressure [56,70,81,120].

   Intravascular factors associated with SEH-IVH include those events which provoke surges in cerebral inflow or compromise outflow of blood

Table 21-4. Categories of neonatal intracranial hemorrhage

1. Subependymal hemorrhage–intraventricular hemorrhage (SEH-IVH)
2. Posterior fossa hemorrhage
   a. Cerebellar
   b. Subdural (SDH)
3. Anterior fossa hemorrhage
   a. Subdural
   b. Intraparenchymal
4. Subarachnoid hemorrhage (SAH)

Table 21-5. Possible etiologic factors associated with SEH-IVH in low-birth-weight infants

Intravascular inflow factors	Intravascular outflow factors	Vascular and extravascular structural factors
Impaired autoregulation [69,70,81,93]	Respiratory distress [15,26,40,65]	Normal regression of germinal matrix [18,19,24,25]
Seizures [49,69]	Pneumothorax [17,45]	Relatively large blood flow to deep cerebral structures (in first half of third trimester) [87]
Manipulation of the infant [81,94]	Congestive heart failure [14]	Hypoxic-ischemic injury to germinal matrix or its vessels [113]
Infusion of hyperosmotic solutions [32,69,91]	Continuous positive airway pressure	
Rapid colloid infusion [31,32,91]	Acute angle of the internal cerebral vein [60]	
Apnea [69,110]		Presence of fibrinolytic enzymes [28]
Large fluctuations in second-to-second cerebrovascular flow velocity [93,117]	Labor/delivery [67]	Poor structural support of germinal matrix vessels [114]
		Abrupt termination of media in arteries proximal to germinal matrix [56,114]
		Abrupt termination of media in arteries proximal to germinal matrix [56,114]
Presence of patent ductus arteriosus [69,72,95]		
		Presence of a bleeding diathesis [3,11,64,102]
Negative intracranial pressure [16]		
Hypertension [30,122] and use of ECMO [13,29,112]		Use of benzyl alcohol as a preservative [46,48]

Key: SEH-IVH = subependymal hemorrhage-intraventricular hemorrhage; ECMO = extracorporeal membrane oxygenation

on the venous side of the matrix circulation. Surges of cerebral blood flow may occur with seizures, episodes of hypoxia, apnea, respiratory distress, rapid infusion of colloid [69], patent ductus arteriosus, extracorporeal membrane oxygenation [13,29,112], and possibly certain caretaking procedures such as tracheal suctioning [81]. Increased venous pressure may be associated with respiratory distress syndrome, pneumothorax, congestive heart failure, certain ventilator parameters such as high continuous positive airway pressure, possibly labor and/or delivery [67], and possibly hyperviscosity. Large second-to-second fluctuations in cerebral blood flow velocity in anterior cerebral arteries as measured by Doppler ultrasonography are significantly associated with development of SEH-IVH [93]. The large measured fluctuations may reflect arterial flow alterations and/or degree of respiratory distress and/or other confounding variables [58,86].

SEH-IVH most often begins as a small hemorrhage, usually petechial, between birth and 48 hours of life [115]. Extravascular factors may act to promote bleeding or extension of bleeding. These factors include the presence of fibrinolytic enzymes within the germinal matrix region [28], thrombocytopenia [3], vitamin K deficiency [11], administration of intravenous flush solutions containing benzyl alcohol as a preservative [46,48], and possibly use of heparin [64]. Occasionally, large hemorrhages develop abruptly.

3. **Clinical presentation.** Clinical symptoms and signs may occur as a result of blood volume loss or neurologic dysfunction (Table 21-6) and depend, in part, on the rapidity of evolution of blood loss. None of the signs is specific for SEH-IVH, although pallor, indicating blood loss, is most useful.

   The clinical presentation depends on the size, site, and rapidity of the hemorrhage. IVH can present as a catastrophic event when blood loss is large and rapid. Presentation can be stuttering with intermittent periods of stabilization when there is a slower evolution of blood loss [118]. A clinically silent presentation may occur in up to 50 percent of cases [62], usually with smaller hemorrhages.

4. **Diagnosis.** Real-time gray scale portable sector ultrasonography is the

Table 21-6. Clinical presentation of SEH-IVH

Blood volume loss		
Signs of blood loss	Laboratory correlates of blood loss	Neurologic dysfunction
		Bulging anterior fontanel
Shock	Metabolic acidosis	Excessive somnolence
Pallor	Low hematocrit	Hypotonia
Respiratory distress	Hypoxemia, hypercarbia and respiratory acidosis	Weakness, seizures
Disseminated intravascular coagulation	Thrombocytopenia and prolongation of both PT and PTT	Temperature instability
Jaundice	Hyperbilirubinemia	Brainstem signs (apnea, lost extraocular movements, facial weakness)

Key: SEH-IVH = subependymal hemorrhage–intraventricular hemorrhage; PT = prothrombin time; PTT = partial thromboplastin time.

method of choice to evaluate infants for the presence of SEH-IVH [5,86,107]. Clinical signs and symptoms, combined with the presence of hemorrhagic cerebrospinal fluid (CSF), were used to make the presumptive diagnosis before ultrasonic evaluations became available. Many premature infants do not tolerate lumbar puncture well, however, and a diagnosis made in this manner can only be presumptive. Although computerized tomographic (CT) scans define the pathologic anatomy of SEH-IVH extremely well, this requires transport of the infant to the machine, and in most circumstances, the stress associated with transport is a relative contraindication to the test. Magnetic resonance imaging (MRI) is both a sensitive and specific manner of identifying SEH-IVH after the first several days of life [75]. The abnormal images persist for up to 3 months after the bleed. However, submitting newborns to MRI testing has the same disadvantages noted for CT scans and requires nonmetallic monitoring wires and equipment for the babies undergoing the test.

There is no universally accepted system for grading hemorrhages, although the systems reported by Papile and Levene are most often cited [65,92] (Table 21-7). Since none of the grading systems is completely satisfactory, however, description of the ultrasonic characteristics of the hemorrhage is most useful [55]. This description should include the following observations:

a. Presence or absence of blood in the germinal matrix
b. Laterality (or bilaterality) of the hemorrhage
c. Presence or absence of blood in a ventricle—location and amount (small, moderate, large)
d. Presence or absence of blood in cerebral parenchyma, with specification of location
e. Presence or absence of ventricular dilatation
f. Presence or absence of other echogenic abnormalities
Echogenic areas of parenchyma, especially white matter, are most often identified in prematurely born babies with SEH-IVH [120] that may develop independently of hemorrhage. Parenchymal echoabnormalities correlate highly with subsequent motor and development deficits [34,35,38,83].

5. Timing of ultrasound examinations. Ultrasound examination should be performed with clinical indications (change in behavior, anemia, shock, bulging fontanelle, change in level of consciousness, or change in respiratory support needs without other explanation) at any time in premature babies. Otherwise, routine ultrasound testing of at-risk premature babies should be performed on day 3. This should be repeated on day 10. Babies with hemorrhages and babies who have had a difficult postnatal course (e.g., RDS, NEC, pneumothorax, sepsis) warrant a "late look" at 3 and possibly 6 weeks, looking for parenchymal echogenic abnormalities. Screening for hydrocephalus also should be undertaken in babies with hemorrhage (see below).

6. Management

a. Prevention. Avoid rapid intravenous administration of osmotically active agents and unnecessary manipulations of the infant [32,91]. Phenobarbital does not prevent development of IVH [57]. Use of indomethacin as a prophylactic agent for development of IVH is controversial, may work differently among babies below and above 1000 gm in birth weight, and requires further clinical studies prior to recommendations for its routine use [23,39,79,116].

Prophylactic use of pancuronium has been reported to reduce the risk of SEH-IVH in specific preselected populations [96]. Prior to recommending routine use of pancuronium, however, studies are needed to affirm the initial study's beneficial effects, to better define the population most likely to benefit from pancuronium, and to evaluate more fully the limitations and risks of prophylactic paralysis.

Table 21-7. Grading system for subependymal hemorrhage–intraventricular hemorrhage

First author	Assessment technique	Grading system	Definitions*
Papile [71]	CT	1	Isolated SEH
		2	IVH without ventricular dilatation
		3	IVH with ventricular dilatation
		4	IVH with parenchymal extension
Krishnamoorthy [53,54]	CT	1	SEH ± blood in less than half of one ventricle
		2	Partial filling of two ventricles or greater than half of one ventricle
		3	Complete filling and distension of both ventricles
		4	Ventricular blood with intraparenchymal hematoma
Mantovani [54]	CT	1	SEH or IVH filling less than 10 percent of ventricles
		2	IVH filling from 10 to 50 percent of ventricles
		3	IVH filling 50 percent or greater of ventricles
Lazzara [47]	CT	Mild	SEH ± one-fourth of AP diameter of ventricles blood-filled
		Moderate	One-fourth to one-half of AP diameter of ventricles blood-filled
		Severe	One-half of AP diameter of ventricles blood-filled
Shankaran [81]	US	Mild	SEH ± small amount of blood in ventricle (normal-sized)
		Moderate	Intermediate amount of blood in enlarged ventricles
		Severe	Filling ventricles forming a cast or intracerebral extension of hemorrhage
Levene [49]	US	1	SEH ± with no inferior or lateral extension of blood beyond most lateral border of ventricles
		2	Downward extension into basal nuclei on at least one side or involvement of caudate to genu of ventricle posteriorly on parasagittal scan
		3	Large hemorrhage with any degree of extension laterally or superiorly into cerebral parenchyma

Key: CT = computerized tomography; SEH = subependymal hemorrhage; IVH = intraventricular hemorrhage; ± = with or without; AP = anteroposterior; US = ultrasound.
*Ventricles are lateral ventricles.

Other prophylactic agents that hold promise but require further study include vitamin E and ethamsylate. These are not recommended currently.

b. Specific treatment. Treatment for SEH-IVH is supportive and is directed at avoiding extension of the hemorrhage. No interventions have been shown conclusively to limit the extent of hemorrhage once it has occurred, although the recommendations for prevention of SEH-IVH (see **a**) are probably applicable. Avoid excessive suctioning and manipulations. Administer osmotically active agents slowly, including albumin, plasma, and blood. Vitamin K administration may be important for those infants who have evidence of abnormalities of coagulation [102] (see Chap. 17). Treat seizures (see Neonatal Seizures above) and hyperbilirubinemia associated with the breakdown of red cells from the hemorrhage (see Chap. 15). Use of ECMO is contraindicated [13]. Infants with SEH-IVH may have low CSF sugar levels in the absence of infection.

In addition to acute cardiovascular and neurologic dysfunction, concomitant or continued cerebral injury may occur because of reduced cerebral perfusion pressure (mean arterial pressure minus intracranial pressure) or because of intermittent ischemia [78,122]. Avoid hypotension (see Chap. 6). Marked elevations in ICP indicate that hydrocephalus likely has occurred.

7. Complications: posthemorrhagic hydrocephalus (PHH)

a. Definition. Hydrocephalus should be differentiated from ventricular dilatation [2]. Hydrocephalus indicates either a state of progressively expanding ventricles or enlarged ventricles and increased ICP (an ICP $>$ 5 cm H_2O) [66,84,106]. In babies without elevations of venous pressure (CPAP, pneumothorax, etc.), a good estimate of intracranial pressure is the vertical distance, measured in centimeters, between the anterior fontanelle and the heart, measured at the point that the anterior fontanelle flattens as you manually tilt the baby up. Ventriculomegaly indicates a static increase in ventricular size without elevated ICP. Some infants may proceed from a state of ventriculomegaly to hydrocephalus after a stable period of 3 months or longer [43].

b. Clinical features. Hydrocephalus can occur immediately following hemorrhage but usually evolves over the weeks following SEH-IVH. It occurs in approximately 25 percent of infants with SEH-IVH and is most readily identified by cranial ultrasound [1,47,89]. Hydrocephalus is more likely to occur with large hemorrhages. Bulging anterior fontanelle, rapidly expanding head circumference, and brainstem signs, including "sunset eyes," are generally late signs [51,118]. Milder clinical signs such as lethargy and lower extremity weakness are often too difficult to evaluate in the ill premature infant; therefore, weekly ultrasonic evaluations until there is clear stabilization of ventricular size are a minimum requirement following development of SEH-IVH. Infants with small hemorrhages, particularly if the hemorrhages are limited to the germinal matrix, may require only a few follow-up scans, whereas infants with ventricular expansion with large volumes of blood may need to be followed for months.

c. Pathophysiology. Hydrocephalus usually occurs because of a combination of factors, including obstruction of CSF outflow through the fourth ventricle or at the base of the brain at the foramina of Luschka and Magendie and impairment of CSF resorption at the arachnoid granulations over the convexity of the brain. If there is complete obstruction of CSF flow at the fourth ventricle or at the base of the brain, the hydrocephalus is noncommunicating. This occurs more often when the hydrocephalus develops rapidly after a massive hemorrhage. Communicating hydrocephalus caused by impaired CSF resorption usually develops gradually.

d. **Management.** Static ventricular dilatation without elevated ICP does not require intervention. Hydrocephalus, however, requires intervention in order to maintain normal cerebral perfusion pressure (CPP) as well as to avoid compression of both periventricular white matter and cerebral arteries, in particular the anterior cerebral arteries [41].

(1) The natural history of PHH is to either (1) progress, occasionally after a period of stabilization, (2) come to an equilibrium of CSF production and efflux at some state of ventricular dilatation, or (3) recede toward normalcy. Since the long-term complication rate of ventricular shunts and their placement exceeds 50 percent [74,76], and since premature infants with PHH are fragile and thus poor surgical risks, avoidance or delay in placement of shunts is often preferred. Serial lumbar punctures with removal of at least 10 ml of CSF is advocated as a means of transiently reducing ventricular pressure and size [33,44,89]. This procedure often enables postponement of definitive shunting and may permit time for an individual patient's hydrocephalus either to come to equilibrium or to recede. The success and required frequency of lumbar punctures should be evaluated by results of opening pressures on lumbar puncture or by manual measure of ICP over the anterior fontanelle (see above) and by repetitive ultrasonic examination. Serial head circumference measures also may be useful. Lumbar puncture opening pressures of less than 80 mm of water for 3 consecutive days in the presence of a static ventricular size are highly predictive of successful management without need for surgery [71]. Serial lumbar punctures will be effective only if the hydrocephalus is at least partially communicating. Serial lumbar punctures have been shown to be an ineffective means of preventing the development of hydrocephalus following SEH-IVH [61].

(2) Surgical intervention is required when hydrocephalus persists despite lumbar puncture treatment for as long as 3 or 4 weeks or with rapid development of raised ICP with florid clinical signs not responsive to lumbar puncture. Surgical intervention can occur in the form of a ventriculoperitoneal shunt or a temporary ventriculostomy with external drainage. Temporary external ventriculostomy need not necessarily be followed by permanent shunt placement [118].

(3) Pharmacologic treatment of PHH with acetazolamide (20 to 100 mg/kg per day), glycerol (8 mg/kg per day), or furosemide (1 mg/kg per day), all divided into q6h doses, has not been studied well enough to advocate it as an alternative initial form of therapy [8,111]. It may be used as an adjunct to lumbar punctures, however, or when other forms of therapy fail and shunting is contraindicated. We usually start with acetazolamide 40 mg/kg per day divided into doses given every 6 hours and furosemide 1 mg/kg per day divided into doses given every 12 hours. The dose of acetazolamide is increased up to 100 mg/kg per day depending on effect. We have not used glycerol. Particular care should be given to blood pressure, fluid, acid–base, and electrolyte status when using these agents. Infants treated with acetazolamide may need treatment with Polycitra (sodium bicarbonate and potassium bicarbonate) to correct electrolyte disturbances. The usual starting dose is 1½ mEq/kg. The dose is then titrated according to response.

8. **Prognosis.** Since longitudinal studies of VLBW infants with SEH-IVH were not feasible until high-resolution portable ultrasound units became available, prognosis of babies with SEH-IVH is only currently becoming available. Approximately 30 percent of babies with SEH-IVH die in the

newborn period, although not necessarily as a result of hemorrhage. Numerous long-term studies are in progress, and some series have been reported [1,52,53,77,88,90,99,100,103,105]. For the most part, these series attempt to correlate the grade of SEH-IVH with degrees of neurologic impairment. The limited data available are conflicting, however, and already have provoked considerable controversy.

Disparate views of the effects of SEH-IVH on outcome may be explained in part by differences in populations studied, variable definitions of abnormality, the timing and nature of evaluations, the use of diverse grading systems, and the lack of consideration of other parenchymal injury.

In general, the more extensive the hemorrhage, the more likely it is that there will be motor or cognitive impairments. When there is major parenchymal hemorrhage or associated parenchymal damage with or without parenchymal hemorrhage, some form of motor impairment is common. Recent studies suggest that ventricular enlargement, either as a static state or as a PHH and parenchymal abnormalities, is most highly predictive of compromised neurologic outcome [54,88,104,116,120].

It is uncertain whether minor abnormalities such as language delay, fine motor disability, learning impairments, and behavioral dysfunctions are related to SEH-IVH or concomitants of SEH-IVH. Some studies suggest that more subtle developmental/educational difficulties may occur in children who have smaller grades of SEH-IVH [88,100,123]. If such disabilities are related to SEH-IVH, it is also uncertain whether the critical prognostic factor is (1) involvement of both germinal matrices or ventricles, (2) development of PHH, (3) cerebral perfusion alterations that may precede, occur with, or follow development of SEH-IVH, (4) associated medical diseases, (5) preexisting predisposition to such problems, or (6) a combination of factors. Delay in shunting also has been associated with poor outcome [21].

B. Posterior fossa hemorrhage

1. **Pathogenesis.** Hemorrhages into the cerebellum or the subdural space of the posterior fossa will often present similar to space-occupying lesions in the posterior fossa. Such hemorrhages usually result from trauma in the full-term infant [121]. In the premature infant, they either result from trauma or may develop as a cerebellar component of germinal matrix hemorrhage [36]. Vertical molding, fronto-occipital elongation, and torsional forces acting on the head during delivery may provoke laceration of dural leaflets of either the tentorium cerebelli or the falx cerebri through which vessels and sinuses course [9]. Laceration may occur with either vertex or breech presentations. Breech presentation also predisposes to occipital osteodiastasis, a depressed fracture of the occipital bone or bones, which may lead to direct laceration of cerebellum or rupture of vessels in the subdural space [87].

2. **Clinical presentation.** When the accumulation of blood is rapid and large, such as occurs with rupture of arterioles, large veins, or sinuses, the presentation follows shortly after birth and evolves rapidly. When the sources of hemorrhage are small veins, there may be few symptoms or signs for up to a week, at which time the hematoma either attains a critical size and imposes on brainstem structures or provokes hydrocephalus [9,101]. Presenting signs may result from (1) the effects of blood volume loss, as with SEH-IVH (see Table 21-6), or (2) neurologic dysfunction caused by increased ICP or, more often, by brainstem dysfunction [9,101]. Seizures are less common [97]. Signs of elevated ICP include bulging anterior fontanel or increasing head circumference, lethargy, and irritability. Head circumference enlargement occurs late, particularly in premature babies. Brainstem signs involve abnormal respirations (including apnea), cranial nerve palsies, nystagmus, and dysconjugate gaze (including skew deviation of the eyes). Hypotonia and vomiting may occur as well [9,73,98,101].

3. **Diagnosis.** The diagnosis should be suspected on the basis of clinical signs and confirmed with a CT scan [9,97,98,101]. Although ultrasound may be valuable in evaluating intracerebellar hematomas, ultrasonic imaging of structures adjacent to bone (e.g., the subdural space) may be inadequate.
4. **Management and prognosis.** Attend to blood volume and cardiovascular status. Excessive hyperbilirubinemia also may occur (see Chap. 15). Open surgical evacuation of clot is the usual management for infants with neurologic signs [9,97,101]. Prognosis for normal development is good with successful surgical evacuation of the hematoma. Fishman et al. [24] recently suggested that when the clinical picture is stable and no deterioration in neurologic function or unmanageable increase in ICP exists, supportive care, using serial CT examinations, should be utilized in the management of cerebellar hematoma instead of surgical intervention.

C. Anterior fossa hemorrhage

1. **Pathogenesis.** Intracerebral hematomas and convexity epidural or subdural hematomas can occur as a result of birth trauma [12,63,121]. Intracerebral hematoma also can occur (1) into necrotic cerebral tissue, such as occurs with periventricular leukomalacia (PVL) and arterial distribution infarction, (2) in association with germinal matrix hemorrhage, either contiguous to or separate from the matrix [4,7,42,63], (3) with exposure to cocaine [109], (4) with persistent pulmonary hypertension [85], (5) with hemophilia [50,108,124] or other bleeding disorders, and (6) rarely due to arteriovenous malformation or aneurysmal rupture. Hemorrhages that occur in the cerebrum may be cortical, in white matter, in thalamus, or in the caudate. Arterial infarcts may occur with coagulopathies (deficiency of protein C, S, or antithrombin III; thrombocytosis; presence of passively transferred lupus and anticardiolipin antibody; hyperviscous state), cardiac lesions (myomas or clots), and exposure to cocaine [109]. Approximately a third of babies greater than 35 weeks' gestation who undergo extracorporeal membrane oxygenation suffer from parenchymal or subarachnoid hemorrhage or hemorrhagic infarction of brain parenchyma. **However, most babies with infarcts and/or hemorrhage do not have a clear predisposing cause** [10,22,37,82]. Such infarcts and hemorrhages may represent emboli seeded from the degenerating placenta.
2. **Clinical presentation.** As with other ICHs in the newborn period, signs may result from blood loss (see Table 21-6) or neurologic dysfunction. With either subdural or intracerebral hematomas, focal neurologic signs predominate. These signs may be obvious or quite subtle and may include lethargy, irritability, focal seizures, hemiparesis, or gaze preference. Sixth nerve dysfunction may occur due to elevated ICP. When the hematoma is large, compression of the third cranial nerve may occur, leading to a dilated and poorly reactive pupil. A small subdural hematoma may be unrecognized clinically and can either resolve or evolve into a chronic subdural fluid collection [119] and can be associated with the development of hydrocephalus.
3. **Diagnosis.** Consider the diagnosis whenever the patient has focal or lateralized signs, including seizures. Hemorrhagic or xanthochromic CSF or both are consistent with the diagnosis, particularly when there are clear signs of elevated ICP to include bulging anterior fontanel or brainstem dysfunction. Lumbar puncture should be deferred unless meningitis is a strong consideration. Definitive evaluation requires CT scan. Ultrasound is a sensitive imaging technique for deep intraparenchymal or intraventricular hemorrhages. It is less sensitive at discerning SDH, although it may demonstrate distortion or shift of the ventricular system as indirect evidence of the more superficial space-occupying lesion.
4. **Management and prognosis.** In general, surgical intervention for subdural hematomas is not required unless there are signs of progressive

increased ICP, progressive worsening of neurologic signs, or signs of herniation. Surgery may take the form of a subdural tap or an open evacuation. There is no specific therapy for intracerebral hematomas. Seizures should be treated. Intracerebral hematoma often results in some form of subsequent motor impairment. Prognosis following SDH is variable, although generally favorable when the hemorrhage does not provoke either cardiovascular compromise or herniation. In addition, hydrocephalus occasionally develops as a late sequela.

D. Subarachnoid hemorrhage (SAH) is a common form of ICH among newborns. Usually, the hemorrhage is trivial and unrecognized. Hemorrhagic or xanthochromic CSF may be the only indication of such a hemorrhage. SAH should be distinguished from subarachnoid extension of blood from an SEH-IVH.

1. **Pathogenesis.** SAH is nearly always the result of the normal trauma associated with the birth process. A role for hypoxia is debated. The source of blood is usually from ruptured bridging veins of the subarachnoid space or from ruptured small leptomeningeal vessels [119]. Occasionally, SAH develops as a result of laceration of the tentorium cerebelli or falx cerebri and may, in this circumstance, be associated with subdural hemorrhage. SAH also can occur as an extension of a cerebral contusion.
2. **Clinical features.** As with other forms of ICH, clinical presentations can occur because of blood loss or neurologic dysfunction (see Table 21-6). Only rarely is the volume loss large enough to provoke catastrophic results. More often neurologic signs manifest as irritability or seizures. Hemiparesis is occasionally seen when there is associated cerebral contusion or hemorrhage [119].
3. **Diagnosis.** The history of seizures and CSF findings suggests the diagnosis. Distinguishing SAH from other forms of ICH may be difficult. With simple SAH, the interictal neurologic state is usually normal, which has led to the designation of "well baby with seizures." The diagnosis, however, must be confirmed with a CT scan. Ultrasonography is not a sensitive technique for identifying a small SAH.
4. **Management and prognosis.** Management of SAH usually requires only symptomatic therapy, such as an anticonvulsant for seizures (see Neonatal Seizures above), and attention to blood volume and cardiovascular status. Treat hyperbilirubinemia. Occasionally, hydrocephalus will develop if the hemorrhage is large. The vast majority of infants do well without recognized sequelae.

References

1. Ahmann, P. A. *Ann. Neurol.* 7: 118, 1980.
2. Allan, W. C. *Am. J. Dis. Child.* 136: 589, 1982.
3. Andrew, M. J. *Pediatrics* 110: 457, 1987.
4. Armstrong, D. *Arch. Dis. Child.* 49: 367, 1974.
5. Babcock, D. S. *A.J.N.R.* 3: 309, 1982.
6. Bandstra, E. S. *Pediatrics* 82: 533, 1988.
7. Barmada, M. A. *Ann. Neurol.* 6: 495, 1979.
8. Bergman, E. *Ann. Neurol.* 4: 189, 1978.
9. Blank, N. K. *Arch. Neurol.* 35: 108, 1978.
10. Cartwright, G. W. *Dev. Med. Child Neurol.* 21: 730, 1979.
11. Chaou, W. T. *J. Pediatr.* 105: 880, 1984.
12. Chaplin, E. R. *Pediatrics* 63: 812, 1979.
13. Cilley, R. E. *Pediatrics* 78: 699, 1986.
14. Cole, V. A. *Arch. Dis. Child.* 49: 722, 1974.
15. Cooke, W. I. *Arch. Dis. Child.* 56: 425, 1981.
16. deCourten, G. M. *Dev. Med. Child Neurol.* 23: 287, 1981.
17. DeLemos, R. A., Tomasovic, J., and Null, D. M., Jr. The Role of Postnatal Factors

in the Premature Infant. Perinatal Intracranial Hemorrhage Conference Syllabus. Washington, D.C., December, 1980. Pp. 63–87.
18. Dobbing, J. *Arch. Dis. Child.* 48: 757, 1973.
19. Dobbing, J. *Nature* 266: 639, 1970.
20. Donn, S. M. *J. Pediatr.* 99: 459, 1981.
21. Etches, P. C. *Pediatr. Neurol.* 3: 136, 1987.
22. Fenichel, G. M. *Arch. Neurol.* 41: 30, 1984.
23. Finer, N. N. *J. Pediatr.* 109: 396, 1986.
24. Fishman, M. A. *Pediatrics* 98: 466, 1981.
25. Friede, R. I. *Developmental Neuropathology.* New York: Springer-Verlag, 1975. Pp. 7–8.
26. Fujimura, M. *Arch. Dis. Child.* 55: 409, 1979.
27. Gilles, F. H., Leviton, A., and Dooling, E. C. (Eds.). *The Developing Human Brain.* Littleton, Mass.: Wright-PSG, 1983.
28. Gilles, F. H. *Biol. Neonate* 18: 426, 1971.
29. Glass, P. *Pediatrics* 83: 72, 1989.
30. Goddard, J. J. *Pediatrics* 96: 1057, 1980.
31. Goddard-Finegold, J. J. *Pediatrics* 100: 796, 1982.
32. Goldberg, R. N. *J. Pediatr.* 96: 1060, 1980.
33. Goldstein, G. W. *Lancet* 1: 512, 1976.
34. Grant, E. G. *A.J.N.R.* 7: 443, 1986.
35. Graziani, L. J. *Pediatrics* 78: 88, 1986.
36. Grunnet, M. L. *J. Pediatr.* 88: 605, 1976.
37. Guekos-Thoni, V. *Helv. Paediatr. Acta* 35: 531, 1980.
38. Guzzetta, F. *Pediatrics* 78: 995, 1986.
39. Hanigan, W. C. *J. Pediatr.* 112: 941, 1988.
40. Harrison, V. C. *Arch. Dis. Child.* 43: 116, 1968.
41. Hill, A. *Pediatrics* 69: 4, 1982.
42. Hill, A. *Pediatrics* 69: 282, 1982.
43. Hill, A. *Pediatrics* 68: 623, 1981.
44. Hill, A. *Ann. Neurol.* 10: 284, 1981.
45. Hill, A. *Pediatrics* 69: 144, 1980.
46. Hiller, J. L. *Pediatrics* 77: 500, 1986.
47. Horbar, J. D. *Pediatrics* 66: 674, 1980.
48. Jardine, D. S. *Pediatrics* 83: 153, 1989.
49. Klein, M. *Pediatr. Res.* 15: 667, 1981.
50. Kletzel, M. A. *Am. J. Dis. Child.* 143: 1107, 1989.
51. Korobkin, R. *Pediatrics* 56: 74, 1975.
52. Kosmetatos, N. *Pediatr. Res.* 13: 536, 1979.
53. Krishnamoorthy, K. S. *Pediatrics* 64: 233, 1979.
54. Krishnamoorthy, K. *Pediatrics* 85: 1027, 1990.
55. Kuban, K. C. *Pediatrics* 74: 358, 1984.
56. Kuban, K. C. *Ann. Neurol.* 17: 539, 1985.
57. Kuban, K. C. *Pediatrics* 77: 443, 1986.
58. Kuban, K. C. *Pediatrics* 82: 548, 1988.
59. Lacey, D. J. *Dev. Med. Child Neurol.* 24: 332, 1982.
60. Larroche, J. C. *Biol. Neonate* 7: 26, 1964.
61. Lazzara, A. *Ann. Neurol.* 10: 291, 1981.
62. Lazzara, A. *Pediatrics* 65: 30, 1980.
63. Leblanc, R. J. *Neurosurgery* 53: 642, 1980.
64. Lesko, S. M. *N. Engl. J. Med.* 314: 1156, 1986.
65. Levene, M. I. *Arch. Dis. Child.* 57: 410, 1982.
66. Levinson, A. *Am. J. Dis. Child.* 32: 208, 1926.
67. Leviton, A. *J. Child Neurol.* in press 1990.
68. Lipman, B. *Pediatrics* 69: 778, 1982.
69. Lou, H. C. *Arch. Neurol.* 37: 585, 1980.
70. Lou, H. C. *J. Pediatr.* 94: 118, 1979.
71. Mantovani, J. F. *J. Pediatr.* 97: 278, 1980.

72. Martin, C. G. *J. Pediatr.* 101: 587, 1982.
73. Martin, R. *Pediatrics* 89: 290, 1976.
74. Matson, D. D. *Neurosurgery of Infancy and Childhood,* 2d Ed. Springfield, Ill.: Thomas, 1969.
75. McArdle, C. B. *Radiology* 163: 387, 1987.
76. Menkes, J. G. *Textbook of Child Neurology.* Philadelphia: Lea & Febiger, 1980.
77. Ment, L. R. *Neurology* 32: A171, 1982.
78. Ment, L. R. *Pediatrics* 68: 763, 1981.
79. Ment, L. R. *J. Pediatr.* 112: 948, 1988.
80. Miall-Allen, V. M. *Pediatrics* 83: 657, 1989.
81. Milligan, D. W. A. *Lancet* 1: 896, 1980.
82. Mitchell, W. *Pediatrics* 65: 35, 1980.
83. Monset-Couchard, M. *Neuropediatrics* 19: 124, 1988.
84. Munro, D. *J.A.M.A.* 90: 1688, 1928.
85. Oelberg, D. *Clin. Pediatr.* 27: 14, 1988.
86. Pape, K. E. *J. Pediatr.* 102: 275, 1983.
87. Pape, K. *Clin. Dev. Med.* 69–70: 1, 1979.
88. Papile, L. A. *J. Pediatr.* 103: 273, 1983.
89. Papile, L. A. *Pediatrics* 97: 273, 1980.
90. Papile, L. A. *Pediatr. Res.* 13: 528, 1979.
91. Papile, L. *Pediatrics* 93: 834, 1978.
92. Papile, L. A. *Pediatrics* 92: 529, 1978.
93. Perlman, J. M. *N. Engl. J. Med.* 309: 204, 1983.
94. Perlman, J. M. *Pediatrics* 72: 329, 1983.
95. Perlman, J. M. *J. Pediatr.* 99: 767, 1981.
96. Perlman, J. M. *N. Engl. J. Med.* 312: 1353, 1985.
97. Ravenel, S. D. *Pediatrics* 64: 39, 1979.
98. Rom, S. *Pediatrics* 93: 486, 1978.
99. Schub, H. S. *Pediatr. Res.* 15: 711, 1981.
100. Scott, D. T. *Ann. Neurol.* 12: 226, 1982.
101. Serfontein, G. L. *Pediatrics* 65: 40, 1980.
102. Setzer, E. S. *Pediatrics* 100: 599, 1982.
103. Shankaran, S. *Pediatrics* 100: 469, 1982.
104. Shankaran, S. *Pediatrics* 114: 109, 1989.
105. Shinnar, S. *N. Engl. J. Med.* 306: 1464, 1982.
106. Sidbury, J. B. *Arch. Pediatr.* 37: 545, 1920.
107. Silverboard, G. *Pediatrics* 66: 507, 1980.
108. Silverstein, A. *Arch. Neurol.* 3: 141, 1960.
109. Spires, M. *Pediatr. Neurol.* 5: 324, 1989.
110. Sims, M. E. *Pediatr. Res.* 15: 681, 1981.
111. Taylor, D. A. *Ann. Neurol.* 10: 297, 1981.
112. Taylor, G. A. *A.J.R.* 153: 355, 1989.
113. Towbin, A. *Am. J. Dis. Child.* 119: 529, 1978.
114. Trommer, B. L. *Pediatr. Res.* 22: 23, 1987.
115. Tsiantos, A. J. *J. Pediatr.* 85: 854, 1979.
116. Vohr, B. R. J. *J. Pediatr.* 115: 296, 1989.
117. Volpe, J. J. *Pediatrics* 72: 589, 1983.
118. Volpe, J. J. *N. Engl. J. Med.* 304: 886, 1981.
119. Volpe, J. J. *Neurology of the Newborn.* Philadelphia: Saunders, 1981.
120. Volpe, J. J. *Ann. Neurol.* 25: 3, 1989.
121. Welch, K. *Dev. Med. Child Neurol.* 28: 156, 1986.
122. Wimberley, P. D. *Acta Paediatr. Scand.* 71: 537, 1982.
123. Williams, M. L. *Dev. Med. Child Neurol.* 29: 243, 1987.
124. Yoffe, G. *J. Pediatr.* 113: 333, 1988.

Perinatal Asphyxia

Evan Y. Snyder and
John P. Cloherty

I. **Definition. Perinatal asphyxia** is an insult to the fetus or newborn due to **lack of oxygen** (hypoxia) and/or **lack of perfusion** (ischemia) to various organs. It is associated with tissue lactic acidosis. If accompanied by hypoventilation, it also may be associated with hypercapnea. The effects of hypoxia and ischemia may not be identical, but they are difficult to separate clinically. Both factors probably contribute to asphyxial injury. Normal blood gases in term newborns are as shown in Table 21-8.

II. **Incidence.** The incidence of perinatal asphyxia is about 1.0 to 1.5 percent in most centers and is usually related to gestational age and birth weight. It occurs in 9.0 percent of infants less than 36 weeks' gestation and in 0.5 percent of infants more than 36 weeks' gestation [19a], accounting for 20 percent of perinatal deaths [24] (or as high as 50 percent of deaths if stillborns are included [21]). The incidence is higher in term infants of diabetic or toxemic mothers; these factors correlate less well in preterm infants. In both preterm and term infants, intrauterine growth retardation and breech presentation are associated with an increased incidence of asphyxia. Postmature infants are also at risk.

III. **Pathophysiology and etiology of asphyxia.** Ninety percent of asphyxial insults occur in the antepartum/intrapartum periods as a result of **placental insufficiency,** resulting in an inability to provide O_2 to and remove CO_2 and H^+ from the fetus. The remainder are postpartum, usually secondary to pulmonary, cardiovascular, or neurologic insufficiency.

During **normal labor** there is reduced blood flow to the placenta, hence decreased O_2 delivery to the fetus. Because there is a concomitant increase in O_2 consumption by both mother and fetus, fetal O_2 saturation falls. Maternal dehydration and maternal alkalosis from hyperventilation may further reduce placental blood flow; maternal hypoventilation may further decrease maternal and fetal O_2 saturation. Some degree of cord compression occurs in many deliveries. Uterine contractions decrease placental blood flow. These normal events cause most babies to be born with little O_2 reserve. Newborns, however, including their central nervous systems (CNS), are fairly resistant to asphyxic damage [12,15,18,21,28,29,38]. Late decelerations are uncommon until pO_2 is less than 20 mmHg and O_2 saturation is less than 31 percent; in the experimental monkey fetus, a decline in heart rate due to this degree of hypoxia could be maintained for several hours without producing encephalopathy [15].

In addition to the normal factors mentioned above, any process which (1) impairs maternal oxygenation, (2) decreases blood flow from mother to placenta or from placenta to fetus, (3) impairs gas exchange across the placenta or at the fetal tissue, or (4) increases fetal O_2 requirement will exacerbate perinatal asphyxia. Such factors include maternal hypertension (either chronic or preeclampsic), maternal vascular disease, maternal diabetes, maternal drug use, maternal hypoxia from pulmonary, cardiac, or neurologic disease, maternal hypotension, maternal infection, placental infarction or fibrosis, placental abruption, cord accidents (prolapse, entanglement, true knot, compression), abnormalities of umbilical vessels, fetal anemia, fetal or placental hydrops, fetal infection, intrauterine growth retardation, and postmaturity.

In the presence of a hypoxic-ischemic challenge to the fetus, reflexes are initiated, causing shunting of blood to the brain, heart, and adrenals and away from lungs, gut, liver, kidneys, spleen, bone, skeletal muscle, and skin ("diving reflex") [18]. In mild hypoxia, there is decreased heart rate, slight increase in blood pressure (BP) to maintain cerebral perfusion, increased central venous pressure (CVP), and little change in cardiac output. As asphyxia progresses with severe hypoxia and acidosis, there is decreased heart rate, decreased cardiac output, and initially increased then falling blood pressure as oxidative phosphorylation fails and en-

Table 21-8. Normal blood gas values in term newborns

	At birth			At age		
	Maternal artery	Umbilical vein	Umbilical artery	10 minutes	30 to 60 minutes (umbilical artery)	5 hours
PO_2	95	27.5	16	50	54	74
PCO_2	32	39	49	46	38	35
pH*	7.4	7.32	7.24	7.21	7.29	7.34

Key: PO_2 = partial pressure of oxygen; PCO_2 = partial pressure of carbon dioxide.
*A scalp pH in labor of 7.25 or above is considered normal (see Chaps. 3 and 5).

ergy reserves become depleted. During asphyxia, anaerobic metabolism produces lactic acid, which, because of poor perfusion, remains in local tissues. Systemic acidosis may actually be mild until perfusion is restored and these local acid stores are mobilized.

A. **Perinatal assessment** of risk includes awareness of preexistent maternal or fetal problems and assessment of changing placental and fetal conditions by ultrasound (e.g., assaying fetal breathing and gross body movements, fetal tone, fetal heart rate reactivity, amniotic fluid volume, fetal and placental blood flow), nonstress tests, and urinary estriols (see Chap. 3).

B. **Perinatal management** of high-risk pregnancies consists of fetal heart monitoring, evaluation of fetal scalp pH, and awareness of the progress of labor and the presence of meconium. The pH is considered a better determinant of fetal oxygenation than pO_2; if a hypoxic-ischemic insult occurs intermittently, the pO_2 may improve transiently, whereas a progressive fall in pH occurs; pH less than 7.0 is good evidence of substantial and prolonged intrauterine asphyxia. (It should be remembered, however, that scalp and cord pH values may be profoundly affected by **maternal** acid–base status.) Abnormalities of fetal heart rate and rhythm plus heavy meconium staining may provide possible supporting evidence of asphyxia but provide no information concerning the severity or duration of the asphyxia. The decision to perform a cesarean section, to augment a vaginal delivery, or to allow labor to progress is the most difficult obstetric decision. Each medical center should have guidelines for intervention in cases of suspected fetal distress (see Chap. 3).

IV. **Delivery room management** (see Chap. 5 for resuscitation, Chap. 6 for shock, and Chap. 13 for meconium aspiration and persistent pulmonary hypertension). A 5-minute Apgar score less than 3 is generally regarded as evidence of asphyxia. A low Apgar score may not indicate asphyxia, however, in preterm or small-for-gestational age infants (see Chap. 5), who are more likely to be hypotonic, have cyanotic extremities, and have diminished responsiveness; a score of 6 to 7 may be maximal for a "normal" preterm infant. Low Apgar scores may be present in **non**asphyxiated infants with (1) depression from maternal anesthesia or analgesics, (2) trauma, (3) metabolic or infectious insults, (4) neuromuscular disorders, and (5) CNS, cardiac, or pulmonary malformations. Further, a low Apgar score, even when a marker of a depressed infant, does not indicate the mechanism for the depression, duration or severity of the specific insult, or the adaptive response of the fetus. A high Apgar score (>6 by 5 minutes), however, speaks compellingly **against** substantial peripartum asphyxia [12].

V. **Postnatal management of asphyxia**

A. **The differential diagnosis of acute asphyxia** in a newborn includes maternal drugs or anesthesia; acute blood loss; acute intracranial bleeding; CNS malformation; neuromuscular disease; cardiopulmonary disease, malformation, or hypoplasia; mechanical impediments to ventilation (airway obstruction, pneumothorax, hydrops, pleural effusion, ascites, diaphragmatic hernia); and infection (including septic shock and hypotension). These problems may be the cause of asphyxia or merely coincident with it. A common presentation is the postmature infant with asphyxia, meconium aspiration, persistent pulmonary hypertension, pneumothorax, and birth trauma. Another common presentation is the premature infant with asphyxia, hyaline membrane disease, and an intracranial bleed. **Intrauterine ischemia,** early in gestation, may present in the newborn as a hypoplastic organ (e.g., lung, gut) or extremity (e.g., sirenomelia), as hydranencephaly, or as a more subtle congenital abnormality of neurocytoarchitecture. Discussion of these entities is beyond the scope of this chapter.

B. **Target organs of perinatal asphyxia and its management** are the brain, heart, lung, kidney, liver, bowel, and bone marrow. In a recent study of asphyxiated newborns [27], 34 percent had no evidence of organ injury, 23 percent had an abnormality confined to one organ, 34 percent involved two organs, and 9 percent affected three organs. The most frequent abnormalities involved the kidney (50 percent), followed by the CNS (28 percent), cardiovascular (25 percent), and pulmonary (23 percent) systems. Often, asphyxiated infants will succumb to dysfunctions of organs other than the CNS (e.g., persistent fetal circulation) while showing minimal evidence of hypoxic-ischemic brain injury. In such instances, the brain was spared at the expense of cardiac output to the affected organ [5]. The degree of asphyxia required to cause permanent neurologic impairment is just below that which is **lethal** from multisystem failure [12].

1. **Hypoxic-ischemic brain injury**
   a. **Pathophysiology. Hypoxic-ischemic brain injury** [3,5,15,28,38] is the most important consequence of perinatal asphyxia. Brief **hypoxia** impairs cerebral oxidative metabolism leading to an increase in lactate, fall in pH, and, given the inefficiency of anaerobic glycolysis to generate ATP, a decrease in high-energy phosphate compounds (first phosphocreatine, then ATP) [3]. The hypoxic brain therefore increases its glucose utilization. Vascular dilation, caused by hypoxia, increases glucose availability for anaerobic glycolysis, but this leads to increased local lactic acid production. The worsening acidosis is ultimately associated with decreased glycolysis, loss of cerebrovascular autoregulation, and diminished cardiac function, which causes local **ischemia** and decreased glucose delivery to the very tissue that has increased its substrate utilization. Local glucose stores therefore become depleted, energy reserves fall further, and accumulated lactic acid remains unremoved. During prolonged hypoxia, more profound cardiac depression occurs (seen as bradycardia), cardiac output falls, cerebral blood flow (CBF) is compromised, and a combined **hypoxic-ischemic insult** produces further failure of oxidative phosphorylation and ATP production. Such energy failure impairs ion pumps (Na^+–K^+ ATPase) with accumulation of Na^+, Cl^-, H_2O, and Ca^{2+} intracellularly and K^+ and excitatory amino acid neurotransmitters (e.g., glutamate, aspartate) extracellularly. The nature of asphyxial damage at the cellular level is presently the subject of intense investigation. Current theories [8] have implicated these **excitotoxic amino acids,** which, through action at glutamate or *N*-methyl-D-aspartate (NMDA) receptors, open ion channels allowing Na^+ and Cl^- to enter a cell, inducing **immediate** neuronal death from the osmolar load. Furthermore, these excitatoxins, by means of direct activation of the NMDA channel (mediated by the phosphoinosotol second messenger system) and/or activation of voltage-dependent Ca^{2+} channels, provoke excessive Ca^{2+} influx, which, in turn, leads to a **delayed** form of neuronal death by (1) activation of undesirable enzyme and second messenger systems (e.g., Ca^{2+}-dependent lipases and proteases), (2) perturbation of mitochondrial respiratory electron chain transport, (3) generation of free radicals and leukotrienes, and (4) depletion of energy stores [28]. Reperfusion of previously ischemic tissue may also promote the formation of excess oxygen free radicals (e.g., superoxide ion, hydrogen peroxide, hydroxyl radical, singlet oxygen), which, when they overwhelm endogenous scavenger mechanisms, may damage cellular lipids, proteins, and nucleic acids and the blood-brain barrier. The degree of hypoxia necessary to produce permanent brain damage in the rat or monkey is close to that which is lethal.

      Grossly, the following lesions may be seen after moderate or severe asphyxia:

      (1) **Focal or multifocal cortical necrosis** (occasionally with cerebral edema) with resultant **cystic encephalomalacia and/or ulegyria** (**attenuation** of depths of sulci), due to loss of perfusion in one or several vascular beds (usually middle cerebral artery) and affecting all cellular elements

      (2) **Watershed infarcts** in boundary zones between cerebral arteries (particularly following severe hypotension) (e.g., (a) **periventricular leukomalacia** in the preterm infant, which reflects poor per-

fusion of periventricular border zones in the centrum semiovale and produces predominantly white matter injury; (b) injury bilaterally to the **parasagittal** superiomedial cortical convexities and subcortical white matter of the term infant; (c) injury to parieto-occipital cortex)

(3) Selective neuronal necrosis, i.e., injury at specific sites to specific cell types (neurons>glia) (e.g., CA_1 region of hippocampus, Purkinje cells of cerebellum, brainstem nuclei)

(4) Necrosis of thalamic nuclei and basal ganglia (status marmoratus), a subtype of selective neuronal necrosis.
The precise pathologic pattern seen in any case is not predictable. However, the longer the asphyxia, the more extensive the involvement. Insults due to **prolonged partial episodes of asphyxia** (e.g., from placental abruption) seem to cause diffuse cerebral (especially cortical) necrosis, while **acute total asphyxia** (e.g., from cord prolapse) seems to spare the cortex and affect primarily brainstem, thalamus, and basal ganglia. In the former instance, seizures and paresis might be expected. In the latter instance, one might see disturbances of consciousness, respiration, heart rate, blood pressure, and temperature control; disorders of tone and reflexes; and cranial nerve palsies. Most cases, however, represent a combination of the two patterns: partial prolonged asphyxia followed by a terminal acute asphyxial event. If diffuse cerebral necrosis and subsequent swelling is severe, increased intracranial pressure (ICP) could theoretically compromise cerebral blood flow (CBF) with further damage to the thalamus and brainstem. Recent data, however, indicate that swelling is an effect from prior, rather than a cause of subsequent, neural damage [9,19] (see **c.7**).

b. The **syndrome of hypoxic-ischemic encephalopathy (HIE)** [5,15,28, 33,38] has a **spectrum of clinical manifestations from mild to severe.** In its most dramatic form, the initial phase lasts about 12 hours after the insult and consists of signs of cerebral dysfunction. The infants are stuporous or comatose, have periodic breathing or irregular respiratory effort (a reflection of bihemispheric dysfunction), are hypotonic, and have lost most complex reflexes (Moro, suck, etc.). They may have roving eye movements while the pupillary responses are intact. Subtle, tonic, or multifocal-clonic seizures occur 6 to 24 hours after the insult in 50 percent of moderate to severely asphyxiated infants. Between 12 and 24 hours there may be apnea requiring respiratory support, reflecting brainstem dysfunction. Severely affected infants have a progressive deterioration in CNS function over 24 to 72 hours following the insult with coma, prolonged apnea, and further brainstem dysfunction (e.g., abnormalities of pupillary reactivity, loss of oculomotor and caloric responses, loss of bulbar function). "Brain death" (see **d**) may ensue between 24 and 72 hours later. In the most severe cases, in which the incidence of death or significant permanent neurologic sequelae is greatest, other organ systems inevitably also display evidence of asphyxial damage. The most striking reduction in blood flow, due to shunting of cardiac output to vital organs, involves the kidneys, particularly the proximal tubule, resulting in acute tubular necrosis. In fact, persistent **oliguria** (<1 ml/kg per hour for the first 36 hours) has recently been found to be significantly associated with severe HIE and poor outcome (90 percent of cases) [26]. This suggests that when the asphyxic insult is severe enough to manifest as persistent oliguria, it is likely the brain also has suffered severe ischemic injury. As previously noted, **the degree of asphyxia required to cause permanent neurologic impairment is just below that which is lethal from multisystem failure.** We also use the **Sarnat clinical stages** to estimate the severity of asphyxial insult to infants more than 36 weeks' gestation [33] (Table 21-9). The sequential appearance and resolution of various transitory clinical signs and their duration over the first 2 postnatal weeks not only indicate the extent and permanence of neurologic impairment but also define clinical categories that have proven fairly accurate for early assessment of prognosis in neonates with HIE [29,29a,33] (e.g., prognosis is good if a neonate does not progress to and/or remain in stage 3 and if total duration of stage 2 is less than 5 days) (see **VI**). Electrodiagnostic tests such as the **electroencephalogram (EEG)** and evoked potentials, in conjunction with these clinical signs, may assist in evaluating and classifying the severity of the damage (see **c.6** and **VI.C**). **Ultrasonic examination** of the brain may reveal hemorrhage (useful in preterm infants) and, less well, the extent of edema (midline shift, ventricular compression). Cranial **computed tomography (CT)** is more useful in assessing the degree of edema, when performed early (2 to 4 days after the insult), and the extent of cerebral injury (encephalomalacia), when performed late (at least 2 to 4 weeks after the insult). There is a correlation between areas of hypodensity and later sequelae in term infants [15]. The CT scan may not be as useful in predicting sequelae in premature infants because the excess water and lower myelin content of the premature brain obscures gray-white differentiation. (In this case, serial ultrasounds may suffice for localizing, for example, periventricular echoes suggestive of periventricular leukomalacia.) CT is useful as well for diagnosing cerebral dysgenesis and malformation and will provide information similar to an ultrasound regarding intracranial bleeding and hydrocephalus. Brain scan with isotope may reveal areas without blood flow [15]. Several studies have documented significant increases ($>$5 IU) in the serum **creatine kinase brain fraction (CK-BB)** at 4 and 10 hours of life (peaking between 6 and 10 days) in asphyxiated infants who ultimately died or developed neurologic sequelae; however, CK-BB also may rise after intraventricular hemorrhage. CK-BB serial determinations were inferior, however, to CT/EEG in prognostic reliability [11].

It should be emphasized that HIE is just one (and not the most common) of a number of etiologies in the differential diagnosis of neurologic dysfunction in the neonate, which also include genetic and structural abnormalities, drugs and toxins, infection, inherited metabolic diseases, trauma, intracranial hemorrhage, and transient homeostatic derangements such as hypoglycemia, hypocalcemia, hyper/hypomagnesemia, hypernatremia, and hypothermia. Asphyxia may be suspected and HIE reasonably included in the differential diagnosis of neonatal coma or neurologic dysfunction if the following have been documented: (1) 5- to 10-minute Apgar score (or, more reliably, 15- to 20-minute Apgar score) less than 3, (2) fetal heart rate of less than 60, (3) prolonged (1 hour) antenatal acidosis, (4) neonatal seizure within the first 24 to 48 hours (though 50 percent of seizures are not asphyxial in character), (5) burst-suppression pattern on EEG, and (6) need for positive-pressure resuscitation greater than 1 minute or greater than 5 minutes until the first cry. Whether **permanent** neurologic sequelae can be **attributed** to HIE is a completely different question and is addressed in **VI.**

c. **Management of hypoxic-ischemic brain injury.** The initial management of hypoxic-ischemic damage in the delivery room is described in Chapter 5. Other specific management consists of supportive care to maintain temperature, perfusion, ventilation, and a normal metabolic state, including glucose, Ca^{2+}, and acid–base balance. Control of seizures is important.

(1) **Oxygen levels** should be kept in the **normal range** by monitoring of transcutaneous or arterial pO_2 or percent O_2 saturation by

pulse oximeter. Hypoxia should be treated with O_2 and/or ventilation. Aminophylline may decrease CBF and should not be used in the initial management of apnea due to asphyxia. Hyperoxia also may cause a decrease in CBF or exacerbate free-radical damage (see also Persistent Pulmonary Hypertension of the Newborn in Chap. 13).

(2) Carbon dioxide should be kept in the **normal range** because hypercapnea may cause cerebral vasodilation, which may cause more flow to uninjured areas with relative ischemia to damaged areas ("steal phenomenon") and extension of infarct size. The excess flow to uninjured areas may furthermore be associated with intracranial hemorrhage (ICH) because of loss of autoregulation of CBF (see Intracranial Hemorrhage above). Excessive hypocapnea may decrease CBF. Hyperventilation is not recommended.

(3) Perfusion. It is important to maintain cerebral perfusion pressure (CPP) within a narrow range. Too little can cause ischemic injury; too much can cause hemorrhage in the areas of damaged blood vessels, with germinal matrix hemorrhage and intraventricular hemorrhage (IVH) in premature infants. Excessive reperfusion of infarcted tissue may cause the infarct to become hemorrhagic because of loss of vascular integrity. Abrupt changes in perfusion and rapid infusions of volume expanders or sodium bicarbonate may be associated with IVH [38]. (There may be a 50 percent decrease in CBF 5 minutes after bicarbonate is administered.) Because cerebrovascular autoregulation is lost, cerebral perfusion entirely reflects systemic blood pressure in a pressure-passive fashion. To maintain cerebral perfusion, a systemic mean arterial pressure (MAP) of 45 to 50 mmHg is usually adequate for term infants, 35 to 40 mmHg for infants weighing 1000 to 2000 gm, and 30 to 35 mmHg for infants weighing less than 1000 gm [9,38]. Conversely, if hypertension develops and persists despite the discontinuation of pressors and the institution of adequate sedation, the systemic blood pressure should **not** be further lowered, since it may be needed to maintain adequate CPP in the face of increased ICP. The following recommendations should be adhered to:

(a) Continuously monitor arterial BP. Continuous central venous pressure monitoring, if possible, (e.g., umbilical venous line with tip in right atrium) to insure there is adequate preload, *i.e.*, that infant is *not* hypovolemic due to vasodilatation or third spacing.

(b) Keep MAP at 45 to 50 mmHg in term infants, 35 to 40 mmHg in 1000- to 2000-gm infants, and 30 to 35 mmHg in $<$1000-gm infants. Keep CVP 5–8 mmHg in term infants and 3–5 mmHg in preterm infants.

(c) Minimize pushes of colloid or sodium bicarbonate, but replace intravascular volume losses as needed to avoid lactic acidosis.

(d) Give volume slowly.

(e) Minimize administered free H_2O (insensible losses plus urine output); however, if urine output is low, first insure that intravascular volume is adequate before fluid restriction.

(f) Judicious use of pressors may help minimize need for colloid in maintaining blood pressure and perfusion.

(g) Monitor ICP if possible.

(4) Glucose (see Neonatal Seizures in Chap. 21). Blood glucose level should be kept at 75 to 100 mg/dl to provide adequate substrate for the brain. Higher levels may lead to (1) elevation of brain lactate, damage to cellular integrity, increased edema and (2) further disturbances in vascular autoregulation [38]. Lower levels may

Table 21-9. Sarnat and Sarnat stages of hypoxic-ischemic encephalopathy (HIE)*

Stage	Stage 1 (mild)	Stage 2 (moderate)	Stage 3 (severe)
Level of consciousness	Hyperalert; irritable	Lethargic or obtunded	Stuporous, comatose
Neuromuscular control:	Uninhibited, overreactive	Diminished spontaneous movement	Diminished or absent spontaneous movement
Muscle tone	Normal	Mild hypotonia	Flaccid
Posture	Mild distal flexion	Strong distal flexion	Intermittent decerebration
Stretch reflexes	Overactive	Overactive, disinhibited	Decreased or absent
Segmental myoclonus	Present or absent	Present	Absent
Complex reflexes:	Normal	Suppressed	Absent
Suck	Weak	Weak or absent	Absent
Moro	Strong, low threshold	Weak, incomplete high threshold	Absent
Oculovestibular	Normal	Overactive	Weak or absent
Tonic neck	Slight	Strong	Absent
Autonomic function:	Generalized sympathetic	Generalized parasympathetic	Both systems depressed
Pupils	Mydriasis	Miosis	Midposition, often unequal; poor light reflex

Respirations	Spontaneous	Spontaneous; occasional apnea	Periodic; apnea
Heart rate	Tachycardia	Bradycardia	Variable
Bronchial and salivary secretions	Sparse	Profuse	Variable
Gastrointestinal motility	Normal or decreased	Increased diarrhea	Variable
Seizures	None	Common focal or multifocal (6 to 24 hours of age)	Uncommon (excluding decerebration)
Electroencephalographic findings	Normal (awake)	Early: generalized low-voltage, slowing (continuous delta and theta) Later: periodic pattern (awake); seizures focal or multifocal; 1.0 to 1.5 Hz spike and wave	Early: periodic pattern with isopotential phases Later: totally isopotential
Duration of symptoms	<24 hours	2 to 14 days	Hours to weeks
Outcome	About 100 percent normal	80 percent normal; abnormal if symptoms more than 5 to 7 days	About 50 percent die; remainder with severe sequelae

*The stages in this table are a continuum reflecting the spectrum of clinical states of infants over 36 weeks' gestational age.

Source: From H. B. Sarnat and M. S. Sarnat, Neonatal encephalopathy following fetal distress: A clinical and electroencephalographic study. *Arch. Neurol.* 33: 696, 1976.

potentiate excitotoxic amino acids and extend infarct size. **Hypoglycemia,** due both to glycogen depletion secondary to catecholamine release and to an unexplained hyperinsulinemic state [9a], is often seen in asphyxiated infants. An initial phase of *hyper*glycemia and hypoinsulinemia (5 to 10 minutes following an acute event, a catecholamine surge inhibits insulin release and stimulates glucagon release, hence glycogenolysis) may be followed within 2 to 3 hours by profound *hypo*glycemia. **Normal glucose infusion rates of 5 to 8 mg/kg per minute may not be sufficient to maintain normoglycemia; rates as high as 9 to 15 mg/kg per minute may be required for short periods.** Because hypoglycemia may be difficult to control without causing fluid overload, concentrated glucose infusions may be necessary by means of a central line (e.g., a "high" umbilical venous line with its tip in the right atrium). Since rapid glucose boluses should be avoided, serum glucose level (via Dextrosticks) should be monitored frequently and adjustments **anticipated.** Glucose infusions should be discontinued slowly to avoid rebound hypoglycemia. **Seizures** may result from hypoglycemia; therefore, if seizures do occur, the possibility of hypoglycemia should be ruled out or treated appropriately before reflexly instituting anticonvulsant therapy (see below). Seizures in such an instance would **not** be used for Sarnat clinical staging.

(5) Temperature should be kept in a **normal range.** Deep hypothermia has not yet proved to be "brain sparing" after asphyxia in humans.

(6) Calcium level should be kept in a normal range. **Hypocalcemia** is a common metabolic alteration in the neonatal postasphyxial syndrome [33]. A subnormal serum Ca^{2+} level will **not** forestall neuronal damage and may only serve to compromise cardiac contractility or cause seizures (see Chap. 24).

(7) Seizures. Seizures should be controlled as described in the section Neonatal Seizures in this chapter. In neonatal HIE, they are typically **focal** or **multifocal** (myelinization and synaptogenesis not having developed sufficiently for generalization of seizures). Seizures occur in about 50 percent of most series [33], characteristically on the first or second day, usually in stage 2, only rarely in stage 3, and almost never in stage 1 (see Sarnat and Sarnat stages, Table 21-9). They may be associated with an increased cerebral metabolic rate, which, in the absence of adequate O_2 and perfusion, may lead to a fall in blood glucose level, an increase in brain lactate level, and a fall in high-energy phosphate compounds. In infants not mechanically ventilated, seizures may be associated with hypoxemia and/or hypercapnia. Abrupt elevations in blood pressure, associated with seizures may contribute to ICH in preterm infants. When seizures are clinically apparent and of typical morphology, an EEG is not necessary to confirm the diagnosis. In infants paralyzed with pancuronium for mechanical ventilation, seizures may be manifested by abrupt changes in blood pressure, heart rate, and oxygenation. An EEG should be obtained in these circumstances. Whether seizures alone, in the absence of metabolic or cardiopulmonary abnormalities, lead to brain injury is controversial [34]. While one should have a low threshold for diagnosing seizures in the setting of HIE, it is no longer felt that asphyxiated infants should be treated prophylactically with anticonvulsants in the absence of clinical seizures (or electrical seizures on EEG in the case of an infant pharmacologically paralyzed). There is actually very little change in ICP during most electrographic seizures [9]. The clinical distinction between multifocal seizures and the "jitteriness" (actually a **rhythmic segmental myoclonus**) seen frequently in stage 1 and even stage 2 HIE is often difficult to make by observation alone. Taking hold of the clonic extremity and changing the tension on the muscle stretch receptor by slightly flexing or extending the joint immediately arrests clonus but does not alter true seizure activity, during which rhythmic convulsive movements continue to be felt in the examiner's hand [33]. When seizures are diagnosed, **phenobarbital,** by convention the first-line drug, should be loaded slowly **20 mg/kg IV to be followed by a maintenance dose of 3 to 5 mg/kg per day.** One should always be vigilant for respiratory depression and/or cardiovascular compromise with hypotension. If the infant is already mechanically ventilated, respiratory depression is not a concern. In non-ICU settings, one may divide the loading dose of phenobarbital, use phenytoin, or leave small, subtle seizures untreated pending transfer to an acute care setting. Phenobarbital, especially at high levels, may itself cause lethargy, stupor, and occasionally brainstem signs. If seizures persist, **phenytoin may be administered slowly as a second drug (20 mg/kg IV loading dose followed by 4 to 5 mg/kg per day maintenance dose).** One should, of course, ascertain that metabolic derangements that may complicate asphyxia and cause seizures have been addressed (e.g., **hypoglycemia, hypocalcemia,** and **hyponatremia**) (see Chap. 24). **Pyridoxine-dependency seizures** and **local anesthetic toxicity** may mimic postasphyxic seizures and should be considered in the differential diagnosis. If seizures nevertheless persist, a **benzodiazepam** (e.g., **lorazepam 0.05 to 0.1 mg/kg per dose IV**) may be given transiently as a third drug. If vascular access cannot be achieved in the non-ICU setting, rectal diazepam, valproate, or paraldehyde may provide a stopgap. (IM phenobarbital is too slowly absorbed and, because it may confound subsequent management, is discouraged.) Seizures in HIE are notoriously difficult to control and often resistant to even aggressive anticonvulsant therapy in the early stages (first 72 hours) of the syndrome. Once levels of conventional anticonvulsants are maximized (phenobarbital to 40 mg/dl, phenytoin to 20 mg/dl), unless there is cardiopulmonary compromise from the seizures, there is often little utility or desirability to eliminating every "twitch" or electrographic seizure [20,34,39]. (There is a growing understanding that even status epilepticus will not extend extant cortical damage or heighten morbidity [20].) For unexplained reasons, even refractory seizures in HIE ultimately "burn themselves out" and cease after approximately 48 hours. **When the infant is stable for 3 to 4 days, all anticonvulsants are weaned except phenobarbital** (the level of which may be allowed to drop to 15 to 20 mg/dl if possible). If seizures have resolved, if the neurologic examination is normal, and if the EEG is normal, anticonvulsants are stopped in the neonatal period (14 days of age). If this is not the case, anticonvulsants are continued for 1 to 3 months. If the neurologic examination is then normal with no recurrent seizures, phenobarbital is tapered over 4 weeks. If the examination is not normal, the advisability of continued anticonvulsant therapy requires consideration of the initial cause of the seizures. The risk of subsequent epilepsy is 100 percent with seizures secondary to cerebral cortical dysgeneses but only 20 to 30 percent after seizures secondary to perinatal asphyxia [39] and essentially nil after seizures secondary to transient metabolic disturbances. Infants with a higher risk of subsequent seizures are those with a persistent neurologic deficit (50 percent risk) and those with an abnormal EEG between seizures (40 percent risk). If the examination is not normal, an EEG is obtained; if there is no electrographic seizure activity, phenobarbital is tapered and discontinued over 4 weeks even with abnormal neurologic signs [39].

(8) Cerebral edema. Devices applied to the anterior fontanel provide noninvasive methods for measuring intracranial pressure (ICP) [9,19,38]. Cerebral edema may be minimized by avoiding fluid overload, although initial resuscitation of an asphyxiated infant and maintenance of cardiovascular stability and cerebral perfusion pressure (cerebral perfusion pressure (CPP) = mean arterial pressure (MAP) minus intracranial pressure (ICP) should always take priority. Two processes may predispose to fluid overload in asphyxiated infants: (1) **syndrome of inappropriate secretion of antidiuretic hormone (SIADH)** (see Chap. 24) and (2) **acute tubular necrosis (ATN)** (see Chap. 26). SIADH, often seen for 3 to 4 days after the insult, is manifested by **hyponatremia** and hypoosmolarity with excretion of an inappropriately concentrated and Na^+-containing urine (elevated urine specific gravity, osmolarity, and Na^+). SIADH should be monitored by daily determinations of serum and urinary Na^+ and osmolarity. Urine output may further be compromised by ATN resulting from shunting of cardiac output away from the kidneys. Persistent oliguria (<1 ml/kg per hour for the first 36 hours of life) has recently been found to provide an index of the severity of asphyxia and risk for neurologic sequelae [26]. **To avoid fluid overload and the exacerbation of cerebral edema, both SIADH and ATN should be managed by limitation of free H_2O administration only to replacement of insensible losses and urine output (usually ~60 ml/kg per day)** (see Fluid and Electrolyte Management of the Newborn in Chap. 24). Before attributing oliguria to SIADH or ATN, rule out prerenal etiologies (hypovolemia, vasodilation) with a 10 to 20 ml/kg fluid challenge followed by a loop diuretic if there is no urine output.

Cerebral edema and increased ICP (>10 mmHg) have actually been determined to be fairly **uncommon** concomitants of perinatal asphyxia [9,19]. When present, they more often reflect extensive prior cerebral necrosis rather than swelling of intact cells, and because they bespeak such extensive cell death, they have a uniformly bad prognosis [19]. They peak 36 to 72 hours after the insult. They are more properly regarded as an **effect** rather than a cause of brain damage. For this reason, one would expect, and indeed the literature has shown, that efforts specifically to reduce cerebral edema or ICP do not affect outcome; neither do ICP elevations reduce cerebral perfusion or introduce any acute functional neurologic disturbances [9,19]. Therefore, such interventions previously explored in the literature as antiedema agents (e.g., high-dose phenobarbital, steroids, mannitol, and other hypertonic solutions) are not employed at our institution. The infant's patent sutures and open fontanel are protective of any acute increases in ICP that might occur [9,19,15]. Our major efforts are devoted to ensuring an adequate cerebral perfusion pressure (CPP) through maintaining an adequate MAP, shown in recent studies to be a more important variable than ICP in ensuring adequate cerebral blood flow (CBF) [9].

(9) Many **brain-sparing, cerebroprotective, and/or infarct-limiting interventions** have been proposed in recent years, many based on the postulated mechanisms of asphyxial damage described earlier (see **a**). Administration of high-dose barbiturates (to decrease cerebral metabolism) and naloxone (for endogenous opioid blockade) have proven ineffective in humans [7,23,31] despite their initial promise in animal models [4,10,14]. Newer possibilities such as (1) antagonists of excitotoxic neurotransmitter receptors [8] (e.g., such NMDA-receptor blockers as dextromethorphan and MK-801), (2) free-radical scavengers [37] (e.g., superoxide dismutase, vitamin E), (3) Ca^{2+} channel blockers [37] (e.g., nifedipine, nicardipine), (4) cyclooxygenase inhibitors (e.g., indomethacin [17]), (5) hypothermia, (6) benzodiazepine receptor stimulation (e.g., midazolam), (7) enhancers of protein synthesis (e.g., dexamethasone), and (8) vasodilators (e.g., prostacyclin), all have a theoretical basis (see **a**), have had conflicting efficacies in experimental animal models, and have not yet undergone any systematic human trials.

d. Brain death in the neonate. In 1987, recommendations for determination of brain death in children and infants more than 7 days of age were proposed by an ad hoc task force committee [1]. The guidelines avoided specific recommendations in infants less than 7 days old, citing lack of published data. Recent data and conclusions from Ashwal et al. [2] have suggested that the current task force guidelines may be extended to include the term infant and the preterm infant greater than 32 weeks' gestation. The clinical diagnosis of brain death is made on the basis of (1) coma, manifested by lack of response to pain, light, or auditory stimulation; (2) apnea, confirmed by documentation of failure to breathe when pCO_2 is greater than 60 mmHg (tested by 3 minutes without ventilator support while continuing 100% O_2 supplementation or for shorter periods if hypotension or bradycardia intervene); (3) absent bulbar movements and brainstem reflexes (including midposition or fully dilated pupils with no response to light or pain and with absent occulocephalic, caloric, corneal, gag, cough, rooting, and sucking reflexes), all normally elicitable by 33 weeks' gestation; and (4) flaccid tone and absence of spontaneous or induced movements (excluding activity mediated at the spinal cord level). If these clinical findings remain unchanged for 24 hours, electrocerebral silence, in the absence of barbiturates (>25 μl/ml), hypothermia (<24°C), or cerebral malformations (e.g., hydranencephaly, hydrocephalus), is confirmatory of brain death. Further, if the initial EEG (done after 24 hours of life) shows electrocerebral silence and the infant remains brain dead for 24 hours, a repeat study is not necessary. Absence of radionuclide uptake (a reliable estimate of CBF) cotemporaneous with initial electrocerebral silence is also associated with brain death. Alternatively, if no radionuclide uptake is demonstrated initially (signifying CBF < 2 mL/min/100 gm) and the infant remains clinically brain dead for 24 hours, a diagnosis of brain death also can be made, even if some EEG activity persists; sensitivity is increased in this regard by repeating the scan in 24 hours and reconfirming no uptake. Term infants clinically brain dead for 2 days and preterm infants brain dead for 3 days do not survive regardless of the EEG or CBF flow status, indicating that determination of brain death in the newborn can be made solely by using clinical criteria over this prolonged period of observation. Therefore, confirmatory neurodiagnostic studies are of value in potentially shortening the period of observation to 24 hours. Phenobarbital levels greater than 25 μg/ml may suppress EEG activity in this age group. The diagnosis of brain death must also be made in the appropriate clinical setting, wherein the cause of coma has been determined and all remediable or reversible conditions eliminated. In isolation, neither EEG alone nor radionuclide flow studies alone are sufficiently sensitive to diagnose brain death; persistent EEG activity and/or prognostically small variations in radionuclide uptake do **not** obviate the diagnosis of brain death in the newborn.

(Unlike in adults or older children, minimal radionuclide uptake may persist in brain-dead neonates, perhaps due to patent sutures, which may moderate acute increases in ICP, which would otherwise diminish CPP to a no-flow state.) Clinical correlation and/or coupled neurodiagnostic studies are necessary. These recommendations take into account all reported cases to date of possible misdiagnosis of brain death. Based on these, the combination of neurologic assessment, an EEG showing electrocerebral silence, and isotope estimation of CBF followed by 24 hours of observation seems valid in deciding that irreversible cessation of brain function has occurred in the preterm and term infant. At present, insufficient information is available to warrant the use of brainstem evoked-response testing for confirmation of brain death in the newborn. In neonates, an additional clinical clue to brain death is a fixed heart rate without decelerations or accelerations. (See Chap. 34 and Table 34-1.)

2. **Cardiac effects of asphyxia** (see Chap. 14)
   a. **Diagnosis.** Infants with perinatal asphyxia may have **transient myocardial ischemia.** These infants usually have had hypoxic stress and 10-minute Apgar scores of less than 4. They develop respiratory distress and cyanosis shortly after birth. They will have signs of congestive heart failure, such as tachypnea, tachycardia, an enlarged liver, and a gallop rhythm. Many infants will have a systolic murmur at the lower left sternal border (**tricuspid regurgitation**), and some will have a murmur at the apex (**mitral regurgitation**). The **chest x-ray** will show cardiomegaly and sometimes pulmonary venous congestion. The **electrocardiogram (ECG)** may show ST depression in the midprecordium and T-wave inversion in the left precordium. A serum **creatine kinase plasma MB isoenzyme** fraction greater than 5 to 10 percent may be present in myocardial damage. The echocardiogram/Doppler will show normal cardiac structures but decreased left ventricular contractions, especially of the posterior wall, and perhaps persistent pulmonary hypertension. It is important to rule out Epstein's disease of the tricuspid valve, pulmonary stenosis, and pulmonary atresia with intact ventricular septum. The ventricular end-diastolic pressures are usually elevated because of poor ventricular function. Some infants will show tricuspid regurgitation with right-to-left shunting at the atrial level. In a recent study of moderately to severely asphyxiated newborns [27], left ventricular (LV) dysfunction occurred in less than 10 percent of infants, while right ventricular (RV) dysfunction was more common (30 percent of infants). Many of these infants will have meconium aspiration syndrome with persistent pulmonary hypertension (see Chap. 13). Of significance, the presence of a fixed heart rate without variation may raise suspicion of clinical brain death.
   b. **Management of the cardiac effects of asphyxia.** The treatment is adequate ventilation with correction of hypoxemia, acidosis, and hypoglycemia. Volume overload must be avoided. (Diuretics may be ineffective if there is concomitant renal failure.) These infants will require continuous monitoring of mean arterial pressure (MAP) (through an arterial line), CVP and mixed venous saturation (possibly through a "high" umbilical venous line in the right atrium), and urine output. Infants with cardiac collapse will require inotropic drugs such as **dopamine** and/or **dobutamine** (see Chap. 6). Some infants in great distress may require afterload reduction with a peripheral beta agonist (e.g., isoproterenol), a peripheral alpha blocker (e.g., phentolamine or tolazoline), or nitroprusside. The prognosis for the heart is good, with most surviving infants having a normal cardiac examination in 3 weeks and a normal ECG in 3 months. If there is severe cardiogenic

shock, the infant usually dies or suffers a severe insult to the brain or other vital organ.

3. **Renal effects of asphyxia.** The asphyxiated infant is at risk for **acute tubular necrosis (ATN)** and for the **syndrome of inappropriate excretion of ADH (SIADH). Urine output, urinalysis, urine specific gravity, and urine and serum osmolarity and electrolytes should be monitored. Measurement of serum and urine creatinine together with serum and urine Na^+** allows calculation of the **fractional excretion of Na^+ (FE_{Na})** and the **renal index** to help confirm a renal insult (see Chapter 26 for diagnosis and management of ATN). Measurement of urinary levels of **beta-2-microglobulin** (B_2), a low-molecular-weight protein freely filtered through the glomerulus and reabsorbed almost completely in the proximal tubule of even immature kidneys, may provide a sensitive indicator of subtle proximal tubular dysfunction [26]. Renal size should be monitored by **ultrasound. Dopamine infusion at 2.5 μg/kg per hour IV may aid renal perfusion.** Oliguria should not be attributed to SIADH or ATN until prerenal etiologies such as hypovolemia or vasodilation have been ruled out (see Chap. 24, Fluid and Electrolyte Management and Chap. 26).
4. **Gastrointestinal effects of asphyxia.** The asphyxiated infant is at risk for bowel ischemia and **necrotizing enterocolitis.** We usually do not feed **severely asphyxiated** infants for 5 to 7 days after the insult (see Chap. 28).
5. **Hematologic effects of asphyxia. Disseminated intravascular coagulation (DIC)** may be seen in asphyxiated infants because of damage to blood vessels. The liver may fail to make clotting factors, and the bone marrow may not produce platelets. Clotting factors (PTT and PT), fibrinogen, and platelets should be monitored and replaced as needed (see Chaps. 17 and 19).
6. **Liver.** The liver may be so damaged (**shock liver**) that it may not provide its basic functions. **Liver function tests** [**transaminases** (SGOT, SGPT), **clotting factors** (PT, PTT, fibrinogen), **albumin, and bilirubin**] should be monitored, and serum **ammonia** level should be measured. Clotting factors should be provided as indicated. Serum **glucose** level should be kept at 75 to 100 mg/dl; glycogen stores have usually been depleted. Drugs that are detoxified by the liver must have their levels monitored closely. If total liver failure occurs, it is usually a bad prognostic sign. The treatment of liver failure is beyond the scope of this text.
7. **Lung.** The pulmonary effects of asphyxia include **increased pulmonary vascular resistance, pulmonary hemorrhage, pulmonary edema** secondary to cardiac failure, and possibly failure of surfactant production with secondary hyaline membrane disease (**Adult respiratory distress syndrome**). Meconium aspiration may be present. Treatment consists of oxygenation and ventilation (and possibly mild alkalinization). The method of ventilation may be different if the primary problem is hyaline membrane disease, persistent pulmonary hypertension, or meconium aspiration (see Chap. 13). Extracorporeal membrane oxygenation (ECMO) provides a recent therapeutic modality in an asphyxiated infant whose CNS appears otherwise intact (see Chap. 13).

VI. **Prognosis of perinatal asphyxia** [6,12,22,29,29a,38]. It is noteworthy that the degree of asphyxia necessary to cause permanent brain damage in experimental animals is quite close to that which causes death [12] (~25 minutes of acute, total asphyxia). Survival with brain damage due to asphyxia is actually uncommon in this model, the extremes of death or intact survival being the most likely outcomes. In humans, too, birth asphyxia severe enough to damage the fetal brain usually kills before or soon after birth. Approximately one-quarter of asphyxiated term newborns will die. The remainder, however, even those with seizures, will overwhelmingly be normal. The only group with significant neurologic impairment will be those who were **severely** asphyxiated yet narrowly escaped death, a relatively small group. Therefore, as in the animal models, death, on one hand, or intact survival, on the other, are more likely outcomes than survival with brain damage. Except in extreme cases where an infant is asphyxiated to near-lethal proportions, if an infant does not die from the asphyxia, then the prognosis is quite favorable for normal neurologic status (including absence of mental retardation and epilepsy) [12].

Given this, no infant will have undergone an asphyxial insult severe enough to cause permanent brain damage without **other organs** being equally severely affected. Thus a diagnosis of asphyxia severe enough to offer a poor prognosis must hinge on **assessment of other systems** in addition to the CNS. A corrollary of this statement is that no neurologic abnormality diagnosed later in childhood (e.g., cerebral palsy) can be ascribed to perinatal asphyxia in the absence of evidence in the perinatal period (including the delivery room) of severe, **multisystemic** asphyxial insult (including severe to moderate HIE with stupor/coma, hypotonia, diminished reflexes, and seizures). Conversely, even when perinatal asphyxia is confirmed, most etiologies of such asphyxia are due **not** to preventable intrapartum events or interventions but to **preexisting,** usually congenital, often subtle (cytoarchitectural) malformations and dysgeneses, neurologic and otherwise [21,25].

A. Outcome [5,6,15,16,20,22,26,27,29,29a,33]. Overall, full-term asphyxiated infants have a mortality of 10 to 20 percent. The incidence of neurologic sequelae in survivors is 20 to 45 percent (approximately 40 percent of these minimal, approximately 60 percent severe); i.e., the **majority will be normal.** Analyzed according to **Sarnat's stages** of severity [33] (Table 21-9), probably a more useful statistic for anticipating outcome for an individual infant, virtually 100 percent of newborns with evidence of mild encephalopathy (stage 1) had normal neurologic outcome; 80 percent of those with moderate encephalopathy (stage 2) were normal neurologically (those who were abnormal exhibiting stage 2 signs over 7 days); and virtually all the children with severe encephalopathy (stage 3) died (one-half) or developed major neurologic sequelae (the other half) (e.g., CP, retardation, epilepsy, microcephaly) [29]. (Preterm infants may have a higher morbidity and mortality at less severe stages because of the high frequency of ICH and problems with other systems.) While the **risk** of cerebral palsy (CP) in the asphyxiated newborn is elevated—5 to 10 percent versus 2 per 1000 in the general population of live births—the actual number is quite small in absolute terms. (Regarding the existence of even subtle school problems among the "neurologically and mentally normal" survivors of HIE, in one study [29a], at 8 years of age, all unimpaired children from the "mild" HIE group and 65 to 82 percent of unimpaired children from the "moderate" HIE group were performing at expected grade level, indistinguishable from a matched peer group.)

The cardiac, renal, gastrointestinal, pulmonary, hepatic, and hematologic problems will usually resolve if the infant survives.

B. Risk of cerebral palsy (CP) [12,21,22,25]. Data from the National Collaborative Perinatal Project (NCPP) and the British National Child Development Study (BNCDS) suggest that perinatal factors of labor and delivery *contribute little to the incidence of mental retardation and seizure.* Only 3 to 13 percent of infants with CP had evidence of intrapartum asphyxia. In support of this assessment is the observation that despite improvements in perinatal care, the incidence of long-term neurologic sequelae has not decreased. The following previously implicated obstetrical events **do not** correlate with CP: oxytocin administration, nuchal cord, midforceps use, and duration of labor. Factors found to be statistically associated with increased risk for development of CP were gestational age less than 32 weeks, fetal heart rate less than 60 beats per minute, breech presentation (although not breech delivery), chorioamnionitis, low placental weight, placental complications, and birth weight less than 2000 gm. Most of these factors, however, reflect preexistent, unpreventable sources of neurologic dysfunction that occur independent of asphyxia but which might also predispose to concomitant asphyxia at birth. (For example, it has recently been postulated that an abnormal CNS may cause otherwise unexplained premature onset of labor and that a fetus with CNS abnormalities might not possess appropriate reflex cardiovascular responses to stress during labor and delivery to ensure proper fetal and placental perfusion [25].) No constant relationship between measures of fetal distress and subsequent long-term neurologic outcome has been demonstrated; i.e., most infants with only **one** of the following predictors do **not** develop CP: meconium staining (98 percent do **not** develop CP), fetal heart rate less than 60 beats per minute (98 percent do **not** develop CP), pH less than 7.1 (no correlation with CP), more than 5 minutes to first cry (98 percent do **not** develop CP), and 10-minute Apgar score less than 3 (83 percent do **not** develop CP). These clearly better reflect clinical status during the perinatal period than they do ultimate long-term outcome. Clustering perinatal events improve prediction of CP; e.g., seizure alone resulted in CP in only 0.13 percent. However, low Apgar score, signs of HIE, and seizures identified a small subgroup in whom the risk for CP was 55 percent. *Most CP, however, is not related to birth asphyxia, and most birth asphyxia does not cause CP.*

C. Indicators of poor outcome. While permanent brain damage from perinatal asphyxia is actually uncommon, are there reliable prognostic indicators of the small subgroup in which this does occur? Within the first 2 weeks of life it is very difficult to offer a prognosis for an individual infant because the present methods of prognostication are so unreliable. Unfavorable signs are (1) severe, prolonged asphyxia [29]; (2) Sarnat stage 3 encephalopathy; (3) seizures of early onset that are difficult to control when accompanied by other signs of asphyxia in multiple systems; (4) elevated ICP (>10 mmHg); (5) persistence of abnormal neurologic signs at discharge (usually for more than 1 to 2 weeks), especially absence of Moro reflex [16]; (6) persistence of extensive hypodensities (cystic encephalomalacia) on CT [3,15] obtained at least 4 weeks after the insult; (7) abnormalities on brain scan [15]; (8) an elevated CK-BB level (>5 IU), although this measure is inferior to CT/EEG in prognostic reliability [11]; and (9) persistent oliguria (<1 ml/kg per hour for the first 36 hours of life) [26]. While a single early Apgar score correlates poorly with acid–base status, which itself correlates poorly with outcome [32], the **extended Apgar score** may help predict outcome. Term infants with Apgar scores of 0 to 3 at 10, 15, and 20 minutes had a mortality of 18, 48, and 59 percent, respectively; in survivors, the CP rates were 5, 9, and 57 percent, respectively [22]. It should be noted that many features of the Apgar score relate to cardiovascular integrity and not neurologic function. (Clearly, if an infant responds in the delivery room by 15 to 20 minutes, it has an excellent chance of being normal; conversely, only a small percentage of infants have a score less than 3 at 20 minutes and survive.) By electrodiagnostic criteria, the neonate with seizures was 50 to 70 times more likely to develop CP than one without seizures; however, more importantly, 70 to 80 percent of infants with neonatal seizures who survived had no CP. Of neonates, however, who required resuscitation (not merely intubation) after 5 minutes of life and subsequently developed seizures, one-half died and almost half the survivors had CP. Simply stated, seizure without depression is not ominous and depression without seizure is not ominous [12,39]. **Background EEG activity** is actually a better indicator of prognosis than ictal patterns per se. Term infants with normal or maturationally delayed interictal EEGs after seizures have an almost 86 percent probability of normal development at 4 years of age. However, interictal background abnormalities such as burst-suppression, low-voltage, or electrocerebral inactivity are associated with poor outcome (30 to 75 percent likelihood) [30]. When EEG records are categorized as of mild, moderate, or marked severity, only markedly abnormal records predict subsequent morbidity or mortality; e.g., 93 percent of neonates with extreme burst-suppression activity had poor outcome [13]. It should be noted that not all neonates who have seizures and later neurologic deficits have those seizures because of asphyxia; often there is concurrent evidence of a metabolic disorder, infec-

tion, or malformation that might predispose to both asphyxia and neurologic deficit. Evoked potentials have not yet proven to be reliable prognosticators [36]. In vivo measurement of decreased high-energy phosphate compounds by phosphorus **magnetic resonance spectroscopy** (i.e., the phosphocreatine: inorganic phosphate ratio or ATP: total phosphorus ratio), indicative of impaired oxidative phosphorylation, may ultimately prove clinically useful as a prognostic tool [3,40]. In a recent prospective study [3] of neonates with significantly reduced ratios, 95 percent died or survived with serious multiple neurologic impairments and had diffuse echodensities on ultrasound. Monitoring CPP by Doppler in the asphyxiated infant may prove of benefit in prognostication. Despite initial enthusiasm that magnetic resonance imaging (MRI) (especially T_1-weighted images) may prove better than CT's anatomic definition of ischemic lesions at an earlier stage, preliminary prospective studies [6a] now suggest that the high water content of the neonatal brain may preclude such detection, indicating very limited clinical usefulness presently, in the neonatal period, for this expensive neuroimaging modality.
In perinatal cardiac arrest, several studies have indicated that if the heartbeat is back within 5 minutes and if the baby is breathing regularly and spontaneously within 30 minutes, the prognosis is good. If this is not the case, the outcome is poor [35].

D. Clinical manifestations of neurologic sequelae. The precise neurologic sequelae one will see following a severe asphyxic insult will reflect the location, identity, and extent of the neural cellular population affected. **Cerebral palsy (CP)** is a nonprogressive motor and/or postural deficit of early onset. The specific types—**pyramidal,** i.e., **spastic quadriplegia** commonly associated with **mental retardation** and **epilepsy; spastic diplegia** (more common in premies) or **hemiplegia; extrapyramidal** (including **dystonic** and **choreoathetoid** types)—are determined by the topography of brain injury. Mixed varieties exist. Focal or multifocal **cortical necrosis,** especially in the distribution of the middle cerebral artery, usually at the depths of sulci, may lead to **pyramidal CP** (unilateral or bilateral spastic hemiplegia or quadriplegia), **focal seizures,** and **mental retardation,** depending on the extent of the damage. A **boundary zone infarct** in a term newborn involving predominantly the parasagittal cortical regions (a watershed between the anterior, middle, and posterior cerebral arteries) may be recognized as weakness of the shoulder girdle and proximal upper extremities. **Auditory, visual-spatial,** or **language** difficulties probably reflect more extensive **parasagittal injury** more laterally and posteriorly in the border zones of the parietal-occipital lobe. In the initially preterm infant, **spastic diplegia** probably represents an ischemic cystic lesion in watershed zones of the periventricular white matter at the angles of the ventricle superior to the germinal matrix (**periventricular leukomalacia**); concomitant **visual impairment** suggests involvement of the optic radiations as well. **Extrapyramidal CP** is probably the long-term clinical correlate of *necrosis* of the basal ganglia and thalamus (**status marmoratus**).

Perinatal Asphyxia

1. Ad Hoc Task Force on Brain Death in Children. *Pediatrics* 80: 298, 1987.
2. Ashwal, S., et al. *Pediatrics* 84: 429, 1989.
3. Azzopardi, D. *Pediatr. Res.* 25: 445, 1989.
4. Baskin, D. S., et al. *J. Neurosurg.* 64: 99, 1986.
5. Brann, A. W. *Pediatr. Clin. North Am.* 33: 451, 1986.
6. Brown, J. K. *Dev. Med. Child Neurol.* 16: 567, 1974.
6a. Byrne, P., et al. *J. Pediatr.* 117: 694, 1990.
7. Chernick, V., et al. *J. Pediatr.* 113: 519, 1988.
8. Choi, D. W. *Trends Neurosci.* 11: 465, 1988.
9. Clancy, R., et al. *Am. J. Dis. Child.* 142: 740, 1988.
9a. Collins, J. E., et al. *Lancet* 1: 311, 1984.

10. Espinoza, M., et al. *Am. J. Physiol.* 256: R1063, 1989.
11. Fernandez, et al. *Acta Paediatr. Scand.* 76: 914, 1987.
12. Freeman, J. M., et al. *Pediatrics* 82: 240, 1988.
13. Grigg-Damberger, M. *Pediatr. Neurol.* 5: 84, 1989.
14. Hartung, J., and Cottrell, J. E. *Anesth. Analg.* 66: 47, 1987.
15. Hill, A., et al. *Clin. Perinatol.* 16: 435, 1989.
16. Ishikawa, T., et al. *Brain Dev.* 1: 48, 1987.
17. Johshita, H., et al. *Stroke* 20: 788, 1989.
18. Low, J. A. *Am. J. Obstet. Gynecol.* 159: 1235, 1988.
19. Lupton, B. A., et al. *Pediatrics* 82: 139, 1988.
19a. MacDonald, H. M. *J. Pediatr.* 96: 898, 1980.
20. Maytal, J., et al. *Pediatrics* 83: 323, 1989.
21. Naeye, R. L., et al. *Am. J. Dis. Child.* 143: 1154, 1989.
22. Nelson, K. B., et al. *N. Engl. J. Med.* 315: 81, 1986.
23. Nussbaum, E., et al. *Pediatrics* 81: 630, 1988.
24. Ohlsson, A., et al. *Am. J. Obstet. Gynecol.* 157: 443, 1987.
25. Painter, M. J. *Pediatr. Neurol.* 5: 137, 1989.
26. Perlman, J. M., et al. *J. Pediatr.* 113: 875, 1988.
27. Perlman, J. M., et al. *Am. J. Dis. Child.* 143: 617, 1989.
28. Raichle, M. E. *Ann. Neurol.* 13: 2, 1983.
29a. Robertson, C. M. T., et al. *J. Pediatr.* 114: 753, 1989.
29. Robertson, C., et al. *Dev. Med. Child Neurol.* 4: 473, 1985.
30. Rowe, R. J., et al. *Electroencephalogr. Clin. Neurophysiol.* 60: 183, 1985.
31. Ruth, V., et al. *J. Pediatr.* 112: 81, 1988.
32. Ruth, V. J., et al. *Br. Med. J.* 297: 24, 1988.
33. Sarnat, H. B., et al. *Arch. Neurol.* 33: 696, 1976.
34. Scher, M. S., et al. *Pediatr. Clin. North Am.* 36: 281, 1989.
35. Steiner, H. *Arch. Dis. Child.* 50: 696, 1975.
36. Stockard, J. E., et al. *Arch. Neurol.* 40: 360, 1983.
37. Thiringer, K., et al. *Pediatr. Res.* 22: 62, 1987.
38. Volpe, J. J. Hypoxic-Ischemic Encephalopathy. In *Neurology of the Newborn,* 2d Ed. Philadelphia: Saunders, 1987. P. 209.
39. Volpe, J. J. *Pediatrics* 84: 422, 1989.
40. Young, R. S. K., et al. *Pediatr. Res.* 20: 581, 1986.

Neural Tube Defects

Lawrence C. Kaplan

I. Definitions and pathology. Neural tube defects (NTDs) comprise one of the most common groups of congenital malformations in newborns, accounting in some centers for over one third of all admissions of children with multiple congenital anomaly syndromes. They represent, however, a heterogeneous group of disorders based on such factors as embryologic timing and the involvement of specific elements of the neural tube and its derivatives [7,9,14]. A recent review of neural tube defects can be found in ref. 19.

A. Types of neural tube defects

1. Primary neural tube defects. These constitute approximately 95 percent of all neural tube defects. They are due to primary failure of closure of the neural tube or possibly disruption of an already closed neural tube between 18 and 28 days' gestation. The resulting abnormality usually consists of two anatomic lesions: an exposed (open or *operta*) neural placode along the midline of the back caudally and, rostrally, the Arnold-Chiari II malformation (malformation of pons and medulla, downward displacement of cerebellum, and fourth ventricle), with aqueductal stenosis and hydrocephalus [20]. On the most severe end of the spectrum is craniorasischisis and anencephaly. The latter is always incompatible with life [15]. Among primary neural tube defects are included the following:

a. **Meningomyelocele.** This is the most common primary neural tube defect. It involves a saccular outpouching of neural elements (neural placode), typically through a defect in the bone and the soft tissues of the posterior thoracic, lumbar, or sacral regions. Structural abnormalities often extend the length of the central nervous system and include hydromyelia, abnormalities of the corpora quadrigemina, the corpus callosum, third and lateral ventricles, and the gyral patterns of the cerebral hemispheres. Hydrocephalus occurs in 84 percent of these children; Arnold-Chiari II malformation occurs in approximately 90 percent. Dura and arachnoid are typically included in the sac (meningo-), which contains visible neural structures (myelo-), and the skin is usually discontinuous over the sac [12].

b. **Encephalocele.** Occipitally, cervically, and more rarely frontally, an outpouching of dura with or without brain. This may vary in size from a few millimeters to many centimeters.

c. **Anencephaly.** In its most severe form, the cranial vault and posterior occipital bone are defective and derivatives of the neural tube are exposed, including both brain and bony tissue. The defect usually extends through the foramen magnum and involves the brainstem.

2. **Secondary neural tube defects.** Five percent of all neural tube defects are secondary neural tube defects resulting from abnormal development of the caudal cell mass late or following primary neural tube closure. This leads to defects primarily in the lumbosacral spinal region. These heterogeneous lesions rarely are associated with hydrocephalus or the Arnold-Chiari II malformation, and the skin is typically intact over the defect [9,12].

a. **Meningocele.** An outpouching of skin and dura without obvious involvement of the neural elements. Bone and contiguous soft-tissue abnormalities may nonetheless occur.

b. **Lipomeningocele.** A lipomatous mass usually in the lumbar or sacral region, occasionally occurring off the midline and typically covered with full-thickness skin. Adipose tissue frequently extends through the defect into the spine and dura and typically adheres extensively to a distorted spinal cord or nerve roots.

c. **Sacral agenesis/dysgenesis, diastematomyelia, myelocystocele.** These and others all may involve varying degrees of bony involvement. While rarely as extensive as primary neural tube defects, neurologic manifestations may be present representing distortion or abnormal development of peripheral nerve structures. These lesions may be inapparent on surface examination (occulta) of the child.

B. **Epidemiology, pathoetiology, and prevention.** In the United States, the overall frequency of neural tube defects is 1 in 2000 live births, and this appears to be decreasing. A well-established increased incidence is known among individuals living in parts of Ireland and Wales (4.2 to 12.5 per 1000), which carries over to descendants of these individuals who live elsewhere in the world [8,18]. This also may be true for other ethnic groups, including Sikh Indians and certain groups in Egypt. The exact cause of failed neural tube closure remains an unknown. Over 95 percent of all neural tube defects occur to couples with no known family history. Etiologies proposed for both primary and secondary neural tube defects are heterogeneous and include such **known** factors as maternal alcohol, aminopterin, thalidomide ingestion, maternal diabetes, prenatal x-irradiation, as well as amniotic band disruption and such **suspected** factors and associations as maternal hyperthermia; hallucinogen, trimethadione, and valproate ingestion; and prenatal exposure to rubella. Both dominant and recessive mendelian inheritance have been documented, and neural tube defects can occur in trisomy 18, triploidy, and Meckel's syndrome, as well as other chromosome disorders. Both zinc and folic acid deficiencies have been proposed as possible etiologies [12]. Controlled, randomized clinical studies of prenatal multivitamin administration to mothers with prior affected offspring suggest a lower recurrence risk than in control groups [16]. The heterogeneity of neural tube defects in particular warrants caution, however, in proposing single or multivitamins as a prevention of these congenital malformations. Primary neural tube defects carry an increased empiric recurrence risk of 1 in 33 for couples with one affected pregnancy and 1 in 10 for those with two affected pregnancies. Affected individuals have a 1 in 25 risk of having one offspring with a primary neural tube defect. Sisters of women with an affected child have a 1 in 100 risk, and sisters of a man with an affected child have a 1 in 300 risk. Brothers of a parent with an affected child have a 1 in 500 risk. Secondary neural tube defects are generally sporadic and carry no increased recurrence risk. In counseling families for recurrence, however, a careful history of drug exposure and/or family history is critical [3].

II. Diagnosis

A. Prenatal diagnosis. This has been greatly enhanced by the combined use of maternal serum alpha fetoprotein (AFP) determinations and prenatal ultrasound, as well as AFP determinations on amniotic fluid where indicated. Maternal serum AFP measured in the second trimester will diagnose 90 percent of fetuses with encephalocele and 80 percent of those with open meningomyelocele. The exact timing of the sample is critical, however. An ultrasound will assist in the assessment of ventricle size and other congenital anomalies, as well as to help confirm the suspected prenatal diagnosis. Prognosis based on prenatal ultrasound remains difficult, however, except in obvious cases of encephalocele or anencephaly [4,11] (see Chap. 3).

B. Postnatal diagnosis. With the exception of some secondary neural tube defects, the diagnosis of most neural tube defects, especially meningomyelocele, is immediately obvious at birth. Sacular masses occasionally confused with these, however, include sacrococcygeal teratomas. These usually occur in the low sacrum.

III. Evaluation

A. History. A detailed family history should be obtained, asking about the occurrence of not only neural tube defects, but also other congenital anomalies or malformation syndromes.

B. Physical examination. A thorough physical examination, including a neurologic examination, is important. Portions of the examination likely to be abnormal are as follows:

1. **General newborn assessment.** Without exception, all newborns with neural tube defects should be evaluated for the presence of congenital heart disease, renal malformation, and structural defects of the airway, GI tract, ribs, and hips. While rare in primary neural tube defects, these can be encountered in the course of subspecialty evaluation and should be at least **considered** before beginning surgical treatment or before discharge from the hospital [6]. In addition, an ophthalmologic examination and hearing evaluation should be planned during the hospitalization or following discharge.
2. **Back.** Inspect the defect and note whether or not it is leaking cerebrospinal fluid (CSF). A sterile glove should be used if a leaking sac is to be touched. In most circumstances, touching the back is not necessary for anyone except the neurosurgeon. The location, shape, and size of the defect should be noted. The size of the cutaneous defect or thin "parchment-like" skin should be observed, although it has little relation to the size of the sac. Often the sac is deflated and has a wrinkled appearance. It is important to note the curvature of the spine and the presence of bony gibbous underlying the defect. Occasionally, there is more than one meningomyelocele in the same child.
3. **Head.** The head circumference should be recorded and plotted daily throughout the first hospitalization. At birth, some infants will have mac-

rocephaly due to hydrocephalus, and still more will develop hydrocephalus after the defect on the back is closed.

4. **Intracranial pressure (ICP).** The ICP can be assessed by palpating the anterior fontanel and tilting the head forward until the midportion of the anterior fontanel is flat. The fontanels may be quite large and the calvarial bones widely separated. (See Intercranial Hemmorrhage, page 381.)
5. **Eyes.** Abnormalities in conjugate movement of the eyes are common and include esotropias, esophorias, and abducens paresis.
6. **Lower extremities.** Look for deformities and evidence of muscle weakness. Abnormalities in the lower extremities, some representing deformations, are common [5,6]. Look at thigh positions and skin folds for evidence of congenital dislocation of the hips. Dislocation of the hips can be diagnosed clinically and by ultrasound (see Chap. 23).
7. **Neurologic examination.** Observe the child's spontaneous activity and response to sensory stimuli in all extremities. Predicting ambulation and muscle strength based on the "level" of the neurologic deficit can be misleading, and very often the anal reflex, or "wink," will be present at birth and absent postoperatively owing to spinal shock and edema. Repeating neurologic examinations at periodic intervals will be more helpful to predict functional outcome than a single newborn examination. Similarly, sensory examination of the newborn can be misleading because of the potential absence of motor response to pinprick. Deep tendon reflexes should be carefully examined (see Table 21-10).
8. **Bladder and kidneys.** Bladder function should be observed, and particular attention should be given to the possibility of inadequate emptying. Examination should include palpating the abdomen for evidence of kidney enlargement. Observe the pattern of urination, and check the child's response to Credé's maneuver by monitoring residual urine in the bladder [1].

IV. Consultation. The care of infants with neural tube defects requires the coordinated efforts of a number of medical and surgical specialists as well as specialists in nursing, physical therapy, and social service. If follow-up is to be by means of a myelodysplasia team, certain protocols may be followed. If not, the following specialties represent the areas needing careful assessment:

A. Specialty consultations

1. **Neurosurgery.** The initial care of the child with a neural tube defect is predominantly neurosurgical. The neurosurgeon is responsible for both assessment and surgical closure of the defect as well as control and treatment of elevated intracranial pressure.
2. **Pediatrics.** A thorough evaluation before surgical procedures are started is important, particularly for the purpose of detecting other abnormalities that might influence surgical risk.
3. **Clinical genetics.** A complete dysmorphology evaluation and genetic counseling should begin during the first hospitalization and be followed up in outpatient visits.
4. **Urology.** A urologist should be consulted early, preferably on the day of birth, because of the risk of obstructive urophathy presenting as early as the first few days of life.
5. **Orthopedics.** Initial assessment of musculoskeletal abnormalities and long-term management of such issues as ambulation, seating, and spine stability are typically responsibilities of a pediatric orthopedic surgeon. Clubfeet frequently encountered in the newborn period should be assessed and may be managed during this hospitalization.
6. **Physical therapy.** A thorough muscle examination should be done as early as possible, and physical therapists should be involved in planning for outpatient physical therapy programs.
7. **Social service.** A social worker familiar with the special needs of children with neural tube defects should meet the parents as early as possible. Children with meningomyelocele may require a considerable amount of

parents' time and resources, thereby placing considerable strain on parents and siblings.

B. Diagnostic tests. The following tests should be done on most children with meningomyelocele during the first hospitalization. Scheduling these tests will vary depending on each situation.

1. **Radiographs**
   a. **Chest.** Rib deformities are common; cardiac malformations also may be identified.
   b. **Spine.** Abnormalities in vertebral bodies, absent or defective posterior arches, and evidence of kyphosis are common [6].
   c. **Hips.** Evidence of dysplasia of hips is common, and some children with neural tube defects are born with dislocated hips. As noted, an ultrasound of the hips can be very helpful to the orthopedic surgeon (see Chap. 23).
2. **Serum creatinine** should be considered if voiding patterns appear initially abnormal. Occasionally, potassium may be elevated in the nonvoiding newborn.
3. **Urodynamic study.** This should be done early in the hospitalization or shortly after discharge to document the status of bladder and urinary sphincter function and innervation and to serve as a basis for comparison later in life [1].
4. **Intravenous pyelogram (IVP).** This will provide detailed information about urinary tract anatomy.
5. **Ultrasound of the urinary tract** is useful to assess possible hydronephrosis and/or structural abnormalities of the upper urinary tract.
6. **Voiding cystourethrogram** is considered if there is an abnormality seen on IVP or urodynamic study or in the setting of a rising serum creatinine level.
7. **Computed tomography (CT) of the head** is usually not necessary before the defect on the back is repaired but generally should be done soon thereafter, even if there is no clinical evidence of hydrocephalus. If ultrasonography is available and can accurately evaluate the presence of hydrocephalus, this may be a useful alternative to an initial CT. Magnetic resonance imaging (MRI) is particularly valuable in assessment of the posterior fossa and syringomyelia but should not necessarily replace CT or ultrasound in the initial assessment period.

V. Selection of an approach to caring for children with neural tube defects

A. Initial general approach. Regardless of the management plan ultimately undertaken, every child with neural tube defects should receive well-planned and consistent care that respects their need for nutrition, comfort, and dignity and honors the right of parents to participate in all decisions regarding that care, including the right to withhold aggressive surgical management. Prognostic criteria, if considered, should guide discussion **not** replace the dialogue that is necessary between parent and care providers. In our experience, discussing "quality of life" is not helpful unless descriptions of possible outcome in concrete and understandable terms based on clinical data are included in that discussion. Parents almost always prefer to hear detail in initial discussions, especially regarding cognitive and functional prognosis. An informed recommendation by a clinician central in the child's care can provide a basis for more frank dialogue but should be made as an entry into discussion [13].

B. Specific selection of care

1. **Supportive care.** This implies no surgical repair of the back or placement of a ventriculoperitoneal shunt but includes nurturing, feeding on demand, and consideration of the child's comfort. The child may die of infection of the open lesion not treated with antibiotics or of complications from hydrocephalus or other congenital malformations. If death appears inevitable, care should be exercised not to prolong undue suffering with such interventions as ventilator support, pressors, etc. Survival without surgery may occur for months or even years. In children who stabilize

(e.g., complete epithelialization of the spinal defect), periodic reassessment of treatment options becomes critical, as does discussion with family. Acceptable options to consider may in fact include placement of a ventriculoperitoneal shunt to arrest progressive hydrocephalus, referral for foster and adoptive care, and alternative feeding techniques.

2. **Aggressive care.** The goal here is habilitation and planning intervention as completely as possible to prevent any further injury to the central nervous system or to prevent morbidity secondary to complications of bladder and bowel dysfunction and progressive orthopedic deformity.
3. **Ethical considerations.** Many physicians, nurses, and other nonmedical personnel hold strong opinions on the treatment of infants born with neural tube defects. Certain concepts need to be considered, especially if selection criteria enter into discussions. Early surgery permits survival of increased numbers of patients with neural tube defects, and most centers cite advances in medical technology and certain societal changes as contributing factors to this. It has been the practice at our institution to identify risk factors that will likely contribute to poor outcome, but not to base management decisions on any set protocol or scoring system. Consulting a hospital ethics committee is recommended to guide in decision making and to help establish a forum to discuss various opinions and treatment options [10,13,21].

VI. Management

A. Initial. The very thin sac is often leaking at birth. The newborn should be kept in the prone position with a sterile saline-moistened gauze sponge over the defect. This reduces bacterial contamination and damage related to dehydration. Intravenous antibiotics (ampicillin and gentamicin) should be administered to diminish the risk of meningitis, particularly that due to group B *Streptococcus*. Children with an open spinal defect can receive a massive inoculation directly into the nervous system at the time of vaginal delivery or even in utero if the placental membranes rupture early. Meningitis is a particularly devastating complication.

B. Surgical treatment. The initial neurosurgical treatment of an open meningomyelocele consists of (1) closing the defect to prevent infection and (2) reducing the elevated intracranial pressure [22]. The back should be closed on the first day of life or as soon thereafter as safely possible to minimize bacterial contamination and the risk of infection. Techniques are available to close rapidly even very large cutaneous defects without skin grafting. Intracranial hypertension can be initially controlled by continuous ventricular drainage (CVD). Typically, once the back is sealed, a ventriculoperitoneal shunt catheter can be placed. Some neurosurgeons may elect to insert the catheter at the time of back closure. If a shunt is to be placed as a second procedure after back closure, careful monitoring of head circumference should be done because intracranial pressure often increases following closure of the back in unshunted patients.

Children whose defect is covered with skin and whose nervous system is therefore not at risk of bacterial contamination can be repaired electively. This may be done at 1 month of age or much later.

C. Parents. Parents must be kept accurately informed of their child's condition. The involvement of multiple specialists heightens the importance of the identification of a primary care provider to coordinate the flow of information [17].

VII. Prognosis

A. Survival. Owing in a large part to various interventions, nearly all children with neural tube defects, even those severely affected, can survive for many years. At the Children's Hospital in Boston, the overall 1-year survival of children admitted with meningomyelocele is 96 percent, and the 10-year survival is 90 percent (computed by life-table technique) [22]. Most deaths occur in the most severely affected children, but sudden infant death syndrome (SIDS) is more common in children with meningomyelocele than in the general population. If children born with spina bifida are approached as if survival is ex-

Table 21-10. Correlation between segmental innervation; motor, sensory, and sphincter function; reflexes; and ambulation potential

Lesion	Segmental innervation	Cutaneous sensation	Motor function	Working muscles	Sphincter function	Reflex	Potential for ambulation
Cervical/ thoracic	Variable	Variable	None	None	—	—	Poor even in full braces
Thoracolumbar	T12	Lower abdomen	None	None	—	—	
	L1	Groin	Weak hip flexion	Iliopsoas	—	—	Full braces, long-term ambulation unlikely
	L2	Anterior upper thigh	Strong hip flexion	Iliopsoas and sartorius	—	—	
Lumbar	L3	Anterior distal thigh and knee	Knee extension	Quadriceps	—	Knee jerk	
	L4	Medial leg	Knee flexion and hip abduction	Medial hamstrings	—	Knee jerk	May ambulate with braces and crutches
Lumbosacral	L5	Lateral leg and medial knee	Foot dorsiflexion and eversion	Anterior tibial and peroneals	—	Ankle jerk	Ambulate with or without short leg braces
	S1	Sole of foot	Foot plantar flexion	Gastrocnemius, soleus, and posterior tibial	—	Ankle jerk	
Sacral	S2	Posterior leg and thigh	Toe flexion	Flexor hallucis	Bladder and rectum	Anal wink	
	S3	Middle of buttock	—	—	Bladder and rectum	Anal wink	Ambulate without braces
	S4	Medial buttock	—	—	Bladder and rectum	Anal wink	

Source: From M. J. Noetzel, Mylomeningocele: Current concepts of management. *Clin. Perinatol.* 6: 318, 1984.

pected, then survival is high. On the contrary, withholding the medical care as part of the program of "selection" will result in lower survival.

B. Motor and intellectual outcome

1. **Motor outcome.** This depends more on a level of paralyses, motivation, and surgical intervention than it does on congenital hydrocephalus. Motor progress is likely to be delayed in most children with neural tube defects, but this can be modified to some degree by appropriate bracing, physical therapy interventions, and monitoring and treatment of **kyphosis** and scoliosis. In addition, such factors as obesity, frequent hospitalizations, tethering of the spinal cord, and decubitus ulcers can contribute to motor delays [12,13]. Table 21-10 is a rough guide to motor, sensory, and sphincter function and ambulation potential.
2. **Intellectual outcome.** Three identifiable subgroups are at risk for mental retardation: (1) those with severe hydrocephalus at birth, (2) those who develop infection in the central nervous system early in life, and (3) those whose intracranial hypertension is not properly controlled. True mental retardation is encountered most commonly in children who have high thoracic level lesions, a history of CNS infection, and hydrocephalus with less than 1 cm of cortical mantle. Formal developmental testing is critical, since visual/perceptual deficits and fine motor difficulties may interfere with intellectual functioning. In addition, complex partial seizures can contribute to impaired intellectual function and should be considered in children, especially school-age children who have lost cognitive milestones. For children whose spinal lesions are at L3 or lower, completion of twelfth grade or beyond has been reported in 85 percent. Overall, the developmental needs of children with neural tube defects should not be discounted. These children require educational and social supports throughout life.

C. Morbidity. The number of hospitalizations, days in the hospital, and the number of operations required are much lower for children with sacral-level lesions and much higher for those with thoracic lesions. Of 132 children consecutively admitted to the Children's Hospital of Boston for whom outcome is known beyond 2 years of age, 12 percent have a "normal" gait, 7 percent have an abnormal gait but require no braces, 38 percent require braces, and 16 percent are only able to sit. For children over 4 years of age, 18 percent have "normal" bladder function, 21 percent receive intermittent catheterization, 42 percent void by Credé's maneuver, and 19 percent have an ileal conduit. In 45 percent of the children over 4 years old, bowel function is reported by parents to be acceptable, and 49 percent report chronic bowel dysfunction, including encopresis. For children over 5 years of age, 45 percent attend regular public schools, and 89 percent of these are felt to be at grade level. Of the 132 children with mylomeningocele, 86 percent live at home with the parents and 4.6 percent live in a skilled nursing facility. Approximately 5 percent of newborns with open neural tube defects develop symptoms related to the Arnold-Chiari II malformation. These pontomedullary symptoms include stridor, ophthalmoplegia, apnea, abnormal gag, and vomiting (often confused with gastroesophageal reflex). These symptoms may all indicate shunt malfunction and frequently disappear without treatment. If they persist, especially in association with cyanosis, the prognosis is poor, with the risk of respiratory failure and death [2]. Posterior fossa decompression and cervical laminectomy are surgical options but are often not successful interventions.

References

1. Bauer, S. B., et al. *J. Urol.* 128: 102, 1982.
2. Charney, E. B., et al. *J. Pediatr.* 111: 364, 1987.
3. Cowchock, S., et al. *Am. J. Med. Genet.* 5: 309, 1980.

4. Crandall, B. F., et al. *Prevention of Neural Tube Defects: The Role of Alpha-Fetoprotein*. New York: Academic Press, 1978.
5. Graham, J. M. *Smith's Recognizable Patterns of Human Deformation*. Philadelphia: Saunders, 1988.
6. Kaplan, L. C. Evaluation of the child with congenital anomalies. In Rubin, I. L. and Crocker, A. C. (Eds.), *Developmental Disabilities: Medical Care for Children and Adults*. Philadelphia, PA: Lea and Febiger, 1989.
7. Khoury, M. J., et al. *Am. J. Epidemiol.* 115: 538, 1982.
8. Laurence, K. M., et al. *Br. J. Prevent. Soc. Med.* 22: 146, 1968.
9. Lemire, R. J., et al. *Normal and Abnormal Development of the Human Nervous System*. Hagerstown, Md.: Harper & Row, 1975.
10. Lorber, J. *J. Med. Ethics* 7: 120, 1981.
11. Macri, J. N., et al. *Obstet. Gynecol.* 59: 633, 1982.
12. McLaughlin, J. F., et al. *J. Perinatol.* 4: 3, 1984.
13. McLaughlin, J. F., et al. *N. Engl. J. Med.* 312: 1589, 1985.
14. Melnick, M., et al. *Am. J. Med. Genet.* 26: 783, 1987.
15. Melnick, M., et al. *Am. J. Med. Genet.* 26: 797, 1987.
16. Mills, J. D. *N. Engl. J. Med.* 321: 430, 1989.
17. Myers, G. J., et al. *A Guide for Helping the Child with Spina Bifida*. Springfield, Ill.: Thomas, 1981.
18. Naggan, L., et al. *N. Engl. J. Med.* 277: 1119, 1967.
19. Noetzal, M. J. *Clin. Perinatol.* 16: 311, 1989.
20. Sieben, R. L., et al. *Neurology* 21: 673, 1971.
21. Tew, B., et al. *Dev. Med. Child Neurol.* 27: 606, 1985.
22. Winston, K. R. *J. Pediatr. Surg.* 13: 303, 1978.

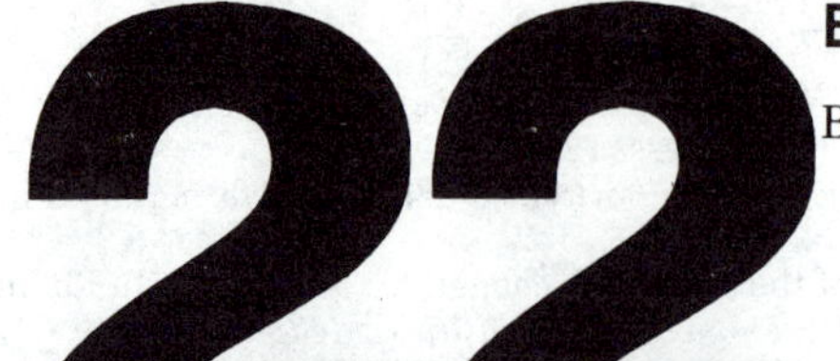

22 Birth Trauma

Brian S. Bradley

I. **Background.** Injuries to the infant resulting from mechanical forces (such as compression or traction) during parturition are grouped under the term **birth trauma.** Factors responsible for mechanical injury may coexist with hypoxic-ischemic insult, and one may predispose the infant to the other.

A. **Incidence.** Between 1970 and 1985, infant mortality resulting from birth trauma fell from 64.2 to 7.5 deaths per 100,000 live births, a remarkable decline of 88 percent [7,8]. This decrease reflects, in part, the technological capability of today's obstetrician to recognize birth trauma risk factors by ultrasound and fetal monitoring prior to attempting a vaginal delivery and the increasing avoidance of potentially injurious instrumentation such as midforceps rotation or vacuum extraction. The accepted alternative has become the cesarean section delivery.

B. **Risk factors.** The process of birth is a blend of compressions, contractions, torques, and tractions. When fetal size, presentation, or neurologic immaturity complicate this event, such intrapartum forces may lead to tissue damage, edema, hemorrhage, or fracture in the neonate. The use of obstetrical instrumentation may further amplify the effect of such forces or may induce injury by itself. Although breech presentation carries the greatest risk of injury, delivery by cesarean section does not guarantee an injury-free infant. The following are associated with an increased risk of birth injury:

1. **Primiparity**
2. **Small maternal stature**
3. **Maternal pelvic anomalies**
4. **Prolonged or extremely rapid labor**
5. **Deep transverse arrest** of descent of presenting part of fetus
6. **Oligohydramnios**
7. **Abnormal presentation** (i.e., breech)
8. **Use of mid-forceps** or vacuum extraction
9. **Versions and extraction**
10. **Very low birth weight infant** or **extreme prematurity**
11. **Fetal macrosomia**
12. **Large fetal head**
13. **Fetal anomalies**

C. **Evaluation.** Recognition of trauma at birth necessitates a careful physical and neurologic examination of the infant to establish whether additional injuries exist. This is also essential in any infant who requires resuscitation in the delivery room when injury may be secretly responsible. Symmetry of structure and function should be assessed as well as such specifics as the cranial nerve examinations, individual joint range of motion, and scalp/skull integrity.

II. **Types of birth trauma**

A. **Head and neck injuries**

1. **Associated with fetal monitoring**

a. **Fetal scalp blood sampling for pH.** This technique has been complicated by a very low incidence of hemorrhage and infection/abscess formation at the site of sampling.

b. **Fetal scalp electrode for fetal heart rate (FHR) monitoring.** Infants are at low risk for site infection or malpositioned electrode (i.e., intraocular).

2. **Cephalhematoma** is a subperiosteal collection of blood secondary to rupture of the blood vessels between the skull and periosteum; its extent will be well delineated by suture lines over days. Occipital cephalhematoma may mimic an encephalocele and require a cranial ultrasound for diagnosis.
   a. **Prognosis and complications.** The extent of hemorrhage may be severe enough to present as anemia and hypotension with secondary hyperbilirubinemia. It may be a focus of infection leading to meningitis or osteomyelitis, particularly when there is a concomitant skull fracture (linear fractures may underlie a cephalhematoma 5 to 20 percent of the time). Skull x-rays should be obtained if there are CNS symptoms, if the hematoma is very large, or if the delivery was very difficult. Resolution occurs over 1 to 2 months, occasionally with residual calcification.
   b. **Management.** Usually observation only. Transfusion and phototherapy may be needed if blood accumulation is significant. The presence of a bleeding disorder should be considered. Infection of the hematoma is rarely present, but if the skin integrity has been broken, aspiration for evaluation of fluid by Gram stain and culture should be considered if it is felt that the risk of infection is high. This is an unusual situation, and we have not yet felt the need to aspirate a cephalhematoma. Aspiration is more likely to increase the risk of infection. Skull x-rays or computerized tomographic (CT) scans are needed for diagnosis of depressed skull fractures.
3. **Subgaleal hematoma** is blood that has invaded the potential space between the skull periosteum and the scalp galea aponeurosis, an area that extends posteriorly from the orbital ridges to the occiput and laterally to the ears.
   a. **Prognosis and complications.** This hematoma is capable of spreading across the entire calvarium; its growth may be insidious and not recognizable for hours or days, or it may present as hemorrhagic shock and even death. The scalp may pit similar to edema; ecchymoses may present periorbitally and/or auricularly. Resorption occurs very slowly.
   b. **Management.** Vigilant observation over days will detect continued growth; scalp pressure dressings may retard extension. Transfusion and phototherapy should be considered for large blood accumulations. Investigation for coagulopathy may be indicated. These hematomas may become infected if the skin has been damaged. If infection occurs, drainage will be required along with antibiotic therapy.
4. **Caput succedaneum** is a serosanguinous, subcutaneous, extraperiosteal fluid collection with poorly defined margins; it may extend across the midline and over suture lines and is usually associated with head molding.
   a. **Prognosis and complications.** Only rarely is this hemorrhage sufficient to alter the hematocrit or cause hyperbilirubinemia. The soft-tissue edema will usually resolve over the first few days postpartum. Rare instances of scalp necrosis with permanent scarring alopecia have been reported [2].
   b. **Management.** Observation only.
5. **Vacuum caput** is a serosanguineous fluid accumulation well defined by the position of the vacuum extractor on the scalp.
   a. **Prognosis and complications.** Significant hemorrhage leading to anemia and jaundice is unusual; the fluid collection typically redistributes within hours after birth. Scalp abrasions and lacerations sometimes leading to local infection are rare.

b. **Management.** Observation is usually adequate, but some infants with vacuum-induced hematomas require treatment for blood loss, hyperbilirubinemia, or infection. The presence of a bleeding disorder should be considered.

6. **Intracranial hemorrhage** (see Intracranial Hemorrhage in Chap. 21)
7. **Skull fracture** may be linear or depressed and involve the frontal, parietal, or occipital bones of the infant skull.
   a. **Prognosis and complications.** The forces responsible for fracture of the skull may be sufficient to cause brain contusions or disruption of blood vessels leading to subcutaneous or intracranial bleeding. Fractures may lie occultly beneath a cephalhematoma or present with seizures, hypotension, or death. Linear fractures are most often asymptomatic. An indentation in the skull may range from inward depression of the outer bony layer without true fracture to a complete disruption of bone. Fractures associated with dural laceration may lead to herniation of meninges and brain, progressing to leptomeningeal cysts.
   b. **Management.** Diagnosis is made with x-rays. Cranial CT scan will show the presence of intracranial hemorrhage or edema. Linear skull fractures without neurologic sequelae heal quickly and require only observation. Depressions of the skull should be evaluated by a neurosurgeon; occasionally, elevation can be made by closed technique without surgery. Fractures should be re-x-rayed at 8 to 12 weeks to look for "growing fractures" or leptomeningeal cysts.
8. **Facial/mandibular fractures** may present as facial asymmetry with ecchymoses, edema, crepitance, respiratory distress, or poor feeding. Dislocation of the cartilaginous nasal septum from its vomerine groove, the most common significant facial injury, will be evident as septal deviation with manual nasal tip compression. Unrecognized/untreated facial fractures may lead to craniofacial deformities, including mandibular hypoplasia and malocclusion, with ocular, respiratory, and mastication problems.
   a. **Management.** Protection of the airway must be the first consideration. A plastic surgeon or otorhinolaryngologist should be consulted immediately and provided with radiographic confirmation of fractures. Cranial CT scan may be helpful in searching for retro-orbital or cribriform plate disruption. Treatment should be initiated before fractures heal, usually by 7 to 14 days.
9. **Ocular injuries.** Retinal and subconjunctival hemorrhages are a common occurrence with vaginal delivery and usually resolve within 24 to 48 hours postpartum without sequelae. Forceps can be responsible for both ocular and periorbital injury. Disruption of Descemet's membrane of the cornea will lead to scarring and eventually to astigmatism and amblyopia. Hyphema, vitreous hemorrhage, local lacerations, palpebral edema, orbital fracture with abnormal extraocular muscle function, and lacrimal gland/duct damage also can occur.
   a. **Management.** Prompt ophthalmologic consultation should always be considered for significant ocular injuries. Follow-up attempts at funduscopic examination may detect the haziness of evolving corneal injury.
10. **Ear Injuries.** Damage to the external pinna may present as hematoma with evolution to a "cauliflower" ear. Lacerations involving the cartilage can develop into refractory perichondritis. Temporal bone injury may lead to middle and inner ear complications such as hemorrhage (seen as hemotympanum) and ossicular disarticulation.
    a. **Management.** Pinna hematomas should be aspirated with a 23-gauge needle before they can organize. Otologic consultation is indicated for external cartilaginous or inner ear involvement.

11. **Sternocleidomastoid (SCM) muscle injury.** Torticollis presenting at birth may be the result of muscle or fascia disruption during delivery. Hematoma formation and fibrosis follow with eventual shortening of the muscle. Significant compromise in surrounding musculoskeletal structures may lead to permanent postural deformities. Although most torticollis is due to abnormal intrauterine position, it may also result from cervical vertebral anomalies.
    a. **Management.** Head tilt and palpable mass in the SCM should alert the examiner to such injury. Passive stretching of the muscle several times each day should be begun promptly; visual and auditory stimulation should encourage infant head movement that stretches the muscle. Recovery over 3 to 4 months is typical (see also Chap. 23).

B. **Cranial nerve, spinal cord, and peripheral nerve injuries** [6]. These may be associated with breech delivery. These injuries result from hyperextension, traction, and overstretching with simultaneous rotation; they may range from localized neurapraxia to complete nerve or cord transection. Compression injury from forceps is rarely involved.

1. **Cranial nerve injuries.** Unilateral branches of the facial (VII) and vagus (X) nerve, in the form of the recurrent laryngeal nerve, are most commonly involved and result in temporary or permanent paralysis.
    a. **Facial nerve injury.** Compression by forceps blades has been implicated in some facial nerve injuries, but most facial nerve palsy is unrelated to trauma.
        (1) **Physical findings**
            (a) **Central nerve injury**—asymmetrical crying facies. The mouth is drawn to the normal side, wrinkles are deeper on the normal side, and movement of the forehead and eyelid is unaffected. The paralyzed side is smooth with a swollen appearance, the nasolabial fold is absent, and the corner of the mouth droops. There is no evidence of trauma on the face.
            (b) **Peripheral nerve injury**—asymmetrical crying facies. Sometimes evidence of trauma is present.
            (c) **Peripheral nerve branch injury**—asymmetrical crying facies. The paralysis is limited to the forehead, eye or mouth.
        (2) **Differential diagnosis**—nuclear agenesis (Möbius' syndrome), congenital absence of facial muscles, unilateral absence of orbicularis oris muscle, intracranial hemorrhage
        (3) **Treatment.** Protect the open eye with patches and "synthetic tears" (methylcellulose drops) every 4 hours. Neurologic and surgical consultation is sought if the condition has not improved in 7 to 10 days.
        (4) **Prognosis.** Electrodiagnostic tests may be useful to predict recovery or potential residual effects. Most infants begin to recover in the first week of life, but full resolution may take several months. Palsy due to trauma will usually resolve or improve. Facial nerve palsy that persists is often due to absence of the nerve. Absence of the orbicularis oris muscle is often confused with facial palsy.
    b. **Recurrent laryngeal nerve injury**
        (1) **Physical findings.** Unilateral abductor paralysis, usually the result of injury to the recurrent laryngeal nerve, presents with a hoarse cry or respiratory stridor. Bilateral vocal cords paralysis may be caused by trauma to both recurrent laryngeal nerves or, more commonly, by a CNS injury such as hypoxia or hemorrhage involving the brainstem. Bilateral paralysis may present with more severe respiratory distress or asphyxia.
        (2) **Differential diagnosis.** Direct laryngoscopy can make the diagnosis and can distinguish vocal cord paralysis from other causes of respiratory distress and stridor in the newborn. Appropriate birth

history (e.g., excess traction on the head during vertex delivery) suggests the diagnosis. In the absence of appropriate history, further evaluation to rule out more unusual etiologies, such as cardiovascular or CNS malformations or a mediastinal tumor, may be considered.

(3) **Prognosis and management.** Infants with unilateral paralysis should be given small, frequent feedings to minimize the risk of aspiration. The paralysis usually resolves within 4 to 6 weeks. Bilateral paralysis may necessitate intubation to maintain the airway. Prognosis for bilateral paralysis is variable; if recovery has not occurred by 6 weeks, tracheostomy is often required.

2. **Spinal cord injuries.** A fetus with a hyperextended head has a high incidence of severe spinal cord injury if delivered vaginally. Infants born with a vaginal breech delivery are also at some risk. Low Apgar scores in the delivery room may reflect injury to the brainstem and/or spinal cord. The infant may be alert, yet flaccid. Cord dural rupture may present as a loud, sharp "snap" heard at the time of delivery. This may occur without vertebral dislocation or damage. Epidural hemorrhage is the most common complication of cord trauma, with edema and temporary denervation subsequent. Motor function will be absent distal to the level of injury with loss of deep tendon reflexes; interruption of peripheral circulatory control may lead to temperature instability. There will be a sensory level if the cord is transected. Constipation and urinary retention may appear.

   a. **Management.** If cord injury is suspected, effort in the delivery room should immediately focus on resuscitation and prevention of further insult. The head should be made immobile relative to the spine and secured on a flat, firm surface with padding of pressure points. A careful neurologic examination and cervical spine x-rays should follow to help rule out other causes of hypotonia or spinal dysraphism. A CT scan, myelogram, or MRI scan may be necessary. Daily neurologic assessment with attention to bowel/bladder function will help to predict long-term outcome.

3. **Cervical nerve root injuries**

   a. **Phrenic nerve palsy (C3, 4, or 5)** is virtually always unilateral and frequently associated with brachial plexus injury. Respiratory distress with ipsilaterally diminished breath sounds may be the presenting signs of diaphragmatic paralysis. This nerve is occasionally damaged by the insertion of chest tubes or by surgery. Congenital absence is rare but occurs.

      (1) **Management.** Diagnosis is confirmed by either ultrasonography or fluoroscopic examination showing diaphragmatic elevation on the affected side with paradoxical (upward) movement during inspiration. Pulmonary toilet to avoid pneumonia should be instituted during the anticipated 1- to 3-month recovery phase. Diaphragmatic plication or phrenic nerve pacing is possible for refractory cases.

   b. **Injuries to the brachial plexus**

      (1) **Physical findings**

         (a) **Injury to the fifth and sixth cervical spinal nerves (Duchenne-Erb paralysis).** The affected arm is adducted and internally rotated with the elbow extended; the forearm is in pronation; and the wrist is flexed. The arm falls limply to the side of the body when passively adducted. The Moro, biceps, and radial reflexes are absent on the affected side. The grasp reflex is intact.

         (b) **Injury to the seventh and eighth cervical and first thoracic spinal nerves (Klumpke's paralysis).** The intrinsic muscles of the hand are affected, and the grasp is absent. The biceps and radial reflexes are present. If the cervical sympathetic fibers of the first thoracic spinal nerves are involved, Horner's syndrome is present.

(c) **Injury to the entire brachial plexus.** The entire arm is flaccid; all reflexes are absent.

(2) **Differential diagnosis**—cerebral injury, bone or soft-tissue injury of shoulder or upper arm

(3) **Diagnosis and management.** X-ray studies should be made of the shoulder and upper arm to rule out bony injury. The chest should be examined to rule out associated phrenic nerve paralysis. Passive movement to maintain range of motion of the affected joints should be delayed until the nerve edema resolves (7 to 10 days). The "Statue of Liberty" splint is not used because of subsequent contractures about the shoulder. Splints may be useful to prevent wrist and digit contractures.

(4) **Complications.** The degree of recovery is difficult to predict in the immediate neonatal period. Definite improvements during the first 1 to 2 weeks predict normal or near-normal function. Lack of improvement by 6 months suggests a permanent deficit. The ultimate length of a permanently denervated limb is markedly shortened. Delayed iris pigmentation or heterochromia iridis may follow Horner's syndrome in the newborn.

C. **Bone injuries** (see also Chap. 23). Fractures are most often seen following breech delivery or with shoulder dystocia in macrosomic infants but are occasionally seen with cesarean delivery. Limb traction and rotation are usually responsible.

1. **Clavicular fracture.** Considered the most common neonatal orthopedic injury, the infant may display a pseudoparalysis on the affected side. Crepitus, palpable bony irregularity, and sternocleidomastoid muscle spasm are other physical findings. Greenstick (incomplete) fractures may be asymptomatic.

   a. **Management.** A chest x-ray will confirm clavicular fracture. Assessment of cervical spine, brachial plexus, or humeral injury also should occur if arm function is diminished. Healing with palpable callus formation occurs in 7 to 10 days, even with displaced fractures, and may make the unaware parent quite anxious when discovered. Arm motion can be limited by pinning the infant's sleeve to the shirt.

2. **Long bone injuries.** Loss of spontaneous arm or leg movement is usually the first sign of humeral or femoral injury, followed by swelling and pain on passive motion. The obstetrician may hear and feel the "snap" of fracture. Orthopedic consultation is important.

   a. **Fractures: management.** Humeral and femoral shaft breaks are usually treatable by splinting; they require closed reduction and casting only when displaced. X-ray will help differentiate fracture from septic arthritis. Radial nerve injury may be seen with humeral fracture. Healing with callus formation occurs over 2 to 4 weeks, with complete recovery expected.

   b. **Epiphyseal displacement: management.** Separation of the humeral or femoral epiphysis occurs at the hypertrophied cartilaginous layer of the growth plate. It is secondary to rotation with strong traction, may be proximal or distal, and may result in limb growth compromise if severe. Initial examination reveals swelling, crepitus, and pain. It may be confused with a dislocation or septic joint. Radiographic plain films are not initially helpful because the epiphysis is not ossified at birth. Metaphyseal displacement may be seen with both separation and septic arthritis. Limb immobilization for 10 to 14 days will allow callus formation. With fractures, treatment of pain should not be neglected.

D. **Intraabdominal injuries** (see Chap. 8, Surgical Problems). These uncommon injuries involve rupture or subcapsular hemorrhage into the liver, spleen, or adrenal gland.

1. **Physical findings.** Presentation may be sudden, with shock and abdominal distension, sometimes accompanied by a bluish discoloration. Hemorrhage confined by the capsule of the liver may present more insidiously, with gradual onset of jaundice, pallor, poor feeding, tachypnea, and tachycardia. Rupture of the hematoma into the abdomen causes discoloration of the abdominal wall and shock.
2. **Diagnosis.** Intraabdominal injuries should be suspected in any newborn with shock, with or without abdominal distension. After a difficult delivery, infants should be followed daily with careful, gentle abdominal palpation and serial determinations of hematocrit level. Abdominal ultrasonography may be useful. Paracentesis is diagnostic in infants with intraperitoneal bleeding.

E. Soft-tissue injuries

1. **Petechiae and ecchymosis** (see Chaps. 17 and 19) are common manifestations of birth trauma in the newborn. The birth history, the location of the lesions, their early appearance without evolution of new lesions, and the absence of bleeding from other sites help in differentiating petechiae and ecchymoses secondary to birth trauma from those caused by coagulopathy or vasculitis. If the etiology is uncertain, studies to rule out coagulation disorders or infectious etiology are indicated. These lesions resolve spontaneously within 1 week. The infant should be observed for signs of anemia or hyperbilirubinemia if the ecchymoses are extensive.
2. **Lacerations and abrasions.** (see Chaps. 7 and 8) May be secondary to fetal monitoring (scalp electrodes) as well as actual injury during the birth process. Deep wounds (e.g., scalpel cuts during cesarean section) may require suturing. Infection is an ever-present risk, particularly with scalp lesions and underlying caput succedaneum or hematoma. Careful cleaning and observation are indicated.
3. **Subcutaneous fat necrosis.** (see Chaps. 7, 8, and 29) Although not detectable at birth, these irregularly shaped, hard, nonpitting, subcutaneous plaques with overlying dusky, red-purple discoloration may be caused by pressure during delivery. They appear during the first 2 weeks of life, usually in large babies, on the cheeks (at the angle of the jaw), arms, back, buttocks, and thighs. These lesions are common; they are usually felt by the mother and cause her concern. They may become calcified and thus appear on x-ray studies. Complete resolution is the rule.

References

1. Curran, J. S. *Clin. Perinatol.* 8: 111, 1981.
2. Donn, S. M. *Clin. Perinatol.* 10: 507, 1983.
3. Faix, R. G. *Clin. Perinatol.* 10: 487, 1983.
4. Fanaroff, A. A., and Martin, R. J. (Eds.). *Neonatal-Perinatal Medicine: Diseases of the Fetus and Infant.* St. Louis: Mosby, 1987.
5. Friedman, E. A. *Clin. Obstet. Gynecol.* 30: 93, 1987.
6. Volpe, J. J. *Neurology of the Newborn,* 2d Ed., Philadelphia: Saunders, 1987.
7. Wegman, M. E. *Pediatrics* 70: 835, 1982.
8. Wegman, M. E. *Pediatrics* 78: 983, 1986.

23 Orthopedic Problems

James R. Kasser
and Paul P. Griffin

This chapter considers common musculoskeletal abnormalities that may be detected in the neonatal period. Consultation with an orthopedic surgeon is often required to provide definitive treatment after the initial evaluation.

I. Torticollis

A. Torticollis is a disorder characterized by limited motion of the neck, asymmetry of the face and skull, and a tilted position of the head. It is usually caused by shortening of the **sternocleidomastoid (SCM) muscle** but may be secondary to muscle adaptation from an abnormal in utero position of the head and neck.

1. The **etiology** of the shortened SCM muscle is unclear; many cases are due to abnormal in utero position, and some may be due to stretching of the muscle at delivery. The result of the latter is a contracture of the muscle associated with fibrosis.
2. **Clinical course.** The limitation of motion is minimum at birth, but increases over the first few weeks. At 10 to 20 days, in cases related to stretching, a mass is frequently found in the SCM muscle. This mass gradually disappears, and the muscle fibers are partially replaced by fibrous tissue, which contracts and limits head motion. Because of the limited rotation of the head, the infant rests on the ipsilateral side of the face in the prone position and on the contralateral side when supine. The pressure from resting on one side of the face and the opposite occipital bone contributes to the facial and skull asymmetry.
3. **Treatment.** Most infants will respond favorably to positioning the head in the direction opposite to that produced by the tight muscle. Padded bricks or sandbags can be used to help maintain the position of the head until the child is able to actively move to free the head. Passive stretching by rotating the head to the ipsilateral side and tilting it toward the contralateral side also may help. The torticollis in most infants resolves by 1 year of age. Patients who have asymmetry of the face and head and limited motion after 1 year should be considered for surgical release of the SCM muscle [1].

B. Torticollis with limited motion of the neck may be due to congenital abnormality of the cervical spine. Some infants with this disorder also have a tight SCM muscle. These infants are likely to have significant limitation of motion at birth. Radiologic evaluation of the cervical spine is necessary to make this diagnosis.

C. A third type of torticollis is associated with congenital asymmetrical contractures of the hip abductor and unilateral metatarsus adduction. The torticollis always subsides spontaneously. Since some infants with this type of torticollis have unilateral hip dysplasia, a roentgenogram or ultrasound examination of the hips should be made if examination reveals tightness in the hip abductors sufficient to cause a pelvic obliquity.

II. Polydactyly

A. Duplication of a digit may range from a small cutaneous bulb to an almost perfectly formed digit. Treatment of this problem is variable.

B. Treatment

1. The small functionless skin bulb without bone or cartilage can be ligated and allowed to develop necrosis for 24 hours, and then the part distal to the suture should be removed. The residual stump should have an antiseptic applied twice a day to prevent infection.
2. When duplicated digits contain bony parts, decision about treatment is more difficult and should be delayed until the patient is evaluated by an orthopedist or hand surgeon.

III. Fractured clavicle (see Chap. 22)

A. The **clavicle** is the site of the most common fracture associated with delivery.

B. Diagnosis is usually made soon after birth, when the infant does not move the arm on the affected side or cries when that arm is moved. There may be tenderness, swelling, or crepitance at the site. Occasionally, the bone is angulated. Diagnosis can be confirmed by radiographic examination. A "painless" fracture discovered by roentgenogram of the chest is more likely a congenital pseudarthorsis (nonunion).

C. The **clinical course** is such that clavicle fractures heal without difficulty. **Treatment** consists of providing comfort for the infant. If the arm and shoulder are left unprotected, motion occurs at the fracture when the baby is handled. We usually pin the infant's sleeve to the shirt and put a sign on the baby to remind personnel to decrease motion of the clavicle. No reduction is necessary. If the fracture appears painful, a wrap to decrease motion of the arm is useful.

IV. Congenital and infantile scoliosis

A. Congenital scoliosis is a lateral curvature of the spine secondary to a failure either of formation of a vertebra or of segmentation. Scoliosis in the newborn may be difficult to detect; by bending the trunk laterally in the prone position, however, a difference in motion can usually be observed. Congenital scoliosis must be differentiated from **infantile scoliosis,** in which no vertebral anomaly is present. Infantile scoliosis often improves spontaneously, although the condition may be progressive in infants who have a spinal curvature greater than 20 degrees. If the scoliosis is progressive, treatment is indicated.

B. Clinical course. Congenital scoliosis will increase in many patients. Bracing of congenital curves is usually not helpful [2,7]. Surgical correction and fusion are frequently indicated before the curve becomes severe. Since many patients with congenital curves have renal or other visceral abnormalities, studies should be done to detect these abnormalities.

V. Congenital dislocation of the hip. Most (but not all) hips that are dislocated at birth can be diagnosed by a careful physical examination (see Chap. 7). Ultrasound examination of the hip is useful for diagnosis in doubtful cases [6]. X-ray examination will not make the diagnosis in the newborn because the femoral head is not calcified but will diagnose an abnormal acetebular fossa seen in hip dysplasia. There are three types of congenital dislocation.

A. The **classic congenitally dislocated hip** is diagnosed by having a positive Ortolani test. The hip is unstable and dislocates on adduction and also on extension of the thigh but readily relocates when the thigh is abducted in flexion. No asymmetry of the pelvis is seen. This type of dislocation is more common in females and is usually unilateral, but it may be bilateral. Hips that are unstable at birth often become stable after a few days. Infant with hips that are unstable after 5 days of age should be treated with a splint that keeps the hips flexed and abducted. The Pavlik harness has been used effectively to treat this group of patients [4].

B. The **teratologic type of dislocation** occurs very early in pregnancy. The femoral head does not relocate on flexion and abduction; that is, the Ortolani test is negative. If the dislocation is unilateral, there may be asymmetry of the gluteal folds and asymmetrical motion with limited abduction. In bilateral cases, the perineum is wide and the thighs give the appearance of being shorter than normal. This may be easily overlooked, however, and requires an extremely careful physical examination. Treatment of the teratologic hip dislocation is by open reduction.

C. The **third type of dislocation** occurs late, is unilateral, and is associated with a **congenital abduction contracture** of the contralateral hip. The abduction contracture causes a pelvic obliquity. The pelvis is lower on the side of the contracture, which is unfavorable for the contralateral hip, and the acetabulum may not develop well. After age 6 weeks, infants with this type of dislocation develop an apparent short leg and have asymmetrical gluteal folds. Some infants will develop a dysplastic acetabulum, which may eventually allow the hip to subluxate. Treatment of the dysplasia is with the Pavlik harness, but after age 8 months, other methods of treatment may be necessary.

VI. **Congenital genu recurvatum,** or hyperextension of the knee, is not a serious abnormality and is easily recognized and treated. It must be differentiated, however, from subluxation or dislocation of the knee, which also may present with hyperextension of the knee. The latter two abnormalities are more serious and require more extensive treatment.

A. **Congenital genu recurvatum** is secondary to in utero position with hyperextension of the knee. This can be successfully treated by repeated cast changes, with progressive flexion of the knee until it reaches 90 degrees of flexion. Minor degrees of recurvatum can be treated with passive stretching exercises.

B. **All infants with hyperextension of the knee** should have a radiographic examination to differentiate genu recurvation from the more serious abnormalities. In congenital genu recurvatum, the tibial and femoral epiphyses are in proper alignment except for the hyperextension. In the subluxed knee with dislocation, the tibia is completely anterior or anterolateral to the femur. The tibia is shifted forward on the femur and is frequently lateral as well. Congenital fibrosis of the quadriceps is frequently associated with the subluxed and dislocated knee, and open reduction is essential, for attempted treatment of the dislocated knee by stretching or by repeated cast changes is hazardous and may result in epiphyseal plate damage.

VII. **Deformities of the feet**

A. **Metatarsus adductus** describes a condition in which the metatarsals rest in an adducted position, but the appearance does not always reveal the severity of the condition. Whether or not treatment is necessary is determined by the difference in the degree of structural change in the metatarsals and tarsometatarsal joint.

1. Most infants with metatarsus adductus have positional deformities that are probably caused by in utero position. The positional type of metatarsus adductus is flexible and can be passively corrected into abduction with little difficulty. This condition does not need treatment.
2. The **structural metatarsus adductus** has a relatively fixed adduction deformity of the forefoot and cannot be abducted passively. The etiology has not been definitely identified but is probably related to in utero position. This is seen more commonly in the first-born infant and in pregnancies with oligohydramnios. Most of the structural types of metatarsus adductus have a valgus deformity of the hindfoot. The structural deformity needs to be treated with manipulation and cast immobilization until correction occurs. Although there is no urgency to treat this condition, it is more easily corrected earlier than later and should be done before the child is of walking age.

B. **Calcaneovalgus deformities** result from an in utero position of the foot that holds the ankle dorsiflexed and abducted. At birth, the top of the foot lies up against the anterior surface of the leg. Structural changes in the bones do not seem to be present. The sequela to this deformity appears to be a valgus or pronated foot that is more severe than the typical pronated foot seen in toddlers. Whether this disorder is treated or not is variable, and no study supports either course. **Treatment** consists of application of a short-leg cast that will keep the foot plantar flexed and inverted. Casts are changed appropriately for growth and maintained until plantar flexion and inversion are equal to those of the opposite foot. Generally, the foot is held in plaster for about 6 to 8 weeks. Feet that remain in the calcaneovalgus position for several months may be more likely to have significant residual **pes valgus;** however, we generally do not treat infants who have this problem.

C. **Congenital clubfoot** is a congenital deformity with a multifactorial etiology. A first-degree relative of a patient with this deformity has 20 times the risk of having a clubfoot than the normal population. The risk in subsequent siblings is 3 to 5 percent. The more frequent occurrence in the first born and association with oligohydramnios suggest an influence of in utero pressure as well. Sometimes clubfoot is part of a syndrome [5]. Infants with neurologic dysfunction of the feet (spina bifida) often have clubfoot.

1. There are three and sometimes four components to the deformity. The foot is in equinus, cavus, and varus, with a forefoot adduction; thus the clubfoot is a talipes equinocavovarus with metatarsal adduction. Each of these deformities is sufficiently rigid to prevent passive correction to a neutral position by the examiner. The degree of rigidity is variable in each patient.
2. **Treatment** should be started early, within a few days of birth. An effective method of treatment consists of manipulation and application of tape casts that are changed every 2 to 3 days. This method allows the nurse or parent to stretch the foot several times a day. After 4 to 6 days of strapping, or when progress in the correction ceases, plaster cast treatment is started and continued until the foot is corrected or until there is no further progress in correction. Another method of treatment is manipulation of the foot and the application of casts, starting at 2 or 3 days of age. If conservative treatment does not successfully correct the deformities, surgical correction will be necessary.

References

1. Ferkel, R. D. *J. Bone Joint Surg.* 65A: 894, 1983.
2. McMaster, J. J. *J. Bone Joint Surg.* 64A: 1128, 1982.
3. Murbarak, S. *J. Bone Joint Surg.* 63A: 1114, 1981.
4. Ramsey, P. L. *J. Bone Joint Surg.* 58A: 100, 1976.
5. Jones, K. L. (Ed.). *Smith's Recognizable Patterns of Human Malformations.* Philadelphia: Saunders, 1988. P. 746.
6. Teele, R. L., and Share, J. C. *Practical Pediatric Ultrasonography.* Philadelphia: Saunders, 1990.
7. Winter, R. B. *J. Bone Joint Surg.* 50A: 1, 1964.

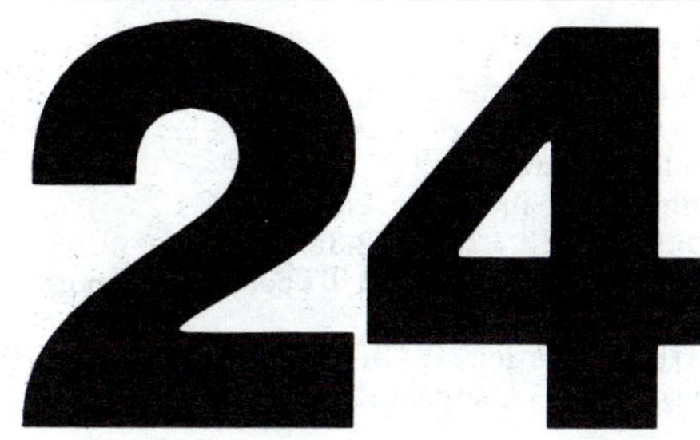

Metabolic Problems

Hypoglycemia and Hyperglycemia

Joan C. Downey and
John P. Cloherty

Hypoglycemia and **hyperglycemia** are common problems in neonates, especially low-birth-weight infants. Both are signs of an underlying pathologic process associated with utilization or production of glucose.

I. **Hypoglycemia.** In the neonate, term or premature, **hypoglycemia** is usually defined as a blood glucose level less than 30 mg/dl [7]. Some infants with blood glucose levels between 30 and 40 mg/dl may have symptoms consistent with hypoglycemia that disappear after glucose administration; thus any blood glucose level less than 40 mg/dl should be a cause for evaluation [30,38,40]. In the newborn, one should use a glucose oxidase method for measuring true glucose rather than methods measuring total reducing substances [10]. Dextrostix* are useful for monitoring glucose; at levels under 40 mg/dl, however, they may be less reliable [12]. False elevations of measured glucose may occur with isopropyl alcohol contamination of samples [17]. Incorrect storage (unsealed container) or outdated shelf life may result in inaccurate results, especially at low blood glucose concentration [22]. For accurate measurements, strict adherence to Dextrostix procedural recommendations is necessary. The Ames Eyetone Instrument* gives an immediate reading of blood glucose level, within ± 5 mg/dl of laboratory whole-blood glucose values [38].

A. **Etiology**

1. **Increased utilization of glucose: hyperinsulinism** [30,33]
    - a. Infants of diabetic mothers (IDMs) (see Maternal Diabetes in Chap. 1)
    - b. **Erythroblastosis** [rebound hypoglycemia after exchange with acid-citrate-dextrose (ACD) blood containing high dextrose levels in these infants with hyperplastic islets of Langerhans] [2,7] (see Chaps. 15 and 20).
    - c. Islet-cell hyperplasia or hyperfunction [13]
    - d. Beckwith-Weidemann syndrome (macrosomia, mild microcephaly, omphalocele, macroglossia, hypoglycemia, and visceromegaly) [13]
    - e. Insulin-producing tumors (nesidioblastosis, islet-cell adenoma, or islet-cell dysmaturity) [13,16,41]
    - f. Maternal tocolytic therapy with beta-sympathomimetic agents [terbutaline, isoxsuprine, albuterol (Salbutamol)] [4,11,34]
    - g. Maternal chlorpropramide therapy (Diabinese) [43]; possibly maternal benzothiadiazides (Chlorothiazide) [37]

*Ames Division, Miles Laboratories, Inc., Elkhart, Ind.

h. Malpositioned UA catheter infusing high glucose concentration into the celiac and superior mesenteric arteries T11–12, stimulating insulin release from the pancreas [42]
i. Rapid taper of high-glucose infusions [25]

2. **Decreased production/stores** [3,7,28,30,32,33]
   a. Prematurity. Incidence: premature SGA, 67 percent; premature LGA, 38 percent [29]
   b. Intrauterine growth retardation (IUGR). Incidence: premature SGA, 67 percent; postterm SGA, 18 percent [29]
   c. Starvation
3. **Increased utilization and/or decreased production or other causes.** Any baby with one of the following conditions is likely to have hypoglycemia; parenteral glucose may be necessary for the management of these infants.
   a. **Perinatal stress**
      (1) Sepsis [26]
      (2) Shock [7,30]
      (3) Asphyxia [5,7,30]
      (4) Hypothermia (increased utilization) [30]
      (5) Islet-cell necrosis [35]
   b. **Exchange transfusion** with heparinized blood that has a low blood glucose level in the absence of a glucose infusion; reactive hypoglycemia after exchange with relatively hyperglycemic CPD blood (citrate-phosphate-dextrose) [7]
   c. **Defects in carbohydrate metabolism** (see Inborn Errors of Metabolism below)
      (1) Glycogen storage disease [7]
      (2) Fructose intolerance [7]
      (3) Galactosemia [7]
   d. **Endocrine deficiency**
      (1) Adrenal insufficiency [7]
      (2) Hypothalamic deficiency [36]
      (3) Congenital hypopituitarism [36]
   e. **Defects in amino acid metabolism** (see Inborn Errors of Metabolism below)
      (1) "Maple syrup" urine disease [7]
      (2) Propionic acidemia
      (3) Methylmalonic acidemia
      (4) Tyrosinemia
   f. **Polycythemia** (possibly due to glucose utilization by the increased mass of red blood cells) [7] (see Chap. 18)
   g. **Maternal therapy with propranolol.** Possible mechanisms include the following:
      (1) Prevention of sympathetic stimulation of glycogenolysis
      (2) Prevention of recovery from insulin-induced decreases in free fatty acids and glycerol
      (3) Inhibition of epinephrine-induced increases in free fatty acids and lactate postexercise [7,8,18]

B. **Diagnosis**
1. **Symptoms** [7,25,30]
   a. **Lethargy, apathy, and limpness**
   b. **Tremors or jitteriness**
   c. **Apnea**
   d. **Cyanosis**
   e. **Seizures, coma**
   f. **Weak or high-pitched cry**
   g. **Poor feeding**
   h. **Some infants may have no symptoms**
2. **Laboratory diagnosis.** Blood glucose level should be routinely measured in infants who have risk factors for hypoglycemia. IDMs usually have hy-

poglycemia in the first day of life and should have frequent early measurements of blood glucose level (see Maternal Diabetes in Chap. 1). Preterm and small for gestational age (SGA) infants should have blood glucose measurements in the first 3 to 4 days of life. Infants with erythroblastosis fetalis should have blood glucose levels measured after exchange transfusions with citrate-phosphate-dextrose (CPD) blood and during exchange with heparinized blood. The symptoms listed in **1** are nonspecific. In order to demonstrate that they are due to hypoglycemia, there should be a blood glucose level of less than 30 mg/dl at the time symptoms are present and correction of the hypoglycemia should result in resolution of the symptoms. When hypoglycemia is prolonged or of uncertain etiology, measurements of insulin, growth hormone, cortisol, adrenocorticotropic hormone (ACTH), thyroxine (T_4), glucagon, plasma amino acids, urinary ketones, reducing substance, amino acids, and organic acids at the time of hypoglycemia may be indicated. This is usually done if the hypoglycemia or need for large glucose infusions lasts over one week.

Some infants with glucose being infused through an umbilical artery line may have normal glucose levels in their feet but hypoglycemic levels in their hands and brain.

3. **Differential diagnosis** [7]. The symptoms mentioned in **1** can be due to many other causes with or without associated hypoglycemia. Some are:
   a. **Adrenal insufficiency**
   b. **Maternal drug use**
   c. **Heart disease**
   d. **Renal failure**
   e. **Liver failure**
   f. **CNS disease**
   g. **Metabolic abnormalities**
      (1) Hypocalcemia
      (2) Hyponatremia or hypernatremia
      (3) Hypomagnesemia
      (4) Pyridoxine deficiency
   h. **Sepsis**
   i. **Asphyxia**
4. **Treatment.** Anticipation and prevention are more important than treatment. (Management of IDMs is discussed under Maternal Diabetes in Chap. 1.)
   a. **Well infants** who are at risk for hypoglycemia (i.e., infants with intrauterine malnutrition) should have their blood glucose levels measured at 3, 6, 12, and 24 hours of age. They should be given early oral or gavage feedings with glucose 10% and water every 2 to 4 hours until the blood glucose level is stable. These infants are then weaned to milk, and their blood glucose levels are monitored for the first 2 days of life. Similarly, early feeding of older premature infants (33 to 36 weeks) often will avoid problems with hypoglycemia.
   b. **Asphyxiated infants** may need parenteral glucose as part of the resuscitative effort in the delivery room. The glucose is often administered through the umbilical vein (care should be taken to avoid a rapid bolus of concentrated glucose solution and to ensure proper placement of the catheter) (see Perinatal Asphyxia in Chap. 21).
   c. **Infants with SYMPTOMATIC hypoglycemia**
      (1) Blood is drawn for whatever tests are indicated (e.g., glucose, insulin). Monitor blood glucose levels every 1 to 4 hours initially.
      (2) **Method A.** Glucose 0.5 to 1.0 gm/kg (as 2 to 4 ml/kg of dextrose 25% in water (25% D/W) is given by rapid IV infusion at the rate of 1 ml per minute (e.g., in a 4-kg infant, 8 to 16 ml of 25% D/W is given over 8 to 16 minutes) [7]. This is followed by a continuous infusion of 4 to 8 mg/kg of glucose per minute. The initial bolus

often results in **hyperglycemia** (lasting more than 1 hour after th infusion).

(3) Method B. Glucose 200 mg/kg per minute is given as 10% D/W over 1 minute (2 ml/kg of 10% D/W over 1 minute), followed by an infusion of 8 mg/kg of glucose per minute (see **c.4**). This metho has a lower incidence of hyperglycemia postinfusion and increase the blood glucose level above hypoglycemic levels within 4 min utes [27,33].

(4) Glucose infusions for maintenance

(a) For most infants, intravenous 10% D/W at daily maintenanc rates will provide adequate glucose. The concentration of th dextrose in the fluids will depend on the daily water requir ment. It is suggested that calculation of both glucose intak (i.e., milligrams of glucose per kilogram per minute) an water requirements be done each day. For example, on th first day the fluid requirements is 80 ml/kg per day, or 0.05 ml/kg per minute; therefore, 10% D/W provides 5.5 mg/kg glucose per minute, and 15% D/W provides 8.12 mg/kg of glu cose per minute.

(b) Some infants with hyperinsulinism and infants with IUG will require 12 to 15 mg/kg of dextrose per minute (often a 15% D/W) [7,33].

(c) The concentration of glucose and the rate of infusion are in creased as necessary to maintain a normal blood glucos level. A central venous catheter may be necessary to give ad equate glucose (15% to 20% D/W) in an acceptable fluid vol ume. Taper glucose to 4 to 6 mg/kg per minute, monitorin glucose levels; then wean slowly while oral feeds are ad vanced [7].

(5) Glucagon 0.1 mg/kg IM (maximum 1.0 mg) may be given intra muscularly in infants with good glycogen stores to mobilize glu cose [7,21] in an emergency until IV dextrose is restored.

(6) Other. Epinephrine, diazoxide, growth hormone, and corticoste roids should be used only in special cases and only after an endo crinologic evaluation. Surgical subtotal pancreatectomy should b considered for nesidioblastosis and islet-cell adenomas [21,41].

II. Hyperglycemia is usually defined as a whole-blood glucose level greater than 12 mg/dl [7] or plasma glucose values greater than 145 mg/dl [28]. This problem i commonly encountered in low-birth-weight premature infants receiving paren teral glucose but is also seen in large premature or term neonates who are sick The major clinical problems associated with hyperglycemia are hyperosmolarit and osmotic diuresis. Hyperosmolarity (each 18 mg/dl rise in blood glucose con centration increases serum osmolality 1 mOsmol/L) of greater than 30 mOsmol/L usually leads to osmotic diuresis. Subsequent dehydration may occu rapidly in small premature infants. The hyperosmolar state, an increase of 25 t 40 mOsmol or a glucose level over 450 to 720 mg/dl, has been associated wit intracranial hemorrhage [33].

A. Etiology

1. **Exogenous parenteral glucose** administration in term normal infants o greater than 6.0 mg/kg of glucose per minute [23] or in preterm infant weighing less than 1100 gm of greater than 6.6 mg/kg of glucose per min ute may be associated with hyperglycemia [28,33].
2. **Exogenous parenteral lipid infusion.** In preterm infants, 10% intralipid at 0.25 gm/kg per hour increased glucose levels 24 percent above baseline at 0.50 gm/kg per hour, glucose levels were increased 65 percent abov baseline owing to enhanced gluconeogenesis secondary to increased fatt acid oxidation [33].
3. **Drugs.** Caffeine and theophylline have been associated with elevations o plasma glucose levels [33]. The mechanism is unknown, but it appear

that depression of insulin release is not a factor. Other drugs associated with hyperglycemia are diazoxide, corticosteroids, and phenytoin [19].

4. **Very low birth weight (VLBW) infants** (<1000 gm), possibly due to variable insulin response, to persistent endogenous hepatic glucose production despite significant elevations in plasma insulin, or to insulin resistance that may in part be due to immature glycogenolysis enzyme systems [33]
5. **Sepsis,** possibly due to depressed insulin release or, in some situations, an endotoxin effect possibly resulting in decreased glucose utilization [19,24]
6. "**Stressed**" premature infants with low birth weight and Apgar scores requiring mechanical ventilation, possibly due to persistent endogenous glucose production, diminished peripheral utilization, or a "relative" insulin deficiency state, but not felt to be due to hypoinsulinemia or hypercortisolemia [28,33]
7. **Hypoxia,** possibly due to increased glucose production in the absence of a change in peripheral utilization [9]
8. **Neonates undergoing surgical procedures,** possibly due to the secretion of epinephrine, glucocorticoids, and glucagon along with the suppression of insulin secretion [1,33]
9. **Transient neonatal diabetes mellitus.** In this rare disorder, infants present with hyperglycemia usually before 15 days of age (range 4 days to 6 weeks). They characteristically are small for gestational age term, have no sex predilection, and a third have a family history of diabetes mellitus. They present with marked glycosuria, hyperglycemia (240 to 2300 mg/dl), polyuria, severe dehydration, acidosis, mild or absent ketonuria, reduced subcutaneous fat, and failure to thrive. Insulin values are either absolutely or relatively low for the corresponding blood glucose elevation. Treatment consists of rehydration, and the majority require insulin (regular 0.5 to 3 units/kg per day SC divided q6h or .01 to 0.1 units/kg per hour by constant infusion). Start with the intravenous dose, then switch to the subcutaneous dose. Monitor serum electrolytes, glucose, and acid–base balance. Repeated plasma insulin values are necessary to distinguish transient from permanent diabetes mellitus. The average length for insulin treatment is 65 days (range 3 days to 18 months). The transient nature of this disorder may be due to delayed or abnormal maturation of the B cell, transiently deficient or delayed insulin secretion, or secretion of an abnormal insulin molecule [7,14,30,39].
10. **Transient hyperglycemia associated with ingestion of hyperosmolar formula.** Clinical presentation may mimic transient neonatal diabetes with glycosuria, hyperglycemia, and dehydration. A history of inappropriate formula dilution is key. Treatment consists of rehydration, discontinuation of hyperosmolar formula, and appropriate instructions for mixing concentrated or powder formula. Insulin has been used briefly but cautiously [20].

B. Treatment. The primary goal is prevention and early detection of hyperglycemia by frequent monitoring of blood glucose levels and urine for glycosuria. If present, evaluation and possible intervention are indicated.

1. Blood is drawn for whatever tests are indicated.
2. Parenteral glucose intake is reduced to 4.0 to 6.0 mg/kg of glucose per minute either by reducing the concentration or rate (or both) of glucose infusion and monitoring the falling blood glucose level. Decrease the glucose concentration by 2 mg/kg per minute every 4 to 6 hours [30,33].
3. Many small infants will be unable to tolerate a certain glucose load (e.g., 6 mg/kg per minute) but will eventually develop tolerance if they are presented with just enough glucose to keep their glucose level high yet not enough to cause glycosuria.
4. Hypotonic fluids (solutions with less than 5% dextrose) should be avoided or used with caution.

5. Exogenous insulin therapy has been used when glucose values exceed 250 mg/dl despite efforts to lower the amount of glucose delivered or when prolonged restrictions of parenterally administered glucose has substantially decreased total caloric intake and the infant is failing to thrive. Caution is exercised because neonates may have an erratic response.
   a. **Continuous insulin infusion** (regular insulin 100 units/ml) .01 to 0.1 units/kg per hour. The rate is adjusted based on hourly Dextrostix results. Monitor potassium level. The tubing is prepped with salt-poor albumin to ensure steady-state insulin delivery. (see Appendix A, Insulin). Monitor for rebound hyperglycemia [15,31]. (See page 553).
   b. **Subcutaneous insulin** 0.10 to 0.20 units/kg every 6 hours. Monitor glucose level at 1, 2, and 4 hours and potassium level [33].

References

1. Anand, K. J. *Pediatrics* 110: 999, 1987.
2. Barrett, C. N. *N. Engl. J. Med.* 278: 1260, 1968.
3. Beard, A. *J. Pediatr.* 79: 314, 1971.
4. Brazy, J. *J. Pediatr.* 94: 444, 1979.
5. Collins, J. E. *Lancet* 2: 311, 1984.
6. Coombs, J. *N. Engl. J. Med.* 275: 236, 1966.
7. Cornblath, M., and Schwartz, R. *Disorders of Carbohydrate Metabolism in Infancy.* Philadelphia: Saunders, 1976.
8. Cottrill, C. *J. Pediatr.* 91: 812, 1977.
9. Cowett, R. *Pediatr. Res.* 20: 408A, 1986.
10. Ek, J. *Acta Paediatr. Scand.* 56: 461, 1967.
11. Epstein, M. *J. Pediatr.* 94: 449, 1979.
12. Frantz, I. *J. Pediatr.* 87: 417, 1975.
13. Gabby, K. H. *N. Engl. J. Med.* 299: 241, 1978.
14. Gantz, J. C. *Adv. Pediatr.* 16: 345, 1969.
15. Goldman, S. *Pediatr. Res.* 14: 50, 1980.
16. Graces, L. *Pediatrics* 41: 789, 1968.
17. Grazaitis, D. *Pediatrics* 66: 221, 1980.
18. Habib, A. *J. Pediatr.* 91: 808, 1977.
19. James, T. *Am. J. Dis. Child.* 133: 645, 1979.
20. Jung, A. L. *Am. J. Dis. Child.* 118: 859, 1969.
21. Kaplan, E. *Surg. Clin. North Am.* 67: 395, 1987.
22. King, G. *Br. Med. J.* 285: 1165, 1982.
23. King, K. *Pediatrics* 44: 381, 1969.
24. Kramer, L. *Am. J. Dis. Child.* 134: 427, 1980.
25. LaFranchi, S. *Pediatr. Clin. North Am.* 34: 961, 1987.
26. Leake, R. *Clin. Pediatr.* 20: 397, 1981.
27. Lilien, L. *J. Pediatr.* 97: 295, 1980.
28. Lilien, L. *J. Pediatr.* 94: 454, 1979.
29. Lubchenco, L. O. *Pediatrics* 47: 831, 1971.
30. Ogata, E. *Pediatr. Clin. North Am.* 33: 25, 1986.
31. Ostertag, S. *Pediatrics* 78: 625, 1986.
32. Pildes, R. *J. Pediatr.* 70: 76, 1967.
33. Pildes, R. *Clin. Perinatol.* 13: 351, 1986.
34. Procianoy, R. *J. Pediatr.* 101: 612, 1982.
35. Roberts, P. *J. Clin. Pathol.* 40: 1206, 1987.
36. Sadeghi-Nejad, A. *J. Pediatr.* 84: 79, 1974.
37. Senior, B. *Lancet* 2: 377, 1976.
38. Sexon, W. *J. Pediatr.* 105: 149, 1984.
39. Sodoyez-Goffaux, F. *J. Pediatr.* 91: 395, 1977.

40. Srinivasan, G. *J. Pediatr.* 109: 114, 1986.
41. Thomas, C. *Ann. Surg.* 185: 505, 1977.
42. Urbach, J. *J. Pediatr.* 106: 825, 1986.
43. Zucker, P. *Pediatrics* 42: 824, 1968.

Hypocalcemia, Hypercalcemia, and Hypermagnesemia

Lewis P. Rubin

Calcium is physiologically important in two general ways. First, **calcium salts in bone** provide structural integrity. Decreased skeletal calcium is a hallmark of neonatal metabolic bone disease (see Metabolic Bone Disease of Prematurity page 446 and Chap. 21, Perinatal Asphyxia). Second, **calcium ions (Ca^{2+}) present in cellular and extracellular fluid (ECF)** are essential for many biochemical processes. Significant aberrations of serum calcium concentrations are observed frequently in the neonatal period. One must evaluate these alterations in light of the normal dynamic changes in serum calcium level that take place during the first week of life. Consequently, a given serum calcium level cannot be interpreted without knowing the newborn baby's postnatal age.

I. Principles of mineral metabolism

A. Laboratory measurement of serum calcium

1. There are three definable fractions of calcium in serum: (1) **ionized calcium** (about 50 percent of serum total calcium), (2) **calcium bound to serum proteins,** principally albumin (about 40 percent), and (3) **calcium complexed to serum anions,** mostly phosphates, citrate, and sulfates (about 10 percent). **Ionized calcium is the only biologically available form of calcium.**
2. For routine clinical purposes, measurement of serum total calcium level usually is adequate. Some clinical laboratories can measure ionized calcium level in microspecimens of anticoagulated blood collected anaerobically. Algorithms for correcting serum total calcium level for alterations in serum albumin concentration and/or pH or for calculating "free" calcium concentrations are not reliable compared with actual measurements of ionized calcium [3,13].
3. Calcium concentration reported as milligrams per deciliter may be converted to molar units by dividing by 4 (e.g., 10 mg/dl converts to 2.5 mmol/L).

B. Hormonal regulation of calcium homeostasis (see Fig. 24-1).

Regulation of serum and ECF ionized calcium concentration within a narrow range is critical for blood coagulation, neuromuscular excitability, cell membrane integrity and function, and cellular enzymatic and secretory activity. The principal calcitropic, or calcium-regulating, hormones are **parathyroid hormone (PTH)** and **1,25-dihydroxyvitamin D [1,25$(OH)_2D_3$].**

1. **PTH.** When ECF ionized calcium level declines, parathyroid cells secrete PTH. PTH (1) mobilizes calcium from bone, (2) increases calcium resorption in the renal tubule, and (3) stimulates renal production of 1,25$(OH)_2D_3$. PTH also mobilizes phosphate from bone and produces significant phosphaturia. Therefore, **PTH secretion causes the serum calcium level to rise and the serum phosphorus level to be maintained or fall.** Newborns in the first 2 days of life may exhibit decreased renal responsiveness to PTH [14].
2. **1,25$(OH)_2D_3$ (calcitriol).** Inactive vitamin D is synthesized in skin exposed to sunlight and is ingested in the diet. The liver then synthesizes **25$(OH)D_3$ (the major storage form of the hormone)** and the kidney synthesizes **the biologically active hormone, 1,25$(OH)_2D_3$.** 1,25$(OH)_2D$ increases intestinal calcium absorption and mobilizes calcium and phosphorus from bone.

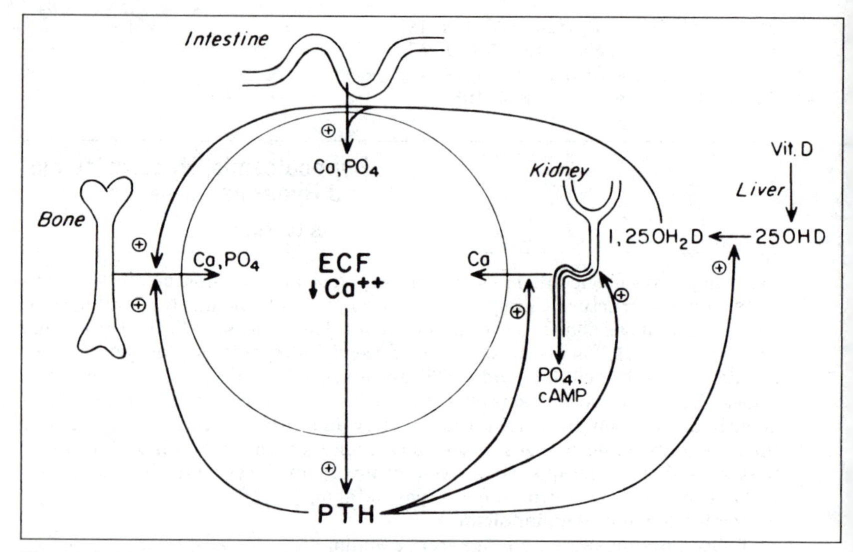

Fig. 24-1. Hormonal regulation of calcium and phosphate by PTH and $1,25(OH)_2D$. Decreased Ca^{2+} stimulates PTH and $1,25(OH)_2D$ secretion. Renal, gastrointestinal, and skeletal mechanisms will increase Ca^{2+}, inhibiting PTH secretion and closing the negative-feedback loop [PTH = parathyroid hormone; $1,25(OH)_2D$ = 1,25-dihydroxyvitamin D; 25(OH)D = 25-hydroxyvitamin D; Ca^{2+} = ionized calcium; PO_4 = inorganic phosphate; ECF = extracellular fluid; cAMP = cyclic adenosine monophosphate]. (From E. M. Brown, *Contemp Issues Nephrol.* 11: 179, 1983.)

3. **Calcitonin.** Calcitonin, secreted by thyroid C-cells, **inhibits bone resorption and has an antihypercalcemic effect.** Its significance for calcium regulation in the human adult is controversial. Calcitonin may play a more important calcitropic role during fetal and/or neonatal development.

C. **Postnatal changes in serum calcium concentrations.** The flow of calcium ions from mother to fetus during the third trimester of gestation is associated with **fetal chronic hypercalcemia.** At birth, the umbilical serum calcium level is elevated (10 to 11 mg/dl) [26]. In healthy term babies, calcium concentrations will decline for the first 24 to 48 hours; the nadir is usually 7.5 to 8.5 mg/dl. Thereafter, calcium concentrations progressively rise to the mean values observed in older children and adults [11]. Serum calcium concentrations in the first 3 days of life are also positively correlated with gestational age [29].

II. **Hypocalcemia.** Neonatal **hypocalcemia** usually is defined as a total serum calcium concentration of less than 7.0 mg/dl and an ionized calcium concentration of less than 4.0 mg/dl.

A. **Etiology of hypocalcemia**

1. **Early-onset hypocalcemia (during the first 3 days)**

a. **Preterm newborns** are born amid the third trimester growth spurt. They are poorly adapted to the cessation of maternal calcium flow and at birth face a calcium crisis. About 50 percent of low-birth-weight infants [29] and **nearly all** very low birth weight (VLBW) infants [31] exhibit total serum calcium levels of less than 7.0 mg/dl by day 2. This hypocalcemia appears to be an exaggeration of the normal term pattern; the nadir occurs by 12 to 24 hours, with little change until 72 hours. The pathogenesis is probably multifactorial. Preterm newborns do mount a PTH response [31], but target-organ responsiveness to PTH may be diminished [14,16]. Even VLBW newborns can synthesize 1,25$(OH)_2$D if vitamin D stores are adequate. Hypercalcitoninemia may be important [27]. High renal sodium excretion in preterm newborns may aggravate calciuric losses [4].

b. **Infants of diabetic mothers (IDMs)** have a 25 to 50 percent incidence of hypocalcemia during the first 24 to 48 hours [23]. The natural history may be similar to that of early neonatal hypocalcemia in preterm infants, or hypocalcemia may persist for several days. Hypercalcitoninemia, hypoparathyroidism, abnormal vitamin D metabolism, and hyperphosphatemia have been implicated, but none has been found consistently. The lower mean maternal and umbilical calcium and magnesium levels associated with diabetes may be important. The macrosomia associated with IDMs also may increase neonatal calcium demands, producing a more profound and prolonged hypocalcemia [7] (see Chap. 1).

c. **Birth asphyxia** is frequently associated with hypocalcemia and hyperphosphatemia, possibly related to renal insufficiency, acidosis, and/or impaired PTH secretion or responsiveness (see Chap. 21, Perinatal Asphyxia, page xxx).

2. **Late-onset hypocalcemia** usually presents at the end of the first week, but onset ranges from the first days to several weeks after birth. The classical syndrome was described in term infants fed **high-phosphate diets.** Contributing factors probably include neonatal immaturity of renal tubular phosphate excretion, hypoparathyroidism, hypomagnesemia, and vitamin D deficiency. Specific etiologies include the following:
   a. **Hypoparathyroidism (most common)**
      (1) **Idiopathic, transient**
      (2) **Congenital.** Parathyroids may be absent in **DiGeorge sequence** (hypoplasia or absence of the third and fourth branchial pouch structures).
      (3) **Maternal hyperparathyroidism** induces transient neonatal hypoparathyroidism.
      (4) **Magnesium deficiency** (including inborn error of intestinal magnesium transport) impairs PTH secretion [1].
   b. **Vitamin D deficiency**
      (1) Secondary to **maternal vitamin D deficiency**
      (2) **Malabsorption**
      (3) **Maternal anticonvulsant therapy** during pregnancy increases metabolism of 25(OH)D.
      (4) **Renal insufficiency** may impair 1,25$(OH)_2$D production.
      (5) **Nephrosis** and **impaired enterohepatic circulation** accelerate losses of 25(OH)D.
      (6) **Hepatobiliary disease** may decrease production of 25(OH)D.
   c. **Miscellaneous**
      (1) Rapid or excessive skeletal mineral deposition ("**hungry bones" syndrome**) may occur in SGA infants or in infants with rickets or hypoparathyroidism who receive aggressive vitamin D therapy.
      (2) **Hyperphosphatemia** is associated with phosphate-rich diets, excessive phosphate administration, renal insufficiency, asphyxia, hypervitaminosis D, hypoparathyroidism, and rhabdomyolysis.
      (3) **Hypoalbuminemia.** Ionized calcium level is unchanged.
      (4) **Alkalosis** and **bicarbonate therapy**
      (5) Rapid infusion of **citrate-buffered blood** (exchange transfusion) chelates ionized calcium.
      (6) **Lipid infusions** may lower ionized calcium level by enhancing calcium-albumin binding [32].
      (7) **Furosemide** produces marked hypercalciuria.
      (8) **Shock** or **sepsis**
      (9) **Hypothyroidism** infrequently is associated with hypocalcemia.

B. Evaluation

1. **Clinical manifestations**
   a. Hypocalcemia increases cellular permeability to sodium ions and increases cell membrane excitability. Signs are usually nonspecific: apnea, seizures, jitteriness, increased extensor tone, clonus, hyperreflexia, and stridor (laryngospasm). Carpopedal spasm and Chvostek's sign are present less frequently.
   b. **Early-onset hypocalcemia in preterm newborns** is usually asymptomatic or clinically mild (30).
   c. **Late-onset syndromes,** in contrast, may present as hypocalcemic seizures.
2. **Laboratory evaluation**
   a. **Suggested schedule for monitoring calcium levels in infants at risk for developing hypocalcemia**
      (1) Preterm infants (>1000 gm): 24 and 48 hours of age
      (2) Preterm infants (≤1000 gm): 12, 24, and 48 hours
      (3) Sick or stressed infants: 12, 24, and 48 hours; then as indicated
      (4) Healthy preterm infants (>1500 gm) and healthy IDMs who begin milk feedings on the first day do not need to be monitored in the absence of signs or symptoms.
   b. An electrocardiographic Q-OTC interval of greater than 0.2 s (due to prolonged systole), when present, is a useful indicator of hypocalcemia.
   c. In other than straightforward early-onset hypocalcemia, obtain calcium, ionized calcium, phosphorus, and magnesium levels. Measurement of albumin, urinary calcium, PTH, vitamin D metabolites, and renal function also may be helpful.
      (1) **Elevated serum phosphorus level** suggests phosphate loading, renal insufficiency, or hypoparathyroidism.
      (2) Magnesium level of 0.8 mg/dl or less strongly suggests **primary hypomagnesemia.**
      (3) Normal to moderately elevated $1,25(OH)_2D$ levels are consistent with hypoparathyroidism.
      (4) Absence of thymic shadow on chest radiograph may suggest DiGeorge sequence.

C. Management

1. **Treatment of hypocalcemia is associated with certain risks,** which are minimized by attention to details.
   a. Rapid IV infusion of calcium can cause sudden elevation of serum calcium level, leading to bradycardia or other dysrhythmias. Intravenous calcium should only be "pushed" for treatment of hypocalcemic crisis (e.g., with seizures).
   b. Extravasation of calcium solutions into subcutaneous tissues can cause severe necrosis and subcutaneous calcifications. Therefore, scrupulous attention to the peripheral IV site is indicated when calcium-containing solutions are infused.
   c. Infusion by means of the umbilical vein may result in hepatic necrosis if the catheter enters a branch of the portal vein.
   d. Rapid infusion by means of the umbilical artery can cause arterial spasms and, at least experimentally, intestinal necrosis [2].
   e. Intravenous calcium solutions are incompatible with sodium bicarbonate, since calcium carbonate will precipitate.
   f. Intravenous infusion of calcium chloride may produce chloride loading and hyperchloremic acidosis in neonates.
2. **Calcium preparations.** We prefer calcium gluconate 10% solution for intravenous (and occasionally oral) use (Table 24-1). Calcium glubionate syrup (Neo-Calglucon) is a convenient oral preparation. However, the high sugar content and osmolality may cause gastrointestinal irritation or diarrhea.

Table 24-1. Common calcium preparations

Preparation	Elemental calcium content (mg/ml)
Calcium gluconate (10% injection)	9.0
Calcium chloride (10% injection)	27.2
Calcium glubionate syrup	23.6

3. **Treatment of early-onset hypocalcemia**
   a. Hypocalcemic preterm infants who have no symptoms and are not ill from any other cause do not require specific treatment. The hypocalcemia should resolve spontaneously by day 3.
   b. If the serum calcium level drops to 6.5 mg/dl or less (usually VLBW newborns), we recommend beginning a continuous calcium infusion with the goal of producing a sustained increase in serum calcium level (7 to 8 mg/dl). A convenient starting dose is 45 mg/kg per day (5 ml/kg per day of calcium gluconate 10%). Bolus infusions are ineffective and hazardous. Prophylaxis or treatment with pharmacologic doses of vitamin D is **not recommended** [12,31].
   c. It may be desirable to prevent the onset of hypocalcemia for newborns who exhibit cardiovascular compromise (e.g., severe RDS, asphyxia, septic shock, PPHN) and require cardiotonic drugs or blood pressure support. Use a continuous calcium infusion, preferably by means of a central catheter, to maintain a total calcium level greater than 7.0 mg/dl and an ionized calcium level greater than 4.0 mg/dl.
4. **Treatment of hypocalcemic crisis with seizures, apnea, or tetany.** Serum calcium level is usually less than 5.0 mg/dl.
   a. **Emergency calcium therapy** consists of 1 to 2 ml of calcium gluconate 10% per kilogram (9 to 18 mg of elemental calcium per kilogram) by IV infusion over 5 minutes.
      (1) Monitor heart rate and the infusion site.
      (2) Repeat dose in 10 minutes if there is no clinical response.
      (3) Following the initial dose(s), maintenance calcium should be given parenterally or orally (see **3.b**).
   b. Symptomatic hypocalcemia unresponsive to calcium therapy may be due to **hypomagnesemia.**
      (1) The preferred preparation for treatment is magnesium sulfate. The 50% solution contains 500 mg, or 4 mEq/ml.
      (2) Correct severe hypomagnesemia ($\leq$1.2 mg/dl) with 0.1 to 0.2 ml of magnesium sulfate 50% per kilogram IV or IM. When administering IV, infuse slowly and monitor heart rate; IM administration may cause local tissue necrosis. The dose may be repeated every 6 to 12 hours. Obtain serum magnesium levels before each dose.
      (3) Maintenance magnesium therapy consists of oral administration of magnesium sulfate 50% 100 mg, or 0.2 mg/kg per day. If there is significant malabsorption, the dose may be increased two- to five-fold.
5. Treatment of specific hypocalcemic syndromes
   a. **Hypocalcemia associated with hyperphosphatemia**
      (1) **Classical late-onset neonatal hypocalcemia** is frequently preventable by ensuring adequacy of maternal vitamin D stores during pregnancy and avoiding high-phosphate diets in infants.
      (2) The goal of therapy is to **reduce renal phosphate load.** Reduce phosphate intake by feeding the infant human milk or a low-phosphorus formula (Similac PM 60/40 or SMA). Mineral contents of some infant diets are shown in Table 24-2.

Table 24-2. Mineral contents of common infant diets

Type of milk	Approximate mineral content	
	Calcium (mg/L)	Phosphorus (mg/L)
Human milk	340	160
Similac PM 60/40	380	190
SMA	425	290
Similac	510	390
Enfamil	470	320
Isomil	710	510
ProSobee	635	500
Similac Special Care 24	1460	730
Enfamil Premature 24	1340	670

(3) Increase the calcium-phosphate ratio of the milk to 4:1 with oral calcium supplements (e.g., 0.5 ml Neo-Calglucon per 30 ml PM 60/40). This will inhibit intestinal absorption of phosphorus. Phosphate binders are generally not necessary.

(4) Gradually wean calcium supplements over 2 to 4 weeks. Monitor serum calcium and phosphorus levels 1 to 2 times weekly.

b. Hypoparathyroid infants are hyperphosphatemic. Use a low-phosphate diet with calcium supplementation (see **5.a.1–4**) and correct vitamin D deficiency if present.

c. Vitamin D disorders

(1) Vitamin D deficiency in neonates is usually treatable with up to 5000 units per day of oral vitamin D_2 (Drisdol, 8000 units/ml), although occasionally higher doses may be required. Wean slowly as deficiency resolves. Frequent assay of serum calcium level is necessary to avoid rebound hypervitaminosis D.

(2) Defects in vitamin D metabolism are treated with vitamin D analogues, e.g., dihydrotachysterol (Hytakerol, DHT), calcitriol (Rocaltrol). The shorter initiation of action and short half-life of these drugs lessen the risk of rebound hypercalcemia.

III. Hypercalcemia. Neonatal hypercalcemia (serum total calcium level greater than 11.0 mg/dl, serum ionized calcium level greater than 5.0 mg/dl) may be asymptomatic and discovered incidentally during routine screening. Alternatively, the presentation of severe hypercalcemia ($\geq$14.0 mg/dl) can be dramatic and life-threatening, requiring immediate medical intervention.

A. Etiology. The physiologic mechanisms that prevent hypercalcemia are inhibition of PTH and $1,25(OH)_2D$ synthesis, which **reduces calcium mobilization from bone, absorption from intestine, and reclamation from kidney.** (The potential pathophysiologic role for calcitonin is unclear.) Elevated serum calcium concentration, therefore, implies inappropriately increased calcium efflux from one of these pools into the ECF.

1. Increased bone resorption

a. Hyperparathyroidism

(1) Congenital hyperparathyroidism associated with maternal hypoparathyroidism usually resolves over several weeks. Decreased availability of maternal calcium for the fetus stimulates the fetal parathyroids.

(2) Neonatal severe primary hyperparathyroidism (NSPHP). The parathyroids are refractory to regulation by calcium [20], producing marked hypercalcemia (frequently 15 to 30 mg/dl) and lack of response to subtotal parathyroidectomy. Milder forms of the disorder probably also occur [25]. NSPHP frequently occurs in **familial hypocalciuric hypercalcemia (FHH)** kindreds (see **3.b**), and it may be the severe, homozygous expression of an FHH gene that is mildly expressed in heterozygotes [18,19].

b. **Hyperthyroidism.** Thyroid hormone stimulates bone resorption and bone turnover [22].

c. **Hypervitaminosis A** accelerates bone resorption [5].

d. **Phosphate depletion** can cause hypercalcemia in preterm infants fed phosphate-poor diets, usually human milk [15,28], or undergoing parenteral nutrition [21]. Low phosphate intake stimulates $1,25(OH)_2D$ production, which mobilizes phosphate and calcium from bone into the ECF.

e. **Hypophosphatasia,** an autosomal-recessive bone dysplasia, produces severe bone demineralization and fractures.

2. **Increased intestinal absorption of calcium**

a. **Hypervitaminosis D** may result from excessive vitamin D ingestion by the mother (during pregnancy) or the neonate. Since vitamin D is extensively stored in fat, intoxication may persist for weeks to months.

3. **Decreased renal calcium clearance**

a. **Thiazide diuretics** can induce or exacerbate hypercalcemia, largely by hypocalciuric effects.

b. **Familial hypocalciuric hypercalcemia (FHH),** an autosomal-dominant disorder, can present in the neonatal period [24]. A dual defect in divalent cation sensing by parathyroid cells (causing parathyroid hyperplasia) and renal tubules (causing hypocalciuria) is proposed.

4. **Uncertain mechanisms**

a. **Idiopathic neonatal/infantile hypercalcemia** occurs in the constellation of **Williams syndrome** (hypercalcemia, supravalvular aortic stenosis or other cardiac anomalies, "elfin" facies, psychomotor retardation) and in a familial pattern lacking the Williams phenotype [17]. Increased calcium absorption has been demonstrated; vitamin D sensitivity [10] and impaired calcitonin secretion [6] are proposed, but controversial mechanisms.

b. **Subcutaneous fat necrosis** is a sequela of trauma or asphyxia. Granulomatous (macrophage) inflammation of the necrotic lesions may be a source of unregulated $1,25(OH)_2D$ synthesis [9].

c. **Acute renal failure,** usually during the diuretic or recovery phase

d. **Acute adrenal insufficiency**

e. **Blue diaper syndrome,** a defect in intestinal transport of tryptophan, causes excretion of water-insoluble blue tryptophan metabolites (indicanuria). The pathogenesis of the hypercalcemia is uncertain [8].

B. **Evaluation**

1. The **clinical manifestations** of severe hypercalcemia (usually hyperparathyroidism) include hypotonia, encephalopathy (lethargy or irritability, occasionally seizures), hypertension, respiratory distress (due to hypotonia and demineralization and deformation of the rib cage), poor feeding, vomiting, constipation, polyuria, hepatosplenomegaly, anemia, and extraskeletal calcifications, including nephrocalcinosis. Mortality is high in untreated cases. Milder hypercalcemia may present as feeding difficulties or poor linear growth.

2. **History**

a. Maternal history of hyper- or hypocalcemia, parathyroid disorders, nephrocalcinosis, and unexplained fetal losses

b. Maternal dietary and drug history (e.g., excessive vitamin A or D, thiazides)

c. Family history of hypercalcemia or FHH

d. Medications (e.g., vitamin A or D, thiazides, antacids)
e. Low-phosphate diet in preterm infants or excessive dietary calcium

3. **Physical examination**
   a. Small for dates (hyperparathyroidism, Williams syndrome)
   b. Craniotabes, fractures (hyperparathyroidism), or characteristic bone dysplasia (hypophosphatasia)
   c. "Elfin" facies (Williams syndrome)
   d. Cardiac murmur (supravalvular aortic stenosis and peripheral pulmonic stenosis associated with Williams syndrome)
   e. Indurated, bluish-red lesions (subcutaneous fat necrosis)
   f. Evidence of hyperthyroidism
   g. Blue discoloration of diaper

4. **Laboratory evaluation**
   a. The clinical history and **serum and urine mineral levels,** e.g., calcium, ionized calcium (if available), phosphorus, and urinary calcium-to-creatinine ratio (U_{Ca}:U_{Cr}), should suggest a likely diagnosis.
      (1) Very elevated serum calcium level (≥15 mg/dl) usually indicates primary hyperparathyroidism or in VLBW infants, phosphate depletion.
      (2) Low phosphorus level indicates phosphate depletion, hyperparathyroidism, or FHH.
      (3) Very low U_{Ca}:U_{Cr} suggests FHH.
   b. Specific **serum hormone levels** [iPTH, 25(OH)D, 1,25$(OH)_2$D] will confirm the diagnostic impression.
   c. **Serum alkaline phosphatase level** increases with increased bone resorption. Very low activity suggests hypophosphatasia (confirmed by increased urinary phosphoethanolamine).
   d. **Radiographs** of hand/wrist may suggest hyperparathyroidism (demineralization, subperiosteal resorption) or hypervitaminosis D (submetaphyseal rarefaction).

C. **Treatment**

1. **Emergency medical treatment**
   a. **Volume expansion with isotonic saline.** Hydration and sodium promote urinary calcium excretion. If cardiac function is normal, infuse normal saline (10 to 20 ml/kg) over 15 to 30 minutes (monitoring blood glucose level), then about 1½ times "maintenance" fluids using, e.g., 5% D/W with 40 to 60 mEq/L sodium chloride and 20 mEq/L potassium chloride.
   b. **Furosemide** (1 mg/kg q6–8h IV) induces calciuria. Since potassium and magnesium may become depleted, monitor and supplement as necessary.
   c. **Inorganic phosphate** may lower serum calcium levels in **hypophosphatemic patients** by inhibiting bone resorption and promoting bone mineral accretion. Parenteral phosphate should be avoided in severely hypercalcemic patients (serum total calcium level greater than 12 mg/dl) unless hypophosphatemia is severe (< 1.5 mg/dl). **Extraskeletal calcification** may occur. Oral phosphate (e.g., Neutra-phos, 200 mg phosphate per milliliter) is preferred. Initial dosage (orally, or in parenteral nutrition) is 3.0 to 5.0 mg/dl.
   d. **Glucocorticoids** are effective in hypervitaminosis A and D and subcutaneous fat necrosis by inhibiting both bone resorption and intestinal calcium absorption; they are ineffective in hyperparathyroidism. Administer cortisone 10 mg/kg per day or methylprednisolone 2 mg/kg per day.

2. **Other therapies**
   a. **Low-calcium, low-vitamin D diets** are an effective adjunctive therapy in hypervitaminosis A or D, subcutaneous fat necrosis, and Williams syndrome. Prolonged use may induce rickets.
   b. **Calcitonin** is a potent inhibitor of bone resorption. The antihypercal-

cemic effect is transient but may be prolonged if glucocorticoids are used concomitantly. There is little reported experience in neonates.

c. **Parathyroidectomy with autologous reimplantation** may be indicated for severe neonatal hyperparathyroidism.

IV. **Hypermagnesemia**

A. **Etiology.** Usually an exogenous magnesium load exceeding renal excretion capacity produces hypermagnesemia.

1. Magnesium sulfate therapy for maternal preeclampsia or preterm labor
2. Administration of magnesium-containing antacids to the newborn
3. Excessive magnesium in parenteral nutrition
4. Magnesium sulfate enemas (contraindicated in newborns)

B. **Diagnosis**

1. Elevated serum magnesium level (normal newborn range 1.6 to 2.8 mg/dl)
2. Hypermagnesemic signs are unusual in term infants if serum magnesium level is less than 6.0 mg/dl. The common curariform effects include apnea, respiratory depression, lethargy, hypotonia, hyporeflexia, poor suck, decreased intestinal motility, and delayed passage of meconium.

C. **Treatment**

1. Often the only intervention necessary is removal of the source of exogenous magnesium.
2. When hypermagnesemic symptoms are severe, an IV calcium infusion may reverse them. (Calcium acts as a magnesium antagonist.)
3. Exchange transfusion, peritoneal dialysis, or hemodialysis are usually not necessary.
4. Begin feedings only after suck and intestinal motility are established.

References

1. Anast, C. S. *J. Clin. Endocrinol. Metab.* 42: 707, 1976.
2. Book, S. B. *J. Pediatr.* 92: 793, 1978.
3. Brown, D. M. *Pediatrics* 49: 841, 1972.
4. Brown, D. R. *Pediatr. Res.* 15: 1100, 1981.
5. Bush, M. E. *Arch. Pathol. Lab. Med.* 108: 838, 1984.
6. Culler, F. L. *J. Pediatr.* 107: 720, 1985.
7. David, L., Glorieux, F. M., Salle, B. L., and Anast, C. S. Human Neonatal Hypocalcemia. In M. F. Molick, T. K. Gray, and C. S. Anast (Eds.), *Perinatal Calcium and Phosphorus Metabolism.* Amsterdam: Elsevier, 1983. Pp. 351–361.
8. Drummond, K. N. *Am. J. Med.* 39: 928, 1964.
9. Finne, P. H. *J. Pediatr.* 112: 792, 1988.
10. Garabedian, M. *N. Engl. J. Med.* 312: 948, 1985.
11. Greer, F. R. *J. Pediatr.* 108: 59, 1982.
12. Koo, W. W. K. *Am. J. Dis. Child.* 140: 1152, 1986.
13. Ladenson, J. H. *J. Clin. Endocrinol. Metab.* 46: 986, 1978.
14. Lanarelli, C. G. *Pediatr. Res.* 7: 329, 1973.
15. Lyon, A. J. *Arch. Dis. Child.* 59: 1141, 1984.
16. Mallett, E. *Biol. Neonate* 33: 304, 1978.
17. Martin, N. D. T. *Arch. Dis. Child.* 59: 605, 1984.
18. Marx, S. J. *N. Engl. J. Med.* 306: 257, 1982.
19. Marx, S. J. *Am. J. Med.* 78: 15, 1985.
20. Marx, S. J. *J. Clin. Endocrinol. Metab.* 62: 445, 1986.
21. Miller, R. R. *J. Pediatr.* 105: 814, 1984.
22. Mundy, G. R. *J. Clin. Invest.* 58: 529, 1976.
23. Noguchi, A. *J. Pediatr.* 97: 112, 1980.
24. Orwell, E. *Pediatrics* 69: 109, 1982.
25. Page, L. A. *J. Pediatr.* 111: 261, 1987.
26. Pitkin, R. M. *Am. J. Obstet. Gynecol.* 133: 781, 1979.
27. Romagnoli, C. *Arch. Dis. Child.* 62: 580, 1987.

28. Rowe, J. C. *N. Engl. J. Med.* 300: 273, 1979.
29. Tsang, R. C. *J. Pediatr.* 82: 423, 1973.
30. Venkataraman, P. S. *Pediatrics* 76: 543, 1985.
31. Venkataraman, P. S. *Am. J. Dis. Child.* 140: 1004, 1986.
32. Zaloga, G. P. *J. Clin. Endocrinol. Metab.* 64: 1010, 1987.

Metabolic Bone Disease of Prematurity

Lewis P. Rubin

Metabolic bone disease occurs in more than 30 percent of infants weighing 1500 gm or less at birth and 50 percent of those weighing less than 1000 gm [4,17,25]. **Osteopenia** ("washed out" or undermineralized bones) develops during the first postnatal weeks. Signs of **rickets** (epiphyseal dysplasia and skeletal deformities) usually become evident in 2 to 4 months or by term-corrected gestational age. The risk of bone disease is greatest for the sickest, most premature infants.

I. Etiology of metabolic bone disease of prematurity

A. Deficiency of calcium and phosphorus is the principal cause. Demands for rapid growth in the third trimester are met by intrauterine mineral accretion rates of 120 to 150 mg/kg of calcium per day and 60 to 120 mg/kg of phosphorus per day [8,28]. Poor mineral intake and absorption after birth result in undermineralized new and remodeled bone.

1. Diets low in mineral content predispose preterm newborns to metabolic bone disease.
   a. Unsupplemented human milk [1,18,24]
   b. Parenteral nutrition [7]
   c. Formulas not designed for use in preterm infants
2. **Furosemide** therapy causes renal calcium wasting.
3. **Renal phosphorus wasting**
   a. Acquired tubular acidosis [3]
   b. The Fanconi syndromes
   c. X-linked hypophosphatemic rickets [6,22] may present in late infancy.
   d. Tumor osteomalacia [27]. Many mesenchymal tumors, including **sclerosing hemangiomas,** produce humoral phosphaturic factors.

B. Vitamin D deficiency. Human milk has a total antirachitic sterol content of only 25 to 50 IU/L [23], insufficient for maintaining normal 25(OH)D levels in preterm infants (400 to 1000 IU per day required) [14]. However, when vitamin D intake is adequate, even very low birth weight newborns can synthesize $1,25(OH)_2D$ [11,20].

1. **Maternal vitamin D deficiency** can cause **congenital rickets.**
2. Inadequate vitamin D intake or absorption produces **nutritional rickets**
3. **Hepatobiliary rickets** results largely from vitamin D malabsorption [15]
4. **Chronic renal failure** (renal osteodystrophy)
5. Chronic use of phenytoin or phenobarbital increases 25(OH)D metabolism.
6. Hereditary pseudo-vitamin D deficiency: type I (abnormality or absence of 1-alpha-hydroxylase activity) or type II [tissue resistance to $1,25(OH)_2D$].

II. Diagnosis

A. Clinical signs include respiratory insufficiency or failure to wean from a ventilator [9], hypotonia, pain on handling due to pathologic fractures, decreased linear growth with sustained head growth, frontal bossing, enlarged anterior fontanel and widened cranial sutures, craniotabes (posterior flattening of the skull), "rachitic rosary" (swelling of costochondral junctions), Harrison's grooves (indentation of the ribs at the diaphragmatic insertions), and enlargement of wrists, knees, and ankles.

B. **Radiographic signs** include widening of epiphyseal growth plates; cupping, fraying, and rarefaction of the metaphyses; subperiosteal new bone formation; osteopenia, particularly of the skull, spine, scapula, and ribs; and occasionally osteoporosis or pathologic fractures.

C. **Laboratory evaluation**

1. **Serum calcium level** (low, normal, or slightly elevated) **and phosphorus level** (low to normal) generally are **not** good indicators of the presence or severity of metabolic bone disease.
2. **Serum alkaline phosphatase level** (an indicator of osteoclast activity) often is correlated with disease severity (>1000 U/L in severe rickets) [10,16]. Note the following:
   a. **Normal neonatal range** may be up to 4 times the adult upper limit [2].
   b. Hepatobiliary disease also elevates alkaline phosphatase level.
   c. Solitary elevated alkaline phosphatase level rarely can occur in the absence of bone or liver disease (transient hyperphosphatesemia of infancy) [19].
3. **25(OH)D_3 levels** are usually low to normal. 25(OH)D_3 is a useful guide for establishing the sufficiency of vitamin D stores; levels are less than 6 ng/ml in severe vitamin D deficiency.
4. **Radiographs.** Routine chest films show osteopenia and sometimes rachitic changes. Wrist or knee films and a skeletal series (pathologic fractures) can be useful.
5. Measurement of **bone mineral content** by photon densitometry remains investigational [12,21].
6. Reserve measurement of 1,25$(OH)_2$D or PTH for complicated or refractory cases.

III. **Prevention and treatment**

A. **Dietary management** (see Chap. 30)

1. **Mineral-fortified human milk or "premature" formulas** are the appropriate diets for preterm infants; their use can prevent and treat metabolic bone disease of prematurity [13,26]. Attempts at reproducing intrauterine mineral accretion rates may be unnecessary and potentially result in complications [5].
2. Use of other diets and specific supplementation with calcium gluconate or glubionate and/or potassium phosphate (93 mg phosphate per milliliter) is less desirable.

B. **Ensure adequate vitamin D stores** by an intake of 400 IU per day (see Chap. 30).

1. **Vitamin D deficiency rickets** is usually treatable with up to 5000 IU per day. Oral calcium supplements may be necessary during therapy, since serum calcium levels may drop precipitously as bone rapidly mineralizes.
2. Defects in vitamin D metabolism may respond better to dihydrotachysterol (DHT) or calcitriol (see Hypocalcemia, page 437).

C. Furosemide-induced renal calcium wasting can be lessened by adding a thiazide diuretic.

D. Avoid nonessential handling and vigorous chest physiotherapy in preterm infants with severely undermineralized bones.

E. Infants receiving mineral modified human milk as "premature" formulas or extra Vitamin D should have periodic monitoring of Ca, PO_4 and alkaline phosphate levels to prevent hypercalcemia. (See Chapter 30.)

References

1. Atkinson, S. A. *J. Pediatr.* 102: 99, 1983.
2. Barnes, D. J. *Proc. Soc. Exp. Biol. Med.* 44: 327, 1949.
3. Brenner, R. J. *N. Engl. J. Med.* 307: 217, 1982.
4. Callenback, J. C. *J. Pediatr.* 98: 800, 1981.
5. Campbell, D. E. *Clin. Perinatol.* 15: 879, 1988.

6. Chan, J. C. M. *J. Pediatr.* 106: 533, 1985.
7. Chessex, P. *J. Pediatr.* 107: 794, 1985.
8. Forbes, G. P. *Pediatrics* 57: 976, 1976.
9. Glasgow, J. F. T. *Arch. Dis. Child.* 52: 268, 1977.
10. Glass, E. J. *Arch. Dis. Child.* 57: 373, 1982.
11. Glorieux, F. H. *J. Pediatr.* 99: 640, 1981.
12. Greer, F. R. *Pediatr. Res.* 17: 259, 1983.
13. Gross, S. J. *J. Pediatr.* 111: 450, 1987.
14. Hillman, L. S. *J. Pediatr.* 106: 981, 1985.
15. Kooh, S. W. *J. Pediatr.* 94: 870, 1979.
16. Kovar, I. *Lancet* 1: 308, 1982.
17. Kulkarn, P. B. *J. Pediatr.* 96: 249, 1980.
18. Laing, I. A. *J. Pediatr.* 106: 265, 1985.
19. Lockitch, G. *J. Pediatr.* 105: 773, 1984.
20. Markestad, T. *Pediatr. Res.* 18: 269, 1984.
21. Minton, S. D. *J. Pediatr.* 95: 1037, 1979.
22. Moncrieff, M. W. *Arch. Dis. Child.* 57: 70, 1982.
23. Reeve, L. E. *Am. J. Clin. Nutr.* 36: 122, 1982.
24. Rowe, J. C. *J. Pediatr.* 104: 112, 1984.
25. Seina, Y. *Arch. Dis. Child.* 56: 628, 1981.
26. Steichen, J. J. *J. Pediatr.* 96: 528, 1980.
27. Weidner, N. *Cancer* 59: 1442, 1987.
28. Ziegler, E. E. *Growth* 40: 329, 1976.

Inborn Errors of Metabolism

John P. Cloherty and Harvey Levy

I. **Clinical indications.** The following are some clinical situations that cause one to suspect an inborn error of metabolism in the newborn. Good reviews of this problem are found in refs. 3, 7, 11, 15, and 17.
   A. A **history of unexplained neonatal deaths** in the family.
   B. **Neonatal signs and symptoms** of weight loss, poor feeding, lethargy, hypotonia, coma, seizures, vomiting, diarrhea, rapid respirations, apnea, dehydration, jaundice, hepatomegaly, unusual color of urine, unusual odor to sweat or urine, coarse facial features, and abnormalities of the skin, hair, eyes, joints, or bones. **Acute symptoms** are those suggestive of sepsis, cardiorespiratory failure, or central nervous system (CNS) disease. **Chronic symptoms** are failure to thrive, neurologic degeneration, and developmental delay.
   C. Onset of the preceding signs and symptoms after an interval of good health, especially in a full-term baby, or onset of symptoms after a change in diet
   D. Progression of these signs and symptoms with no evidence of infection, CNS hemorrhage, or other congenital or acquired defects
   E. Lack of relief of signs and symptoms with usual therapy
   F. Metabolic acidosis, hyperammonemia, hypoglycemia, lactic acidosis, ketonuria, reducing substances in the urine, or abnormal liver function tests (SGOT, SGPT, PT, PTT)
   G. Other causes of these symptoms such as sepsis, central nervous system bleed, or blood loss should be considered. An ultrasound or CT of the head may show brain edema in metabolic disease. An EEG may be abnormal but not show a specific pattern. Some patterns such as burst-suppression, which often suggest a poor prognosis after asphyxia, may be reversible in metabolic disease.

II. **Clinical problems associated with metabolic disease in the newborn**
   A. **Feeding difficulties or vomiting** is associated with many metabolic diseases but is most prominent with the following:
      1. **Protein intolerance,** such as the organic acidemias or the hyperammonemia syndromes

2. **Carbohydrate intolerance,** such as galactosemia or hereditary fructose intolerance
3. The **adrenogenital syndrome**

B. **Hepatomegaly** is prominent in the following:
1. **Disorders of carbohydrate metabolism,** such as galactosemia, hereditary fructose intolerance, or glycogen storage diseases
2. **Hereditary tyrosinemia**
3. **Alpha-1-antitrypsin deficiency**
4. **Organic acidemias** in association with acidosis
5. **Urea cycle disorders** in association with hyperammonemia
6. **Lysosomal disorders** such as Wolman's disease and on occasion mucolipidosis
7. **Peroxisomal disorders** such as Zellweger's syndrome, hyperpipecolic acidemia, and neonatal adrenoleukodystrophy
8. **Disorders of fatty acid metabolism**

C. **Abnormal coarse facial features** are often seen in the following:
1. **Peroxisomal disorders** (Zellweger's syndrome, neonatal adrenoleukodystrophy, rhizomelic chondrodysplasia)
2. **Pyruvate dehydrogenase deficiency**

D. **Seizures** are seen in the following (see Chap. 21, Seizures, page 370):
1. **Glycogen storage disease** (hypoglycemia)
2. **Galactosemia**
3. **Hereditary fructose intolerance**
4. **Maple syrup urine disease**
5. **Congenital lactic acidosis**
6. **Vitamin D–resistant rickets**
7. **Organic acidemias**
8. **Urea cycle disorders**
9. **Hyperglycinemia**
10. **Pyridoxine dependency**

E. **Other neurologic conditions** [decreased tone and reflexes (with or without seizures)]
1. **Nonketotic hyperglycemia**
2. **Hypophosphatasia**
3. **Organic acid disorders**
4. **Urea cycle defects**
5. **Zellweger's disease**

F. **Cardiac enlargement and failure** are seen in the hepatorenal type of tyrosemia, the organic acidemias, and after the newborn period in carnitine deficiency.

G. **Jaundice** (see Chap. 15)
1. **Elevated indirect bilirubin**
   a. Inborn errors of red blood cell metabolism, such as pyruvate-kinase deficiency or glucose-6-phosphate dehydrogenase (G-6-PD) deficiency.
   b. Galactosemia (early)
   c. Crigler-Najjar syndrome
   d. Gilbert's syndrome
   e. Hypothyroidism
2. **Elevated direct bilirubin**
   a. Rotor's syndrome
   b. Dubin-Johnson syndrome
   c. Galactosemia (late)
   d. Hereditary fructose intolerance
   e. Alpha-1-antitrypsin deficiency
   f. Hereditary tyrosinemia

H. **Hepatic dysfunction** as manifested by jaundice, hepatomegaly, coagulopathy, hepatocellular dysfunction, elevated liver enzymes, hypoglycemia, or hyperammonemia

1. **Galactosemia**
2. **Hereditary tyrosinemia**
3. **Nieman-Pick, type A**
4. **Glycogen storage disease type IV**
5. **Neonatal hemochromatosis**

I. **Hypoglycemia**
1. **Galactosemia**
2. **Hereditary fructose intolerance**
3. **Glycogen storage disease**
4. **Glycerol intolerance**
5. **"Maple syrup" urine disease**
6. **Organic acidemias**
7. **Hereditary tyrosinemia**
8. **Any illness with liver dysfunction**

J. **Metabolic acidosis**
1. **Organic acidemias**
2. **Maple syrup urine disease**
3. **Fatty acid oxidation disorder**
4. **Glycogen storage disease**
5. **Hereditary fructose intolerance**
6. **Renal tubular acidosis** (see Chap. 26)
7. **Cytochrome oxidase defects**
8. **Multiple carboxylase deficiency**

K. **Ketosis**
1. **Maple syrup urine disease**
2. **The organic acidemias**

L. **Hyperammonemia**
1. **The organic acidemias** (with metabolic acidosis)
2. **The hyperammonemia syndromes** (see **III.E**).

M. **Abnormal odor to sweat or urine**
1. **Ketosis**—sweet odor due to acetone
2. **Maple syrup urine disease**—maple syrup odor due to branched-chain ketoacids
3. **Isovaleric acidemia**—sweaty feet odor due to isovaleric acid
4. **Tyrosinemia**—rancid butter odor due to alpha-ketogammamethiolbutyrate
5. **Beta-methylcrotonyl–coenzyme A deficiency**—cat's urine odor due to beta-hydroxyisovalerate
6. **Trimethylaminuria**—rotten fish odor due to trimethylamine

N. **Reducing substances in urine** (with the involved compound)
1. **Diabetes mellitus** (glucose)
2. **Essential fructosuria** (fructose)
3. **Fanconi syndrome** (glucose)
4. **Galactokinase deficiency** (galactose)
5. **Galactosemia** (galactose)
6. **Hereditary fructose intolerance** (glucose, fructose)
7. **Pentosuria** (xylulose)
8. **Renal glycosuria** (glucose)
9. **Severe liver disease** with secondary galactose intolerance (galactose)

O. **Positive ferric chloride reaction in urine** (with the color of the reaction)
1. **Phenylketonuria** (green)
2. **Tyrosinemia** (green, fading rapidly)
3. **"Maple syrup" urine disease** (gray-green)
4. **Histidinemia** (blue-green)
5. **Alkaptonuria** (dark brown)
6. **Ketosis** (light green)
7. **Melanoma** (black)

8. **Pheochromocytoma** (blue-green)
9. **Formiminotransferase deficiency** (gray-green)
10. **Drug intoxication** (purple, red-brown, or green)
11. **Conjugated hyperbilirubinemia** (green)

III. Inborn errors of metabolism that are potentially lethal in the newborn

A. Galactosemia [11]

1. **Symptoms**
   a. Jaundice (mostly unconjugated in the first week, thereafter increased conjugated)
   b. Hepatomegaly
   c. Lethargy
   d. Weight loss
   e. Gram-negative sepsis
   f. Cataracts
   g. Hypoglycemia
2. **Diagnosis**
   a. In galactosemia, after the ingestion of milk (lactose), the urine is positive for reducing substance (Clinitest), but it is negative for glucose (glucose-oxidase dipstick test).
   b. Assay of blood for galactose-1-phosphate uridyltransferase (Beutler test) on filter-paper "PKU" blood specimen
   c. Assay of urine for galactose
   d. Abnormal liver function tests (SGOT, SGPT, PT, PTT)
3. **Treatment.** Elimination of lactose from the diet is the primary treatment.

B. Hereditary fructose intolerance

1. **Symptoms.** Problems after eating sucrose (such as in soy formulas) or fructose include the following:
   a. Vomiting
   b. Hypoglycemia
   c. Seizures
   d. Coma
   e. Hepatomegaly
   f. Jaundice
   g. Sepsis
2. **Diagnosis**
   a. Hypoglycemia after ingestion of sucrose or fructose
   b. Intravenous fructose tolerance test
   c. Measurement of hepatic fructose-1-phosphate aldolase activity
3. **Treatment.** Elimination of fructose and sucrose from the diet

C. Branched-chain ketoaciduria (maple syrup urine disease)

1. **Signs and symptoms**
   a. Lethargy
   b. Poor feeding
   c. Episodes of decreased muscle tone alternating with increased tone
   d. Seizures
   e. Coma
2. **Diagnosis**
   a. Maple syrup odor to urine and body
   b. Metabolic acidosis
   c. Ketoacidosis
   d. Green-gray urine color with the ferric chloride test
   e. Urine test with 2,4-dinitrophenylhydrazine for abnormal ketoacids
   f. Blood test for leucine by bacterial inhibition assay
   g. Plasma amino acid analysis
   h. Measurement of branched-chain decarboxylase in leukocytes or skin fibroblasts
3. **Treatment.** Dietary, vitamins

D. Organic acidemias: methylmalonic acidemia, propionic acidemia, isovaleric acidemia, and other organic acidemias

1. **Signs and symptoms**
   a. Poor feeding
   b. Vomiting
   c. Lethargy
   d. Coma
   e. Hypotonicity
   f. Spasticity
   g. Seizures
2. **Diagnosis**
   a. Metabolic acidosis
   b. Ketoacidosis
   c. Hyperammonemia
   d. Hypoglycemia
   e. Urine methylmalonic acid by paper chromatography
   f. Gas-liquid chromatography of urine for organic acids
   g. Plasma and urine amino acid analysis for increased glycine
3. **Treatment** involves reversal of metabolic acidosis and dietary therapy with administration of vitamins appropriate for the disorder.

E. Hyperammonemia syndromes [5,8,18]

1. **Urea cycle disorders including:**
   a. Carbamyl phosphate synthetase deficiency (CPS)
   b. Ornithine transcarbamylase deficiency (OTC)
   c. Argininosuccinate synthetase deficiency (citrullinemia) (AS)
   d. Argininosuccinate lyase deficiency (AL)
   e. Arginase deficiency
   f. *N*-acetylglutamate synthetase deficiency
2. **Disorders of branched-chain amino acid metabolism including** (see **III.D**):
   a. β-ketothiolase deficiency
   b. Isovaleric acidemia
   c. Methylmalonic acidemia
   d. Propionic acidemia
3. **Severe perinatal asphyxia**
4. **Total parenteral nutrition**
5. **Liver failure**
6. Rare miscellaneous disorders
   a. Congenital lysine intolerance
   b. Syndrome of hyperornithinemia-hyperammonemia-homocitrullinuria (HHH)
   c. Lysinuric protein intolerance
   d. Syndrome of Rett (hyperammonemia-cerebral atrophy)
   e. Hyperlysinemia with lysine-induced crisis
   f. Short-chain acyl-coenzyme A dehydrogenase deficiency
7. **Transient hyperammonemia** of a severe degree has been described in **premature infants.** This is manifest by respiratory distress in the first day of life, coma by the second day of life, and an elevated ammonia level with a normal anion gap. There is often a mildly elevated citrulline [9].
   a. **Signs and symptoms**
      (1) Feeding difficulties
      (2) Irritability
      (3) Lethargy
      (4) Hypotonicity
      (5) Coma
      (6) Convulsions
   b. **Diagnosis.** An approach to the diagnosis is found in ref 9.
      (1) Hyperammonemia

(2) Blood gases, electrolytes, bicarbonate, amino acids, organic acids, carnitine, lactate, pyruvate

(3) Urine ketones, amino acids, organic acids, and orotic acid

8. **Treatment** [4,6,17] of hyperammonemia from urea cycle defects involves four elements:

a. **Control production of ammonia** by stopping protein intake and providing enough calories to prevent tissue catabolism.

b. **Removal of excess ammonia** can be done by peritoneal dialysis and, if possible, hemodialysis. Hemodialysis is the treatment of choice. Exchange transfusion should only be used in an emergency on a temporary basis when dialysis is not immediately available.

c. **Provision of alternate pathways** for nitrogen excretion by giving sodium benzoate, sodium phenylacetate, or anginine.

d. Any cause of catabolism such as infection or asphyxia should be treated.

Infants with transient hyperammonemia of the premature may respond to repeated exchange transfusions and intravenous glucose and lipids to decrease catabolism of protein.

F. Nonketotic hyperglycinemia

1. **Signs and symptoms**

a. Lethargy

b. Poor feeding

c. Seizures

d. Hypotonicity

e. Death

2. **Diagnosis** is by plasma and spinal fluid amino acid analysis for elevated glycine.

3. **Treatment.** Anticonvulsants, benzoate

G. Infant of maternal PKU [1,13]

1. **Signs and symptoms**

a. Microcephaly

b. Low birth weight

c. Dysmorphic facies

d. Congenital heart disease (12 to 15 percent)

2. **Diagnosis** is by plasma amino acid determination for phenylalanine or PKU **on the mother.**

3. **Treatment.** Supportive for baby; counseling to mother about dietary treatment during future pregnancies.

H. Pyridoxine-dependent convulsions

1. **Symptom**—seizures

2. Test for therapeutic responses (see Neonatal Seizures in Chap. 21)

3. **Treatment** involves pyridoxine (see Neonatal Seizures in Chap. 21)

I. Cystic fibrosis

1. **Symptom**—intestinal obstruction by meconium ileus

2. **Diagnosis**—sweat test

3. **Treatment** is with respiratory therapy, antibiotics, diet, sodium replacement, and pancreatic enzymes.

4. Carrier testing and prenatal diagnosis are now available.

J. Adrenogenital syndrome (see Chap. 25)

1. **Diagnosis**

a. Vomiting, dehydration, hyponatremia, and hyperkalemia

b. Ambiguous genitalia

2. **Treatment** involves fluid and electrolyte therapy as well as corticosteroids.

IV. Management of infants with a suspected metabolic disorder

A. When a sibling died of a suspected metabolic disorder, the following steps should be taken:

1. **Preliminary considerations**

a. There should be a prenatal discussion of possibilities, and the parents and relatives should be screened for possible clues.
b. Intrauterine diagnosis by measurement of abnormal substances in the amniotic fluid or by enzyme assay of fibroblasts obtained by amniocentesis should be considered (see Chaps. 3 and 11).
c. Old hospital charts and postmortem material should be reviewed.
d. The baby should be delivered in a facility equipped with a laboratory capable of performing many sophisticated tests.

2. **Initial evaluation** includes a careful physical examination, seeking any of the signs described in **I.B.** Careful examination of the eyes, skin, and liver should be performed. Blood tests for glucose, pH, carbon dioxide, electrolytes, liver function, ketones, ammonia, lactate, pyruvate, organic acids, amino acids, and very long chain fatty acids should be done. Urine should be examined for color, odor, sediment, ketones, and reaction to ferric chloride. Urinary amino acids and organic acids should be analyzed. Spinal fluid amino acids should be analyzed (e.g., hyperglycinemia has increased spinal fluid glycine with blood glycine only slightly elevated). All nonmetabolic causes of symptoms such as anoxia or infection should be excluded. All abnormal substances found in the blood or urine should be identified, and appropriate enzyme assays on red blood cells, white blood cells, skin fibroblasts, or liver tissue should be performed.
3. **Sophisticated tests.** Amino acid, organic acid, or blood and urine analysis by column chromatography, thin-layer or paper chromatography, or gas chromatography and mass spectrometry should be performed by personnel who are aware of their uses and limitations. These tests should be performed on cord blood and blood and urine obtained from the baby at 12, 24, and 48 hours of age.
4. **Initial feedings**
    a. During the first 24 hours, the infant may be fed dextrose 5% to 10% and dextrose polymer (Polycose*) as tolerated.
    b. After 24 hours, the baby is given fat in the form of medium-chain triglycerides to prevent protein catabolism and possible accumulation of toxic by-products (Nil Prote† contains glucose, emulsifiable fat, minerals, and vitamins).
    c. If the tests performed at 48 hours are all negative, protein is introduced in the form of breast milk or any low-protein milk.
    d. The tests are repeated after 48 hours of protein intake. If no abnormalities are found (as would be expected in 75 percent of offspring from those who carry genes for autosomal-recessive disorders), the child may be cautiously fed. If metabolic abnormalities are found, the specific problem should be identified and appropriate diet or vitamin treatment started.

B. When an infant has signs or symptoms of metabolic disease (see **I.B**), he or she should be managed as follows:
1. Tests as in **A.2** and **A.3** should be performed.
2. The response to hemodialysis, peritoneal dialysis, or exchange transfusion should be evaluated.
3. The baby should be fed a simple diet as in **A.4** until the evaluation is complete; one should attempt to give adequate calories to prevent catabolism. This may involve giving intravenous glucose in high doses with added insulin if necessary (see Chap. 24, Hypoglycemia and Hyperglycemia). Often 150 kcal/mg per day will be needed. This often can only be obtained with enteral feedings. In pyruvate dehydrogenase deficiency, excess glucose is contraindicated. In these cases, give lipid and enough glucose to keep the blood sugar level normal. Lipids may be used to prevent

*Ross Laboratories, Columbus, Ohio.
†Product 80056, Mead Johnson Laboratories, Evansville, Ind.

protein catabolism. Other medications are sometimes used (see specific disorders).

V. **Postmortem diagnosis.** If an infant is dying or has died from what may be a metabolic disease, it is very important to make a specific diagnosis in order to help with genetic counseling. Sometimes families that will not permit a full autopsy will allow the collection of some specimen that may help in diagnosis. Specimens that should be collected are the following:

A. **Blood**—both clotted and heparinized. The specimen should be centrifuged and the plasma frozen.

B. **Urine**—refrigerated

C. **Spinal fluid**—refrigerated

D. **Skin biopsy** for fibroblast culture to be used for chromosomal analysis or enzyme assay. Two samples should be taken from a well-perfused area in the torso. The skin should be well cleaned, but any residual cleaning solution should be washed off with sterile water. The skin can be placed in sterile saline until special tubes are available.

E. **Liver.** Premortem liver biopsies as well as generous postmortem samples should be "flash frozen" to provide better enzyme analysis and preserve structure.

F. **Other.** Sometimes other tissue such as skeletal muscle, cardiac muscle, brain, and kidney should be preserved.

Infants who die with what may be a metabolic disease should have photographs and a full skeletal radiologic screening done. A full autopsy should be done. Information on the proper handling of the tissue should be obtained from one of the regional information centers (see **VII**).

VI. **Prenatal diagnosis** (see Chaps. 3 and 11)

A. **Amniocentesis during second trimester**

1. Analysis of fluid (methylmalonic acidemia, nonketotic hyperglycinemia)
2. Enzyme analysis of cultured cells from amniocentesis or chorionic villus biopsy
3. Fetal liver biopsy

B. **Detectable disorders** include galactosemia, "maple syrup" urine disease, organic acidemias, urea cycle disorders, homocystinuria, hyperglycinemia, and tyrosinemia. This is a rapidly changing area. Consult with your regional center as to what disorders are detectable (see Chap. 11).

VII. **Regional information centers**

A. **New England:**

New England Regional Newborn Screening Program
State Laboratory Institute
305 South Street
Jamaica Plain, MA 02130
(617) 522-3700, ext. 165

B. **Mid-Atlantic states:**

Pediatric Genetics Clinic
1004 CMSC
Johns Hopkins Hospital
Baltimore, MD 21205
(301) 955-3701

C. **Southeast:**

Emory Genetic Clinic
Emory University School of Medicine
2040 Ridgewood Drive, NE
Atlanta, GA 30322
(404) 329-5731

D. **Southwest:**

Department of Pediatrics
University of Texas Medical School
P.O. Box 20708
Houston, TX 77025
(713) 792-4784

E. Pacific states:
Medical Genetics Clinic
Children's Hospital of Los Angeles
P.O. Box 54700
Los Angeles, CA 90054
(213) 669-2152

F. Northwest:
PKU and Metabolic Birth Defects Center
University of Oregon Health Sciences Center
P.O. Box 574
Portland, OR 97297
(503) 225-8344

G. Rocky Mountain area:
Inherited Metabolic Disease Clinic
University of Colorado Health Sciences Center
4200 East Ninth Avenue
Denver, CO 80262
(303) 394-7195

H. Midwest:
Metabolic Clinic
Waisman Center on Mental Retardation and Human Development
1500 Highland Avenue
Madison, WI 53706
(608) 263-5993

Routine screening. Massachusetts routinely screens filter-paper blood specimens on all newborns for phenylketonuria, maple syrup urine disease, homocystinuria, galactosemia, hypothyroidism, sickle cell disease, congenital adrenyl hyperplasia, and toxoplasmosis. See ref. 2 for an article on newborn screening.

References

1. American Academy of Pediatrics. *Pediatrics* 76: 313, 1985.
2. American Academy of Pediatrics Committee on Genetics. *Pediatrics* 83: 449, 1989.
3. Ampola, M. G. *Clin. Perinatol.* 3: 1, 1976.
4. Batshaw, M. L. *J. Pediatr.* 97: 893, 1980.
5. Batshaw, M. L. *N. Engl. J. Med.* 306: 1387, 1982.
6. Batshaw, M. L. *Enzyme* 38: 242, 1987.
7. Burton, B. K. *Pediatrics* 79: 359, 1987.
8. Donn, S. M., et al. *Pediatr. Rev.* 5: 203, 1983–1984.
9. Hudak, M. L. *J. Pediatr.* 107: 712, 1985.
10. Levy, H. L. Genetic Screening. In H. Harris and N. Hirsch (Eds.), *Advances in Human Genetics,* Vol. 4. New York: Plenum, 1975.
11. Levy, H. L. Inborn Errors in Metabolism. In M. E. Avery and H. W. Taeusch (Eds.), *Diseases of the Newborn.* Philadelphia: Saunders, 1984.
12. Milunsky, A. (Ed.). *Genetic Disorders of the Fetus: Diagnosis, Prevention and Treatment.* New York: Plenum, 1979.
13. Rohr, F. J. *J. Pediatr.* 110: 391, 1987.
14. Scriver, C. R. *J. Pediatr.* 113: 495, 1988.
15. Scriver, C. R., Beaudet, A. L., Six, W. S., and Valle, D. (Eds.). *The Metabolic Basis of Inherited Disease,* 6th Ed. New York: McGraw-Hill, 1989.
16. Shih, V. E. Homozygote Screening in Disorders of Amino Acid Metabolism. In A. Milunsky (Ed.), *The Prevention of Genetic Disease and Mental Retardation.* Philadelphia: Saunders, 1975.
17. Vidailhet, M., and Morali, A. Inborn Errors of Metabolism. In L. Stern and P. Vent (Eds.), *Neonatal Medicine.* New York: Masson, 1988.
18. Oski, F. A., and Stockman, J. A., III (Eds.). *Yearbook of Pediatrics.* Chicago: Year Book Medical Publishers, 1987. P. 22.

Fluid and Electrolyte Management of the Newborn

Charles F. Simmons, Jr.

Support of the term and premature newborn provides the clinician with unique problems in fluid and electrolyte management. Dramatic changes in body composition, integument, renal and neuroendocrine function accompany the transition from fetal to extrauterine life. The increasing survival of very low birth weight (VLBW) infants is due in part to improved fluid and electrolyte management, and we must acknowledge that small margins for error exist in our sickest infants.

I. **Principles of water and electrolyte metabolism.** It is essential that clinicians understand the underlying principles of fluid and electrolyte therapy. Each infant's unique requirements can be determined only by careful ongoing assessment of clinical and laboratory status.

   A. **Compartmentation of total-body water.** Total-body water is divided into **intracellular fluid (ICF)** and **extracellular fluid (ECF)** compartments (see Fig. 30-2). ECF is, in turn, composed of intravascular and interstitial fluid. When evaluating fluid and electrolyte therapy, the ECF is the most readily assessed compartment. The goals of fluid and electrolyte therapy are (1) to maintain an appropriate ECF volume, which is determined primarily by total-body sodium and (2) to maintain appropriate ICF and ECF osmolality, determined by the amount of total-body water relative to solutes [15].

   B. **Changes in total-body water at birth.** In term infants, a diuresis of total-body water and ECF occurs after birth. This normal process results in a weight loss of 5 to 10 percent [6,8,9]. This diuresis also may be desirable in the preterm infant, since excessive parenteral fluid and sodium administration may be detrimental in this population [2,5,16]. With decreasing gestational age, ECF comprises an increasing proportion of birth weight (see Fig. 30-2). VLBW infants may therefore lose a greater percentage of birth weight (5 to 15 percent) during the first week of life to attain ECF proportions equivalent to the term infant.

   C. **Renal and hormonal maturation.** Renal function matures with advancing gestational age. Urine can be a source of great variation in water and electrolyte losses. Premature infants exhibit numerous aspects of immature sodium and water homeostasis: (1) glomerular filtration is decreased, (2) maximal proximal and distal tubule sodium reabsorption is reduced, (3) renal capacity for concentration and dilution of urine is diminished, and (4) bicarbonate reabsorption and potassium and hydrogen ion secretion are decreased [10,11]. This state of renal immaturity leads to less tolerance of challenges to water and electrolyte balance (see Chap. 26).

   D. **Extrarenal sources of water and electrolyte loss.** Insensible water loss (IWL) in VLBW infants can exceed 150 ml/kg per day when accompanied by use of radiant warmers, phototherapy, loss of skin integrity, or extreme prematurity [3,4,7,13,17] (Table 24-3). Other sources of fluid loss, such as cerebrospinal fluid (ventriculostomy drainage or repeated lumbar punctures), stool (diarrhea or ostomy drainage), nasogastric tubes, and thoracostomy tubes, should be quantitated, characterized, and replaced if significant.

II. **Assessment of fluid and electrolyte status**

   A. **History.** An infant's fluid and electrolyte status at birth partially reflects maternal hydration and drug administration. The use of oxytocin, diuretics, and hypotonic IV fluid may lead to maternal and fetal hyponatremia.

   B. **Physical examination**

      1. **Body weight.** Acute changes in total-body water lead to changes in total-body weight. Body weight should usually be assessed at least once per day. Of note, the final distribution of water in body compartments also reflects the distribution of total-body solutes and vascular permeability

Table 24-3. Insensible water loss*

Birth weight (gm)	IWL (ml/kg/day)
750–1000	82
1001–1250	56
1251–1500	46
>1501	26

Key: IWL = insensible water loss.
*Values were derived from refs. 3, 4, 7, 13, and 17 and are mean IWL for infants in incubators during the first week of life. IWL is **increased** by phototherapy (approximately 40 percent), radiant warmers (approximately 45 percent), and fever. IWL is **decreased** by the use of humidified gas with respirators and heat shields in incubators.

characteristics. Thus acute changes in body weight may not reflect changes in intravascular volume. For example, intravascular volume contraction despite increased body weight and interstitial edema can accompany neuromuscular paralysis or peritonitis.

2. **Skin.** Abnormalities of ECF volume can lead to changes in skin turgor, tension of the anterior fontanel, moistness of mucous membranes, and peripheral or periorbital edema. These physical findings, however, are not sensitive indicators of fluid or electrolyte imbalance.
3. **Cardiovascular.** Tachycardia can result from a reflex increase in cardiac output but can be observed in ECF depletion (decreased preload) or ECF excess (e.g., congestive heart failure). **Delayed capillary refill time** (reperfusion after pressure-induced skin blanching) can signify reduced cardiac output, and **hepatomegaly** can suggest an increased ECF volume. **Blood pressure changes** occur late in the sequence of events that follow reduced cardiac output.

C. Laboratory evaluation

1. **Serum electrolytes and plasma osmolarity** reflect composition and tonicity of ECF.
2. **Urine electrolytes and specific gravity** can reflect renal capacity to concentrate or dilute urine and reabsorb or excrete sodium. If the patient's hydration and ECF tonicity are normal, urine electrolytes do not correlate well with replacement needs.
3. **Urine output** falls with ECF depletion (dehydration), often to less than 1 cc/kg per hour. In neonates with immature renal function, urine output may not decrease despite ECF volume depletion.
4. **Fractional excretion of sodium (FE-Na)** is determined after measuring sodium (Na) and creatinine (Cr) concentrations in urine and plasma:

$$\text{Percent filtered sodium excreted} = \frac{\text{excreted Na}}{\text{filtered Na}} \times 100$$

$$= \frac{\text{urine Na} \times \text{plasma Cr}}{\text{urine Cr} \times \text{plasma Na}} \times 100$$

Determination of this value aids evaluation of the oliguric newborn; values less than 1 percent suggest oliguria due to prerenal factors that reduce renal blood flow, such as hypovolemia or poor cardiac output. Values greater than 2.5 percent occur with acute renal failure and in infants receiving diuretics. FE-Na is frequently greater than 2.5 percent in infants less than 32 weeks' gestation and is thus not helpful in evaluating oliguria in the very premature infant.

5. **Blood urea nitrogen (BUN) and serum creatinine** determinations provide indirect information about ECF volume and glomerular filtration.

Values in the early postnatal period reflect placental clearance of these molecules.

6. **Arterial pH, carbon dioxide tension (PCO_2), and sodium bicarbonate** determinations can provide indirect evidence of intravascular volume depletion, since poor tissue perfusion leads to high-anion-gap metabolic acidosis (lactic acidosis).

III. **Management of fluids and electrolytes.** The goal of initial fluid **management** is to allow initial loss of ECF over the first 5 to 6 days of life, reflected by weight loss, while maintaining normal tonicity and intravascular volume, reflected by blood pressure, heart rate, urine output, serum electrolytes, and pH.

A. **The term infant.** Body weight should decrease by 5 to 10 percent over the first 5 to 6 postnatal days. Subsequently, fluids should be adjusted such that changes in body weight are consistent with caloric intake. Maldistribution of body water (e.g., edema) should be monitored. Sodium is not usually required in the first 24 hours unless ECF expansion is necessary.

B. **The premature infant.** Body weight may be allowed to decrease 5 to 15 percent over the first 5 to 6 postnatal days. Tables 24-4 and 24-5 represent a management strategy developed for infants housed in humidified incubators [10]; increased fluid administration rates are needed for infants under radiant warmers. Fluids should then be adjusted to maintain a stable weight until an anabolic state is achieved and growth occurs. Fluid and electrolyte status should be reassessed frequently during the first 2 days of postnatal life in order to refine requirements. Physical examination, urine output and specific gravity, and serum electrolyte determinations may be required as frequently as every 6 to 8 hours in infants who weigh less than 1000 gm. Losses of water through skin and urine may approach 200 cc/kg per day, which can represent up to **one-third of total-body water per day.** Sodium should not be added to IV fluids in the first 24 hours unless ECF volume loss exceeds 5 percent of body weight per day.

IV. **Approach to disorders of sodium and water balance.** Abnormalities may be grouped into disorders of **tonicity** and **ECF volume.** The conceptual approach to a patient with a disorder of tonicity (e.g., hyponatremia) depends on whether a state of normal ECF (euvolemia), ECF depletion (dehydration), or ECF excess (edema) coexists.

A. **Isonatremic disorders**

1. **Dehydration**

a. **Predisposing factors** frequently involve equivalent losses of sodium and water, such as thoracostomy, nasogastric or ventriculostomy drainage, or third-space losses that accompany peritonitis, gastroschisis, or omphalocele. Renal sodium and water losses in the VLBW infant can lead to hypovolemia despite normal body tonicity.

b. **Diagnosis.** Dehydration is manifested by weight loss, decreased urine output, and increased urine specific gravity. Infants less than 32

Table 24-4. Fluid therapy for the premature infant (day 1)*

Birth weight (kg)	Fluid volume (ml/kg/day)	Dextrose	Sodium
>1.5	50–60	10	None
1.0–1.5	60–70	10	None
0.75–1.0	80–100†	5–10	None

*Note that these infants were in humidified incubators. Infants under radiant warmers usually require higher initial fluid rates.
†Very low birth weight infants frequently require even greater rates of fluid administration.
Source: From J. M. Lorenz et al., Water balance in very low birth weight infants: Relationship to water and sodium intake and effect on outcome. *J. Pediatr.* 101: 423, 1982.

Table 24-5. Fluid therapy for the premature infant (after day 1)*

Increase Fluids if:
Infant loses more than 2 to 5 percent of body weight per day or more than 10 to 15 percent at any time
Urine output is less than 0.5 ml/kg per hour over an 8-hour period
Decrease Fluids if:
Infant loses less than 1 to 3 percent of body weight per day or gains excessive weight after 8 to 15 percent of body weight is lost
Sodium Administration:
When sodium concentration is less than 140 mEq/L, begin sodium (1 to 3 mEq/L) when fluids are increased
If sodium concentration is less than 135 mEq/L, begin sodium even if fluid intake is not increased
Increase Sodium Concentration if:
Serum sodium concentration is less than 135 mEq/L and no weight gain
Serum sodium concentration is less than 140 mEq/L and weight loss is greater than 2 to 5 percent per day
Decrease Sodium Concentration if:
Serum sodium concentration is greater than 140 and no weight loss
Serum sodium concentration is greater than 135 mEq/L and weight gain

*If signs of extracellular fluid volume excess or depletion exist, of if the serum sodium concentration changes by more than 5 mEq/L in an 8-hour period, refer to text for further management.

Source: From J. M. Lorenz et al., Water balance in very low birth weight infants: Relationship to water and sodium intake and effect on outcome. *J. Pediatr.* 101: 423, 1982.

weeks' gestation may not demonstrate oliguria in response to hypovolemia. Poor skin turgor, tachycardia, hypotension, metabolic acidosis, and increasing BUN may coexist. A low FE-Na (<1 percent) is consistent with dehydration, although this is usually only seen in infants beyond 32 weeks' postconceptual age.

c. **Therapy.** Sodium and water administration should be liberalized to correct the deficit and then adjusted to equal maintenance plus ongoing losses.

2. **Edema**

a. **Predisposing factors** include excessive administration of isotonic crystalloid or colloid, CHF, sepsis, and neuromuscular paralysis.

b. **Diagnosis.** Edema is most easily manifest in the eyelids and extremities. Increased weight and hepatomegaly may accompany edema.

c. **Therapy.** Restriction of sodium is necessary (excess total-body sodium), as well as water, depending on the subsequent electrolyte response.

B. **Hyponatremic disorders** (Table 24-6). Factitious hyponatremia due to hyperlipidemia or hyperosmolar hyponatremia due to osmotic agents should be initially considered. True hypo-osmolar hyponatremia can then be established and evaluated.

1. **Hyponatremia due to ECF volume depletion**

a. **Predisposing factors** include diuretics, osmotic diuresis (glycosuria), VLBW with renal water and sodium wasting, adrenal or renal tubular salt-losing disorders, gastrointestinal losses (vomiting, diarrhea), and third-space losses of ECF (skin sloughing, early necrotizing enterocolitis).

b. **Diagnosis.** Decreased weight, poor skin turgor, tachycardia, rising BUN, and metabolic acidosis suggest the diagnosis. If renal function

Table 24-6. Hyponatremia

Clinical diagnosis	Etiology	Therapy
ECF volume excess	Congestive heart failure Neuromuscular blockade (pancuronium) Sepsis	Water restriction
ECF volume normal	SIADH Pain Opiates Excess intravenous fluids	Water restriction
ECF volume deficit	Diuretics Congenital adrenal hyperplasia Severe glomerulotubular imbalance (immaturity) Renal tubular acidosis Gastrointestinal losses Necrotizing enterocolitis (third-space loss)	Increased sodium administration
Factitious hyponatremia	Hyperlipidemia	
Hypertonic hyponatremia	Mannitol Hyperglycemia	

Key: ECF = extracellular fluid; SIADH = syndrome of inappropriate antidiuretic hormone secretion.

is mature, decreased urine output, increased specific gravity, and a low FE-Na exist.

c. **Therapy.** If possible, reduce ongoing losses. Liberalization of sodium and water intake will replete deficits and allow for maintenance plus ongoing losses.

2. **Hyponatremia with normal ECF volume**
   a. **Predisposing factors** include excess IV fluids and the syndrome of inappropriate antidiuretic hormone secretion (SIADH). Factors that may cause SIADH include pain, opiate administration, intraventricular hemorrhage (IVH), asphyxia, pneumothorax, and positive-pressure ventilation.
   b. **Diagnosis.** Weight gain without edema suggests the diagnosis. The infant who has received excess IV fluids without SIADH should demonstrate appropriately low urine specific gravity and high urine output. SIADH leads to **decreased urine output** and **increased urine osmolarity.** Urinary sodium excretion usually reflects sodium intake and thus may not contribute to the evaluation. The diagnosis of SIADH presumes no volume-related stimulus to ADH release exists, such as from reduced cardiac output or abnormal renal, adrenal, or thyroid function.
   c. **Therapy.** Water restriction is the therapy for SIADH unless (1) serum sodium concentration is less than approximately 120 mEq/L or (2) neurologic signs such as obtundation or seizure activity develop. In these instances, furosemide 1 mg/kg IV q6h can be initiated while replacing urinary sodium excretion with hypertonic NaCl (3%). This strategy leads to loss of free water with no net change in total-body sodium. Fluid restriction alone can be utilized once serum sodium concentration exceeds 120 mEq/L.
3. **Hyponatremia due to ECF volume excess**
   a. **Predisposing factors** include sepsis with decreased cardiac output,

late necrotizing enterocolitis, CHF, abnormal lymphatic drainage, and neuromuscular paralysis.

b. **Diagnosis.** Weight increase with edema is suggestive of this diagnosis. Decreasing urine output, rising urine specific gravity and BUN, and a low FE-Na are often present in infants with mature renal function. The cardiac examination may be abnormal.

c. **Therapy** should be directed toward ameliorating the underlying disorders. Water restriction can help alleviate hypotonicity. Sodium restriction may be required, and efforts to improve cardiac output may be beneficial.

C. **Hypernatremic disorders**

1. **Hypernatremia with normal or deficient ECF volume**

a. **Predisposing factors** include VLBW infants with increased renal and insensible water loss. Skin sloughing can accelerate water losses. ADH deficiency secondary to IVH can exacerbate renal water losses.

b. **Diagnosis.** Weight loss, tachycardia and hypotension, and metabolic acidosis can occur. Decreasing urine output and rising urine specific gravity may develop. Urine may be dilute if central or nephrogenic diabetes insipidus is present. **Hypernatremia in the VLBW infant in the first 24 hours of life is almost always due to free-water deficits.**

c. **Therapy.** The rate of free-water administration should be increased. If signs of ECF depletion or excess develop, sodium intake also should be adjusted. The development of hypernatremia does not necessarily imply excess total-body sodium.

2. **Hypernatremia with ECF volume excess**

a. **Predisposing factors** include excessive administration of isotonic or hypertonic fluids. Hypernatremia and edema can be pronounced in infants predisposed to sodium retention because of reduced cardiac output.

b. **Diagnosis.** Weight increase with edema is suggestive of this diagnosis. The infant may exhibit normal heart rate, blood pressure, and urine output and specific gravity and an elevated FE-Na.

c. **Therapy.** Reduce the rate of sodium administration by reducing the sodium concentration of fluids, restricting the rate of fluid administration, or both.

V. **Oliguria** may be defined as the presence of less than 1 ml/kg per hour of urine flow. Although delayed micturition in a healthy infant is not of concern until 24 hours after birth, assessment of urine output in a critically ill infant should be established by 8 to 12 hours of age, using urethral catheterization if necessary. Diminished urine output may reflect abnormal prerenal, renal parenchymal, or postrenal factors (Table 24-7). The most common causes of acute renal failure in the neonate are asphyxia, sepsis, and severe respiratory illness. It is important, however, to exclude other etiologies in an infant with oliguria [1,14].

A. **History and physical examination.** The maternal and infant history should be assessed for maternal diabetes (renal vein thrombosis), birth asphyxia, or oligohydramnios (Potter's syndrome). Force of the infant's urinary stream (posterior urethral valves), rate and nature of fluid administration and urine output, and the use of nephrotoxic drugs (aminoglycosides, indomethacin, furosemide) should be evaluated. **Physical examination** should determine blood pressure and ECF volume status; evidence of cardiac disease, abdominal masses, or ascites; and the presence of any congenital anomalies associated with renal abnormalities (e.g., Potter's syndrome, epispadias).

B. **Diagnosis**

1. **Initial laboratory examination** should include urinalysis and BUN, creatinine, and FE-Na determinations. Although sometimes diagnostic, these values often serve as a baseline for further management.

2. **Fluid challenge,** consisting of a total of 20 ml/kg of normal saline or albumin 5%, is administered as two 10 ml/kg per hour infusions. This approach is utilized if no suspicion of structural heart disease or CHF exists.

Table 24-7. Oliguria

Prerenal	Renal parenchymal	Postrenal
Decreased inotropy	Acute tubular necrosis	Posterior urethral valves
	Ischemia (hypoxia, hypovolemia)	
Decreased preload	DIC	
	Renal artery or vein thrombosis	Neuropathic bladder
Increased peripheral resistance	Nephrotoxin	
	Congenital malformation	Prune-belly syndrome
	Polycystic disease	
	Agenesis	Uric acid nephropathy
	Dysplasia	

Key: DIC = disseminated intravascular coagulation.

Decreased cardiac output not responsive to ECF expansion may require the institution of inotropic/chronotropic pressor agents. Dopamine at a dose of 1 to 5 μg/kg per minute may increase renal blood flow and at a dose of 2 to 15 μg/kg per minute may increase total cardiac output. These effects may augment glomerular filtration and urine output.

3. **If no response to fluid challenge occurs,** diuresis may be attempted with **furosemide** 2 mg/kg IV. **Mannitol** 0.5 kg IV **slowly** over 1 to 2 hours may induce an osmotic diuresis without great increases in serum osmolality.
4. Patients who are unresponsive to increased cardiac output and diuresis should be evaluated with abdominal ultrasound to define renal, urethral, and bladder anatomy. Intravenous pyelography, renal scan, angiography, or cystourethrography may be required to clarify suspected abnormalities (see Chap. 26).

C. Management. Prerenal causes of oliguria should continue to respond to increased cardiac output. Postrenal obstruction requires urologic consultation, with possible urinary diversion and surgical correction. If parenchymal acute renal failure is suspected, a regimen of fluid and electrolyte management must be instituted to avoid excessive ECF expansion and electrolyte abnormalities. Any reversible causes of declining glomerular filtration rate (GFR) such as administration of nephrotoxic drugs should be eliminated, if possible.

1. **Monitoring** should consist of daily weights, input and output, BUN and creatinine, and serum electrolytes.
2. **Fluid restriction.** Insensible fluid loss plus urine output should be replaced. Potassium should be withheld unless hypokalemia develops. Sodium should be administered to replace urinary losses unless edema develops.
3. **Drug dosage** and frequency should be adjusted for drugs that rely on renal excretion. Measurement of serum drug concentrations frequently aids the adjustment of dosing intervals.
4. **Peritoneal or hemodialysis** may be indicated in patients who have progressive decline in GFR with complications related to ECF volume or electrolyte abnormalities (see Chap. 26).

VI. Metabolic acid–base disorders

A. Normal acid–base physiology. Acidosis results from excessive loss of buffer or from an increase of volatile or nonvolatile acid in the extracellular space. Normal sources of acid production include the metabolism of proteins containing sulfur and phosphate as well as hydrogen ion released from bone mineralization. Intravascular buffers include bicarbonate, phosphate, and intracellular hemoglobin. Maintenance of normal pH depends on excretion of volatile acid (e.g., carbonic acid) from the lungs, skeletal exchange of cations for hydrogen, and renal preservation of bicarbonate. The contribution of the kidneys to acid–base balance includes resorption of the filtered load of bicarbonate, secretion of hydrogen ions as titratable acidity (e.g., $H_2PO_4^-$), and excretion of ammonium ions.

B. Metabolic acidosis (see Inborn Errors of Metabolism Chap. 24, page 448)

1. **The anion gap.** Metabolic acidosis can be caused by accumulation of acid or by the loss of buffering equivalents. Determination of the anion gap will assist in distinguishing which of these two processes led to the development of metabolic acidosis. Sodium, chloride, and bicarbonate are the primary ions of the extracellular space and exist in approximately electroneutral balance. The difference between the sodium concentration and the sum of the chloride and bicarbonate concentrations, commonly known as the **anion gap,** reflects the unaccounted for anion composition of the ECF. Thus acidosis caused by accumulation of organic acids results in an increased anion gap, whereas acidosis due to loss of buffer does not increase the anion gap. The normal range of values for the anion gap in the neonate is 5 to 15 mEq/L and varies directly with the serum albumin concentration.
2. **Metabolic acidosis associated with an increased anion gap (>15 mEq/L).** These disorders (Table 24-8) include renal failure, inborn errors of metabolism, lactic acidosis, late metabolic acidosis, and toxin exposure. Lactic acidosis is most commonly due to diminished tissue perfusion and resultant anaerobic metabolism in infants with asphyxia or severe cardiorespiratory disease. Late metabolic acidosis typically occurs during the second or third week of life in premature infants ingesting formula containing high concentrations of casein. An increased acid load is produced by the metabolism of sulfur-containing amino acids in casein and by increased hydrogen ion release due to the rapid mineralization of bone. Inadequate hydrogen ion excretion by the kidney of the premature infant results in acidosis.
3. **Metabolic acidosis associated with a normal anion gap (<15 mEq/L).** These disorders are usually due to a loss of buffer by means of the renal or gastrointestinal systems (Table 24-8). Premature infants less than 32 weeks' gestation frequently manifest a proximal or distal renal tubular acidosis (RTA). Distal RTA is suggested if the urine pH is persistently greater than 7.0 in an infant with metabolic acidosis. A urinary pH of less than 5.0 documents normal distal tubule hydrogen ion secretion but does not establish the ability of the proximal tubule to reabsorb a normal filtered load of bicarbonate. Infusion of sodium bicarbonate in infants with a proximal RTA will result in a urinary pH greater than 7.0 prior to attaining a normal serum bicarbonate concentration (22 to 24 mEq/L).

Table 24-8. Metabolic acidosis

Increased anion gap (>15 mEq/L)	Normal anion gap (<15 mEq/L)
Acute renal failure	Renal bicarbonate loss
Inborn errors of metabolism	Renal tubular acidosis
Lactic acidosis	Acetazolamide
Late metabolic acidosis	Renal dysplasia
Toxins (e.g., benzyl alcohol)	Gastrointestinal bicarbonate loss
	Diarrhea
	Cholestyramine
	Small bowel drainage
	Dilutional acidosis
	Hyperalimentation acidosis

4. **Therapy.** Whenever possible, therapy should be directed at correcting the underlying cause of metabolic acidosis. Lactic acidosis due to low cardiac output or to decreased peripheral oxygen delivery should be treated with specific measures. The use of a low-casein formula may obviate late metabolic acidosis. The treatment of metabolic acidosis not accompanied by an increased anion gap should focus on decreasing the rate of bicarbonate loss (e.g., decreased small bowel drainage) or the provision of buffer equivalents. Intravenous sodium bicarbonate or sodium acetate (which is compatible with calcium salts) are most commonly used for this purpose if the arterial pH is less than 7.25. The bicarbonate deficit may be estimated from the following formula:

   Deficit = 0.4 × body weight × (desired bicarbonate − actual bicarbonate)

   The changing dynamics of acid–base balance, however, require reassessment of the infant's acid–base status at regular intervals. The ability of the infant to tolerate the sodium load and to metabolize acetate are important variables that require careful monitoring of subsequent acid–base status.

C. **Metabolic alkalosis.** The etiology of metabolic alkalosis can often be clarified by determining the urinary chloride concentration. Alkalosis accompanied by ECF depletion is associated with decreased urinary chloride, whereas states of mineralocorticoid excess are usually associated with increased urinary chloride (Table 24-9). Therapy is almost always directed toward correction of the underlying disorder.

VII. **Disorders of potassium balance.** Potassium is the fundamental intracellular cation. Of note, serum potassium concentrations (3.5 to 5.5 mEq/L) do not reflect total-body potassium stores, since the distribution of extracellular and intracellular potassium is also dependent on the pH of body compartments. An increase of 0.1 pH units in serum results in approximately a 0.6 mEq/L fall in serum potassium concentration due to an intracellular shift of potassium ions. Total-body potassium is regulated by the balance of potassium intake (normally 1 to 2 mEq/kg per day) and potassium excretion through the urine and GI tract.

A. **Hypokalemia** can lead to arrhythmias, ileus, renal concentrating defects, and obtundation in the newborn.

1. **Predisposing factors** include nasogastric or ileostomy drainage, chronic diuretic use, and renal tubular defects.
2. **Diagnosis** is made by determining serum and urine electrolytes and pH and an ECG to detect possible conduction defects (prolonged QT interval and U waves).
3. **Therapy** should focus on reducing abnormal renal or gastrointestinal losses of potassium and gradually increasing oral or parenteral potassium salts as needed.

Table 24-9. Metabolic alkalosis

Low urinary chloride (<10 mEq/L)	High urinary chloride (>20 mEq/L)
Diuretic therapy (late)	Bartter's syndrome with mineralocorticoid excess
Correction of chronic respiratory acidosis	Alkali administration
Nasogastric suction	Massive blood product transfusion
Vomiting	Diuretic therapy (early)
Secretory diarrhea	Hypokalemia

B. Hyperkalemia can result in malignant arrhythmias in the newborn, including ventricular fibrillation (see Chap. 14).

1. **Predisposing factors** include medication errors, hemolytic anemia, congenital adrenal hyperplasia, renal failure/oliguria, and extreme prematurity.
2. **Diagnosis** is based on determination of nonhemolyzed serum and urine electrolytes, as well as serum pH and calcium concentrations. An ECG can demonstrate signs of prolonged PR interval, prolonged QRS, and eventually ventricular tachycardia/fibrillation.
3. **Therapy** should include a reduction in potassium intake, acute elevation of pH (hyperventilation and/or administration of 1 to 2 mEq/kg sodium bicarbonate), and administration of 0.1 cc/kg calcium chloride 10% IV. In the event of severe, life-threatening hyperkalemia, administration of a glucose/insulin infusion can be instituted. (See Hypoglycemia and Hyperglycemia in Chap. 24.) The use of cation exchange resins (Kayexalate) may be useful in infants less than 32 weeks' gestation, despite the obligate sodium load and irritation of bowel mucosa from rectal administration of the resin slurry.

VIII. Common clinical situations

A. VLBW infant. Increased free-water loss through integument and urine often leads to hypernatremia and the need for increased rates of parenteral fluid administration. In addition, impaired glucose tolerance also can lead to hyperglycemia, necessitating reduced rates of parenteral glucose infusion (see Hypoglycemia and Hyperglycemia in Chap. 24). This combination frequently leads to administration of reduced dextrose concentrations (below 5%) in parenteral solutions. One should avoid the infusion of parenteral solutions containing less than 200 mOsmol/L (i.e., less than 3% D/W) in order to minimize local osmotic hemolysis and thus reduce renal potassium load. Hyperkalemia in the VLBW infant is often a combination of a shift from intracellular to extracellular potassium, reduced peripheral glucose and potassium uptake in insulin-sensitive tissues, and reduced renal excretion of potassium [10]. The use of insulin infusions to treat hyperkalemia in the VLBW infant is sometimes necessary but can be extremely difficult to properly titrate, increasing the risk of iatrogenic hypoglycemia. The use of cation exchange resin (Kayexalate) for treatment of hyperkalemia can be useful in infants less than 32 weeks' gestational age despite the obligate sodium load and frequent irritation of bowel mucosa by rectal administration.

B. Bronchopulmonary dysplasia (see Chronic Lung Disease in Chap. 13). Chronic lung disease that requires diuretic therapy often leads to hypokalemic, hypochloremic metabolic alkalosis. These infants frequently have previously established chronic respiratory acidosis with metabolic compensation. Vigorous diuresis can lead to total-body potassium depletion and contraction of ECF volume, thus exacerbating a superimposed metabolic alkalosis. If the alkalosis is severe, alkalemia ($pH > 7.45$) can supervene and result in central hypoventilation. The physician should gradually reduce sodium and potassium loss induced by diuretics and increase potassium intake by administration of potassium chloride (up to 1 mEq/kg per day). Rarely, administration of ammonium chloride (0.5 mEq/kg) may be required to treat the metabolic alkalosis.

References

1. Anand, S. K. *Pediatr. Clin. North Am.* 29: 791, 1982.
2. Bell, E. F. *N. Engl. J. Med.* 302: 598, 1980.
3. Bell, E. F. *J. Pediatr.* 96: 452, 1980.
4. Bell, E. F. *J. Pediatr.* 96: 460, 1980.
5. Brown, E. R. *J. Pediatr.* 92: 982, 1978.
6. Cheek, D. B. *Pediatrics* 28: 861, 1961.

7. Fanaroff, A. A. *Pediatrics* 50: 236, 1972.
8. Fink, C. W. *Pediatrics* 26: 397, 1960.
9. Fisher, D. A. *Am. J. Dis. Child.* 106: 137, 1963.
10. Gruskay, J. *J. Pediatr.* 113: 381, 1988.
11. Leake, R. D. *Clin. Perinatol.* 4: 321, 1977.
12. Lorenz, J. M. *J. Pediatr.* 101: 423, 1982.
13. Norman, M. E. *Pediatrics* 63: 475, 1979.
14. Okken, A. *Pediatr. Res.* 13: 1072, 1979.
15. Rahman, N. *Clin. Perinatol.* 8: 241, 1981.
16. Skorecki, L. *Am. J. Med.* 70: 77, 1981.
17. Stevenson, J. G. *J. Pediatr.* 90: 257, 1977.
18. Wu, P. Y. K. *Pediatrics* 54: 704, 1974.

25 Ambiguous Genitalia in the Newborn

Mary Deming Scott

I. Background

A. Definition. The term **ambiguous genitalia** applies to any infant with a confusing appearance of the external genitalia, including (1) any full-term infant who has a phallus and bilateral cryptorchidism, (2) any infant with unilateral cryptorchidism and hypospadias, or (3) any infant who has penoscrotal or perineoscrotal hypospadias, even if the testes are descended. In these cases, sex cannot be determined from external appearance, and a thorough evaluation is required.

B. Assignment of a sex for rearing. Speed in the determination of the sex to be used in rearing an infant is essential for the parents' peace of mind.

1. Sex for rearing of children with ambiguous genitalia should have less to do with chromosomes than with the actual anatomy and functional endocrinology. A team approach between pediatric endocrinologist and pediatric surgeon is generally necessary. Comments such as "It looks like a boy" or "We have to wait for chromosomes" should be avoided. Initial hasty statements by unthinking professionals can haunt families until their children reach adulthood and can have profound psychosocial consequences [2].
2. **All babies with severe hypospadias** should be examined by the pediatric endocrinologist to rule out partial testosterone resistance, which would be a contraindication to rearing the child as a male (see **IV.C**), and to provide information for genetic counseling for future pregnancies.
3. The birth of a baby with ambiguous genitalia is a social emergency. If the stretched phallic length is less than 25 mm at birth, it is unlikely to be adequate in adulthood despite the best efforts of the most skilled surgeon (Fig. 25-1). The parents of such an infant should be informed that the child's genitalia are "incompletely formed," but that "she" will be able to function well as a female after reconstructive surgery and hormonal support.

C. Normal sexual development. A timetable of sexual development is given in Figure 25-2 and Table 25-1. Sex determination progresses in stages. At fertilization, a **genetic sex** is determined, and this in turn determines **gonadal sex.** The testis determining factor is located on the short arm of the Y chromosome [4]. 46,XX males and 46,XY females are created by aberrent X–Y interchange during paternal meiosis [8]. A region necessary for spermatogenesis has been localized to the proximal long arm of the Y chromosome. Gonadal differentiation and sex hormone secretion affect internal genital tract development and external genital development, and a **phenotypic sex** is established at the end of the first trimester [5]. **Psychologic sex** identity is formed by sociologic imprinting within a few years after birth. Prenatal hormonal secretion may have psychologic implications. At puberty, hopefully, the appearance of secondary sex characteristics reinforces gender identity.

II. Nursery evaluation of a newborn with ambiguous genitalia

A. History

1. Family history of hypospadias, cryptorchidism, or infertile aunts.

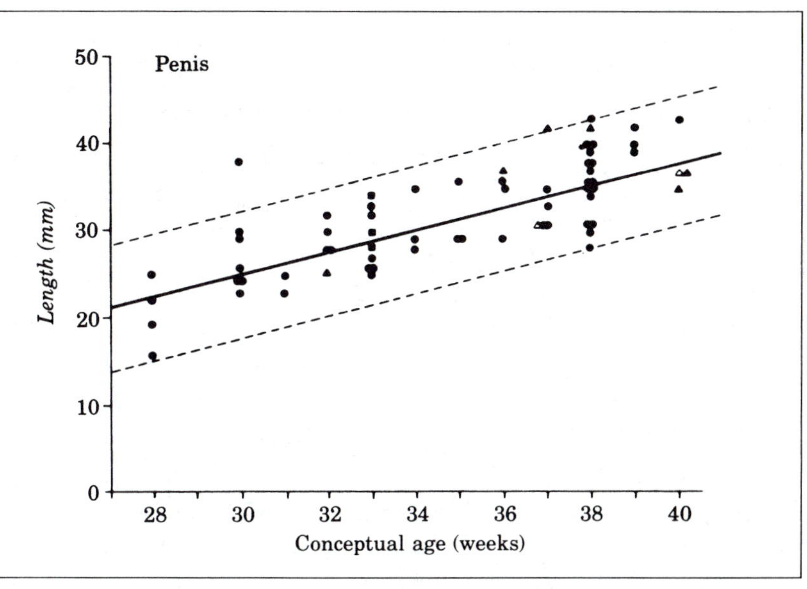

Fig. 25-1. Stretched phallic length of 63 normal premature and full-term infants (●), showing lines of mean ± 2 standard deviations. Correlation coefficient is 0.80. Superimposed are data for two small-for-gestational-age infants (Δ), seven large-for-gestational-age infants (▲), and four twins (■), all of whom are in the normal range. (From K. W. Feldman and D. W. Smith, Fetal phallic growth and penile standards for newborn male infants. *J. Pediatr.* 86: 395, 1975.)

2. Maternal drug exposure in pregnancy (progestogens, testosterone, phenytoin, and aminoglutethimide).
3. Repeated deaths in the neonatal period of other children born to the parents (adrenogenital syndrome).
4. **Placental insufficiency. Human chorionic gonadotropin (HCG)** initiates the synthesis of testosterone in the fetal testes.

B. Physical examination

1. The examiner should note phallic size, position of the urethral orifice, any fusion of the labia or scrotum, and the descent and size of the gonads.
2. Bimanual rectal examination may reveal a palpable uterus in the midline.
3. The examiner should seek associated congenital anomalies; if any are present, the **chromosome 13 deletion syndrome** should be considered.
4. If the child has a uterus and vagina and if the external genitalia would necessitate a several-stage hypospadias repair, the child should be reared as a female.

C. Diagnostic tests [1]. A pelvic ultrasound should determine if a uterus and ovaries are present. The examiner should obtain chromosomes. Quinacrine stains of white cells for Y-body fluorescence are quick but not completely accurate. R^-, C^-, and Q^- banding and G-11 staining may reveal anomalies of the Y chromosome [3].

III. XX females with genital ambiguity. If chromosomes are XX, the diagnosis is (1) true hermaphroditism, (2) adrenogenital syndrome (due to 21-hydroxylase deficiency, 11-hydroxylase deficiency, or 3-beta-hydroxysteroid dehydrogenase deficiency), or (3) maternal drug ingestion or masculinizing tumors in the mother or

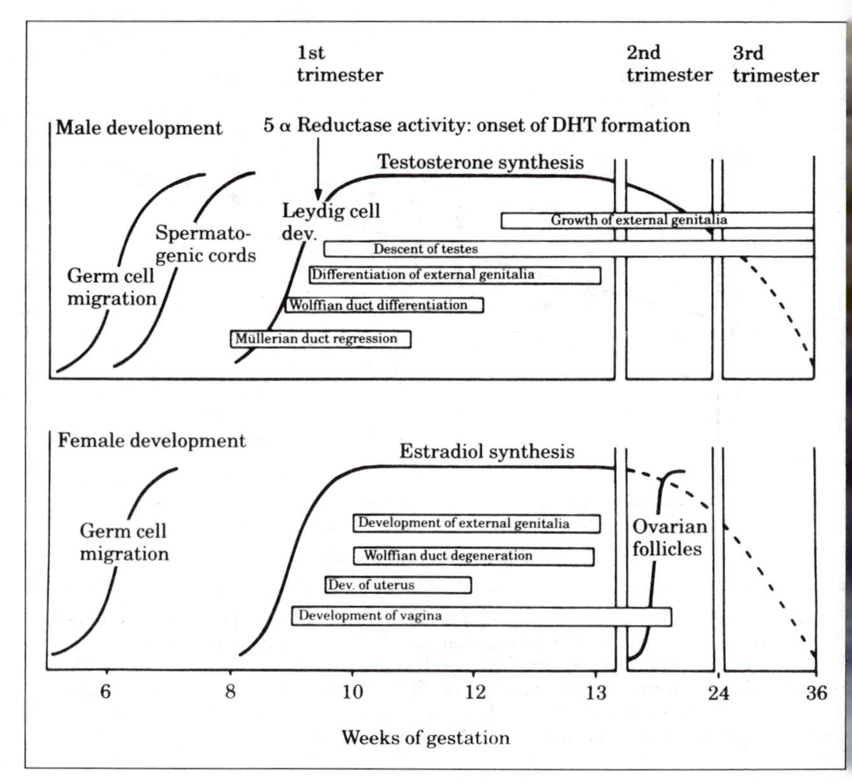

Fig. 25-2. Role of gonadal hormones in development of sexual phenotypes (DHT = dihydrotestosterone; Dev. = development). (From J. D. Wilson et al., Relation between differentiation of gonads and anatomic differentiation of human male and female embryos. *Hum. Genet.* 58: 78, 1981.)

fetus. If excessive androgens are present before 12 weeks of gestation, labial fusion may occur; after the first trimester, however, clitoral hypertrophy will be the only sign of excessive androgen exposure.

A. A **17-hydroxyprogesterone (17-OHP)** level, 17-OH pregnenolone level, dehydroepiandrosterone level, testosterone level, and 24-hour urine determination for 17-ketosteroids should be obtained. In 90 percent of girls with adrenogenital syndrome, the 17-OHP level will be elevated (see review by New et al. [7]). Worldwide newborn filter-paper screening programs for 17-hydroxyprogesterone show an incidence of 1 per 14,554 births, varying by country. Salt-losers outnumber non-salt-losers by 3:1. The male-to-female sex ratio is 1:1. False-positive results occur in sick, premature, and low-birth-weight infants, with a false-positive rate of up to 0.19 percent and a recall rate of up to 0.2 percent. Normal values must be determined for each individual program, since they depend on the filter-paper thickness and radioimmunoassay used [9].

B. If laboratory investigations are normal, ultrasound of the adrenals and ovaries may reveal a masculinizing tumor. Laparotomy or gonadal biopsy (or both) may be required to diagnose the rare true hermaphrodite.

IV. XY chromosomes. Even if chromosomes are XY, the parents should not be hastily told that the child is a boy. Rearing the child as a female may still be appropriate.

Table 25-1. Timetable of sexual development

Days after conception	Events of sexual development
19	Primordial germ cells migrate to the genital ridge
40	Genital ridge forms an undifferentiated gonad
44	Müllerian ducts appear; testes develop
62	Müllerian inhibitor (from testes) becomes active
71	Testosterone synthesis begins (induced by placental chorionic gonadotropin)
72	Fusion of the labioscrotal swellings
73	Closure of the median raphe
74	Closure of the urethral groove
77	Müllerian regression is complete

A. Diagnostic possibilities

1. **Chromosomal disorders**
   a. **True hermaphroditism (10 percent are XY, 10 percent are mosaic, and 80 percent are XX).** Sex assignment should be based on external genitalia. Generally, with the presence of a patent uterus and vagina, these patients should be raised as girls. Two-thirds of them will menstruate.
   b. **Mixed gonadal dysgenesis.** This disorder usually has a 46,X–46,XY chromosomal complement. Genitalia may range from predominantly male to completely female, and a uterus and fallopian tube are generally present. HCG stimulation tests should be done to evaluate gonadal function. **Gonadal neoplasia (gonadoblastoma)** may arise in the first 20 years of life in up to 20 percent of these children; therefore, streak gonads should always be removed in infancy.
   c. **XY gonadal dysgenesis.** Infants with XY gonadal dysgenesis fail to masculinize owing to incomplete failure of testicular differentiation. The genitalia usually appear female, but clitoromegaly may occur and streak gonads are present. Up to 30 percent of patients with XY gonadal dysgenesis will develop gonadoblastoma or dysgerminoma, so streak gonads should be extirpated. The uterus and vagina function well.
2. **Male pseudohermaphroditism** [12,13,15,17,18]. Some possible defects in male genital development are listed in Figure 25-3 and in Tables 25-2 and 25-3. These include the following:
   a. **Hereditary disorders**
      (1) Enzyme defects in testosterone synthesis (autosomal recessive) [11]
      (2) Partial end-organ resistance to testosterone (X-linked recessive, incomplete testicular feminization)
      (3) Adrenogenital syndrome (autosomal recessive) [7,16]
      (4) Defects in testosterone metabolism (autosomal recessive). A review of male pseudohermaphroditism by Saenger [15] is recommended.
   b. **Nonhereditary**
      (1) Maternal drug ingestion (progesterone, phenytoin)
      (2) Placental insufficiency

B. Further **tests** in a baby with XY chromosomes will determine the infant's ability to snythesize testosterone and convert it to dihydrotestosterone.

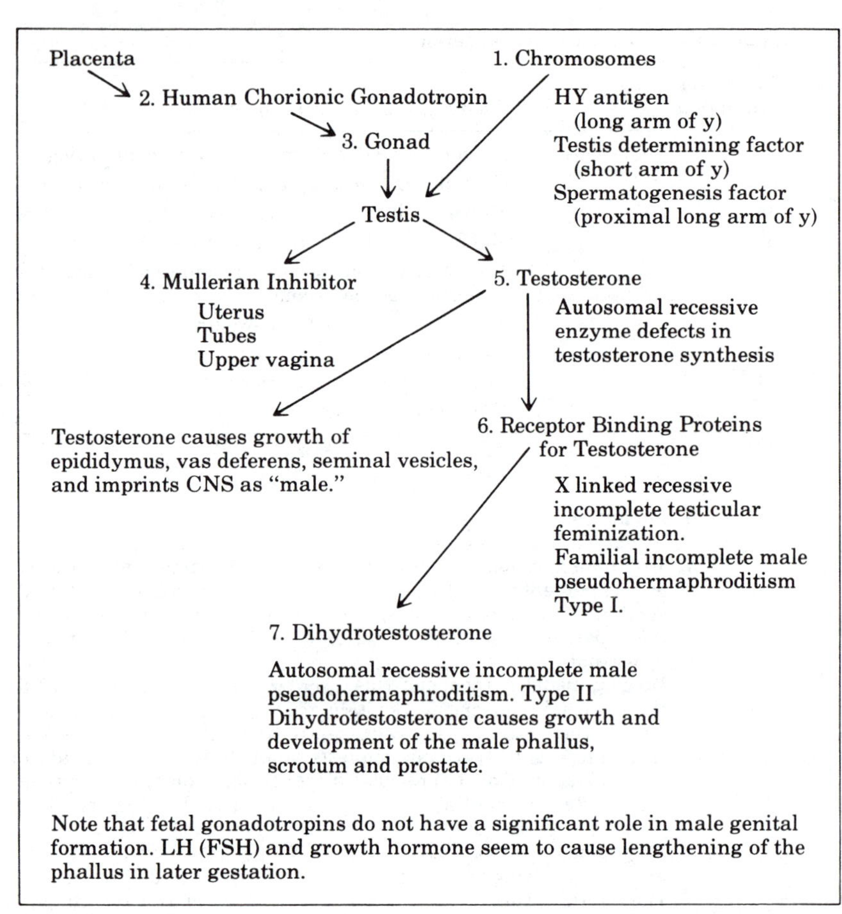

Fig. 25-3. Possible defects in male genital development. Note that fetal gonadotropins do not have a significant role in male genital formation. Luteinizing hormone (follicle-stimulating hormone) and growth hormone seem to cause lengthening of the phallus in later gestation (CNS = central nervous system).

Table 25-2. Causes of male pseudohermaphroditism

Abnormal gonadal differentiation
Mixed gonadal dysgenesis
True hermaphroditism
Abnormal gonadal function
Placental or fetal pituitary gonadotropin deficiency
Leydig-cell agenesis
Congenital anorchia (vanishing testes syndrome)
Abnormalities of antimüllerian hormone synthesis or action (persistent oviduct syndrome)
Defective testosterone synthesis
Abnormal testosterone metabolism
5-Alpha-reductase deficiency
Abnormal testosterone action
Testicular feminization (complete or incomplete)

Source: Modified from P. Saenger, Pseudohermaphroditism. *Pediatr. Ann.* 10: 15, 1981.

1. **Initial tests.** Blood is obtained for follicle-stimulating hormone, leutinizing hormone, testosterone, dihydrotestosterone, dehydroepiandrosterone, androstenedione, cortisol, and 17-OHP. Urine is obtained for 17-ketosteroids.
2. After blood and urine samples have been obtained, 500 IU of HCG is given intramuscularly for 3 days. Repeat tests are then performed on urine for 17-ketosteroids and on blood for the tests mentioned in **1.** Serum sodium and potassium levels should be monitored periodically for the first several weeks of life if the infant is discharged before a diagnosis of salt-losing adrenogenital syndrome is ruled out.

C. Testosterone resistance. If these tests show initial high levels of testosterone that do not increase when HCG is given, the infant probably has incomplete testicular feminization (androgen resistance). **Such children must never be raised as males** because they will never masculinize adequately (despite hormone therapy) and will feminize at adolescence.

References

1. Alsever, R. N., and Gotlon, R. W. *Handbook of Endocrine Tests in Adults and Children*. Chicago: Year Book Medical Publishers, 1978.
2. Donahoe, P. K. *Pediatr. Clin. North Am.* 23: 361, 1976.
3. Drummond, B. M., et al. *J. Pediatr.* 113: 469, 1988.
4. Editorial. *Lancet* 2: 1008, 1976.
5. Edman, C. D. *Obstet. Gynecol.* 49: 208, 1977.
6. Feldman, K. W. *J. Pediatr.* 86: 395, 1975.
7. New, M. I., et al. Congenital Adrenal Hyperplasia and Related Conditions. In J. B. Stanbury and J. B. Wyngaarden (Eds.), *The Metabolic Basis of Inherited Disease*, 5th Ed. New York: McGraw-Hill, 1983. Pp. 973–1000.
8. Page, D. C. Sex Reversal: Deletion Mapping of the Male-Determining Function of the Human Y Chromosome. In *Molecular Biology of Homo Sapiens* (Cold Spring Harbor Symposium on Quantitative Biology). New York: Cold Spring Harbor Press, 1986.
9. Pang, S., et al. *Pediatrics* 81: 866, 1988.
10. Parks, J. S. Intersex. In W. B. Kaplan (Ed.), *Clinical Pediatric and Adolescent Endocrinology*. Philadelphia: Saunders, 1982. Pp. 327–450.
11. Peterson, R. E. *Am. J. Med.* 62: 170, 1977.

(Cont. on page 476.)

Table 25-3. Undermasculinization of the genetic male

	Defects in adrenal and testis			Defects in testis		Defects in end-organ response			
								Testicular feminization	
	20, 22-Desmolase	3-Beta-HSD	17-Alpha-reductase	17, 20-Desmolase	17-KS reductase	Transient defects	5-Alpha-reductase	Partial	Complete
External genitalia	Ambiguous $F > M$	Ambiguous $M > F$	Ambiguous $F > M$	Ambiguous $F > M$	Ambiguous $F > M$	Ambiguous $F > M$	Ambiguous $M > F$	Ambiguous $M > F$	Female
Müllerian ducts	No uterus or fallopian tubes, since Müllerian-inhibiting factor production is normal								
Wolffian ducts	Variably present, depending on severity of enzymatic defect						Epididymis and vas	Abnormal	None
Gonads	Testes in scrotal, inguinal, or abdominal locations								
Fertility	Impaired due to low intratesticular testosterone level					Possible	Possible	Possible	No
Tumors	Possibly increased incidence, but difficult to evaluate due to small numbers of patients with precise diagnoses						Rare	Rare	Various types: 4 percent at 20 years, 33 percent at 50 years

Puberty									
Virilization	Possible	Common	Possible	Possible	Possible	Common	Common	Sparse	No
Breasts	No	Common	Possible	Possible	Common	Rare	No	Common	Yes
Karyotype	46,XY by definition in undermasculinized genetic males								
Inheritance	AR	AR	AR	AR or XL	AR	?AR	AR	XL	XL
Elevated plasma steroids	None	17-Hydroxy-pregneno-lone, androstene-diol	Corticos-terone	17-Hydroxy-proges-terone	Androstene-dione, estrone	None	High testos-terone-to-dihy-drotes-tosterone ratio	Testos-terone, estradiol	Testosterone
Additional features	Salt loss	Salt loss	Hyperten-sion	None	None	None	Sparse sexual hair		

Key: 3-beta-HSD = 3-beta-hydroxysteroid dehydrogenase; KS = ketosteroids; F = female; M = male; AR = autosomal recessive; XL = X-linked.
Source: Modified from J. S. Parks. Intersex. In W. B. Kaplan (Ed.), *Clinical Pediatric and Adolescent Endocrinology*. Philadelphia: Saunders, 1982, P. 327.

12. Prader, A. *Pediatr. Ann.* 3: 57, 1974.
13. Roberts, C. J. *Br. Med. J.* 1: 768, 1973.
14. Saenger, P. *J. Pediatr.* 104: 1, 1984.
15. Saenger, P. *Pediatr. Ann.* 10: 15, 1981.
16. Shackleton, C. H. *Pediatrics* 49: 198, 1972.
17. Walsh, P. C. *N. Engl. J. Med.* 291: 944, 1974.
18. Wilson, J. D. *N. Engl. J. Med.* 290: 1097, 1974.

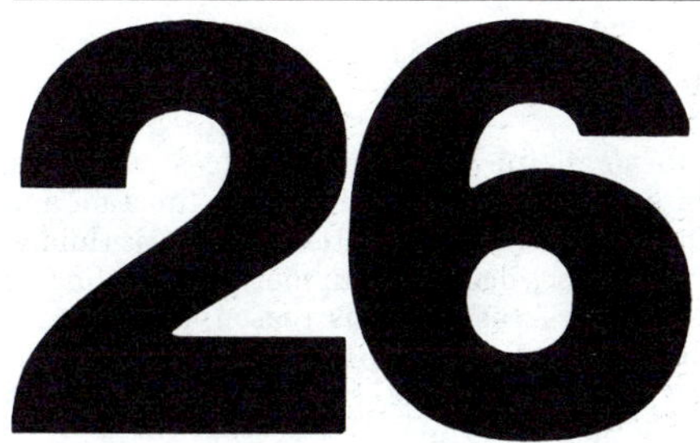

Renal Conditions in the Newborn Period

Julie R. Ingelfinger

I. **Background.** Familiarity with renal embryology and functional development is necessary for understanding kidney problems arising in the newborn period. These problems are also influenced by changing body fluid and electrolyte requirements following birth [6,7] (see Fluid and Electrolyte Management of the Newborn in Chap. 24).

II. **Embryology and physiology** [5,6,9]

A. **The kidney.** The human kidney evolves through the embryologic formation and differentiation of three mesodermal structures. The first two, the **pronephros** and **mesonephros,** regress rapidly but are important to the proper development of the **metanephros,** which develops into the final infant kidney. The pronephros forms a series of tubules, which are the anlage of the mesonephros. In turn, the mesonephros, appearing in the fourth week, gives rise to the ureteric bud. The mesonephros partially disappears during the third month of gestation in the female. In the male, however, the mesonephric tubules and duct system persist, forming portions of the reproductive system—the epididymis, the vas deferens, and the ejaculatory duct. Important points include the following:

1. From the fifth week of gestation, the metanephros forms secretory components of the kidney and the mesonephros forms excretory components.
2. Growth of the ureteric bud dorsally is followed by induction of mesenchymal cells of the nephrogenic ridge to form the secretory portion of the metanephric, or definitive, kidney. Although later development of secretory and excretory portions is largely independent, interaction between the ureteric bud and the metanephric blastema is necessary for proper induction of nephron formation.
3. The **nephrons** in each kidney (1 million) elongate by cellular proliferation, followed by dichotomous branching. The coalescence of the third to fifth generations of branching produces the renal pelvis and major calyces; inward prolapse forms the renal papillae, with a renal collecting tree draining the collecting ducts that empty into each ampulla.

B. **Abnormal development results in significant urologic malformations.**

1. Persistence of the mesonephros can result in aberrant ureters emptying into the persistent mesonephric (Wolffian) duct.
2. Failure of ureteric bud development or division may lead to renal agenesis or to ureteric atresia with multicystic dysplasia.
3. Interference with mesonephric formation in the male may be followed by lack of testicular development in association with renal agenesis. Later obstruction to lower urinary tract development results in megaureter with dysplastic kidney. In the female, such interference may be followed by unilateral renal agenesis and uterine abnormalities.
4. New nephrons form up to the thirty-sixth week of gestation. No new nephrons form after this time, although maturation continues to approximately 12 years of age. Nephrogenesis proceeds in a centrifugal manner; the deeper zones are the most mature. The newborn infant therefore has

a juxtamedullary kidney. The limitations of this kidney are reviewed in Table 26-1.

5. Although urine first forms at the twelfth week of gestation, abnormal embryogenesis may interfere with evolution of renal function and urine formation in utero. Normally, urine contributes to amniotic fluid volume. Failure of urine excretion causes decreased amniotic fluid volume, resulting in direct pressure on the fetus. For this reason, a baby with renal agenesis may have abnormal (so-called Potter) facies and limb-positioning defects. Pulmonary hypoplasia is associated with, and may be partially due to, small amniotic fluid volume.

III. **Renal function in the newborn** differs from that in older children [2,6–8,10–12].

A. During fetal life, the placenta regulates fluid and electrolyte homeostasis, although urine flow may be greater than 200 ml per day. Prenatal renal blood flow (RBF) constitutes a small fraction of cardiac output (CO) (RBF/CO = 0.03 at 20 weeks compared to placental blood flow/CO = 0.4 to 0.5 or adult RBF/CO = 0.2 to 0.3).

B. Following birth, the loss of placental blood flow is followed by a rapid increase in renal blood flow and glomerular filtration rate (GFR). Table 26-2 describes normal renal function in the newborn. The assessment of renal function in the first 2 to 4 weeks of life should also consider nonrenal factors:

1. The expanded extracellular fluid (ECF) volume, which diminishes rapidly over the first 2 weeks of life
2. The solute load of infant feedings
3. The possible contributions of nonrenal medical problems in the neonatal period (e.g., cardiac failure, "leaky" capillaries)

Table 26-1. Limitations of neonatal kidney function*

Limitation	Therapeutic considerations
Low GFR	Decreased GFR; thus decreased filtration of substances handled by the glomerulus
Juxtamedullary preponderance with renal blood flow predominantly to deep nephrons	Decreased water excretory ability; increased sodium retention and potassium excretion
Glomerulotubular balance with low insulin-to-glucose clearance fraction and normal filtration fraction	Close attention to sodium and water administration (see Fluid and Electrolyte Management of the Newborn in Chap. 24)
Enzyme immaturity and decreased tubular transport of some compounds	Check doses of medications, ions, and sugars
Acidification mechanisms immature; functional decrease in titratable acidity; probable decrease in ammonia excretion and low tubular maximum for bicarbonate	Avoid acid loading
Concentrating defect with maximum concentration 700 to 800 mOsmol/L	Note this fact in solute administration

Key: GFR = glomerular filtration rate.
*The reader is referred to M. A. Holliday, T. M. Barratt, R. L. Vernier, *Pediatric Nephrology*. Baltimore: Williams & Wilkins, 1987, pp. 900–944.

Table 26-2. Normal values of renal function*

Function	Age						
	Premature	Full-term	2 weeks	8 weeks	1 year	Adult	Age of maturation (months)
Glomerular filtration rate (ml/min/1.73 m^2)	13–58	15–60	~50	63–80	120	420	12–18
Renal plasma flow [*para*-aminohippuric acid clearance (ml/min/1.73 m^2)]	120–150	140–200		300	425	630	3–6
Distal tubular transport							
Concentrating ability (mOsmol/L)	480	800	900	1200	1400	1400	3–6
Diluting capacity (mOsmol/L)	25–30						
Proximal tubular resorption [tubular maximum glucose (mg/min/1.73 m^2)]		60		170		300	12–24
Excretion [tubular maximum *para*-aminohippuric acid (mg/min/1.73 m^2)]		16		50		75	12–18
Bicarbonate threshold	14–16	21	21.5	—	22.5		24–28
Acidification	Limited			Mature			2
Urine volume (ml/24 h)	1–3 ml/kg/h	15–60	250–400	250–400	500–600		

*Kidney length is normally 5 to 7 cm, but it correlates best with length of the infant rather than with gestational age. In premature infants, plasma creatinine levels are approximately 1.0 to 1.4 mg/dl, which is higher than in normal full-term infants.

C. During the first weeks of life, the ability to concentrate urine increases rapidly as the solute load increases. Early concentration to levels above 600 to 700 mOsmol/L may occur during severe stress (e.g., persisting hypovolemia or hypoplasia of the left side of the heart). The immature kidney has a limited ability to excrete solutes and electrolytes. This limitation rarely becomes a clinical problem in the normal infant.

1. Because the newborn's metabolism is largely directed toward growth, most protein and electrolyte intake is utilized in building new tissue and contributes little to the excretory load.
2. In situations of stress, however, the immature kidney is less adequate than the mature kidney in maintaining homeostasis. The sick neonate has poor tolerance for salt loss, water deprivation, or catabolic stress from vomiting, diarrhea, or infection; the imbalance between intake and output may create an urgent clinical problem [4,6]. The immature kidney may not tolerate various medications [5].

IV. Diagnosis

A. History

1. **Family history.** Newborn renal disease is more likely when there is a family history of urinary tract anomalies, hereditary nephritis, polycystic kidney disease, or medullary cystic disease. Careful screening of the newborn is also indicated in families who have a history of inherited or genetic diseases associated with renal abnormalities (Table 26-3). A history of tubular disorders (e.g., Fanconi syndrome, cystinuria) in siblings or parents will alert one to a similar disturbance in the newborn.
2. **Obstetric history.** Clues from the obstetric history associated with renal disease in the newborn include oligohydramnios or the presence of a fetal abdominal mass, leading to obstruction of labor or difficult delivery.
   a. **Severe oligohydramnios** is frequently associated with aplasia or dysplasia of the kidneys or with lower urinary tract obstruction.
   b. Extremely large masses may be found in polycystic disease of the kidney, massive hydronephrosis, or tumors.
   c. **Sonographic studies** during gestation may detect infants with renal abnormalities (see **VIII**).

B. Physical examination may reveal abnormal renal contour or a palpable abdominal mass (0.8 percent of neonates). Other general findings may reveal a syndrome with a renal component (Table 26-3).

1. The **technique of the abdominal examination** is important. Several methods can be used for palpation of the abdominal contents.
   a. From the supine position, the infant's upper torso may be lifted upward while the examiner's hand palpates deeply over the anterior abdominal wall.
   b. Alternatively, one hand may be positioned dorsally, with the fingers spread from the lower ribs to the pelvis on one side, while the other hand is used to palpate deeply. In this second method, the middle fingers of the dorsally positioned hand are used to push upward, raising the kidney or other contents toward the palpating hand. This second method allows the two hands to entrap the kidney; with a slight lateral movement, the surface of the kidney can be felt as it slips out of the trap.
   c. A third method involves positioning the fingers of one hand dorsally, as in **b,** but palpating deeply with the thumb of the same hand, sliding the thumb cephalad to caudad.
2. **Findings.** Particular attention should be paid to any inequality of size or abnormality of position of either kidney. If a mass is felt, it should be defined as either unilateral or bilateral and as having a smooth or bosselated surface. Attempts should be made to determine whether a mass is in the kidney or whether it is independent in the abdominal cavity. A large lower midline ballotable mass suggests bladder distention secondary to urethral valves, ureterocele, urachal cyst or bladder dysfunction

Table 26-3. Syndromes with renal components that are identifiable in the neonatal period or during gestation

Syndrome	General features	Renal abnormalities
Skeletal Malformations		
Spina bifida	Meningomyelocele	Double ureter, horseshoe kidney, hydronephrosis
Hemihypertrophy	Hemihypertrophy	Wilms' tumor, hypospadias
Potter's syndrome	Abnormal facies; lung, cardiac, and skeletal anomalies	Renal agenesis
Meckel's syndrome	Encephalocele, polydactyly	Polycystic kidneys
Cerebrohepatorenal syndrome (Zellweger's syndrome)	Hepatomegaly, glaucoma, brain anomalies, chondrodystrophy	Polycystic kidneys
Jeune syndrome	Thoracic asphyxiating dystrophy	Medullary necrosis, proteinuria, hydronephrosis, horseshoe kidneys
VATER syndrome	Vertebral abnormalities, anal atresia, tracheoesophageal fistula, radial dysplasia	Renal dysplasia
VACTERL syndrome	Same as VATER, plus additional cardiac and limb abnormalities	Renal dysplasia
MURCS syndrome	Müllerian duct aplasia, cervicothoracic somite dysplasia	Renal aplasia
Visceral Abnormalities		
Prune belly	Hypoplasia of abdominal muscles, cryptorchidism	Urinary tract dysplasia
Tuberous sclerosis	Tuberous sclerosis, adenoma sebaceum	Cystic kidneys, kidney tumors
Beckwith-Wiedemann syndrome	Macroglossia, hypoglycemia	Renal dysplasia, nephroblastoma
Facial or Eye Abnormalities		
Oculocerebrorenal syndrome (Lowe's syndrome)	Cataracts, rickets, mental retardation	Proximal tubular defects
Aniridia-Wilms	Aniridia, cryptorchidism	Wilms' tumor
Johanson-Blizzard syndrome	Hypoplastic alae nasi, hypothyroidism, deafness	Hydronephrosis, caliectasis
Meckel-Gruber syndrome (dysencephalia splanchnocystica)	Encephalocele, polydactyly, cryptorchidism, cardiac anomalies, liver disease	Polycystic kidneys
Melnick-Fraser syndrome (branchio-otorenal [BOR] syndrome)	Preauricular pits, branchial clefts, deafness	Renal dysplasia

Table 26-3 *(continued)*

Syndrome	General features	Renal abnormalities
Oral-facial-digital (OFD) syndrome, type I	Oral frenula and clefts, hypoplastic alae nasi, digital asymmetry (cross-linked, lethal in male)	Renal microcysts
Chromosomal Abnormalities		
Down syndrome (trisomy 21)	Abnormal facies, brachycephaly, congenital heart disease	Cystic kidney and other renal abnormalities in 7 percent
Turner syndrome	Small stature, congenital heart disease, amenorrhea, XO sex chromosomes	Horseshoe kidney; duplications and malrotations of the urinary collecting system occur in 60 percent
Trisomy 13 (Patau's syndrome)	Abnormal facies, cleft lip and palate, congenital heart disease	Cystic kidneys and other renal anomalies in 60 percent
Trisomy 18 (Edwards' syndrome)	Abnormal facies, abnormal ears, overlapping digits, congenital heart disease	Cystic kidneys, horseshoe kidney, or duplication occurs in 70 percent
Partial trisomy 10q	Abnormal facies, limb and cardiac abnormalities	Renal abnormalities
Triploidy syndrome	Abnormal facies, cardiac defects, hypospadias and cryptorchidism in male, brain anomalies	Renal anomalies
Metabolic Abnormalities		
Galactosemia	Cataracts, hepatic injury, brain damage	Renal tubular dysfunction
Glycogen storage disease (von Gierke's disease)	Hypoglycemia, hepatomegaly	Renal tubular dysfunction
Hereditary tyrosinemia	Failure to thrive, fever, hepatomegaly	Renal tubular dysfunction
Congenital Infection		
Congenital rubella	Cataracts, cardiac anomalies, deafness, microcephaly	Various renal anomalies, renal artery stenosis with late hypertension
Miscellaneous Syndromes		
Rokitansky sequence	Failure of paramesonephric ducts; vaginal atresia, absent or hypoplastic uterus	Renal hypoplasia, agenesis, or double ureters
Rubinstein-Taybi's syndrome	Broad thumbs and toes, slanted palpebral fissures, hypoplastic maxilla	Renal anomalies

from narcotics or neurologic problems. Assessment may be made by catheterization after preparation is made for management of postobstructive diuresis.

C. Investigations. If the physical examination raises the suspicion of renal disease, a urinalysis and imaging evaluation may be indicated.

1. **Urinalysis**
   a. **Method of collection.** One should select the method of urine collection that will provide the most useful information.
      (1) **Suprapubic bladder aspiration** is the most reliable method to document urinary tract infection. However, when the presence or absence of red blood cells (RBCs) in urine is a consideration in the differential diagnosis (see **V.B**), suprapubic collection is inappropriate.
      (2) **Bladder catheterization** is used in the infant who fails to pass urine by 36 to 48 hours and who has no evidence of hypovolemia or circulatory compromise to explain decreased urine output (see **V.A**). Infection can result from the passage of a catheter, however.
      (3) **Bag collection of urine** is adequate for most studies (e.g., levels of amino acids and protein, presence of blood, glycosuria, viral cultures, and sediment examination).
   b. **Specific studies.** In addition to standard analysis for specific gravity (or osmolality), pH, glucose, protein, and sediment, other studies may be required. Tests for non-glucose-reducing substances (Clinitest), sugar chromatography, tests for ketones, and ferric chloride screening are used to evaluate inborn metabolic abnormalities (see Inborn Errors of Metabolism in Chap. 24).
2. **Ultrasound** can delineate most abdominal masses. **Doppler studies** may be utilized to assess renal artery flow. Excretory urograms should not be done unless ultrasound is unavailable or inconclusive. Indications for sonographic study include the following:
   a. Perineal or anal anomalies
   b. Decreased abdominal wall musculature ("prune belly")
   c. Gonadal dysgenesis
   d. Hypospadias
   e. Increased blood urea nitrogen (BUN) or creatinine
   f. Incomplete voiding
   g. Suspicion of inferior vena cava thrombosis or renal vein thrombosis
   h. Abdominal masses
3. **Intravenous pyelography (IVP)** may be helpful in further delineating known sonographic abnormalities yet is rarely useful in the immediate newborn period owing to the neonate's limited concentrating ability and difficulty excreting an osmolar load. IVP is no longer an imaging study of first choice for evaluation of newborn renal anomalies or function.
4. **Voiding cystourethrography** should be performed in infants with obstructive uropathy or hydronephrosis or who have had urinary tract infection.
5. **Renal scanning by radionuclide techniques.** Scanning is useful to demonstrate the position and relative function of renal tissue, even when renal function is less than can be shown within the limits of resolution of standard contrast techniques. Renograms and scintigrams may be performed using technetium-99m–iron ascorbate, tin, technetium-99m–diethylene triamine pentacetic acid (DPTA), and provide vascular flow and function data. Parenchymal function may be assessed with technetium-99m–dimercaptosuccinic acid, which is resorbed by renal tubules.
6. **Chemistry and renal clearance studies.** Serum chemistries and clearance studies define the degree of metabolic imbalance and the status of renal function (see Table 26-2 and **V.D**). Creatinine levels at birth (about 0.8 mg/dl) reflect maternal renal function and fall to about 0.5 mg/dl by 5

to 7 days and to 0.3 to 0.4 mg/dl by 9 days. Glomerular filtration rate ma be estimated by the following formula:

$$\frac{0.40 \times \text{length (cm)}}{\text{creatinine level (premature infants)}}$$

or

$$\frac{0.45 \times \text{length (cm)}}{\text{creatinine level (term infants)}}$$

V. Common clinical renal problems

A. Failure to pass urine (Table 26-4). The normal neonate has 6 to 44 ml of urin in the bladder at birth and may not void for the first 48 hours of life; howeve 17 percent of newborns void in the delivery room, and 92 percent void by 2 hours.

1. Major stresses that may cause delay in voiding

a. Perinatal anoxia or hemorrhage

b. Limited fluid intake from poor feeding

c. Increased fluid losses due to phototherapy or radiant warmers

2. Failure to pass urine by 48 hours may be secondary to (1) an inability t form urine or (2) an obstruction to urinary flow [6,11].

a. Inability to form urine

(1) Circulatory insufficiency, caused by either hypovolemia or hyp tension

(2) Inadequate fluid intake

(3) Bilateral renal agenesis

(4) Acute tubular necrosis

(5) Bilateral renal vein thrombosis

(6) Congenital nephrotic syndrome

(7) Congenital nephritis

(8) Pyelonephritis

b. Obstruction to urinary flow

(1) Posterior urethral valves

(2) Megacystis-megaureter syndrome

Table 26-4. Causes of acute renal failure in the neonate

Prerenal*	Renal parenchymal	Obstructive
Hypotension	Hypoperfusion related to:	Urethral obstruction
Septic shock	Hypoxia	Posterior urethral valve
Maternal hemorrhage	Respiratory Distress Syndrome	Stricture
Twin-twin transfusion	Sepsis	Diverticulum
Surgical	Diarrhea	Ureterocele
Cardiac disease	Dehydration	Ureteropelvic obstruction
Congestive failure	Hemorrhage	Ureterovesical obstruction
Asphyxia	Shock	Extrinsic tumors
Dehydration	Surgical procedures	Neurogenic bladder
	Thromboembolic disease	Megacystis-megaureter
	Venous	
	Arterial	
	Disseminated intravascular coagulation	
	Nephrotoxins	

*May progress to renal parenchymal failure.

(3) Urethral stricture
(4) Urethral diverticulum
(5) Neurogenic bladder
(6) Ureterocele
(7) Tumors
(8) Hypertrophy of the verumontanum

3. **Management.** Bladder catheterization will determine (1) if urine is present but outflow is obstructed or (2) if urine has not been formed. Sonographic, radiologic, or urologic evaluation is done as indicated to confirm a diagnosis so that therapy can be implemented.

B. **Hematuria** is uncommon in newborns. Red staining of the diaper can be due to either RBCs or urates. When such stains are noted, a urinalysis should be obtained. If red blood cells are found, a careful analysis of the sediment is the first step to differentiate glomerular disease (in which red cell casts are present) from nonglomerular causes.

1. **Causes of hematuria.** Gross hematuria is seen most commonly in hemorrhagic disease, but is also common in renal vein thrombosis. Other causes of gross and microscopic hematuria include the following:
   a. Microscopic hematuria following hyperosmolar loads (e.g., glucose or sodium bicarbonate given through an umbilical artery catheter)
   b. Obstructive uropathy
   c. Cortical and medullary necrosis
   d. Renal artery thrombosis
   e. Infection
   f. Congenital malformations
   g. Blood dyscrasias
   h. Renal stones
   i. Drugs and nephrotoxins
   j. Trauma
   k. Congenital neoplasms (Wilms' tumor and neuroblastoma)
2. **Evaluation.** If RBC casts are present, evaluation for glomerulonephritis should be made. The presence of a flank mass necessitates further evaluation for an obstructive anomaly, neoplasm, or venous thrombosis. Renal ultrasound, IVP, voiding cystourethrogram (VCUG), cystoscopy, renal arteriography, or renal scan may be necessary to confirm the diagnosis.

C. **Urinary tract infection (UTI)** must be suspected in any infant, especially a male, who is not gaining weight, is feeding poorly, is jaundiced, or has any other nonspecific signs or symptoms of sepsis, such as poor temperature control, poor color, diarrhea, or vomiting (see Chap. 12).

1. **Diagnosis** is confirmed by culture of urine obtained by suprapubic bladder aspiration. Approximately 70 percent of cases are due to *Escherichia coli*; infections caused by *Klebsiella, Pseudomonas,* and *Proteus* are less common, and gram-positive organisms are rare. Blood cultures should be obtained because septicemia may frequently be present in newborns, either secondary to UTI or as a cause of hematogenous bacterial spread to the kidney.
2. **Treatment** is initiated parenterally while one is awaiting the results of cultures. Antibiotic coverage with ampicillin and gentamicin is usually begun; the treatment is adjusted when the sensitivity testing is available.
3. **Urinary tract anomalies.** When a UTI is present in an infant under 1 year of age, an underlying urinary tract anomaly will be found in 55 percent of males and in 35 percent of females. All infants with documented UTI should have a sonogram to assess renal size and configuration. A VCUG after the infection is under control is essential to determine whether or not reflux is present. In the infant with sepsis, the sonogram or a renal scan should be performed early in the course of infection to rule out obstruction. An IVP may be done if ultrasound is not available or if the VCUG or sonogram is abnormal. Further evaluation (e.g., cystoscopy) should be done if the radiographic studies reveal an anomaly, and only by

a urologist with newborn experience. Newborns with urinary infectio should be treated with antibiotics until the above studies are complete and known to be negative.

D. Acute renal failure (ARF) in the newborn may be secondary to prerenal, pa renchymal, or obstructive disorders [5,7]. Medications such as indomethaci and captopril have been implicated [12].

1. **Causes** of renal failure are listed in Table 26-4.
2. **Management and diagnosis** should proceed hand in hand. Confirm ol guria (urine flow <0.5 ml/kg per hour).
   - **a.** Seek prerenal or obstructive causes because they are readily rever ible or correctable (see Table 26-4).
     - **(1)** If obstruction is the cause of ARF, examine the infant for evidenc of a mass (see **IV.B**). Catheterize the bladder with a no. 5 or 8 feeding tube, and perform an ultrasonic examination. If an ol struction is found, consult a urologist who is skilled with ne nates.
     - **(2)** To rule out prerenal failure, give fluid challenge (10 to 20 ml/k body weight) over 1 to 2 hours **if there is no heart failure or cli ical volume overload.** Give furosemide (Lasix), 1 mg/kg IV. N response suggests parenchymal failure.
     - **(3)** Table 26-5 gives indices helpful in distinguishing renal failu from parenchymal failure in the term newborn. Determination microproteins in urine may be helpful [3,4].
   - **b. Management of renal failure** should include reduction of excreto load. Extrarenal routes of excretion should be utilized.
     - **(1) Fluid** should be limited to 400 ml/m² of body area per day (inse sible water loss; see Table 24-3 on page 458) plus urine replac ment for the preceding day. It is often convenient to replace urir output over 8-hour intervals.
     - **(2) Sodium** should be limited to 0.3 mEq/kg per day.
     - **(3) Potassium** (see page 465) A low-potassium formula or potassiun free solutions should be used. Hyperkalemia (potassium > 6 mE L) is treated as follows:
       - **(a) Sodium polystyrene sulfonate (Kayexalate),** administere rectally in a dose of 1.0 to 1.5 gm/kg (dissolved in normal sa line at 0.5 gm/ml saline) or orally in a dose of 1.0 gm/kg (di solved in dextrose 10% in water). The enema is inserted 1 t 3 cm using a thin silastic feeding tube. If possible, we avoi using Kayexalate in low birth weight infants [8]. 1 gm resi removes 1 mEq potassium. A calcium exchange resin may b used when hypernatremia is present.

Table 26-5. Renal failure indices in newborns

Test	Hypoperfusion (prerenal failure)	Parenchymal diseas
U_{Na} (mEq/L)	10–50	30–90
U/S_{Na}	0.23 ± 0.14	0.45 ± 0.22
U/S_{cr}	29.2 ± 1.6	9.7 ± 3.6
RFI	1.3 ± 0.8	11.6 ± 9.6
FE_{Na}	0.9 ± 0.6	4.3 ± 2.2

Key: U_{Na} = urinary sodium; U/S_{Na} = ratio of urine to serum sodium; U/S_{cr} = ratio of urin to serum creatinine; RFI = renal failure index, which is $(U_{Na})/(U/S_{cr})$;FE_{Na} = fractional ex cretion of sodium, which is (Na excreted/Na filtered) × 100 = $(U_{Na}/S_{Na})/(U_{cr}/S_{cr})$ × 100.
Source: From O. P. Mathew et al. Neonatal renal failure: usefulness of diagnostic indices. *Pe diatrics* 65:57, 1980.

(b) **Calcium.** Give 1.0 to 2.0 ml/kg of calcium gluconate 10% over 2 to 4 minutes, while monitoring the electrocardiogram (ECG). (See Chap. 24.)

(c) **Sodium bicarbonate,** 1 mEq/kg, will decrease serum potassium by 1 mEq/L.

(d) **Glucose and insulin.** Begin with a bolus of regular human insulin (0.05 units per kilogram) and dextrose 10% in water (2 ml/kilogram) followed by a continuous infusion of dextrose 10% in water at 2–4 ml/kilogram per hour and human regular insulin (10 units/100 ml) at 1 ml/kg per hour. The blood glucose level is monitored frequently. The ratio should be 1 or 2 units of insulin to 4 gm of glucose. (See Chap. 24.)

(e) **Furosemide** 1 mg/kg is given when renal function is adequate because kaliuresis as well as natriuresis occurs with this diuretic.

(f) **Dialysis** is performed when hyperkalemia cannot be controlled by the measures listed in **(a)–(e).**

(4) **Phosphorus** is restricted by using a low-phosphate formula (e.g., Similac PM 60/40* or SMA†).

(5) **Protein** is limited to 0.5 gm/kg per day as essential amino acids; this amount is increased as tolerated.

(6) Limit drugs that are renally excreted, and modify dosages for renal failure. Obtain drug levels of potential nephrotoxins.

c. Supplemental nutrients

(1) **Calcium** 150 to 200 mg/kg per day of elemental calcium is given orally.

(2) **Bicarbonate** 4 mEq/kg per day is given to correct acidosis.

(3) **Vitamin D_2 (calciferol)** is given in a dose of 500 to 1000 units per day. Monitor calcium levels. Calcitriol (vitamin D_3) generally is not used, since preparation is in gel and dosing is too difficult.

(4) **Calories and protein** are provided in supplemental oral preparations such as AMIN-Aid§, Polycose,* or Controlyte.¶ In infants with complicated courses already on hyperalimentation, however, calories and protein are provided in the daily solution (see Chap. 30).

(5) **Parenteral hyperalimentation** may be indicated for patients who have prolonged renal failure (see Chap. 30).

d. Dialysis is used to replace the function of the kidneys. Dialysis of newborn infants requires modification of equipment to monitor small changes in volume and weight. It is best performed in centers experienced in the use of such techniques in a small child. Although transplantation has been attempted in the newborn, it is generally unsuccessful.

(1) **Clinical indications for dialysis**

(a) Rapidly rising BUN accompanying severe oliguria

(b) Severe and persistent acidosis not necessarily secondary to renal failure. Dialysis allows correction of acidosis by administration of large amounts of bicarbonate, as well as by removal of large amounts of ammonia, while definitive diagnosis is made of a metabolic abnormality.

(c) Renal failure associated with salt and water overload

(d) Uncontrolled hyperkalemia

*Ross Laboratories, Columbus, Ohio.
†Wyeth Laboratories, Philadelphia, Pa.
§McGaw Laboratories, Santa Ana, Calif.
¶Doyle Pharmaceutical Company, Minneapolis, Minn.

(2) Biochemical indications for dialysis
- **(a)** An increase in BUN of greater than 30 mg/dl per day
- **(b)** BUN greater than 65 mg/dl in the presence of acidosis
- **(c)** Renal failure with acidosis and bicarbonate less than 10 mEq/L
- **(d)** Acidosis combined with continuing hyperkalemia or hypocalcemia (or both).

e. A plan for **long-term therapy** includes a firm diagnosis (with biopsy if applicable), radiologic definition of the anatomic structures, and monitoring of function (including protein loss, creatinine clearance, BUN, urine sediment, and levels of sodium, potassium, chloride, and carbon dioxide or pH).

E. Abdominal masses (see Chap. 27)

1. Diagnosis of an abdominal mass depends on the history and physical examination, supplemented by sonography as the first test. IVPs may not be necessary. The definition of a mass of renal or urinary tract origin is as follows:

a. Unilateral masses

(1) Types
- **(a)** Multicystic dysplasia
- **(b)** Hydronephrosis
- **(c)** Tumors (congenital, mesoblastic, nephroma, Wilms tumor)
- **(d)** Renal vein thrombosis
- **(e)** Renal cyst

(2) Differential diagnosis
- **(a)** Ovarian cyst or mass
- **(b)** Reduplication cyst of the gut
- **(c)** Liver or gall bladder masses
- **(d)** Neuroma

(3) Differential testing
- **(a)** Sonography, occasionally IVP
- **(b)** Urinalysis, including test for hematuria
- **(c)** Urine sediment
- **(d)** Vanillylmandelic acid excretion, urinary catecholamines, cystathionine
- **(3)** Renal scan

b. Bilateral masses

(1) Types
- **(a)** Bilateral hydronephrosis
- **(b)** Polycystic disease (infantile or adult)
- **(c)** Megacystis-megaureter
- **(d)** Renal vein thrombosis
- **(e)** Leukemic infiltrate (this is rare)

(2) Differential testing—sonography, nuclide scans, CT scans, VCUG, IVP

c. Midline masses

(1) Types
- **(a)** Obstructive uropathy, including obstructed bladder, posterior urethral valves, and megacystis-megaureter syndrome
- **(b)** Urachal cyst

(2) Differential diagnosis
- **(a)** Hydrocolpos
- **(b)** Hydrometrocolpos

(3) Differential testing and examination
- **(a)** The bladder should be felt and percussed.
- **(b)** Rectal examination should be performed.
- **(c)** Genitalia should be examined for imperforate hymen or vaginal atresia.

(d) Catheterization should be performed and the mass reevaluated.

(e) **Tests** include sonography, IVP, VCUG, CT scans, and panendoscopy.

2. **Therapy.** After diagnosis, therapy is basically surgical. If obstructive lesions are present, care should be exercised when correcting fluid deficits and metabolic abnormalities. Deficits are best repaired using Ringer's lactate or balanced saline solution. Once adequate circulation is established, correction of the underlying abnormality can proceed. The serum calcium level determines how quickly acidosis can be corrected, since acidosis protects against the tetanic effects of hypocalcemia. After relief of the obstruction, severe depletion of sodium and water may result from the "release" diuresis produced.

   a. **Careful replacement of fluid and electrolytes** and close monitoring of the infant are necessary. We use a solution of 0.25 isotonic saline with sodium bicarbonate (20 to 30 mEq/L) and potassium (10 to 30 mEq/L) added, depending on urinary electrolyte losses. Fluid is administered at twice the maintenance rate for 2 hours; it is then adjusted according to the hourly urinary output.

   b. **Hypertension** (see **VII**) should be controlled preoperatively in hydronephrosis and renal vein thrombosis. If renal vein thrombosis is treated medically with anticoagulation, hypertension should be controlled as well. Hydralazine 0.25 mg/kg parenterally (maximum 1 to 4 mg/kg per day) may be used to lower blood pressure initially and for maintenance. Nifedipine, nitroprusside, or diazoxide may be used for rapid lowering of blood pressure in severe hypertension (see Table 26-6).

   c. **Fluid and sodium restriction and diuretics** may be necessary to control potential fluid overload in infantile polycystic disease of the kidney.

F. **Metabolic acidosis** (see Chap. 24). The most common causes of metabolic acidosis are poor renal perfusion, hypoxemia, renal or adrenal disease, and gastrointestinal losses. In the premature infant, metabolic acidosis also may be due to late metabolic acidosis of prematurity.

1. **Late metabolic acidosis of prematurity.** In the slowly growing premature infant, acidosis also may occur as a result of formula feeding with a high amount of protein or with a usual protein load (3 gm/kg per day).

   a. **Cause.** The most likely cause of this acidosis is a disproportion between the rate of endogenous acid production and renal excretion, leading to a net positive acid balance with a decreased growth rate. Since the acidosis will limit growth, the disproportion is perpetuated.

   b. **Treatment.** Therapy with sodium bicarbonate (2 to 4 mEq/kg per day) for 1 or 2 days and decreased protein feeding (10% D/W for 24 hours) is usually effective. As soon as growth begins, the acidosis resolves and alkali supplementation is no longer required.

2. **Renal tubular acidosis.** Late metabolic acidosis of prematurity must be differentiated from renal tubular acidosis (congenital or acquired).

   a. **Renal tubular acidosis** is defined as the inability to produce an acid urine in response to acid stress, either spontaneously or under experimental loading. It occurs in the following forms:

      (1) The proximal lesion is associated with bicarbonate wasting (type II).

      (2) The distal or "classic" variety is associated with the inability to excrete hydrogen ions (type I).

      (3) An incomplete or mixed tubular acidosis may be seen in obstructive uropathy and in hereditary fructose intolerance.

      (4) Secondary forms of proximal tubular acidosis (bicarbonate wasting) may be seen in Fanconi syndrome, cystinosis, Lowe's syn-

Table 26-6. Antihypertensive agents in early infancy[1] (see Appendix A)

Medication[2]	Dose (parenteral or oral)	Comment
Sodium nitroprusside (Nipride)	0.4 μg/kg/min IV, NOF	Check isothiocyanate levels
Diazoxide	2–5 mg/kg IV, NOF	Unpredictable in degree of blood pressure control; follow blood sugar; watch for fluid accumulation
Hydralazine (Apresoline)	0.15 mg/kg IM or IV or 0.25 mg/kg/day q4–6h	Preserves renal blood flow; may increase heart rate
Alpha-methyldopa (Aldomet)	2–4 mg/kg IV or IM or 10 mg/kg/dose in 3 or 4 doses	May cause generally depressed state
Propranolol (Inderal)[4,5]	1.5 mg/kg/day PO	May cause bronchospasm
Captopril (Capoten)[4]	0.01–0.3 mg/kg/day PO	May cause marked oliguria, hyperkalemia or renal failure
Furosemide (Lasix)[3]	0.25–1 mg/kg/dose PO or IV	May potentiate above agents; may cause hypercalciuria
Nifedipine Procardia®[4]	0.5–1.0 mg, sublingual	Limited experience in newborns

Key: NOF = no oral form.
[1]Resperine, guanethidine, and other "older" agents are primarily of historic interest. Experience is limited with newer beta blockers, clonidine, and prazosin.
[2]Suggested order of agents: mild hypertension: furosemide or other diuretic, adding hydralazine or methyldopa or oral propranolol; moderate hypertension: captopril, nifedipine ± diuretic; severe hypertension: nitroprusside, labetalol, nifedipine, diazoxide.
[3]For other diuretic doses, see Chap. 14.
[4]Not approved for children, and doses approximate at best.
[5]Dosage for other beta blockers and for labetalol unknown.

drome, and tyrosinosis (which may be either congenital or a result of parenteral nutrition).

b. Treatment. The initial therapy involves the correction of the acidosis and reestablishment of growth, followed by definitive testing with acid loading. Therapy is started with 2 to 3 mEq/kg per day of sodium bicarbonate in divided doses; this amount is increased if necessary. This dose will be sufficient to correct the deficit in babies with distal renal tubular acidosis; however, in those with the proximal tubular lesion, larger amounts are needed because of urinary bicarbonate losses in addition to the dietary acid load.

G. Neonatal ascites occurs rarely; it may be secondary to congenital nephrotic syndrome, congenital syphilis, or urine extravasation from the genitourinary tract in obstructive disease. Nephrotic syndrome is indicated when urinalysis shows an active sediment with oval fat bodies and proteinuria. Radiology and appropriate laboratory tests further aid in the differential diagnosis (see Chap. 15).

H. Urologic and nephrologic syndromes. Table 26-3 reviews the findings of the more commonly occurring syndromes associated with renal abnormalities. Radiographic studies should be performed to determine the presence of a renal anomaly that may need correction. Since infants with these problems frequently develop UTIs, routine urine cultures are helpful in management. Further evaluation of renal tubular function should be pursued when indicated.

Table 26-7. Normal blood pressure in premature infants (birth weight 600 to 1750 gm)*

	600 to 999 gm		1000 to 1249 gm		1250 to 1499 gm		1500 to 1750 gm	
Day	S (± 2 SD)	D (± 2 SD)	S (± 2 SD)	D (± 2 SD)	S (± 2 SD)	D (± 2 SD)	S (± 2 SD)	D (± 2 SD)
1	37.9 (17.4)	23.2 (10.3)	44 (22.8)	22.5 (13.5)	48 (18.0)	27 (12.4)	47 (15.8)	26 (15.6)
3	44.9 (15.7)	30.6 (12.3)	48 (15.4)	36.5 (9.6)	59 (21.1)	40 (13.7)	51 (18.2)	35 (10.0)
7	50.0 (14.8)	30.4 (12.4)	57 (14.0)	42.5 (16.5)	68 (14.8)	40 (11.3)	66 (23.0)	41 (24.0)
14	50.2 (14.8)	37.4 (12.0)	53 (30.0)		64 (21.2)	36 (24.2)	76 (34.8)	42 (20.3)
28	61.0 (23.5)	45.8 (27.4)	57 (30.0)		69 (31.4)	44 (26.2)	73(5.6)	50 (9.9)

Key: S = systolic; D = diastolic; SD = standard deviation.
*Blood pressure was obtained by the Dinamap method.
Source: Modified from J. R. Ingelfinger, L. Powers, and M. F. Epstein, Blood pressure norms in low-birth-weight infants: Birth through four weeks. *Pediatr. Res.* 17: 319A, 1983.

I. Other gross malformations involving the urinary tract (e.g., exstrophy of the bladder) will occur sporadically. Consultation with a pediatric urologist is indicated for early planning of necessary correction and follow-up.

VI. **Circumcision** is primarily a socially established procedure rather than a medical one. It is indicated medically only in instances in which adhesions of the foreskin or tight phimosis leads to urinary retention. The pros and cons of circumcision are discussed in Chapter 8. It is important to avoid circumcision under the following circumstances:

A. In cases of **hypospadias,** since the tissue may be necessary for surgical repair

B. In cases of **ambiguous genitalia,** until the sex for rearing is determined

C. In the presence of **bleeding disorders**

VII. **Blood pressure** (see Chap. 6) in the newborn is lower than in later infancy and in the premature is related to weight and gestational age [1,10].

A. During fetal life, blood pressure is low and is related to placental blood flow and to fetal circulation.

B. Following birth, blood pressure is low and appears to be stable, rising gradually over the first 6 to 8 weeks. Table 26-7 shows normal blood pressure in the first 4 weeks of life in premature infants; Table 26-8 shows normal blood pressure in term infants at 1 week and at 6 weeks of age.

C. Since normal blood pressure levels vary according to size and gestational age, **hypertension** may be defined by persistent elevation of blood pressure greater than 2 standard deviations above the mean.

1. Clues as to the **etiology of hypertension** may be found in the obstetric history (e.g., maternal diabetes predisposing to thrombotic disease) and perinatal events. Renal thromboembolic phenomena complicating umbilical artery catheters occur frequently and should be considered when an infant develops hypertension. A record of recent volume expansion or administration of medications that could cause hypertension may help elucidate the etiology. Causes of hypertension in the neonatal period are listed in Table 26-9).

2. The **symptoms and signs** of hypertension in infancy are nonspecific and include cardiorespiratory difficulties, neurologic abnormalities (irritability, convulsions), gastrointestinal distress, failure to thrive, or fever. Abdominal mass, unequal upper or lower extremity pulses, edema, oliguria, or polyuria may occur. Physical examination for renal size (see **IV.B**) is helpful. Examinations of upper and lower extremity blood pressures are necessary to exclude coarctation of the aorta in hypertensive infants. Careful neurologic, ophthalmologic, and cardiac examination is helpful in looking for end-organ damage.

3. **Laboratory studies** should be directed at finding a cause of hypertension (see Fig. 26-1). Antihypertensive therapy should be administered for sustained hypertension not related to volume expansion or drug administration. Doses are found in Table 26-7.

VIII. **Renal abnormalities in the fetus** [3,6,9,14]

A. **Diagnosis** of potentially treatable congenital defects in the fetus is becoming more common. Renal abnormalities may be detected during maternal ultra-

Table 26-8. Normal blood pressure in term infants*

Day	S	± 2 SD
7	74	± 22
42	96	± 20

Key: S = systolic; SD = standard deviation.
*Blood pressure was obtained by the Doppler method.
Source: Modified from M. de Swiet, P. Fayers, and E. A. Shinebourne, Systolic blood pressure in a population of infants in the first year of life: The Brompton study. *Pediatrics* 65: 1028, 1980.

Table 26-9. Causes of hypertension in neonatal period

Iatrogenic or Accidental Causes
Phenylephrine eye drops
Nosedrops
Steroids
Umbilical artery catheter accidents
Vascular Causes
Coarctation of the aorta
Renal artery stenosis
Renal artery accidents
Occlusion
Aneurysm
Renal vein thrombosis
Segmental hypoplasia
Renal Causes
Infantile-type polycystic kidney disease
Nephritides
Acute or chronic renal failure
Tumors
Neuroblastoma
Wilms' tumor (nephroblastoma)
Ganglioneuroma
Leiomyoma
Pheochromocytoma
Endocrine Causes
Congenital adrenal hyperplasia
Cushing's syndrome
Neurologic Causes
Intraventricular hemorrhage
Cerebral angioma
Subdural hemorrhage
Infections
Rubella (vascular problems)
Perinephric abscess
Pulmonary Causes
Associated with bronchopulmonary dysplasia
Miscellaneous
Closure of abdominal wall defects
Associated with ECMO

sonic examinations. Abnormalities that may be found include Potter's syndrome, hydronephrosis, renal cysts, hydroureteromegacystis, and renal tumors (see Table 26-3).

B. The best **management** of these prenatally detected conditions is uncertain. A suggested approach is as follows:

1. **Hydronephrotic kidney.** If poor function is suspected and the condition is bilateral, or if there is a solitary kidney, obstruction should be relieved as soon as possible. Some physicians believe this should be done by early delivery, after fetal lung indices are mature, or by in utero decompression. If hydronephrosis is unilateral, or is bilateral but with good function, appearance of the kidneys should be followed by ultrasound and the hydro-

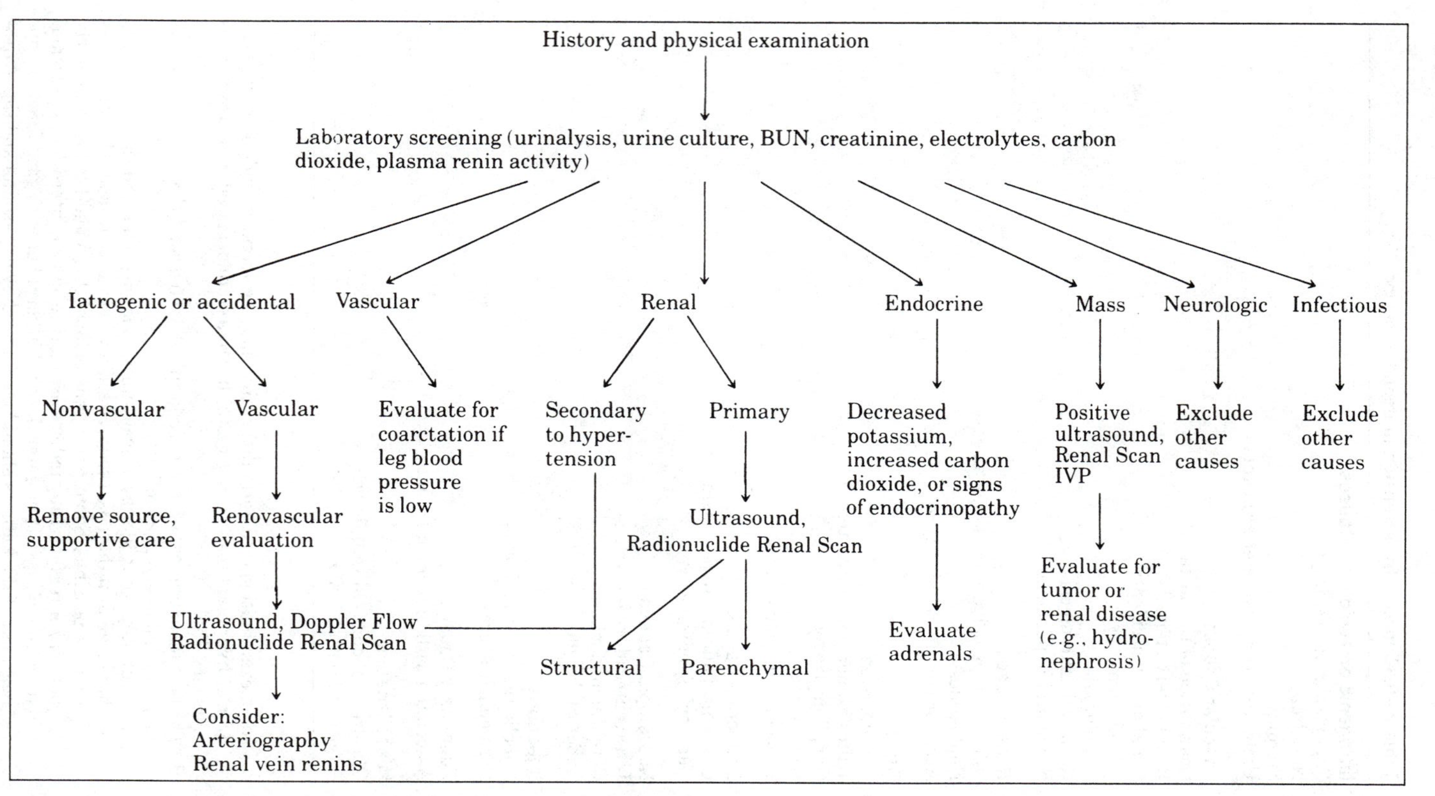

Fig. 26-1. Evaluation of hypertension in newborns (BUN = blood urea nitrogen; IVP = intravenous pyelogram). (Adapted from J. R. Ingelfinger (Ed.), Hypertension in the first year of life. In *Pediatric Hypertension*. Philadelphia: Saunders, 1982. Pp. 229–240.)

nephrosis is corrected after delivery at term. Poor function is suspected if there is severe oligohydramnios, or if the anatomy of the kidneys is severely distorted. Fetal surgery for congenital hydronephrosis is reviewed by T. L. Pinckert and M. S. Golbus in *Clinics in Perinatology* 15: 948, 1988.

2. **Multicystic-dysplastic-agenetic kidney.** If the kidneys appear to have very little parenchyma, fetal outcome is likely to be poor, especially if there is no response to furosemide (assessed by appearance of urine in fetal bladder). If the renal abnormality is unilateral, it may be corrected as needed after delivery.
3. **Polycystic kidneys.** (Prenatal chromosomal detection of autosomal-dominant form is possible also.) Renal function should be tested after birth.
4. **Tumors.** There are as yet no definite guidelines for prenatal treatment.

C. The outcome following identification of these abnormalities in the fetus is uncertain. The ethical issues of the fetus as patient will need to be resolved.

IX. **Renal problems in the very ill neonate.** The very sick neonate frequently requires therapy that may interfere with or exceed renal functional capacity. Furthermore, toxic drug levels can occur if the dosage is not tailored to the low level of renal function in the newborn.

A. **Antibiotics** used may cause nephrotoxicity, especially aminoglycosides and cephalosporins.

B. **Tolazoline,** sometimes used as a pulmonary vasodilator, is an alpha-sympatholytic agent and may induce oliguric renal failure due to systemic hypotension and consequent renal hypoperfusion.

C. **Indomethacin,** or other prostaglandin inhibitors used for pharmacologic closure of ductus arteriosus, may cause oliguria, decrease in GFR, and decreased fractional excretion of sodium and chloride.

D. **Captopril,** angiotensin-I-converting enzyme, should be used in low doses and with caution, since oligoanuria has been reported with this agent (see **VII**).

E. **Contrast agents** used for radiography are hyperosmolar and contain a large amount of sodium (1300 to 1940 mOsmol/kgH_2O).

1. Contrast agents should be used only after adequate hydration; consider nonionic contrast agents.
2. These agents are associated with renal vein thrombosis, hypoperfusion, ischemia, and acute tubular necrosis.

F. **Evaporative water loss** through the skin may be increased in very small babies. **Phototherapy** further increases insensible water loss. Failure to account for this fluid can lead to ARF.

G. **ECMO (extracorporeal membrane oxygenation)** may be associated with acute renal failure and hypertension. Hemodialysis through the apparatus is possible.

References

1. Adelman, R. D. *Clin. Perinatol.* 15: 567, 1988.
2. Arant, B. S. *Pediatr. Nephrol.* 1: 308, 1987.
3. Burghard, R., et al. *Pediatr. Nephrol.* 1: 574, 1987.
4. Cole, J. W., et al. *Pediatrics* 76: 958, 1985.
5. Guignard, J.-P., and Gouyon, J.-B. *Biol. Neonate* 53L: 248, 1988.
6. Kim, M. S., and Mandell, J. Renal function in the fetus and neonate. In L. R. King (Ed.), *Urologic Surgery in Neonates and Young Infants.* Philadelphia: Saunders, 1988.
7. Oh, W. *Biol. Neonate* 53: 230, 1988.
8. Ohlsson, L., and Hosking, M. *Eur. J. Ped.* 146: 571, 1987.
9. Robillard, J. E., and Nakamura, K. T. *Biol. Neonate* 53: 210, 1988.
10. Skalina, M. E. L., et al. *Am. J. Perinatol.* 3: 235, 1986.
11. Springate, J. E., et al. *Pediatr. Rev.* 9: 51, 1987.
12. Tack, E. D., and Perlman, J. M. *J. Pediatr.* 112: 805, 1988.
13. Vanpee, M., et al. *Acta Paediatr. Scand.* 77: 191, 1988.
14. Grupe, W. *PCNA* 34: 629, 1987.

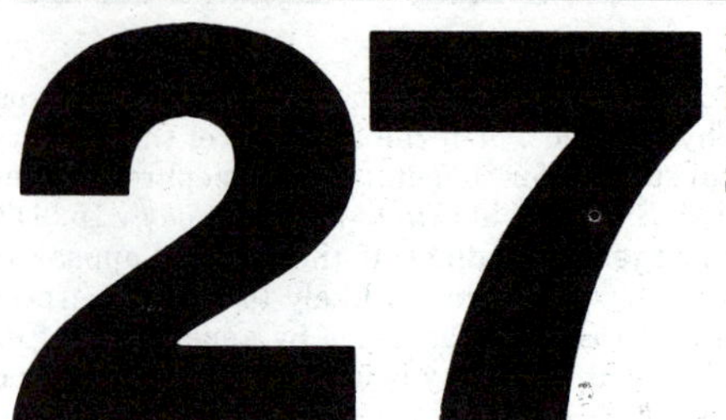

Surgical Emergencies in the Newborn

Steven A. Ringer

I. Fetal manifestations

A. Polyhydramnios (amniotic fluid volume greater than 2 liters) occurs in 1 in 1000 births.

1. **Gastrointestinal obstruction** (including esophageal atresia) is the most frequent surgical cause of polyhydramnios. Measurement of bile acid concentration in amniotic fluid may differentiate a lesion above the ampulla of Vater (in which bile acids are absent) from those below the ampulla (in which bile acids are present) [6] (see **X.D**).
2. **Other causes** of polyhydramnios include abdominal wall defects (omphalocele and gastroschisis), anencephaly, diaphragmatic hernia, tight nuchal cord, fetal death, inability of the fetus to swallow, inability of the fetus to concentrate urine, and maternal diabetes.
3. All mothers with suspected polyhydramnios should have an ultrasonic examination. In experienced hands, these studies are the method of choice for the diagnosis of intestinal obstruction, abdominal wall defects, and diaphragmatic hernia [3], as well as abnormalities leading to an inability of the fetus to swallow.
4. If an obstructing intestinal lesion is diagnosed antenatally and there is no evidence of dystocia, vaginal delivery is acceptable. Pediatric surgical consultation should be obtained prior to delivery.

B. Dystocia may result from fetal intestinal obstruction, abdominal wall defect, genitourinary anomalies, or fetal ascites (see **D**).

C. Meconium peritonitis

1. A **plain film of the abdomen** will show scattered calcific shadows. Most congenital lesions causing intestinal obstruction (see **VI.A**) have, on occasion, produced meconium peritonitis [19].
2. **Meconium peritonitis** is often associated with an antenatal perforation of the intestinal tract.

D. Fetal ascites (see **IX.D**). Fetal ascites is usually associated with urinary tract anomalies (lower urinary tract obstruction due to posterior urethral valves). Other causes are hemolytic disease of the newborn, any severe anemia (e.g., alpha-thalassemia), peritonitis, thoracic duct obstruction, cardiac disease, hepatic or portal vein obstruction, hepatitis, and congenital infection (e.g., syphilis or TORCH infections; see Chap. 12) as well as other causes of hydrops fetalis (see Chap. 15). After birth, ascites may be seen in the congenital nephrotic syndrome. **Prenatal ultrasound** is important in light of recent advances of fetal surgery, which might allow decompression of either the bladder or a hydronephrotic kidney and can save renal parenchyma (see Chaps. 3 and 26).

E. Oligohydramnios is usually associated with intrauterine growth retardation, postmaturity, or fetal distress, but it may indicate absent kidneys (Potter's syndrome; see Chap. 26) or amniotic fluid leak.

II. Postnatal manifestations

A. Respiratory distress (see **IV** and **V.** and Chaps. 5 and 13)

1. **Choanal atresia.** If bilateral, the baby is unable to breath nasally (see **V.E**).
2. Laryngotracheal clefts (see **V.D**)

3. Tracheal agenesis
4. Esophageal atresia with or without tracheoesophageal fistula (TEF) (see **III**)
5. Diaphragmatic hernia (see **IV**)
6. Congenital lobar emphysema
7. Cystic adenomatoid malformation of the lung
8. Biliary tracheobronchial communication (extremely rare)

B. Scaphoid abdomen

1. Diaphragmatic hernia (see **IV**)
2. Esophageal atresia without TEF (see **III**)

C. Excessive mucus and salivations before first feeding—esophageal atresia (see **III**)

D. Pneumoperitoneum

1. **Perforated stomach** is associated with large amounts of free intraabdominal air. At times it is necessary to aspirate air from the abdominal cavity to relieve respiratory distress prior to definitive surgical repair. The lesion is associated with localized ischemia of the stomach and requires simple closure [25].
2. **Perforated Meckel's diverticulum** in the newborn is associated with free intraabdominal air.
3. **Perforated appendix** is associated with free intraabdominal air in the newborn.
4. Air from a pulmonary air leak may dissect into the peritoneal cavity in infants on ventilators.
5. Any perforation of the bowel may cause pneumoperitoneum (see Chap. 28).

E. Gaseous distension has a rapid onset in the left upper quadrant when there is complete duodenal obstruction. Lower obstruction causes more generalized distension, which varies with location. Gaseous distension may occur where there is esophageal atresia with tracheoesophageal fistula (see **III**). In the normal infant, the progression of the air column seen on x-ray of the abdomen is as follows: **1 hour** after birth the air is past the stomach into the upper jejunum; **3 hours** after birth it is at the cecum; by **8 to 12 hours** after birth it is at the rectosigmoid. The movement of air through the bowel is slower in the premature infant.

F. Vomiting. The causes of vomiting can be differentiated by the presence or absence of bile. The presence of bile-stained vomit in the newborn should be treated as a life-threatening emergency, with at least 20 percent of such infants requiring surgical intervention immediately after evaluation. Surgical consultation should be obtained immediately.

1. **Bile-stained vomitus.** Intestinal obstruction may result from the following:
   a. Malrotation with or without volvulus
   b. Atresias—duodenal, jejunal, ileal, colonic
   c. Annular pancreas
   d. Hirschsprung's disease
   e. Aberrant superior mesenteric artery
   f. Preduodenal portal vein
   g. Peritoneal bands—persistent omphalomesenteric duct
   h. Bile-stained vomitus is occasionally seen in infants without intestinal obstruction. In these cases the bile-stained vomiting will only occur one or two times.
2. **Non-bile-stained vomitus**
   a. Overfeeding (feeding excessive volume)
   b. Milk or formula intolerance
   c. Sepsis
   d. Central nervous system (CNS) lesion
   e. Lesion above ampulla of Vater
      (1) Pyloric stenosis

(2) Upper duodenal stenosis
(3) Annular pancreas (rare)

G. **Failure to pass meconium** can occur in sick babies with decreased tone and in premature infants. It also may be the result of the following disorders:
1. Imperforate anus
2. Functional intestinal obstruction (see **VII**)

H. **Failure to develop transitional fecal stools** after the passage of meconium
1. Volvulus
2. Malrotation

I. **Hematemesis and bloody stools**
1. Necrotizing enterocolitis (most frequent cause of hematemesis and bloody stool in premature infants; see Chap. 28)
2. Gastric and duodenal ulcers (due to stress) and Cushing-Rokitansky-type ulcer (e.g., CNS disease, meningitis, kernicterus, and CNS tumors)
3. Coagulation disorder (see Chap. 17)
4. Disseminated intravascular coagulation (DIC) (see Chap. 17)
5. Duodenal stenosis
6. Meckel's diverticulum
7. Duplications of the small intestine
8. Volvulus
9. Intussusception
10. Polyps, hemangiomas
11. Cirsoid aneurysm
12. Maternal blood
    a. **Maternal blood** is sometimes swallowed by the newborn during labor and delivery. This can be diagnosed by an Apt test performed on blood aspirated from the infant's stomach (see **X.C** and Chap. 16).
    b. In breast-fed infants, if blood obtained from the infant's stomach is adult blood, inspection of the mother's breasts or having the mother express milk from her breasts may reveal the source of blood. If the stomach is aspirated before a feeding and no blood is found, the baby should then nurse and the stomach should be aspirated after the feeding to document the breast as the source of the blood.

J. **Abdominal masses** [12] (see **IX.F**)
1. Genitourinary anomalies (see **IX.D**)
2. Tumors (see **IX.E**)
3. Distended bladder

K. **Birth trauma** (see Chap. 22)
1. Lacerated solid organs—liver, spleen
2. Spinal cord transection with quadriplegia

III. **Esophageal atresia** may occur with or without TEF.

A. At least 85 percent of infants with esophageal atresia have TEF. They may present with respiratory distress due to (1) airway obstruction secondary to excess secretions, (2) abdominal distension and diaphragmatic elevation, or (3) both. Respiratory distress also can occur from the reflux of gastric contents up the distal esophagus into the lung by way of the fistula. Excessive salivation and vomiting soon after feedings are often the first clue in the nursery.

B. **Esophageal atresia** is diagnosed by the inability to pass a catheter into the stomach; the diagnosis is confirmed by x-ray studies showing the catheter coiled in the upper esophageal pouch. Plain x-rays may demonstrate a distended blind upper esophageal pouch filled with air that is unable to progress into the stomach. Some infants may have associated vertebral anomalies of the cervical or upper dorsal spine. Pushing 50 cc of air into the catheter under fluoroscopic examination may show dilatation and relaxation of the upper pouch, thus avoiding contrast studies.

C. Rarely, esophageal atresia may occur without a TEF or with the fistula connecting with the upper esophagus. No gastrointestinal gas will be seen on x-ray examination, and the abdomen is scaphoid. Respiratory difficulties are less acute. Diagnostic maneuvers are the same as in **B.**

D. Infants who have a TEF without esophageal atresia (H-type fistula) are rare and usually present after the neonatal period. These infants have a history of frequent pneumonias or respiratory distress temporally related to meals. This disorder can often be demonstrated with a nonionic water-soluble contrast medium (Omnipaque) and cinefluoroscopy. The definitive examination is combined fiberoptic bronchoscopy and esophagoscopy with passage of a fine balloon catheter from the trachea into the esophagus. The H-type fistula is usually high in the trachea (cervical area).

E. Babies with esophageal atresia with or without TEF are often of low birth weight. Approximately 21 percent of these babies are premature (five times the normal incidence), and 19 percent are small for gestational age (eight times the normal incidence). Other anomalies may be present, including the syndrome of vertebral and vascular defects, imperforate anus, TEF with esophageal atresia, renal dysplasia, renal defects (VATER syndrome), and chromosomal anomalies [2].

F. A **multiple end-hole suction catheter (Replogle)** should be placed in the proximal pouch and put under intermittent suction at the time the diagnosis is made. Prior to transportation of an infant with esophageal atresia with TEF, a suction cannula must be placed in the proximal pouch. Guidelines for intubation are the same as in other types of respiratory distress (see Chap. 39, sec. **VI**). If intubation is required, ventilation should be at an increased rate with low pressure to prevent gastric and intestinal distension. In the usual TEF, the fistula to the trachea is near the carina. Care must be taken to avoid accidental intubation of the fistula. If possible, it is best to avoid mechanical ventilation of these babies until the fistula is closed because the abdomen may become very distended. The baby should be transported in the upright position (at about 45 degrees) to diminish gastroesophageal reflux. Surgical therapy usually involves immediate placement of a gastrostomy tube. As soon as the infant can tolerate further surgery, the fistula is divided, and primary repair of the esophagus is performed. Many infants with esophageal atresia are premature or have other defects that make it advisable to delay primary repair. They will need careful nursing care to prevent aspiration and total parenteral nutrition to allow growth until repair. We usually do the primary repair when the infant's weight is 2000 gm. **Mechanical ventilation** and nutritional management may be difficult in these infants because of the TEF. This problem has occasionally forced us to do the repair before the infant is 2000 gm. If the infant has cardiac disease requiring surgery, it is usually best to repair the fistula before cardiac surgery; if not, the postoperative ventilatory management will be very difficult.

IV. Diaphragmatic hernia (DH)

A. Respiratory distress associated with a scaphoid abdomen and development of bowel sounds in a hemithorax are pathognomonic of DH. The most common site is left hemithorax, with the defect in the diaphragm being posterior (foramen of Bochdalek in 70 percent of infants). DH also can occur on the right, with either an anterior or a posterior defect.

B. The **incidence** of DH is 1 in 4000. Fifty percent of these hernias are associated with other malformations, especially neural tube defects, cardiac defects, and intestinal malrotation. Some families have been described with recurrence of DH. DH has been associated with trisomy 18, 45 XO, and deletion of the small arm of the number 27 chromosome. It has been reported as part of Goldenhar, Beckwith-Wiedemann, Pierre Robin, Goltz-Goulen, and the rubella syndromes [31].

C. Symptoms. Infants with large DHs may present at birth with cyanosis, respiratory distress, a scaphoid abdomen, decreased or absent breath sounds on the side of the hernia, and heart sounds displaced to the side opposite the hernia. Small hernias, right-sided hernias, and substernal hernias of Morgagni may have a more subtle onset, manifested by feeding problems and mild respiratory distress.

D. **Diagnosis.** The diagnosis is confirmed by x-ray. If the child is in no distress, the x-ray should be done after all tubes and lines are in place. A radioopaque marker should be placed on one side of the chest to aid interpretation of the x-ray. The diagnosis is often made prenatally by ultrasonic studies, which may be precipitated by the occurrence of polyhydramnios [2]. Diagnosis earlier in gestation because of some fetal symptom (e.g., polyhydramnios) may be correlated with poorer prognosis. However, a prenatal diagnosis should lead to delivery in a center equipped to handle the problem to optimize chances for survival as much as possible. If delivery before term is likely, fetal lung maturity should be assessed by determinations of the lecithin-sphingomyelin (L/S) ratio and saturated phosphatidylcholine (SPC) in amniotic fluid. If these indices are immature, maternal therapy with beta-methasone should be given (see Chap. 13).

E. **Treatment.** A large sump nasogastric tube should be inserted immediately at the time of diagnosis. If assisted ventilation is required, it should be given by means of endotracheal tube. Bag and mask ventilation is contraindicated. All infants requiring transport should be intubated. Care must be taken with assisted ventilation to keep inspiratory pressures low to avoid damage or rupture of the contralateral lung. Umbilical venous and arterial lines should be placed as rapidly as possible. Pancuronium 0.1 mg/kg IV should be given. The pancuronium should be repeated if there is any muscular activity; it is often required every hour. Fentanyl 3 μg/kg IV is given as needed for sedation. It may need to be repeated hourly. **The fentanyl should be given only after paralysis with pancuronium.**

F. **Surgical repair** is through either the abdomen or the chest, with reduction of intestine into the abdominal cavity. DH is frequently associated with intestinal malrotation. Small babies may require abdominal mesh if the abdominal cavity is too small for the intestines.

G. Despite modern advances, mortality from diaphragmatic hernia remains very high, approaching 50 percent. Although repair of the defect itself is relatively straightforward, the underlying pulmonary hypoplasia and pulmonary hypertension are largely responsible for overall mortality (see Persistent Pulmonary Hypertension in Chap. 13).

Avoidance of hypoxia and acidosis will aid in minimizing pulmonary hypertension, and initial oxygen tension (PO_2) and carbon dioxide tension (PCO_2) after institution of therapy are predictive of prognosis. Newer therapies, including extracorporeal membrane oxygenation, offer the promise of improved survival [11] (see ECMO in Chap. 13).

V. **Other mechanical causes for respiratory difficulty**

A. **Congenital lobar emphysema (CLE)** may be due to a malformation, a cyst in the bronchus, or a mucous or meconium plug in the bronchus. These lesions cause air trapping, compression of surrounding structures, and respiratory distress. There may be a primary malformation of the lobe (**polyalveolar lobe**). Overdistension from mechanical ventilation may cause lobar emphysema. Extrinsic pressure on a bronchus also may cause obstruction. CLE usually affects the upper and middle lobes on the right and the upper lobe on the left. Diagnosis is by chest x-ray.

Elective intubation of the opposite bronchus may decompress the lobe if overinflation is thought to be the cause and if the infant can tolerate it. When the tube is withdrawn to the trachea after 8 to 12 hours, the lobar emphysema may not recur. Occasionally, selective suctioning of the bronchus on the side of the lesion may remove obstructing mucus or meconium and resolve the pulmonary problem. Treatment of acquired lobar emphysema (from inflammation of a bronchus) has been described with dexamethasone 0.5 mg/kg per day for 3 days [17]. If the child is symptomatic and conservative measures fail, the child should undergo an operation. Bronchoscopy should be performed to remove any obstructing material or rupture a bronchogenic cyst; if this procedure fails, the involved lobe should be resected.

B. **Cystic adenomatoid malformation of the lung** may be confused with a DH. Respiratory distress is related to the effect of the mass on the uninvolved lung. This malformation can cause shifting of the mediastinal structures [1].

C. **Vascular rings.** The symptomatology of vascular rings is related to the architecture of the ring. Both respiratory (stridor) and gastrointestinal symptoms (vomiting, difficulty swallowing) may occur, depending on the anatomy of the ring. Barium swallow is diagnostic.

D. **Laryngotracheal clefts.** The length of the cleft determines the symptoms. The diagnosis is made by instillation of contrast material into the esophagus and is confirmed by bronchoscopy. Very ill newborns should go for immediate bronchoscopy without contrast studies.

E. **Tracheal agenesis.** This rare lesion is suspected when a tube cannot be passed down the trachea and the infant is ventilated by way of bronchi coming off the esophagus. Diagnosis is by contrast material in the esophagus and by endoscopy.

F. **Choanal atresia.** Respiratory distress in the delivery room is associated with bilateral lesions. Infants are obligate nose breathers until approximately 4 months of age. An oral airway is satisfactory initial treatment. Definitive therapy includes burrowing a hole through the bony plate, which can be accomplished with a laser, if available.

G. **Robin anomaly (Pierre Robin syndrome)** consists of a hypoplastic mandible associated with a midline cleft palate. Airway obstruction often occurs secondary to the tongue occluding the airway. Forcibly pulling the tongue forward will relieve the obstruction. The neonate is best cared for in the prone position. These infants often improve after placement of nasopharyngeal or endotracheal tubes. If the infant can be helped for a few days, he or she will sometimes adapt, and aggressive procedures can be avoided. Button procedures have been utilized to avoid a tracheostomy (this procedure is rarely indicated). A gastrostomy may be necessary for feeding, but a specialized feeder (Breck) can be used to feed the child.

H. **Laryngeal web.** This is a web occluding the larynx. Perforation of the web by an endotracheal tube may be lifesaving.

VI. **Mechanical intestinal obstruction** [23]. The most critical lesion to rule out is malrotation with volvulus. All patients with suspected intestinal obstruction should have a nasogastric sump catheter placed prior to transport.

A. **Congenital mechanical obstruction**

1. **Intrinsic**
   - a. Atresia
   - b. Stenosis
   - c. Hypertrophic pyloric stenosis
   - d. Meconium ileus (may occur in two forms)
     - (1) Associated with cystic fibrosis
     - (2) A rare form (familial or nonfamilial) that is not associated with cystic fibrosis [7]
   - e. Cysts within the lumen of the bowel
   - f. Imperforate anus

2. **Extrinsic**
   - a. Malrotation with or without midgut volvulus
   - b. Volvulus without malrotation
   - c. Congenital peritoneal bands with or without malrotation
   - d. Incarcerated hernia (premature infants)
   - e. Annular pancreas
   - f. Duplications of the intestine
   - g. Aberrant vessels, usually the mesenteric artery or preduodenal portal vein

h. Hydrometrocolpos
i. Obstructing bands—persistent omphalomesenteric duct

B. **Acquired mechanical obstruction**
1. Intussusception
2. Peritoneal adhesions
a. After meconium peritonitis
b. Idiopathic
3. Mesenteric thrombosis
4. Meconium and mucous plugs
5. Necrotizing enterocolitis (acute and secondary to scarring and healing)
6. Formation of abnormal intestinal concretions not associated with cystic fibrosis

VII. **Functional intestinal obstruction** constitutes the major cause of intestinal obstruction seen in any neonatal unit.

A. **Immaturity of large bowel** [15]

B. **Defective innervation (Hirschsprung's disease)** [14]

C. **Paralytic ileus**
1. Induced by maternal drug ingestion
a. Narcotics
b. Hexamethonium bromide
c. Hypermagnesemia due to prenatal use of magnesium sulfate [26]
2. Sepsis
3. *Pseudomonas* enteritis

D. **Meconium plug syndrome**

E. **Endocrine disorders**
1. Hypothyroidism
2. Adrenal insufficiency

F. **Intrinsic defects in the bowel wall**

G. **Other disorders** (e.g., sepsis, CNS disease, necrotizing enterocolitis)

VIII. **Other disorders associated with intestinal obstruction**

A. **Duodenal atresia** in 70 percent of cases is associated with other malformations, including Down syndrome, cardiovascular anomalies, and such other gastrointestinal anomalies as annular pancreas, esophageal atresia, malrotation of the small intestine, small bowel atresias, and imperforate anus.
1. There may be a history of polyhydramnios.
2. Prenatal diagnosis by ultrasound is possible.
3. The concentration of bile acids in the amniotic fluid may be increased if the obstruction is below the bile ducts [6].
4. Vomiting of bile-stained material usually begins a few hours after birth.
5. Abdominal distension is limited to the upper abdomen.
6. The infant may pass meconium in the first 24 hours of life; then bowel movements cease.
7. Aspiration of the stomach returns greater than 30 ml of gastric contents prior to feeding.
8. A plain x-ray of the abdomen will show air in the stomach and upper part of the abdomen ("double bubble") with no air in the small or large bowel.
9. The neonate may be jaundiced in the presence of intestinal obstruction.
10. Preoperative management includes nasogastric suction. Contrast radiographs of the upper intestine are not mandatory preoperatively.

B. **Pyloric stenosis** typically presents with nonbilious vomiting after 2 to 3 weeks of age, but it has been seen in the first week of life. The infant will have a large stomach on x-ray examination; little or no gas is found below the duodenum. Often the pyloric mass cannot be felt in the newborn. The infant may have associated jaundice and hematemesis. An upper GI series is diagnostic. Real-time ultrasonography is used increasingly in diagnosis.

C. **Meconium ileus** is a frequent cause of meconium peritonitis [4]. In most other obstructions, flat and upright x-ray films will demonstrate fluid levels. This is not the case in meconium ileus if fetal perforation has not occurred. Instead, the distended bowel may be granular in appearance or may show tiny bubbles mixed with meconium.

1. No meconium will pass through the rectum, even after digital stimulation.
2. Rare cases (both familial and nonfamilial) have occurred that were not associated with cystic fibrosis but displayed the clinical picture and x-ray findings described in **C** [7].
3. A sweat test should be performed (see **X.E** for pitfalls).
4. Tests of stool trypsin activity are negative in cystic fibrosis, but they are also negative in all types of complete obstruction (see **X.F**).
5. Contrast enemas can be both diagnostic and therapeutic. Meglumine diatrizoate (Gastrografin) can be used in an adequately hydrated neonate. NA diatrizoate (Hypaque) also may be used. Both these contrast agents are hypertonic. The baby should be well hydrated, and fluids should be run at 2 to 3 times maintenance. The Gastrografin is often diluted 1:4 before use.
6. If the diagnosis is certain and the neonate stable, repeat enemas with a hyperosmolar, ionic contrast material (Gastrografin or Hypaque) may be used to relieve the impaction.
7. Nasogastric suction should be used to prevent further distension.
8. Distal atresias can accompany meconium ileus and require surgical therapy.
9. Surgical therapy is required if an enema with meglumine diatrizoate fails to relieve the obstruction.

D. Imperforate anus is often associated with other anomalies such as esophageal atresia with or without TEF and is a component of the VATER syndrome. Infants with imperforate anus may pass meconium if a rectovaginal or rectourinary fistula exists; in these infants, the diagnosis may be missed.

There are two types of imperforate anus: low and high. In females, 80 percent of cases of imperforate anus are of the low type, in males, 50 percent are low.

1. **Low imperforate anus.** The rectum has descended through the puborectalis sling and exists on the perineum as a fistula.
   a. Meconium may be passed into the vagina.
   b. Meconium may be visualized on the perineum. In males it may be found in the rugal folds of the scrotum.
   c. Perineal fistulas may be dilated to temporarily relieve intestinal obstruction and allow passage of meconium.
2. **High imperforate anus.** The rectum ends above the puborectalis sling. No perineal fistula is present. The fistula may enter the urinary tract or vagina.
   a. The presence of meconium particles in the urine is diagnostic of a rectovesical fistula. Vaginal examination with a nasal speculum or cystoscope may reveal a fistula.
   b. A cystogram may show a fistula and the level of rectal descent. Injection of dye into the most distal portion of the pouch may show the level of rectal descent. Use of the Wangensteen-Rice technique of taking AP and lateral films in the upside-down position at 48 hours of age may be misleading if the distal rectum is filled with meconium [10].
   c. Ultrasound is often helpful in defining the level of distal rectum.
   d. Temporary colostomy is necessary in all neonates with high imperforate anus with or without fistula.

E. Volvulus with or without malrotation of the bowel [10]

1. Malrotation may be associated with other gastrointestinal abnormalities such as diaphragmatic hernia, annular pancreas, and bowel atresias.
2. If this condition develops during fetal life, it may cause a large midabdominal calcific shadow seen on x-ray examination; this results from calcification of meconium in the segment of necrotic bowel.
3. After birth there is a sudden onset of bilious vomiting in an infant who

has had some normal stools. If the level of obstruction is high, there may not be much abdominal distension.

4. Signs of shock and sepsis are often present.
5. Plain x-rays will show a dilated small bowel.
6. If a malrotation is present, barium enema may show failure of barium to pass beyond the transverse colon or may show the cecum in an abnormal position.
7. Demonstration of absent or abnormal position of the ligament of Treitz confirms the diagnosis of malrotation. An upper GI series for localization of the ligament of Treitz is the most reliable diagnostic study for malrotation.
8. Malrotation as the cause of intestinal obstruction is a surgical emergency because intestinal viability is at stake.

F. **Annular pancreas** may be nonobstructing but associated with duodenal atresia or stenosis. It presents as a high intestinal obstruction.

G. **Hydrometrocolpos**

1. The hymen bulges.
2. Accumulated secretions in the uterus may cause intestinal obstruction by bowel compression.
3. Meconium peritonitis or hydronephrosis may occur.
4. Edema and cyanosis of the legs may be observed.
5. If hydrometrocolpos is not diagnosed at birth, the secretions will decrease, the bulging will disappear, and the diagnosis will be missed until puberty.

H. **Meconium and mucous plug syndrome.** This disorder is seen in premature babies, infants of diabetic mothers, and sick babies (see also **C**); it also may be caused by (1) functional immaturity of the bowel with a small left colon, as seen in infants of diabetic mothers, (2) meconium or mucous plug, or (3) Hirschsprung's disease (see **I**), which should always be considered when a newborn has difficulty passing stools. **Treatment** consists of glycerine suppository and ½ normal warm saline enemas (5 to 10 ml/kg) and digital stimulation. Normal stooling pattern should follow evacuation of a plug. Contrast enema with a hyperosmolar contrast material may be both diagnostic and therapeutic.

I. **Hirschsprung's disease** [4,10,14] should be suspected in any newborn who fails to pass meconium spontaneously by 24 to 48 hours after birth and who develops distension relieved by rectal stimulation. This is especially so if the infant is not premature or is not the infant of a diabetic mother or has the problems seen in **VII.** The diagnosis should be considered until future development shows sustained normal bowel function.

1. Parents taking home a newborn suspected of having Hirschsprung's disease must understand the importance of immediately reporting obstipation, diarrhea, poor feeding, distension, lethargy, or fever. A toxic megacolon may be fatal.
2. Barium enema frequently does not show the characteristic transition zone in the neonate. Suction rectal biopsy can be helpful if ganglion cells are found in a submucosal zone, thereby ruling out Hirschsprung's disease.
3. Histochemical tests show an increase in acetylcholine. Formal full-thickness rectal biopsy is the definitive method for diagnosis.
4. Obstipation can be relieved by gentle rectal irrigations with warm saline.
5. Neonates require colostomy when diagnosis is made. Definitive repair is postponed until the infant is between 8 and 12 months of age or weighs between 7.5 and 9.0 kg.

IX. **Other surgical problems**

A. **Appendicitis** is extremely rare in newborns. Its presentation may be that of pneumoperitoneum. The appendix usually perforates prior to the diagnosis; therefore, the baby may present with intestinal obstruction, sepsis, or even DIC related to the intraabdominal infection. Rule out Hirschsprung's disease.

B. Omphalocele [10]. **The sac may be intact or ruptured.** The diagnosis is often made by prenatal ultrasound. Cesarean section may prevent rupture of the sac.

1. **Intact sac. Emergency treatment** includes the following:
   - **a.** Nasogastric sump suction
   - **b.** Cover sac with ointment [povidone-iodine (Betadine)] or petrolatum-impregnated gauze.
   - **c.** Wrap sac on abdomen with Kling gauze so as to support intestinal viscera on the abdominal wall.
   - **d.** Thoroughly wrap the neonate to prevent heat loss.
   - **e.** Saline-soaked gauzes are unnecessary and may contribute to heat loss.
   - **f.** There should be no attempt made to reduce the sac because this may cause rupture of the sac, interfere with venous return from the sac, and cause respiratory distress.
   - **g.** A reliable intravenous line should be placed in an upper extremity.
   - **h.** Start broad-spectrum antibiotics (ampicillin and gentamicin).
   - **i.** Arrange a surgical consultation; definitive surgical therapy should be delayed until the baby is thoroughly resuscitated. Monitor temperature and pH. In the presence of other more serious abnormalities (respiratory or cardiac), definitive care can be postponed as long as the sac remains intact.
2. **Ruptured sac**
   - **a.** Nasogastric sump suction
   - **b.** Place a saline-soaked gauze over the exposed intestine, and then wrap the baby in a dry, sterile towel to prevent heat loss.
   - **c.** Monitor temperature and pH.
   - **d.** Start a reliable intravenous line.
   - **e.** Start broad-spectrum antibiotics (ampicillin and gentamicin).
   - **f.** Arrange emergency surgical treatment to cover intestine.
   - **g.** Bowel viability may be compromised with a small defect and an obstructed segment of eviscerated intestine. Prior to transfer, the defect must be enlarged in these circumstances by incising the abdomen cephalad or caudad to relieve the strangulated viscera.
3. Omphalocele may be associated with other anomalies such as chromosomal defects, malrotation of the colon, congenital heart disease, or extrophy of the cloaca. A careful search must be made for associated problems.

C. Gastroschisis [10], by definition, contains no sac and the intestine is eviscerated.

1. Nasogastric sump suction
2. Monitor temperature and pH.
3. Cover exposed intestine with saline-soaked gauze, and wrap the baby in a dry, sterile towel to prevent heat loss.
4. Start a reliable intravenous line.
5. Get immediate surgical evaluation.
6. Ten percent of cases of gastroschisis have intestinal atresia. Other anomalies should be searched for.

D. Renal disorders (see Chap. 26)

1. **Genitourinary abnormalities** should be suspected in babies with abdominal distension, ascites, flank masses, persistently distended bladder, poor nutrition, bacteriuria, or pyuria. All male infants, and especially those displaying symptoms, should be observed for voiding patterns. Normal voiding is forceful; voiding occurs by 24 hours in 92 percent of term babies and in 90 percent of premature babies (it occurs by 48 hours in 99 percent of normal babies).

a. Posterior urethral valves [18] may cause obstruction.
b. Spontaneous pneumomediastinum or pneumothorax in infants not being given ventilatory assistance has been associated with obstructive urinary tract disease.

2. **Renal vein thrombosis.** Hematuria with a flank mass suggests the diagnosis of renal vein thrombosis.
   a. Renal ultrasound will initially show a large kidney on the side of the thrombosis. In time the kidney will become small.
   b. A renal scan will show no function on the affected side.
   c. **Treatment** in the past was usually nephrectomy. Thrombectomy has been advocated by some in bilateral renal vein thrombosis [28]. Treatment in most centers now consists of supporting the patient medically and avoiding operative treatment. Heparin is not usually used by us in this disorder but has been advocated by some (see Chap. 26).
3. **Extrophy of the bladder** ranges from an epispadias to complete extrusion of the bladder on the abdominal wall. Currently, most centers are attempting bladder turn-in within the first 48 hours of life.
   a. **Management of extrophied bladder preoperatively**
      (1) Moist, fine-mesh gauze or vaseline-impregnated gauze to cover the exposed bladder
      (2) Intravenous pyelogram (IVP) is not required preoperatively, although renal ultrasound is useful.
      (3) Transport to facility for definitive care within 48 hours.
   b. **Management of extrophied bladder intraoperatively.** Surgical management of an extrophied bladder includes turn-in of the bladder to preserve bladder function. The symphysis pubis is approximated. The penis is lengthened. Iliac osteotomies are not necessary if repair is accomplished within 48 hours. No attempt is made to make the bladder continent at this procedure.
4. **Cloacal exstrophy** is a complex gastrointestinal and genitourinary anomaly that includes vesicointestinal fissure, omphalocele, extrophied bladder, hypoplastic colon, imperforate anus, absence of vagina in females, and microphallus in males.
   a. **Preoperative management**
      (1) **Genetic counseling.** It is surgically easier to rear the child as a female, regardless of genotype.
      (2) Nasogastric suction relieves partial intestinal obstruction. The baby stools through a vesicointestinal fissure that is often partially obstructed.
      (3) A series of complex operations is required in stages to achieve the most satisfactory results.
   b. **Surgical management**
      (1) Initial procedure includes division of vesicointestinal fissure and establishment of fecal and urinary stomas.
      (2) The bladder can be closed during the initial procedure if the baby is stable.
      (3) Subsequent procedures are designed to reduce the number of stomas.

E. **Tumors** [9,12]
   1. **Neuroblastoma** is the most common malignant neonatal tumor, making up about 50 percent of neonatal malignant tumors. It may be massive or minute, irregular, and stony hard. There are many sites of origin; the adrenal-retroperitoneal area is the most common. This tumor can, on rare occasions, cause diarrhea or hypertension by the release of tumor byproducts, especially catecholamines or vasointestinal peptides. Tests should be performed to determine levels of catecholamines and their metabolites. Calcifications can often be seen on plain radiographs. Ultrasound is the most useful test.

2. **Wilms' tumor** is the second most common malignant tumor in the newborn. It presents a smooth, flat mass and may be bilateral. One should palpate gently to avoid rupture. Ultrasound is the most useful diagnostic test.
3. **Teratomas.** These are the most common tumor in the neonatal period. They are most commonly found in the sacrococcygeal area. Some will be in the retroperitoneal area, and some will arise in the ovaries. They may arise anywhere. Approximately 10 percent contain malignant elements. Prenatal diagnosis is often made by ultrasound. After delivery, rectal examination, ultrasound, CT, MRI, as well as serum for alphafetoprotein and beta-HCG are used in evaluation. Calcifications are often seen in x-ray. Excessive heat loss, platelet trapping, and dystocia are often seen.
4. **Sarcoma botryoides.** This grapelike tumor arises from the edge of the vulva or vagina. It may be small and thus be confused with a normal posterior vaginal tag. IVP is an important test preoperatively, especially to avoid confusing the lesion with an obstructing ureterocele.
5. **Other tumors**
   a. Hemangiomas
   b. Lymphangiomas
   c. Hepatoblastomas
   d. Hepatoma
   e. Hamartoma
   f. Nephroma
   g. Hepatoblastoma

F. Abdominal masses

1. Renal masses (see **IX.D** and Chap. 26), polycystic kidneys, multicystic dysplastic kidney, hydronephrosis, renal vein thrombosis
2. Tumors (see **IX.E**)
3. Adrenal hemorrhage
4. Ovarian tumor or cysts
5. Pancreatic cyst
6. Choledochal cyst
7. Hydrometrocolpos
8. Mesenteric or omental cyst
9. Intestinal duplications

G. Inguinal hernia. Inguinal hernia is found in 5 percent of premature infants weighing under 1500 gm. It is more common in small for gestational age infants and male infants [20]. In females the ovary is often in the sac. In general, in premature infants, hernias that are easily reducible and are causing no problems are repaired shortly before discharge home. We have occasionally had well-instructed parents bring their babies home to be admitted later for repair. This method of management has had poor results on occasion but has not been fully evaluated. Infants with pulmonary disease, such as bronchopulmonary dysplasia, are often best repaired as a later time when their respiratory status has improved. In a term infant, repair should be scheduled when the diagnosis is made. If the hernia is incarcerated, sedation, steady firm pressure, and elevation of the feet usually reduce the hernia. If a hernia has been incarcerated, it should be repaired as soon as the edema is gone. Inguinal hernia repair is the most common operation performed on premature infants. It may be a difficult operation and should be performed by an experienced pediatric surgeon. We have the infant's primary nurse and neonatologist go to the operating room with the infant to assist in the details of intraoperative management (see **XII**). The postoperative care is usually done by this same team.

X. Tests

A. X-ray examinations. Flat and upright x-ray studies of the abdomen usually suffice. A cross-table lateral x-ray is done to see free air in the abdomen.

1. **Barium enema** may sometimes (but not always) be diagnostic in suspected cases of Hirschsprung's disease. It may reveal microcolon in com-

plete obstruction of the small intestine and may show a narrow segment in the sigmoid in the meconium plug syndrome due to functional immaturity.

2. **Barium swallow** with Gastrografin may be used to demonstrate H-type TEF without esophageal atresia.
3. Some infants with Hirschsprung's disease will have problems passing barium after a barium enema. Gentle rectal saline washes are helpful in removing trapped air and barium.
4. In patients with suspected malrotation, a combination of contrast studies may be necessary. A barium enema may show malposition of the cecum. In combination with air or contrast media, an upper GI series will determine the presence or absence of the normally placed ligament of Treitz. Neonates with intestinal obstruction presumed secondary to malrotation require urgent surgery to relieve possible volvulus of the midgut.

B. **Abdominal ultrasonography** is the preferred method of evaluating abdominal masses in the newborn. It is useful for defining the presence of masses, together with their size, shape, and consistency. This modality can be used to assess the presence of kidneys [30].

C. **Apt test** differentiates maternal from fetal blood. A small amount of bloody material is mixed with 5 ml of water and centrifuged. One part 0.25 normal sodium hydroxide is added to five parts of pink supernatant. The fluid remains pink in the presence of fetal blood but rapidly becomes brown if maternal blood is present.

D. **Amniotic fluid bile acid concentration** uses amniotic fluid. It is not a simple test, but it can be set up as a routine laboratory procedure. The method is described in ref. 6.

E. **Sweat test** for cystic fibrosis will not be accurate if less than 100 mg of sweat is collected. It may be necessary to repeat the test when the infant is 3 to 4 weeks old if inadequate sweat is collected. Prenatal testing for cystic fibrosis is available.

F. **Test for stool trypsin activity.** Unfortunately, a negative result is not diagnostic of cystic fibrosis, since in any type of complete bowel obstruction the stool will be without enzyme activity. The method involves making 1:5 and 1:10 dilutions of meconium or stool and placing them on the gelatin side of undeveloped x-ray films. They should be incubated at 37°C for 1 hour. If trypsin activity is present, the gelatin will be dissolved.

G. **Computerized tomography (CT)** is an excellent modality to evaluate abdominal masses as well as their relationship to other organs. Contrast enhancement can outline intestine, blood vessels, kidneys, ureter, and bladder.

H. **IVP** use should be restricted to evaluating genitourinary anatomy if other modalities (ultrasound and contrast CT scanning) are not available. The IVP dye is poorly concentrated in the newborn.

I. **Renal scan** can determine the function of the kidney. This is especially useful in assessing complex genitourinary anomalies and in evaluating the contribution of each kidney to renal function.

J. **MRI** is useful to better define the anatomy and location of masses.

XI. **Management**

A. **Bilious vomiting and abdominal distension**

1. Gastric suction with a sump catheter is mandatory if intestinal obstruction is suspected. All babies with presumed intestinal obstruction should be transported with a nasogastric suction catheter in place. A catheter-tip syringe (Becken-Dickinson catheter-tip 60-ml syringe no. 5664) should be available to continuously aspirate gastric contents. Failure to decompress the stomach could lead to gastric rupture, aspiration, or respiratory compromise secondary to diaphragmatic compression. This is especially important in infants who are to be transported by air ambulance, since loss of cabin pressure may be associated with rupture of an inadequately drained viscus.

2. **Shock, dehydration, and electrolyte imbalance** should be treated if present, or measures should be taken to prevent these problems. The baby should be resuscitated with the appropriate fluids and electrolytes (see Fluid and Electrolyte Management of the Newborn in Chap. 24 and ref. 13).
3. **Antibiotics** are used if there is suspicion of volvulus or any question about bowel integrity; broad coverage is indicated (ampicillin and gentamicin are preferable).
4. **Studies** that should be performed include the following:
   - **a.** Hematocrit
   - **b.** Electrolytes
   - **c.** Blood gases and pH
   - **d.** Clotting studies (e.g., prothrombin time, partial thromboplastin time, and platelet count)
   - **e.** Continuous monitoring of oxygen saturation, blood pressure, and urine output is often indicated.

B. Nonbilious vomiting with distension. Many babies with nonbilious vomiting and distension will respond to glycerin suppositories, half-strength saline enemas (5 ml/kg body weight), rectal stimulation with a soft rubber catheter, or a combination of these measures. It is important to rule out other nonfunctional causes of distention. Limited feedings, stimulation to the rectum, and care for the general condition of the baby will solve most of these problems. Plain x-ray studies are helpful. Barium enema should be used with caution because it may be difficult to evacuate the barium.

C. Vomiting without distension

1. If the baby's general condition is good, feedings of dextrose and water should be attempted. If these are tolerated, milk should be given again. If vomiting recurs, the baby should be given a trial of nonmilk formula. If this is successful, a trial of a milk formula should be undertaken in 2 weeks.
2. The mechanics of feeding the baby should be observed. Rapid feeding, difficult burping, and excessive volumes are all causes of nonbilious vomiting without distension.
3. The functional and mechanical causes must be ruled out.

D. Masses. The following steps may be taken for the diagnosis of the cause of abdominal masses:

1. X-ray examination of the chest and abdomen with the infant supine and upright
2. Abdominal ultrasonography
3. Contrast-enhanced CT
4. MRI
5. Determination of the level of catecholamines and their metabolites
6. Complete blood count and urinalysis
7. Angiography—venous and arterial
8. Surgical consultation

XII. Intraoperative management

A. Monitoring devices

1. Temperature probe
2. Electrocardiogram (ECG)
3. Arterial cannula to monitor blood gas and pressure. Transcutaneous PO_2 ($PtcO_2$) (see Blood Gas Monitoring in Chap. 13) is helpful but can be inaccurate when anesthetic agents that dilate skin vessels are used.
4. Pulse oximetry [8]

B. Well-functioning IV line. In babies with omphalocele or gastroschisis, the IV line needs to be in the upper extremity or neck.

C. Maintenance of body temperature

1. Warmed operating room
2. Humidified, warmed anesthetic agents

3. Cover exposed parts of the baby, especially the head.
4. Warmed prepping solution, blood, and fluids used intraperitoneally

D. Fluid replacement

1. Replace lost blood with warmed packed cells if the loss is greater than 15 percent of total blood volume.
2. Replace ascites loss milliliter per milliliter to maintain pressure.
3. The neonate loses approximately 5 ml of fluid per kilogram for each hour that the intestine is exposed. This should be replaced by Ringer's lactate or fresh-frozen plasma.

E. Anesthetic management of the neonate is reviewed in ref. 27.

F. Postoperative pain management is discussed in ref. 29.

G. Postoperatively, newborn fluid requirement is two-thirds standard maintenance for the first 24 to 48 hours, plus continuing losses which must be replaced.

References

1. Adzick, N. S. *J. Pediatr. Surg.* 20: 483, 1985.
2. Atwell, J. D. *J. Pediatr. Surg.* 8: 825, 1974.
3. Benacerraf, B. R., and Adzick, N. X. *Am. J. Obstet. Gynecol.* 156: 573, 1987.
4. Chawls, W. J. *J. Perinatol.* 8: 62, 1988.
5. Cohen, M. D. *Pediatrics* 59: 587, 1982.
6. Deleze, G. *Pediatrics* 59: 647, 1977.
7. Dolan, T. F., Jr. *J. Pediatr. Surg.* 9: 821, 1974.
8. Dziedzic, K. *J. Perinatol.* 16: 177, 1989.
9. Gale, G. B. *Pediatrics* 70: 409, 1982.
10. Guzzetta, P. C. Surgery of the Neonate. In G. B. Avery (Ed.), *Neonatology,* Philadelphia: Lippincott, 1987.
11. Hendren, W. H., and Lillehei, C. W. *N. Engl. J. Med.* 319: 86, 1988.
12. Hartman, G. E., and Shocat, S. J. *Clin Perinatol* 16: 123, 1989.
13. John, E. M. *Clin. Perinatol.* 16: 219, 1989.
14. Kleinhause, S., et al. *J. Pediatr. Surg.* 14: 588, 1979.
15. Lequesne, G. W. *Radiol. Clin. North Am.* 13: 331, 1975.
16. Mequid, M. *Surg. Gynecol. Obstet.* 139: 541, 1974.
17. Mohsini, K. *J. Pediatr.* 111: 901, 1987.
18. Mooney, J. K. *J. Urol.* 113: 272, 1975.
19. Neuhauser, E. B. D. *Am. J. Radiol.* 51: 421, 1944.
20. Plevey, K. J. *Pediatrics* 77: 246, 1986.
21. *Problems of Neonatal Surgery: Forty-Ninth Ross Conference.* Columbus, Ohio: Ross Laboratories, 1963.
22. Ringer, S. A., and Stark, A. S. *Clin. Perinatol* 16: 23, 1989.
23. Rowe, M. I., Foreword. *Clin. Perinatol.* 5: 1, 1978.
24. Schaffer, A. J., and Avery, M. E. *Diseases of the Newborn,* 3d Ed. Philadelphia: Saunders, 1971.
25. Shaw, A. *Surgery* 58: 561, 1985.
26. Sokal, M. M. *N. Engl. J. Med.* 286: 823, 1972.
27. Sukhani, R. *Clin. Perinatol.* 16: 43, 1989.
28. Thompson, I. M. *J. Urol.* 113: 396, 1975.
29. Truog, R. *Clin. Perinatol.* 16: 61, 1983.
30. Wilson, D. A. *Am. J. Dis. Child.* 136: 147, 1982.
31. Wolff, G. *Hum. Genet.* 54: 1, 1980.

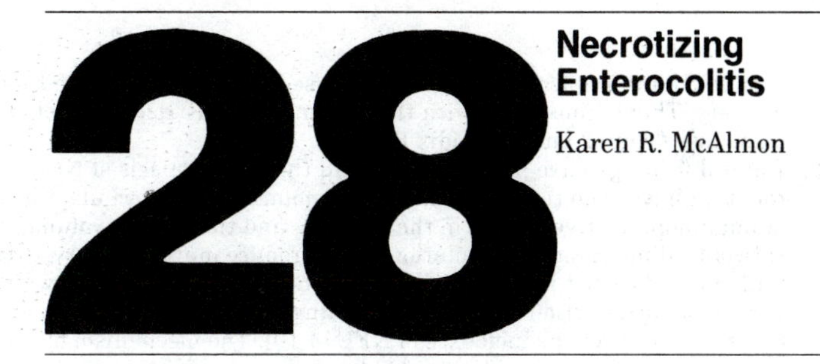

Necrotizing Enterocolitis

Karen R. McAlmon

I. **Background. Necrotizing enterocolitis (NEC)** is a syndrome of acute intestinal necrosis. The etiology of NEC is unknown, and our understanding of the pathophysiology is largely speculative. Its pathogenesis, however, is probably complex and multifactorial. Current clinical practice is directed toward prompt, early diagnosis and rapid institution of proper intensive care management [4,5]. Kliegman and Walsh [10] have published an excellent review of necrotizing enterocolitis. Walsh also has published a recent review [21].

A. **Epidemiology.** NEC is the most common serious surgical disorder among infants in a neonatal intensive care unit (NICU) and is a significant cause of neonatal morbidity and mortality.

1. The **incidence** of NEC varies from center to center and from year to year within centers. There are endemic and epidemic occurrences. In most centers, NEC occurs in 2 to 5 percent of all NICU admissions. If infants who die early are excluded and only infants who have been fed included, the incidence is approximately 15 percent [10].
2. Sex, race, geography, climate, and season all appear to play no determining role in the incidence or course of NEC [4].
3. **Prematurity** is the single greatest risk factor. The mean gestational age of infants with NEC is 30 to 32 weeks, and the infants are generally appropriate for gestational age. Between 7 and 10 percent of infants are full-term. The mean age at onset is 12 days, and the mode is 3 days. More than 98 percent of infants have been fed prior to the onset of this disease [12,13,20].
4. The overall **mortality** is 30 to 40 percent regardless of surgical or medical intervention. The mortality for infants weighing 1.0 kg or less is greater than 80 percent.
5. Case-controlled epidemiologic studies have revealed that almost all previously described risk factors for NEC, including maternal disorders (e.g., toxemia), the infant's course [e.g., asphyxia, patent ductus arteriosus (PDA)], and the type of management (e.g., umbilical artery catheterization), simply describe a population of high-risk neonates. No maternal or neonatal factors other than prematurity are known to increase the risk of NEC [12,20].
6. Birth-weight-specific weekly attack rates reveal that the time period for risk of NEC declines as gestational age increases. Thus the postnatal age at onset of NEC is inversely proportional to the gestational age at birth. These data may indicate that NEC represents an insult to the gastrointestinal tract that depends on maturation of specific enteric functions [22].

B. **Pathogenesis**

1. The **causes** of NEC are not well defined. A leading hypothesis is that NEC results from the deleterious effects of intestinal microflora on an injured or ischemic enteric mucosa in the presence of a luminal substrate. The mucosal injury may result from several different processes, including asphyxia and ischemia secondary to shunting of blood flow away from the gut. The specificity of this process is unknown [4]. NEC has been seen in

some term infants whose mothers have used cocaine around the time of delivery. This is consistent with the known vasoconstrictive effect of cocaine (see Chap. 2 and Appendix B).

2. Enteral feedings have been implicated in the pathogenesis of NEC. Factors that have been considered include osmolality of the formula, the lack of immunoprotective factors in the formula, and the timing, volume, and rate of feeding. Hypertonic solutions may produce mucosal injury. Breast milk alone does not protect against NEC. Some studies have shown that very slow introduction of feedings avoiding large day-to-day volume increases may lower the incidence of NEC [4,10]. The mechanism by which excessive volumes predispose to the development of NEC is not known.
3. The microbiologic flora involved in NEC are not unique but represent the predominant bowel organisms present in the infant at the time of disease onset. Bacterial and viral agents have been included in the microbial picture that is sometimes associated with NEC. As yet none has been proven to be causal.
4. **Pathologic examination** of tissue from surgery or autopsy cases indicates that the terminal ileum and ascending colon are the most frequently involved areas. This finding has implications for long-term sequelae (see **IV**). The pathologic lesions of coagulative necrosis without exaggerated cellular infiltrate are identical to those seen in older children and adults with acute intestinal necrosis [3].

II. Diagnosis. Early diagnosis of NEC is the most important factor in determining outcome. This is accomplished by careful clinical observation for nonspecific signs in infants who are at risk to develop NEC.

A. Clinical characteristics. There is a broad spectrum of disease manifestations. The clinical features of NEC can be divided into systemic and abdominal signs. Most infants have a combination of findings.

1. **Systemic signs**—respiratory distress, apnea or bradycardia (or both), lethargy, temperature instability, irritability, poor feeding, hypotension (shock), decreased peripheral perfusion, oliguria, bleeding diathesis [4,13,17]
2. **Abdominal (enteric) signs**—abdominal distension, abdominal tenderness, gastric aspirates (feeding residuals), vomiting (bilious or hematemesis or both), ileus (decreased or absent bowel sounds), abdominal wall erythema or induration, persistent localized abdominal mass, ascites, and bloody stools [4,13,17]
3. The **course** of the disease varies among infants. Most frequently, it will appear (1) as a fulminant, rapidly progressive presentation of signs consistent with intestinal necrosis and sepsis or (2) as a slow, paroxysmal presentation of abdominal distension, ileus, and possible infection. The latter course will vary with the rapidity of therapeutic intervention and require consistent monitoring and anticipatory evaluation [4] (see **III**).

B. Differential diagnosis

1. **Pneumonia and sepsis** are common in this population and frequently are associated with an abdominal ileus. The abdominal distension and tenderness characteristic of NEC will be absent, however.
2. Surgical abdominal catastrophes occurring in this population include malrotation with obstruction (complete or intermittent), malrotation with midgut volvulus, intussusception, ulcer, gastric perforation, and mesenteric vessel thrombosis (see Chap. 27). The clinical presentation of these disorders may overlap with that of NEC. Occasionally, the diagnosis is made only at the time of exploratory laparotomy.
3. **Infectious enterocolitis** is rare in this population but must be considered if diarrhea is present. *Campylobacter* species have been associated with bloody diarrhea in the newborn. These children lack any other systemic or enteric signs of NEC.
4. Severe forms of inherited metabolic disease (e.g., galactosemia with *Esch-*

erichia coli sepsis) may lead to profound acidosis, shock, and vomiting and may initially overlap with some signs of NEC.

5. **Feeding intolerance** is a common but ill-defined problem in premature infants. Despite adequate gastrointestinal function *in utero,* some premature infants will have periods of gastric residuals and abdominal distension associated with advancing feedings. Differentiation of this problem from NEC is difficult at times. Cautious evaluation by withholding enteral feedings and administering intravenous fluids and antibiotics for 72 hours may be indicated until this benign disorder can be distinguished from NEC.

C. **Laboratory features.** No laboratory tests are specific for NEC; nevertheless, some tests are valuable in confirming diagnostic impressions.

1. **Roentgenograms.** The abdominal roentgenogram will often reveal an abnormal gas pattern consistent with ileus. Both anteroposterior (AP) and cross-table lateral or left lateral decubitus views should be included. These films may reveal bowel wall edema, a fixed-position loop on serial studies, appearance of a mass, pneumatosis cystoides intestinalis, portal or hepatic venous air, pneumobilia, or pneumoperitoneum [5,6].
2. **Blood studies.** Thrombocytopenia, persistent metabolic acidosis, and severe refractory hyponatremia are the most common triad and help to confirm the diagnosis.
3. **Analysis** of stool for the presence of blood and carbohydrate has been used to detect infants with NEC based on changes in intestinal integrity. Although grossly bloody stools may be an indication of NEC, occult hematochezia does not correlate well with NEC [19]. Carbohydate malabsorption, as reflected in a positive stool Clinitest, can be a frequent and early indicator of NEC within the setting of signs noted in **A.**
4. **New diagnostic methods** including (1) upper GI series with metrizamide contrast studies may detect gaseous blebs before they are detectable on plain films [8] and (2) ultrasound to detect microbubbles of gas within the portal vein that are below the detection of plain films may aid in the diagnosis of NEC. However, they are not yet routine and are not currently used in our NICUs. The hydrogen breath test, which was initially thought to be promising, is too nonspecific to be beneficial.

D. **Additional considerations in the diagnosis**

1. Since early features are often nonspecific, a high index of suspicion is the most reliable approach to early diagnosis. The entire picture of history, physical examination, and laboratory features must be considered in the context of the particular infant's course. Isolated signs or laboratory values often indicate the need for a careful differential diagnosis, despite the obvious concern with NEC [4,7].
2. **Diarrhea** is an uncommon presentation of NEC in the absence of bloody stools. The presence of this sign should point away from NEC.
3. **Roentgenographic findings** can often be subtle and confusing. For example, perforation of an abdominal viscus will not always cause pneumoperitoneum, and conversely, pneumoperitoneum does not necessarily indicate abdominal perforation from NEC. Careful serial review of the roentgenograms with a pediatric radiologist is indicated to assist in interpretation and to plan for further appropriate studies.

III. Management

A. **Immediate medical management.** Treatment should begin promptly when signs suggestive of NEC are present. Therapy is based on the institution of intensive care measures and the anticipation of potential problems [4,7].

1. **Respiratory.** Rapid assessment of ventilatory status (physical examination, arterial blood gases) should be made, and supplemental oxygen and mechanical ventilatory support should be provided as needed.
2. **Cardiovascular.** Rapid assessment of circulatory status (physical examination, blood pressure) should be made, and circulatory support should

be provided as needed. We use fresh-frozen plasma (dose 10 ml/kg), since this is also a good source of clotting factors (see **6**). Pharmacologic support may be necessary; in this case, we use low doses of dopamine (3 to 5 μg/kg per minute) to optimize the effect on splanchnic and renal blood flow. Impending circulatory collapse will often be reflected by poor perfusion and oxygenation, even though arterial blood pressure may be maintained. Intraarterial blood pressure monitoring will often be necessary, but the proximity of the umbilical arteries to the mesenteric circulation precludes the use of these vessels. In fact, any umbilical artery catheter should be promptly removed. We use radial and tibial artery catheters placed percutaneously or by cutdown. Further monitoring of central venous pressure (CVP) may become necessary if additional pharmacologic support of the circulation or failing myocardium is needed. We avoid using central venous catheters until blood cultures are negative (see **4**); if necessary, either a jugular venous or subclavian catheter can be placed to measure CVP.

3. **Metabolic.** Severe metabolic acidosis will generally be responsive to volume expansion but may require treatment with sodium bicarbonate (dose 2 mEq/kg q6–8h). The blood pH should be carefully followed; in addition, serum electrolytes and liver function tests should be measured. Blood glucose level should be followed closely.
4. **Nutrition.** All gastrointestinal feedings should be discontinued, and the bowel should be decompressed by suctioning through a nasogastric tube. Parenteral nutrition should be initiated through a peripheral vein as soon as possible, with the aim of providing 90 to 110 cal/kg per day once both amino acid solutions and Intralipid are tolerated. Central venous hyperalimentation may be necessary to provide adequate calories in the very low birth weight infant in whom venous access can be a problem. We wait to place a central catheter for this purpose until the blood cultures are negative for 3 days, during which time adaptation to peripheral hyperalimentation can take place.
5. **Infectious disease.** Blood, urine, stool, and cerebrospinal fluid (CSF) should be obtained, examined carefully for indications of infection, and sent for culture and sensitivity. We routinely begin broad-spectrum antibiotics as soon as possible, utilizing a penicillin (usually ampicillin) and an aminoglycoside to cover most enteric flora. Stool should be tested for aminoglycoside-resistant organisms. If abdominal perforation has occurred, coverage of anaerobic bacteria should be added. We use clindamycin for this purpose. In a randomized study, routine use of clindamycin in infants with pneumotosis, intraportal gas, or both did not reduce the frequency of intestinal gangrene or perforation [6]. Antibiotic therapy can be adjusted based on culture results, but only 40 percent of blood cultures will be positive, necessitating continued broad coverage in most cases. Treatment is maintained for 7 to 14 days depending on the severity at the initial presentation [10]. There is no evidence to suggest that enteral antibiotics play a role in the treatment of NEC [8].
6. **Hematologic.** Analysis of the complete blood count and differential, with examination of the blood smear, is always indicated. We use platelet transfusions to correct severe thrombocytopenia and packed red blood cells to maintain the hematocrit above 40 percent. Neutropenia may be severe, and in extreme cases we treat this with whole blood exchange transfusion, although some advocate use of white blood cell (WBC) transfusion (see Chaps. 12 and 20). The prothrombin time, partial thromboplastin time, and platelet count should be evaluated for evidence of disseminated intravascular coagulation. Fresh-frozen plasma is used to treat coagulation problems. In addition, we administer vitamin K to these infants (see Chap. 30), since they are not fed enterally for a prolonged period.

7. **Renal.** Oliguria will often accompany the initial hypotension and hypoperfusion of NEC; careful evaluation of urine output is essential. In addition, serum blood urea nitrogen (BUN) and creatinine levels should be followed as well as serum and urine electrolytes and plasma osmolality. Daily urinalysis will help to monitor for early evidence of glomerulotubular injury. Impending renal failure from acute tubular necrosis, coagulative necrosis, or vascular accident must be anticipated, and fluid therapy must be adjusted accordingly.
8. **Neurologic.** Evaluation of the infant will be difficult given the degree of illness, but one must be alert to the problems of associated meningitis and intraventricular hemorrhage. Seizures may occur secondary to either of these problems or from the metabolic perturbations associated with NEC. These complications must be anticipated and promptly recognized and treated.
9. **Gastrointestinal.** Physical examination and serial roentgenograms are used to assess ongoing gastrointestinal damage. Unless either perforation occurs or full-thickness necrosis precipitates severe peritonitis, the management of this system will be medical. The evaluation for surgical intervention, however, is an important and complex management issue (see **B**).
10. **Family support.** Any family of an infant in the NICU may be overwhelmed by the crisis. Infants with NEC present a particular challenge, because the disease is often a sudden deterioration for "no apparent reason." Furthermore, the impending possibility of surgical intervention and the high mortality and uncertain prognosis make this situation most difficult for parents. Careful anticipatory sharing of information must be utilized by the staff to establish a trusting alliance with the family.

B. Surgical intervention [7,15,17]

1. **Prompt consultation** should be obtained with a pediatric surgeon. This will allow the surgeon to become familiar with the case prior to intervention and will provide the staff with an additional evaluation by another skilled individual.
2. **Gastrointestinal perforation** is generally agreed on as an indication for intervention. Perforation occurs in 20 to 30 percent of patients and is usually seen 12 to 48 hours after onset of NEC, although it can occur later. In some cases, the absence of pneumoperitoneum on the abdominal radiograph can delay the diagnosis [16]. In these cases, paracentesis may aid in establishing the diagnosis. In general, an infant with increasing abdominal distension, an abdominal mass, a worsening clinical picture despite medical management, or a persistent fixed loop on serial roentgenographic studies may have a perforation and may require operative intervention.
3. **Full-thickness necrosis of the gastrointestinal tract** may require surgical intervention, although, in the absence of perforation, this condition is difficult to document. In most cases, the infant with bowel necrosis will have signs of peritonitis, such as ascites, abdominal mass, abdominal wall erythema, or induration. Improvement may not occur until the necrotic bowel is surgically removed. Paracentesis may help to identify these patients before perforation occurs [16].
4. At surgery, peritoneal fluid can be examined for signs of infection, and bowel can be obtained to examine for pathologic confirmation. Cultures of peritoneal fluid should be sent. All sites of diseased bowel should be noted, regardless of whether removal is indicated or not. If there is extensive involvement, a "second look" operation should be done within 48 to 72 hours to determine if any areas that appeared necrotic are actually viable. The length and areas of removed bowel should be recorded. If large areas are resected, the length and position of the remaining bowel should be noted, since this will affect long-term outcome.

C. **Long-term management** [14,17]. Once the infant has been stabilized and effectively treated, feedings can be reintroduced. We generally begin this process after 2 weeks of treatment by stopping nasogastric decompression. If infants can tolerate their own secretions, feedings are begun very slowly while parenteral alimentation is gradually tapered. No data are available on the best method or type of feeding. We sometimes use an elemental lactose-free formula. The occurrence of strictures may complicate feeding plans. The incidence of recurrent NEC is 4 percent and does not appear to be related to any type of management. Recurrent disease should be treated as before and will generally respond as during the first episode. If surgical intervention was required and an ileostomy-colostomy created, some feel that reanastamosis should optimally occur before discharge from the hospital.

IV. **Prognosis** [1,10,17,18]. Few detailed and accurate studies are available on prognosis. In uncomplicated cases of NEC, long-term prognosis is comparable with that of their cohort of other low-birth-weight infants. NEC requiring surgical intervention may have more serious sequelae, including increased morbidity and mortality secondary to infection, respiratory failure, parenteral nutrition–associated hepatic disease, rickets, and significant developmental delay.

A. **Sequelae** from NEC can be directly related to the disease process or to the long-term NICU management often necessary to treat the disease. Gastrointestinal sequelae include strictures, which occur in up to 20 percent of patients and are most common in the large bowel; enteric fistulas; short bowel syndrome following surgical treatment; malabsorption and chronic diarrhea; dumping syndromes related to loss of terminal ileum and ileocecal valve; fluid and electrolyte losses with rapid dehydration, which may occur via ileostomy; and hepatitis or cholestasis related to long-term hyperalimentation. Metabolic sequelae include failure to thrive, metabolic bone disease, and problems related to CNS function in the very low birth weight infant.

B. **Prevention of NEC is the ultimate goal.** Unfortunately, this can best be accomplished only by preventing premature birth. If prematurity cannot be avoided, glucocorticoids may be of potential benefit. Premature infants whose mothers received prenatal glucocorticoid therapy to accelerate lung maturation had a significantly decreased incidence of NEC compared with the control group [2]. Neither prophylaxis with enteral antibiotics nor feeding of breast milk alone will prevent NEC. Very slow introduction of feedings may be a useful approach [3], but more data are required, including the possible harmful effects of this nutritional approach.

References

1. Abassi, S., et al. *J. Pediatr.* 104: 550, 1984.
2. Bauer, C. R., et al. *Pediatrics* 73: 682, 1984.
3. Bounous, G. *Gastroenterology* 82: 1457, 1982.
4. Brown, E. G., et al. *Pediatr. Clin. North Am.* 29: 1149, 1982.
5. Egan, E. A. Neonatal Necrotizing Enterocolitis. In E. Lebenthal (Ed.), *Textbook of Gastroenterology and Nutrition in Infancy.* New York: Raven Press, 1981. P. 979.
6. Faix, R. G., et al. *J. Pediatr.* 112: 271, 1988.
7. Gregory, J. R., et al. *Am. J. Surg.* 141: 562, 1981.
8. Hansen, T. N., et al. *J. Pediatr.* 97: 836, 1980.
9. Keller, M. S., et al. *Am. J. Dis. Child.* 139: 713, 1985.
10. Kliegman, R. M., et al. *Curr. Probl. Pediatr.* 17: 213, 1987.
11. Kliegman, R. M., et al. *N. Engl. J. Med.* 310: 1093, 1984.
12. Kliegman, R. M., et al. *J. Pediatr.* 100: 440, 1982.
13. Kliegman, R. M. *Am. J. Dis. Child.* 135: 603, 1981.
14. Kliegman, R. M. *Am. J. Dis. Child.* 135: 608, 1981.
15. O'Neill, J. A. *Surg. Clin. North Am.* 61: 1013, 1981.

16. Rickets, R. R. *Am. Surg.* 52: 61, 1986.
17. Schullinger, J. N., et al. *Am. J. Dis. Child.* 135: 612, 1981.
18. Stevenson, D. K., et al. *Pediatrics* 66: 925, 1980.
19. Stiles, A. D. *Pediatr. Res.* 18: 1525, 1984.
20. Stoll, B. J., et al. *J. Pediatr.* 96: 447, 1980.
21. Walsh, M. C. *Pediatr. Rev.* 9: 219, 1988.
22. Wilson, R., et al. *Am. J. Dis. Child.* 136: 814, 1982.

29 Dermatology

John P. Hubbell, Jr.

I. Transient cutaneous lesions

A. Milia. Many infants, especially those born at term, have multiple pearly white or pale yellow papules or cysts. These cysts are known as **milia** and are scattered about on the face, especially the nose, chin, and forehead. Histologically milia are epidermal cysts (up to 1 mm in diameter) developing in connection with the pilosebaceous follicle. They will exfoliate and disappear within the first few weeks of life. No treatment is necessary.

B. Sebaceous gland hyperplasia is similar to milia, but the lesions are smaller, more numerous, and usually confined to the nose, upper lip, and chin. These lesions are present mainly in full-term babies and, like milia, they disappear within a few weeks after birth.

C. Mongolian spots are pigmented lesions most often found at birth. They are present in more than 90 percent of Indian, Oriental, and black infants. Mongolian spots are frequently found in infants of Mediterranean and Latin backgrounds and are occasionally seen in those of Northern European background. The area most commonly involved is the lumbosacral region, but the upper back, shoulders, arms, buttocks, legs, and face are occasionally included. The lesions may be small or large, grayish blue or bluish black in color, and irregularly round in shape; they are never elevated or palpable. Mongolian spots occur as the result of an infiltration of melanocytes deep in the dermis. Although they frequently fade as the child gets older, this is probably the result of decreasing transparency of the overlying skin rather than a true disappearance of the lesion. They present no known danger.

D. Macular hemangiomas. These lesions are very common, occurring in up to 50 percent of normal newborn infants. They most commonly occur on the bridge of the nose, the forehead, the upper eyelids, and the nape of the neck. Macular hemangiomas are flat, pale pink in color, and irregular in shape. They also tend to disappear with age, although lesions at the base of the neck persist longer than others. Again, they are of no consequence except for the occasional cosmetic worry.

E. Erythema toxicum. The rash of erythema toxicum, which usually appears on the first or second day of life, is a scattering of macules, papules, and even some vesicles, usually occurring on the trunk but frequently on the extremities and face as well. The condition is not serious and is self-limited, but it may cause alarm when papules and vesicles are numerous, especially when the lesions are considered to be pustular.

1. If the vesicles are opened and the contents smeared, stained with Wright's stain, and examined microscopically, they are found to contain almost exclusively eosinophils. Cultures are sterile except for an occasional contaminant such as *Staphylococcus epidermidis*.
2. The **cause** of erythema toxicum is not really known, although some allergic or immediate hypersensitivity reaction is suspected.
3. Although erythema toxicum may occur in 50 to 70 percent of full-term babies in a nursery, this figure decreases as the gestational age decreases. Infants less than 1500 gm in weight or less than 30 weeks' gestational

age rarely exhibit erythema toxicum. No treatment is known to be effective; however, none is needed.

F. **Transient neonatal pustular melanosis** is a benign, self-limited cutaneous disorder of newborn infants recently described by a group from Israel [4]. The condition occurred in about 10 infants in a series of over 4000 examined. In all cases, the lesions were present at birth and consisted of small papules, crusted vesicles, and hyperpigmented spots. The "scale detachment sign" is considered diagnostic. Cultures of pustules and crusts were all negative, and lesions healed without scarring.

G. **Trauma** (see Chap. 22). Various forms of contusions, abrasions, and ecchymoses occur as the result of forces associated with delivery.

1. **Caput succedaneum** is a collection of edema and frequently small or large hemorrhages in the skin of the scalp over the presenting part. Similar areas may appear over buttocks, scrotum, or vulva in breech presentations. The edema usually disappears in a day or two, but the ecchymosis may take longer; if the ecchymosis is large, it may contribute to hyperbilirubinemia.
2. **Forceps application and extraction,** especially if forceps rotation is required, may lead to varying degrees of trauma to the skin and subcutaneous tissues of the face, neck, and scalp. **Abrasions and ecchymoses** from forceps are quite common and of no serious consequence, except as a possible path of entry for infection. Occasional deeper lacerations may need surgical repair, however, and injury to the facial nerve may result.
3. **Subcutaneous fat necrosis.** Small, firm, movable masses can occur over bony prominences of mandible or zygoma as the result of pressure, usually from forceps. These lumps are often not discovered for several days, and then may persist for weeks. They eventually disappear without treatment.
4. Areas of **pressure necrosis** of the scalp (similar to subcutaneous fat necrosis) can occur over the parietal bosses. These masses occasionally break down and drain, and they may become secondarily infected, thereby necessitating antibiotic treatment.
5. **Sucking blisters** may be present at birth, usually on a hand or wrist (sometimes both). They may be filled with clear fluid, or they may be open and in the process of healing. Some may even be so old as to be more like calluses than blisters. Observations of fetuses in utero by ultrasonography show that they do suck frequently, and may suck on any part that comes easily to the mouth. Treatment is not necessary.
6. **Bruising and abrasions** of the legs and feet caused by difficult breech extraction are now largely lesions of the past. Although these usually clear with remarkable rapidity, the resorption of blood breakdown products from the tissues may lead to an elevation of serum bilirubin.
7. **Ecchymosis** of the back, buttocks, and feet has resulted from overvigorous physical stimulation as part of resuscitation; fortunately, this is seldom seen in the modern nursery.
8. **Small puncture wounds** (sometimes multiple) of the scalp are new lesions that result from advances in medical care. The puncture wounds are caused by the placement of an internal monitoring electrode or by the sampling of fetal blood to detect fetal distress. These lesions are usually insignificant, but occasionally they may lead to superficial infection. Similar wounds, or scars of wounds, may also result from amniocentesis needles.

II. Developmental abnormalities of skin

A. **Skin dimples and sinuses** may occur on any part of the body, but they are most common over bony prominences such as the scapula, knee joint, and hip. They may be simple depressions in the skin (of no pathologic significance) or actual sinus tracts connecting to deeper structures.

1. In the sacral area, the **pilonidal dimple or sinus** may be connected to the lower end of the central nervous system (CNS); in some cases, this may lead to serious infection. Occasionally, a dimple, sometimes accompanied by a nevus or hemangioma, may signify an underlying spinal disorder such as diastematomyelia.
2. **Dermal sinuses or cysts** along the cheek or jaw line, or extending into the neck, may represent remnants of the branchial cleft structures of the early embryo.
   a. The more common dermal sinus is the **preauricular sinus,** which is a leftover from the first branchial cleft. It appears in the most anterior upper portion of the tragus of the external ear. Preauricular sinuses may be unilateral or bilateral; they usually require no treatment unless secondary infection develops, in which case surgical excision is recommended. In the author's experience, preauricular sinuses rarely cause problems in the newborn period.
   b. **Sinuses or cysts in the sides of the neck** usually arise from the second branchial cleft. They may or may not open into the mouth or pharynx.
   c. **Cysts or sinuses in the anterior midline of the neck** arise from the thyroglossal duct. Many of these are not detected in the newborn period, and they may never cause problems. Surgical removal is the usual solution if the size, appearance, or location of the lesion poses a problem.

B. **Cutaneous appendages**
1. **Auricular tags**—bits of skin and subcutaneous tissue attached to the external ear, or just anterior to it—are common. They are quite variable in size, have very small to quite broad attachments, and may be single or multiple. Most can be removed simply by ligating the base.
2. Less frequently, such appendages occur on other areas of the body, such as the chest or the extremities.
   a. In some cases, **supernumerary digits** are little more than skin tags; however, they may be fully developed digits (i.e., with bone, cartilage, and nail). (See Chap. 23.)
   b. **Supernumerary nipples** are another example of duplication of skin appendages. These may be unilateral or bilateral; they appear below the original nipple, on the anterior chest wall, in the same vertical line. No treatment is needed for this anomaly, unless cosmetic reasons dictate removal in a female after puberty.
3. **Redundant skin** also may be considered an anomaly. This usually occurs as loose folds of excess skin in the posterior neck. It is a common finding in some chromosomal disorders, such as trisomy 18, Down syndrome, trisomy 13, and especially Turner syndrome.

C. **Hemihypertrophy** is a condition in which one side of the body is larger than the other. The asymmetry is often apparent at birth, but it becomes more and more obvious as growth takes place.
1. The **skin** is only one of many systems involved, and anomalous development of the extremity on the larger side is frequent. The skin on the hypertrophied side usually feels thicker and may sweat more. The hypertrophied side is also more prone to the development of anomalies such as nail defects, hypertrichosis, pigmentation abnormalities, nevi, and vascular anomalies.
2. **Asymmetry of the face** may be more striking than that of the rest of the body, especially with involvement of the eye and the tongue. Treatment is for both cosmetic and symptomatic reasons.
3. **Mental retardation,** occasionally with seizures, occurs in some of these patients. Children with hemihypertrophy are also more prone to the development of embryonal tumors of the kidney, adrenal, and liver.

D. **Aplasia cutis (congenital absence of skin)** is seen most frequently in the midline of the posterior scalp. It is usually a round, punched-out lesion 1 or 2 cm in diameter that is present at birth. The area is devoid of hair; it is sometimes covered with a thin membrane and is sometimes crusted and weeping. Rarely, other parts of the body may be involved, but the scalp is the most common site. Treatment is simply protection from trauma and infection; healing is usually slow. Plastic surgical repair might be considered for the rare occasion when the scar cannot be adequately covered by growing hair.

III. Vascular disorders and malformations

A. Nevus flammeus (port-wine stain) (see **I.D**)

B. Sturge-Weber syndrome

1. Recently, a retrospective study of port-wine stains of the face was made. Of the three trigeminal sensory areas, only involvement of area V1 the ophthalmic area, was accompanied by neuro-ocular involvement (Sturge-Weber syndrome). When the skin lesions occurred only in the maxillary (V2) and/or mandibular (V3) areas, no ocular or intracranial lesions were found. When coverage of the ocular (V1) area was complete (high-risk group), 60 percent had central nervous system (CNS) lesions [1].

C. Capillary and cavernous hemangiomas

1. Kasabach-Merritt syndrome (thrombocytopenia)

2. Diffuse neonatal hemangiomatosis

3. Blue rubber bleb nevus syndrome

4. Riley-Smith syndrome

D. Cutis marmorata telangiectica congenita (congenital generalized phlebectasia)

E. Familial annular erythema

F. Periarteritis nodosa

G. Disorders of lymphatic vessels

1. Lymphangiomas (simple, lymphangioma circumscriptum, and cavernous lymphangioma)

2. Cystic hygroma

3. Lymphedema

4. Milroy's disease (congenital hereditary lymphedema)

H. Purpura may result from one of these conditions:

1. Infectious disorders such as TORCH infections (see Chap. 12) or bacterial infections

2. Giant hemangioma with thrombocytopenia

3. Congenital leukemia

4. Congenital Letterer-Siwe disease

5. Immune disorders (isoimmune thrombocytopenia) (see Chap. 19)

6. Maternal drug ingestion

7. Congenital megakaryocytic hypoplasia (see Chap. 19)

8. Inherited thrombocytopenias (see Chap. 19)

9. Coagulation defects (see Chap. 17)

IV. Pigmentation abnormalities

A. Diffuse hyperpigmentation

1. Melanism

2. Progressive familial hyperpigmentation

3. Congenital Addison's disease

4. Fanconi syndrome

5. Generalized hereditary lentiginosis

6. Androgen excess

B. Localized hyperpigmentation

1. Flat lesions

a. Café-au-lait spots occasionally occur in newborn infants; these lesions are somewhat darker in color in black infants than in whites. Many appear after birth as the infant grows older. A few small spots are of little or no significance, but larger ones (or increasing numbers) may indicate the presence of neurofibromatosis. A biopsy may reveal differences in the appearance of melanosomes within the melanocytes.

The presence of giant pigment granules is characteristic of neurofibromatosis (see **b**).

b. **Neurofibromatosis (von Recklinghausen's disease),** a hereditary disease resulting from an autosomal gene, is mainly characterized by the development of multiple mixed neural and fibrous tumors in late childhood and adolescence. The café-au-lait spots that eventually develop in over 90 percent of patients are occasionally present at birth, but they usually develop during the first year of life. Neurofibromatosis should be strongly suspected in any newborn infant with more than three café-au-lait spots (especially if any of the spots is larger than 3 cm).

c. **Albright's syndrome** is characterized in the newborn by the presence of a large, very irregular, ragged pigmented area, as much as 9 to 12 cm in extent. Other features, appearing later, are bony lesions and endocrine disorders.

d. **Junctional nevi** are brown or black in color and are flat to slightly raised; they are present at birth. Junctional nevi are composed of nests of cuboidal cells with melanocytes and occur at the border of the dermis and epidermis. They are benign lesions, needing no treatment unless excision is desired for cosmetic reasons.

e. **Peutz-Jeghers syndrome.** At birth, individuals with this condition show multiple, scattered hyperpigmented macules, especially around the nose and mouth, but also on the hands and fingers, and frequently on the mucous membrane of the mouth. The more serious part of the syndrome appears later, with the development of polyposis of the small bowel and subsequent episodes of intussusception.

2. **Raised lesions**

a. **Giant hairy nevus (bathing trunk nevus).** These lesions, present at birth, may be huge (involving 20 to 30 percent of the body surface); they are leathery to hard in consistency and brown to black in color, with a large amount of hair. Other pigmentary abnormalities are frequently present on the remaining skin. Occasionally, deeper structures, including the central nervous system (CNS), may be involved as well. Surgical removal, although sometimes an extremely difficult procedure, is indicated, not only for the obvious cosmetic reason but also because a significant number of these lesions (>10 percent) progress to malignant melanoma.

b. **Compound nevi** are very similar to junctional nevi in that they are composed of melanocytes. Compound nevi tend to be larger, however, and are often hairy; they involve the dermis as well as the epidermis. Treatment involves surgical removal if technically feasible at age 5 or 6 because of the possibility of a later change to a malignant lesion in compound nevi present at birth.

c. **Other raised lesions.** Epidermal nevi, blue nevi, and juvenile melanoma are other forms of raised lesions that are rarely seen in the newborn; they require no treatment except occasional diagnostic excision.

C. **Hypopigmentation**

1. **Albinism** is a hereditary disease caused by an autosomal recessive gene that leads to a defect in tyrosinase activity. This defect, in turn, produces a pronounced defect in pigment production throughout the body. The defect is most noticeable in the skin, the hair, and the eyes (iris). No treatment is effective; the infants must be protected from ultraviolet light.

2. **Piebaldism,** also known as **partial albinism,** is probably caused by an autosomal-dominant gene with decreased penetrance. In this condition the skin and hair are involved in a patchy way, with some areas being hypomelanotic and some normal. A white "forelock" of hair, as in Waardenburg's syndrome, is a feature of this disorder.

3. **Vitiligo** is characterized by patchy areas of decreased or absent pigmentation. The lesions are occasionally present at birth, but may develop in

later infancy or childhood. The characteristic appearance under the microscope shows few or no melanocytes present in the junctional layer.

4. **White spots (tuberous sclerosis).** The typical white spot seen in tuberous sclerosis is small (2 to 3 cm in length at most), is usually seen on the trunk and buttocks, and is variable in number. The lesion differs from the lesion of vitiligo in that melanocytes are present in fair to good numbers, but the melanosomes are poorly pigmented. In fair-skinned infants, it may be difficult to demonstrate the white macule without the use of a mercury lamp (Wood's lamp) fitted with a filter that restructures its emission to 3600 Å. Many infants with tuberous sclerosis also have one or more café-au-lait spots.
5. **Waardenburg's syndrome and Chédiak-Higashi syndrome** are other examples of inherited conditions in which pigmentary deficits form part of the clinical picture but are not primarily responsible for the problems associated with the disease. The main problems in these disorders are immune deficiencies in Chédiak-Higashi syndrome and congenital deafness in Waardenburg's syndrome.

V. **Scaling disorders**

A. Harlequin fetus (ichthyosis)
B. Ichthyosis vulgaris
C. Sex-linked ichthyosis
D. Nonbullous congenital ichthyosiform erythroderma
E. Bullous congenital ichthyosiform erythroderma
F. Ichthyosis linearis circumflexa
G. Erythrokeratodermia variabilis
H. Other syndromes with scaling
    1. Netherton's syndrome
    2. Sjögren-Larsson syndrome
    3. Rud's syndrome
    4. Conradi's syndrome
    5. Refsum's syndrome
    6. Tay's syndrome
I. **Keratoderma of palms and soles**
    1. Tylosis
    2. Mutilating keratoderma
    3. Progressive keratoderma
    4. Mal de Meleda
    5. Papillon-Lefèvre syndrome
J. Psoriasis.
K. **Zinc deficiency** [1,4,5] has recently been determined to be a leading cause, or perhaps *the* cause, of **acrodermatitis enteropathica**; therefore, a more complete discussion is presented here. The condition previously was considered to be a hereditary autosomal recessive disorder; however, recent reports document remarkable response to intravenous or oral doses of zinc sulfate only slightly in excess of the recommended daily requirement. In the newborn period, zinc deficiency has been reported almost exclusively in infants receiving total parenteral nutrition with solutions containing either no zinc or inadequate amounts. Most infants have had increased zinc losses in gastric or ileostomy fluids and increased requirements due to sepsis. There have been a few reports of zinc deficiency occurring in otherwise healthy breast-fed infants whose mother's milk, for unknown reasons, was exceptionally low in zinc content.

    The **skin lesions** of acrodermatitis enteropathica may be dry or moist; they are scaling and impetiginous and appear primarily around the nose, mouth and perineum, as well as around ostomy wounds. They frequently spread to adjacent areas and especially to the fingers and toes. The condition is often accompanied by severe diarrhea, irritability, and failure to thrive despite theoretically adequate nutritional intake. Sepsis is frequently associated with acrodermatitis enteropathica. Response to zinc therapy is prompt and dramatic.

Guidelines established by the American Medical Association Department of Foods and Nutrition [5] suggest that term babies receive 0.1 mg/kg per day of zinc, and that premature infants (low birth weight) of less than 3 kg receive 0.3 mg/kg per day. Current formulas, as well as human milk, contain zinc in the range of 0.35 mg/dl, which should be adequate under most circumstances. Human milk is also believed to contain a factor that enhances the absorption of zinc from the gastrointestinal tract (see Chap. 30).

L. **Neonatal lupus erythematosus** may occur in infants born to mothers with systemic lupus erythematosus (SLA). Skin lesions typical of discoid lupus, dry, scaly and reddened areas, may appear on face, trunk, or extremities or may be present at birth. Congenital heart block occurs in about half the affected infants and is the only complication resulting in significant morbidity and mortality. If persistent, the heart block may require implementation of a permanent pacemaker [4].

VI. **Vesicobullous eruptions**
- A. **Hereditary causes (nonscarring)**
  1. Epidermolysis bullosa simplex
  2. Epidermolysis bullosa lethalis
  3. Bullous eruption of hands and feet (Cockayne-Weber's syndrome)
- B. **Hereditary causes (scarring)**
  1. Epidermolysis bullosa dystrophica (dominant)
  2. Epidermolysis bullosa dystrophica (recessive)
- C. Congenital porphyria
- D. Incontinentia pigmenti
- E. Juvenile dermatitis herpetiformis
- F. **Infiltrative diseases**
  1. **Mast cell diseases**
     - a. Mastocytosis
     - b. Urticaria pigmentosa
  2. Histiocytosis X
- G. **Infections**
  1. **Bacterial infections**
     - a. Staphylococcal infections
       - (1) Bullous impetigo
       - (2) Ritter's disease
     - b. *Pseudomonas* infections
     - c. Listeriosis
     - d. Syphilis (congenital)
  2. **Viral infections**
     - a. Varicella-zoster
     - b. Herpes infections
     - c. Rubella
  3. Candidal infections
  4. Toxoplasmosis

VII. **Skin care** in the newborn period must be given careful consideration. Because the skin is a protective organ and because any break in integrity may create an opportunity for infection, care should involve cleaning that will both offer protection and prevent infection (see Chap. 8).
- A. There should be minimum manipulation of the skin to
  1. Prevent heat loss
  2. Prevent trauma
  3. Prevent exposure of the infant to agents that may have potentially harmful side effects (e.g., hexachlorophene)
- B. **Bathing**
  1. The infant should be bathed only when the body temperature is stable.
  2. Water and a mild nonmedicated nonabrasive soap should be used, and the baby should be rinsed well.

3. In small premature infants, the skin should be bathed only with sterile water, and should be gently patted dry.

C. **Umbilical cord care** involves exposure of the cord to air and application of alcohol to the cord 2 times per day to aid drying and possibly to prevent infection. Topical antimicrobial agents may also be applied, although this may delay the drying process because of the petroleum jelly base used with these agents. Use of these agents may encourage the emergence of bacteria that are resistant to multiple antibiotics (see Chap. 8).

D. Infants who have an extremity immobilized or who have casts or intravenous arm boards should be watched for signs of pressure necrosis of the skin.

E. **Endotracheal tubes and catheters** placed in umbilical or peripheral vessels should be secured in place by adhesive tape on the skin that has been prepared with benzoin tincture. When this tape is removed, the edge of the tape is lifted and the skin-adhesive interface is wiped with an adhesive tape remover* while the tape is peeled back. The adhesive tape remover should be washed off the skin after the tape is removed.

F. Less important equipment can be attached to the skin by paper tape or by a hypoallergenic cloth tape,† which is less adherent.

G. **Topical agents** applied to the skin of infants may be absorbed and have systemic effects. Agents should not be used on newborn skin without attention to possible toxic effects from absorption.

References

1. Enjoiras, O., Riche, M. C., and Merland, J. J. *Pediatrics* 76: 48, 1985.
2. Herson, V. C. *Am. J. Dis. Child.* 135: 968, 1981.
3. Jacobs, A. H. *Pediatr. Clin. North Am.* 25: 189, 1978.
4. McLure, A. B., Weston, W. L., and Lee, L. A. *Ann. Intern. Med.* 106: 518, 1987.
5. Palma, P. A. *Pediatrics* 69: 801, 1982.
6. Schaller, J. Dermatology. In M. E. Avery and L. R. First (Eds.), *Pediatric Medicine.* Baltimore: Williams & Wilkins, 1989.
7. Shils, M. E. *J.A.M.A.* 241: 2051, 1979.
8. Solomon, L., and Esterly, N. Neonatal Dermatology. In *Major Problems in Clinical Pediatrics,* Vol. 9. Philadelphia: Saunders, 1973.

*Clinipad adhesive tape remover contains 1,1,1-trichloroethane, petroleum naphtha, and hexadecyl alcohol. Available from the Clinipad Corporation, Guilford, CT 06437.

†Dermicel. Available from Johnson & Johnson Products, Inc., Patient Care Division, 501 George Street, New Brunswick, NJ 08903.

30 Nutrition

Jean B. Crouch and
Lewis P. Rubin

The newborn infant rapidly adapts from a relatively constant intrauterine supply of nutrients to intermittent feedings of milk. The normal newborn diet, which is high in fat, disaccharide, and mineral content, sustains a doubling of birth weight by about 5 months. Preterm infants and infants with many medical or surgical conditions, however, commonly exhibit impaired sucking or absorption or may have increased energy and/or nutrient needs. The clinician is challenged to design individualized nutritional support programs that will enable these babies with special needs to grow and develop appropriately. Considerations include the suitability of enteral and/or parenteral nutrition, choice of specific diet, and choice of feeding methods. The application of several basic principles simplifies these tasks.

I. Principles of nutritional support

A. Growth of the fetus and newborn

1. **Growth patterns.** During the third trimester, the intrauterine growth curve is sigmoid and can be described by logistic equations. [61] (Fig. 30-1). **From about 24 weeks to 37 to 39 weeks, growth is exponential, increasing at a rate of approximately 15 gm/kg fetal weight per day, or 1.5 percent of fetal weight per day.** Growth slows at 37 to 39 weeks. After birth, the term newborn loses about 5 percent of birth weight, largely from loss of body water. Breast-fed term newborns should regain birth weight by 10 days and then grow rapidly (about 20 gm per day), albeit less rapidly than during intrauterine growth.
2. **Body composition** changes during development (Fig. 30-2). Total-body water (TBW), distribution of water between the intracellular and extracellular fluid, and deposition of fat and glycogen are dependent on gestational age, body weight, and postnatal age. Water constitutes about 90 percent of weight at 24 weeks and 70 percent at term. The term infant normally has sufficient glycogen and fat to meet energy demands during the relative starvation that may occur during the first few days of extrauterine life. In contrast, extremely preterm infants rapidly deplete their limited endogenous nutrient stores, becoming hypoglycemic and catabolic unless substrates and energy are provided.

B. Nutritional goals for preterm infants. Attainment of normal growth and development is the goal of neonatal nutrition. To this end, artificial formula diets for **term** infants tend to mimic the **nutrient content** of human milk or use it as a standard. For preterm infants, however, a logical and widely accepted approach uses **intrauterine growth and nutrient accretion rate data as reference standards for assessing growth** and nutrient requirements [2,13,23].

II. Nutrient requirements. Estimated nutrient needs of the normal newborn are summarized in the *Recommended Dietary Allowances (RDAs)* published by the Food and Nutrition Board of the National Academy of Sciences (Table 30-1). The RDAs for the first 6 months of life generally are extrapolated from the average nutrient intakes of healthy breast-fed infants or from the amounts of nutrients required to prevent disease states, such as vitamin D deficiency. Recommended intakes for nutrients about which less information is available (e.g., trace ele-

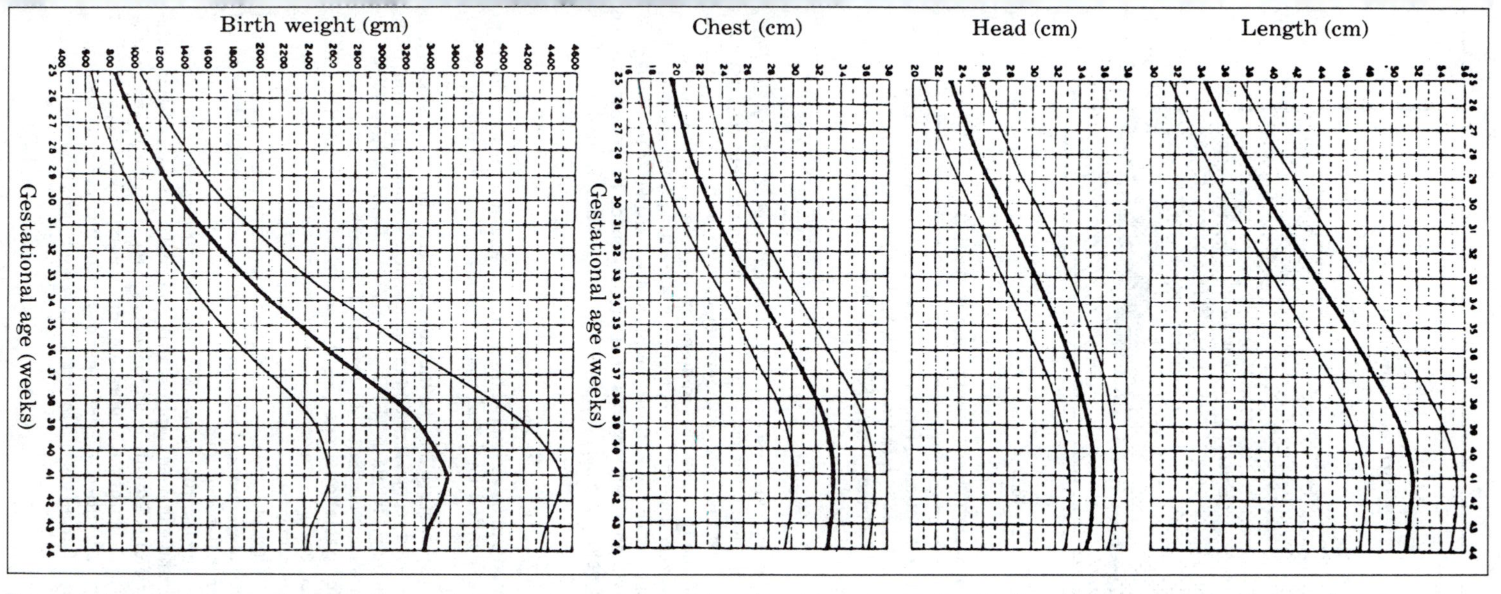

Fig. 30-1. Smoothed curve values for the mean (plus or minus 2 standard deviations) measurements of birth weight, chest and head circumference, and crown-heel length made on 300 infants of known gestational age. (From R. H. Usher and F. H. McLean, Intrauterine growth of live-born Caucasian infants at sea level. Standards obtained from measurements in 7 dimensions of infants born between 25 and 44 weeks of gestation.)

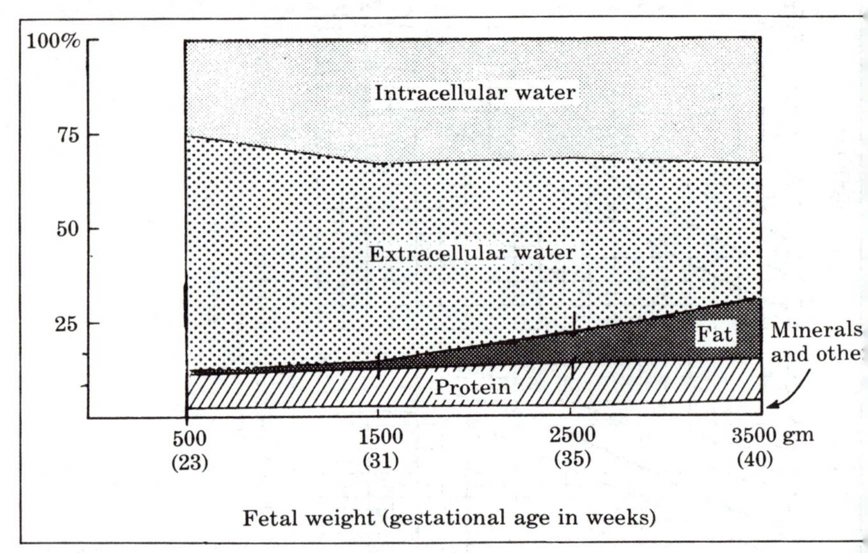

Fig. 30-2. Body composition in relation to fetal weight and gestational age. (From H. S. Dweck, *Clin. Perinatol.* 2: 183, 1975; data from E. M. Widdowson, Growth and Composition of the Fetus and Newborn. In N. S. Assali (Ed.), *Biology of Gestation,* Vol. 2. New York: Academic Press, 1968.)

ments and some vitamins) are described as *Estimated Safe and Adequate Daily Dietary Intakes* (Table 30-1). Estimations for energy and nutrient requirements for preterm infants must take into consideration decreased absorption, lower nutrient reserves, and the requirements imposed by a greater growth velocity.

A. **Energy.** The average energy content of human milk is 67 kcal/dl. Healthy term babies appear to grow well with intakes of at least 80 to 90 kcal/kg per day. **Low-birth-weight (LBW) infants have greater needs in order to sustain greater growth velocity.** Energy intake (E_{intake}) may be estimated as follows (Table 30-2):

$$E_{intake} = E_{stored} + E_{expended} + E_{excreted}$$

1. **Energy stored** can be estimated from fetal fat and protein accretion data.
2. **Energy is expended** for basal metabolism, activity, thermoregulation, and growth.
   a. Energy expenditure may be **increased** by cold, infection, surgery, or the increased respiratory and metabolic activity accompanying bronchopulmonary dysplasia (BPD) or congestive heart failure (CHF).
   b. Cold stress can be limited by control of the ambient temperature.
   c. **Small for gestational age (SGA) newborns** also frequently require increased energy intakes owing to elevated resting metabolic needs and higher energy costs of synthesis of new tissue [11].
3. **Energy excreted** is increased in preterm infants owing to poor fat and carbohydrate digestion and absorption and in infants with short bowel syndrome or malabsorption.

These estimates suggest that preterm infants who are maintained in a thermoneutral environment need approximately 50 kcal/kg per day for **maintenance of body weight. Growth,** including energy stored in new tissue and the energy cost of tissue synthesis, requires an additional 5 to 6 kcal/gm of weight gain. Hence a growth rate of 15 gm/kg per day **theoretically** requires 50 kcal/kg per day (maintenance) plus 75 to 90 kcal/kg per day (growth), which equals

Table 30-1. Recommended daily dietary allowances for infants

				Fat-soluble vitamins				Water-soluble vitamins							Minerals and trace elements						
Infant age (years)	Weight (kg)	Kcals	Protein (gm)	Vitamin A (μg RE)[a]	Vitamin D (μg)[b]	Vitamin E (mg α-TE)[c]	Vitamin K (μg)	Vitamin C (mg)	Thiamine (mg)	Riboflavin (mg)	Niacin (mg NE)[d]	Vitamin B_6 (mg)	Folacin (μg)	Vitamin B_{12} (μg)	Calcium (mg)	Phosphorus (mg)	Magnesium (mg)	Iron (mg)	Zinc (mg)	Iodine (μg)	Selenium (μg)
0.0–0.5	6	kg × 108	kg × 2.2	375	7.5	3	5	30	0.3	0.4	5	0.3	25	0.3	400	300	40	6	5	40	10
0.5–1.0	9	kg × 98	kg × 1.6	375	10	4	10	35	0.4	0.5	6	0.6	35	0.5	600	500	60	10	5	50	15

Estimated Safe and Adequate Daily Dietary Intakes of Selected Vitamins and Minerals[e]

	Vitamins		Trace elements[f]				
Infant age (years)	Biotin (μg)	Pantothenic acid (mg)	Copper (mg)	Manganese (mg)	Fluoride (mg)	Chromium (μg)	Molybdenum (μg)
0–0.5	10	2	0.4–0.6	0.3–0.6	0.1–0.5	10–40	15–30
0.5–1	15	3	0.6–0.7	0.6–1.0	0.2–1.0	20–60	20–40

[a]Retinol equivalents: 1 retinol equivalent = 1 μg retinol or 6 μg β-carotene. See text for calculation of vitamin A activity of diets as retinol equivalents.
[b]As cholecalciferol: 10 μg cholecalciferol = 400 IU of vitamin D.
[c]α-Tocopherol equivalents: 1 mg of D-α-tocopherol = 1 α-TE. See text for variation of allowances and calculation of vitamin E activity of the diet as α-tocopherol equivalents.
[d]Niacin equivalent: 1 NE is equal to 1 mg of niacin or 60 mg of dietary tryptophan.
[e]Because there is less information on which to base allowances, these figures are not given in the main table of RDA and are provided here in the form of ranges of recommended intakes.
[f]Since the toxic levels for many trace elements may be only several times usual intakes, the upper levels for the trace elements given in this table should not be habitually exceeded.
Source: Food and Nutrition Board, National Academy of Sciences–National Research Council, 1989.

Table 30-2. Estimates of average daily energy requirements in preterm infants

		kcal/ kg/day
Maintenance (energy expended)	Resting metabolic rate*	45–60
	Activity	5–10
	Thermoregulation	5–10
Energy cost of growth (energy expended and stored)	Synthesis	10–25†
	Storage†‡	20–30
Energy excreted		10–30
TOTAL		95–165

*Resting metabolic rate is estimated from basal metabolic rate and an irreducible amount of minimal physical activity in a thermoneutral environment.
†Data from clinical studies vary widely.
‡Calculated for an average weight gain of 15 gm/kg/per day.
Source: Modified from J. C. Sinclair et al., Supportive management of the sick neonate. *Pediatr. Clin. North Am.* 17: 863, 1970; O. G. Brooke et al., Energy retention, energy expenditure, and growth in healthy immature infants. *Pediatr. Res.* 13: 215, 1979; B. L. Reichman et al., Partition of energy metabolism and energy cost of growth in the very low-birth-weight infant. *Pediatrics* 69: 446, 1982.

125 to 140 kcal/kg per day. In practice, lesser energy intakes (90 to 120 kcal/kg per day) may sustain intrauterine growth rates if activity and cold stress are minimal and fat is well absorbed or if parenteral nutrition is used. Sick or stressed infants may require greater intakes. A recommended upper limit of energy intake is about 165 kcal/kg per day [23]. Above this value, energy may not be adequately utilized, producing fat deposition but not necessarily faster or better growth.

B. **Water** (see Chap. 24). **The first step in nutritional support is to determine the infant's water requirements.** These requirements depend on gestational age, postnatal age, and environmental conditions. Term infants fed ad libitum typically ingest milk at a rate of at least 150 ml/kg per day. During the first week, VLBW newborns may require fluid intakes of more than 200 ml/kg per day because of their increased urinary and insensible water losses. Environmental factors (phototherapy, radiant warmers, low humidity) also increase insensible losses and thus increase water requirements. Conversely, restriction of water intake may be necessary for infants with RDS or BPD, congestive heart failure or PDA, or renal insufficiency. These babies will need diets with **increased caloric density** in order to meet energy requirements.

C. **Protein**

1. **Digestion and absorption.** Up to 3 months of age, peptic activity is low and minimal protein digestion occurs in the stomach. However, intraluminal digestion of proteins by pancreatic proteases and mucosal brush border and cytosolic peptidases is relatively efficient, even in preterm babies.
2. **Amount of protein.** The RDA for protein for term infants during the first 6 months of life is 2.2 gm/kg per day. We recommend intakes of 3.5 to 4 gm/kg per day enterally and **2.5 to 3.5 gm/kg per day** parenterally for LBW infants. Lower protein intakes may not support nitrogen retention or growth. Higher intakes have been associated with potentially deleterious metabolic consequences (azotemia, metabolic acidosis, elevated plasma and urine amino acid levels) [50,52], poor neurodevelopmental outcomes [28], and lack of significant augmentation of "true" growth rate, although retention of water and minerals may appear to enhance weight

gain [38]. It is also important that **energy intake be adequate for optimal utilization of dietary protein.** When energy intake is low, dietary protein cannot be utilized fully for tissue synthesis, causing decreased nitrogen retention and azotemia. When dietary energy available for growth is adequate, the same protein intake produces greater weight gain and nitrogen retention. **We recommend that 7 to 16 percent of daily calories be derived from protein.**

3. **Type of protein.** Precipitation of whole milk at pH 4.0 to 5.0 produces a large curd, **casein** (high in proline, methionine, phenylalanine and tyrosine content and cysteine-poor), and a suspension of more easily digestible **whey** proteins.
   a. **Human milk,** considered the highest-quality protein source for human infants, **is whey-predominant** (whey-casein ratio of 60:40) and, consequently, contains relatively little methionine, phenylalanine, and tyrosine. The relatively high cysteine content and very low methionine-cysteine ratio of human milk are adapted to newborns' limited capability to convert methionine to cysteine. Human milk is also an unusually rich protein source for taurine, an amino acid important in brain development and the conjugation of bile acids.
   b. **Cow's milk is casein-predominant** (whey-casein ratio of 18:82). Commercial cow's milk–based formulas are made more easily digestible by heat treatment. They may be supplemented with whey protein, cysteine and taurine to simulate human milk protein more closely.
   c. **All standard commercial formulas** sustain adequate growth and nitrogen retention in healthy term babies. However, several amino acid pathways are not completely developed in preterm infants [51]. When fed casein-predominant milk diets, these babies can develop elevated plasma levels of methionine, phenylalanine, and tyrosine [41], hyperammonemia, and acidosis. Furthermore, several additional amino acids may be essential for preterm infants, e.g., cysteine, taurine, and glycine.

D. **Fat.** Approximately 50 percent of dietary energy in human milk and most commercial formulas is derived from fat. Fat intakes greater than 60 percent of total calories may lead to ketosis.

1. **Dietary fat has several metabolic fates,** including the following:
   a. An **energy source** via the cellular metabolism of fatty acids
   b. An **energy store** as deposition of triglyceride in adipose tissue
   c. A **structural component** of cellular membranes, myelin, surfactant, etc.
   d. A **precursor for physiologically active substances,** e.g., phosphoinositides, prostaglandins, and leukotrienes.
2. **Linoleic acid** and related unsaturated C_{18}, C_{20}, and C_{22} compounds are **essential fatty acids (EFAs),** required for synthesis of structural components and physiologically active substances, and must be provided in the diet. It is recommended that all infant formulas supply at least 3 percent of total energy as linoleic acid (300 mg per 100 kcal) [3]. Long chain polyunsaturated fatty acids (C_{20}–C_{22}) are essential to brain development and are available in human milk, but not in formula or parenteral fat [32a]. Preterm infants are more vulnerable than term infants to **EFA deficiency** because of inefficient fat absorption, increased fat requirements for rapid brain growth and myelinization, and limited adipose reserves. **VLBW infants should be provided with an enteral or parenteral EFA source by the end of the first week of life.**
3. **Fat digestion** is largely determined by intraluminal concentrations of lipases and bile acids. In the newborn, digestion is initiated by lingual lipase acting in the stomach and continues in the duodenum by pancreatic lipases and a bile salt–activated lipase present in human milk. Bile salts act as emulsifiers, decreasing fat particle size (micelle formation) and in-

creasing the surface area exposed to lipolysis. Fat absorption is limited by the following:

a. **Type of fatty acids.** Triglycerides containing palmitic acid esterified at the 2 position (the predominant form present in human milk) are better absorbed than other esters. In general, unsaturated fatty acids are better absorbed than saturated fatty acids. **Medium-chain triglycerides (MCTs)** are more easily digested and absorbed than long-chain fatty acids. MCTs are absorbed directly into the portal circulation and are not dependent on concentrations of lipases or bile salts. However, **MCTs do not contain EFAs.**

b. **Bile salt deficiency** occurs in prematurity and cholestasis. Duodenal bile acid concentrations are decreased in preterm infants owing to ineffective ileal resorption of bile acids and reduced synthesis. Feeding with human milk can increase preterm total bile acid concentration and bile acid pool size [36,66].

c. A high fat intake may interfere with calcium absorption.

d. **Heat treatment of human milk** destroys its lipolytic activity.

E. **Carbohydrate.** Nearly all carbohydrate in mature human milk (about 7 g/dl, 40 percent of total calories), cow's milk (about 5 g/dl, 30 percent of calories), and cow's milk–based formulas is lactose. Generally, intestinal mucosal disaccharidase activity increases rapidly after the twentieth week of gestation and is very active by the twenty-eighth week [29]. Lactase activity rises more slowly but increases in response to preterm birth. Glycosidases, which act on glucose polymers, are active in very preterm infants; hence these polymers are well tolerated by these babies. Since glucose polymers contribute fewer osmotic particles per unit volume of formula than monosaccharides, equivalent energy can be provided at lower osmolality.

F. **Minerals**

1. **Sodium, potassium, chloride**

a. **Approximate dietary requirements for sodium, potassium, and chloride** are 2 to 3 mEq/kg per day. Requirements may be considerably higher in very preterm infants (birth weight < 1000 gm) because of significant renal loss of electrolytes.

b. **Human milk** contains about 0.7 mEq/dl of sodium, which is often **not** sufficient to meet the needs of VLBW infants. Therefore, preterm formulas contain 1.5 to 2.25 times more sodium than human milk or standard formulas.

2. **Calcium.** About 99 percent of body calcium is located in bone. Prolonged deficiency of dietary calcium or abnormal intestinal or renal calcium losses eventually demineralize bone, causing osteopenia and rickets (see Chap. 24).

a. The calcium present in human milk (30 to 35 mg/dl) is well-absorbed by healthy preterm infants.

b. Preterm infants are especially susceptible to calcium deficiency. Third-trimester calcium accretion (120 to 150 mg/kg per day) is greater than the amount of calcium that a preterm infant can ingest from human milk, even if absorption were maximal. Therefore, breast-fed preterm infants require mineral supplementation to support normal bone mineralization.

3. **Phosphorus** (see Chap. 24). Inorganic phosphate is distributed mostly in bone (80 percent) and muscle (9 percent). Human milk contains 12 to 15 mg/dl of phosphate. The intrauterine accretion rate is about 75 to 85 mg/kg per day. Therefore, phosphate requirements are greater in preterm than term babies, and dietary supplementation for breast-fed preterm babies is necessary.

4. **Magnesium** is an abundant intracellular cation, a constituent of bone matrix, and a cofactor for many enzymes. The intrauterine accretion rate for magnesium is approximately 3 to 4 mg/kg per day. Human milk (4 mg/dl)

and commercial formulas (4 to 10 mg/dl) can provide sufficient magnesium for the needs of preterm infants.

5. **Iron** performs many biological functions, e.g., as an oxygen carrier in heme.
   a. Iron stores accrued during late gestation should protect the term infant from iron deficiency until mid-infancy. Human milk, although a relatively iron-poor food source (about 100 μg/dl), markedly enhances iron absorption.
   b. Preterm babies have diminished iron stores. These babies can become rapidly depleted of iron when active erythropoiesis resumes, sometimes as early as 6 to 8 weeks after birth. However, feeding iron-fortified formulas increases vitamin E requirements and therefore puts preterm infants at risk for developing hemolytic anemia secondary to vitamin E deficiency [68]. Section **III.C.4** suggests schedules for iron supplementation. Iron supplementation may not be indicated in infants receiving frequent blood transfusions.

G. **Vitamins.** Vitamins are essential cofactors for normal metabolism that cannot be synthesized endogenously in sufficient amounts. The water-soluble vitamins generally function as cofactors in enzymatic reactions. Toxicities are unusual because of high renal clearance and low storage capacity. The fat-soluble vitamins (A, D, E, and K) subserve many roles in cellular metabolism. Greater storage in tissues is possible, and the potential for toxic overdose is well-recognized.

1. **Vitamin A** (retinol), a fat-soluble alcohol, is a component of rhodopsin, modulates epithelial cell differentiation, and may be especially important for rapidly growing or renewing tissue. The RDA for retinol (birth to 6 months of age) is 375 μg per day (see Table 30-1), based on average intakes of normal infants fed human milk. VLBW infants, on the other hand, have virtually no hepatic reserves of retinol and are particularly susceptible to vitamin A deficiency. Low serum retinol levels have been observed in infants with bronchopulmonary dysplasia [35a].
2. **Vitamin B complex** includes B_1 (thiamine), B_2 (riboflavin), B_3 (niacin), B_5 (pantothenic acid), B_6 (pyridoxine), B_8 (biotin), and B_{12} (cobalamin). Requirements for term and preterm infants appear to be met by standard and preterm proprietary formulas. **Vitamin B_{12} deficiency** (megaloblastic anemia, glossitis, neurologic symptoms) can occur in unsupplemented breast-fed infants of women who are strict vegetarians (vegan diet) [34] and infants who have had terminal ileal resections. In LBW infants fed fresh or frozen/thawed human milk, there is no evidence that other specific vitamin B complex deficiency syndromes occur, although riboflavin and pyridoxine levels may become depleted. Heat treatment of human milk inactivates thiamine.
3. **Vitamin C** (ascorbic acid) functions in conversion of folate to folacin, collagen biosynthesis, iron absorption and transport, and tyrosine metabolism. It has been suggested that formula-fed preterm infants should receive more vitamin C (20 to 50 mg per day) than infants fed human milk in order to prevent hypertyrosinemia and to enhance iron absorption [55].
4. **Vitamin D** (calciferol) is a precursor for calcium-regulating sterol hormones (see Chap. 24). It is synthesized from cholesterol in skin exposed to sunlight (ultraviolet light), but adequate levels generally require a dietary source as well. The new recommended intake for term infants is 300 IU per day; 400 IU per day for preterm infants appears to be adequate. Vitamin D deficiency can cause **rickets** (see pages 437, 446).
5. **Vitamin E** (D-alpha-tocopherol) is a fat-soluble, naturally occurring antioxidant. When incorporated into cell membranes, vitamin E prevents peroxidation of unsaturated cell membrane phospholipids.
   a. **Vitamin E requirements.** The level of dietary **polyunsaturated fatty acids (PUFA)** influences cell membrane fatty acid composition. Increased cell membrane PUFA content enhances membrane suscepti-

bility to free-radical oxidative damage. Consequently, the dose of vitamin E necessary to prevent lipid peroxidation is directly related to dietary PUFA content. **Iron** catalyzes cell lipid oxidation through the generation of free radicals. Iron also interferes with vitamin E absorption from the gut. Therefore, dietary supplementation of iron further increases vitamin E requirements. The vitamin E–PUFA (mg:gm) ratio of human milk is 0.7:1.1. All commercial infant formulas provide a vitamin E–PUFA ratio of greater than 0.4, sufficient to prevent lipid peroxidation.

b. Preterm infants have increased vitamin E requirements.

(1) Body stores are low.

(2) Fat malabsorption in preterm infants limits the absorption of fat-soluble vitamins, including Vitamin E.

(3) Preterm diets (either based on human milk or commercial preterm formulas) have high PUFA content for improved fat absorption.

(4) **Vitamin E deficiency** has been reported in preterm infants fed diets with low vitamin E–PUFA ratios. The manifestations are mild generalized edema, mild hemolytic anemia, and thrombocytosis [53] (see Chap. 16).

(5) Preterm infants receiving supplemental oxygen are at increased risk for oxidative tissue damage.

c. Vitamin E supplementation

(1) The recommended daily intake of vitamin E for LBW infants is 0.7 IU (0.5 mg of D-alpha-tocopherol) per 100 kcal and at least 1.0 IU of vitamin E per gram of linoleic acid [4]. In addition, oral administration of 5 to 25 IU per day of alpha-tocopherol acetate has been suggested [4,18]. We generally do not supplement vitamin E beyond the amount provided by appropriate preterm food sources and a multivitamin preparation (see **III.C.2.e**). This schedule provides approximately 5 IU/kg per day parenterally and 5 to 10 IU/kg per day enterally, 10- to 20-fold the weight-adjusted RDA for term infants (0.5 IU/kg per day). We also do not routinely supplement iron for babies who are less than 6 weeks old. Similar schedules have produced vitamin E sufficiency in VLBW infants [32].

(2) Pharmacological doses of vitamin E (up to 100 IU per day) have been proposed for the prevention and/or treatment of several diseases of preterm infants believed to be related to oxygen toxicity, including retinopathy of prematurity, bronchopulmonary dysplasia, intraventricular hemorrhage, and anemia of prematurity [48] (see Chap. 38). However, prolonged high serum levels of vitamin E (>5 mg/dl) and use of intravenous vitamin E preparations in VLBW infants have been associated with sepsis and necrotizing enterocolitis [37,43]. At present, there is no proven benefit for pharmacologic doses of vitamin E. Suggested safe serum levels in preterm babies are 1 to 2 mg/dl (23 to 46 μmol/L) [49].

6. Vitamin K is required for the hepatic synthesis of coagulation factors II (prothrombin), VII, IX, and X. Administration at birth of vitamin K (0.5 to 1.0 mg IM) can prevent hemorrhagic disease of the newborn. We provide repeated weekly doses of vitamin K (0.5 to 1.0 mg IM or IV) for infants who receive prolonged courses of broad-spectrum antibiotics and do not receive parenteral nutrition (which in our NICUs contains at least 60 μg/dl) (see Chap. 17).

7. Folate (folacin compounds), usually considered with B-complex vitamins, participates in the synthesis of amino and nucleic acids. **Fresh** human milk (folate is unstable to heat or light) provides folate at about 5 to 10 μg/kg per day for breast-fed infants.

a. **Folate deficiency** in infants is associated with megaloblastic anemia (a late sign), leukopenia, thrombocytopenia, growth retardation, and delayed CNS maturation or degeneration [20]. Folate deficiency is usually caused by malabsorption or insufficient dietary intake.

b. Preterm infants appear to have greater needs for folate than term infants because of lower body stores at birth and their increased postnatal cell division and body growth. Megaloblastic anemia due to folate deficiency has been described in preterm infants [63]; 50 to 65 μg of folate per day normalizes serum folate levels and blood cell morphology [20] in these babies.

H. **Trace elements** are constituents of metalloenzyme complexes and are cofactors in numerous metabolic processes.

1. The **zinc** concentration of human milk falls throughout lactation from 800 μg/dl in colostrum to 80 μg/dl at 4 to 7 months [57]. Standard infant formulas contain approximately 300 to 500 μg/dl. Zinc is accumulated at an intrauterine rate of approximately 265 μg/kg per day during the third trimester [57]. Preterm infants absorb zinc inefficiently, and when fed unsupplemented human milk, they can develop zinc deficiency [45]. Consequently, preterm formulas are designed with a high zinc content (810 to 1200 μg/dl), and fortifiers for human milk contain zinc. Recommendations for parenteral intakes are 250 μg/kg per day for term infants and 400 μg/kg per day for VLBW infants [30].

2. **Copper** is accumulated at an intrauterine rate of about 50 to 60 μg/kg per day during the third trimester [57]. Current recommendations for copper intake to prevent copper deficiency in preterm infants are at least 90 μg per 100 kcal per day [6] enterally and 20 μg/kg per day parenterally [30].

3. Requirements for other trace elements (**chromium, manganese, molybdenum**) are under investigation.

I. **Carnitine** is a modified amino acid with a quarternary amine structure. Carnitine facilitates transport of long-chain fatty acids across mitochondrial membranes. It is synthesized from lysine and methionine as well as ingested preformed in human milk and cow's milk–based formulas. Carnitine is not present in soy-based formulas or parenteral nutrition solutions. Synthesis may be deficient in prematurity, and carnitine deficiency has been implicated as a possible cause of the prolonged metabolism of parenteral lipids in preterm babies [56].

III. Infant diets

A. **Human milk** is the preferred complete diet for term infants. Women who choose to express milk for prolonged periods for their preterm or sick infants will require ongoing support and advice from the NICU staff (see Chap. 31).

1. **Alternatives to breast-feeding or, when appropriate, supplementation of human milk** should be considered in the following instances:

   a. Parental choice
   b. Lack of milk availability due to maternal absence or illness
   c. Presence of certain maternal diseases (e.g., active tuberculosis or HIV infection)
   d. Maternal medications for which breast-feeding is contraindicated (see Appendix C)
   e. Small preterm infants and infants with special nutrient needs
   f. See Table 30-3.

2. The **composition of human milk** and human neonatal physiology are mutually adapted (see Table 30-4).

   a. Human milk contains an average energy density of 67 kcal/dl (20 kcal/30 ml); protein, 0.9 to 1.3 gm/dl (about 7 to 10 percent of total calories); fat, 3.8 to 4.5 gm/dl (about 50 percent of calories); and carbohydrate, 6.8 gm/dl (about 40 percent of calories). Human milk is readily digested, absorbed, and metabolized.

Table 30-3. Indications for use of infant formulas

Clinical condition	Suggested formula	Rationale
Allergy to cow's milk protein or soy protein	Pregestimil or Nutramigen	Protein hydrolysate due to protein sensitivity
Bronchopulmonary dysplasia	High-energy, nutrient-dense	Increased energy requirement, fluid restriction
Cholestasis, biliary atresia	Portagen	Impaired intraluminal digestion and absorption of long-chain fats
Chylothorax (persistent)	Portagen	Decrease lymphatic absorption of fats
Congestive heart failure	SMA, Enfamil; high-energy formula	Lower sodium content; increased energy requirement
Constipation	Standard formula, increase sugar (Polycose)	Mild laxative effect
Cystic fibrosis	Portagen, Pregestimil	Impaired intraluminal digestion and absorption of long-chain fats
Diarrhea		
Chronic nonspecific	Standard formula	Appropriate distribution of calories
	Soy formula	If malabsorbing lactose
Intractable	Pregestimil	Impaired digestion of intact protein, long-chain fats, and disaccharides
Galactosemia	Soy formula	Lactose free
Gastroesophageal reflux	Standard formula	Thicken with 1 tablespoon of cereal per ounce; small, frequent feedings
GI bleeding (due to cow's milk protein intolerance)	Soy-free or other cow's milk–free formula	Milk protein intolerance
Hepatic insufficiency	Portagen	Impaired intraluminal digestion and absorption of long-chain fats
Hypoparathyroidism, late-onset hypocalcemia	PM 60/40	Low phosphate content
Lactose intolerance	Soy formula	Impaired digestion or utilization of lactose
Lymphatic anomalies	Portagen	Impaired absorption of long-chain fats
Necrotizing enterocolitis	Pregestimil (when feeding is resumed)	Impaired digestion
Renal insufficiency	PM 60/40	Low phosphate content, low renal solute load

Source: Modified from J. Gryboski and W. A. Walker, *Gastrointestinal Problems in the Infant,* 2d Ed. Philadelphia: Saunders, 1983.

b. Several factors may alter the composition of human milk:
   (1) The mother's health and nutritional status
   (2) Protein, sodium, mineral, immunoglobulin content, etc. are highest in colostrum, intermediate in transitional milk, and lowest in mature milk.
   (3) "Hindmilk" (milk expressed at the end of a feeding) has a higher fat content and lower protein content than "foremilk."
   (4) Milk of women delivering prematurely differs from milk of women delivering at term (see **4.c**).
c. Human milk has many properties that are not reproduced by current artificial formulas, including the following:
   (1) **Anti-infective factors**—leukocytes, immunoglobulins (especially secretory IgA), lactoferrin, lysozymes, and complement. Serious infections may be less frequent in breast-fed infants [33].
   (2) **Growth and differentiation factors,** e.g., epidermal growth factor, which may promote intestinal maturation
   (3) **Enzymes,** e.g., bile salt–stimulated lipase

   Freezing human milk destroys the cells. Heat sterilization destroys most of the above-listed bioactive proteins.

3. Our protocol for **collection and storage of human milk** is outlined in Chapter 31 (sec. **IV.A** and **B**).
4. We routinely supplement human milk for preterm infants.
   a. The psychological benefits for mothers who desire to provide a milk supply for their preterm babies are obvious. However, the necessity to express milk by pump, possibly for many weeks, can be a daunting and frustrating task. It is essential that physicians and nurses offer frequent counsel and assistance.
   b. Fresh or frozen/thawed human milk contains potentially important anti-infective and trophic factors for preterm infants.
   c. Preterm breast milk (i.e., milk expressed by mothers of preterm infants) may contain more protein, sodium, chloride, and magnesium than term breast milk. However, these findings are inconsistent [7,31], and composition varies from batch to batch.
   d. Generally, human milk for preterm infants requires nutritional supplementation, e.g., Enfamil Human Milk Fortifier (HMF) (Mead Johnson) or Similac Natural Care (Ross) (Table 30-5). Protein deficiency, rather than insufficient energy retention per se, can cause poor growth in human milk-fed preterm babies [19]. Mineral deficiency causes metabolic bone disease (see Chap. 24). Addition of a fortifier to human milk raises energy, protein, mineral, and vitamin contents to levels more appropriate to the needs of preterm infants.

B. **Infant formulas.** In the United States, the Committee on Nutrition of the American Academy of Pediatrics provides specific guidelines for the composition of infant formulas [2]. Artificial formulas approximate human milk in terms of energy density and distribution of calories among protein, fat, and carbohydrate. Table 30-4 enumerates the composition of commonly available formulas. Many infant formulas are derived from modified cow's milk. **Cow's milk itself is not an appropriate diet for young infants** because of the high renal solute load, high protein (3.3 gm/dl) and casein content, high proportion of saturated fats, poor mineral bioavailability, and increased risk for sensitization to milk proteins. Formula selection should be based on an infant's gestational age, energy needs, digestive and absorptive capacities, and disease entities.

1. **Standard (modified cow's milk–based) formulas,** designed for healthy term infants, are altered in order to approximate human milk by (1) adding carbohydrate, (2) partial or complete replacement of butter fats by various combinations of vegetable oils, and (3) use of demineralized whey. Currently available modified cow's milk formulas, except for Similac, are whey-predominant. Vitamin and mineral contents of these formulas are

Table 30-4. Human milk and formula composition

Formula (distributor)	kcal/30 ml	Protein, gm/dl	Fat, gm/dl	Carbohydrate, gm/dl	Minerals, mg/dl			Electrolytes, mEq/dl			Vitamins, IU/dl			Folate, mg/dl	Osmolality, mOsmol/kg	Renal solute load, mOsmol/L†
					Ca	P	Fe*	Na^+	K^+	Cl^-	A	D	E			
Breast milk (Composition varies)	20–22	1.1	4.5	7.1	33	15	0.03	0.8	1.4	1.1	250	2.2	0.18	5.0	290-300	75
Standard Cow's Milk–Based Formulas																
Similac 20 (Ross)	20	1.5	3.6	7.2	51	39	0.15 (1.2)	0.8	1.9	1.3	203	41	2.0	10	300	100
Enfamil (Mead Johnson)	20	1.5	3.8	6.9	46	32	0.11 (1.3)	0.8	1.8	1.2	210	41.5	2.1	10.5	300	98
SMA (Wyeth)	20	1.5	3.6	7.2	42	28	0.15 (1.2)	0.7	1.4	1.2	200	40	0.95	5.0	300	91
Similac 24 (Ross)	24	2.2	4.3	8.5	73	56	0.18 (1.5)	1.2	2.7	1.9	244	49	2.4	12	380	146
Enfamil 24 (Mead Johnson)	24	1.8	4.5	8.3	56	38	0.13 (1.5)	1.0	2.2	1.4	251	50	2.5	13	360	117
SMA 24 (Wyeth)	24	1.8	4.3	8.6	50.5	33.5	0.18 (1.4)	0.8	1.7	1.3	240	48	1.1	6.0	364	110
Soy Formulas																
Isomil (Ross)	20	1.8	3.7	6.8	71	51	1.2	1.4	1.9	1.2	203	41	2.0	10.0	240	116
Prosobee (Mead Johnson)	20	2.0	3.6	6.8	63	50	1.3	1.0	2.1	1.6	208	41.5	2.1	10.5	200	127
Nursoy (Wyeth)	20	2.1	3.6	6.9	60	42	1.2	0.9	1.8	1.1	200	40	1.0	5.0	296	122

Preterm Formulas‡																
Similac Special Care (Ross)	24	2.2	4.4	8.6	146	73	0.3 (1.5)	1.5	2.7	1.9	552	122	3.2	30	300	149
Enfamil Premature (Mead Johnson)	24	2.4	4.1	8.9	134	68	0.2	1.4	2.3	2.0	970	220	3.7	29	300	153
SMA "Preemie" (Wyeth)	24	2.0	4.4	8.6	75	40	0.3	1.4	1.9	1.5	240	48	1.5	10	280	128
Specialized Formulas																
Pregestimil (Mead Johnson)	20	1.9	3.8	6.9	63	42	1.3	1.4	1.9	1.6	250	51	2.5	10.5	320	125
Nutramigen (Mead Johnson)	20	1.9	2.6	9.1	63	42	1.3	1.4	1.9	1.6	208	42	2.1	10.5	320	125
Portagen (Mead Johnson)	20	2.4	3.2	7.8	63	48	1.3	1.6	2.2	1.6	530	53	2.1	10.5	220	152
Similac PM 60/40 (Ross)	20	1.6	3.8	6.9	38	19	0.15	0.7	1.5	1.1	203	41	2.0	10.0	280	96
Similac 27 (Ross)	27	2.5	4.8	9.6	82	64	0.2	1.4	3.1	2.1	274	55	2.7	14.0	430	164
SMA 27 (Wyeth)	27	2.0	4.9	9.7	57	38	0.2	0.9	1.9	1.4	270	54	1.3	7.0	416	123

Key: Ca = calcium; P = phosphorus; Fe = iron; Na^+ = sodium; K^+ = potassium; Cl = chloride.
*In instances where high and low Fe formulations are available, the low Fe value appears.
†Estimated renal solute load = [Protein (gm) × 4] + [Na(mEq) + K (mEq) + Cl (mEq)].
‡20 kcal/30ml formulations are also available.

Table 30-5. Oral dietary supplements

Nutrient	Supplements		Human milk (100 ml)* (approximate value)	
	Enfamil Human Milk Fortifier (Mead Johnson) per 4 packets	Similac Natural Care (Ross) per 100 ml	Plus 4 packets Enfamil HMF (Mead Johnson) per 100 ml	Diluted 1:1 with Natural Care (Ross) per 100 ml
Energy (kcal)	14	81	81	77
Protein (gm)	0.7	2.2	1.73	1.6
Fat (gm)	<0.1	4.4	4.0	4.2
Carbohydrate (gm)	2.7	8.6	9.9	7.9
Minerals				
Calcium (mg)	90	171	118	100
Phosphorus (mg)	45	85	59	50
Magnesium (mg)	—	10	3.5	6.8
Sodium (mEq)	0.3	1.5	1.1	1.1
Potassium (mEq)	0.4	2.7	1.8	2.0
Chloride (mEq)	0.5	1.1	1.7	1.5
Zinc (mg)	0.71	1.9	0.83	0.7
Copper (μg)	80	203	105	114
Manganese (μg)	9	10	9.4	5.3
Vitamins				
A (IU)	780	552	1003	388
D (IU)	210	122	212	62
E (IU)	3.4	3.2	3.6	1.7
K (IU)	9.1	10	9.3	5.1
Thiamine (μg)	187	203	208	112
Riboflavin (μg)	250	503	285	269
Niacin (μg)	3100	4060	3220	2105
Pantothenate (μg)	790	1543	970	862
Pyridoxine (μg)	193	203	213	112
Biotin (μg)	0.81	30	1.2	15.2
Vitamin B_{12} (μg)	0.21	0.45	0.25	0.25
Vitamin C (mg)	24	30	28	17
Folate (μg)	23	30	28	18

*Source: Milk-based and soy-based infant formulas for feeding infants in the hospital, Ross Laboratories, Columbus, Ohio, 1989.

generally greater than those of human milk in order to compensate for decreased absorptive efficiency. Standard formulas have an energy density of 67 kcal/dl (20 kcal/30 ml), equivalent to breast milk; 81 kcal/dl (24 kcal/30 ml) formulations are also available for feeding infants with increased energy or nutrient needs (e.g., increased energy expenditure or need for catch-up growth) or infants taking limited fluid volumes.

2. **Soy protein–based lactose-free formulas** were developed for infants with intolerance to cow's milk protein or lactose. The soy protein is supplemented (e.g., with methionine) to improve its biologic quality. Carbohydrate is provided as glucose polymers (corn syrup solids) and/or sucrose. The fat composition of these formulas is similar to that of standard milk-based formulas. The growth and nitrogen retention of term infants fed soy and cow's milk formulas are equivalent.
   a. Soy formulas are recommended for use in the following instances (see Table 30-3):
      (1) **Secondary lactose intolerance** (e.g., following gastroenteritis), **primary lactase deficiency,** and **galactosemia**
      (2) Allergy or intolerance to cow's milk protein or prophylaxis for potentially allergic infants (with a family history of atopy)
      (3) Term infants when families do not desire use of animal protein formulas
   b. We do **not** recommend soy formulas for routine use in preterm infants because of the following:
      (1) Phytate-protein-mineral complexes may impair mineral absorption and may lead to hypophosphatemia and metabolic bone disease.
      (2) Growth and nitrogen retention may be inadequate.
      (3) The vitamin content is low relative to estimated needs.
3. **Preterm formulas** are designed to meet the nutritional and physiologic needs of the preterm infant. The common features of preterm formulas include the following:
   a. **Whey-predominant, taurine-supplemented protein** that is better tolerated and produces a more normal plasma amino acid profile than casein-predominant protein
   b. Carbohydrate mixtures of 40 to 50 percent lactose and 50 to 60 percent **glucose polymers** to compensate for a relative lactase deficiency
   c. Fat mixtures containing approximately 50 percent **MCTs** to compensate for limited pancreatic lipase secretion and small bile acid pools
   d. Higher concentrations of electrolytes, minerals, vitamins, and protein to meet increased needs associated with rapid growth velocity, poor absorption, and limited fluid tolerance
   e. These formulas are available as 67 and 81 kcal/dl (20 and 24 kcal/oz).
4. **Specialized formulas** have been designed for use in a variety of congenital and neonatal disorders, including allergy, malabsorption syndromes, and several inborn errors of amino acid, organic acid, urea, and carbohydrate metabolism [12,39] (see Table 30-3). The formulas described below are those commonly used in neonatal special care. These products were **not** designed for use in preterm infants and therefore do not contain sufficient nutrients to meet the special needs of this population. Preterm infants fed these formulas require vigilant nutritional monitoring and assessment for mineral and multivitamin supplementation.
   a. **Pregestimil** is a **readily digestible** formula designed for infants with disorders of digestion and absorption. The protein is casein, which is enzymatically hydrolyzed to free amino acids and small peptides and treated to reduce allergenicity. Fat is provided as 60 percent MCT oil. The carbohydrate source is primarily glucose polymers. It is high in fat-soluble vitamins and essential fatty acids. We frequently use Pregestimil for term infants (and for short intervals for preterm infants)

with short bowel syndrome or those recovering from conditions associated with impaired intestinal function.

b. **Nutramigen** was originally developed as a hypoallergenic formula containing the same protein hydrolysates as Pregestimil. It is lactose- and sucrose-free. Nutramigen can be useful in the management of patients with protein allergies or lactose intolerance.

c. **Portagen** was designed to meet the needs of patients who cannot efficiently digest or absorb conventional dietary fat or have certain lymphatic anomalies or disruptions. Portagen contains only slightly less fat than standard formulas, but 85 percent of its total fat content is provided as MCTs. Corn oil (containing linoleic acid) is added to provide essential fatty acid requirements. Portagen contains casein-based protein and carbohydrate comprised of approximately 75 percent glucose polymers and 25 percent sucrose. Portagen is useful for the nutritional management of infants with significant **fat malabsorption** (steatorrhea) due to pancreatic insufficiency (e.g., cystic fibrosis), bile salt deficiency (e.g., severe cholestasis, uncorrected extrahepatic biliary atresia), small bowel resection, or lymphangiectasia. We also use Portagen for babies with persistent chylothorax in order to minimize chylomicron formation and decrease thoracic duct flow [46].

d. **Similac PM 60/40** was one of the earliest developed cow's milk–based whey-predominant (whey-casein ratio of 60:40) formulas. It has a **low sodium and phosphate content.** PM 60/40 and SMA are similar, but PM 60/40 is not available for routine home use for healthy babies. It is useful in the management of infants with the following conditions:

(1) Renal insufficiency requiring sodium and potassium restriction and a low renal solute load

(2) Hypoparathyroidism (see Chap. 24).

Both these conditions cause hypocalcemia and hyperphosphatemia. We generally prefer Similac PM 60/40 to SMA for these babies because of its higher calcium-phosphorus ratio (2:1 versus 1.5:1).

e. **Similac 27** and **SMA 27** are high-energy (90 kcal/dl, 27 kcal/30 ml) products. These formulas have similar carbohydrate (lactose), protein (whey-predominent), and fat compositions, but Similac 27 is significantly higher in protein, electrolyte, and mineral content than SMA 27. SMA 27 is a concentrate of SMA 20, whereas Similac 27 is formulated by adjusting protein and ash contents in order to limit renal solute load and by augmenting the calcium and phosphate contents. These products may be useful for fluid-restricted infants with congestive heart failure or bronchopulmonary dysplasia.

C. **Nutrient and multivitamin supplementation.** Many ill and preterm infants require supplementation of specific dietary components (see pages 437, 446).

1. **Major nutrients.** The oral dietary supplements listed in Table 30-6 are available for use in infants.

a. We use **MCT oil** supplementation (up to approximately 55 percent of total dietary calories from fat) as a convenient and usually well-tolerated source of additional energy. For example, the addition of about 0.25 ml MCT oil per 30 ml of formula increases the energy content by about 2 kcal/30 ml.

b. Polycose is hydrolyzed by maltase and theoretically is more efficiently absorbed than are lactose and sucrose. If supplemented at more than 4 kcal/30 ml of formula, Polycose may increase intestinal motility or cause diarrhea in some infants.

c. The use of either fat or carbohydrate supplements to increase dietary energy content above 4 kcal/30 ml will significantly decrease the protein-energy ratio, possibly with deleterious effects (see **II.C.2**). Therefore, in general, we first increase caloric density by concentration of formula to 24 kcal/30 ml and then add MCT oil and/or Polycose in increments of 2 kcal/30 ml as needed.

Table 30-6. Oral dietary supplements available for use in infants

Nutrient	Product	Source	Energy content
Fat	MCT oil (Mead Johnson)	Medium chain triglycerides	8.3 kcal/gm 7.7 kcal/ml
	Corn oil	Long-chain triglycerides	9 kcal/gm 8.4 kcal/ml
Carbohydrate	Polycose (Ross)	Glucose polymers	4 kcal/gm 8 kcal/tsp (powder) 2 kcal/ml (liquid)
Protein	Casec (Mead Johnson)	Calcium caseinate	3.7 kcal/gm 5.8 kcal/tsp
	Promod (Ross)	Whey concentrate	4.2 kcal/gm 5.7 kcal/tsp

d. For infants who require protein supplementation, Promod (1 gm protein per teaspoon) or Casec (1.3 gm protein per teaspoon) is available.

e. Human milk fortifiers (HMF) (see **III.A.4.d**). Although designed for human milk-fed preterm infants, these products can be useful additives to human milk or formulas for some infants with increased protein, energy, and mineral requirements and/or restricted fluid intakes.

2. Vitamins. Liquid drop preparations currently available in the United States for infants contain either vitamins A, C, and D or vitamins A, C, D, thiamine, riboflavin, niacin, B_6, B_{12}, and E. These preparations are available with or without **iron** and/or **fluoride.** Folate is not included in liquid multivitamin preparations because it is relatively unstable in solutions. Polyvisol (1 ml) contains

Vitamin A, 1500 IU	Niacin, 8 mg	Vitamin C, 35 mg
Thiamine, 0.5 mg	Pyridoxine, 0.4 mg	Vitamin D, 400 IU
Riboflavin, 0.6 mg	B_{12}, 2 mcg	Vitamin E, 5 IU

We use the following guidelines for vitamin supplementation:

a. All newborns receive vitamin K at birth.

b. There is no conclusive evidence that healthy, breast-fed infants of **well-nourished** mothers require vitamin supplementation, provided that sunlight exposure is adequate for vitamin D synthesis.

c. Healthy, term infants who consume average volumes of commercial formulas do **not** require vitamin supplementation.

d. Conditions producing **fat malabsorption** (e.g., severe cholestasis, short bowel syndrome, and cystic fibrosis with pancreatic insufficiency) will produce malabsorption of fat-soluble vitamins (A, D, E, and K) and may impair water-soluble vitamin absorption. Therefore, depending on the severity of fat malabsorption, we provide one to two times the usual daily dose of a multivitamin preparation (e.g., Polyvisol 1 to 2 ml per day) and periodically screen for the presence of deficiency states.

e. In our NICUs, we provide vitamin supplementation to preterm babies in order to meet recommended intakes, particularly with respect to vitamin D (400 IU per day) and folate (50 to 65 μg per day) [48]. We use the supplementation schedule shown in Table 30-7, which assumes a formula intake of about 150 cc/kg per day.

f. We begin vitamin supplementation as soon as the infant is receiving full volume feedings.

Table 30-7. Typical vitamin supplementation schedule for preterm babies*

Food source	Body weight	Polyvisol (ml/day)	Folate (μg/day)
Human milk + 4 pks HMF/100 ml	<1000 gm	0.5	25
Human milk alone	All preterm infants	1.0	50
Enfamil Premature 24	<1000 gm	0.5	25
Similac Special Care 24	<1000 gm	1.0	25
	1000–2500 gm	0.5	0
Nonpreterm formulas	All preterm infants, term infants at nutritional risk	1.0	25

*Goal: 200 mg/kg/day calcium; 100 to 200 mg/kg/day phosphorus. See pages 437 and 446.

g. Multivitamin preparations can markedly increase the osmolality of infant feedings [22]. We recommend limiting the concentration of supplements to 0.5 ml/30 ml formula in order to minimize increases in osmolality.

3. Iron. Iron deficiency anemia is the most common hematologic disorder of infancy (see Chap. 16). Its causes include preterm birth or low birth weight, perinatal hemorrhage, presence of nuchal cord at birth [58], low dietary iron, and chronic intestinal blood loss from exposure to cow's milk protein.

a. We use iron-fortified formulas for term infants who are not breast-fed.

b. We consider **prophylactic iron supplementation in preterm babies** starting at 6 to 8 weeks after birth. Elemental iron 2 to 4 mg/kg per day can be provided by an iron-fortified formula (1.2 to 1.8 mg/dl) or FerinSol (25 mg/ml).

c. Iron deficiency anemia is **treated** with elemental iron 6 mg/kg per day.

4. Fluoride. We recommend fluoride supplementation (0.25 mg per day) for the following:

a. Exclusively breast-fed term infants when the mother drinks spring or well water or when the community water supply contains less than 0.3 ppm of fluoride [5].

b. Term infants fed formula diluted with nonfluoridated water.

IV. Enteral feeding methods. The feeding method chosen for each infant should be individualized on the basis of gestational age, clinical condition, and extrauterine adaptation. Very sick or VLBW infants may not tolerate any enteral feedings for prolonged periods. Whenever possible, however, the enteral route is preferred to parenteral nutrition. Enteral feeding is generally safer, less expensive, more nutritionally complete (since more is known about enteral requirements), and more physiologic [65]. Moreover, lack of enteral feedings, despite parenteral nutrition, can lead to intestinal mucosal atrophy.

A. Breast and bottle feedings. Normal breast-feeding behavior in term infants is described in Chapter 31. In preterm infants, breast-feeding or feeding by a soft nipple specifically designed for preterm babies often is possible by 32 to 34 weeks' gestational age, when coordination of suck and swallow may be present. Considerations for bottle feeding include the following:

1. Temperature. The milk can either be warmed to body temperature or offered at room temperature.

2. Position. The hungry infant should be held in a comfortable, secure position, either reclining or sitting in the feeder's lap. The bottle should be held so that the air rises to the upturned bottom and the infant sucks in milk and no air through the nipple. The bottle should never be "propped" for a young infant; the benefit derived from cuddling and close body contact is as important as caloric intake.

3. **Schedule**
    a. **Bottle feedings** can either be offered on a schedule of every 3 or 4 hours (the usual practice in a busy hospital nursery) or on a more flexible demand schedule.
    b. The initial bottle feeding is sterile water. If water is tolerated without aspiration or regurgitation, the infant can be rapidly advanced to full-strength formula or breast milk.

B. Gavage (orogastric tube) feeding

1. **Candidates for gavage feeding** include the following:
    a. Infants less than 32 weeks' gestational age
    b. Preterm infants who expend significant energy in the process of nippling may require a combination of breast (or bottle) and gavage feedings.
    c. Infants with high respiratory rates may sometimes be gavage fed, although enteral feedings are usually withheld if the respiratory rate exceeds 75 breaths per minute.
    d. Infants with impaired suck and swallow mechanisms.
        (1) Encephalopathy, e.g., due to anoxia, intracranial hemorrhage, hyperbilirubinemia, meningoencephalitis, cerebral dysgenesis
        (2) Hypotonia, e.g., due to trisomies and a variety of other syndromes, congenital muscular dystrophy, anterior horn cell disease, hypothyroidism
        (3) Maxillofacial abnormalities, e.g., due to choanal atresia, cleft lip and palate, macroglossia, retro- or micrognathia
2. **Method**
    a. With the infant's head placed to the side, a no. 5 or 8F polyethylene feeding tube is passed through the nose or mouth; the distance from the nose to the ear to the xiphoid should first be marked on the tube. The catheter position is checked by auscultation over the stomach when air is injected.
    b. After placement of the catheter, residual gastric aspirate is checked. The volume is recorded, and the aspirate is returned. This prevents metabolic complications resulting from continued acid and electrolyte removal.
    c. A measured amount of fluid is poured into a syringe attached to the gastric tube and is allowed to drip in by gravity. The feeding is **never** injected under pressure.
    d. When the tube is removed, it is pinched closed to avoid dripping fluid into the pharynx.
3. **Feeding schedule** (see **IV.E** for feeding VLBW infants)
    a. The **volume** of fluid ordered depends entirely on the estimated stomach volume. Undistended stomach volume varies from 3 ml in the 800-gm neonate to 40 ml in the 4000-gm neonate.
    b. The **written order** for gavage feeding should include the type of formula, the frequency and volume of the initial feedings, and the increments of feedings to be given over the next 12 to 24 hours.
    c. When the gastric residual measured before the feeding is greater than expected, the residual should be returned to the stomach and the planned feeding reduced by that volume. Should residuals persist, one should look for the presence of other signs of gastrointestinal or systemic illness. Positioning the infant in the prone position after feedings may facilitate stomach emptying, thereby reducing gastric residual.
    d. **Sterile water** is recommended for the initial feeding because, in the event of aspiration, dextrose 5% in water (5% D/W) is as irritating to

the lungs as formula. Once formula is introduced, increase strength and volume by the recommended increments (see **IV.E.4**) until fluid and caloric requirements are met.

C. Continuous nasogastric (NG) feedings

1. **Candidates for continuous NG feeding.** We reserve continuous feeding through an indwelling NG tube for infants who do not tolerate intermittent gavage (e.g., gastric distension or regurgitation).
2. **Method**
   a. A no. 5F polyethylene feeding tube is passed through the nose into the stomach in the same manner as for intermittent gavage. With an indwelling NG tube, extreme care must be taken to tape the tube securely to the infant's nose and head; otherwise, manipulation of the infant or tube could dislodge the tube into the esophagus or pharynx, where infusion of formula could cause aspiration.
   b. Formula is administered at a constant slow rate **by pump.**
3. **Feeding schedule** is similar to that for gavage feeding of the infant weighing less than 1000 gm (see **IV.E.4**), except that the formula is delivered at a constant rate by pump, starting at 0.5 to 1.0 ml per hour.
   a. The indwelling NG tube is changed every 12 to 24 hours. Extension tubing from pump to gastric tube is changed every 8 to 12 hours.
   b. A fresh supply of formula or breast milk is flushed through the pump and tubing every 3 or 4 hours.
   c. **Gastric residuals** are checked every 2 to 4 hours. Adjustments in subsequent feedings are the same as those made with intermittent gavage feedings. Residual volumes should not exceed the volume of feeding given per hour.
   d. Feedings may be advanced by 0.5 to 1.0 ml per hour every 8 to 12 hours, until full volume is attained.

D. Continuous transpyloric feedings

1. **Candidates for transpyloric feedings.** Transpyloric feedings by means of indwelling nasoduodenal or nasojejunal tubes are an alternative to continuous NG feedings for infants who cannot tolerate intragastric nutrition owing to gastric retention or regurgitation.
2. **Method**
   a. A Silastic mercury-tip feeding tube, or a length approximately equal to the distance from the tip of the infant's nose to the knee, is passed in the same manner as for gavage feeding. Ultrasound guidance facilitates transpyloric passage.
   b. Alternatively, the infant may be placed on his or her right side and the tube allowed to migrate through the pylorus into the duodenum. This is usually accomplished within 10 minutes to 3 hours.
   c. The position of the tube is verified by a pH reading greater than 5 and by the yellow color of the aspirate; verification by radiograph may, on occasion, be necessary.
3. **Feeding schedule.** The same formulas and feeding schedules are used as for continuous nasogastric feedings. Formula is administered at a constant slow rate by pump, starting at 0.5 to 1.0 ml per hour.
   a. The constant rate of administration should be advanced gradually by 0.5 to 1.0 ml every 8 to 12 hours, up to the full fluid and caloric requirements of the infant.
   b. **Orders** should include volumes, rates of administration, and infusion pump settings. Care should be taken not to deliver excessively rapid or large volumes to the intestine, and observations for abdominal distension and diarrhea should be made regularly.
   c. **Gastric residuals** should be checked every 4 hours; presence of formula in the stomach may indicate a malpositioned tube, intestinal obstruction, or ileus.
   d. The indwelling nasojejunal tube is not changed routinely. Connecting tubing and formula supplies are changed as in continuous NG feeding.

E. Special considerations for feeding preterm infants

1. It is uncertain whether intragastric or transpyloric feedings are more metabolically advantageous for VLBW infants. Consequently, preferences for different feeding methods and schedules vary considerably among NICUs [17]. In our NICUs, intermittent gavage is more frequently the feeding method of choice for VLBW infants. When a baby does not tolerate intermittent gavage, we first attempt continuous NG feeding and then, if necessary, utilize continuous transpyloric feeding.
2. **Initiation of feeding**
   a. We routinely begin enteral feedings on day 1 for nondistressed, larger preterm infants (>1500 gm, >32 weeks).
   b. For nondistressed infants weighing 1000 to 1500 gm at birth, enteral feedings are withheld for the first 12 to 24 hours. We then begin intermittent gavage if there is no cardiovascular instability, respiratory distress, significant apnea, or evidence of asphyxia.
   c. We do not begin feedings for acutely ill infants during the first postnatal days.
   d. Some extremely small intrauterine-growth-retarded infants can safely be fed earlier than more premature infants of the same weight.
3. **Choice of feeding interval**
   a. A 3-hour feeding schedule is suggested for infants with birth weights less than 1500 gm, hyperbilirubinemia, hypoglycemia, asphyxia, or a past history of feeding intolerance.
   b. A 4-hour feeding schedule is suitable for most other infants.
4. **Feeding schedule**
   a. An initial volume of 25 to 35 ml/kg per day is given divided over a 3- to 4-hourly feeding schedule.
   b. The first feeding is sterile water.
   c. Generally, breast milk or formula concentration is increased before volume.
      (1) For infants weighing less than 1500 gm, we avoid "testing" feeding tolerance by feedings of 5% D/W, since the osmolality (250 mOsmol/L) exceeds that of dilute formula (e.g., quarter-strength Premature Enfamil = 61 mOsmol/L).
      (2) Breast milk or preterm formula is increased in concentration from quarter-strength to full-strength over 6 to 24 hours depending on birth weight and tolerance.
   d. A conservative approach is to increase the amount of each feeding each day by 1 to 5 ml in babies weighing less than 1000 gm, 2 to 10 ml in babies weighing 1000 to 1500 gm, and 5 to 25 ml in babies weighing 1500 to 2000 gm. Volume may be advanced more quickly once feedings are well established.
   e. Intravenous fluid and nutrient intakes must be adjusted downward as enteral feeding increases.

F. Feeding intolerance, gastroesophageal reflux, and gastrointestinal dysmotility

1. **Signs** of feeding intolerance in the newborn include poor suck, swallowing difficulties, choking, vomiting, abdominal distension, gastric stasis or gastroparesis, and reducing substances or blood in the stool (see Chaps. 27 and 28)
2. **Associations**
   a. Persistent or severe feeding intolerance may indicate NEC, sepsis, or metabolic abnormalities (see Chaps. 12, 24, 27, and 28).
   b. Functional feeding intolerance and gastric stasis frequently are associated with prematurity [35], CNS or neuromuscular disease, repaired esophageal atresia, and BPD.
3. **Symptomatic gastroesophageal reflux (GER)** often complicates oral feedings for these babies and may lead to apnea, airway obstruction, and failure to grow.

a. GER, a **physiological event** in infancy, decreases in frequency as lower esophageal sphincter pressure gradually rises over the first several months. **Pathologic,** or **symptomatic, GER,** caused by a breakdown of the gastroesophageal antireflux barrier, may be defined as an abnormally frequent passage of gastric contents into the esophagus. Pathologic GER is frequently associated with delayed gastric emptying and eosphageal motility disorders [27,40].

b. **Signs** of pathologic GER, especially in preterm infants, include those mentioned above, as well as increased pulmonary secretions, episodes of pulmonary deterioration, apnea or airway obstruction, refusal to eat, irritability, arching, and failure to grow.

4. **Treatment for symptomatic GER and gastric stasis**

a. Positioning the infant is a simple and frequently effective maneuver. LBW infants reflux less frequently when prone than when placed on the left or right side. The prone position with the head elevated about 30 degrees is preferred for infants with symptomatic GER [44]. Upright positioning in "achalasia chairs" may actually exacerbate GER.

b. Frequent feedings with small volumes can decrease gastric distension.

c. Thickening feedings with cereal may be effective.

d. **Esophagitis** can potentiate GER. Antacids or H2 antagonists (cimetidine) diminish gastric acid and may relieve esophagitis.

e. Metoclopramide, a dopamine antagonist, promotes gastric emptying and stimulates upper gastrointestinal tract tone.

(1) Persistent functional feeding intolerance, even in preterm babies and term infants with neuromuscular disease, may respond to metoclopramide 0.03 to 0.1 mg/kg per dose PO.

(2) Metoclopramide toxicity can produce extrapyramidal reactions (especially dystonia-dyskinesia) and methemaglobinemia [39,60].

f. Transpyloric feeding (see **D**).

g. Persistent clinically compromising GER may require fundoplication.

V. **Parenteral nutrition. Parenteral nutrition (PN)** refers to the intravenous delivery of energy and nutrients. This method of nutritional support is indicated for infants who for extended periods cannot meet energy and nutrient needs enterally.

A. **Indications for PN**

1. Owing to the complexity, risks of complications, and expense, **PN should be reserved for infants in whom adequate enteral diets are not possible.** Very short term parenteral nutrition has no clear benefits, particularly for larger neonates with greater energy and nutrient reserves. Parenteral nutrition **should** be considered for infants who are metabolically stable and who are

a. ≤1800 gm and not expected to receive significant enteral nutrition for more than 3 days

b. >1800 gm and not expected to receive significant enteral nutrition for more than 5 to 7 days

2. **Choice between peripheral and central PN.** PN solutions can be infused into peripheral veins or a central vein, usually the vena cava. Central PN allows the use of more hypertonic solutions but incurs greater risks.

a. It is possible to support growth, even fetal growth rates [14], by the use of **peripheral parenteral nutrition with a fat emulsion,** thereby avoiding the complications associated with prolonged use of central venous catheters.

b. Placement of a central venous catheter is warranted under the following circumstances:

(1) An anticipated extended period (e.g., ≥2 weeks) of "bowel rest," such as occurs, for example, in some postoperative infants and infants with necrotizing entercolitis

(2) Nutritional requirements exceeding the capabilities of peripheral PN. Significantly increased energy demands, especially combined

with decreased fluid volume tolerance, may necessitate concentrating dextrose greater than 10% to 12.5% D/W.

(3) Anticipated imminent lack of peripheral venous access

(4) The stress associated with frequent placement of peripheral venous catheters in VLBW infants may significantly increase metabolic needs.

B. Nutritional goals

1. Preterm infants who receive 60 kcal/kg per day of intravenous glucose and 2.5 gm/kg per day of amino acid solution show a positive nitrogen balance [8]. Higher energy intakes improve nitrogen retention and spare endogenous fat reserves.
2. In general, parenteral nutrition can support growth at slightly lower energy intakes than usually is possible with feedings, since energy is not lost in absorption and digestion.
3. Intrauterine accretion rates provide practical guidelines for estimating appropriate parenteral nutrient intakes. These goals must be individualized for patient needs. For example, infants subjected to metabolic stress, such as postoperative neonates, may require more energy and protein.

C. Nutrient sources

1. **Carbohydrate** (see Chap. 1 and Chap. 24A). Glucose (dextrose) is the carbohydrate source for intravenous solutions. The glycerol present in lipid emulsions also makes a small caloric contribution.
   a. Intravenous dextrose has an energy density of **3.4 kcal/gm** (owing to water of hydration).
   b. The osmolality of glucose limits the concentrations that can be infused safely by means of peripheral vein to 10% to 12.5% D/W. We use concentrations up to 12.5% D/W for umbilical arterial infusions and up to 25% D/W for central venous infusions.
   c. The signs of **glucose intolerance** are hyperglycemia, hyperosmolality, and secondary glycosuria and osmotic diuresis. The quantity of dextrose that an infant will tolerate varies, especially with gestational age.
   d. It is helpful to refer to dextrose infusions in terms of milligrams of glucose per kilogram per minute, which expresses the total glucose load and takes into account infusion rate, dextrose concentration, and patient weight. Figure 30-3 is a nomogram for easily interconverting glucose infusion units.
      (1) Term infants usually tolerate initial infusions of 7 to 8 mg/kg per minute and can be rapidly increased to 11 to 14 mg/kg per minute without displaying glucose intolerance.
      (2) **Glucose tolerance is related to gestational age,** owing in part to decreased peripheral glucose utilization and to persistent hepatic glucose production despite hyperglycemia secondary to hepatic insensitivity to insulin. LBW infants usually tolerate an initial infusion rate of 6 to 8 mg/kg per minute and a gradual increase up to 11 to 14 mg/kg per minute. At this level, hyperglycemia becomes prevalent [16]. VLBW infants may develop significant and persistent hyperglycemia if infusion rates exceed 6 to 7 mg/kg per minute, equivalent to 10% D/W infused at about 100 ml/kg per day.
      (3) As the rate of glucose infusion increases, both metabolic rate (oxygen consumption) and carbon dioxide production rise as carbohydrate is converted to fat. Thus very high glucose infusion rates may compromise infants with lung disease by increasing oxygen consumption and carbon dioxide production; these effects can be limited by replacing **some** carbohydrate with fat.
2. **Protein.** Crystalline amino acid solutions provide the nitrogen source in PN.
   a. The energy density of amino acids is 4 kcal/gm.
   b. Two pediatric amino acid formulations are commercially available in

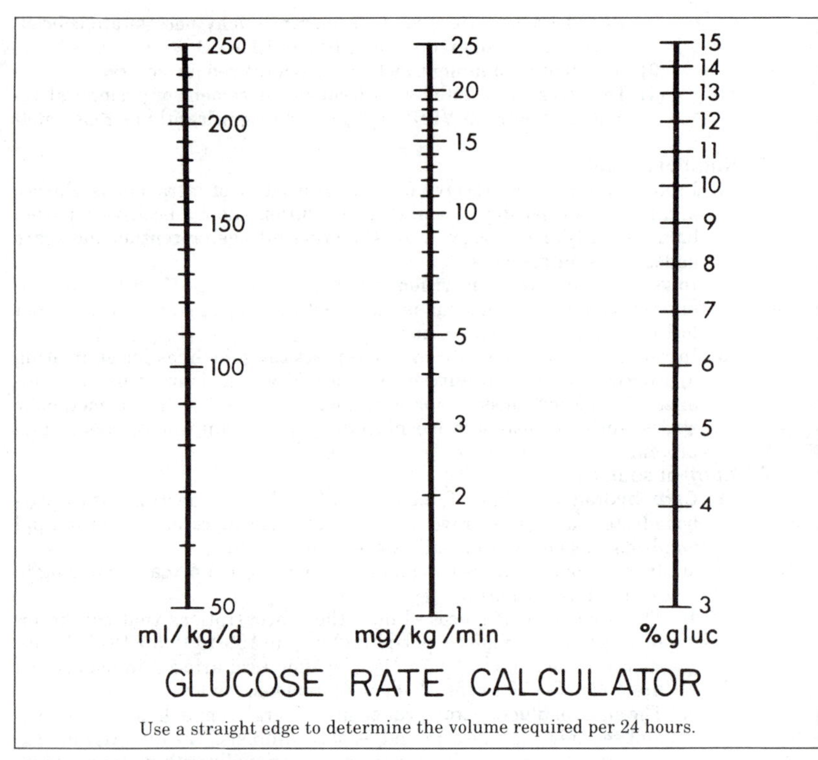

Fig. 30-3. Interconversion of glucose infusion units. (From M. H. Klaus and A. A. Fanaroff (Eds.), *Care of the High-Risk Neonate,* 2d Ed. Philadelphia: Saunders, 1979. P. 430.)

the United States (Aminosyn-PF, Abbott Laboratories, and Troph amine, McGaw). These solutions are designed to produce a plasma amino acid pattern that approximates the postprandial plasma o healthy, milk-fed neonates. In theory, these products are bette adapted to the needs of newborns than are standard adult amino acid solutions, which are based on the composition of egg albumin.

c. The optimal amino acid composition for neonatal PN is yet to be de fined. Nevertheless, the available pediatric formulations produce ni trogen retention and growth, and they are metabolized well, as mea sured by plasma amino acid concentrations and hormonal responses [15]. No products specifically designed for preterm infants are cur rently available.

d. Standard PN solutions contain 0.5 to 2.0 gm of amino acids per deciliter.

3. Fat. Soybean oil–based Intralipid (Cutter Medical) and Soyacal (Alpha Therapeutic) and safflower oil–based Liposyn (Abbott Laboratories) are the currently available lipid emulsions.

a. 10% lipid emulsions have an energy density of 1.1 kcal/ml (0.9 kcal from lipid and 0.2 kcal from glycerol and phospholipid stabilizer); 20% lipid emulsions yield 2.0 kcal/ml.

b. Lipid emulsions are made approximately isotonic (280 to 330 mOsmol/ml) by the addition of glycerol. The lipid particles resemble chylomicrons in size, appearance, composition, and metabolism.
c. Lipid emulsions contain essential fatty acids (EFAs), including linoleic acid. **Neonatal EFA requirements can be met by infusing a lipid emulsion at a rate of 0.5 to 1.0 gm/kg per day.**
d. By providing nonprotein calories as fat and glucose rather than as glucose alone, one prevents fatty acid deficiency, lowers endogenous carbon dioxide production, and promotes protein sparing.
e. Since fatty acids potentially can displace **bilirubin** from albumin binding sites, the safety of intravenous fat emulsions during neonatal hyperbilirubinemia has been questioned. At low infusion rates, displacement is not significant [62]. When the serum unconjugated bilirubin level exceeds half the projected exchange transfusion level, we limit the lipid infusion rate to 1 gm/kg per day.

4. **Electrolytes**
   a. Sodium and potassium concentrations may be adjusted daily to meet individual needs. Electrolytes are added by the pharmacy at the time of preparation.
   b. **Metabolic acidosis** in VLBW infants may be treated by increasing the proportion of anions provided as acetate.
5. **Calcium, phosphorus, and magnesium** (see Chap. 24). The amount of calcium and phosphate that can be administered intravenously is limited by the precipitation of calcium phosphate. Unfortunately, the variables that determine calcium and phosphate compatibility in parenteral solutions are complex [25,26,64], and what constitutes maximal safe concentrations is controversial. We use the following guidelines:
   a. **Calcium.** Our standard solution contains 30 mg/dl (1.5 mEq/dl) of elemental calcium.
   b. **Phosphate.** Approximately 21 mg/dl of phosphate is **routinely** added to solutions as 1.0 mEq potassium phosphate (0.68 m*M* phosphate; 1 m*M* phosphate = 31 mg).
   c. These standard mineral concentrations provide **only about a third of the daily intrauterine accretion rates for calcium and phosphorus.** Therefore, preterm infants receiving prolonged TPN are at **risk for metabolic bone disease** (see Chap. 24).
   d. Metabolic bone complications can be diminished by increasing the mineral content of PN solutions to **50 to 60 mg/dl of calcium and 40 to 45 mg/dl of phosphate.**
      (1) The calcium-phosphate ratio should be about 1.3:1 by weight (1:1 molar).
      (2) These suggested greater intakes of calcium and phosphate for preterm infants should be given through a central venous line and not a peripheral vein [30].
   a. **Magnesium.** Magnesium 0.3 to 0.6 mEq/dl is added to solutions. Higher concentrations (1.0 mEq/dl) in our NICUs have been associated with hypermagnesemia and intestinal dysmotility in VLBW infants.
6. **Vitamins and trace elements**
   a. Recommendations for intravenous vitamin intakes for infants and children, including **preterm** infants, have been recently revised. The current vitamin formulation (MVI Pediatric, Armour) does not maintain blood levels of all vitamins within an acceptable range for preterm babies [30]. Therefore, there is an urgent need for a multivitamin preparation designed specifically for these infants. Table 30-8 provides guidelines on how to best use the available formulation for term and preterm infants.
   b. **Trace metal parenteral requirements** have been estimated for pre-

Table 30-8. Suggested intakes of parenteral vitamins in infants

Vitamin	Estimated needs: Term infants (dose/day)	Estimated needs: Preterm infants (dose/kg/day)	Forty percent of a single-dose vial MVI Pediatric (Armour) per kilogram of body weight	1.5 cc MVI Pediatric per 100 ml PN administered at a rate of 150 ml/kg per day*
Lipid Soluble				
A (μg)†	700	500	280	315
D (IU)†	400	160	160	180
E (IU)†	7	2.8	2.8	3.2
K (μg)	200	80	80	90
Water Soluble				
Thiamine (mg)	1.2	0.35	0.48	0.54
Riboflavin (mg)	1.4	0.15	0.56	0.63
Niacin (mg)	17	6.8	6.8	7.65
Pantothenate (mg)	5	2.0	2.0	2.25
Pyridoxine (mg)	1.0	0.18	0.4	0.45
Biotin (μg)	20	6.0	8.0	9.0
Vitamin B_{12} (μg)	1.0	0.3	0.4	0.45
Vitamin C (mg)	80	25	32	36
Folate (μg)	140	56	56	63

*Assumes 150 cc/kg is the average PN administration rate.
†700 μg retinol equivalent = 2300 IU; 7 mg α-tocopherol = 7 IU; 10 μg vitamin D = 400 IU.
Source: From H. L. Greene et al., Guidelines for the use of vitamins, trace elements, calcium, magnesium, and phosphorus in infants and children receiving total parenteral nutrition. *Am. J. Clin. Nutr.* 48: 1324, 1988.

term infants [59]. Trace elements preparations are added to provide the following concentrations per 100 ml:

Zinc, 200 μg
Copper, 20 μg
Chromium, 0.2 μg
Manganese, 5 μg
Selenium 1.5 μg

These standard additions are designed to meet the needs of infants receiving about 150 ml/kg per day of parenteral nutrition. Significantly different fluid requirements or altered rates of excretion necessitate modifications.

c. Copper and manganese are eliminated in **bile.** Therefore,
  (1) Caution is required in administering intravenous copper to infants with impaired biliary excretion, including infants with TPN cholestasis.
  (2) Manganese should be withheld when cholestatic liver disease is present [30].

d. At present, several potentially important micronutrients are not contained in neonatal parenteral nutrition solutions, including carnitine, iodide, and molybdenum.

D. Schedules for PN. A suggested schedule for TPN follows. It should be modified according to the requirements and tolerance of each infant and tapered as enteral feeding begins. Convenient daily nutrient calculations appear in Table 30-9.

1. Dextrose

a. 6 to 8 mg/kg per minute (10% D/W at a rate of approximately 80 to 120 ml/kg per day) is generally well-tolerated initially.

b. Advance by about 2 mg/kg per minute every 24 hours either by increasing dextrose concentration (e.g., 7.5% D/W to 10% D/W) or by increasing infusion rate. The upper limit of tolerance is usually 11 to 14 mg/kg per minute.

c. Newborns with birth weights less than 1000 gm may have fluid requirements in excess of 200 ml/kg per day. These infants are also relatively intolerant to the standard neonatal dextrose infusions.

(1) When hyperglycemia is particularly severe or persistent, an **insulin** infusion may be useful [9]. We initiate an infusion of short-acting insulin at a rate of 0.01 to 0.05 unit/kg per hour. The

Table 30-9. Nutritional calculations

Intravenous Intake

Carbohydrate

________ (% dextrose) × ________ (ml/day of solution) × 0.034 kcal/gm = ________ (total CHO kcal/day)

Example: Dextrose 10% at 150 ml per day = 51 kcal/day

Protein

________ (% amino acid) × ________ (ml/day of solution) × 0.040 kcal/gm = ________ (total protein kcal/day)

Example: 2.5% amino acid solution at 150 ml per day = 15 kcal/day

Fat 10% Intralipid ________ (ml/day of solution) × 1.1 kcal/ml = ________ (total kcal fat/day)

Example: 10% intralipid at 24 ml/day = 26.4 kcal/day

20% Intralipid ________ (ml/day of solution) × 2.0 kcal/ml = ________ (total kcal fat/day)

Example: 20% Intralipid at 24 ml/day = 48 kcal/day

Total intravenous kcals/day =

________ (total CHO kcal) + ________ (total protein kcal) + ________ (total fat kcal)

Enteral Intake

(________ (Basic formula kcal/oz) + ________ (Additive kcal/oz))

× ________ (ml/day of solution) × 1 oz/30 ml = ________ (total kcal day)

Example: Similac 24 kcal/oz with 2 kcal/oz polycose and 2 kcal/oz MCT oil at 150 ml/day = [24 kcal/oz + 2 kcal/oz + 2 kcal/oz] × 150 ml × 1oz/30ml = 140 kcal/day

Caloric Content of Ingredients

Dextrose = 3.4 kcal/gm	Polycose = 2 kcal/ml (liquid)
Protein = 4.0 kcal/gm	Polycose = 8 kcal/5 ml (powder)
10% Intralipid = 1.1 kcal/ml	MCT oil = 7.7 kcal/ml
20% Intralipid = 2.0 kcal/ml	HMF = 3.5 kcal/package

insulin dose is titrated to maintain blood glucose concentrations between 100 and 150 mg/dl. A convenient initial solution is 10 units of insulin/kg in 100 ml of fluid (0.1 unit/cc). The IV tubing first should be thoroughly flushed with the solution (see pages 436, 628).

(2) For the smallest preterm infants, on rare occasions we use 2.5% D/W with sodium, potassium, calcium salts or amino acids to adjust osmolality. The risk of hemolysis and hyperkalemia sometimes associated with this approach must be weighed against the risk of swings in glucose level that sometimes accompany insulin infusion.

2. Protein

- **a.** Begin with 0.5 to 1.0 gm/kg per day, usually a 1.0 gm/dl solution for larger infants and a 0.5 gm/dl for VLBW infants.
- **b.** Advance by 0.5 to 1.0 gm/kg per day to 2.5 to 3.0 gm/kg per day.

3. Fat

- **a.** Begin with 0.5 to 1.0 gm/kg per day (e.g., 5 to 10 ml/kg per day of a 10% lipid emulsion).
- **b.** Advance as tolerated by 0.5 gm/kg for larger infants or 0.25 gm/kg for VLBW infants every 12 to 24 hours up to 3 gm/kg per day.
- **c.** We do not exceed 1.0 gm/kg per day when the unconjugated **bilirubin** level exceeds half the projected exchange transfusion level.
- **d.** We generally infuse lipid emulsions over 24 hours per day.

E. Peripheral alimentation procedures

1. The amino acid–dextrose and fat solutions can be infused together through either a plastic catheter (no. 22 or 24F) or a scalp vein needle.
2. Dextrose and amino acids are mixed in the same bottle, which is then connected to the distal end of an infusion line with a 0.22-μm in-line air-eliminating filter.
3. The lipid emulsion is connected with the infusion line beyond the filter through the upper portion of a T-connector or Y-connector.
4. Infusion pumps are required to maintain a constant rate of intravenous fluid administration.
5. We recommend that the entire infusion set, including tubing up to the intravenous needle, be changed every 72 hours, except for the lipid emulsion tubing, which is changed every 24 hours. The intravenous needle ideally should be replaced every 48 hours. Parenteral solutions and lipid emulsions are changed daily.
6. **Medications** are **not** given in PN solutions. The PN catheter is flushed with saline, and the medication is then infused in a compatible intravenous solution.
7. All solutions are prepared in the pharmacy under laminar flow hoods.
8. We do **not add** heparin to peripheral alimentation solutions, although at some centers heparinization of peripheral lines is routine [1].
9. Mineral, vitamins, and trace elements are added as outlined in **C.5–6.**
10. **Either** 10% **or** 20% fat emulsions may be used in peripheral venous lines.

F. Central alimentation procedures

1. The catheter may be placed percutaneously or by venous cut-down (see Chap. 39). We prefer to use very thin no. 1.9F Silastic catheters for central venous access in VLBW infants. For larger infants, no. 2.7F catheters (e.g., Cook, Broviac) may be used. We avoid larger double-lumen catheters because of the association with superior vena cava syndrome and vessel wall erosion.
2. The catheter is inserted through the antecubital, saphenous, internal or external jugular, or subclavian vein or, less frequently, through the umbilical or femoral vein. The catheter should be threaded so that the tip lies at the junction of the right atrium and the superior or inferior vena cava.
3. We try to avoid using **umbilical arterial catheters** to infuse parenteral

nutrition solutions in VLBW neonates. The disadvantages of this route are (1) the incidence of arterial thrombosis is high, (2) the catheter needs to be entered for blood sampling, and (3) we usually do not provide any enteral feeding while an umbilical arterial catheter is in place. The difficulty of maintaining peripheral access frequently necessitates use of umbilical artery catheters for parenteral nutrition, however.

4. Solutions are infused by pumps through Y- or T-connectors, as with peripheral alimentation (see **E**).
5. Because of the increased risk of infection with central alimentation catheters, the continuity of the central line should **not** be broken for blood drawing, medication infusion, or blood transfusion.
6. All solutions are prepared in the pharmacy under laminar flow hoods.
7. **Heparin** is added at a concentration of 0.5 unit/ml of solution.

G. Complications

1. PN-associated **cholestatic hepatitis** [55] (see Chap. 15) is common and more often transient than progressive. Experimentally, even short-term PN can reduce bile flow and bile salt formation.
   a. Risk factors include prematurity, duration of PN administration, duration of fasting (since lack of enteral feeding also produces bile inspissation and cholestasis), underlying disease, infections, and narcotic administration.
   b. Recommended **management** includes the following:
      (1) Evaluate other possible causes of hepatic dysfunction.
      (2) Attempt enteral feeding slowly and decrease PN. Even "token" feedings may stimulate bile secretion.
      (3) Reduce the amino acid infusion to the lower end of the recommended range, particularly if the infusion rate has exceeded 3 gm/kg per day.
      (4) Decrease dextrose infusion rates. High rates may produce steatosis.
      (5) Continue lipid infusion, maintaining serum triglyceride (TG) concentrations of 150 mg/dl or less.
2. **Cholelithiasis.** Risk factors include prolonged fasting, ileal disease, ileal resection, and exposure to opiates or anticholinergic drugs.
3. **PN-associated hepatic steatosis.** PN enhances hepatic fatty acid synthesis and decreases TG secretion. Experimentally, steatosis is associated with glucose overfeeding [54]. Substituting intravenous lipid for some dextrose-derived calories can decrease hepatic fat accumulation.
4. **Metabolic bone disease** (see Chap. 24)
5. **Metabolic abnormalities**
   a. Azotemia, hyperammonemia, and hyperchloremic metabolic acidosis have become uncommon since introduction of the current crystalline amino acid solutions. Term infants usually tolerate amino acid infusions of up to 3.0 gm/kg per day without overt metabolic derangements.
   b. VLBW newborns may develop **metabolic acidosis** even at low amino acid infusion rates (1.0 to 1.5 gm/kg per day). Treatment is either a temporary decrease of the amino acid infusion rate (e.g., 0.5 gm/kg per day) or a temporary substitution of acetate for chloride anions in the solution.
6. Metabolic disturbances related to **lipid emulsions**
   a. **Hyperlipidemia and hypercholesterolemia.** The incidence is inversely related to gestational age. Treatment is a decrease in infusion rate sufficient to normalize serum lipid levels.
   b. **Abnormalities in pulmonary gas diffusion** have been reported [10, 47]. The problem may be minimized by avoidance of hyperlipidemia. Intravenous lipid should be used with caution in situations of severe pulmonary insufficiency and hypoxemia.

Table 30-10. Schedule for metabolic monitoring of infants receiving intravenous alimentation

Measurement	Frequency of measurement
Blood	
Glucose, electrolytes, including total carbon dioxide or pH	Daily for 2 to 3 days, then twice weekly
Blood urea nitrogen, creatinine, calcium, phosphorus, magnesium, total protein, albumin, transaminases, (ALT, AST), bilirubin, alkaline phosphatase, cholesterol, triglycerides, hematocrit	Weekly or every other week
Urine	
Specific gravity, reducing substances, total volume	Daily

c. Alveolar macrophage and pulmonary vascular lipid deposits [60]. The short- and long-term clinical significance is uncertain.
d. Possible impairment of bactericidal defenses [24,67]
e. Decreased platelet adhesion has been reported. Use of lipid emulsions is contraindicated if severe thrombocytopenia or abnormal bleeding is present.
f. Acute reactions (respiratory distress, cyanosis, fever, rash, vomiting) are associated with older formulations no longer available.

VI. **Nutritional assessment.** The clinical and laboratory evaluation of growth and metabolic stability is an essential part of nutritional support.

A. **Growth (anthropometric) parameters.** Under most circumstances, we recommend measurement of body weight **daily** and body length and head circumference **weekly** for **all** infants requiring hospitalization.

1. Data for preterm infants should be recorded on a percentile grid for intrauterine growth or for growth of preterm infants (see Fig. 30-1).
2. Data for term infants or preterm infants with a postmenstrual age greater than 40 weeks are recorded on National Center for Health Statistics (NCHS) growth charts (1976).
3. **The growth chart is the single most useful tool for the assessment of nutritional status.**

B. **Metabolic parameters. All** babies receiving PN as well as babies who are fed enterally but are at **high nutritional risk** are monitored according to the schedule indicated in Table 30-10.

C. **Indications of inappropriate or inadequate nutrition**

1. Inadequate energy intake—poor growth
2. Excessive protein intake—elevated BUN level, metabolic acidosis
3. Inadequate protein intake—low BUN level, low albumin level
4. Inadequate mineral (calcium and/or phosphate) intake or vitamin D deficiency—elevated alkaline phosphatase level (with normal direct bilirubin level) and low or normal levels of serum calcium and phosphorus
5. Fat intolerance—elevated TG level, elevated cholesterol level
6. Cholestasis (associated with PN and/or fasting)—elevated direct bilirubin level, alkaline phosphatase level and transaminase level

References

1. Alpan, G. *Pediatrics* 74: 375, 1984.
2. American Academy of Pediatrics, Committee on Nutrition. *Pediatrics* 57: 278, 1976.
3. American Academy of Pediatrics, Committee on Nutrition. *Pediatrics* 58: 218, 1976.
4. American Academy of Pediatrics, Committee on Nutrition. *Pediatrics* 60: 519, 1977.
5. American Academy of Pediatrics, Committee on Nutrition. *Pediatric Nutrition Handbook*. 1979.
6. American Academy of Pediatrics, Committee on Nutrition. *Pediatrics* 75: 976, 1985.
7. Anderson, D. M. *Am. J. Clin. Nutr.* 37: 810, 1983.
8. Anderson, T. L. *Pediatrics* 94: 947, 1979.
9. Binder, N. D. *J. Pediatr.* 114: 273, 1989.
10. Brano, Y. W. *Pediatrics* 78: 79, 1986.
11. Brooke, O. G. *Pediatr. Res.* 13: 215, 1979.
12. Caballero, B. *Clin. Nutr.* 4: 85, 1985.
13. Canadian Pediatric Society, Committee on Nutrition. *Can. Med. Assoc. J.* 124: 1301, 1981.
14. Cashore, W. J. *Pediatrics* 56: 8, 1975.
15. Chessex, P. *J. Pediatr.* 106: 111, 1985.
16. Cowett, R. M. *Pediatrics* 63: 389, 1979.
17. Churella, H. R. *Pediatrics* 76: 243, 1985.
18. Dallman, P. R. *J. Pediatr.* 85: 742, 1974.
19. DeCurtis, M. *Arch. Dis. Child.* 62: 830, 1987.
20. Elk, J. Folic acid and vitamin B_{12} requirements in premature infants. In R. Tsang (Ed.), *Vitamin and Mineral Requirements in Premature Infants*. New York: Marcel Dekker, 1985.
21. Elsas, L. J. Nutrition support of inherited metabolic diseases. In M. E. Shils and V. R. Young (Eds.), *Modern Nutrition in Health and Disease*, 7th Ed. Philadelphia: Lea & Febiger, 1988.
22. Ernst, J. A. *Pediatrics* 72: 347, 1983.
23. European Society of Paediatric Gastroenterology and Nutrition, Committee on Nutrition of the Preterm Infant. *Nutrition and Feeding of Preterm Infants*. Oxford: Blackwell Scientific, 1987.
24. Fischer, G. W. *Lancet* 2: 819, 1980.
25. Fitzgerald, K. A. *Am. J. Hosp. Pharm.* 43: 88, 1986.
26. Fitzgerald, K. A. *Am. J. Hosp. Pharm.* 44: 1396, 1987.
27. Fonkalarud, E. W. *Am. J. Surg.* 154: 11, 1987.
28. Goldman, H. I. *J. Pediatr.* 85: 764, 1974.
29. Grand, R. J. *Gastroenterology* 70: 790, 1976.
30. Greene, H. L. *Am. J. Clin. Nutr.* 48: 1324, 1988.
31. Gross, S. J. *J. Pediatr.* 99: 389, 1981.
32. Gross, S. J. *J. Pediatr.* 106: 635, 1985.

32a. Hamosh, M. Fat needs for term and preterm infants. In Tsang, R. and Nichols, B. (Eds.) *Nutrition During Infancy*. Philadelphia: Hanley and Belfus, 1988.

33. Heird, W. C. Nutritional requirements and methods of feeding low birth weight infants. In L. Gluck (Ed.), *Current Problems in Pediatrics*, Vol. 3. Chicago: Year Book Medical Publishers, 1977.
34. Higginbottom, M. C. *N. Engl. J. Med.* 299: 317, 1978.
35. Hrabovsky, E. E. *J. Pediatr. Surg.* 21: 583, 1986.

35a. Husted, V. A. *J. Pediatr.* 105: 610, 1984.

36. Jarvenpau, A. L. *Pediatrics* 72: 677, 1983.
37. Johnson, L. *Pediatrics* 75: 619, 1985.
38. Kagan, B. M. *Am. J. Clin. Nutr.* 25: 1153, 1972.

39. Kearns, G. L. *Pediatrics* 82: 364, 1988.
40. Lebenthal, E. *J. Pediatr. Gastroenterol. Nutr.* 4: 1, 1985.
41. Malloy, M. H. *Semin. Perinatol.* 3: 315, 1979.
42. Merritt, R. J. *J. Pediatr. Gastroenterol. Nutr.* 5: 9, 1986.
43. Montane, W. J. *Pediatrics* 78: 591, 1986.
44. Orenstein, S. R. *J. Pediatr.* 103: 534, 1983.
45. Parker, P. H. *Am. J. Dis. Child.* 136: 77, 1982.
46. Peitersen, B. *Acta Paediatr. Scand.* 66: 121, 1977.
47. Pereira, G. R. *J. Pediatr.* 66: 26, 1980.
48. Phelps, D. L. *Am. J. Clin. Nutr.* 46: 187, 1987.
49. Poland, R. L. *Lett. Pediatr.* 77: 787, 1986.
50. Raiha, N. C. R. *Pediatrics* 57: 659, 1976.
51. Raiha, N. C. R. *Adv. Nutr. Res.* 3: 173, 1980.
52. Rassin, D. K. *J. Pediatr.* 90: 356, 1977.
53. Ritchie, J. A. *N. Engl. J. Med.* 279: 1185, 1968.
54. Sax, H. C. *Surgery* 100: 697, 1986.
55. Schanler, R. J. The water-soluble vitamins C, B_{12}, B_2, B_6 and niacin. In R. Tsang (Ed.), *Vitamin and Mineral Requirements of Premature Infants.* New York: Marcel Dekker, 1985.
56. Schmidt-Sommerfeld, E. *J. Pediatr.* 100: 260, 1982.
57. Shaw, J. C. L. *Am. J. Dis. Child.* 133: 1260, 1979.
58. Shepperd, A. J. *Am. J. Dis. Child.* 139: 71, 1985.
59. Shils, M. E. *J.A.M.A.* 241: 2037, 1979.
60. Shulman, R. J. *Pediatrics* 79: 99, 1987.
61. Sparks, J. W. *Semin. Perinatol.* 8: 74, 1984.
62. Stahl, G. E. *Clin. Perinatol.* 13: 133, 1986.
63. Strelling, M. K. *Arch. Dis. Child.* 54: 271, 1979.
64. Venkataraman, P. S. *J. Pediatr. Gastroenterol. Nutr.* 2: 640, 1983.
65. Walker, W. A. *Manual of Pediatric Nutrition.* Philadelphia: W.B. Saunders, 1985.
66. Watkins, J. B. *Gastroenterology* 85: 793, 1983.
67. Wheeler, J. G. *J. Pediatr. Gastroenterol. Nutr.* 4: 453, 1985.
68. Williams, M. L. *N. Engl. J. Med.* 292: 887, 1975.
69. Wilson, C. M. *J. Pediatr. Gastroenterol. Nutr.* 6: 640, 1987.

31 Breast-Feeding

Jeanne W. Driscoll

I. **Breast-feeding** is an art and a skill. It requires maternal confidence and consistent information. As the technology of lactation advances, it is imperative that the health care team continues to promote and nurture the art. Two good reviews of breast-feeding are found in refs. 8 and 9.

II. **Prenatal preparation** [6,12] includes a discussion of infant feeding initiated by the obstetrician, nurse-midwife, or obstetric nurse to allow the parents to make an informed decision. The pregnant woman should be encouraged to read the literature available on breast-feeding [5,16] as well as talk with other women who have nursed their babies. Nipple assessment should be made to determine nipple protractility, and nipple preparation should begin in the twenty-eighth week of pregnancy.

III. **Postpartum management** [11]. The hospital experience sets the stage for successful lactation. Health care providers must provide support, encouragement, and consistent information regarding the process of lactation and breast-feeding skills. The mother needs confidence in herself to allow both the physiologic and the psychologic processes to develop and mature. Although it is often assumed that breast-feeding is a natural, instinctive process, it is the combination of the baby's reflexes and the mother's learned behavior that facilitates the process.

A. **Physiology of lactation.** When the placenta is delivered, estrogen and progesterone levels fall, causing prolactin levels to rise in the mother. Prolactin, a hormone secreted from the anterior pituitary gland, stimulates the production of milk in the alveoli cells of the breasts. Although the milk is made under the influence of prolactin, the ability to eject the milk is a conditioned response. The **letdown reflex,** the key factor in successful nursing, takes place when the baby comes to the breast and begins to suckle. Nerve endings in the nipple-areola area stimulate the posterior pituitary, which in turn secretes oxytocin. **Oxytocin** causes the myoepithelial cells in the alveoli cells and lactiferous sinuses to contract and eject the milk. The "hindmilk" that is ejected after the letdown is rich in fats and nutrients. Because the pituitary gland is controlled by the hypothalamus gland, the letdown reflex is influenced by fear, stress, pain, anxiety, and the environment.

B. **Guidelines for beginning breast-feeding**

1. The baby should be nursed as soon as possible after birth.
2. The baby should be nursed every 2 to 3 hours or on demand, whichever comes first, during the day and on demand during the night.
3. Supplementation with glucose water or formula (or both) is generally not recommended for healthy full-term infants [11].
4. Both breasts should be used at each feeding, starting on the breast that was used to end the previous feeding.
5. We recommend nursing on each breast for 7 to 10 minutes with additional time added to each feeding as long as it is comfortable for the mother. The letdown reflex in a new mother may take 3 to 5 minutes to occur; consequently, less than 3 minutes of sucking time per breast can lead to faulty conditioning and ineffective letdown.

C. **Positions for nursing a baby.** Several positions are possible for nursing a baby comfortably in the postpartum period. These positions include the traditional "Madonna position" and the "football hold," both of which allow the mother to sit, as well as a lying-down position, with the mother lying on her side. See refs. 5 and 16 for details of these techniques.

D. **Latching on.** The position of the nipple in the baby's mouth is important in the prevention of sore nipples and cracks. The baby's gums must be about 0.5 to 1.0 cm behind the nipple-areola junction in order to milk the lactiferous sinuses effectively.

E. **Common problems in the postpartum period** include nipple discomfort ("sore nipples"), hemorrhagic nipple tips, engorgement, plugged ducts, mastitis, and cracked nipples. Except when infection is suspected, care for these conditions is mostly supportive, and nursing should be continued.

F. **Special situations**

1. **Cesarean delivery.** Breast-feeding should be encouraged, although the mother may require additional help initially.
   a. The mother should nurse as soon as possible after delivery, preferably while the regional anesthesia is still in effect.
   b. The mother should nurse every 2 to 3 hours in the day, with assistance as needed by the nurse or the baby's father.
   c. Analgesics should be given as needed. Relaxation breathing techniques may help decrease pain.
   d. The mother should be encouraged to sleep when the baby sleeps.
   e. The "football hold" position for nursing will prevent the infant from inadvertently kicking the incision.
2. **Jaundice** [2]. In the healthy full-term infant, breast-feeding can be continued in the event of physiologic hyperbilirubinemia. If the baby has a poor suck and is lethargic, the woman can pump her breasts and give the baby her milk in a bottle. This method will help ensure that the baby receives adequate fluid and nutrition while the mother is processing her milk in a physiologic manner (see Chap. 15).
3. **Multiple births.** Women can nurse multiple babies, since the supply of breast milk will increase to meet the additional demand. Detailed suggestions are found in refs. 7 and 9. General guidelines for twins are (1) both breasts should be used at each feeding, (2) each baby can have his or her own breast, and (3) the babies can be fed simultaneously (or the hungriest baby can be fed first on both breasts and then the twin fed on both).

G. **Maternal concerns** for successful breast-feeding include the following:

1. A supportive environment
2. Nutritional requirements
   a. The nursing mother must add 500 to 600 calories to her prepregnant nutritional requirements. Foods should be high in iron, calcium, protein, and vitamins A, C, and D.
   b. All foods can be tolerated in moderation, and variety should be encouraged.
3. **Fluid requirements**
   a. Between 8 and 10 large glasses of fluid (300 to 360 ml each) should be consumed daily. Some studies suggest that ingestion of quantities of cow's milk by the mother is related to colic and allergic reactions in the baby [6,12].
   b. Caffeine-containing beverages should be limited.
   c. Although an occasional glass of wine or beer can be consumed, alcohol in excess may inhibit the letdown reflex.
4. **Medications.** Most medications taken by the mother will appear in the milk, although rarely is breast-feeding contraindicated (see Appendix C).
5. **Rest.** Since both the physiologic recovery of the postpartum mother and lactation require rest, the nursing mother should be encouraged to sleep or rest when the baby sleeps.

6. The nursing mother should wear a well-fitted bra without plastic liners to avoid stretching of the Cooper's ligaments that support the breast tissue.
7. **Infections.** Some viral infections may be transmitted by breast-feeding (see Chap. 12).

H. **Baby behaviors.** Babies have to learn how to nurse, and their mothers have to learn how to breast-feed. The baby's reflexes, including rooting, sucking, and swallowing, combined with the mother's learned behaviors make a successful experience.
1. **Suck-swallow rhythm.** The baby will develop his or her own style, although the general pattern is one of suck, suck, suck, pause, swallow. The mother must observe this behavior and not expect continuous sucking-swallowing coordination.
2. **Normal behavior** during the first 6 weeks of breast-feeding includes the following:
   a. Nursing every 2 to 3 hours or on demand in the day, and nursing only on demand at night. The baby should nurse at least every 5 hours at night and every 3 hours in the day during the first few weeks.
   b. The baby will urinate clear, odorless urine 8 to 12 times in 24 hours. This indicates adequate intake if the baby is receiving only breast milk.
   c. The baby will pass a soft, yellow, seedy stool after most feedings [11]. The totally breast-fed baby rarely gets constipated.
3. **Growth spurts.** There are predictable times when the breast-fed baby will want to nurse frequently for 24 to 48 hours. This allows milk production to increase in response to the increased demand during growth spurts. The spurts occur at 7 to 10 days, 3 to 6 weeks, and 12 weeks.
4. **Sleepy baby.** This is a common complaint during the first 1 or 2 days after birth. The sucking urge is at its peak for the first 2 to 3 hours after birth and then declines during the recovery period after birth. Most babies will begin to nurse well again at about 24 to 36 hours after birth. Others must be awakened for every feeding.

IV. **Separation of the mother and infant** [3,13,14]. When the mother of either a premature infant or an infant who requires intensive care chooses to provide breast milk during separation, the health care team must provide consistent information and support. The goal is first to maintain milk production and then to initiate feeding at the breast when the infant's condition has sufficiently improved.

A. **Use of a breast pump**
1. **Selection of a breast pump**
   a. **Electric pumps** are the most efficient, especially when combined with manual expression.
   b. **Recommended manual pumps** are the Medela Manual Electric and the Lloyd-B or Lupuco pump (see Appendix 31A). We do not recommend the handheld suction-type bulb pumps for expression during separation or long-term pumping.
2. **Pumping routines**
   a. Pumping should begin within 24 hours after delivery.
   b. The mother should pump in a position that is comfortable for her in order to promote the letdown reflex.
   c. Techniques for conditioning the mother to have letdown with a pump include the following:
      (1) Massaging the nipple-areola area for several minutes prior to pumping and sitting in the same room or chair for each pumping
      (2) Thoughts that promote relaxation should be encouraged.
      (3) The mother should pump after holding, stroking, or seeing her baby.
      (4) It is helpful to have a picture of the baby near the pump and to use sensory cues, such as a diaper or a blanket from the baby's crib.

(5) Oxytocin nasal solution (Syntocinon nasal spray, Sandoz Pharmaceuticals, East Hanover, N.J.), may be helpful for several pumping sessions to initiate the letdown and increase the mother's self-confidence in her ability to produce milk. It is best not to recommend its continual usage [6].

d. Pumping should be done every 2 to 3 hours in the day and once at night when awake. Alternating sides at 5-minute intervals several times tends to encourage multiple letdowns and increase production.

e. It is common for milk production to decrease because of stress related to the infant's condition and because of long-term pumping. Maternal fatigue and inadequate fluid intake and rest patterns can contribute to this problem. When the baby begins to nurse at the breast, the supply will increase.

B. Storage of milk. Milk must be collected in a sterile collection bottle using scrupulously clean technique. The milk can be stored in plastic and is best if used fresh [6].

1. Fresh breast milk can be refrigerated for 24 hours.
2. Breast milk can be stored for approximately 6 months in a freezer with a temperature of −18°C.
3. Milk should be kept cool during transport from the mother's home to the hospital.
4. Frozen milk is thawed by holding the bottle under warm water for 5 to 10 minutes and then shaking. It should not be boiled or placed in a microwave oven, since the effects of these types of warming are unknown.

C. Breast-feeding in the neonatal intensive care unit. In general, premature infants will breast-feed as their age increases and as their reflexes develop. The baby's mother needs support and encouragement while this process happens. Since the infant's first response at the breast is not predictive of later reactions to sucking opportunities, and since infants become more willing to suck after a week or more of trial time, hasty decisions should not be made about the feasibility of relactation [1].

1. When the baby's condition is stable and he or she can be held, the mother should hold the baby close to her naked breast to smell, lick, or nuzzle.
2. Feeding the baby by gavage or bottle while the mother is holding him or her near her naked breast will promote rooting reflexes and will encourage the hormonal letdown reflex, which will increase the mother's milk production.
3. **Bringing the baby to the breast to suck**

a. The mother should massage her breast and nipple-areola area to promote letdown and to increase nipple protrusiveness.

b. The baby is held in the "football hold"; he or she is supported on a pillow and is brought up to the breast.

c. A small amount of milk is expressed into the baby's mouth; when his or her mouth is open, the nipple-areola is inserted. The nipple must be aimed at the baby's hard palate to stimulate sucking.

d. In the first nursing session, most babies will suck two or three times, pull away, arch their backs, and cry, probably because they are used to the automatic flow of milk from a rubber nipple (if this has been used). The ideal situation is to encourage breast-feeding, coupled with gavage feedings, before introducing rubber nipples. If the mother is anxious, her letdown reflex is inhibited and the baby receives no milk. Since this is common, it should be anticipated and the mother warned. Frequent supervised practice sessions at the breast are useful, lasting 5 to 10 minutes per side, if this is well tolerated by the infant. The mother must not expect significant weight gains after these practice sessions. The infant receives his or her usual feeding after the time spent at the mother's breast.

D. Discharge planning and follow-up. When the infant is ready for discharge, the mother must have clear, written instructions regarding the relactation process. The process of relactation generally takes 2 to 3 weeks. Two methods have been used successfully to accomplish relactation.

1. **Relactation with a supplemental bottle.** This method involves the gradual weaning of the infant from supplemental feedings given after each nursing [3,14]. One method of accomplishing this is as follows: When the mother and infant arrive home, they should be encouraged to go to bed to become reacquainted in their own environment. The infant should be nursed at each feeding. After each nursing, the infant is supplemented the prescribed amount of stored breast milk or formula in a bottle, and the amount taken is recorded. The bottle feedings should be done by another adult, rather than the mother, if possible. While the infant is being bottle-fed, the mother can pump for 5 minutes at a time (two or three times at each breast), both to obtain fresh breast milk for the supplements and to increase production. The infant will take decreasing amounts of the supplement at each feeding. When the amount of supplement taken decreases by about half, the supplement is then offered after every other feeding. As the infant continues to take less supplement, it should be offered after every third nursing. This process is continued until supplementation is no longer required. Each situation must be individualized, and ongoing support and supervision must be provided.
2. **Relactation with Nursing Supplementer** (see Appendix 31A) [1,6,12]. This device is worn by the mother during the feeding session and consists of a plastic reservoir filled with 60 to 120 ml of breast milk or formula. A capillary tube leads from the reservoir to the mother's nipple-areola area. While the baby sucks at the breast, the tube is in place above the nipple under the baby's hard palate. The baby's sucking draws the supplementary feeding into his or her mouth. This method ensures infant nutrition while increasing the mother's milk supply and allows the baby to suckle at the breast rather than with a rubber nipple. When the mother's milk supply is sufficient, the baby is weaned from the Nursing Supplementer.
3. **Follow-up** is done by the pediatrician or pediatric nurse-practitioner after discharge. Many women may require daily reassurance and support. Referring these women to other nursing mothers who have breast-fed premature babies can provide additional support.

References

1. Auerbach, K. G., et al. *Pediatrics* 65: 236, 1980.
2. Auerbach, K. G., et al. *Clin. Perinatol.* 14: 89, 1987.
3. Driscoll, J. W., et al. *Neonatal Network* 8: 18, 1985.
4. Hopkinson, J. M., et al. *Pediatrics* 88: 815, 1988.
5. Huggins, K. *The Nursing Mother's Companion.* Boston: The Harvard Common Press, 1986.
6. Lawrence, R. A. *Breast-Feeding: A Guide for the Medical Profession.* St. Louis: Mosby, 1985.
7. McBride, M. C., et al. *Clin. Perinatol.* 14: 109, 1987.
8. Lawrence, R. *Clin. Perinatol.* 14: 1, 1987.
9. Lawrence, R. *Pediatr. Rev.* 11: 163, 1989.
10. Meier, P., et al. *Am. J. Matern. Child Nurs.* 12: 97, 1987.
11. Neifert, M. R., et al. *Contemp. Pediatr.* 2: 26, 1986.

12. Neville, M., and Neifert, M. R. *Lactation: Physiology, Nutrition and Breast-Feeding*. New York: Plenum, 1983.
13. Steichen, J. J., et al. *Clin. Perinatol.* 14: 131, 1987.
14. Walker, M., and Driscoll, J. W. *Breast-Feeding Your Premature or Special Care Baby*. Weston, Mass.: Lactation Associates (254 Conant Road, Weston, Mass. 02193), 1986.
15. Walker, M. *Am. J. Matern. Child Nurs.* 12: 270, 1987.
16. Wossner, C., Lauwers, J., and Bernard, B. *Breast-Feeding Today: A Mother's Companion*. Garden City Park, N.Y.: Avery Publishing Group, 1987.

Appendix 31A: Equipment for Breast-Feeding

Breast Shells (Milk Cups)

Medela Breast Shells
Medela, Inc.
457 Dartmoor Drive, P. O. Box 386
Crystal Lake, IL 60014
800-435-8316

Nursing Supplementer

Supplementer Nutrition Systems
Medela, Inc.
457 Dartmoor Drive
Crystal Lake, IL 60014

Lact-Aid Nursing Trainer
Lact-Aid International, Inc.
P. O. Box 1066
Athens, TN 37303

Breast Pumps

Manual:

Medela Manual/Electric Breastpump
Medela, Inc.
457 Dartmoor Drive
Crystal Lake, IL 60014

Lloyd-B
Lopuco
1615 Old Annapolis Road
Woodbine, MD 21797

Battery:

Gentle Expressions
Healthteam
625 Montrose Avenue
South Plainfield, NJ 07080

Almeda/Egnell
412 Park Avenue
Cary, IL 60013

Electric:

Egnell, Inc.
412 Park Avenue
Cary, IL 60013

(continued)

Medela, Inc.
457 Dartmoor Drive
Crystal Lake, IL 60014

NUK nipples
Reliance Products Corporation
Woonsocket, RI 02895

32 Temperature Control

Michael Fant and
John P. Cloherty

I. Heat production. Thermoregulation in the adult is achieved by both metabolic activity and muscular activity (shivering). During fetal life, these mechanisms in the mother are responsible for maintaining fetal body temperature. Once delivered, however, neonates must adapt to their relatively cold environment by the production of heat metabolically, as they are not able to generate an adequate shivering response. Term newborns have a highly specialized brown fat (their primary source of thermogenesis), which is highly vascularized and innervated by sympathetic neurons. When the infant faces a cold stress, there is increased production of norepinephrine, which acts locally in the brown fat to stimulate lipolysis. Most of these **free fatty acids (FFA)** are reesterified or oxidized; both reactions produce heat. Hypoxia or beta-adrenergic blockade decreases this response to cold stress [10].

II. Temperature maintenance

A. Problems in premature babies. Most infants who are provided with reasonable warmth are able to maintain a normal temperature without sacrificing calories needed for growth. Premature infants have special problems that put them at a disadvantage in temperature maintenance.

1. There is a larger skin surface area for the weight of the infant.
2. There is decreased subcutaneous fat, and thus less insulation.
3. There are less well-developed brown fat stores, and therefore less ability to mobilize norepinephrine and FFAs.
4. The premature infant is unable to take in enough calories to provide nutrients for thermogenesis.
5. Oxygen consumption is limited in some premature babies because of pulmonary problems.

B. Cold stress. Premature infants who are subjected to acute episodes of hypothermia respond with peripheral vasoconstriction, leading to anaerobic metabolism and metabolic acidosis. This may cause pulmonary vessel constriction, leading to further hypoxia, anaerobic metabolism, and acidosis. This hypoxia further compromises the infant's response to cooling. The premature baby is therefore at great risk for hypothermia and its sequelae (i.e., hypoglycemia, metabolic acidosis, increased oxygen consumption). These problems place the premature infant at greater risk with respect to other determinants of neonatal morbidity and mortality [2,5,7].

The more common problem facing the premature infant is the **caloric loss from unrecognized chronic cold stress,** resulting in excess oxygen consumption and failure to gain weight.

III. Mechanisms of heat loss. Neonates exchange heat with the environment in four basic ways.

A. Radiation. Radiant heat loss represents the dissipation of heat from the baby to a colder object in his or her environment.

B. Conduction represents heat loss from the infant to the surface on which the baby lies. Heat loss via this route is generally minimum, due to the low thermal conductivity of the infant's bedding.

C. Convection. Heat is lost from skin to moving air. The amount lost is dependent on air speed and temperature.

Table 32-1. Neutral thermal environmental temperatures

Age and weight	Temperature*	
	At start (°C)	Range (°C)
0–6 hours		
Under 1200 gm	35.0	34.0–35.4
1200–1500 gm	34.1	33.9–34.4
1501–2500 gm	33.4	32.8–33.8
Over 2500 gm (and >36 weeks' gestation)	32.9	32.0–33.8
6–12 hours		
Under 1200 gm	35.0	34.0–35.4
1200–1500 gm	34.0	33.5–34.4
1501–2500 gm	33.1	32.2–33.8
Over 2500 gm (and >36 weeks' gestation)	32.8	31.4–33.8
12–24 hours		
Under 1200 gm	34.0	34.0–35.4
1200–1500 gm	33.8	33.3–34.3
1501–2500 gm	32.8	31.8–33.8
Over 2500 gm (and >36 weeks' gestation)	32.4	31.0–33.7
24–36 hours		
Under 1200 gm	34.0	34.0–35.0
1200–1500 gm	33.6	33.1–34.2
1501–2500 gm	32.6	31.6–33.6
Over 2500 gm (and >36 weeks' gestation)	32.1	30.7–33.5
36–48 hours		
Under 1200 gm	34.0	34.0–35.0
1200–1500 gm	33.5	33.0–34.1
1501–2500 gm	32.5	31.4–33.5
Over 2500 gm (and >36 weeks' gestation)	31.9	30.5–33.3
48–72 hours		
Under 1200 gm	34.0	34.0–35.0
1200–1500 gm	33.5	33.0–34.0
1501–2500 gm	32.3	31.2–33.4
Over 2500 gm (and >36 weeks' gestation)	31.7	30.1–33.2
72–96 hours		
Under 1200 gm	34.0	34.0–35.0
1200–1500 gm	33.5	33.0–34.0
1501–2500 gm	32.2	31.1–33.2
Over 2500 gm (and >36 weeks' gestation)	31.3	29.8–32.8
4–12 days		
Under 1500 gm	33.5	33.0–34.0
1501–2500 gm	32.1	31.0–33.2
Over 2500 gm (and >36 weeks' gestation)		
4–5 days	31.0	29.5–32.6
5–6 days	30.9	29.4–32.3
6–8 days	30.6	29.0–32.2
8–10 days	30.3	29.0–31.8
10–12 days	30.1	29.0–31.4

Table 32-1 *(continued)*

Age and weight	Temperature*	
	At start (°C)	Range (°C)
12–14 days		
Under 1500 gm	33.5	32.6–34.0
1501–2500 gm	32.1	31.0–33.2
Over 2500 gm (and >36 weeks' gestation)	29.8	29.0–30.8
2–3 weeks		
Under 1500 gm	33.1	32.2–34.0
1501–2500 gm	31.7	30.5–33.0
3–4 weeks		
Under 1500 gm	32.6	31.6–33.6
1501–2500 gm	31.4	30.0–32.7
4–5 weeks		
Under 1500 gm	32.0	31.2–33.0
1501–2500 gm	30.9	29.5–35.2
5–6 weeks		
Under 1500 gm	31.4	30.6–32.3
1501–2500 gm	30.4	29.0–31.8

*In their version of this table, Scopes and Ahmed [13] had the walls of the incubator 1 to 2°C warmer than ambient air temperatures. Generally speaking, the smaller infants in each weight group will require a temperature in the higher portion of the temperature range. Within each time range, the younger infants require the higher temperatures.
Source: From M. Klaus and A. Fanaroff, The Physical Environment. In *Care of the High Risk Neonate*. Philadelphia: Saunders, 1973. Chap. 4.

D. **Evaporation.** Evaporative loss depends primarily on air velocity and its relative humidity. Wet infants in the delivery room are especially susceptible to heat loss via this route.

IV. **Neutral thermal environment.** Heat loss can be minimized by keeping infants in a neutral thermal environment. This is defined as the thermal condition at which heat production (as measured by oxygen consumption) is minimum yet core temperature is within the normal range [1]. Table 32-1 gives neutral thermal environment temperatures.

V. **Treatment to prevent heat loss**

A. **Healthy infant**

1. The infant should be dried and wrapped in a warmed blanket immediately after birth.
2. Any examination in the delivery room should be done under radiant heaters. A skin probe with servocontrol to keep the skin temperature at 36.5°C (97.7°F) should be used for prolonged examinations.
3. A cap or other head covering is very useful in preventing significant heat loss through the scalp.
4. If the baby's temperature is stable, he or she can be placed in a crib with blankets.

B. **Sick infant**

1. The infant should be dried.
2. Heated incubators should be used for transporting the baby.
3. Radiant warmers should be used during procedures.
4. Sick or premature infants should be kept in a neutral thermal environment by servocontrolled incubators that keep skin temperature at 36.5°C (97.7°F). The incubator should be kept at a neutral thermal temperature

if a skin probe cannot be used because of damage to the skin of small prematures.

5. Servocontrolled open warmer beds may be used for very sick infants when access is important. The use of plastic tenting (Saran Wrap) over the baby has been shown to be most effective in preventing both convection heat loss and insensible water loss [4].
6. A small, clear plastic heat shield around small infants will prevent convection heat loss by limiting air movement. It will also prevent body heat from radiating to cold walls because the shield will be heated by the incubator air. This may help prevent apnea related to sudden changes in temperature [6,12]. Clothing the baby helps but sometimes makes observation difficult.

VI. Hazards of temperature control methods

A. Hyperthermia. Servocontrolled warmers can generate excess heat and cause severe hyperthermia if the probes become detached from the infant's skin. Temperature alarms are subject to mechanical failure.

B. Undetected infections. Servocontrol may mask the hypothermia or hyperthermia seen with infection. A record of both environmental and core temperatures, along with observation for other signs of sepsis, will help one detect this problem.

C. Dehydration. Radiant heaters are a cause of increased insensible water loss [15]. By measuring **radiant power density (RPD)** and monitoring the weight and surface area of the infant, it is possible to estimate the insensible water loss due to radiant warming in a predictable manner [3].

References

1. Adamson, K., Jr. *J. Pediatr.* 66: 495, 1965.
2. Anagnostakis, D. *Am. J. Dis. Child.* 136: 602, 1982.
3. Baumgart, S. *Pediatr. Res.* 15: 1495, 1981.
4. Baumgart, S. *J. Pediatr.* 99: 948, 1981.
5. Chessell, J. M. *Arch. Dis. Child.* 45: 539, 1970.
6. Dailey, J. R. *Pediatrics* 43: 510, 1969.
7. Day, R. L. *Pediatrics* 34: 171, 1965.
8. Hill, J. *J. Physiol.* 149: 346, 1959.
9. Klans, M., and Fanaroff, A. (Eds.). The Physical Environment. In *Care of the High Risk Neonate.* Philadelphia: Saunders, 1973. Pp. 58–76.
10. Moore, R. E. *Fed. Proc.* 22: 920, 1963.
11. Perlstein, P. M. *Pediatrics* 54: 411, 1974.
12. Perlstein, P. H. *N. Engl. J. Med.* 282: 461, 1970.
13. Scopes, J. *Arch. Dis. Child.* 47: 417, 1966.
14. Sinclair, J. *Pediatr. Clin. North Am.* 17: 158, 1970.
15. Williams, P. R. *Am. J. Dis. Child.* 128: 511, 1974.

33 Neonatal Transport

Steven A. Ringer and
Linda J. VanMarter

I. The establishment of a formalized approach to **neonatal transport** was a logical extension of the high-risk regionalization program of the early 1970s. Regionalization of high-risk perinatal services was advocated following studies [8,12] that linked preventable perinatal mortality with the smallest obstetric delivery services. Grants from the Robert Wood Johnson Foundation were instrumental in establishing the first regionalization programs [7]. Subsequently, Paneth [10] and others [3,4] showed overall and birth-weight-specific mortality to be lower in level III hospitals compared with level I or II facilities. The substantial proportion of deaths seen in the first few hours of life in infants born in level I and II hospitals [9] underscored the importance of high-risk maternal transfers [5], as well as the need for a mechanism for providing expert neonatal care to infants born in community hospitals. This prompted the present era of neonatal transport services [2,4] made possible by portable technology and mobile level III hospital teams trained in the principles of neonatal care. See MacDonald and Miller for a good general review [6].

II. General philosophy of neonatal transport. The goals of a transport team extend beyond the concept of bringing the necessary personnel and equipment to the infant as quickly as possible to begin intensive care. The team should function as an extension of the referral hospital. Medical intervention should be limited to rapid, accurate assessment and stabilization prior to transport. This includes, when appropriate, triage of the patient and notification of necessary subspecialists at the referral hospital. **Care of the parents** should include both complete information and anticipatory guidance concerning the probable course of disease. The **educational experience** for both referring physicians and the members of the transport team should be carefully structured and reinforced.

- **A. Transport personnel.** The team should consist of at least two individuals, experienced in neonatal intensive care, who are competent to make decisions and perform necessary procedures. Our team consists of a transport physician and a nurse. The American Academy of Pediatrics recommends that transport physicians should be at or beyond the third year of pediatric training. Other team compositions are used elsewhere, but our system promotes collaborative practice that draws on the skills of both members. Required technical expertise includes intravenous cannulation, arterial and venous catheter placement, tracheal intubation and chest tube placement, as well as a familiarity with the indications for and dosages of emergency medications.
- **B. Medications and supplies** (Tables 33-1 and 33-2). Required medications and supplies for the initial treatment of the infant should be carried by the transport team and should be arranged in an easily accessible kit (e.g., in a multicompartment tackle box).
- **C. Equipment** (Table 33-3). Required equipment should allow the team to function as a portable NICU. All equipment should function through the use of battery power as well as standard ac current.
- **D. Transport vehicle.** The transport vehicle must be ready to leave on short notice. Many hospitals own and maintain their own vehicles, to provide the rapid access that such a system offers. We use a contracted commercial ambulance company. A vehicle and staff are rapidly available, even when several

Table 33-1. Medications used by transport personnel

Albumin 5%	Fentanyl
Antibiotics	Fresh-frozen plasma
Ampicillin	Furosemide
Clindamycin	Heparin
Gentamicin	Isoproterenol
Oxacillin	Lidocaine
Penicillin	Lorazepam
Phytonadione (Aquamephyton)	Magnesium sulfate
Atropine	Morphine
Calcium gluconate	Naloxone
Dexamethasone	Normal saline
Dextrose 50% in water	Pancuronium
Dextrose 10% in water	Paralydehyde
Diazepam	Phenobarbital
Diphenylhydantoin (Dilantin)	Phenytoin
Digoxin	Prostaglandin E_1 (on ice)
Dobutamine	Sodium bicarbonate
Dopamine	Sterile water
Epinephrine	Tolazoline

Table 33-2. Supplies used by transport personnel

Airways	Lubricating ointment
Alcohol	Masks
Antiseptic skin preparation solution (an iodophor)	Needles: 18, 22, 26 gauge
Armboards	Oxygen tubing
Benzoin	Replogle nasogastric tube
Betadine ointment	Scalpel blades, no. 11
Blood culture bottles	Sterile gloves
Blood filtration set	Sterile gown
Butterfly needles: 21, 23, 25 gauge	Sterile Kelly clamp
Chest tubes: 10 and 12F, and connectors	Sterile swabs
Clipboard with transport data forms, permission forms, progress notes, and booklet for parents describing NICU	Stopcocks
Culture tubes	Suction catheters: 8 and 10F and traps
Dextrostix	Suture material (silk 3-0, 4-0, on curved needle)
Endotracheal tubes: 2.5, 3.0, 3.5, 4.0 mm	Syringes: 1, 3, 10, 20, 30, 50 ml
Feeding tubes: 5 and 8F	Tape: adhesive, paper, and plastic
Gauze pads (2 × 2, 4 × 4 inch)	T-connectors
Heimlich valves	Thermometer
Intravenous catheters: 22 and 24 gauge	Tubes for blood specimens (red, green, and purple top)
Intravenous tubing and buret	Umbilical catheters: 3.5 and 5F
Lancets	Urine collection bags
	Venisection tray
	Water bags for water bed

Key: NICU = neonatal intensive care unit.

Table 33-3. Equipment for transport

Adaptors necessary for plugging devices into both hospital and vehicle power
Anesthesia bag with manometer
Chest tube placement tray
Doppler and blood pressure cuff
Flashlight
Full oxygen tank and compressed air tank
Heart rate and blood pressure monitors with fully charged batteries plus required leads and transducers
Infusion pumps (two) with fully charged batteries
Instant camera and film
Laryngoscope, no. 0 and 1 blades, extra bulbs, and batteries
Magill forceps
Oxygen analyzer
Stethoscope
Suction machine with fully charged battery
Temperature monitor and probe
Transcutaneous oxygen or oxygen saturation monitor and calibration equipment with fully charged batteries
Transillumination light
Transport incubator or radiant warmer with fully charged battery
Umbilical arterial catheterization tray

vehicles are needed simultaneously. The vehicle must be large enough to accommodate the team and equipment and be equipped with adequate oxygen, compressed air, and electrical supplies. Except when geographic distance is great, ground transportation is usually preferable to air transport. Referral of infants from islands or from long distances (greater than 100 miles) merits consideration of air transport.

E. Transport. Optimal transport of ill infants involves the use of different skills than does care within the NICU. These are evident during each phase of the process.

1. Request for transport

a. Referring hospitals and physicians must be made aware of the availability of the transport team, including information on its composition and any policies (age group covered, attendance at deliveries, and so on) that determine whether a specific request is appropriate.

b. Incoming calls should be referred to the neonatologist on call. Pertinent information about the patient should be compiled rapidly. Information requested should include heart rate, respiratory rate, blood pressure, serum glucose level, risk of sepsis, adequacy of oxygenation, and specific recommendations should be made on procedures, tests, or institution of support measures. In addition to providing medical consultation, we request copies of maternal and infant records, x-rays, and samples of maternal blood. The placenta also may be required for examination. An estimate should be given of the anticipated time until arrival of the team.

c. At the same time, the team should be alerted, and all supplies and equipment should be assembled and checked, reconfirming the check made by the last team using the equipment.

d. Transportation must be arranged by notifying the ambulance service.

2. **Anticipation**
   a. The assembled team must be informed about the patient. Specific plans and anticipation of potential problems and the appropriate solutions to them are outlined and discussed with the neonatologist prior to leaving the referral center.
   b. Other appropriate services (e.g., cardiology, surgery, neurosurgery) should be informed or consulted before the team leaves. Adequate communication is critical for successful and expedient transports.
3. **Evaluation.** On arrival at the referring hospital, the team members should briefly discuss the case with the referring physician and then evaluate the infant's condition. If additional tests are considered, the value of the information must be balanced against the time required to obtain it. If the results will not alter care during the transport, the time is wasted. During evaluation, appropriate monitoring devices are attached to the patient.
4. **Stabilization.** The goal of the team is to rapidly transfer an infant who is in stable condition. While it is important to minimize the turnaround time, maximizing stability is the first priority.
   a. **Airway.** A thorough assessment of the adequacy of the infant's airway includes anticipation of possible events during transfer. A patient who might or might not require tracheal intubation could be closely observed if already in a NICU; while on transport, any possibility that the infant may need tracheal intubation mandates that this procedure be done prior to leaving the referring hospital.
   b. **Respiratory support.** After assessing and/or establishing the airway, support with supplemental oxygen, mechanical ventilation, or both should be initiated as required. The adequacy of support should be gauged by clinical evaluation, appropriate degree of chest movement, and transcutaneous oxygen measurements. Repeated sampling of blood for determination of blood gases is often too time consuming or impossible. We use oxygen saturation monitors to measure oxygenation during transport. The possibility of air leaks should always be considered. If pneumothorax is present, a chest tube should be inserted and connected to a drain. The use of a Heimlich one-way valve is usually more convenient for transport than is a standard water-seal apparatus. Establishment of an airway and adequate respiratory support ensures that **hypoxia** and **hypercarbia** are avoided.
   c. **Vascular access.** Every infant requiring transport should have some form of vascular access. A peripheral intravenous cannula is often adequate, but special circumstances may make central venous or arterial access necessary, usually by means of the umbilical vessels. Use of the time required for umbilical arterial catheter placement is justified **only** when it is deemed the **only safe** and **stable** vascular access route available. The need for monitoring of arterial blood gases is not an indication since no blood gas determinations are available in the ambulance.
   d. **Temperature stabilization.** The infant must be maintained in an appropriate thermal environment during evaluation and stabilization. If the referring hospital's equipment is not adequate, the transport incubator should be used. **Hypothermia** must be avoided or corrected (see Chap. 32).
   e. **Metabolic and hemodynamic stabilization.** Correction and/or prevention of metabolic abnormalities (specifically **hypoglycemia**) and hemodynamic instability (primarily **hypotension**) is largely accomplished through attention to temperature and cardio-respiratory abnormalities. Glucose infusions are given to maintain normal serum levels. Volume expanders such as albumin 5% or pressors, such as dopamine, may be administered by slow infusion to improve blood pressure and peripheral perfusion.

f. **Antibiotic therapy.** Any infant born with significant risk factors for infection or an infant whose illness cannot be definitively ascribed to a noninfectious etiology should be rapidly evaluated for infection, including blood and other appropriate cultures. Broad-spectrum antibiotics should be administered.

g. **Specialized stabilization therapy for special problems** [11].

(1) **Anemia** (see Chap. 16). A variety of conditions may result in anemia in the newborn, including twin-to-twin transfusion, perinatal hemorrhage, and hydrops fetalis. Acute hemorrhage may not be reflected in the hematocrit for several hours but is suggested by history and clinical presentation. In such cases, cross-matching of blood for transfusion should begin at the referral hospital while the transport team is en route. Emergently ill infants should be transfused with non-cross-matched type O-negative cells until other blood is available.

(2) **Congenital diaphragmatic hernia** (see Chap. 27). In infants in whom congenital diaphragmatic hernia is suspected, we perform immediate endotracheal intubation and place a nasogastric tube to prevent gaseous distension of herniated viscera during respiratory support. Such infants should be well sedated (usually with fentanyl) and be given pancuronium. Mechanical ventilation is accomplished at high rates and the lowest possible peak pressures in order to avoid air leak. Close attention to adequate oxygenation and avoidance of acidemia are mandatory.

(3) **Abdominal wall defects** (see Chap. 27). Both omphalocele and gastroschisis are treated by placement of a nasogastric tube and immediate wrapping of exposed viscera with warm, sterile saline-soaked gauze. An outer wrapping with a plastic bag or plastic wrap will decrease heat and insensible water losses. Associated abnormalities are common with omphalocele, including hypoglycemia in the Beckwith-Wiedeman syndrome, as well as cardiac, genitourinary, and skeletal defects.

(4) **Tracheoesophageal fistula and esophageal atresia** (see Chap. 27). Positive pressure ventilation should be avoided if possible in order to avoid overdistension of the gastrointestinal tract. It is sometimes possible to safely ventilate by advancing the tip of the endotracheal tube past the opening of the fistula, but this approach risks selectively intubating a single mainstem bronchus. In all cases, a Replogle-type (sump) tube should be placed gently in the esophageal pouch to minimize the risk of aspiration.

(5) **Neural tube defects** (see Chap. 21). These should be carefully wrapped in warm saline-soaked gauze and plastic wrap for protection and to minimize heat and fluid loss, as well as to prevent contamination with stool.

(6) **Hydrops fetalis.** In addition to evaluation and treatment of any associated anemia, effusions found in any of several locations frequently must be rapidly treated. Respiratory embarrassment due to pleural effusions or ascites can be relieved through immediate thoracentesis followed by chest tube placement drainage. Similarly, drainage can reverse the circulatory compromise caused by a sizable pericardial effusion. Cardiotonic and vasopressor agents may be required to support cardiac output.

(7) **Cyanotic congenital heart disease** (see Chap. 14). When this is a possible diagnosis, prostaglandin E_1 (PGE_1) must be available on transport, and administration should be initiated at the referring hospital. Apnea, hyperthermia and hypotension are common side effects of PGE_1. Prophylactic endotracheal intubation is usually warranted for transport of an infant who requires prostaglandin infusion.

5. **Parents.** Following evaluation and initial stabilization, a team member should talk with the family. Parental anxiety is understandably high; even a relatively minor illness appears much more serious if it means that the infant must be separated from his or her parents and be taken to a distant, unknown hospital. Such fears can be minimized by a thorough discussion of the infant's problems and prognosis, as well as an explanation of the plan of care during the transport itself. Brief directions to the referral center and the location of the NICU are helpful, as is a list of the specific personnel who will care for the baby and their phone numbers. After the infant is placed in the transport incubator, we bring the infant to visit the parents on the way to the ambulance. We also try to leave a picture of the infant with the parents.
6. **Transport.** Before leaving on the return trip, the medical and nursing team at the receiving NICU is notified. If the infant's condition will require subspecialty or surgical care, these physicians should be contacted as well. Careful anticipation of problems before leaving the referring hospital will decrease the likelihood of emergency procedures being necessary while en route. If, despite these precautions, a sudden deterioration occurs, it is usually best to stop the transport vehicle while interventions are made.

F. **Air transport** [1]. Ground transportation is usually the preferred route for infant transport over short distances, but on occasion, the long distances involved or referrals from an island hospital make air transport a better alternative. A decreased ability to accurately monitor a patient's clinical status during flight (owing to noise or vibration) can be partially offset by anticipatory institution of therapy (e.g., intubation for otherwise debatable indications) and additional monitoring devices (e.g., pulse oximetry). However, the limited space and access to the patient make acute interventions very difficult, if not impossible. If air transports are done regularly by the team, all personnel must have additional training in proper and safe operating procedures in and around the types of aircraft used. Additionally, two physiologic phenomena must be considered.

1. **Partial pressure of oxygen.** Oxygen comprises about 21 percent of air. The barometric pressure drops as altitude increases, leading to a net decrease in oxygen tension. This is important even in pressurized-cabin aircraft, because pressure is usually maintained at a level equal to 8000 to 10,000 ft above sea level. To correct for this, $F\text{IO}_2$ must be increased to result in an adequate PaO_2. The easiest and most expeditious way to monitor and adjust $F\text{IO}_2$ is to employ transcutaneous monitoring techniques. In lieu of this, the PaO_2 is estimated from the alveolar gas equation, which can be simplified to [13]

$$PaO_2 = F\text{IO}_2\,(P_B - 47) - \frac{PaCO_2}{R}$$

where PaO_2 = arterial PO_2
$F\text{IO}_2$ = fraction of inspired oxygen
P_B = barometric pressure (assume = 760 mmHg at sea level)
47 = vapor pressure of water at 37°C
$PaCO_2$ = arterial PCO_2
R = respiratory quotient

If one assumes a $PaCO_2$ of 40 mmHg and an R of about 1, the simplified equation is employed to calculate the necessary $F\text{IO}_2$ for maintenance of PaO_2 for a given change in barometric pressure. The barometric pressure in the aircraft cabin is available from the flight crew. Use of Table 33-4 is a rapid way to do this. Thus an infant who requires a fractional concentration of inspired oxygen ($F\text{IO}_2$) equal to 0.40 to maintain arterial oxy-

Table 33-4. F_{IO_2} required to maintain a constant PaO_2 at increasing altitude

	Altitude (ft)										
	Sea level	2000	4000	6000	8000	10,000	12,000	14,000	16,000	18,000	20,000
	0.21	0.23	0.24	0.27	0.29	0.31	0.34	0.37	0.41	0.45	0.49
	0.30	0.32	0.35	0.38	0.41	0.45	0.49	0.53	0.59	0.64	0.71
	0.40	0.43	0.47	0.51	0.55	0.60	0.65	0.71	0.78	0.85	0.94
F_{IO_2}	0.50	0.54	0.58	0.63	0.69	0.75	0.81	0.89	0.98		
	0.60	0.65	0.70	0.76	0.83	0.99	0.98				
	0.70	0.76	0.82	0.89	0.96						
	0.80	0.86	0.94								
	0.90	0.97									
	1.00										

Key: F_{IO_2} = fractional concentration of inspired oxygen; PaO_2 = arterial oxygen tension genation (PaO_2) at sea level will require an FIO_2 of 0.55 at 8000 ft above sea level (see Table 33-4). The changing oxygen requirement may be easily compensated for by increasing the FIO_2 to maintain a constant oxygen saturation. If oxygen saturation monitoring is not available, one can determine what FIO_2 is required at sea level and read across the corresponding line in Table 33-4 to determine the appropriate FIO_2 at any altitude.

2. **Gas expansion.** As barometric pressure decreases, gases trapped in closed spaces will expand. Even small pneumothoraces or normal gaseous distension of the intestinal tract may become clinically significant and should be drained or vented before transport. All infants undergoing air transport should have a nasogastric tube placed prior to takeoff.

G. **Posttransport responsibilities.** The team is responsible for accurately and completely conveying pertinent information to the care team. Complete documentation of history, physical examination, and the clinical course is necessary. In addition, documentation of issues and problems surrounding the transport will permit careful analysis of the data. This has an impact on research concerning transports and ensures continued improvement in the quality of care.

References

1. American Academy of Pediatrics. *Pediatrics* 78: 943, 1986.
2. Chance, R. *J. Pediatr.* 93: 662, 1978.
3. Gortmaker, S. *Am. J. Obstet. Gynecol.* 152: 517, 1985.
4. Hood, J. *Crit. Care Med.* 11: 419, 1983.
5. Levy, D. *Obstet. Gynecol.* 57: 500, 1981.
6. MacDonald, M. G., and Miller, M. K. (Eds.). *Emergency Transport of the Perinatal Patient.* Boston: Little, Brown, 1989.
7. McCormick, M. *J.A.M.A.* 253: 799, 1985.
8. *National Study of Maternal Care.* Chicago: American College of Obstetrics and Gynecology, 1970.
9. Paneth, N. *Pediatrics* 73: 854, 1984.
10. Paneth, N. *N. Engl. J. Med.* 307: 149, 1982.
11. Ringer, S. A. *Clin. Perinatol.* 16: 23, 1989.
12. Ryan, G. *N. Engl. J. Med.* 296: 228, 1977.
13. Thibeault, D. *Neonatal Pulmonary Care.* Norwalk, Conn.: Appleton-Century-Crofts, 1986. P. 125.

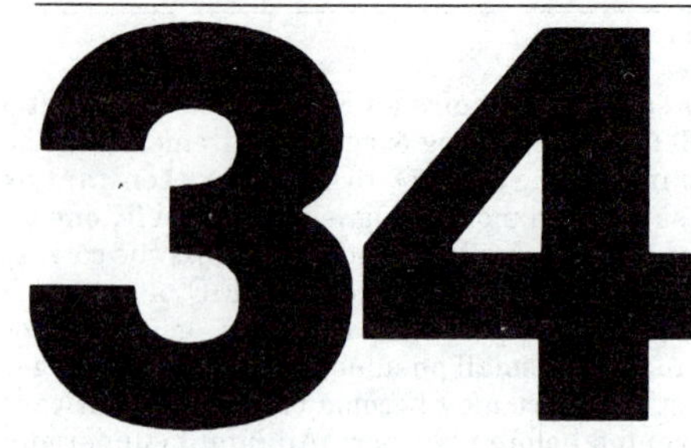

Decision Making and Ethical Dilemmas

Michael F. Epstein

Newborn intensive care units (NICUs) can be viewed as areas that specialize in decision making. Everyday at each bedside, hundreds of decisions are made about ventilator settings, fluids and electrolytes, nutrition, antibiotics, laboratory tests, radiographs and many other matters related to patient care. Systems are clearly in place; expectations are specific and shared by all professional groups and families. This smoothly functioning apparatus, however, is occasionally stressed to its limits when a particular group of decisions is raised for consideration—decisions about instituting, withholding, or withdrawing life-supporting therapy.

These decisions are much more frequently faced in the NICU than in the context of a regular medical or surgical unit. Mortality rates of 10 to 15 percent in referral NICUs are common. Issues such as extreme prematurity, multiple congenital anomalies, severe depression at birth, and chronic ventilator dependency regularly occur, and caregivers are faced with difficult choices. Physicians, nurses, and parents sometimes struggle to first identify these choices and then to identify a process for making decisions between difficult choices.

This chapter will not attempt an overview of biomedical ethical theories or their application in the NICU. Rather, it will suggest an approach to making decisions. It will focus on process and less so on substance. Since these questions inevitably are asked by parents or house officers rotating through a NICU, even if the senior physicians and staff nurses have settled on an approach, it is important to be able to explain the process. This is immeasurably aided by a written policy and procedure indicating a consensus on this issue by physicians and nurses who work in the NICU. The effort to reach consensus on such a policy/procedure is perhaps as important as the document itself, but both have great value. The effort to reach consensus allows the caregivers to explore and discuss not just the "facts and literature" upon which, for example, decisions to resuscitate 24-week premature infants are made, but it also allows and encourages a discussion of values and beliefs that of necessity play a critical role in addressing ethically troubling issues of care. In our pluralistic society where there is no national religion and where many laws differ from state to state, the influence of individual values, beliefs, and moral accountability is maximized. The opportunity to discuss these questions at a time and place distant from a specific patient will ease the process for all involved when the actual case needs a decision.

The following suggestions may prove helpful in the clinical setting as the caregivers and families face these difficult decisions:

1. Develop a written set of guidelines and procedures for addressing difficult decisions regarding patient care. Focus on process (who, when, where) as well as on substance (how). Identify areas of consensus as well as those of disagreement. Identify your guiding principles, e.g., focus on best interests of child, parents are equal partners in decision making, quality of life is a relevant factor in these decisions, etc. Have these guidelines available in the NICU and have them included in orientation of new nursing and medical staffs.
2. Identify common decision models and situations (e.g., extreme prematurity, complex multiple malformations, severe asphyxia), and develop a series of multidisciplinary rounds or conferences to discuss these issues. Develop a consen-

sus on the group's values and its tolerance for differences. Develop models for discussion and a facility for managing these complex problems. Establish trust between the professionals so that at least the caregivers are prepared when these situations arise.

3. Identify resources that the primary caregivers and parents can call on if desired. What are the roles of social service, hospital chaplains, hospital legal counsel? Is there an ethics committee or infant care committee at your hospital? What is its role? What policies already exist in your hospital regarding DNR ("Do not resuscitate") or withdrawal of life support? What is your department's or division's policy regarding these issues? What do the professional codes of ethics of the AMA and ANA say regarding these issues? What are the laws—federal as well as state—where you practice?
4. A special effort needs to be made to define the role of parents in these issues. Are parents the formal decision makers, partners with the caregivers, or the passive recipients of predetermined decisions? Who communicates with families and under what circumstances?
5. Decisions should be based on the most accurate, up-to-date, and available essential medical information. Good ethics starts with good facts. Consult widely, and take the necessary time to accumulate the data. Do not set **certainty** as your goal—it is almost never achievable in the NICU. A reasonable degree of medical certainty is achievable—as the weight of the decision's consequences increases, so will the rigor of the requirement for a reasonable degree of certainty. Uncertainty will never be totally eliminated.
6. Decision making optimally should be broad based and as free from temporal urgency as possible. **Broad based** means relevant caregivers, family members, and others as defined by "responsibility for the patient's well-being." A resident who is on another team is not relevant. A nurse who does not know the baby or family but who will be caring for the baby tonight is. Some grandparents are relevant; others are not. The primary physician, nurse, and parents determine the group.
7. Decision making must start out by identifying options and then using the agreed-on guidelines with the principles that are caregivers in the unit have agreed on to choose among the options. Most units identify the best interests of the child and the application of a benefit/burden calculus as an operating procedure. Guidelines on how to determine the best interests and evaluate benefits/burdens should already have emerged from meetings, rounds, and discussions among the medical and nursing staffs.
8. Individual caregivers must feel capable of removing themselves from patient care responsibility if their moral sense or conscience is in conflict with the decision of the primary team and the parents.
9. Parents and caregivers must have the opportunity to appeal decisions regarding care to another individual, e.g., the NICU medical director, hospital lawyer, or group of individuals, such as the ethics committee, the courts, etc.

Decision making in the NICU when it applies to life and death decisions in morally ambiguous situations can create terribly uncomfortable dilemmas. A dilemma exists when equally forceful moral arguments support opposite courses of action. People of good conscience and fine moral character can disagree. Medical facts can be uncertain. Parents and even caregivers can be immobilized by emotion. Yet decisions must be made. No system will result in 100 percent certainty that the "right" decision will always be made; however, a system that is inclusive rather than exclusive, systematic and purposeful rather than haphazard and rushed, and is built on an approach that anticipates these issues, discusses them, establishes a procedure for approaching them, and involves consensus and trust is a system most likely to result in acceptable decisions.

One controversial area that has been extensively examined in recent years is the definition of **brain death** in newborns, a group specifically excluded by the President's Commission for the Study of Ethical Problems in Medicine in its 1981 publication, ***Defining Death.*** At least partially stimulated by a nationwide shortage of organs for transplantation in critically ill children, many neonatologists and neurologists have tried to define brain death criteria for the newborn. In

Table 34-1. Criteria for determination of brain death in newborns

History
Determination of proximate cause for coma
Absence of remediable or reversible conditions

Physical Examination
Coma—complete loss of consciousness, vocalization, and volitional activity.
Absence of brainstem function:
- Midposition or fully dilated, unresponsive pupils
- Absence of spontaneous eye movements
- Absence of bulbar musculature movement (no corneal, gag, cough, suck, or root reflexes)

Apnea confirmed by standardized apnea testing
Flaccid tone

Laboratory Testing
EEG showing electrocerebral silence for 30 minutes
Cerebral radionuclide angiography or contrast angiography demonstrating lack of visualization of cerebral circulation.

Source: From American Academy of Pediatrics, Criteria for determination of brain death in the newborn. *Pediatrics* 80: 298, 1987.

1987, the American Academy of Pediatrics in consultation with several other professional groups identified such criteria [1] (Table 34-1). These criteria have been debated and discussed widely, and concerns have been raised on both sides of this issue by those who believe they are too restrictive and by those who believe the criteria are too lax and inclusive. (See Chap. 21.)

The discussion continues, but as of this time, two observations appear relevant. For the first time we have a series of diagnostic observations and studies that can lead to a widely supported and officially sanctioned diagnosis of brain death in the neonate. These criteria are cumbersome and onerous, necessitating the support of the infant for at least 7 days after delivery and the performance of expensive and complex studies (EEG, angiogram, or radionuclide scans). Second there are almost no infants who currently meet these criteria. In the three NICUs of the Joint Program in Neonatology, with over 16,000 deliveries per year and more than 500 neonatal transports per year, we have identified no infant in the last 3 years who met the Academy's definition of brain death.

The burden to the infant, the family, and the NICU of waiting several days and employing extensive high-tech testing has been clearly stated by the group at Loma Linda, who attempted to apply these criteria to anencephalic infants on a clinical research protocol [2].

The next few years of experience with these criteria should provide further information for this important issue. In the meantime, caregivers are left with guidelines, not rules, for this very important medical decision.

References

1. American Academy of Pediatrics. *Pediatrics* 80: 298, 1987.
2. Peabody, J. L., et al. *N. Engl. J. Med.* 321: 344, 1989.

35 Developmentally Supportive Interventions

Gretchen Lawhon and
Alexandra Melzar

The challenge of neonatal caregivers is to minimize the stressful aspects of intensive care in an effort to optimize the long-term developmental outcome of the newborn. There is increasing concern regarding the environmental iatrogenic effects of neonatal intensive care. A recent study by Als et al. [3] showed dramatic improvement in the outcome of infants when behavioral observation was used in restructuring the environment and modifying the caregiving techniques. Special care nurseries should have a specially trained professional who is not a direct caregiver and whose function is to observe the interaction between infants, parents, caregivers, and their environment. This will allow changes to be made to benefit all individuals [13].

I. **Individualized developmentally supportive care.** In order to provide developmentally supportive care to each newborn, the primary team assesses the newborn's current level of neurointegrative functioning [1] and incorporates this information into a collaborative approach to caregiving (see Fig. 35-1).

   A. **Primary team.** For each newborn, a specific primary nurse, physician, and social worker are identified within 24 hours of admission.

   B. **Collaborative practice.** In addition to the daily rounds at the bedside, each newborn's primary team meets on a regular basis, thus creating a milieu that fosters both cooperation and communication. The resulting individualized plan of care for each newborn is documented and referred to by all other caregivers in the intensive care unit.

II. **Enhancement of physical environment.** It has been observed that the immature nervous system of the premature infant is stressed by the nursery environment [7]. The premature infant is unable to selectively process input; thus large amounts of tactile, auditory, visual, and kinesthetic stimuli may be overloading or stressful for the infant.

   A. **Overall newborn intensive care unit environment.** Providing developmentally supportive care requires the reduction of environmental onslaught to the newborn [8,14].

      1. **Light.** The alternative to bright overhead lighting is individualized bedside controlled lighting with dimmer capacity. The degree of lighting in the room should be necessary to provide critical care for an infant without impinging on the needs of other infants.

      2. **Noise.** Owing to the potentially dangerous sound levels in the NICU [4,10], infants are transferred from warming tables into isolettes as soon as possible. The auditory impact on each infant should be evaluated and kept to a minimum. This includes noise from conversation, phones, doors, wastebaskets, intercoms, and extraneous mechanical devices, including isolette motor noise [5].

   B. **Infant's individual bed space.** If the infant must be on the warming table, rounds are held away from the bedside and the infant is protected from the environment by a plastic wrap or a light blanket. When premature infants are stable, they should be moved to isolettes as soon as possible. The isolette may be covered with a heavy blanket to reduce light and noise. Proper cardiac and respiratory monitoring ensures the safety even of infants on respirators. Those infants who have been assessed as acutely sensitive to environmental stimuli are located in less hectic areas, away from sinks, doors, and heav traffic patterns.

III. Enhancement of direct caregiving to the environment. Immediately upon ad mission, the infant's flexed posture is supported with blanket rolls, nesting, anc or swaddling. The practice of providing hands-on containment replaces the use c any physical restraints during procedures. Prone or sidelying position improve physiologic functioning and therefore is preferred over the supine position [11 Clothing infants and the use of personal linen encourages parent-infan attachment.

A. Timing and sequence of interventions. The primary team coordinates an schedules all the interventions for a 24-hour period into clusters of caregiving This provides periods of rest-promoting sleep and optimal growth. Each inter vention is evaluated and assessed as to its necessity for that infant. Care giving is scheduled on either a 3- or 4-hourly interval, based on both the in fant's pulmonary needs and feeding tolerance. Each infant's caregivin schedule is coordinated with the family visiting routine.

B. Feeding patterns. Infants are fed on a 3- or 4-hourly bolus feeding patter unless otherwise indicated by special problems. Indwelling versus intermit tent gavage insertion is individualized, as well as initiation of breast/bottl feeding. Nonnutritive sucking is encouraged for self-consolation and wit feeding [2,6,12].

C. Bathing practices. The most fragile infants are bathed no more than twice week, avoiding soap and other drying agents. When the individual infant i assessed to be able to handle tub bathing, it is done with warm water and ful immersion. As soon as possible, bathing becomes a parenting activity.

D. Transition facilation. In addition to providing brief periods of rest and recov ery between manipulations, the infant is put in a comfortable position an calmed following caregiving. Individualized self-consoling efforts are encour aged, such as sucking, grasping, and hand-to-mouth/face behaviors [3]. Thi necessitates using oversized oxyhoods and early use of nasal cannulas.

E. Sleep organization. When approaching the sleeping infant for caregiving, quiet, gentle manner is used in an effort to minimize the stress of sleep dis ruption. Previously described self-consoling behaviors are encouraged an reinforced to promote sleep maturation. When the infant has fallen asleep careful attention is directed at maintaining and protecting the sleep state.

F. Organization of attention/interaction. As the alert state emerges, it is neces sary to ensure protection from the environment and very gradually cultivat beginning alerting behaviors. Caregiver interactions are titrated individuall depending on behavioral cues of the newborn [2]. Interactive experiences ar planned separate from unpleasant manipulations to enhance parent-infan interaction.

IV. Enhancement of parent-infant interaction. In the course of admission, parent are given a packet containing information on the organization of the intensiv care unit and relevant explanations of intensive care. Parent participation is en couraged and supported throughout the infant's hospitalization. The inclusion o parents as members of the primary team facilitates the transition to parentin and increases parental confidence.

A. Provision of knowledge. Information concerning each newborn is communi cated not only informally at the bedside, but through regularly scheduled fam ily meetings with the primary team. Other methods of teaching parents ar the use of audiovisual aids and the parent support group.

B. Utilization of behavioral assessment. Teaching parents about their infant' behavior guides their interaction with their infant and gives them confidenc in caregiving [9]. Infants are assessed before, during, and after usual care giving utilizing the observation sheet (Fig. 35-1) to document individual be haviors. This behavioral assessment is integrated into the infant's plan c care. An example of how this form is used is seen in ref. 9.

C. Discharge planning. Throughout the infant's hospitalization, the primar team models caregiving, thus supporting parents' increasing confidence an

OBSERVATION SHEET Name: ______________ Date: __________ Sheet Number ________

			Time:				
			0-2	3-4	5-6	7-8	9-10
Resp:	Regular						
	Irregular						
	Slow						
	Fast						
	Pause						
Color:	Jaundice						
	Pink						
	Pale						
	Webb						
	Red						
	Dusky						
	Blue						
	Tremor						
	Startle						
	Twitch Face						
	Twitch Body						
	Twitch Extremities						
Visceral/ Resp:	Spit up						
	Gag						
	Burp						
	Hiccough						
	BM Grunt						
	Sounds						
	Sigh						
	Gasp						
Motor:	Flaccid Arm(s)						
	Flaccid leg(s)						
	Flexed/ Tucked Arms	Act.					
		Post.					
	Flexed/ Tucked Legs	Act.					
		Post.					
	Extend Arms	Act.					
		Post.					
	Extend Legs	Act.					
		Post.					
	Smooth Mvmt Arms						
	Smooth Mvmt Legs						
	Smooth Mvmt Trunk						
	Stretch/Drown						
	Diffuse Squirm						
	Arch						
	Tuck Trunk						
	Leg Brace						
Face:	Tongue Extension						
	Hand on Face						
	Gape Face						
	Grimace						
	Smile						

		Time:				
		0-2	3-4	5-6	7-8	9-10
State:	1A					
	1B					
	2A					
	2B					
	3A					
	3B					
	4A					
	4B					
	5A					
	5B					
	6A					
	6B					
	AA					
Face (cont.):	Mouthing					
	Suck Search					
	Sucking					
Extrem.:	Finger Splay					
	Airplane					
	Salute					
	Sitting On Air					
	Hand Clasp					
	Foot Clasp					
	Hand to Mouth					
	Grasping					
	Holding On					
	Fisting					
Attention:	Fuss					
	Yawn					
	Sneeze					
	Face Open					
	Eye Floating					
	Avert					
	Frown					
	Ooh Face					
	Locking					
	Cooing					
	Speech Mvmt.					
Posture:	(Prone, Supine, Side)					
Head:	(Right, Left, Middle)					
Location:	(Crib, Isolette, Held)					
Manipulation:						
	Heart Rate					
	Respiration Rate					
	$TcPO_2$					

H.Als 1981 2002 02 1M (12/83)

Fig. 35-1. Observation Sheet for Neonatal Behavioral Assessment

competence. Prior to discharge, parents have gained a clear understanding of their newborn infant's current behavioral development and methods of facilitating further maturation.

References

1. Als, H. *Infant Mental Health Journal* 3: 229, 1982.
2. Als, H. *Physical and Occupational Therapy in Pediatrics* 6: 3, 1986.
3. Als, H., Lawhon, G., Brown, E., et al. *Pediatrics* 78: 1123, 1986.
4. American Academy of Pediatrics. *Pediatrics* 54: 476, 1974.

5. Cohen, M. *Am. J. Matern. Child Nurs.* 9: 324, 1984.
6. Field, T., Ignatov, E., Stringer, J. B., et al. *Pediatrics* 70: 381, 1982.
7. Gorski, P., Hole, W., Leonard, C., et al. *Pediatrics* 72: 198, 1983.
8. Klaus, M., et al. The Physical Environment. In M. Klaus and A. Fanaroff (Eds.), *Care of the High Risk Neonate.* Philadelphia: Saunders, 1986.
9. Lawhon, G., and Melzar, A. *J. Perinat. Neonat. Nurs.* 2: 56, 1988.
10. Long, J. G., Lucey, J. F., and Philip, A. G. S. *Pediatrics* 64: 143, 1980.
11. Martin, R. J. *Pediatrics* 63: 528, 1979.
12. Measel, C. P., and Anderson, G. C. *J. Obstet. Gynecol. Neonat. Nurs.* 8: 265, 1979.
13. Neonatal Individualized Developmental Care and Assessment Program, Directed by Heidelise Als, Ph.D., Neurobehavioral Infant and Child Studies, The Children's Hospital, Boston, Mass.
14. Rushton, C. *Neonatal Network* 4: 21, 1986.

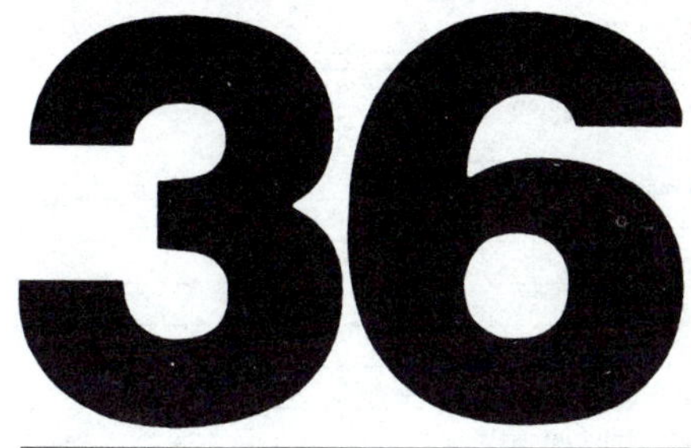

Management of Neonatal Death, Bereavement, and Bereavement Follow-Up

Stephanie J. Skoolicas,
F. Sessions Cole, and
Denise Poirier Maguire

I. **Purpose.** The goal of family management is to establish and reinforce a memory of the infant to facilitate successful grieving. To meet the individual needs of the grieving family, we have used a multidisciplinary approach to the management of bereavement and infant death follow-up. The responsible health care team consists of a primary physician, primary nurse, and a social worker (if involved). Bereavement follow-up provides the opportunity to discuss the events that led to the infant's death and implications for future pregnancies, explain autopsy results, evaluate the need for community referrals, and explore the psychologic effects of grieving on the family unit.

II. **Management of the family with a critically ill infant.** The primary physician and nurse should collaborate to establish an alliance of trust with the parents. They must discuss medical issues at the parents' level of understanding, including uncertainty of outcome. Interventions include the following:

   A. Establish a primary care team that meets regularly to discuss medical and nursing management and make plans for family management.

   B. Meet frequently with parents, provide consistent information, and help them interpret medical data.

   C. Acknowledge and validate the family's and caregivers' loss of control and the inability of the infant to achieve the parents' expectations.

III. **Management of the family around the time of an infant's death.** The primary team frankly anticipates the child's death with the family, preserves the child's dignity, and reinforces the family's importance to the child. Interventions include the following:

   A. Assess the ability of the family to cope with the infant's impending death.

   B. Aggressively support the need for the family to be with the infant at the time near death, provide adequate time and place for the family to hold the infant, and acknowledge and validate the individual needs of each family member at the time of the infant's death.

   C. Reinforce the family's positive role during the infant's life.

   D. Discuss the technical aspects of the infant's death in a simple, slow manner.

   E. Offer the option of autopsy, and underscore its importance and limitations.

   F. Establish an expectation of continuing contact with the family.

      1. Provide the family with a bereavement booklet (see references).

      2. Encourage the family to utilize bereavement support groups in their community.

      3. Verbalize expectation of telephone contact by primary team within first 2 weeks.

      4. Present the bereavement follow-up meeting as standard care following an infant death.

IV. **Management of the family after the death of an infant.** The primary physician and nurse work to foster a sharing and understanding attitude of the family unit toward the infant's death. At the same time, each family's stage of grieving should be assessed, and the family should be helped to understand their grieving process. Interventions include the following:

   A. Establish a coordinator within the primary team who will document the care of the family (see documentation tools, Figs. 36-1 and 36-2).

Bereavement Follow-Up Tool

Infant name:________________

Medical record no.:________________

Date of birth:________________

Date of death:________________

Gestational age:________________

Age of death:____(hrs)____(days)

Route of delivery___(C/S)___(NVD)

Amniocentesis?________Yes No

Abdominal ultrasound?____Yes No

Words used to describe death______

____

____

Diagnosis:________________

Names: Mother__________Age___

Father__________Age___

Address:________________

____

Telephone________________

Marital status:___S___M___D___Sep

Occupation: Mother____________

Father____________

Ethnicity: Mother____________

Father____________

Primary RN____________ ID No.________

Primary MD____________ ID No.________

Ethnicity: RN________________

MD________________

Social worker?________________Yes No

Name of worker____________ ID No.________

Community referrals________________None

__________RN/MD________Social

Family involvement at time of death________

____

____

____

Predeath conference?________________Yes No

Postdeath conference?________________Yes No

Did mother hold the infant?____________Yes No

Did father hold the infant?____________Yes No

Autopsy permission?____________Yes No

Bereavement package given?________Yes No

Pictures taken?________________Yes No

Religion: Mother________________

Father________________

Siblings' names and ages________________

____

Record of telephone contact

Date	Call initiated by	Purpose of call

Fig. 36-1. Bereavement follow-up tool (C/S = cesarean delivery; NVD = normal vaginal delivery; S = single; M = married; W = widowed; D = divorced; SEP = separated.)

B. The physician or nurse who has never been involved in a bereavement follow-up should seek support from the appropriate resource individuals prior to initiating the follow-up meetings.

C. The team initiates telephone contact with the parents within 1 week of the child's death. To assess their state of grief when preliminary autopsy results are available, a family meeting should be scheduled to discuss results. In general, this meeting takes place at 4 to 6 weeks, but it can be earlier or later depending on the needs of the individual family. Involvement of additional family members and referring care providers should be encouraged.

D. To evaluate this approach to bereavement, we use two forms (see Figs. 36-1 and 36-2) to gather data and assess results.

E. The team assesses each family's understanding of autopsy results, each family member's stage of grieving, and the need for further follow-up or referral to community resources.

F. The team communicates news of the death to the referring obstetrician, pediatrician, nursing personnel, and social worker (if involved) by telephone and by letter.

Clinical Review Meeting Record

Review date: ____________________ Location: ____________________

Persons present: ____

____

Check if completed:

_______Review of medical records

_______Autopsy report

_______Implications for future pregnancies

_______Referral to bereavement support group

Another meeting planned? ____

Progress notes: Assessments

____

____

____

Fig. 36-2. Clinical review meeting record. This tool is used to document parental reactions and interactions following their infant's death.

G. Forums such as multidisciplinary rounds, team care conferences, and nursing support groups should be used to help find solutions to family problems pertaining to the infant's death.

References

1. Arnold, J. H., Gemma, P. B. Working with Families. In *A Child Dies: A Portrait of Family Grief.* Rockville, Md.: Aspen Systems, 1983. Pp 135–149.
2. Carr, D., and Knupp, S. *J. Obstet. Gynecol. Neonat. Nurs.* 14: 130, 1985.
3. Childbirth and Parent Education Association of Madison for the Bereaved Parents Support Group. *A Booklet for Bereaved Parents.* Boston: Joint Program in Neonatology, The Children's Hospital, Brigham & Women's Hospital, and Beth Israel Hospital, 1982.
4. Cordell, A., and Apolito, R. *J. Obstet. Gynecol. Neonat. Nurs.* 10: 281, 1981.
5. Estok, P., and Lehman, A. *Birth* 10: 17, 1983.
6. Hodge, D., and Graham, P. *Neonatal Network* 4: 11, 1985.
7. Kavanaugh, R. *Facing Death.* New York: Penguin Books, 1972.
8. Klaus, M. H., and Kennel, J. H. Caring for Parents of an Infant Who Dies. In *Maternal-Infant Bonding.* St. Louis: Mosby, 1976. Pp. 209–239.
9. Lindemann, E. *Am. J. Psychiatry* 101: 141, 1944.
10. Maquire, D. P., Skoolicas, S. J. Developing a Bereavement Follow-Up Program. *J. of Perinatal and Neonatal Nursing.* 2(2):67–77.
11. Walwork, E., and Ellison, P. *Clin. Pediatr.* 24: 14, 1985.

37 Follow-Up

Marie C. McCormick

I. Overview. Systematic **follow-up care** of the neonatal intensive care unit (NICU) graduate may serve several purposes. Each of these activities has the goal of ensuring the best possible outcomes for current and future NICU graduates.

A. Activities of follow-up program

1. **Management of sequelae associated with prematurity.** As smaller and smaller infants survive through advances in NICU care, the risk of chronic sequelae rises. At discharge, many infants will still be experiencing symptoms related to conditions including bronchopulmonary dysplasia, necrotizing enterocolitis, intraventricular hemorrhage, and seizures. Although symptoms related to most of these problems will resolve over the first 2 years of life, medical management beyond the skills of many primary care practitioners may be required [1].
2. **Consultative assessment and referral.** Irrespective of the presence of specific morbidity, NICU graduates require sophisticated systematic surveillance for the emergence of a variety of problems [2], requiring referral to and coordination of multiple preventive and rehabilitative services.
3. **Monitoring outcomes.** As with mortality rate, information on the health problems and service use of NICU graduates is integral to the ongoing assessment of the effect of such services generally and to the counseling of parents regarding the individual child's future [3].

B. Structure of a follow-up program

1. The **population** requiring follow-up will depend on the experience of the individual NICU and the availability and quality of community resources. Most programs use as criteria some combination of birth weight and specific complications. The criteria must be explicit and well understood by all members of the team, and mechanisms must be developed for identifying and referring children to ensure continuity of care. We currently target all graduates who weigh 1500 gm or less at birth.
2. **Schedule of visits** somewhat depends on the needs of the child and community resources. Most programs recommend a visit within a few weeks following discharge to assess the transition from the NICU to home. If not dictated by symptomatic problems, future visits are scheduled to assess progress in key activities. In the absence of acute care needs, we assess patients routinely at 6-month intervals.
3. Since the focus of the follow-up program is the enhancement of function of the child and family, **personnel** must have a broad range of skills. These include clinical expertise in the management of the sequelae of prematurity, neurologic and cognitive diagnostic assessment, familiarity with more general pediatric problems as they relate specifically to the premature infant, the ability to manage the child with complex medical, motor, and cognitive problems, and knowledge of the availability and access to community programs. (See refs. 4 and 5 for other approaches.)
4. The **methods** for assessing the progress of individual children depend on the need for direct assessment by health professionals and the quality of primary care and early intervention services in the community. A variety of indirect approaches now exist for children with few problems and ade-

quate community resources that provide information needed to NICU programs at minimal inconvenience to parents [6].

II. Overview of health status of very low birth weight (VLBW) infants. Over the past 20 years, the infant mortality rate in the United States has declined dramatically. A major factor in this decline has been increasing survival of VLBW infants. This increase in survival has not resulted in an increased proportion of children with severe handicapping, although changes in absolute numbers of children surviving with such conditions are uncertain. The majority of NICU survivors will be free of severe handicaps, although substantial postdischarge intervention may be required to ensure optimal outcomes [2,7]. Appropriate follow-up requires a broad-based conceptualization of outcome, its developmental progression and age-appropriate assessment, and management techniques. We consider health status to include (1) specific conditions or types of morbidity, (2) the effects of health problems on the usual activities of daily living, and (3) mental or social health or both. We are also concerned about how problems in these areas affect the child, as well as impact on the family and other social units [9].

III. Specific conditions or types of morbidity

A. Neurologic problems

1. **Definition and prevalence.** Intracranial events are a major cause of mortality in the neonatal period and a source of long-term morbidity. Severe neurologic problems include significant cerebral palsy, major seizure disorders, hydrocephalus, sensorineural loss (blindness and deafness), and severe mental retardation (IQ less than 70, generally due to a specific deficit) [7]. The risk of such handicap increases with decreasing birth weight: 26 percent of those weighing less than 800 gm, 17 percent of those weighing 750 to 1000 gm, and 11 percent of those weighing 1000 to 1500 gm. Thus 10 to 15 percent of surviving children born weighing less than 1500 gm, will be severely handicapped, a percentage that has not changed appreciably for about 20 years. Less severe, relatively common neurologic abnormalities are also seen in infancy. These include changes in muscle tone (increased and decreased) of various muscle groups and muscle weaknesses leading to ptosis and strabismus. In older children, high rates (30 to 50 percent) of minor neurologic abnormalities, fine motor coordination difficulties, and perceptual problems have been reported, although their functional significance is uncertain [9]. The risk of neurologic problems is increased by extreme prematurity, intracranial hemorrhage, periventricular leukomalacia or cyst formation, severe asphyxia, severe IUGR, and prolonged sequelae such as BPD.
2. **Assessment.** For techniques of surveillance for intracranial hemorrhage and retinopathy of prematurity in the NICU, see Chapters 21 and 38. All infants should have ophthamologic examinations and hearing assessments with evoked potentials prior to discharge. Vision and hearing screening should be repeated in the follow-up program for those with normal findings at discharge and for the emergence of new findings such as strabismus, recurrent otitis, or language delay. Detection of neuromuscular problems in infancy requires careful neurologic examinations [4]. For children beyond this first year of life, specific subscales of routine developmental or intelligence tests are used for assessment.
3. **Management.** Both long-term and transient motor problems in infancy require assessment and treatment by physical therapists. Infants with sensorineural handicap require coordination of appropriate clinical specialty services and developmental programs. Consultation with the schools and participation in the development of an educational plan are important in addressing problems in older children.

B. Respiratory problems (see Chronic Lung Disease in Chap. 13)

1. **Definition and prevalence.** Residual respiratory problems in the NICU graduate include chronic lung disease, recurrent apnea, and airway obstruction. Later in childhood, NICU graduates may experience higher rates of reactive airway disease. The proportion of children discharged

with bronchopulmonary dysplasia varies among different units from 5 to 35 percent [11,12], although most will have resolved their symptoms by age 2 years [1]. The exact prevalence of those with reactive airway disease in childhood is uncertain.

2. The elements of **assessment** include the following:
   a. **Respiratory effort**—resting respiratory rate, use of accessory muscles, prolonged expiratory phase or expiratory wheezing, the presence of adventitious sounds (rales)
   b. **Oxygenation**—periodic measurement of hemoglobin or hematocrit, pulse oximetry, arterial blood gases, or both
   c. **Pharmacotherapy**—serum levels of drugs when appropriate, monitoring for side effects, e.g., electrolytes with diuretics
   d. **Physical growth** (see **IV. A**)
3. **Management** techniques include the use of bronchodilators, fluid restriction, diuretics, adequate caloric intake to ensure weight gain, chest physiotherapy, and oxygen when needed [4]. Instruction is provided to parents in monitoring respiratory rate, use of apnea monitors, use of CPR, and avoidance of respiratory irritants (e.g., smoking). For older children, asthma management protocols may be needed.

C. Other health problems

1. **Definition and prevalence.** VLBW survivors experience higher rates of more general morbidity than children of higher birth weights, but the specific conditions and the relationship to prematurity remain to be established. For example, VLBW infants are four times more likely to be rehospitalized during the first year than normal-birth-weight infants, with 30 to 50 percent having at least one rehospitalization by age 3 years [13,15]. About half this medical care can be attributed to sequelae of prematurity [14], and some includes surgery for common problems of higher prevalence in premature infants, such as hernias and strabismus. After the first year, hospitalization is less likely to relate to perinatal events. The risk of illness not requiring hospitalization is not well established, but a predisposition to infectious problems such as otitis may occur [16]. Considerable controversy surrounds the risk of VLBW infants for injury, accidental or intentional [17,18]. At least through the first year, no increase in risk is seen for injuries in general [18]. Intentional injury or child abuse may be more frequent in NICU graduates, but the data are subject to a number of criticisms [17]. The risk of morbidity among older children is currently being examined.
2. **Detection and management.** The increased risk of morbidity for VLBW infants requires access to high-quality pediatric care. This is both most important and most problematic for infants from disadvantaged families, where the risk conferred by low birth weight is compounded by the risks associated with poverty. Primary care provided to these infants should include the completion of recommended immunizations on a schedule consistent with chronologic age (not corrected for duration of gestation), annual influenza shots for children with pulmonary problems, and consideration of earlier administration of bacterial vaccines (*Pneumococcus.*) in selected patients [19].

IV. Limitations in usual activities of daily living. The concept of limitations in daily living has been developed to capture the personal impact of health problems. For infants, important daily activities include physical growth, psychosocial development, and the degree to which greater difficulty is encountered or increased help is needed than is normal for age in routine things like feeding, elimination, or achieving regular sleep patterns. As children grow older, the scope of activities broadens to include play, sports, and participation in school and work activities.

A. Physical growth

1. **Definition and prevalence of problems.** The normal growth patterns of premature infants are being established. One or more periods of rapid,

"catch-up" growth generally occur during the first 3 years of life, such that only about 20 percent of VLBW infants are below the third percentile by age 3 years [20,21]. The pattern of growth favors head growth followed by gains in weight and height. By school age, average head size is normal for age, whereas height and weight may fall in the range of less than the fiftieth percentile (but in a range that is normal for age) [9,21]. Those at risk for poor growth include infants with chronic disease, malformations and environmental deprivation (nonorganic failure to thrive) [20].

2. **Detection.** Routine measurements of growth should be made and plotted on standard curves; percentiles for both chronologic age and age corrected for duration of gestation should be recorded. In addition, monitoring for iron deficiency anemia is recommended.
3. **Management** of growth includes a careful history of feeding practices and amount and types of food. For children with chronic illnesses, aggressive management with high-calorie formulas may be needed. In addition, careful attention to appropriate supplements is needed, such as iron, vitamins, and fluoride.

B. Psychosocial development

1. **Definition and prevalence.** The psychosocial development of VLBW infants has attracted a great deal of attention. Most often their progress is assessed using some form of intelligence or development quotient (IQ or DQ) on an established scale. VLBW infants tend to average somewhat lower on such scales than normal-birth-weight infants but still within the normal range [22,23]. The percentage of infants with scores less than 68 to 70 (below two standard deviations) is between 5 and 20 percent in different studies; the lower the birth weight, the higher is the proportion of infants seen in this range (but still the minority) [22,23]. Most of these studies reflect the status of children less than 2 years of age. Among older children, the percentage severely affected (i.e., in the same range) appears to be the same, but the percentage with school failure or school problems is as high as 50 percent in some studies [9]. Although such children may have average IQ scores, greater variation in performance on subscales is seen [24].

   Children at greater risk for developmental problems include those surviving at extremely low birth weight; those with evidence of intracranial problems such as hemorrhage, leukomalacia, and shunting required for hydrocephalus; those with severe chronic sequelae such as bronchopulmonary dysplasia; and those with severe intrauterine growth retardation. The developmental problems related to these risk factors may emerge relatively early. Toward the end of the second year, problems related to environmental factors, such as the socioeconomic disadvantage that increased the risk of low birth weight, also may contribute to delayed development [24,25]. The risk factors for school problems in the presence of normal IQs are still being established.
2. **Detection.** Detection involves routine inquiry concerning the achievement of developmental milestones with periodic assessment using established scales or scores. For screening purposes in primary care, the Denver Developmental Screening Instruments [26] provide a useful starting point, although they must be used with caution in premature infants. However, their use does not substitute for periodic assessment by a trained developmental psychologist using well-standardized, more diagnostic observational instruments such as the Bayley Scales of Infant Development [27], the Stanford Binet [28], or the WISC-R [29], depending on the age of the child. School functioning may be assessed with standard scales such as the Woodcock-Johnson [20]. Ramey et al. [31] have reviewed the most frequently used assessment approaches. For specific areas of performance, or for children with sensorineural handicaps, special testing by experienced assessors is needed.

3. **Management.** Management requires coordination of a variety of the peutic modalities and health professionals over a period of time. Early physical therapists may provide regimens to enhance normal motor act ities necessary for other aspects of development. Specialists in infant a preschool development may provide programs of activities for parents enhance acquisition of developmental skills, especially for parents wi limited experience. More intensive interventions based on intense curr ula used in conjunction with home visits and educational day care ha proven successful in enhancing development but remain expensive many communities [32]. At school age, careful coordination in the pla ning of individual educational plans is needed. Such coordination a community-based programs are being fostered by national legislati (PL94-142, and PL99-457) [33,34].

C. **Other activities**

1. **Definition and prevalence.** Parents report a variety of problems f VLBW infants. Such infants may be difficult to feed, requiring prolong periods to finish a meal and more frequent feedings. Problems in regul tion of state may result in difficulty in establishing sleeping pattern over- and underreaction to stimuli, and perceptions of temperamental d ficulties. Abnormal patterns of parent-infant interaction may be set that exacerbate the situation. The exact prevalence and risk factors f these problems is still being established, although anecdotal experien suggests that they are fairly frequent but may not be revealed witho specific questions. In one study [35], 35 percent of VLBW preschool su vivors were described as experiencing limits in activities due to health
2. **Detection.** Few established scales of documented clinical utility are avai able. For the most part, detection relies on sensitive inquiry with suff cient time to elicit problems.
3. **Management.** For many parents, reassurance that such problems are re atively frequent among premature infants and may represent their "no mal" pattern is sufficient. For others, specific management technique psychotherapy, and parent support groups may be indicated.

V. **Emotional and behavioral health**

A. **Overview.** Routine consideration of emotional and behavioral issues in chil health is a relatively recent phenomenon. The recognition of the contributio of problems in this area emerged only with the control of the acute infectiou conditions that dominated childhood morbidity until only recently and is ca tured in discussions of the new morbidity. Most current information relates t behavior problems.

B. **Behavior problems**

1. **Definition and prevalence.** Because children often lack the ability to com municate their emotions, early specialists in child mental health relie on the presence of aberrant behaviors to signal mental health problem Such behaviors included those thought to be associated with increase aggression or withdrawal. On standardized measures of behavior, abou 15 percent of general populations of preschool children have abnorma scores (7 to 10 percent severely affected), with recent evidence suggestin that such abnormalities are associated with a high risk of future problem such as delinquency. Data on VLBW infants are limited but suggest tha such infants are at increased risk for behavior problems related to hyper activity [37]. Risk factors for behavior problems also include stress on th family and maternal depression [36].
2. **Detection.** In the United States, the most commonly used scales are thos developed by Achenbach to elicit parental concerns and those develope by Connors to elicit teacher reports [36]. The youngest children for whic such standardized scales are available are aged 2 years.
3. **Management.** Management depends on the nature of the problem and th degree of disruption that is caused. Some problems may be managed wit

special educational programs; others may involve referral to appropriate psychotherapy services, medication, or both.

VI. **Overall perceived health or rating of health.** Self-rating of health or, in the case of children, parental rating of health has proven a powerful predictor of health care use in general populations. Anecdotal evidence beginning with Green and Solnit's observations [38] on the vulnerable child syndrome suggest that VLBW infants may be perceived as less healthy than their peers, largely as a result of the experiences and parental anxiety related to the neonatal period rather than because their current health status, and these suggestions have recently been confirmed [39]. Such disproportionate concern is associated with inappropriate health care use for relatively trivial illness and may be associated with developmental problems [40]. The prevalence and risk factors for such parental overconcern are being established using recently developed measures. Recent studies indicate that maternal perceptions of child health are releated to birth weight and may be elicited using relatively simple questions such as, How do you rate your child's health?

VII. **Family and social impact**

A. **Overview.** With the increased survival of increasingly smaller infants, the assessment of the effect on society of these survivors has been extended to include such outcomes as the financial and other burdens associated with caring for these infants that may fall to the family or to the medical care or the educational systems. As yet, however, the data are rudimentary.

B. **Definition and prevalence.** Most attention has focused on the costs of initial hospitalization, with much less information on subsequent medical care. However, a recent estimate [15] indicates that the monthly costs for medical services for VLBW infants until age 3 may average 3 to 200 times that of a healthy term child (i.e., $60 to $1200 versus $22 to $26 respectively). This estimate may well be an underestimate, since the study did not assess the full range of direct and indirect costs that may be associated with caring for such infants [49]. In particular, parents may be more stressed by the burden rather than the financial outlay [36].

C. **Detection and management.** Without specific questions, the stresses of caring for such children may be minimized by parents. Careful nursing and social work evaluations are needed to elicit difficulties and to plan additional support where appropriate and available. Such support covers a broad range of activities, including parent support groups, individual parental counseling, visiting nurse and other home health referrals, respite care, and financial aid through Medicaid, Supplemental Social Security, and WIC (Special Supplemental Food Program for Women, Infants, and Children).

VIII. **Summary.** The initial hospitalization at birth in the NICU may represent the first phase of a prolonged period of medical care of varying intensity. The special needs and available resources are still in the process of being defined. However, maintenance and consolidation of the gains in the NICU may require equally assiduous postdischarge monitoring and intervention.

References

1. Hack, M., Rivers, A., and Fanaroff, A. A. *J. Dev. Behav. Pediatr.* 4: 243, 1983.
2. McCormick, M. C. *N. Engl. J. Med.* 312: 82, 1985.
3. Ellwood, P. M. *N. Engl. J. Med.* 318: 1549, 1988.
4. Ballard, R. A. *Pediatric Care of the ICN Graduate.* Philadelphia: Saunders, 1988.
5. Feldman, W., and Pari, C. (Eds.): *Neonatal Follow-Up Programs in Canada: Report of the Seventh Canadian Ross Conference in Paediatrics.* Montreal: Ross Laboratories, 1988.
6. Hutch, L. M. M., Johnson, M. A., and Morley, R. *Arch. Dis. Child.* 64: 1394, 1989.
7. *Neonatal Intensive Care for Low Birthweight Infants: Cost and Effectiveness*

(Health Technology Case Study 38). Washington: Congress of the United States, Office of Technology Assessment, 1987.
8. Eisen, M. et al. *Conceptualizations and Measurement of Health for Children in the Health Insurance Study* (R-2313-HEW). Santa Monica, Calif.: The Rand Corporation, 1980.
9. McCormick, M. C. *J.A.M.A.* 261: 1767, 1989.
10a. Georgieff, M. K., et al. *Pediatrics* 77: 659, 1986.
10b. Georgieff, M. K., et al. *Pediatrics* 77: 664, 1986.
11. Avery, M. E., et al. *Pediatrics* 79: 26, 1987.
12. Horbar, J. D., et al. *Pediatrics* 82: 554, 1988.
13. McCormick, M. C., Shapiro, S., and Starfield, B. H. *Pediatrics* 66: 991, 1980.
14. Hack, M. et al. *Am. J. Dis. Child.* 135: 263, 1981.
15. Shankaran, S., et al. *Pediatrics* 81: 372, 1988.
16. Bowman, E., and Yu, V. Y. H. *Early Hum. Dev.* 18: 165, 1989.
17. Leventhal, J. M. *Pediatrics* 68: 684, 1981.
18. McCormick, M. C., Shapiro, S., and Starfield, B. H. *Am. J. Dis. Child.* 135: 159, 1981.
19. *Report of the Committee on Infectious Disease,* 20th Ed., Elk Grove Village, Illinois American Academy of Pediatrics, 1988. P. 41.
20. Hack, M., et al. *Am. J. Dis. Child.* 138: 370, 1984.
21. Binkin, N. R., et al. *Pediatrics* 82: 828, 1988.
22. Hoy, E. A., Bill, J. M., and Sykes, D. H. *Int. J. Behav. Dev.* 11: 37, 1988.
23. Aylward, G. P., et al. *J. Pediatr.* 115: 515, 1989.
24. Hunt, J. V., Cooper, B. A. B., and Tooley, W. H. *Pediatrics* 82: 596, 1988.
25. Collaborative Group on Antenatal Steroid Therapy. *J. Pediatr.* 104: 259, 1984.
26. Frankenberg, W. K., et al. *J. Pediatr.* 112: 560, 1988.
27. Bayley, N. *Manual for the Bayley Scales of Infant Development.* New York: Psychological Corporation, 1969.
28. Terman, L. M., and Merrill, M. A. *Stanford-Binet Intelligence Scale: Manual for the Third Revision* (Form L-M). Boston: Houghton-Mifflin, 1973.
29. Wechsler, D. *Wechsler Intelligence Scale for Children.* New York: Psychological Corporation, 1974.
30. Woodcock, R. W., and Johnson, M. B. *Woodcock-Johnson Psycho-Educational Battery.* Allen, Texas: DLM Teaching Resources, 1977.
31. Ramey, C. T., et al. *Topics in Early Childhood Special Education.* 1: 5, 1982.
32. Infant Health and Development Program. JAMA 263: 3035, 1990.
33. Palfrey, J. S. *J. Pediatr.* 97: 417, 1980.
34. DeGraw, C., et al. *J. Pediatr.* 113: 971, 1988.
35. McCormick, M. C., et al. *J. Dev. Behav. Pediatr.* 7: 217, 1986.
36. Benasich, A. A., Brooks-Gunn, J., and McCormick, M. C. Behavioral Problems in the Two- to Five-Year-Old: Measurement and Prognostic Ability. Unpublished manuscript, 1989.
37. Gortmaker, S. L., McCormick, M. C., and Sobol, A. M. *J. Dev. Behav. Pediatr.* 10: 266, 1989.
38. Green, M., and Solnit, A. J. *Pediatrics* 34: 58, 1964.
39. Perrin, E. C., et al. *Pediatrics* 83: 355, 1989.
40. Levy, J. C. *Pediatrics* 65: 956, 1980.
41. McCormick, M. C., et al. *J. Clin. Epidemiol.* 41: 323, 1988.
42. McCormick, M. C., et al. *Am. J. Dis. Child.* 141: 393, 1987.
43. McCormick, M. C., and Richardson, D. Long Term Costs of VLBW Survivors of Neonatal Intensive Care. In H. W. Taeusch, R. Ballard, and M. E. Avery (Eds.), *Schaeffer and Avery's Diseases of the Newborn,* 7th Ed. Philadelphia: Saunders, 1991.

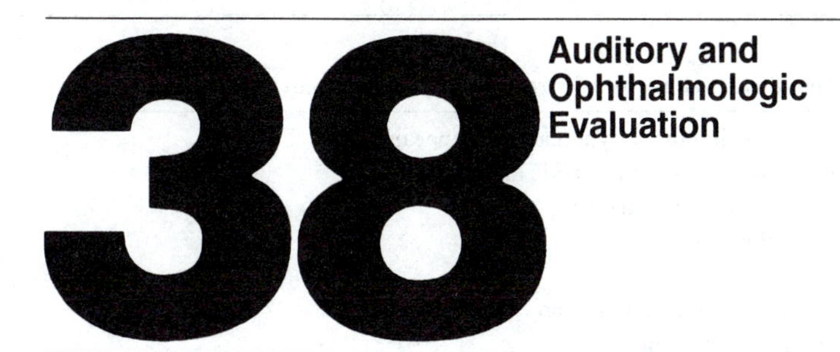

38 Auditory and Ophthalmologic Evaluation

Retinopathy of Prematurity

Susan Hall Guttentag

I. Background. Retinopathy of prematurity (ROP) is an alteration of the normal retinal vascular development seen often in premature infants whose retinas have not fully developed [1]. Approximately 7 percent of infants weighing less than 1250 gm develop ROP, and it is estimated that 500 infants per year are left blind as a result of ROP [5,9]. Not unexpectedly, the incidence of ROP decreases with increasing birth weight and gestational age [5].

II. Pathogenesis

A. Normal development [5]. The normal retina develops through a series of stages, reaching maturity at 42 to 43 weeks postconception. Spindle-cell migration begins at the optic disk at 16 weeks' gestational age and is complete by 29 weeks. Photoreceptor development lags behind spindle-cell migration. Miller cells interact with glial cells to promote vitamin A transport to the developing retina by means of retinol-binding protein. Inner retinal vasoformation then follows the path of spindle-cell migration until vascularization is complete.

B. Possible mechanisms of injury [5,8]

1. Increased numbers of gap junctions have been noted between spindle cells exposed to hypoxia or hyperoxia. This results in developmental arrest.
2. Developing retinal vessels respond to hypoxia and/or hyperoxia by vasoconstricting, decreasing blood flow to the developing retina.
3. Factors promoting neovascularization are secreted by spindle cells and other cell lines.
4. Myofibroblasts invade the vitreous and then exert traction on the retina that can lead to detachment.

C. Risk factors. Many factors have been associated with the development of ROP in premature infants [1,10] (Table 38-1). Those receiving the most attention focus on oxidant injury and antioxidant deficiency states, such as vitamin E (see below) [1,5].

III. Clinical presentation. Because there are no early signs or symptoms of developing ROP, early examination by indirect ophthalmoscopy is necessary. Later stages of ROP may be evident as leukocoria, the appearance of a fibrous membrane behind the lens. This finding prompted the use of the term **retrolental fibroplasia** in the first descriptions of this disease [1,3,7].

IV. Diagnosis. All infants less than 34 weeks' estimated gestational age exposed to oxygen or other risk factors should be examined by indirect ophthalmoscopy by 4 to 6 weeks of age to detect early progression with the hope of early intervention. We examine all infants with birth weight less than 1250 gm regardless of risk factors. Reexamination should occur every 2 weeks until vascularization is complete, although more frequent examinations may be warranted if progression is accelerating [4]. A standard form has been developed to facilitate uniformity in reporting ROP [3] (Fig. 38-1). Information is collected regarding the location, extent, and severity of retinal changes and then is classified based on a schema

Table 38-1. Risk factors for retinopathy of prematurity

Risk factors
Hyperoxia, hypoxia, hypercarbia, hypocarbia
Metabolic acidosis, metabolic alkalosis
Apnea requiring ventilatory support
Blood transfusions
Sepsis
Intraventricular hemorrhage
Vitamin E deficiency
Multiple birth
Bright-light exposure

devised by the Committee for the Classification of Retinopathy of Prematurity and the International Committee for the Classification of the Late Stages of Retinopathy of Prematurity in 1984 and 1988, respectively [3,7].

A. Categories

1. **No ROP.** This diagnosis requires the presence of a mature vascular pattern complete to the ora serrata.
2. **Immature, at risk.** Avascular zones still exist on the premature retina with transition to the vascular zone.
3. **ROP.** Active neovascularization is present, stable, or regressing.

B. Classification

1. **Location.** The retina is divided into three concentric zones originating at the optic disk and proceeding outward (see Fig. 38-1), just as normal retinal vascular growth proceeds from the disk to the ora serrata. Zone 1 is adjacent to the optic disk and is the most posterior location.
2. **Extent of disease.** The retina is divided as the hours of a clock. The right eye nasal area is at 3 o'clock, as is the left eye temporal region.
3. **Severity.** The degree of abnormal vascular response is grouped into stages. In general, there is an orderly evolution from less involved to more severe disease. Staging does not take into account the rate of progression.
   Stage 1: A demarcation line exists between the vascular and avascular zones, representing an early vascular shunt.
   Stage 2: The vascular shunt is ridgelike, elevated above the plane of the retina.
   Stage 3: Neovascularization has invaded the vitreous. This may produce scars that place traction on the retina or optic disk.
   Stage 4: A subtotal retinal detachment has occurred. These are further subdivided into extrafoveal (4A) and those including the fovea (4B).
   Stage 5: Previously referred to as **retrolental fibroplasia (RLF),** this refers to total retinal detachment. The detached retina takes on a funnel-like appearance with anterior and posterior elements that are open or closed.
4. **Plus disease.** This is an additional designation that refers to vascular dilation and tortuosity of the peripheral retinal vessels.

V. Prognosis. The prognosis for visual acuity relates to the stage to the disease. Most of stage 1 and 2 ROP will regress, although progression is unpredictable until vascularization is complete. These stages have been associated with a higher incidence of refractive errors, amblyopia, and strabismus. Stage 3 ROP often results in a high incidence of refractive errors requiring corrective lenses, as well as strabismus. Late retinal detachments and vitreous hemorrhages have also been known to occur [6]. The degree of functional vision as a result of stage 4 ROP depends on the subclass. Since the macula is uninvolved in stage 4A, the prognosis for functional vision is good. Conversely, the prognosis for functional vision is poor in stage 4B ROP owing to the involvement of the macula. In either

Retinopathy of Prematurity (ROP) Ophthalmic Examination Record*

BIOGRAPHICAL DATA

Name ______________________ Hospital # __ __ __ __ __ __ __

Birthdate (MM/DD/YY) __ __/__ __/__ __ Sex (M=1, F=2) __

Birthweight (grams) __ __ __ __ Gestational Age (weeks) __ __

Multiple Births (Single=1, Twin=2, Triplet=3) __

EXAMINATION

Date of Exam __ __/__ __/__ __ Examiner's Initials or # __ __ __

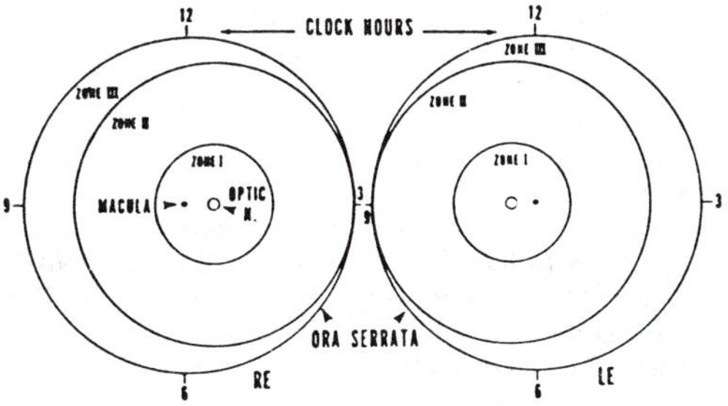

12 ← CLOCK HOURS → 12

ZONE III ZONE II ZONE I

9 MACULA OPTIC N. 3 9 3

ORA SERRATA

6 RE 6 LE

ZONE
Mark with 'X'

Z 1 ☐ Z 2 ☐ Z 3 ☐ Z 1 ☐ Z 2 ☐ Z 3 ☐

STAGE AT CLOCK HOURS

Blank=normal
1=Demarcation line
2=Ridge
3=2+Extraret prolif
4=3+Retinal detach
9=No information

(Grids for clock hours 12, 11, 10, 9, 8, 7, 6 / 12, 1, 2, 3, 4, 5, 6 — three for each eye)

Mark highest stage at every clock hour

☐ If Stage 3: 1=mild, 2=moderate, 3=severe ☐

☐ If Stage 4: 1=exudative, 2=tractional, 3= combined ☐

Other Findings
Mark with 'X'

O.D.			O.S.
☐	A	Dilatation/tortuosity posterior vessels	☐
☐	B	Iris vessel dilatation	☐
☐	C	Pupil rigidity	☐
☐	D	Vitreous haze	☐
☐	E	Hemorrhages	☐

Cicatricial RLF (Reese, 1953)
Mark with 'X'

O.D.			O.S.
☐	I.	Small mass opaque tissue in periphery without detachment	☐
☐	II.	Larger mass opaque tissue in periphery with localized detachment	☐
☐	III.	Larger mass in periphery with traction fold to disc	☐
☐	IV.	Retrolental tissue covering part of pupil	☐
☐	V.	Retrolental tissue covering entire pupillary area	☐

COMMENTS:

____
Signature

*Format permits complete recording of detailed examination results both graphically employing retinal drawing and numerically for later analysis if desired.

Fig. 38-1. Scheme of retina of right eye (*RE*) and left eye (*LE*) showing zone borders and clock hours exployed to describe location and extent of retinopathy of prematurity. Retinopathy of prematurity ophthalmic record.

subclass, acute-angle glaucoma may develop. Finally, the prospect of functional vision in stage 5 ROP is very poor at this time [1,3,7].

VI. **Management**

A. **Prevention**

1. **General measures.** The prevention of premature births would drastically reduce the incidence of ROP. Until that goal is achieved, high-risk groups should receive early ophthalmologic examinations with follow-up examination at intervals appropriate to the severity of the disease [5]. Oxygen therapy should be monitored to maintain a PO_2 greater than 50 mmHG and less than 70 mmHg and O_2 saturations of 90 to 95 percent [2].
2. **Vitamin E** (see Chap. 30). The evidence for vitamin E supplementation is conflicting. Although vitamin E deficiency does predispose to ROP, supplementation beyond sufficiency gives no added protection and may be associated with toxic side effects. Vitamin E serum levels should be maintained at 0.8 to 3.5 mg/dl, and levels greater than 3.5 mg/dl should be avoided because of their association with adverse effects (NEC, IVH, sepsis). This can be accomplished by using commercial premature formulas, all of which contain 20 to 35 mg vitamin E per 100 kcal, or breast milk, which, although it contains less vitamin E (2.3 mg/100 kcal), is a more bioavailable source. However, specialized formulas such as Nutramigen and Pregestamil may not meet infant needs; if prolonged use of such a formula is anticipated, vitamin E levels should be routinely monitored. Current parenteral nutrition formulations contain adequate vitamin E to meet infant needs. Further supplementation should be considered only if vitamin E deficiency has been proven and if serum levels can be monitored during therapy. Finally, simultaneous administration of iron supplements may result in decreased bioavailability and deficiency of vitamin E [9] (see Chap. 30).

B. **Specific treatment**

1. **Cryotherapy.** Preliminary results of the Multicenter Trial demonstrated a significant (48.5 percent) reduction in unfavorable outcome in treated versus control eyes with advanced ROP. As a result, further enrollment in the study was ended with the recommendation that cryotherapy was an effective mode of therapy. The procedure can be done under topical, local, or general anesthesia, with or without sedation or paralysis. The cryoprobe is applied to the external surface of the eye until an indentation of the retina is observed by indirect ophthalmoscopy. This area is then frozen by the probe until whitening of the retina is observed. Subsequent contiguous areas are frozen until the entire anterior avascular retina has been treated, avoiding any vascularized areas that can bleed into the vitreous upon freezing. Again, close follow-up is required in the event that progression continues and further cryotherapy is required [4].
2. **Retinal reattachment.** While still experimental, in the future, retinal reattachment may provide limited functional vision for those infants with stage 5 ROP (RLF).

References

1. Bancalari, E., et al. *Pediatrics* 79: 663, 1987.
2. Committee for the Classification of Retinopathy of Prematurity. *Pediatrics* 74: 127, 1984.
3. Cryotherapy for Retinopathy of Prematurity Cooperative Group and the National Eye Institute. *Pediatrics* 81: 697, 1988.
4. DeVoe, W. M. *Semin. Perinatol.* 12: 373, 1988.
5. Gong, A. K., et al. *Pediatrics* 83: 422, 1989.

6. International Committee for the Classification of the Late Stages of Retinopathy of Prematurity. *Pediatrics* 82: 37, 1988.
7. Machemer, R. *Ophthalmology* 92: 1000, 1985.
8. Phelps, D. L., et al. *Pediatrics* 79: 489, 1987.
9. Ricci, B., and Calogero, G. *Pediatrics* 82: 193, 1988.

Hearing Loss in Neonatal Intensive Care Unit Graduates

Susan Hall Guttentag

I. Definition. NICU graduates are at high risk of developing sensorineural hearing loss. This commonly refers to a 55-dB hearing loss that is associated with significant functional handicaps (i.e., hearing aids, special educational requirements, articulation abnormalities) [1].

II. Incidence. From 1.5 to 9.0 percent of low-birth-weight infants requiring neonatal intensive care will develop a sensorineural hearing loss, although the extent of impairment varies greatly. The risk-factor combination of low birth weight and neonatal seizures carries with it a 28.6 percent incidence of sensorineural impairment [1].

III. Risk factors [1,5]

- **A.** Birth weight under 1800 gm or gestational age under 35 weeks
- **B.** CNS insult
  1. Hypoxic-ischemic injury
  2. Intracranial hemorrhage
  3. Neonatal seizures
  4. Infection (meningitis)
- **C.** Otologic damage
  1. Inner ear hemorrhage
  2. Hyperbilirubinemia (high enough to meet criteria for exchange transfusion)
  3. Ototoxic drugs (aminoglycosides, diuretics)
  4. Congenital viral infection or toxoplasmosis
  5. Persistent pulmonary hypertension
  6. Hyperventilation, respiratory alkalosis
- **D.** Malformation of ear, palate, lip, face or neck
- **E.** Family history of hearing loss since childhood

IV. Auditory brainstem responses (ABR, BAER). At present, the ABR is the most reliable screening tool for the evaluation of hearing loss in the NICU graduate. Electrodes are placed on the mastoid process behind the ear and on the forehead in the midline, just below the hairline. Earphones are either held or allowed to rest on the ear to be tested, and 33 clicks per second for a total of 2000 are emitted from the earphones. The waveform recorded becomes more well defined with increasing gestational age. The auditory threshold, the minimum intensity for a recognizable wave V, decreases with increasing gestational age [6]. Thresholds 20 dB higher than expected at a given postconceptional age raise the suspicion of a hearing loss [4,6,8].

V. Screening recommendations [2,6,8]

- **A.** Infants at risk should have an ABR done prior to discharge. We currently screen infants with the risk factors in **III.** We do not screen term infants treated with aminoglycosides if they were only treated for 72 hours and the serum antibiotic levels were in the therapeutic range. If infants were treated for 7 days, we test hearing even if medication levels were acceptable. If hospitalization is prolonged, testing can be done at 40 weeks' postconceptional age. Since auditory brainstem responses depend on the maturation of the auditory system, abnormal tests obtained while the infant is at a postconceptional age less than 40 weeks may reflect immaturity. At BWH, 10 percent of infants screened have abnormal ABRs. On follow-up, 25 percent of this group has significant neurosensory hearing impairment. In one study, only 3 of 128 (2.3 percent) infants who had abnormal ABRs prior to NICU discharge had a serious hearing impairment on follow-up assessment at more than 3 months' corrected age [7]. Therefore, screening too early may cause needless parental anxiety.

We usually screen sick or premature infants just prior to discharge. If the testing is abnormal, we rescreen them at 40 weeks' postconceptional age or 1 month later. Term infants who are screened because of antibiotic use are usually screened after 2 weeks of age to eliminate transient perinatal problems (maternal anesthesia, medication) that may interfere with the test.

B. All infants with abnormal screening ABRs should have follow-up testing (repeat ABR, behavioral testing, Crib-O-Gram) by 6 months of age.

C. Infants with neonatal seizures or evidence of neurodevelopmental delay, regardless of results of ABR before discharge, also should be retested by 6 months of age.

D. Infants with persistently abnormal test results require close supervision by an audiologist and otolaryngologist. Early intervention programs geared to optimize aural/oral skills acquisition should be instituted.

VI. Prognosis. Prognosis depends largely on the degree of impairment. Abnormalities in auditory threshold may be predictive of language delays [3,4,8].

References

1. Bergman, I. *J. Pediatr.* 106: 95, 1985.
2. Duara, S. *J. Pediatr.* 108: 276, 1986.
3. Kramer, S. *J. Pediatr.* 83: 385, 1989.
4. Lary, S. *J. Pediatr.* 107: 593, 1985.
5. Nield, T. A. *Pediatrics* 78: 417, 1986.
6. Roberts, J. L. *J. Pediatr.* 101: 257, 1982.
7. Rothberg, J. L. *Pediatrics* 98: 106, 1981.
8. Stein, L. S. *J. Pediatr.* 103: 447, 1983.

Procedures

39 Common Procedures

Steven A. Ringer

Procedures are a necessary but potentially risk-laden part of newborn intensive care. The person who performs these techniques in an efficient, nontraumatic way contributes to the ultimate well-being of the infants under his or her care. Good supervision is important as skills are being acquired and as procedures are being done for the first time. Procedures should be carried out as quickly as is safely possible, because the extensive handling of a baby, the possible interruption of heat source, and some degree of nutritional deprivation can be devastating to the baby's outcome. In addition, we use "universal precautions," including gloves and barriers to the eyes, to protect the operator from exposure to blood and bodily fluids that may be contaminated with infectious agents. Some commonly used procedures are discussed here. For a more extensive description, including less frequently used procedures, see ref. 5.

I. **Blood drawing.** The preparations for withdrawing blood depend somewhat on the particular blood studies that are required.

A. **Capillary blood** is drawn when there is no need for many serial studies in close succession.

1. **Applicable blood studies** include hematocrit, blood glucose levels (using Dextrostix or other methods), electrolyte levels, and occasionally blood gas studies.
2. **Techniques**
   a. Better results will be obtained if the extremity to be used is warmed to increase peripheral blood flow.
   b. If only a small quantity of blood is required, a lancet is probably adequate for 3 or 4 drops of blood. If more blood is necessary, a no. 11 scalpel blade should be used, resulting in increased blood flow and a more accurate determination of laboratory values.
   c. When a **capillary puncture of the foot** is performed, the operator should use the lateral side of the sole of the heel, avoiding previous sites if possible.
   d. Capillary blood can be obtained from the side of the fingers (distally) as well.
   e. The skin should be cleaned carefully with povidone-iodine and alcohol before puncture to avoid infection of soft tissue or underlying bone.

B. **Catheter blood samples**

1. **Umbilical artery or radial artery catheters** are often used for blood samples, especially for blood gas studies.
2. **Techniques**
   a. The infusion tubing is clamped proximal to the T-connector, and a small needle is inserted into the injection port. Blood is allowed to flow back through the catheter and needle into a gauze pad until all infusate is cleared from the line. The minimal volume (0.5 ml) of diluted blood is discarded.
   b. For **blood gas studies,** a 1-ml syringe, rinsed with 0.5 ml of heparin, is used to withdraw the sample. The line is then cleared with a small volume of saline flushing solution.
   c. The line must be adequately cleared of infusate prior to withdrawing samples to avoid false readings.

C. **Venous blood** for blood chemistry studies, blood cultures, and other laboratory studies is usually obtained from either the antecubital vein, the external jugular vein, or the saphenous vein. For blood cultures, the area should be cleaned with an iodine-containing solution; if the position of the needle is directed by using a sterile gloved finger, the finger should be cleaned in the same way. A new sterile needle should be used to insert the blood into the culture bottles.

II. **Bladder tap**

A. Since bladder taps are most often performed as part of a workup on an infant with suspected sepsis, a sterile specimen is crucial. Careful cleaning with iodine and alcohol solution over the prepubic region is essential.

B. **Technique.** Bladder taps are done with a 5- to 10-ml syringe attached to a 22 or 23 gauge needle or to a 23 gauge butterfly needle. One should try to determine before the tap that the baby has not recently urinated. One technique is as follows:

1. The pubic bone is located by touch.
2. The needle is placed in the midline, just superior to the pubic bone.
3. The needle is slid in, aimed at the infant's coccyx.
4. If the needle goes in more than 3 cm and no urine is obtained, one should assume that the bladder is empty and wait before attempting again.

III. **Intravenous therapy.** Insertion and management of intravenous catheters requires great care. As in older infants, hand veins are used most often.

A. **Scalp vein**

1. The vein is usually visualized by combing hair away. Shaving the scalp is infrequently necessary and is often upsetting to parents.
2. Generally, 24-gauge IV cannulas are used. Scalp vein needles, 23 to 27 gauge, are acceptable.
3. A rubber-band tourniquet placed around the scalp proximal to the vein is quite useful.
4. If multiple attempts at placement are unsuccessful, one should obtain help if possible.

B. **Foot and ankle veins.** The method of placement of intravenous lines in foot or ankle veins is similar to that in the older infant. The site should be prepared and the limb held and manipulated as required for optimal positioning. Careful palpation should allow identification of a vein, but transillumination also may be useful.

IV. **Arterial punctures** are usually carried out by using the radial artery; occasionally, the temporal, brachial, or posterior tibial artery is used. **Radial artery punctures** are most easily done using transillumination to assist in location of the vessel. The radial artery is visualized and entered with the bevel of the needle up and at a 15-degree angle against the direction of flow. The artery is transfixed, and then the needle is slowly withdrawn and the syringe filled. A 23- to 25-gauge scalp vein needle is most often used.

V. **Lumbar puncture** (see Chap. 12)

A. **Technique**

1. The infant should be placed in the lateral decubitus position or in the sitting position with legs straightened. The assistant should hold the infant firmly at the shoulders and buttocks so that the lower spine is curved. Neck flexion should be avoided so as not to compromise the airway [17].
2. A sterile field is prepared and draped with towels.
3. A 22- to 24-gauge spinal needle with a stylet should be used. Use of a no. 25 butterfly needle may introduce skin into the subarachnoid space.
4. The needle is inserted in the midline into the space between the fourth and fifth lumbar spinous processes. The needle is advanced gradually in the direction of the umbilicus, and the stylet is withdrawn frequently to detect the presence of spinal fluid. Usually a slight "pop" is felt as the needle enters the subarachnoid space.

5. The **cerebrospinal fluid (CSF)** is collected into three or four tubes, each with a volume of 0.5 to 1.0 ml.

B. **Examination of the spinal fluid.** CSF should be inspected immediately for turbidity and color. In many newborn infants the CSF may be mildly xanthochromic, but it should always be clear.

1. **Tube 1.** Cell count and differential should be performed on the unspun fluid in a counting chamber. The unspun fluid should be stained with methylene blue; it should be treated with concentrated acetic acid if there are numerous red blood cells (RBCs). A Gram's stain and a Wright's stain should be done on the centrifuged sediment.
2. **Tube 2** should be sent for culture and sensitivity studies.
3. **Tube 3.** Glucose and protein determinations should be obtained.
4. **Tube 4.** The cells in this tube also should be counted if the fluid is bloody. The fluid can be sent for latex fixation tests for infectious agents.

C. **Information obtainable**

1. When the CSF is collected in three or four separate containers, an **RBC count** can be done on the first and last tubes to see if there is a difference between these specimens in the number of RBCs/mm^3. With traumatic taps, the final tube will have fewer RBCs than the first. CSF in the newborn may normally contain up to 600 to 800 RBCs/mm^3.
2. **White blood cell (WBC) count.** The normal number of WBCs/mm^3 in newborn infants is a matter of controversy. We accept up to 5 to 8 lymphocytes or monocytes as normal if there are no polymorphonuclear WBCs. Others accept as normal up to 25 WBCs/mm^3, including several polymorphonuclear cells. Data obtained from high-risk newborns without meningitis by Sarff, Platt, and McCracken [11] (Table 39-1) show 0 to 32 WBCs/mm^3 in term infants and 0 to 29 WBCs/mm^3 in preterm infants with about 60 percent polymorphonuclear cells to be within the normal range. Higher WBC counts are generally seen with gram-negative meningitis than with

Table 39-1. Cerebrospinal fluid examination in high-risk neonates without meningitis

Determination	Term	Preterm
White blood cell count (cells/mm^3)		
No. of infants	87	30
Mean	8.2	9.0
Median	5	6
Standard deviation	7.1	8.2
Range	0–32	0–29
±2 Standard deviations	0–22.4	0.25.4
Percentage of polymorphonuclear cells	61.3%	57.2%
Protein (mg/100 ml)		
No. of infants	35	17
Mean	90	115
Range	20–170	65–150
Glucose (mg/100 ml)		
No. of infants	51	23
Mean	52	50
Range	34–119	24–63
Glucose in cerebrospinal fluid divided by blood glucose (%)		
No. of infants	51	23
Mean	81	74
Range	44–248	55–105

Source: From L. D. Sarff, L. H. Platt, and G. H. McCracken, Cerebrospinal fluid evaluation in neonates: Comparison of high-risk neonates with and without meningitis. *J. Pediatr.* 88: 473, 1976.

group B streptococcal disease; as high as 50 percent of the latter group will have 100 WBCs/mm^3 or less. Because of the overlap between normal infants and those with meningitis, the presence of polymorphonuclear leukocytes in CSF deserves careful attention. Ultimately, the diagnosis depends on culture results and clinical course.

3. Data on glucose and protein levels in CSF from high-risk newborns are shown in Table 39-1. The CSF glucose level is about 80 percent of the blood glucose level for term infants and 75 percent for preterm infants. If the blood glucose level is high or low, there is a 4- to 6-hour equilibration period with the CSF glucose.
   The normal level of CSF protein in newborns falls in a wide range. In full-term infants, levels below 100 mg/dl are acceptable. In premature infants, the acceptable level can be as high as 180 mg/dl [2]. Values for high-risk infants are shown in Table 39-1. The level of CSF protein in the premature infant appears to be related to the degree of prematurity.

VI. Intubation

A. Endotracheal intubation. In most cases an infant can be adequately ventilated by bag and mask so that endotracheal intubation can be done as a controlled procedure. In an emergency and in the delivery room, oral intubation is usually quicker and easier. In the neonatal intensive care unit, when mechanical ventilation is necessary, we routinely use nasotracheal intubation with a Portex polyvinyl chloride tube, although others may prefer the oral route [13].

1. **Tube size and length.** The correct tube size (see Chap. 5, sec. **11.C.5**) and length (Fig. 39-1) [4] can be estimated from the infant's weight.

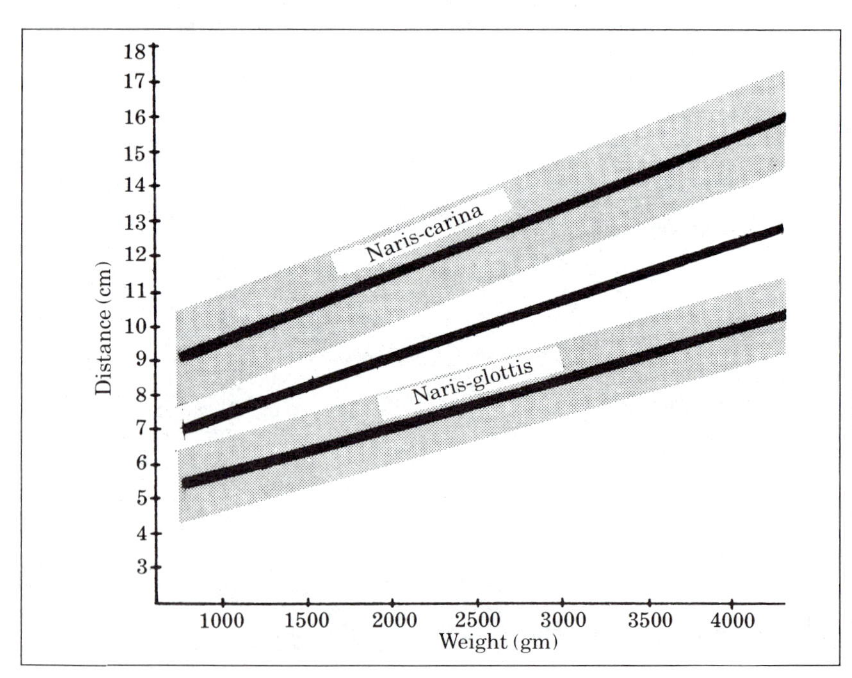

Fig. 39-1. The relation of naris-carina and naris-glottis distance with body weight. The middle line represents the distance from naris to midtrachea. (Modified from J. Coldiron, Estimation of nasotracheal tube length in neonates. *Pediatrics* 41: 823, 1968. Copyright American Academy of Pediatrics, 1968.)

2. **Technique**
   a. The baby's head should be slightly lifted anteriorly with the baby's body aligned straight. The operator should stand looking down the midline of the body.
   b. The **laryngoscope** is held between the thumb and first finger of the left hand, with the second and third fingers holding the baby's chin and stabilizing the head. Pushing down on the larynx with the fifth finger of the left hand (or having an assistant do it) may help to visualize the vocal cords.
   c. The laryngoscope blade is passed into the right side of the mouth and then to the midline, swinging the tongue out of the way. It should be advanced into the vallecula. Keeping the infant's head straight will aid in visualization of the vocal cords.
   d. The **endotracheal tube** is held with the right hand and inserted between the vocal cords to about 2 cm below the glottis. During nasotracheal intubation, Magill forceps can be useful in guiding the tube appropriately. If a finger is pressing on the trachea, the tube can be felt passing underneath.
   e. The anatomic structures of the larynx and pharynx have different appearances. The esophagus is a horizontal muscular slit; it should never be accidentally or mistakenly intubated if this is kept clearly in mind. The glottis, in contrast, consists of a triangular opening formed by the vocal cords meeting anteriorly at the apex. This orifice lies directly beneath the epiglottis, which is lifted away by gentle upward traction with the laryngoscope.
   f. The **tube position** is checked by auscultation of the chest to ensure equal aeration of both lungs and observation of chest movement with positive-pressure inflation. If air entry is poor over the left chest, the tube should be pulled back until it improves. Endotracheal tubes with metal rings molded in the distal end are now available. Tube position is checked using a special handheld sensor unit (Trach-Mate System, C.R. Bard, Inc., Tewksbury, Mass.).
   g. Observation of the patient and monitoring of the heart rate are mandatory. Electronic monitoring with an audible pulse rate frees personnel to attend to other tasks. If bradycardia is observed, especially if accompanied by hypoxia, the procedure should be stopped and the baby ventilated with bag and mask. An anesthesia bag attached to the tube adapter can deliver oxygen to the pharynx during the procedure or free-flow O_2 at 5 liters/minute can be given from a tube placed 1/2 inch from the infant's mouth.
3. **Intubation in the delivery room** is usually temporary, and the tube can be held in place by hand. For prolonged ventilation, the tube should be taped securely in place; the position of the tube is checked by x-ray studies or the sensor unit mentioned above.
4. **Commonly observed errors**
   a. Too much attention may be given to the procedure and not enough to the baby.
   b. The baby's neck may be excessively extended. Slight flexion will sometimes allow better visualization of the vocal cords.
   c. The infant's upper gums may be lacerated by excessive pressure of the laryngoscope blade.
   d. The tip of the laryngoscope blade is tilted upward instead of traction being exerted parallel to the handle.
   e. The tube may be inserted too far and into the right mainstem bronchus.

C. **Nasal CPAP.** Continuous distending pressure can be applied using nasal prongs as part of the ventilator circuit. These are simple to insert and are usually held on by a Velcro-fastened headset.

VII. Thoracentesis and chest tube placement (see Air Leak in Chap. 13)

VIII. Vascular catheterization (see Fig. 39-2 for diagrams of the newborn venous and arterial systems)

A. Types of catheters

1. **Umbilical artery catheters** are used (1) for frequent monitoring of arterial blood gases, (2) as a stable route for infusion of parenteral fluids, and (3) for continuous monitoring of arterial blood pressure.
2. **Radial artery catheters** are used in our NICUs when frequent blood gas monitoring is still required and an umbilical artery catheter is contraindicated, cannot be placed, or is removed because of complications. Radial artery catheters must not be used to infuse alimentation solution or medications. They require that the infant be kept restricted with an armboard in place.
3. **Umbilical vein catheters** are used for exchange transfusions, monitoring of central venous pressure, infusion of fluids (when passed through the ductus venous and near the right atrium), and for emergency vascular access for infusion of fluid, blood, or medications.

Fig. 39-2. A. Diagram of the newborn umbilical venous system (SVC = superior vena cava; RA = right atrium; FO = foramen ovale; RV = right ventricle; IVC = inferior vena cava; DV = ductus venosus; PS = portal sinus; L = liver; PV = portal vein; UV = umbilical vein). **B.** Diagram of the newborn arterial system, including the umbilical artery (LCCA = left common carotid artery; LSA = left subclavian artery; DA = ductus arteriosus; MPA = main pulmonary artery; H = heart; A = aorta; SMA = superior mesenteric artery; RRA = right renal artery; LRA = left renal artery; IMA = inferior mesenteric artery; RCIA = right common iliac artery; RUA = right umbilical artery; LCIA = left common iliac artery; RHA = right hypogastric artery; REIA = right external iliac artery). (From J. A. Kitterman, R. H. Phibbs, and W. H. Tooley, Catheterization of umbilical vessels in newborn infants. *Pediatr. Clin. North Am.* 17: 898, 1970.)

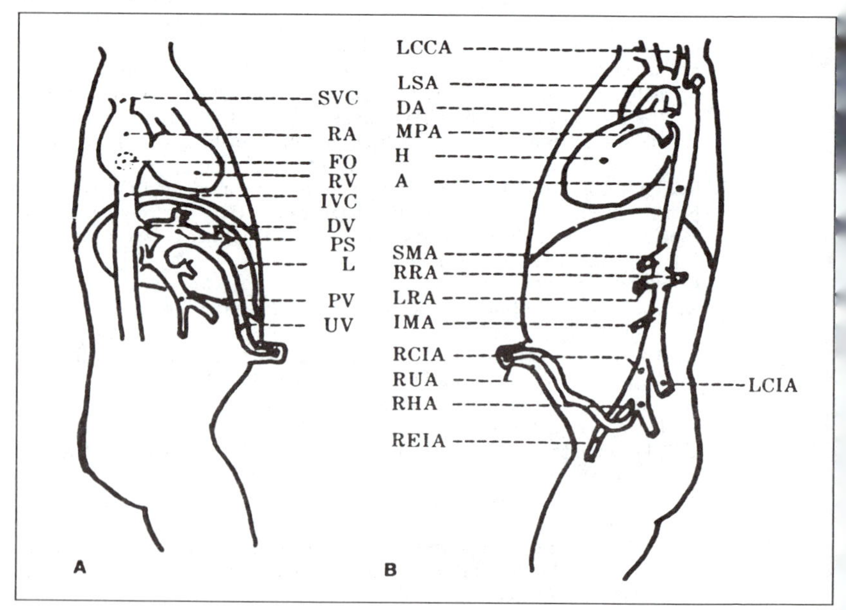

4. **Central venous lines,** used largely for prolonged hyperalimentation and occasionally to monitor central venous pressure, also can be placed percutaneously through the external jugular, subclavian, basilic, or saphenous veins. [5,6]

B. Umbilical artery catheterization

1. **Guidelines.** In general, only seriously ill infants should have an umbilical artery catheter placed. If only a few blood gas measurements are anticipated, peripheral arterial punctures should be performed together with transcutaneous oxygen monitoring, and a peripheral intravenous route should be used for fluids and medications.
2. **Technique**
   a. **Sterile technique is used.** Before preparing cord and skin, make external measurements to determine how far the catheter will be inserted (Figs. 39-3, 39-4, and 39-5). In a high setting, the catheter tip is between the eighth and tenth thoracic vertebrae; in a low setting, the tip is between the third and fourth lumbar vertebrae.
   b. The cord and surrounding area are washed carefully with an antiseptic solution, and the abdomen is draped with sterile towels. Avoid burns caused by allowing excess solution to remain on the skin, including the back.
   c. Umbilical tape is placed around the base of the cord, not the skin surrounding the umbilicus. If the latter technique is used, the tie must be loosened after the procedure. The tape is used to gently constrict

Fig. 39-3. Localization of umbilical artery catheters. The crosshatched areas represent sites in which complications are least likely. Either site may be used for placement of the catheter tip.

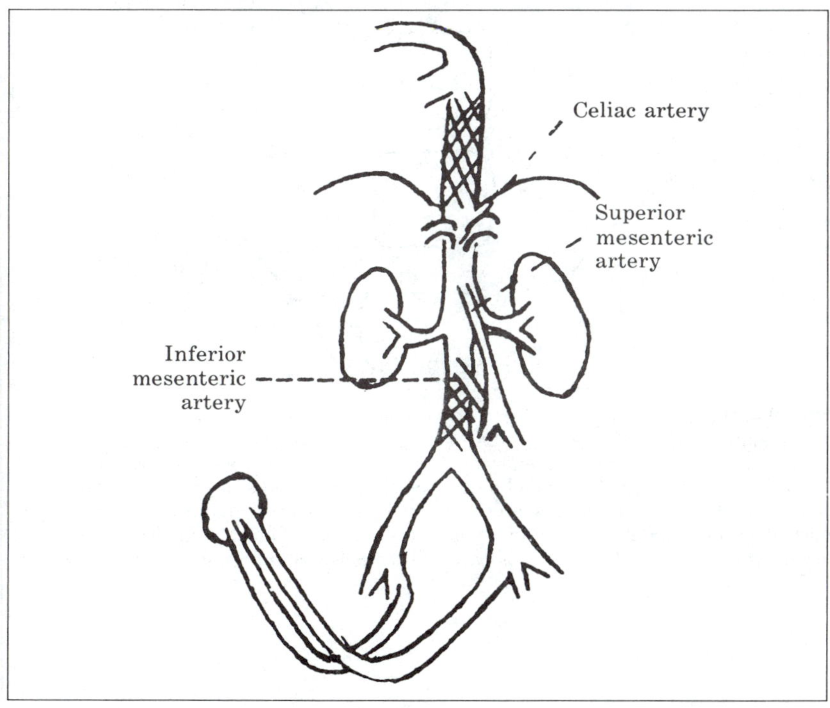

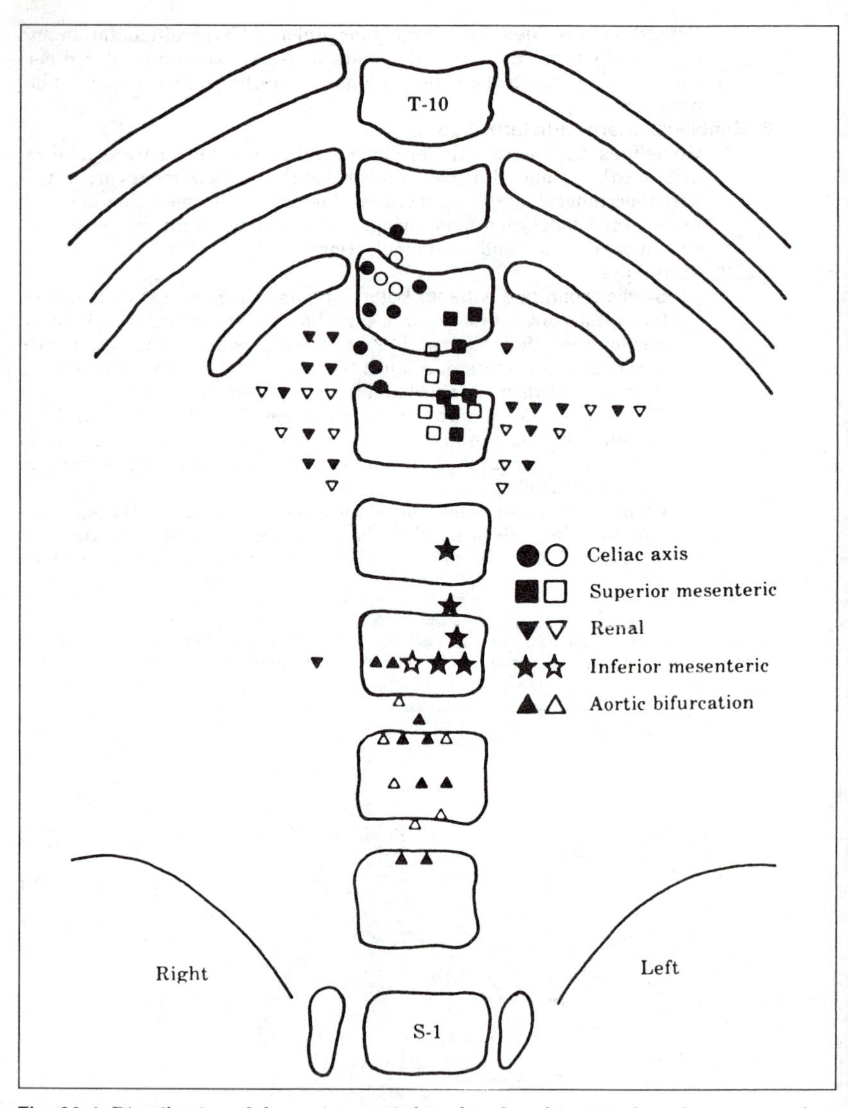

Fig. 39-4. Distribution of the major aortic bunches found in 15 infants by aortography as correlated with the vertebral bodies. Filled symbols represent infants with cardiac or renal anomalies (or both); open symbols represent those without either disorder. Major landmarks appear at the following vertebral levels: diaphragm, T12 interspace; celiac artery, T12; superior mesenteric artery, L1 interspace; renal artery, L1; inferior mesenteric artery, L3; aortic bifurcation, L4. (From D. L. Phelps et al., The radiologic localization of the major aortic tributaries in the newborn infant. *J. Pediatr.* 81: 336, 1972.)

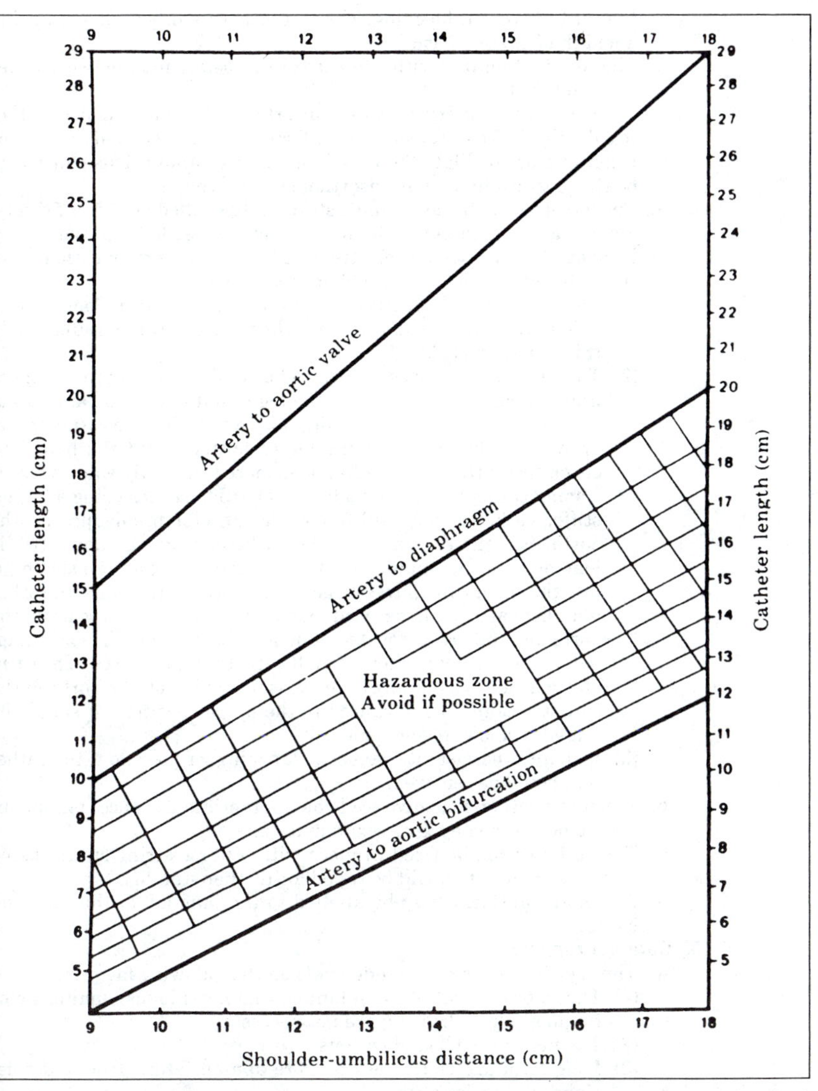

Fig. 39-5. Distance from shoulder to umbilicus measured from above the lateral end of the clavicle to the umbilicus, as compared with the length of the umbilical artery catheter needed to reach the designated level. (From P. M. Dunn, Localization of the umbilical catheter by post-mortem measurement. *Arch. Dis. Child.* 41: 69, 1966.)

the cord to prevent bleeding. The cord is cut cleanly with a scalpel to a length of 1.0 to 1.5 cm.

d. The cord is stabilized with a forceps or hemostat, and the two arteries are identified.

e. The closed tip of an iris forceps is inserted into the lumen of an artery to a depth of 0.5 cm. Tension on the forceps is released, and the forceps is left in place to dilate the vessel for about 1 minute. This pause may be the most useful step in insertion of the catheter.

f. The forceps is withdrawn, and a sterile saline-filled no. 3.5 or 5F polyvinyl chloride catheter with an end-hole is threaded into the artery. In about 5 to 10 percent of attempted umbilical artery catheterizations, one of the following problems may occur:

(1) The catheter will not pass into the abdominal aorta. Sometimes a double-catheter technique will allow successful cannulation in this situation [12].

(2) The catheter may pass into aorta but go downstream to one of the iliac arteries and then down the leg or out one of the arteries to the buttocks. There may be difficulty advancing the catheter and cyanosis or blanching of the leg or buttocks (lift the baby and check the buttocks). This happens more frequently when there is a small catheter (3.5) and a large baby. Sometimes using a larger, stiffer catheter (5.0) will allow the catheter to advance up the aorta. Sometimes removing the catheter from the aorta (while leaving it in the umbilical artery), twirling it, and reinserting it into the aorta will allow it to go up the aorta. If this fails, the other umbilical artery can be tried. Sometimes the catheter goes up the aorta and then reverses itself and goes back down. This may happen in a large baby when a small catheter (3.5) is used. The catheter may also go out any of the vessels coming off the aorta. If the catheter cannot be advanced to the proper position, it should be pulled to a low line or removed.

(3) If there is persistent cyanosis, blanching, or poor flow, the catheter should be removed.

g. When the catheter is advanced the appropriate distance, placement should be checked by x-ray examination.

h. The catheter can be fixed in place with a purse-string suture using silk thread, and it should be taped for further stability.

i. Antibiotic ointment may be applied to the junction of the cord and catheter.

3. Catheter removal

a. Timing of catheter removal depends on the following factors:

(1) The improvement of the infant so that continuous monitoring or frequent blood drawing are not necessary

(2) The presence of complications

(3) Long-term arterial access is more appropriately done using peripheral arteries [10].

b. Method of catheter removal. The catheter is removed slowly over a period of 30 to 60 seconds, allowing the umbilical artery to go into spasm at its proximal end while the catheter is still occluding the distal end. This usually prevents profuse bleeding. Old sutures should be removed.

4. Dangers of umbilical artery catheterization. Significant morbidity can be associated with complications of umbilical artery catheterization [3,8]. These complications are mainly due to vascular accidents, including thromboembolic phenomena to the kidney, bowel, legs, or rarely to the spinal cord. These may be manifest as hematuria, hypertension, signs of necrotizing enterocolitis or bowel infarction, and cyanosis or blanching of skin of back, buttocks, or legs. Other complications seen are infection, disseminated intravascular coagulation (DIC), and vessel perforation.

Close observation of the skin, monitoring of the urine for hematuria, measuring blood pressure, and following the platelet count may give clues to complications. These complications are indications for catheter removal.

a. We frequently do ultrasonic examination of the aorta to see thrombi in infants who are under 1500 gm in weight, infants requiring prolonged umbilical artery catheterization, and infants in whom we are concerned about complications. If thrombi are observed, the catheter is removed.

b. If there are small thrombi without symptoms or only increased blood pressure, we usually remove the catheter and monitor for DIC, follow the aorta and renal vessels by ultrasound examination and treat hypertension if necessary (see Chap. 26). If there are any embolic signs and loss of pulses, coagulopathy, and no intracranial hemorrhage, we consider heparinization, maintaining the PTT at double the control value. If there is a large clot with total occlusion of a leg, we consider the use of fibrinolytic agents and/or surgery [16].

c. **Blanching of a leg** following catheter placement is probably the most common complication noted clinically. The opposite leg should be warmed, and it should be observed for one hour. If the vasospasm resolves, the catheter may be left in place. If there is no improvement, the catheter should be removed.

d. **Use of heparin for anticoagulation to prevent clotting.** Whether or not the use of heparin in the infusate decreases the incidence of thrombotic complications is not known. Our practice is to use dilute heparin 0.25 to 0.5 unit/ml of infusate.

5. **Placement of the catheter.** There is little helpful information to support preferentially either high or low placement of umbilical artery catheters. One study found a higher complication rate in the group with the catheter tip at L3 to L4, compared with T7 to T8, owing to more episodes of blanching and cyanosis of one or both legs [9]. There was no difference between the high and low position groups in the rate of complications requiring catheter removal. Renal complications and emboli to the bowel are probably more common with lines at T7 to T8 while low lines (L3 to L4) have complications such as cyanosis or blanching of the leg, which are easier to observe.

6. **Indwelling time.** The incidence of complications associated with umbilical artery catheterization appears to be directly related to the length of time the catheter is left in place [7,14].

7. **Infection and use of antibiotics.** A trial of the use of antibiotics while umbilical artery catheters were in place revealed no more infection from the catheter alone than when antibiotics were withheld [1]. In infants who have umbilical artery catheters in place, we use antibiotics whenever infection is suspected and after appropriate cultures have been obtained.

C. **Umbilical vein catheterization** (see Figs. 39-2 and 39-6).

1. **Guidelines.** We use umbilical vein catheterization for exchange transfusions and emergency vascular access; in these cases, the venous catheter is replaced by an umbilical artery catheter or an intravenous catheter as soon as possible. In critically ill infants, we also use an umbilical vein catheter to monitor central venous pressure.

2. **Technique**

a. The site is prepared as for umbilical artery catheterization after determining the appropriate length of catheter to be inserted (Fig. 39-6).

b. Umbilical tape is placed around the base of the cord so that one is ready to control bleeding, and the cord is cut to a length of 1.5 cm or less.

c. Any clots seen are removed with a forceps.

d. The catheter is prepared by filling it with heparinized saline, 1 unit of heparin per milliliter of saline, with an attached syringe. The cath-

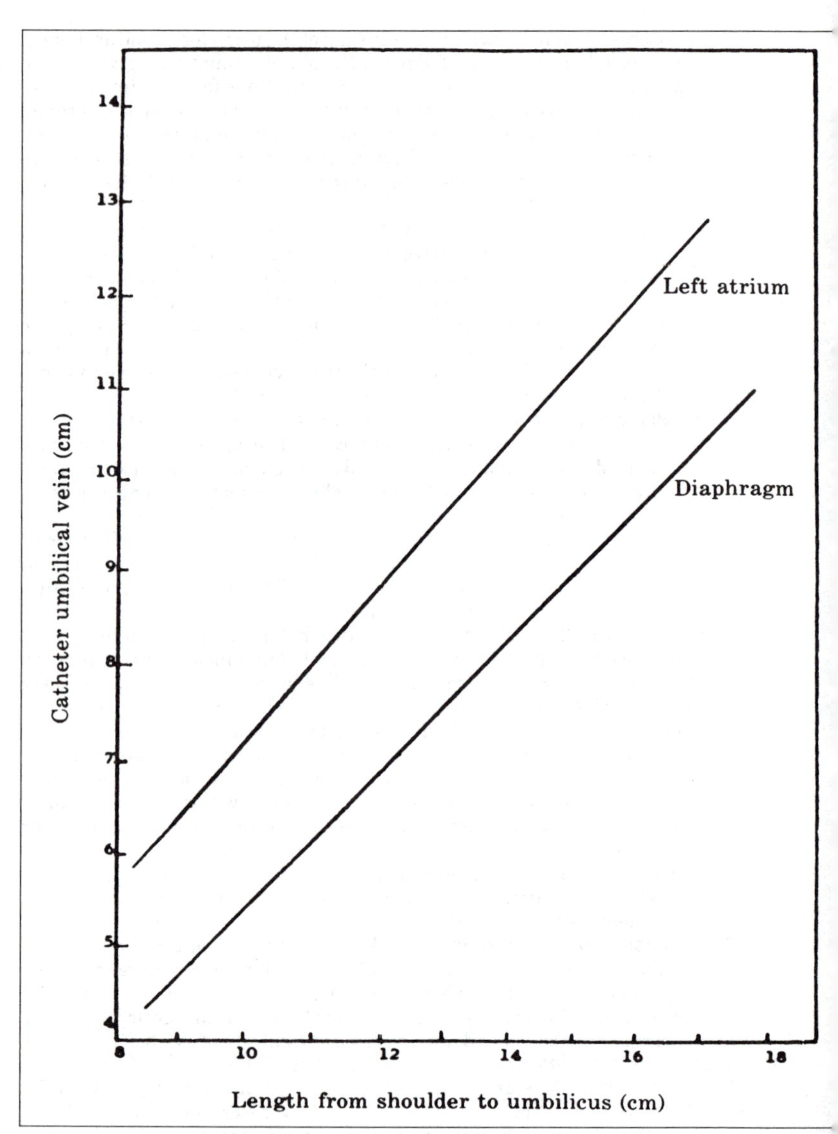

Fig. 39-6. Catheter length for umbilical vein catheterization. The catheter tip should be placed between the diaphragm and the left atrium. (From P. M. Dunn, Localization of the umbilical catheter by post-mortem measurement. *Arch. Dis. Child.* 41: 69, 1966.)

eter should never be left open to the atmosphere because negative intrathoracic pressure could cause an air embolism.

e. The catheter is inserted while gentle traction is exerted on the cord. Once the catheter is in the vein, one should try to slide the catheter cephalad just under the skin, where the vein runs very superficially. If the catheter is being placed for an exchange transfusion, it should be advanced only as far as is necessary to establish good blood flow. If the catheter is being used to monitor central venous pressure, it should be advanced through the ductus venosus into the inferior vena cava and its position verified by x-ray.

f. Only isotonic solutions should be infused until the position of the catheter is verified by x-ray studies. If the catheter tip is in the inferior vena cava, hypertonic solutions may be infused.

D. **Percutaneous radial artery catheterization** [15]. An indwelling radial artery catheter is often a useful alternative to umbilical artery catheterization for monitoring blood gas levels and blood pressure. Some information suggests greater safety than umbilical arterial catheterization.

1. **Advantages**
   a. Accessibility (when the umbilical artery is inaccessible or has been used for a long period)
   b. Reflection of preductal flow (if the right radial artery is used)
   c. Avoidance of thrombosis of major vessels, which is sometimes associated with umbilical vessel catheterization
2. **Risks** are usually small if the procedure is performed carefully, but infection, air embolus, inadvertent injection of incorrect solution, and arterial occlusion may occur.
3. **Equipment** required includes a 22- or 24-gauge intravenous cannula with stylet, a T-connector, heparinized saline flushing solution (0.5 to 1.0 units heparin per milliliter of solution), and an infusion pump.
4. **Method of catheterization**
   a. The adequacy of the ulnar collateral flow to the hand must be assessed. The radial and ulnar arteries should be simultaneously compressed, and the ulnar artery should then be released. The degree of flushing of the blanched hand should be noted. If the entire hand becomes flushed while the radial artery is occluded, the ulnar circulation is adequate. A high-intensity light may be used to view both the radial and ulnar arteries.
   b. The hand may be secured on an arm board with the wrist extended, leaving all fingertips exposed to observe color changes.
   c. The wrist is prepared with an iodine-containing solution, and the site of maximum arterial pulsation is palpated.
   d. The IV cannula is inserted through the skin at an angle less than 30 degrees to horizontal and is slowly advanced into the artery. Transillumination may help delineate the vessel and its course. If the artery is entered as the catheter is advanced, the stylet is removed and the catheter is advanced in the artery. If there is no blood return, the artery may be transfixed. The stylet is then removed, and the catheter is slowly withdrawn until blood flow occurs; then it is advanced into the vessel.
5. **Caution.** Only heparinized saline, at a rate not exceeding 2 ml per hour, is infused in the line.

D. **Percutaneous central venous catheterization.** Useful for long-term venous access for IV fluids, particularly hyperalimentation.

1. **Subclavian vein catheterization.** Useful in infants greater than 1200 gm
   a. **Equipment** required includes a 3.0F catheter with introducer needle and guidewire. Double-lumen 4.0F catheters may be used in larger infants (>2.5 kg).
   b. **Technique.** The infant is sedated and placed supine with a roll between the scapulae. The head is turned to the side of insertion. The

shoulders should drop posteriorly. The skin is prepared with an iodine-containing solution and infiltrated with local anesthetic. The introducer needle is inserted through the skin and immediately beneath the clavicle, a third of the way from shoulder to midline. The needle should be almost parallel to the chest wall and aimed at the sternal notch. When blood flow is established, the guidewire is passed and the catheter is placed over the wire. Catheter position is determined by radiograph. The catheter tip should lie at the junction of the superior vena cava and right atrium.

2. **Peripheral or jugular vein catheterization.** Useful in infants weighing less than 1500 gm, as small as 500 gm or less.
   a. **Equipment** required includes a 1.9F silicone catheter cut to the appropriate length, an introducer needle, and iris forceps.
   b. **Technique.** An appropriate vein of entry is selected. This may be an external jugular, basilic, or greater saphenous vein. Percutaneous access is preferred over a cut-down technique [6]. The site is prepared with an iodine-containing solution, and the introducer needle inserted into the vein until free blood flow occurs. The silicone catheter is inserted through the needle with forceps and is slowly advanced the predetermined distance for central venous positioning. The introducer needle is removed, the extra catheter length is coiled on the skin near the insertion site, and the site is covered with transparent surgical covering. Catheter tip position at the junction of the vena cava and right atrium is confirmed by radiograph. Some physicians inject a small amount of isotonic contrast material to make visualization easier.
   c. **Complications** are rare but include infection, thrombosis, and thrombophlebitis.

References

1. Bard, H. *Arch. Dis. Child.* 48: 630, 1973.
2. Bauer, C. H. *J. Pediatr.* 66: 1017, 1965.
3. Cochran, W. D. *Pediatrics* 42: 769, 1968.
4. Coldiron, J. *Pediatrics* 41: 823, 1968.
5. Fletcher, M. A., McDonald, M. G., and Avery, G. B. (Eds.). *Atlas of Procedures in Neonatology.* Philadelphia: Lippincott, 1983.
6. Gilhooly, J., Lindenberg, J., and Reynolds, J. W. *Pediatrics* 78: 636, 1986.
7. Gupta, J. M. *Arch. Dis. Child.* 43: 382, 1968.
8. James, L. S. Complications Arising from Catheterization of the Umbilical Vessels In *Problems of Neonatal Intensive Care Units: Report of the Fifty-ninth Ross Conference on Pediatric Research.* Columbus, Ohio: Ross Laboratories, 1969. P. 36.
9. Mokrohisky, S. T. *N. Engl. J. Med.* 299: 561, 1978.
10. Randel, S. N., Tsang, B. H., Wung, J. T., et al. *Am. J. Dis. Child.* 141: 848, 1987.
11. Sarff, L. D. *J. Pediatr.* 88: 473, 1976.
12. Schreiber, M. D. *J. Pediatr.* 104: 768, 1984.
13. Spitzer, A. R. *J. Pediatr.* 100: 806, 1982.
14. Symansky, M. R. *J. Pediatr.* 80: 820, 1972.
15. Todres, I. D. *J. Pediatr.* 87: 273, 1975.
16. Vailas, G. N. *J. Pediatr.* 109: 101, 1986.
17. Weisman, L. E. *Am. J. Dis. Child.* 137: 1077, 1983.

Appendixes

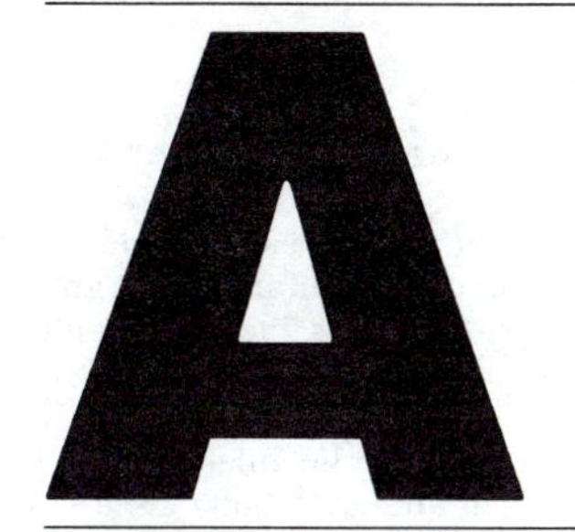

Medications Used in the Newborn*†

Celeste M. Marx and
Jonathan H. Cronin

I. Antimicrobial agents (see Chap. 12)

acyclovir

8 to 10 mg/kg per dose IV is given every 8 hours for treatment of herpesvirus infections. Common adverse reactions include renal dysfunction and phlebitis. Serum creatinine level should be closely monitored, and the dose should be administered over at least 1 hour. Acyclovir should be used for documented herpesvirus infections as well as in those patients which are deemed at high risk. It is also used for varicella infections (see Chap. 12).

amikacin

7.5 mg/kg is given by IV infusion q12h to newborn infants over 35 weeks' gestational age (G.A.), less than 1 week old and q8h to those 1 week or more of age. Infants 30–34 weeks' G.A. get 10 mg/kg q24h under 1 week of age then 7.5 mg/kg q12h. Infants under 29 weeks G.A. get 7.5 mg/kg q24h under 1 week of age then 10 mg/k q24h. Dose adjustment should be made based on serum level monitoring. The desirable level 1 hour after the end of a 20-minute infusion is 20 to 30 μg/ml; the serum level immediately prior to the dose should be 5 to 10 μg/ml. Renal function should be monitored and auditory function assessed.

amphotericin B

Intravenously (slow drip): The initial 0.25 to 0.5 mg/kg daily dose is diluted in 5% D/W to at least 1.0 mg per 10 ml. Daily dosage is increased by 0.25 mg/kg per day every other day until the maximum daily dose of 1 mg/kg per day is reached. Daily dose may need to be reduced if flucytosine is also used. Treatment for 4 to 6 weeks is necessary, with a total dose of 25 to 35 mg/kg. The dose should be infused over an extended period; although the manufacturer recommends a 6-hour period, shorter infusions (i.e., 2 hours) are well tolerated. Amphotericin should be used only in severe disseminated fungal infection. Renal and hematologic toxicity may be seen. Allergic reactions (e.g., chills, fever) may be prevented by antihistamine or antipyretic pretreatment or concomitant hydrocortisone administration. There are many problems with the use of this drug, and little data on its use in the newborn are available (see manufacturer's package insert). These recommendations are an adaptation of the experience with adults. Protect IV tubing and bottle from light with foil. (See package insert for directions.)

Topically: Applied as 2% ointment (in liquid petrolatum 95%, polyethylene 5%).

ampicillin

50 to 100 mg/kg per dose IM or IV is given q12h to newborns less than 1 week old and q8h to newborns more than 1 week old. When treating suspected meningitis, 75 to 100 mg/kg per dose is given q6h. Higher doses may be needed in the treatment of *Listeria* meningitis but are rarely indicated for other infections. When higher doses are used, monitoring for interstitial nephritis should be done.

***Package inserts should be read for all medications to get information on method of administration, adverse reactions, monitoring and drug incompatibilities.**
†Prober, L. The use of antibiotics in neonates weighing less than 1200 gms. Pediatr. Inf. Dis. J. 9:119, 1990.

bacitracin

Topically: Applied as ointment, 500 units/gm q4–8h.

carbenicillin disodium

100 mg/kg is given q12h IV or IM during the first week of life for all newborns. After 7 days of age, this dose is given q8h for infants 2000 gm or less and q6h for infants over 2000 gm. Adverse reactions include anaphylaxis, platelet dysfunction, and electrolyte abnormalities.

cefazolin

40 mg/kg per day is given in two divided doses by IM injection or as a 30-minute IV dose to infants under 2000 gm. Infants over 2000 gm and over 7 days of age should get 60 mg/kg per day divided q6–8h. The manufacturer does not recommend its use in newborns. Monitor for eosinophilia. Elevation of aspartate aminotransferase level may be seen.

cefoperazone

A 25 to 50 mg/kg dose is given by IM injection or as a 30-minute IV infusion q12h to infants in the first week of life. Eosinophilia may be observed.

cefotaxime

Active against gram-negative bacteria except *Pseudomonas.* Not effective against group B strep, pneumococcus, *Listeria,* and other gram-positive aerobic organisms. To be used with ampicillin in suspected gram-negative sepsis or meningitis. The dose is: under 2000 gm and under 7 days of age: 100 mg/kg per day divided q12h; under 2000 gm and over 7 days of age: 150 mg/kg per day divided q12h; over 2000 gm and under 7 days of age: 100 mg/kg per day divided q12h; and over 2000 gm and over 7 days old: 150 mg/kg per day divided q8h. For meningitis, give 200 mg/kg per day divided q6h.

cefoxitin

30 mg/kg given IM or by IV injection over 30 minutes q8h has been observed to provide acceptable blood levels and clinical efficacy in premature and term newborns.

ceftriaxone

50 to 100 mg/kg per dose given IM or IV q24h for premature infants less than 1 week of age and q12h for premature infants greater than 1 week old and for term infants less than 7 days old. This new third-generation cephalosporin has excellent penetration into the CSF, bile, and lung. Ceftriaxone may interfere with vitamin K metabolism, so the prothrombin time (PT) should be monitored. Poor activity against *Pseudomonas,* enterococci, methicillin-resistant staphylococci, and *Listeria.* There is recent evidence that ceftriaxone may displace bilirubin from albumin. Therefore, this drug should be used judiciously in jaundiced neonates.

cefuroxime

100 mg/kg per day divided q12h. For meningitis, use 200 mg/kg per day divided q12h.

cephalothin (Keflin)

20 mg/kg per dose given IM or by IV injection over 30 minutes q8h for newborns less than 1 week old and q6h for those older than 1 week. There are little data on the toxicity of this agent in the newborn. Cephalothin does not penetrate the cerebrospinal space reliably; disk sensitivity testing may not correlate with clinical efficacy.

Note: Adverse reactions of the preceding cephalosporins include blood dyscrasias, hepatic and renal dysfunction, thrombophlebitis, and hypersensitivity reactions.

chloramphenicol (Chloromycetin)

Avoid use if other options available. The third-generation cephalosporins have decreased the need for chloramphenicol. A single IV infusion of 25 mg/kg per day over 30 minutes is given to all infants less than 2 weeks old or to low-birth-weight infants (<2000 gm) of any age being treated for **sepsis**; 50 mg/kg per day in two divided doses is given by 30-minute IV infusion to all newborns 2 weeks to 1 month of age, but also including newborns less than 2000 gm being treated for **meningitis.**

Because newborns and infants display widely varying abilities to eliminate chloramphenicol, it is critically important to monitor serum concentrations. Peak blood level is seen 45 minutes to 4 hours after the dose because of a delay in metabolic activation of the succinate salt. Owing to the drug's long half-life, it is best to draw a postdose serum level 3 hours after the dose; this level should be 10 to 20 μg/ml. Predose levels may aid in allowing pharmacokinetic dose adjustment. Infants with meningitis should be treated with doses calculated to keep serum levels near 20 μg/ml. Metabolism takes place in the liver, resulting in an inactive form that is excreted in the urine with some active drug. Assays specific for active drug must be used for therapeutic drug monitoring. Toxic effects, such as cardiovascular collapse ("gray baby" syndrome) are seen with serum levels in excess of 50 μg/ml. Reversible bone marrow suppression may be seen; the manifestations are increased serum iron concentration, increased saturation of iron-binding capacity, decreased hematocrit, mild thrombocytopenia, mild leukopenia, and vacuolization of bone marrow elements. These effects are generally reversible when the drug is discontinued and are not usually seen with blood levels less than 25 μg/ml. Infants on chloramphenicol should have weekly determinations of hematocrit, reticulocyte count, platelet count, white cell count, differential, and serum iron level. The dreaded side effect of chloramphenicol-induced aplastic anemia occurs in 1 in 40,000 persons exposed to the drug; this is 15 times the spontaneous incidence of aplastic anemia. It is not dose-related and may occur at any time (even months to years after the drug is stopped). If absolutely necessary, the oral route may be used; bioavailability appears to be adequate.

clindamycin phosphate

Clindamycin does not penetrate the cerebrospinal space reliably. The following doses provide generally recommended serum levels of clindamycin in newborns:

Premature infants less than 1 month of age: 15 mg/kg per day in three divided doses.

Full-term infants less than 1 week of age: 15 mg/kg per day in three divided doses.

Infants older than 28 days or greater than 3.5 kg: 20 mg/kg per day in four divided doses

Pseudomembranous colitis is an uncommon but serious side effect caused by the suppression of normal gastrointestinal flora.

colistin sulfate

15 mg/kg per day PO divided into doses given q6h. Used for enteropathogenic strains of *Escherichia coli* as an alternate to neomycin therapy. Only very limited absorption occurs in the intact gastrointestinal tract.

erythromycin

Orally (estolate): 40 mg/kg per day in four divided doses.

Intravenously (lactobionate): 30 to 40 mg/kg per day in three or four divided doses. This drug is used primarily for *Chlamydia* infections in neonates, and adverse effects include intrahepatic cholestasis as well as interfering with the clearance of theophylline, digoxin, and carbamazepine.

Ophthalmic (0.5% ointment): Fill conjunctival sac qid for infection and once for prophlaxis against ophthalmia neonatorum.

5-flucytosine (Ancobon) (5-FC)

50 to 200 mg/kg per day PO divided q6h for treatment of fungal infections.

Comment: There is limited experience in newborns. Dose should be reduced in renal failure. Bone marrow suppression should be monitored. When serum levels are followed, they are maintained from 50 to 80 μg/ml. When used in combination with amphotericin B, the daily dose of amphotericin may need to be reduced.

gamma globulin [immune serum globulin (ISG) (Human)]

Preventive dose of ISG in measles exposure is 0.25 ml/kg IM. When exposure to hepatitis A is likely (particularly if the mother has hepatitis), a dose of 0.15 ml/kg of ISG is administered IM (see Chap. 12). As replacement therapy for hypogammaglobulinemic infants, the usual dose is 100 mg/kg per month (equal to 0.6 ml/kg per month) IV or IM. The dose for treatment of ITP or alloimmune thrombocytopenia is 400 mg/kg per day IV infused over 6 hrs. for 5 days (see Chap. 19).

gentamicin

Term newborns receive 2.5 mg/kg per dose q12h up to 1 week of age and q8h thereafter. Pharmacokinetic studies show that 2.5 mg/kg per dose q18h generally produces acceptable serum levels for premature newborns less than 35 weeks' gestational age and that 2.5 mg/kg per dose once daily is appropriate for premature infants less than 28 weeks' gestational age. Gentamicin should be given IM or as an IV infusion over 30 minutes. Optimal serum levels are 4 to 8 μg/ml 1 hour after the end of the dose infusion or injection; levels should be less than 2 μg/ml immediately preceding the dose. Levels should be monitored on the second day of treatment (before and after the third dose) and then twice weekly. Doses should be reduced when renal function is impaired; the first two doses should not be reduced to "load" the patient. Serum creatinine level should be measured every 4 days. Impaired hearing and vestibular function have been reported with the use of gentamicin. Infants under 26 weeks' gestation should have levels monitored before and after the second dose.

Note: The manufacturer recommends a maximum dose of 6 mg/kg per day.

hepatitis B immune globulin (HBIG)

Newborn infants whose mothers are hepatitis B antigen (HbsAg)–positive are given 0.5 ml of HBIG in the delivery room or within 12 hours of birth (see Chap. 12).

hepatitis B vaccine (HBV)

0.5 ml (10 μg) IM is administered within 7 days of birth and again at 1 and 6 months of age. HBV may be given at the same time as HBIG, but it should be given in a separate site (see Chap. 12).

isoniazid

10 to 20 mg/kg per day PO is given in a single daily dose (see Chap. 12).

kanamycin sulfate

Newborns less than 7 days old

Less than 2000 gm body weight: 7.5 mg/kg q12h IM or by slow IV infusion over at least 20 minutes

More than 2000 gm body weight: 10 mg/kg q12h IM or by slow IV infusion over at least 20 minutes

Newborns over 7 days old

Less than 2000 gm body weight: 10 mg/kg q12h

More than 2000 gm body weight: 10 mg/kg q8h

Comment: These doses exceed the manufacturer's recommendations, but are effective and safe. To reduce the risks of nephrotoxicity, doses should be adjusted to provide serum levels 1 hour after the dose infusion of 15 to 25 μg/ml. Serum trough levels 30 minutes prior to next dose should be under 10 μg/ml. An attempt should be made to keep the total dose received at less than 500 mg/kg. Serum creatinine level should be measured every 4 days.

ketoconazole

2.5 to 5.0 mg/kg per day PO every 24 hours for treatment of *Candida* and other disseminated fungal infections. Treatment is required for 7 to 14 days. CSF penetration is poor, so an alternative antifungal agent should be used for CNS infections. Common adverse reactions are gastrointestinal intolerance and liver dysfunction.

methicillin (see oxacillin sodium)

metronidazole (Flagyl)

Manufacturer's recommendations of 7.5 mg/kg PO or IV q12h for children may not provide adequate serum levels in infants. For both term and preterm newborns, it has been proposed that an initial dose of 15 mg/kg be given, followed by 7.5 mg/kg q12h after 48 hours in the preterm newborn and after

24 hours in the term newborn. A serum level of 8 μg/ml is therapeutic with good CSF penetration.

mezlocillin

75 mg/kg per dose is given IV over 30 minutes or IM to preterm newborns in the first week of life, q12h to older prematures or term newborns in the first week of life, and q8h to older term newborns.

neomycin

100 mg/kg per day PO is given in divided doses. Premature newborns or full-term newborns less than 1 week old are given doses q12h; full-term newborns more than 1 week old are given doses q6h. Ototoxicity has been described after oral administration. Neomycin is not used parenterally in the newborn.

netilmicin (Netromycin)

The manufacturer recommends that this aminoglycoside be given in doses of 4.0 to 6.5 mg/kg per day as 2.00 to 3.25 mg/kg q12h to newborns up to 6 weeks of age. Infants older than 6 weeks receive 5.0 to 8.0 mg/kg per day in divided doses q8–12h. Pharmacokinetic studies of preterm infants in the first week of life indicate benefit from an initial loading dose of 3 mg/kg, followed by 2 mg/kg q12h. After 1 week of age, 3 mg/kg q8h is tolerated. Netilmicin is given IM or as a 30-minute IV infusion.

Comment: Dosing should be individualized to provide peak serum levels of 6 to 10 μg/ml 30 minutes after the dose. Postdose levels in excess of 16 μg/ml and predose levels in excess of 4.0 μg/ml should be avoided. Renal function should be monitored for signs of toxicity and for dose adjustments. This drug is potentially ototoxic.

nystatin

Orally: 100,000 to 200,000 units q6h for thrush.

Topically: Applied as 2% ointment (in liquid petrolatum 95%, polyethylene 5%) three or four times daily.

oxacillin sodium

50 mg/kg per day divided q12h for infants under 2000 gm and under 7 days old; 75 mg/kg per day divided q8h for infants under 2000 gm and over 7 days old; 75 mg/kg per day divided q8h for infants over 2000 gm and under 7 days old; and 100 mg/kg per day divided q6h for infants over 2000 gm and over 7 days old. These doses are doubled for meningitis and severe systemic infections. **Note:** Because it has less protein-binding ability, methicillin is probably the preferred penicillinase-resistant agent to use in newborns. The doses are identical to those of oxacillin.

Comment: The IV route (as a 10-minute infusion) is preferred; IM injection may lead to sterile abscess formation. The most common adverse reaction is interstitial nephritis.

penicillin G potassium aqueous

50,000 to 100,000 units/kg per day IM or IV in divided doses is given q12h to premature and full-term newborns less than 1 week of age and q6–8h to full-term infants more than 1 week of age. For infants with meningitis, the dose is 100,000 to 150,000 units/kg per day in infants under 1 week of age and 150,000 to 250,000 units/kg per day in infants over 1 week. In group B streptococcal infection, the dose is 200,000 to 250,000 units/kg per day.

penicillin G procaine

50,000 units/kg per day IM as a single daily dose for premature or full-term newborns.

piperacillin

50 to 100 mg/kg per dose IV or IM q12h for premature infants less than a week old, q8h for premature infants more than 1 week old and term babies less than 7 days old, and q6h for term infants greater than 7 days of age. Liver and renal dysfunction can occur as well as eosinophilia.

pyrimethamine

2 mg/kg per day for 72h then 1 mg/kg per day PO divided q12h for 4 weeks.

Comment: For toxoplasmosis, 5 mg of folinic acid should be given twice a week during treatment with pyrimethamine; sulfadiazine is often used concurrently.

ribavirin

1 vial of ribavirin (6 gm/100 cc) is diluted in 30 cc of sterile water and given by continuous aerosol for 12 to 18 hours per day for 3 to 7 days for treatment of respiratory syncytial viral infections. Efficacy is increased if given early in the course of the disease. **Note:** This drug is a teratogen, so its administration by pregnant caregivers must be avoided.

rifampin

10 to 20 mg/kg per day PO divided q12h should be used in combination with other agents in the treatment of TB. Effective against *Neisseria* and staphylococci. There is not much neonatal experience (see TB, Chap. 12).

silver nitrate

1 drop silver nitrate solution 2% in each eye (prophylaxis against gonococcal ophthalmia) (see Bacterial Infections, Chap. 12).

streptomycin

30 mg/kg per day IM divided into two to four doses. Rarely used except for tuberculosis.

sulfadiazine

Orally: 50 to 120 mg/kg per day divided into four to six doses

Subcutaneously or intravenously: 50 to 100 mg/kg per day divided into two to four doses

Comment: Slow renal clearance may lead to excessively high blood levels. Contraindicated in the presence of jaundice. Used with pyrimethamine against *Toxoplasma gondii* infections in dose of 120 mg/kg per day (see Chap. 12).

sulfisoxazole

Orally: 100 mg/kg per day in four equal doses

Intramuscularly or intravenously: 50 to 75 mg/kg per day in four equal doses

Comment: In premature newborns or in the presence of jaundice, sulfisoxazole may interfere with the binding of bilirubin by albumin. Sulfonamides are rarely recommended as therapy for newborns except as topical ophthalmic treatment of inclusion-body conjunctivitis.

tetracycline hydrochloride

50 mg/kg per day PO, IM, or IV; administered in four divided doses PO or in two or three divided doses by injection. Topically as ointment applied tid (see Chap. 12).

Comment: Systemic tetracycline may stain teeth and retard bone growth and is rarely indicated in the treatment of the newborn.

ticarcillin

For newborns less than 2000 gm, a dose of 75 mg/kg IM or IV is given q12h when less than 1 week of age and q8h for those older than 1 week. For newborns weighing more than 2000 gm, 75 mg/kg IM or IV is given q8h for the first week of life and 100 mg/kg is given q8h thereafter.

tobramycin

See **gentamicin**; the same dosage, serum-level guidelines, and toxicities apply.

vancomycin

This drug is primarily used in the treatment of methicillin-resistent staphylococci and *Staphylococcus epidermidis* infections. Newborns less than 1 week old receive 30 mg/kg per day divided q12h. Babies more than 1 week old receive 45 mg/kg per day divided q8h. After 1 month of age, the dose is 45 to 60 mg/kg per day divided q6h. Vancomycin is potentially ototoxic. Renal toxocity is rare, except when used in combination with aminoglycosides. Neutropenia and phlebitis have been seen.

Comment: Serum levels should be monitored to allow quantitative dose adjustment. Optimum levels are 25 to 40 μg/ml at the end of the 1-hour dose infusion, 20 to 30 μg/ml 0.5 to 1 hour later, and approximately 5 to 10 μg/ml prior to the next dose. Premature newborns frequently require dose reduction. Infants under 29 weeks of age should get 15 mg/kg per dose every 24 hours. Levels should be checked before and after doses 2 and 3. Monitor serum creatinine level.

vidarabine

15 to 30 mg/kg per day IV infused over 12 hours is used to treat documented HSV infections. This drug may cause blood dyscrasias and hepatic dysfunction. It is gradually being replaced by acyclovir.

Ophthalmic (3% ointment): Apply to conjunctival sac q3h for treatment of HSV keratoconjunctivitis.

II. **Cardiovascular drugs** (see also Chaps. 6, 14, and 26)

captopril

0.1 to 0.4 mg/kg per dose PO q6–24 hours is the dose used in neonates. Infants require 0.5 to 0.6 mg/kg per day divided q6–24h. Adverse side effects include hypotension, neutropenia, and rash. **Comment:** Adjust dose in patients with renal failure.

chlorothiazide

20 to 40 mg/kg per day PO divided q12h

Comment: Chlorothiazide is used for maintenance diuresis; serum potassium levels should be monitored.

defibrillation

Approximately 2W - seconds/kg with a maximum of 10 W·s per infant

digoxin

IV total digitalizing dose:

Newborns less than 1000 gm receive 15 μg/kg.
Newborns 1000 to 1400 gm receive 15 to 20 μg/kg.
Newborns 1500 to 1999 gm receive 23 μg/kg.
Newborns 2000 to 2500 gm receive 25 μg/kg.
Heavier or term newborns receive 30 μg/kg.
Term infants (older than 1 month) receive 45 μg/kg.

This total digitalizing dose is divided into three doses that are given at 6- to 8-hour intervals.

Maintenance dose: One-fourth of digitalizing dose is given daily in two divided doses PO, IM, or IV.

Comment: When PO or IM routes are used, dose should be increased by one-third. Digoxin toxicity is common in premature newborns, even at recommended doses. Serum levels usually are between 1 and 2 ng/ml, but because serum levels do not correlate well with efficacy or toxicity, electrocardiographic monitoring of PR intervals should be performed (see Chap. 14).

dobutamine

5 to 10 μg/kg per minute is infused IV for cardiogenic or septic shock. A higher dosage may be required; maximum dose is 40 μg/kg per minute (see Chaps. 6, 13 (Persistent Pulmonary Hypertension), and 14). This drug has more specific beta-1-adrenergic activity compared with dopamine. **Preparation of infusion:** 15 mg in 50 cc infused at a rate in cubic centimeters per hour equal to the patient's body weight in kilograms will deliver 5 μg/kg per minute. In the newborn, to keep the volume of infusate low, make it two times more concentrated or four times more concentrated for 10 to 20 μg/kg per minute.

dopamine

2 to 30 μg/kg per minute is infused IV, as needed, to maintain blood pressure. For cardiogenic and septic shock, the dose-response effects of dopamine that are known in adults have not been proven in neonates.

Comment: Dopamine is used in infants with low cardiac output.

Manufacturer's note: The safety and efficacy of dopamine in infants have not been established. Extravasation of IV infiltrates of dopamine solutions should be treated by reinfiltrating the area with 1 mg/ml of phentolamine (Regitine) in normal saline (see Chaps. 6, 13, and 14). Preparation of infusion is identical to that for dobutamine.

epinephrine (see **VI,** page 631)

furosemide (Lasix)

1 mg/kg per dose up to a maximum dose of 2 mg/kg IV or IM

For maintenance only: 1 to 4 mg/kg per day divided into two or three doses, PO or IM. Owing to poor bioavailability, some infants may require even higher doses.

Comment: Calciuresis occurs, thereby increasing the risk of nephrolithiasis and osteopenia. Hypokalemia and hypochloremia may develop. Furosemide is potentially ototoxic, especially in patients with BPD.

hydralazine hydrochloride (see Chap. 26)

Dose in hypertensive crisis: 0.1 to 0.5 mg/kg slow IV push; the dose is increased by 0.1 mg/kg q6h until the desired effect is attained. The maximum dosage is variable; the range is 1 to 4 mg/kg per day.

Maintenance dose: 0.7 mg/kg per day PO in divided doses given q6h. This dose is increased up to 2 to 5 times as needed (see Chap. 26).

hydrochlorothiazide

4 to 5 mg/kg per day in divided doses given q12h PO

Comment: This drug is used for maintenance diuresis; potassium levels should be monitored.

indomethacin (Indocin)

0.2 mg/kg per dose is given q12h for three doses, IV, to a maximum dose of 0.6 mg/kg per course.

Comment: Transient oliguria, hyponatremia, hyperkalemia, hypoglycemia, and decreased platelet aggregation may occur. Relative contraindications include thrombocytopenia, active bleeding, or recent intraventricular hemorrhage (see Chap. 14).

isoproterenol hydrochloride (see Chap. 6)

Intravenously: 0.1 to 0.5 μg/kg per minute is infused to treat bradycardia and/or poor cardiac output. The rate of infusion should be adjusted according to the heart rate. **Preparation of infusion:** 0.5 mg in 50 cc infused at a rate in cubic centimeters per hour equal to the patient's body weight in kilograms will deliver 0.1 μg/kg per minute. Tachyphylaxis is common.

Nebulizer: 0.1 to 0.2 cc/dose diluted in 2 cc of normal saline q4–6h prn for bronchospasm

lidocaine hydrochloride

For treatment of ventricular arrhythmias, lidocaine should be diluted in 5% D/W to a concentration of 0.5 to 1.0 mg/ml; 0.5 to 2 mg/kg is given IV over 5 to 10 minutes while the heart rate and rhythm are monitored. This dose may be repeated after 10 minutes if necessary to a maximum of 5 mg/kg. IV infusion 10 to 50 μg/kg per minute. **Preparation of solution:** Place 20 mg (1 ml) in 100 ml of 5% dextrose in water. Infusion of 3 to 15 ml/kg per hour will deliver 10 to 50 μg/kg per minute. Be prepared for bradycardia and hypotension. Contraindicated in severe heart block. Widening of QRS interval by more than 0.2 sec or ventricular bradycardia suggests toxicity.

alpha-methyldopa (Aldomet)

10 mg/kg per dose or 30 mg/kg per day IV

Comment: Monitor hemolysis, leukopenia, and liver enzymes (see Chap. 26).

morphine

0.1 to 0.2 mg/kg per dose IV or IM for analgesia as well as treatment for tetralogy of fallot spells. Repeat as needed usually q3 to 4h. Side effects of respiratory depression can be reversed quickly by the administration of naloxone.

nitroprusside sodium

Starting dose is 0.4 μg/kg per minute IV, increased as needed to control severe hypertension. This drug also has been used for pulmonary hypertension.

Comment: Monitor thiocyanate levels with prolonged use (see Chap. 26), and make sure infusion is protected from light.

procainamide hydrochloride

1.5 to 2.0 mg/kg (1% solution 10 mg/ml) diluted in IV drip and titrated over 10 to 30 minutes. This dose is repeated in 30 minutes if needed.

Comment: Procainamide is used in refractory supraventricular tachycardia and ventricular arrhythmias (see Chap. 14).

propranolol hydrochloride

0.05 to 0.15 mg/kg IV over 10 minutes; this may be repeated in 10 minutes and then given q8h for maintenance if needed. The PO dose is 0.5 to 1.0 mg/kg per day in three or four divided doses.

Comment: Propranolol is used for ventricular tachycardias, supraventricular arrhythmias, hypoxic spells, and hypertension. Signs of toxicity include hypotension and bronchospasm. Congenital (low output) congestive heart failure and bronchospasm are relative contraindications.

prostaglandin E_1

0.05 to 0.1 μg/kg per minute per continuous IV infusion to keep the ductus arteriosus patent in patients with ductal dependent congenital heart disease. Initial dose may be decreased by increments of 0.01 μg/kg per minute depending on the patient's response. Side effects include fever, apnea, bradycardia, hypotension, seizures, and decreased platelet function. **Note:** Use only when persons skilled in neonatal resuscitation are immediately available (see Chap. 14).

quinidine

2.0 to 4.0 mg/kg IM q2–4h for four or five doses. Total daily dosage is 10 to 30 mg/kg.

Comment: IV administration is not recommended. Quinidine is used with digitalis for refractory supraventricular tachycardia; it is occasionally used for ventricular arrhythmias. The ECG should be checked before each dose. If the QRS interval is over 0.1 sec or increases by more than 0.02 sec, the medication should be discontinued and dose revision considered (see Chap. 14).

spironolactone

1.0 to 3.0 mg/kg per day PO divided q12h

Comment: Spironolactone can cause hyponatremia and potassium intoxication. It is used in chronic congestive heart failure, systemic hypertension, and bronchopulmonary dysplasia. The drug is used alone or in combination with thiazides.

Manufacturer's warning: Spironolactone has been shown to cause tumors in chronic toxicity studies in rats. Unnecessary use of this drug should be avoided.

tolazoline hydrochloride

1 to 2 mg/kg is given over 30 minutes, followed by 0.16 mg/kg per hour for each 1 mg/kg of loading dose administered IV through a scalp vein.

Comment: Hypotension may result. Volume expanders should be prepared before treatment is started (see Persistent Pulmonary Hypertension in Chap. 13, page 233). Other adverse reactions include cutaneous flushing, GI bleeding, and thrombocytopenia.

tromethamine (THAM)

Initial dose equal to one-fourth body weight in kilograms times base deficit is followed by repeated doses as indicated by arterial blood gases. Maximum 24-hour dosage is 40 ml/kg.

III. Drugs for volume expansion (treatment for shock; see also Chap. 6)

albumin, human serum, 25%

Dilute with saline to 5% solution and give 10 ml/kg per dose IV over 10 minutes.

Caution: Cardiac overload may occur in asphyxiated infants. Hypoxia should be corrected; then repeated doses of albumin are given as needed.

blood, colloid, plasma, normal saline, or lactated Ringer's solution

10 ml/kg/dose IV, and repeat as needed.

IV. Drugs for seizures (see also Neonatal Seizures in Chap. 21)

diazepam (Valium)

0.1 to 0.3 mg/kg q2min up to a total dose of 1.0 mg/kg, or for continuous seizures, 0.1 to 0.3 mg/kg IV as a bolus followed by 0.3 mg/kg per hour as IV infusion diluted in saline (0.1 mg/ml).

Comment: There is a risk of circulatory collapse and respiratory failure.
Manufacturer's note: The efficacy and safety of parenteral diazepam have not been established in the neonate.

glucose
0.5 to 1.0 gm/kg IV (equal to 2 to 4 ml/kg of glucose 25%). Some authors recommend a "minibolus" of 200 mg/kg in order to avoid excess insulin secretion and rebound hypoglycemia (see Hypoglycemia in Chap. 24).

lorazepam (Ativan)
0.05 to 0.1 mg/kg per dose IV has been used for status epilepticus or sedation. If there is no response, repeat dose in 15 minutes. Maintenance dose is dependent on response but is often 0.05 mg/kg IV q6–24h. Subsequent doses are given every 8 to 12 hours based on clinical response. Most common adverse effect is respiratory depression, especially when used with other anticonvulsants.

magnesium sulfate
A 20% solution is used or made by mixing 1 ml of magnesium sulfate 50% injection with 1.5 ml sterile water or saline. Then 0.2 ml/kg of the 20% solution (equals 40 mg magnesium sulfate per milliliter) is given IM as needed. For IV use, injection is diluted to 1% by mixing 1 ml of 50% injection with 49 ml sterile water or saline; then 10 to 20 ml/kg (equals 100 to 200 mg magnesium sulfate per kilogram) is given over 1 hour. Blood pressure should be monitored

paraldehyde
0.2 ml/kg IV, PO, or rectally
Comment: Paraldehyde is used for persistent seizures. IV use carries the risk of pulmonary hemorrhage, right ventricular dilatation, and circulatory collapse. Injection should be diluted with several volumes of saline prior to infusion. Avoid IM use; sterile abscesses or necrosis may occur at the injection site. Dilute drug for rectal use with double volume of mineral oil to decrease irritation.

phenobarbital
Dose for immediate effect: 10 mg/kg IV over 10 minutes or IM. May be repeated one or two times at 20- to 30-minute intervals as a loading dose.
Maintenance dose: 2.5 to 5.0 mg/kg per day IV, IM, or PO for newborns. Adjust dose based on therapeutic effect and serum levels of 15 to 40 μg/ml.

phenytoin (Dilantin)
Dose for immediate effect: 10 mg/kg IV over 5 to 15 minutes. May be repeated once in 20 to 30 minutes as a loading dose.
Maintenance dose: 5 to 8 mg/kg per day IV. IM forms are unreliably absorbed. Some infants require much higher IV doses to maintain optimal neonatal serum levels of 5 to 20 μg/ml. Because of capacity-limited metabolism, dose increases may result in much greater serum level increases than expected. Therefore, increases in serum level should be achieved by giving additional partial loading doses (1 mg/kg for each 1 mg/dl increase in serum level desired), followed by small increases in the maintenance dose (0.5 to 1.0 mg/kg per day). Steady state may not be reached for weeks after a dose increase. If needed for maintenance, oral administration (5 to 10 mg/kg per day in q4–6h doses) may achieve adequate serum levels.

pyridoxine
50 mg IV as a single diagnostic dose

V. Miscellaneous drugs

acetaminophen
5 mg/kg per dose is given PO or rectally q4h when used in newborns.

acetazolamide (Diamox)
5 mg/kg per day IV or PO divided into three equal doses for diuresis. 50 to 100 mg/kg per day divided q6–8h to reduce CSF production (see Chap. 21, Intracranial Hemorrhage).

aminophylline (see **theophylline**)

caffeine citrate

A loading dose of 10 mg/kg caffeine base (20 mg/kg caffeine citrate) is followed by 2.5 mg/kg caffeine base daily in a single dose. When serum concentrations are monitored, optimal levels are 5 to 20 μg/ml. Adverse effects include GI disturbances, tachycardia, and agitation. (See Chap. 13, Apnea.)

calcium glubionate (Neo-Calglucon)

Contains 23 mg elemental calcium per milliliter. Supplement premature infants to a total intake of 150 mg/kg per day of calcium, including content of feedings. Gradually increase dose to full supplement, divided into feedings, to avoid osmotic diarrhea from syrup base. (See Chap. 24, Hypocalcemia.)

chloral hydrate

10 to 40 mg/kg per dose is given PO or rectally q6–8h as required. Maximum daily dose is 50 mg/kg per day. May irritate mucous membranes. Severe chloral hydrate toxicity has been described in premature infants unable to metabolize the drug (Laptook A. R. *Pediatr. Pharmacol.* 4: 161, 1984).

cholestyramine

240 mg/kg per day is given PO in three divided doses. To avoid interference with absorption, oral medications should not be given closer than 1 hour before or 6 hours after cholestyramine.

cimetidine

2 to 10 mg/kg per day is given PO or IV in three divided doses to premature infants; 15 to 20 mg/kg per day in divided doses q6h for term infants.

Comment: Because of limited experience with the use of this drug in newborns and because of concern over endocrinologic toxicities, use should not be routine. Requires dosage reduction in renal dysfunction to avoid CNS side effects. It also may interfere with platelet function. Reduce theophylline dose by half if used with cimetidine.

corticotropin (ACTH)

3 to 5 units/kg per day IM in four divided doses

cortisone acetate

For replacement therapy: 15 to 25 mg/m^2 per day; in newborns, 1 mg/kg per day PO in three equal doses. The dose is doubled at times of stress.

For pharmacologic therapy: 10 mg/kg per day

desoxycorticosterone acetate (DOCA)

2 mg the first day and 0.5 to 1.0 mg each day thereafter for a full-term baby. Fludrocortisone has largely replaced this product.

dexamethasone

0.5 to 1.0 mg/kg per day IM or IV divided q6–8h for treatment of CNS or airway edema. For BPD, several drug regimens have been proposed. Commonly, 0.5 mg/kg per day for 3 days, 0.3 mg/kg per day for 3 days, 0.1 mg/kg per day for 3 days, 0.05 mg/kg per day for 3 days, and 0.01 mg/kg per day for 3 days have been used. (See Chap. 13, Chronic Lung Disease.) All the doses are intravenous and divided bid. Major side effects include hyperglycemia, hypertension, fluid overload, and potential infectious complications.

diazoxide

10 to 15 mg/kg per day PO in two or three divided doses for hypoglycemia unresponsive to glucose infusion. May displace bilirubin from albumin. Hypertrichosis, hyperglycemia, hyperosmolar coma, and transient cataracts have been seen with prolonged use. 1 to 2 mg/kg per dose IV over 30 seconds is used for acute hypertension. May be repeated in 20 minutes if necessary.

edrophonium chloride (Tensilon)

As Tensilon test for myasthenia gravis, 0.04-mg test dose is given by slow IV push and is followed by 0.16 mg/kg after 1 minute. Antidote for reactions is 0.01 to 0.04 mg/kg atropine by IV push.

fentanyl

1-4 μg/kg per dose IV or IM q2–4h prn for analgesia and/or sedation. May also be given by a continuous IV infusion of 0.5 to 5 μg/kg per hour. 10 to 50 μg/kg per dose is used in anesthesia for surgical procedures.

Comment: This new narcotic has similar side effects to morphine: respiratory depression, bradycardia, bronchoconstriction, and ileus. These are most often seen in doses greater than 5 μg/kg. The advantage of fentanyl is that it has less histamine effects. Muscle rigidity can occur. Withdrawal symptomatology has been described in patients treated for prolonged periods.

fludrocortisone (Florinef)

For replacement therapy: 0.025 to 0.2 mg per day PO. This medication has generally replaced desoxycorticosterone acetate in the treatment of chronic mineralocorticoid deficiency.

glucagon

30 μg/kg IM or IV; the dose may be repeated after 6 to 12 hours. 300 μg/kg IM or IV in infants of diabetic mothers (see Chap. 1).

heparin

To keep intraarterial or IV lines open: 0.5 to 1.0 unit/ml in flushing and parenteral solutions, depending on the infusion rate.

For heparinization:

Initial dose: 50 units/kg IV

Maintenance dose: 5 to 35 units/kg per hour IV. The dose is titrated to yield a clotting time of 20 to 30 minutes or two to three times the clotting time before the heparin was administered. Dose can be monitored by the partial thromboplastin time (PTT).

hydrocortisone

For adrenal crisis: As hydrocortisone sodium succinate, 3 to 10 mg/kg per day IM or IV in four equal doses

For long-term maintenance therapy: 15 to 25 mg/m^2 per day or 1 mg/kg per day PO in the newborn

insulin

Used to keep blood sugar normal in very low birth weight infants with inability to tolerate glucose. Used in hyperkalemia (see Chaps. 24 and 26). Regular insulin 0.01 to 0.1 unit/kg per hour by IV infusion pump. Flush tubing with 50 ml of the insulin solution prior to infusing to reduce adsorption loss and improve delivery. Titrate dose according to blood sugar level. Adding albumin 0.3 gm/100 ml of solution may decrease adsorbtion of insulin by the plastic tubing. Intermittent dosage is rarely used but is 0.1 to 0.2 unit/kg q6h S.C.

iron

Treatment of iron deficiency: 6 mg/kg per day elemental iron PO

Prevention of iron deficiency: 2 mg/kg per day PO

Comment: Fer-In-Sol delivers 2.5 mg elemental iron per 0.1 ml. Dropper is calibrated to 0.3 and 0.6 ml (see Chap. 16).

magnesium sulfate

For treatment of hypomagnesemia, 25 to 50 mg magnesium sulfate per kilogram (equals 0.05 to 0.10 ml of 50% solution) is administered IM or IV at 4- to 8-hour intervals. For IV use, the solution should be diluted to 1% (add 1 ml 50% injection to 49 ml saline or sterile water) and infused over 1 hour. For IM injection, dilute measured 50% solution dose with 1.5 times the volume of sterile water or saline to make a 20% injection and give 0.2 ml/kg of 20% solution.

Maintenance dose: 1 mEq is added to each 100 ml of IV fluid; daily intake is 0.25 to 0.50 mEq/kg.

medium-chain triglyceride (MCT) oil

1 to 8 ml over 24 hours PO divided into feedings is the usual dose. Increase gradually to avoid diarrhea. For small premature infants, total fat calories and percentage fat in diet must be determined. MCT oil provides 7.7 cal/ml (see Chap. 30).

meperidine (Demerol)

1.0 to 1.5 mg/kg per dose PO or IM q4h as needed.

methylene blue

0.1 to 0.2 mg/kg in a 1% solution IV (given slowly)

Comment: Methylene blue is used as treatment for methemoglobinemia (see Chap. 14).

metoclopramide (Reglan)

0.1 to 0.3 mg/kg per day in three divided doses has been used for management of feeding intolerance. There is limited experience in newborns to support efficacy. Dystonic reactions may occur.

morphine sulfate

0.1 to 0.2 mg/kg is given IV, SC, or IM q2–4h. Infants treated for more than a short course (i.e., 3 days) should have the dose gradually weaned to avoid withdrawal symptoms.

opium

To provide optimal effect, use diluted deodorized tincture of opium; 1 ml is added to 24 ml sterile water. Dosage for management of withdrawal is 0.8 to 2.0 ml/kg per day PO of this neonatal opium solution divided into six equal doses. Calibrate dropper to convert dose to drops, if desired (see Chap. 2).

pancuronium bromide (Pavulon)

Initial dose of 0.10 to 0.20 to achieve neuromuscular paralysis. Following this, 0.05 to 0.10 mg/kg is given every 90 minutes to 4 hours as needed to maintain paralysis. Tachycardia may be seen. Increased effect seen in hypothermia, acidosis, renal dysfunction, hypokalemia, hypermagnesemia, or with concomitant use of aminoglycosides (see Chap. 13). Reversed by neostigmine (0.04 to 0.08 mg/kg IV plus atropine 0.02 mg/kg IV).

phosphate supplement (Neutra-Phos-A)

Reconstituted solution contains 250 mg phosphorus per 75 ml or 3.3 mg/ml. Supplement premature infant feeds to total intake of 75 mg/kg per day of phosphorus including content of feedings. Gradually increase dose to full supplement to prevent diarrhea. Supplement also provides 0.1 mEq sodium and 0.1 mEq potassium per milliliter. (See Chaps. 24 and 30.)

potassium chloride

1 to 2 mEq/kg per day PO divided into feedings or by slow IV infusion. Concentration should not exceed 3 mEq/dl IV fluid.

prednisone

2 mg/kg per day is given PO.

protamine sulfate

1.0 mg is given IV for each 1.0 mg (100 units) of heparin administered in the preceding 4 hours.

sodium polystyrene sulfonate resin (Kayexalate)

1 gm/kg PO or 1.0 to 1.5 gm/kg rectally q6h. Give as a solution in saline (0.5 gm Kayexalate in 1 ml q saline). Monitor hypocalcemia and hypomagnesemia (see Inborn Errors of Metabolism, Chap. 24 and Chap. 26, page 486).

theophylline

In the management of apnea of prematurity, doses are as follows:

IV therapy: Aminophylline is given in a dose of 7.0 to 8.0 mg/kg (equal to 5.6 to 6.9 mg/kg theophylline) as a loading dose when rapid attainment of plasma levels is desired. This does is infused over 15 to 20 minutes IV.

Maintenance therapy: Aminophylline is given IV at a dose of 2.5 to 8.0 mg/kg per day in divided doses; theophylline is given at a dose of 2.0 to 6.5 mg/kg per day PO in divided doses. Generally, efficacy is seen with every q8–12h dosing because of long elimination half-life. For convenience and oral tolerance, some prefer to administer small doses more frequently. Older infants may require much higher doses. For safety in the presence of capacity-limited metabolism, dose increases should be limited to a 25 percent increase over the previous dose.

Comment: The optimal theophylline serum level for reduction in number and severity of apneic and bradycardia spells is 4 to 15 μg/ml. When a loading dose is not given, it takes several days to reach a full steady-state serum level. Dosage should not be adjusted prior to the fourth day after a dose is instituted. If apnea is severe prior to this time, a serum level should be drawn, and if low, a partial bolus should be given; 0.5 to 1.0 mg/kg theophylline IV (0.6 to 1.2 mg/kg aminophylline PO) is given for each 1 μg/ml that the plasma level is lower than desired. Serum levels should be drawn whenever toxicity is suspected (e.g., with tachycardia, seizures, jitteriness, feeding intolerance). For routine monitoring, post-dose levels are taken 1 hour after the dose infusion or 2 hours after the oral dose (see Apnea in Chap. 13).

thyroid hormone (levothyroxine, Synthroid)

Initial dose is 10 μg/kg per day; generally 0.025 or 0.050 mg is given daily (see Chap. 1).

tubocurarine

0.2 mg/kg IV push; 50% of this dose is then given as needed.

Comment: Tubocurarine is not often used in the newborn.

vecuronium

0.1 mg/kg IV push for paralysis. Repeat as needed every 1 to 2 hours for skeletal muscle relaxation in infants on mechanical ventilation.

verapamil

0.1 to 0.2 mg/kg is infused slowly over 1 to 2 minutes. If antiarrhythmic response in inadequate, this dose may be repeated in 30 minutes.

Comment: Use for supraventricular tachycardia. Monitor the ECG continuously for signs of sinus bradycardia, atrioventricular blockade, or asystole. Hypotension may occur in neonates, especially with prolonged infusion; calcium gluconate administration may be antidotal (see Chap. 14).

vitamins (see Chap. 30)

vitamin A

600–1500 units per day PO

vitamin B_1 (thiamine)

Preventive dose: 0.5 to 1.0 mg per day PO in premature babies

Therapeutic dose: 2 to 5 mg per day PO

vitamin C (ascorbic acid)

Preventive dose: 25 to 50 mg per day PO; 50 mg per day in premature babies

Therapeutic dose: 100 mg q4h PO or IM

vitamin D

400 to 1000 IU per day PO

vitamin E (Aquasol E) (see Chaps. 30 and 38)

25 IU per day PO for prevention of hemolysis

Comment: Aquasol E is very hyperosmolar and should be diluted in at least an equal volume of formula or sterile water for administration.

folic acid (Folacin)

1 mg per week PO

Requirement for term infant: 50 μg per day

vitamin K_1 oxide

Preventive dose: 1.0 mg IM at birth; 0.5 mg if baby is less than 1500 gm

Therapeutic dose: 1 to 2 mg q4h IV or IM (see Chap. 17).

VI. Drugs for resuscitation (see also Chaps. 5 and 6)

atropine (0.4 mg/ml)

0.01 to 0.03 mg/kg per dose IV rapid push, IM, SQ, or endotracheally, given as needed q3min. Preanesthetic dose for infant under 5 kg: 0.04 mg/kg per dose. Maximum total dose is 0.04 mg/kg.

calcium gluconate 10%

Emergency dose: 1 to 2 ml/kg per dose (9 to 18 mg/kg per dose of elemental calcium) IV over 10 minutes; up to 5 ml in premature newborns and up to 10 ml in term babies may be needed.

Maintenance dose: 30 to 80 mg/kg per day of elemental calcium mixed into compatible IV fluids or PO divided into doses q4h.

Comment: 1 ml of calcium gluconate injection 10% contains 9 mg of calcium or 0.46 mEq (see Chap. 24 for discussion of hypocalcemia).

epinephrine

1 to 2 ml of 1:10,000 solution (0.1 to 0.2 ml/kg) (if premixed not available, dilute 1 ml of 1:1000 with 9 ml normal saline). Dose is given IV or intratracheally and repeated as needed. For shock, 0.1 μg/kg per minute (maximum 1 μg/kg per minute). **Preparation of infusion:** 0.5 mg in 50 cc infused at a rate in cubic centimeters per hour equal to the patient's body weight in kilograms will deliver 0.1 μg/kg per minute. **Do not use undiluted 1:1000 epinephrine IV, intratracheally, or intracardiac.**

glucose

The emergency dose is 0.5 to 1.0 gm/kg or 2 to 4 ml of glucose 25% IV.

naloxone

0.1 mg/kg per dose. Naloxone is available in a strength of 0.4 mg/ml, and the use of neonatal naloxone (Narcan 0.02 mg/ml) is no longer recommended (*Pediatrics* 83: 803, 1989). Give IV or intratracheally (SC or IM is occasionally given).

Comment: Naloxone effect lasts approximately 4 hours. It may be repeated as needed and does not cause respiratory depression. Do not give naloxone to infants of drug-addicted mothers because it may precipitate acute withdrawal.

sodium bicarbonate

1 to 3 mEq/kg per dose (use only half-strength solution for newborns (0.5 mEq/ml) or 2 to 6 ml/kg per dose of half-strength solution).

Comment: If half-strength bicarbonate is not available, full-strength should be diluted with an equal volume of dextrose 10% and administered at a rate not faster than 1 mEq/kg per minute (equal to 0.5 ml/kg per minute).

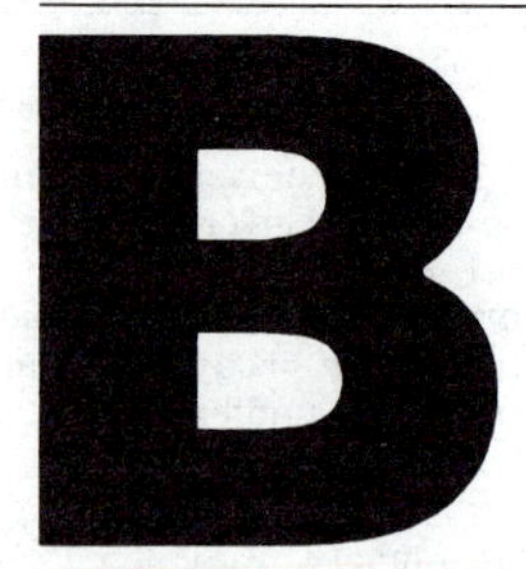

Effect of Maternal Drugs on the Fetus

Celeste M. Marx and
Cheryl A. Stoukides

I. Introduction

A. In most instances, the **risk** of adverse fetal effects from drugs taken by the mother is not known. Properly designed scientific studies cannot be performed ethically, since they would require that women take drugs when they do not need them in order to eliminate the confounding effect of maternal disease or disorder. Thus current investigational methods (retrospective analysis, cohort studies, and case reports) often cannot differentiate the cause of a malformation or other adverse outcome. When a problem occurs in association with a history of maternal drug ingestion, any of the following can be the cause [44,209,324]: A review of fetal damage exposure is found in ref. 481.

1. The drug itself
2. The maternal disease state (e.g., diabetes, maternal infection, or environmental toxicity)
3. Preexistant physical factors (e.g., amniotic bands) producing deformation or disruption
4. Unrecognized illness (e.g., unrecognized viral illness)
5. An already anomalous pregnancy may have produced symptoms that led to drug ingestion.
6. Genetic aberration
7. A spontaneous malformation rate of 2 to 3 percent, a stillbirth risk of 1 percent, and a spontaneous abortion rate of 10 percent
8. Other or unknown cause. In addition, maternal drug histories are extremely unreliable, and findings often depend on how the interview was conducted [42].

B. Teratogenic effects. Because of tremendous variability in maternal elimination and drug disposition characteristics, very little predictivity comes from knowing the maternal dose. Timing of drug exposure is important. Drugs taken when the embryo is extremely undifferentiated are unlikely to produce physical malformation unless the drug persists in the body or alters the gametes. The most critical period for the induction of physical defects is believed to be 15 to 60 days after conception. Because the timing of this event is rarely known with certainty, however, one cannot exclude the possibility of malformation in any clinical situation. Drugs taken after organogenesis can affect the growth and development of the fetus. The brain, in particular, continues to grow and develop in the latter trimesters and beyond. A drug taken during gestation also can act as a transplacental carcinogen. In short, there is no "guaranteed safe" time for a pregnant woman to take a drug [159,181].

C. Even when a drug is associated with a statistically significant increase in the risk of a birth defect, the actual risk may remain low. For example, a birth defect that naturally occurs in 1 in 1,000,000 births may be made 1000 times more likely by drug exposure and still would be seen in only 0.1 percent of drug exposures. A real example of this is with phenytoin exposure: This drug produces a 200 to 400 percent increase in the risk of common birth defects (cleft lip, heart defects); however, 85 percent of children born to women who take phenytoin are normal or have only minor effects of exposure [5]. Numerical risks cannot be stated with certainty for most drugs because the data have been collected retrospectively. Where a risk is stated, the value should be interpreted with caution. For a given pregnancy, studied risk may not accurately reflect the risk to that fetus; genetic factors may have a strong influence on susceptibility to certain teratogens.

D. New information about the effects of drugs and other chemical agents on the fetus. **Manufacturers' recommendations and package inserts should be checked before the fetus is exposed to these agents.**

II. Analgesics

A. Acetaminophen [58,68,85,251,396]. Acetaminophen crosses the placenta but has not been implicated as a teratogen. Neonatal renal failure, fatal at 8 weeks of life, was reported in association with maternal ingestion of 1.3 gm daily or more; no renal biopsy was performed to establish the etiology. A woman who ingested 22.5 gm of acetaminophen at 36 weeks' gestation was treated with acetylcysteine and had a normal delivery at term.

B. Acetylsalicylic acid (aspirin) [30,78,248,396,398,448]. Salicylates readily cross the placenta and can depress maternal urinary estriol excretion. Delayed onset and prolonged duration of labor have been noted. Despite evidence of anomalies in rodents, the widespread use of aspirin noted in many surveys and the lack of evidence of an increased risk of malformations would indicate that it is not an important human teratogen. Birth defects associated with its use are skeletal and heart defects, cleft lip and palate, hypospadias, and cyclopia; these reports are not unexpected in light of the drug's ingestion in up to 69 percent of pregnancies. Some investigators have noted that aspirin may inhibit spontaneous abortion of an already malformed fetus. Aspirin ingestion within 5 days of delivery has been associated with an increased risk of excessive bleeding for both the mother and the infant. Platelet dysfunction has been described (see Chap. 17). There may be an association between high-dose maternal aspirin and the syndrome of pulmonary hypertension in the newborn (see Chap. 13, Persistent Pulmonary Hypertension).

C. Butorphanol (Stadol) [190,354]. Butorphanol is a synthetic opioid agent that does not appear to produce any greater effect on Apgar scores or Scanlon neurobehavioral tests than meperidine (Demerol) in equianalgesic dosage; both drugs are used for labor pain. Presumed depression due to butorphanol may be reversed with naloxone. The ratio of fetal to maternal serum concentrations has been stated to be 0.4 to 1.4:1.0, averaging 0.9:1.0.

D. Meperidine (Demerol) [29,190,236,303,307,367]. When meperidine is given to laboring women, their infants may display depression for up to 4 days on tests of neurobehavior. This effect is most pronounced from 0.5 to 4 hours after the dose, with peak effect at 2 to 3 hours. The toxicity is greater in the premature or asphyxiated baby. The accumulation of normeperidine metabolite (which has greater respiratory depressant and convulsant properties) continues to increase to peak at 20 to 36 hours after the dose. The depressant effects are reversible with naloxone. No teratogenic effects have been identified.

E. Pentazocine (Talwin) (see **IX**) [367]

F. Propoxyphene (Darvon) (see **IX**) [466]

III. Anesthetics [15,51,71,72,127,223,433,503] (see Chap. 4). A cause-effect relationship between chronic occupational anesthetic exposure and reproductive failure (infertility, miscarriage, and anomalies) has not been established. The methodology of the studies that have indicated an increased risk for male and female workers exposed to anesthetics has been strongly criticized. For patients who require surgery in the first or second trimesters, an increased risk of spontaneous abortion, but not congenital malformations, has been reported. The risk of central nervous system (CNS) and respiratory depression is related to duration of exposure. Induction-to-delivery times that exceed 8 minutes are associated with a significantly greater chance of acidosis or low Apgar score at 1 minute (see Chap. 4).

A. Atropine (anesthetic premedication) [212,328]. Atropine undergoes rapid placental transfer with significant fetal uptake after administration of 0.01 mg/kg IV or IM to the mother. Fetal levels are 24 to 87 percent of maternal levels, depending on the time after injection. Thus direct effect on fetal heart rate may be seen, with onset within 5 minutes and persisting for more than 1 hour.

B. **halothane** [490]. Halothane is known to produce abnormal products of cell division and to alter deoxyribonucleic acid (DNA) synthesis in vitro, but rodent studies of teratogenesis have not demonstrated a consistent effect of malformation.

C. **Local anesthetics** [23,88]. With all routes of administration of local anesthetics except spinal, the infant is exposed to small concentrations of the agent. No one agent has been consistently proved to produce the least effect on neonatal neurobehavior. Transient hypotonia, lasting up to 12 hours, may be observed after epidural anesthesia. The CNS effects associated with toxicity may be more profound in asphyxiated infants. Direct injection of local anesthetic agents into the fetal scalp is associated with severe neonatal toxicity.

D. **Nitrous oxide** [180]. Although wives of dentists exposed to higher concentrations of nitrous oxide have been reported to show greater abortion rates than wives of nonexposed dentists, the study design (survey) limits the utility of the data. No increase in anomalies has been reported. When nitrous oxide is used in labor in analgesic doses, no adverse effect on neonatal neurobehavior has been seen.

E. **Scopolamine** [124,293]. Transplacental scopolamine toxicity was documented in an infant after the administration of multiple doses to the mother during labor; the last dose had been given 1 hour prior to delivery. Tachycardia and lethargy responded to physostigmine administration. Delayed onset of breathing and crying has been reported in 10.3 percent of infants given scopolamine and meperidine in one study. A similar experience was observed after the use of cyclopentolate. Meperidine alone generally produces these effects less often.

F. **Skeletal muscle relaxants** [87,291]. Despite a high degree of ionization, muscle relaxants cross the placenta in small amounts without demonstrated effect on the fetus. For pancuronium (Pavulon), the ratio of cord to maternal serum concentrations averaged 0.22:1.00 at delivery, with evidence for fetal uptake. Vecuronium 0.04 mg/kg given to the mother produces fetal levels that are 11 percent of maternal levels at delivery.

G. **Thiopental** [301]. Infants whose mothers are exposed to thiopental metabolize and eliminate the drug rapidly, as well as adults do.

IV. **Anticoagulants**

A. **Heparin** [171]. Because heparin is such a large molecule and should not cross the placenta, direct teratogenicity should not occur. Maternal complications of heparin use such as bleeding also may be seen. Other problems are usually related to the underlying maternal disease not the heparin. These data are drawn from a review of 135 pregnancies. An increased risk of anomalies was not seen.

B. **Warfarin** [171,230,440]. Warfarin use during pregnancy is associated with (1) an embryopathy (stippled epiphyses, chondrodysplasia punctata, hypoplastic nasal bridge, growth retardation) and (2) an increased risk of CNS abnormality. A 1980 review [171] of 423 published cases with warfarin exposure in pregnancy revealed 29 cases of embryopathy. All the affected infants were exposed between 6 and 9 weeks' gestation. Eight percent of all infants exposed during this period were affected; half had no severe disability. CNS effects were seen in 3 percent of infants exposed to warfarin; these effects included mental retardation (31 percent), blindness (12 percent), deafness (12 percent), and seizures (4 percent). Mental retardation was seen only in those infants who were exposed to warfarin in the second or third trimesters, indicating a late effect. The authors estimated that if coumarin derivatives are used during gestation, one-sixth of pregnancies will result in an abnormal live-born infant, one-sixth will be miscarried, and at most two-thirds will have a normal outcome. A more recent review of 40 women in South Africa [230] agrees with these estimates. The proposed mechanism of the embryopathy is an interference with calcium-binding, vitamin K–dependent osteocalcin activity.

V. Anticonvulsants

A. Ethosuximide (Zarontin) [231]. See discussion under **Trimethadione.** In one mother-infant pair, the fetal and maternal serum concentrations were similar at delivery. No anomalies were observed, and the newborn eliminated the drug with a half-life of 41 hours. The mother had been receiving ethosuximide and primidone.

B. Phenobarbital [5,96,143,186,454]. Phenobarbital has been linked, in a few reports, to a syndrome of dysmorphic facies (wide-set eyes, depressed nasal bridge, and ptosis, with mild to moderate growth retardation). Neonatal withdrawal, hypocalcemia, and coagulation defects have been associated with its use near term. The glucuronyl transferase enzyme system may be induced by small doses close to term. The American Academy of Pediatrics' Committee on Drugs has advised that pregnant women should not be switched from effective anticonvulsant therapy with phenobarbital (or phenytoin) to other anticonvulsants about which the teratogenicity data are even less complete; the risk of seizures and resultant hypoxia for both the mother and the fetus likely outweigh the risk of the drugs. The likelihood of a normal child is approximately 90 percent, although the risk of congenital malformations and mental retardation is 2–3 times normal.

C. Phenytoin (Dilantin) [3,5,10,40,92,94,143,186,232,347]. Phenytoin embryopathy is well established. The fetal hydantoin syndrome (FHS) consists of (1) dysmorphic facies (broad, low nasal bridge; epicanthic folds; short, upturned nose; ptosis; strabismus; hypertelorism; prominent and slightly malformed ears; wide mouth or prominent lips), (2) hypoplasia of the distal phalanges and nails, (3) intrauterine and postnatal growth retardation with microcephaly, and (4) mental or motor retardation. The risk of this full syndrome has been estimated at 11 percent of exposed fetuses, and that of minor components of the syndrome in up to 31 percent more, although not all researchers agree with these numbers. Cardiac defects have also been reported in association with FHS. There is some indication that the risk of congenital defects is increased when phenytoin levels are excessive. Genetic factors appear to be important in determining susceptibility to the teratogenic effects, as indicated by discordant expression in genetically distinct twins and triplets. Recent reports note an increased risk of neuroblastoma in children affected with FHS. Cataracts and other vascular anomalies also have been described as occurring with the syndrome (see page 632).

Neonatal hemorrhage due to the competitive inhibition of clotting factor synthesis by phenytoin also has been seen. Onset is generally in the first few hours of life, independent of the administration of vitamin K at birth. There have been some claims that antenatal treatment of the mother with oral vitamin K may reduce the risk of bleeding; however, vitamin K is not effective treatment of the neonate who has a hydantoin-induced bleeding. Clotting factors (fresh-frozen plasma) should be given (see Chap. 17).

D. Primidone (Mysoline) [5,54,125,143,163,273,313,316,364,395]. In a review of 270 cases of antenatal primidone exposure, no consistent trend in teratogenicity was shown; these cases were often complicated by exposure to other known teratogenic anticonvulsants and by poor seizure control. Phenobarbital is a metabolite of primidone; consequently, the infant is at risk for the adverse effects associated with barbiturates, including withdrawal seen in the second and third weeks after delivery. Anomalies associated with the use of primidone are dysmorphic facies (hirsutism, broad nasal bridge, epicanthic folds, hypertelorism, antimongoloid slant eyes, anteverted nares, and small mandible), phalangeal hypoplasia, growth retardation, microcephaly, and cardiac defects. One reported case of possible embryopathy was criticized for its phenotypic similarity to a genetic disorder, Noonan's syndrome.

E. Valproic acid (Depakene) [22,37,91,114,315,422]. Subsequent to the statement in an editorial in the *British Medical Journal* [22] that valproic acid may be the preferred agent for use in pregnancy, a statistically significant increased risk of neural tube defects (spina bifida) to 1 percent has been reported. There are many case reports of anomalies associated with valproate use, but these are frequently complicated by other anticonvulsant use or by poor seizure control. In a report of eight pregnancies in which only valproic acid was taken, growth retardation, diastasis recti abdominis, inguinal hernia, hemangiomas, telangiectasia, supernumerary nipples, odd-looking ears, and hypertelorism were associated minor anomalies. Hyperbilirubinemia was more common in children of mothers who were treated with valproic acid. No cardiac defects were seen. Hyperglycinemia may be seen and can obscure screening for aminoacidopathies.

VI. Anti-infectives

A. Acylovir [173,242,299]. Animal studies show no fetal toxicity or teratogenicity. Safety and efficacy have not been established for use of acyclovir any time during pregnancy.

B. Amphotericin B [16,129,279,320,351,399]. The medical literature documents seven pregnancies in which systemic antifungal therapy was required. One spontaneous abortion and two preterm deliveries (due to preeclampsia and antepartum hemorrhage) were reported complications. These are not necessarily drug-related. At delivery of one of the term infants, cord blood levels were found to be equal to maternal concentrations (2.60 μg/ml). The amniotic fluid contained a concentration of 0.08 μg/ml. There is extensive experience with the use of amphotericin in neonates with fungal sepsis (see Chap. 12).

C. Aminoglycosides [320]. The major concern with the administration of these agents during pregnancy is the eighth cranial nerve toxicity that has been seen in patients receiving direct therapy. Several case reports of fetal and neonatal ototoxicity have been reported with the use of aminoglycosides. The potential for enhancing pharmacologic neuromuscular blockage is also a concern for infants delivered under general anesthesia or requiring therapeutic paralysis.

D. Ciprofloxacin, norfloxacin. Although there are no reports of the use of these agents during pregnancy, these agents are known to cause arthropathies in animals, and the agents are not recommended for use in children whose skeletal growth is incomplete.

E. Gentamicin [84,216,217,486]. When an 80-mg dose is administered IM, lower serum levels are achieved in pregnant women compared with nonpregnant women. Cord serum levels range from 0.25 to 1.68 μg/ml, with a peak level at 1 hour and 20 minutes after injection. This is significantly lower than those levels achieved in maternal serum or amniotic fluid but exceeds the minimum inhibitory concentration for many organisms. These values are drawn from single-dose studies in which the maternal peak concentration was only 2 μg/ml in one study and 7.9 μg/ml in another. When the same dose was followed by a constant infusion of 18.5 μg per hour to women at 18 to 23 weeks' gestation, fetal central venous serum concentrations were 21 to 37 percent of those in maternal serum, similar to the relationship observed in term infants.

F. Neomycin [362]. Neomycin reduces maternal estriol excretion. No anomalies have been reported in association with its use. Little, if any, neomycin is absorbed from the intact gastrointestinal tract.

G. Pentamidine [77,137]. There is one study of placental transfer of drug. Pentamidine was injected into the maternal circulation. Minimal placental transfer to fetus was reported, with significant concentrations in the placenta. Another letter describes cautions when the drug is inhaled. Pentamidine was used in pregnant health care personnel. Pentamidine may work as a folic acid antagonist; other folic acid antagonists (Methotroxate) are associated with problems in the developing fetus.

H. Streptomycin [100,429]. A review of 16 years' experience in 87 patients who received streptomycin for at least 1 month during pregnancy showed that of 30 women and 33 children available for follow-up testing, 3 mothers and 3 children had defective hearing; in two of these cases both mother and child were affected. The children's deafness was high-tone and did not interfere with their normal activity. A control mother-child pair who did not receive streptomycin but were tested also displayed high-tone hearing loss. No vestibular dysfunction was found. There is some speculation that a familial factor may influence susceptibility. A larger retrospective review by the Centers for Disease Control (CDC) that spanned 203 pregnancies from 1948–1979 found that one in six fetuses exposed to streptomycin as a part of combination therapy developed some hearing loss or vestibular effect. Some profound social and educational consequences were described.

I. Antimalarials

1. **Chloroquine** [122,178,268,386,467]. Chloroquine is known to cross the placenta, appear in fetal blood and urine, and accumulate in fetal tissues. Some case reports document no anomalies. Four pregnancies showed a variety of malformations, however, including congenital deafness, gait instability, chorioretinitis, hemihypertrophy, and spontaneous abortion.
2. **Hydroxychloroquine (Plaquenil)** [320]. As with chloroquine, some normal children have been born to women who have received hydroxychloroquine in pregnancy. There is no specific information on risks of this therapy or on associated anomalies.
3. **Quinine** [283]. Placental transfer is rapid. This medication may have an oxytocic or toxic effect, leading to abortion. There are some case reports of ear, eye, heart, kidney, and limb anomalies in exposed fetuses. Congenital deafness, thrombocytopenia, esophageal atresia, hydrocephaly, and mental retardation have been reported.

J. Antiparasitic agents

1. **Crotamiton 10% (Eurax)** [164]. For the treatment of scabies. No data on the use of this agent in pregnancy. No adverse reactions have been reported. This is a safer alternative to lindane.
2. **Lindane (gamma benzene hydrochloride, Kwell)** [155,164]. The manufacturer has indicated that some absorption does occur after topical use of the lotion or shampoo. In animal studies there is no evidence of fetotoxicity, although mean litter weight is decreased and increased evidence of embryo loss is found. There have been no reports of anomalies associated with the use of lindane in pregnancy; therefore, no estimate of the risk from its use can be stated. This is potentially toxic; choose an alternate agent.
3. **Mebendazole (Vermox)** [89,308]. The manufacturer has collected data on 174 pregnancies during which mebendazole was ingested. Forty-two women elected to terminate their pregnancy because of adverse effect on animal fetuses. Of the 132 patients remaining, 96 percent proceeded to a normal, full-term delivery. The 6 remaining infants displayed the following anomalies: capillary hemangiomas (three infants), cleft palate (one), esophageal atresia and imperforate anus (one), absent digits on one hand (one of the children with a hemangioma), and talipes equinovarus (in a child with a positive family history). After a review of the timing of ingestion and the incidence of these disorders, it was stated that the possibility that mebendazole was causal was remote. A review on intestinal parasites in pregnancy recommends treatment only when the parasite poses a public health problem or causes clinical disease in the patient. If necessary the agent may be used for wipworm (*Trichuris teichiurae*).
4. **Paromomycin** [235,388]. Paromomycin is an aminoglycoside antibiotic that is used for *Giardia lamblia* infection (giardiasis). Two patients with severe giardiasis (one in the first trimester, one in the second trimester) were treated with paromomycin 500 mg tid × 10 days. Each subject delivered a normal baby. Little is known about the teratogenic potential of paromomycin if absorbed; however, given the alternative agents (metronidazole, quinacrine, furazolidin), if treatment is necessary during pregnancy (patient is severely symptomatic), parcmomycin is probably the drug of choice.

5. **Pyrethrins, piperonyl butoxide (A-200, RID, RTC)** [164]. For the treatment of pediculosis pubis. Although there are no data on the use of this agent in pregnancy, no adverse reactions are reported. Probably a safe alternative to lindane.
6. **Thiabendazole** [89]. No reports of human thiabendazole teratogenicity exist. A group of pregnant women with intestinal parasites received 50 mg/kg. No adverse effects were seen in the fetus. A review on intestinal parasites in pregnancy recommends treatment when the parasite poses a public health problem or causes clinical disease in the patient. If necessary the agent may be used for hookworm (*Strongyloides stercoralis*).

K. **Antituberculars** [429] (see Chap. 12). A report from the CDC reviewing two U.S. Public Health Service trials and the medical literature revealed 1480 pregnancies in which drug therapy was given. Ninety-four percent of pregnancies resulted in apparently normal infants. Only 2.89 percent of gestations were associated with birth defects, in accordance with the expected spontaneous malformation rate. Therefore, the benefit of treatment has been stated to outweigh the risk.

1. **Ethambutol** [330,411]. There is no evidence of an increased risk of congenital malformations. Long-term follow-up of children exposed in utero shows no adverse effects on growth or development. Cord blood samples drawn at delivery, 30 hours after the last dose of ethambutol showed a cord to maternal ratio of 0.75:1.00 (4.1 to 5.5 μg/liter).
2. **Ethionamide** [356]. A single study reports evidence of heart, CNS, and skeletal system anomalies; others dispute this association.
3. **Isoniazid** [298,320,429]. The CDC survey [429] described isoniazid as "the safest drug to use during pregnancy." As the agent with the most extensive clinical use, it can be seen that in 95 percent of 1480 pregnancies in which isoniazid was used alone or in combination, the outcome was a normal infant. Only slightly more than 1 percent of fetuses or infants were abnormal, although many of the abnormalities suggested CNS toxicity.
4. **Rifampin** [320,429]. Although there was no evidence of an increased risk of malformation from in utero exposure to rifampin in the CDC review, the number of exposed pregnancies was low (442). A limb reduction defect was observed in three pregnancies.

L. **Cephalosporins and cephamycins**

1. **Cefazolin (Ancef, Kefzol)** [34,95]. Cefazolin has been detected at inhibitory concentrations in fetal blood after materal administration at up to 20 weeks' gestation. Levels in first trimester after a 500 mg dose IM were lower than those observed in the second and third trimesters.
2. **Cefotaxime (Claforan)** [208]. After the administration of a single 1-gm IV dose during the second trimester of pregnancy, fetal serum levels ranged from 0.9 to 6.5 μg/ml. No consistent relationship between maternal and fetal concentrations was observed. Fetal levels ranged from nondetectable at 1 hour after injection, with a concomitant maternal level of 5.9 μg/ml, to 106 percent of maternal serum level of 6.1 μg/ml at 2.75 hours after injection. After repeated doses, the fetal serum levels did not change, although maternal values were higher. Cefotaxime was detected in most tissues, although rarely in the spleen and brain of the fetus. Fetal cerebrospinal fluid (CSF) levels were of similar magnitude to serum levels in the single-dose study and lower after multiple dosing.
3. **Cefoxitin (Mefoxin)** [104,134]. After a single 1-gm IM dose, a mean peak cord serum level of 15.1 μg/ml was detected 45 minutes after injection. Fetal samples remained above 1 μg/ml for 370 minutes. No constant relationship was determined for the maternal-fetal ratio, although fetal levels were generally lower.
4. **Cefuroxime (Zinacef)** [348]. Cefuroxime crosses the placenta rapidly after an IV dose of 750 mg. Levels as high as 11 μg/ml can be seen by 1 hour after injection. No consistent relationship between maternal and fetal levels can be described. Cord serum levels can remain above 1.7 μg/

ml for as long as 4 hours after injection. Cefuroxime is detectable in the amniotic fluid 48 minutes after injection, and concentrations may accumulate to exceed concurrent maternal serum levels.

5. **Cephalexin (Keflex)** [112]. After the maternal administration of 1 gm PO, fetal concentrations appear to rise gradually, peaking within 2 hours after ingestion, exceeding maternal concentrations by 3 hours after the dose, and being eliminated at a rate similar to that in the mother thereafter. Fetal serum levels are likely to exceed minimum inhibitory concentrations for sensitive gram-positive and gram-negative organisms for at least 6 hours after the dose.
6. **Cephalothin (Keflin)** [306]. When a single 1-gm IM dose of cephalothin is given to women in labor, the drug may appear in the fetus as soon as 14 minutes after injection. Fetal levels tend to be much lower (6 to 20 percent) than maternal values until maternal levels fall below 8 μg/ml.

M. Chloramphenicol (Chloromycetin) [387,416,488]. Transplacental passage of chloramphenicol occurs, but a constant relationship between maternal and fetal concentrations has not been found. Measured fetal serum levels have ranged from undetectable to 106 percent of concurrent maternal level, all within 5 hours of delivery. Chloramphenicol does not appear to cause malformations. Do not use if another alternative is available (see Appendix A).

N. Clindamycin (Cleocin) [351,485]. Clindamycin crosses the placenta and achieves minimum inhibitory concentrations for many organisms in the fetus after repeated PO doses. It has been seen to accumulate in the fetal liver. After a 60-mg IV dose to the mother at term pregnancy, cord clindamycin levels are up to 46 percent of concurrent maternal level and are in the therapeutic range; peak cord concentrations of 3 μg/ml occur approximately 20 minutes after the injection. Clindamycin cannot be detected in the amniotic fluid within the first hour after injection. No congenital malformations have been associated with its use.

O. Erythromycin [350]. Erythromycin appears to cross the placenta unpredictably when administered PO during the second trimester. Fetal plasma levels are 5 to 20 percent of concurrent maternal plasma levels. Fetal liver tissue may contain higher concentrations than fetal plasma. No anomalies have been reported (see Syphillis, Chap. 12).

P. Methenamine salts [500]. Methenamine depresses maternal urinary estriol excretion.

Q. Metronidazole [32,346,377]. Despite multiple review articles that state that metronidazole is contraindicated for pregnant women, there is no evidence of increased incidence of abortion or prematurity. Four anomalies were observed in infants of 55 mothers treated with metronidazole in the first trimester. A 10-year follow-up of treated women has shown no excess cancer risk; a concern about carcinogenicity had formed the basis for prohibiting this drug during pregnancy. These data are controversial. One author has stated, "although metronidazole is apparently free of teratogenic potential . . . its administration during the first trimester of pregnancy should be avoided."

R. Miconazole (Monistat) [297]. Limited information is available. Miconazole is absorbed from the vagina. Although there is no evidence of teratogenic effects, it is prudent to avoid use in the first trimester. The manufacturer reports that in 487 treated pregnancies, follow-up on 446 is available without evidence of adverse effect on the fetus.

S. Nitrofurantoin [343,344]. Nitrofurantoin crosses the placenta but only reaches low levels. It is rapidly cleared by the newborn. The use of nitrofurantoin in the second and third trimesters is not associated with fetal harm, except in the case of glucose-6-phosphate dehydrogenase (G-6-PD) deficiency (see **XXII**).

T. Penicillins

1. **ampicillin** [84,115,233,349]. Although serum levels are lower in pregnant women compared with nonpregnant women, ampicillin crosses the placenta to reach therapeutic levels in the fetus. Levels are equal after 90

minutes; thereafter, fetal plasma levels are higher than maternal plasma levels. The amniotic fluid contains significant levels of the drug from 30 minutes up to 43 hours after injection. After 1 gm of ampicillin IV, concentrations in cord and neonatal serum have been estimated to exceed the minimum inhibitory concentration for *Escherichia coli* for approximately 4 hours and for *Listeria monocytogenes* and Lancefield group B *Streptococcus* for at least 8 hours. Maternal urinary estriol excretion is depressed. No congenital anomalies have been reported.

2. **Carbenicillin** [115]. After 4 gm is administered IM during the second trimester, cord blood levels are approximately 80 percent of concurrent maternal values (60 μg/ml and 73 μg/ml, respective averages). Carbenicillin concentrations of 5 to 10 μg/ml are seen in the aminiotic fluid and 30 to 45 μg/ml in the placental tissue at delivery 2 hours after the injection. No adverse fetal effect has been reported.
3. **Methicillin** [115,265]. Doses of 0.5 to 1.0 gm IV result in rapid fetal transfer and produce cord serum levels of 0.2 to 2.4 μg/ml up to 2 hours after injection. Maximum fetal to maternal serum level ratio is 0.63.
4. **Mezlocillin** [425]. Transplacental passage has been documented after administration of 2 to 5 gm of mezlocillin IV. No adverse fetal effect was reported. At 20 minutes after injection, fetal levels of 15 to 20 percent of maternal values were seen; maternal and fetal levels were equal at 2.5 hours. The mezlocillin was completely gone from the neonatal urine by 40 hours after delivery.

U. **Povidone-iodine (Betadine)** [243,477]. The vaginal application of povidone-iodine gel results in rapid absorption of iodine. Fetal exposure by means of rinsing of scalp-electrode monitor sites with povidone-iodine solution (1 to 2 percent) results in elevated neonatal iodine concentrations and elevated thyroid-stimulating hormone and lower thyroxin concentrations on the third and fifth days of life, although values had normalized by the fourteenth day of life.

V. **Sulfonamides** [25,33,110,136,320,368]. The sulfonamides cross the placenta rapidly and reach equivalent concentrations in the fetus and the mother. Some sulfonamides can displace bilirubin from binding sites and may lead to kernicterus if the drug is used near delivery. Sulfadiazine appears, from in vitro studies, to have little of this potential. A recent review of 94 pregnancies in which sulfadiazine prophylaxis against rheumatic fever was given through gestation demonstrated that nine of the infants developed clinical jaundice during the neonatal course [25]. There was no clinical evidence to suggest that kernicterus was developing in any of the babies; no gross neurologic deficits were noted on follow-up examinations. No pathologic examinations or sensitive neurologic tests were performed. Indirectly measured unconjugated bilirubin is not an accurate method of assessing free (toxic) bilirubin concentrations. Sulfonamides should not be near the time of delivery. Sulfonamides should not be used in G-6-PD-deficient patients (see **XXII**).

W. **Sulfamethoxazole-trimethoprim combination** [33,368]. Since trimethoprim is now available as a single agent, it is possible to avoid the use of the sulfonamide component of combination products (Bactrim, Septra) in women close to term. Trimethoprim is known to cross the placenta and produce concentrations in fetal serum and tissues that are equal to those in maternal serum and amniotic fluid. The combination with sulfamethoxazole has been used in early pregnancy with no apparent increase in the risk of fetal anomalies. The combination should not be used in patients with G-6-PD deficiency. Trimethoprim use may result in falsely increased serum creatinine levels, which do not reflect a true decrease in renal function.

X. **Tetracyclines** [150,176,239]. The tetracyclines reach cord levels that are 50 to 60 percent of the levels in maternal blood. They selectively concentrate in the teeth (chelating calcium), producing tooth discoloration, enamel hypoplasia, and a tendency to caries. Both deciduous and permanent teeth can be involved. The tetracyclines have also been shown to depress skeletal growth in premature infants. Use during the first trimester has resulted in bone fluorescence and cataracts in the newborn. Pregnant women appear to be particularly susceptible to tetracycline-induced hepatotoxicity (acute fatty liver, which may be fatal).

VII. Cardiovascular medications

A. Acetazolamine (Diamox) [82,412,417,482]. Acetazolamine is known to induce a unique postaxial forelimb defect in rats, *CBA/J* mice, and hamsters. This effect has not been consistently demonstrated in rhesus monkeys or reported in humans. Clinical trials of acetazolamide in late pregnancy complicated by preeclampsia did not show an increase in fetal mortality. Neonatal dehydration and sacrococcygeal teratoma have been separately reported. Outcome of the use of this agent in epileptic gravidas is confounded by associated ingestion of anticonvulsants with known adverse fetal effects.

B. Captopril, enalapril [108,224,234,353,413]. In a case report of a woman who took captopril for severe renovascular hypertension and who elected to terminate her pregnancy, examination of the fetus revealed limb defects and skull malformation. Causality is not established. Animal studies demonstrate a high fetal wastage (up to 60 percent), but no evidence of teratogenicity. There is a report of congenital renal dysgenesis in the offspring of a woman who took captopril during pregnancy. Enalapril has been reported to cause acute renal failure in a neonate and fetal anuria. In a survey of 22 women taking captopril and 9 taking enalapril, angiotension-converting enzyme inhibitors were implicated in fetal death or growth retardation, preterm delivery, and patent ductus arteriosus.

C. Chlorthalidone (Hygroton) [310]. Drug levels in the fetus reach approximately 15 percent of maternal blood concentrations. Infants of four women treated for preeclamptic toxemia with 50 mg daily suffered no reported adverse reactions.

D. Diazoxide [428]. Both acute IV and chronic PO diazoxide therapy have been associated with neonatal hyperglycemia. Neonatal alopecia has been reported occasionally.

E. Digoxin [177,189,219,337,380]. Digoxin readily crosses the placenta and reaches levels in fetal blood that are generally similar to those found in the mother; maternal serum concentrations following standard doses are frequently found to be very low. Conversion of fetal tachyarrhythmias has occasionally occurred during maternal digoxin administration. Digoxin is generally thought not to be a teratogen and does not appear to influence fetal weight or course of pregnancy.

F. Diltiazem [352]. In the rat model, diltiazem is noted to accumulate up to 4 times the maternal concentrations.

G. Dipyridamole (Persantine) [258]. Administration of dipyridamole to 12 pregnant women revealed no compromise of uteroplacental blood pool despite a decline in the cardiac blood pool reflective of decreased cardiac output.

H. Disopyramide (Norpace) [249,419]. The use of disopyramide during pregnancy has been associated with an oxytocic action. Use in the third trimester has not been noted to produce growth retardation. Fetal levels at delivery have been measured at 39 percent of maternal serum level 6 hours following a PO dose.

I. Furosemide (Lasix) [64,342,475,476]. Furosemide crosses the placenta, and fetal urination in close temporal relation to the maternal dose has been observed ultrasonographically. A decrease in the maternal blood volume may have an adverse effect on placental perfusion. No fetal anomalies have been associated with its use. There is the potential for neonatal electrolyte imbalances, although the clinical significance of these has been questioned. There is tremendous variability in cord blood concentrations after administration of furosemide to women at various times prior to delivery. Neonatal concentrations tended to be of the same order of magnitude as those of the mother, but varied from 17 to 545 percent of concurrent maternal level in one study [491]. The elimination half-life in those neonates ranged from 6.8 to 96 hours, inversely correlated with gestational age.

J. **Hydralazine** [48,254,275,494,497]. Hydralazine reaches levels in the fetus that are comparable with, or higher than, those achieved in the mother. Decreased neonatal blood pressure and hypothermia have been reported. Although neonatal thrombocytopenia has been associated with maternal use of hydralazine, the increased incidence of thrombocytopenia in infants of hypertensive mothers must be considered in critically evaluating this report. Both the benefit to the mother and placental perfusion must be considered when hydralazine is given. The fetal heart rate may change with maternal dosing if altered perfusion is induced.

K. **Hydrochlorothiazide** [9,28,48,61,146,497]. The initiation of thiazide diuretics in advanced pregnancy may be associated with a sharp decrease in placental perfusion. Neonatal hyponatremia and hypokalemia have been reported in a case study and were attributed to hydrochlorothiazide. The relationship of thiazides to neonatal thrombocytopenia is questionable; this condition is often seen when the mother is severely hypertensive, even without the use of thiazides. Transfer of the drug to the fetus is indicated by cord plasma levels that reach 10 to 80 percent of simultaneous maternal levels. Thiazide diuretics may decrease urinary estriol excretion.

L. **Lidocaine** [237,480,501]. Lidocaine appears rapidly in fetal circulation after maternal administration (<1 minute). Levels in fetal plasma at delivery are generally less than those of the mother, but the active metabolites are generally found in equal amounts in mother and child. Newborns exposed to epidural local anesthetics may have depressed scores of motor organization, including tone, for 12 to 48 hours after delivery.

M. **Magnesium sulfate** [165,470]. In general, magnesium sulfate is used as an anticonvulsant in preeclamptic women in the third trimester. The magnesium ion crosses the placenta easily, and neonatal hypermagnesemia may be seen. Symptoms of respiratory depression, hypotonia, ileus, and hypocalcemia have been reported but do not correlate with the newborn's serum level unless the magnesium sulfate infusion was prolonged enough to allow full distribution (>24 hours).

N. **Methyldopa (Aldomet)** [205,294,335,492]. Infants whose mothers require methyldopa display systolic blood pressures that are slightly but significantly lower than control infants on the first and third days of life. Methyldopa crosses the placenta to reach levels in fetal serum that are equal to maternal concentrations. The newborn is able to conjugate and excrete the agent slowly after delivery; methyldopa is measurable in neonatal serum for up to 5 days. Because of a report in which the infants of women who were treated with methyldopa starting at 16 to 20 weeks' gestation were seen to have lower mean head circumferences than an untreated control groups' infants, there was some concern that this indicated an adverse effect of methyldopa on development. In follow-up at 4 years of age, the exposed children were developing normally, and the treated group actually scored higher on mental and motor tests.

O. **Nitroglycerin** [430]. Carefully controlled infusions of nitroglycerin have been used to normalize elevated maternal blood pressures during anesthesia for cesarean section. This use of nitroglycerin is not reportedly associated with neonatal depression or hypotension. Nitroglycerin would be expected to cross the placenta easily because of its low molecular weight and uncharged state.

P. **Nitroprusside** [253]. When nitroprusside infusions are used to control maternal blood pressure, there is concern regarding the potential for thiocyanate toxicity in the fetus and newborn. Certainly, the short-term benefit to the mother is to be considered when this titratable agent is selected for acute use.

Q. **Prazosin** [392]. When eight women with uncontrolled hypertension in the third trimester were given prazosin, blood pressure response was good. One of the eight infants showed hypoglycemia and hypocalcemia after delivery at term; all patients also received atenolol. Infant follow-up examinations at 6 to 30 months were entirely normal. It was concluded that prazosin was safe and effective to use when a beta blocker alone failed.

R. Procainamide (Pronestyl) [106,256]. Conversion of fetal tachyarrhythmias has been reported after maternal administration of procainamide. There is great variability in the ratio of fetal to maternal serum concentrations, ranging from 28 percent to approximately 140 percent. The *N*-acetylated active metabolite of procainamide is also expected to cross the placenta and provide fetal effect.

S. Propranolol and other beta blockers [36,48,49,80,107,119,145,245,262,270, 288,327,351,372,393,394,456,457,497]. Most case reports of the use of these agents describe their effects in late pregnancy. Occasional reports of their use in the first trimester for essential hypertension do not reveal a teratogenic effect. There has been some controversy regarding separation of the effects of chronic maternal hypertension on the fetus (e.g., growth retardation, prematurity, and platelet count depression) from those of the medication.

1. **Propranolol** administration has been associated with symptoms of bradycardia, hypoglycemia, and respiratory depression in the neonatal period; the maternal need for this agent may outweigh these transient and manageable effects. An inconsistent relationship between beta-blocker use and intrauterine growth retardation has been described; intrauterine growth retardation is not a common result. Fetal serum levels are similar to those seen in the mother and may rise after delivery, indicating redistribution from tissue stores [80,270,361,394].
2. **Metoprolol.** Metoprolol levels in newborn cord blood approximate those of the mother and may rise after delivery, indicating redistribution from tissue stores [262].
3. **Nadolol.** Treatment of a woman with immunoglobulin A (IgA) nephropathy and hypertension with nadolol and triamterene (Dyazide) throughout pregnancy was associated with neonatal bradycardia and hypoglycemia. Newborn serum nadolol levels were in the adult therapeutic range at birth and rose by 12 hours after delivery, similar to the pattern seen with propranolol and metoprolol. The long duration of action and lack of cardioselectivity may make nadolol one of the less desirable beta blockers for management of hypertension in pregnancy [49].

T. Quinidine sulfate [187]. A woman with idiopathic ventricular tachycardia who conceived during quinidine sulfate maintenance therapy was kept on the drug throughout the pregnancy and delivered a small but normal infant. Cord serum level was 82 percent of concomitant maternal serum level at delivery, 10 hours after the last PO dose. Neonatal thrombocytopenia and an ototoxic effect also have been reported in association with quinidine use.

U. Spironolactone (Aldactone) [296]. An article in the Italian medical literature questions whether or not spironolactone may be safely used in pregnancy because of its antiandrogenic effects. A case is reported in which administration of the drug on days 13 to 21 of gestation was associated with feminization of a male fetus.

V. Verapamil [113,222,336,446,447]. Verapamil has been administered as a labor suppressant at a dose of 2 μg/kg per minute by infusion, with the mean fetal serum level observed to be 51.4 percent of the mean maternal level.

VIII. Antineoplastic agents [21,154,403]. Evaluation of reports of pregnancy outcome after chemotherapy is hampered by the small number of cases. A survey of 30 pregnancies that occurred after aggressive therapy or that were complicated by treatment after the first trimester ($n = 7$) or during the first trimester ($n = 1$) revealed that 10 elective abortions were performed. Two spontaneous abortions were seen, and the 18 remaining infants were born at term and were normal. The heterogeneity of this group makes analysis of the safety of specific treatments impossible. It is now clear that chemotherapy does not provide an invariable contraceptive effect. Up to 40 percent of infants are of low birth weight, and more infants are born prematurely than at full term; whether these factors are due to drug therapy or maternal disease state is unknown.

A. Prior chemotherapy [38,193,194,271,277,423,479]. Much of the literature on the reproductive capacity of people who have received cancer chemotherapy in the past is anecdotal. There is no clear evidence of an increased risk of fetal loss or malformation after prior cancer chemotherapy. Long-term follow-up of the offspring to evaluate the risk of carcinogenesis has not been done. A few case reports note various anomalies (laparoschisis, hypopituitarism), but these are not known to occur more often than by chance. A 1978 report stated that women who had received both chemotherapy and radiation prior to conception were more likely to produce abnormal offspring, and the wives of previously treated men were more likely to miscarry than controls; a criticism of the method by which statistical significance was decided has cast doubt on the findings.

B. Alkylating agents

1. **Busulfan** [43,98]. The use of busulfan in the first trimester has been associated with two malformed infants (one premature infant with microophthalmia, corneal opacities, cleft palate, cytomegaly, streak ovaries and neonatal death and one with anomalous spleen and liver and neonatal death). One normal fetus, one premature infant, and 16 normal term infants were delivered after first-trimester exposure. One case of pyloric stenosis was observed among the normal infants. With later use one infant with intrauterine growth retardation and liver and kidney anomalies and nine normal infants have been reported. In four of the first-trimester exposures, chemotherapy was also given later in pregnancy.
2. **Cyclophosphamide (Cytoxan)** [21,154,166]. First-trimester cyclophosphamide use has been associated with anomalous extremities (four toes or no toes), single coronary artery, palatal anomalies, inguinal hernias and, in combination drug therapy, neonatal leukopenia. One normal premature infant and four normal term infants were born after second- or third-trimester exposure.
3. **Mechlorethamine (nitrogen mustard)** [154,284]. Six case reports of the use of mechlorethamine in the first trimester reported no malformations or adverse effects. Use in the second trimester with procarbazine and vinblastine was associated with abnormality of the feet (four toes and webbing). Causality is not determined.

C. Cytarabine (Ara-C, cytosien arabinoside) [111,154,261,300,318,341,354,478]. This antimetabolite is the subject of several reports documenting the lack of harm to the fetus when administered in the second or third trimester. Ten normal infants have been born after exposure at this time. Splenomegaly, electrolyte disturbances, prematurity, anemia, intrauterine fetal demise, and chromosomal abnormalities have been reported after use of cytarabine in late pregnancy as part of combination chemotherapy, but a responsible agent has not been identified. Although eight normal infants have been born to women treated with cytarabine in the first trimester (or have been electively aborted), other pregnancies have produced infants with defects, including digital and limb anomalies, bilateral microtia, and atresia of the external auditory canals. These anomalies are similar to those induced by administration of cytarabine to pregnant mice. The sensitive time for production of these defects in the human fetus has been estimated to be 4 to 8 weeks' gestation.

D. Dactinomycin [154]. No adverse effects have been attributed to dactinomycin use in the second and third trimesters (three reported pregnancies).

E. Daunorubicin [74,154,458]. One child whose mother had been treated at 29 weeks' gestation required resuscitation at birth 7 weeks later. His hematocrit was 25 percent, but the remainder of the blood count was normal. His mother also had been given cytarabine, vincristine, and ribiazone. Two intrauterine fetal deaths, two premature births, and five normal infants are recounted after use in late pregnancy. Splenomegaly, anemia, and electrolyte disturbances are reported after combination chemotherapy including daunorubicin.

F. **Doxorubicin (Adriamycin)** [74,458]. There has been some speculation that the apparent lack of fetal toxicity (seven normal infants, three of whom were born prematurely) was due to failure of doxorubicin to cross the placenta; it is now clear that transplacental passage does occur.

G. **5-Fluorouracil** [204,434,438]. After use in the first trimester, spontaneous abortions, normal delivery, and, in one case where radiation therapy and tetracycline also were given, bilateral radial aplasia, absent thumbs, duodenal aplasia, and imperforate anus with kidney anomalies have been reported. Fluorouracil intoxication in the newborn has reportedly been seen after use during the second trimester.

H. **6-Mercaptopurine (6-MP)** [93,98,102,154,240,319]. Several case reports document an apparent high incidence of prematurity (5 of 11 cases reported) and infant mortality (3 of 11 cases) after first-trimester use. Anomalies have been seen only after use with radiation and busulfan or aminopterin.

I. **Methotrexate** [39,93,102,154,240,319]. Because of the severe craniofacial anomalies observed after use of a related drug, aminopterin, other antimetabolites such as methotrexate, 5-FU, and 6-MP have been routinely proscribed. It has been stated in one review that as many as half of all fetuses exposed to methotrexate may have cranial or digital malformations. Of 11 reported pregnancies, 7 infants were normal. One infant with cushingoid appearance and one with leukopenia also have been reported. Two other infants have cranial malformations with and without digital anomalies, after first-trimester use.

J. **Methylnitrosourea** [203]. Administration of this agent to pregnant mice has resulted in focal cerebellar damage in the offspring.

K. **Procarbazine** [39,103,147,154,206,284]. The use of procarbazine during the first trimester of four pregnancies did not appear to produce anomalies. Hemangiomas on the extremities were seen in a fifth-first-trimester exposure. In two other cases in which procarbazine was used with other agents (nitrogen mustard and vinca alkaloids), problems included a therapeutically aborted fetus with small, malpositioned kidneys and a miscarried fetus with four toes on each foot and webbing.

L. **Thioguanine (6-TG)** [102,154,261]. The administration of this agent in combination with cytarabine early in two successive pregnancies was associated with bilateral absence of the medial toes and fingers in one of the babies. Cytarabine alone has been associated with limb malformations. Normal infants have resulted from nine 6-TG–exposed pregnancies (three during the first trimester). Reported adverse outcomes of combination chemotherapy include intrauterine fetal demise, splenomegaly, trisomy C (second-trimester use only), and anemia with electrolyte imbalance.

M. **Vinca alkaloids** [39,93,102,111,154,206,240,255,284,318,319,329,341]. In four case reports in which oral vinblastine alone was given in the first trimester, no abnormal infants were born. One infant with four toes and webbing on each foot was miscarried after first-trimester use of vinblastine with procarbazine and nitrogen mustard. Use of these agents during the second or third trimester did not have any adverse effect on two pregnancies. From a review of vincristine use in combination therapy for Hodgkin's disease, no increased risk of fetal loss was apparent. Four of five combination exposures during the first trimester resulted in normal fetuses or infants; the fifth fetus had small, malpositioned kidneys (therapeutic abortion). Later-trimester use of vincristine has been associated with leukopenia (one case), electrolyte imbalance with anemia (one case), prematurity (three cases), cushingoid appearance (one case), splenomegaly, and normal infants (nine) and fetuses (one).

IX. **Drugs of habit or abuse** (see also Chap. 2)

A. **Alcohol (ethanol)** [69,81,141,175,207,334,384,444,445,450,453]. Heavy alcohol ingestion is associated with a syndrome [fetal alcohol syndrome (FAS)] of prenatal or postnatal growth retardation, developmental delay or intellectual impairment, and a characteristic facies with at least two of the following three elements: microcephaly, micro-ophthalmia, or flattened maxillary area. Associated defects have included skeletal, joint, and cardiac malformations. The risk to children born of mothers who drink heavily [>90 ml (3 oz) of absolute alcohol daily] is stated to be 30 to 50 percent. FAS has been reported in a child born to a woman who ingested the alcohol through a proprietary cough preparation. Elements of the syndrome have been noted after lesser amounts of alcohol intake. The danger of light drinking [<30 ml (1 oz) of absolute alcohol daily] has not been established and should not be overstated. A small cohort study of intake of less than 45 ml of absolute alcohol daily did not show a difference in newborn weight or incidence of the FAS anomalies. Similarly, a German study of 7535 pregnancies, 353 complicated by moderate alcohol ingestion, did not demonstrate a poorer growth or psychomotor development up to age 3 years in the exposed group. No absolutely safe amount of alcohol consumption is known. Neonatal withdrawal has been described (see Chap. 2). When used as a tocolytic agent, alcohol has been associated with a neonatal death from intoxication and with an increased risk of respiratory distress. Neural tube defects have been induced in animals and observed in humans after alcohol use in early pregnancy, but an increased risk of major malformations in general has not been proved.

B. **Caffeine** [162,191,257,302,339,383]. Although reports of teratogenicity of high-dose caffeine in rats led the U.S. Food and Drug Administration in 1980 to advise women to reduce their intake of caffeine during pregnancy, in subsequent studies, its effects (i.e., low birth weight and prematurity) were more commonly seen in infants born to women who drank more than four cups of coffee daily. These effects were not sustained when use of tobacco was controlled for. The fetus can be born with significant caffeine levels (up to 12 μg/ml) after maternal ingestion of 290 ± 230 mg per day of caffeine (approximately 3.5 ± 2 cups of coffee daily). Although these figures are well below levels associated with newborn toxicity (50 μg/ml), a respiratory stimulant effect may be seen. Interestingly, the capacity of pregnant women near term to metabolize caffeine is severely restricted (to as much as 33 percent) relative to their postpartum capacity.

C. **Cocaine** [127,267,418,507]. Eye and skeletal defects have been induced in mice but not in rats. The disposition of cocaine in the pregnant mouse demonstrates deposition in fetal tissues at concentrations less than maternal levels; the uterus and placenta were noted to concentrate cocaine. Because of the dramatic cardiovascular effects on maternal blood pressure and the potential for constriction of uterine blood vessels, fetal growth retardation may be seen. A neonatal withdrawal syndrome has been described. Abruptio placentae has been seen after reported cocaine use; causality is not proved. Premature delivery, infarcts, low birth weight, and decreased head circumference have been reported in newborns exposed to cocaine in utero.

D. **LSD (lysergic acid diethylamide)** [62,149,182,269,504]. Because of reports demonstrating chromosomal breakage in leukocytes of users of LSD, there was concern that it could be a strong teratogen. Although there are many case reports of limb-reduction defects, anencephaly, anophthalmia, chromosomal anomalies, and exstrophy of the bladder, there are many case reports of normal infants born to women who have ingested LSD prior to or during gestation. Very small studies describe 17 to 21 percent abnormal newborns, but no definite conclusion regarding the risk of LSD can be made. These case reports are based on the presumed ingestion of LSD, the identity or purity of which should always be questioned.

E. **Marijuana** [139,167,338,437]. Adverse effects on duration of labor and fetal distress have been reported in studies with incompletely matched controls; these findings were not verified in a study of 420 middle-class white women with a user rate of 3 percent. A shorter mean gestation and decreased maternal weight gain were seen. Babies of women who smoked more than five marijuana cigarettes weekly during gestation demonstrated marked tremors, startles, and altered responses to visual stimuli at 2 to 4 days of age; this effect had attenuated by 30 days. No developmental difference was discernible at 1 year of age in children born to women who smoked two or more marijuana cigarettes daily while pregnant. No increase in malformations has been observed, despite indirect evidence that would indicate an increased risk of fetal wastage and congenital anomalies, in addition to increased numbers of chromosomal breaks in leukocytes of marijuana smokers.

F. Narcotics (see also Chap. 2)

1. **Heroin** [41,76,132]. Heroin use is not associated with production of physical malformations. It is associated with an increased risk of low birth weight (nearly one-half of infants weight < 2500 gm). Heroin use may induce maturity of the lung and liver and produce a withdrawal syndrome in the first 24 to 72 hours after delivery. There is an increased risk of behavioral disturbances, including hyperactivity; the mechanism and specific cause of this problem are not known.
2. **Methadone** [76,132,332,381,385]. Methadone maintenance is prescribed for pregnant women to decrease the stress that unreliable heroin dosing and uncontrolled withdrawal in utero produces in the fetus. The risk of neonatal withdrawal is higher than with heroin (75 to 90 percent versus 60 percent); withdrawal may be more protracted and later in onset, with a second exacerbation frequently seen. The risk of severe withdrawal is less for infants of mothers maintained on 20 mg or less daily. Women on methadone should be tapered extremely gradually (i.e., tapered in 5-mg decrements weekly or every 2 weeks) and only in the second trimester to avoid increased risk of miscarriage or intrauterine fetal death. Occasionally, neonatal withdrawal does not begin until 2 to 4 weeks after delivery. There is no reported increase in the risk of major malformations, but the drug is often not started until the second or third trimester. Methadone maintenance, as an alternative to continued illicit narcotic use and its attendant lifestyle, can improve pregnancy outcome and decrease the risk of complications when administered as part of a comprehensive care program. Children of methadone-maintained mothers have been reported to have a greater incidence of microcephaly, but moderate to heavy alcohol use was seen in 15 percent of the methadone-treated mothers studied. Tone discrepancies, developmental delay, poor fine-motor coordination, lower Bailey scores, and a higher incidence of otitis media were seen in the same study. Because of the multifactorial nature of neurobehavior, the cause (drug or environment) of these observations is not known, and such studies are fraught with methodologic problems that confound interpretation of their results.
3. **Pentazocine (Talwin)** [157,229]. Pentazocine readily crosses the placenta. Cord blood levels have been reported at 1 μg/ml, dropping to 0.5 μg/ml by 24 hours after delivery. With prolonged use of pentazocine during pregnancy, infant withdrawal may be seen, usually presenting in the first 48 hours of life. For a description of the withdrawal syndrome, see Chapter 2.
4. **Propoxyphene (Darvon)** [466]. Propoxyphene readily crosses the placenta. The infant's serum may show higher levels of the drug and its metabolite than does maternal serum. Several cases have been reported of withdrawal in infants following prolonged use. No congenital abnormalities have been seen. These infants appear normal at birth, but by 3 to 14 hours of age they may exhibit withdrawal. The symptoms generally decrease by the third or fourth day, and the babies are normal by the fifth day of life.
5. **Phencyclidine (PCP)** [158,443]. After maternal use of PCP, infants have been reported to undergo protracted withdrawal. The etiology of pre-

sumed cerebral palsy in one infant was not apparent and was questionably a drug effect.

G. **Polydrug abuse** [57,188,331]. Despite the known health risks of the lifestyle associated with polydrug abuse, congenital abnormalities are apparently not seen with increased frequency in this group. Low birth weight, prematurity, and low Apgar scores are more common than in non-drug-using controls. Elevated platelet counts in the second week of life, persisting for several months, were reported in 33 infants born to women using methadone plus other drugs. A second peak of platelet count was reported at 10 weeks and resolved by 16 weeks of age (approximately).

H. **Tobacco smoking** [52,99,109,188,264,286,287,290,305]. Cigarette smoking is associated with an increased incidence of growth retardation, perinatal mortality, placenta previa, abruptio placentae, possible increased incidence of cleft lip, and it may impair oxygen exchange across the placenta. Follow-up data on children of smoking mothers raise questions of possible long-term detrimental effects, such as growth retardation and developmental delay. Maternal smoking is known to increase fetal thiocyanate levels, to induce placental metabolism, and to elevate amniotic fluid catecholamines. These elevations may be due to an indirect effect, producing fetal hypoxia, or by a direct effect of nicotine on the fetus. One study suggests that stopping smoking 6 weeks before gestation may be beneficial.

X. **Gastrointestinal medications**

A. **Antacids** [407]. In one small retrospective study, antacids as a group were more commonly ingested (5.9 percent) by mothers of anomalous babies than by mothers of normal infants (2.6 percent). However, no one antacid was more likely to have been taken, no causality may be inferred, and no further studies have substantiated an increased risk.

B. **Atropine and belladonna alkaloids** [73,160,161,220]. When taken in large amounts or when given parenterally prior to anesthesia, atropinic agents can decrease beat-to-beat variability in fetal heart rate and mask the effect of vagal stimulation on the fetal heart. Maternal-fetal transfer of parenteral atropine has been seen to produce a fetal to maternal serum ratio of 0.24 to 0.81:1.00.

C. **Cholestyramine (Questran)** [60]. No adverse fetal effect has been reported from the use of cholestyramine in pregnancy. Malabsorption of fat-soluble vitamins should not occur when less than 20 to 30 gm of cholestyramine is administered daily.

D. **Cimetidine (Tagamet) and Ranitidine (Zantac)** [7,151,156,281,499,508]. Cimetidine administered in the third trimester for peptic ulcer disease has been reported to be associated with transient neonatal liver dysfunction in one case and with a preterm but normal child in another. Long-term effects have not been studied, and earlier use has not been examined. This is of concern because of reports of hypoandrogenization in adult rats exposed to cimetidine in utero and as neonates. Despite its efficacy in managing hyperparathyroid states, cimetidine does not appear to affect calcium placental transfer in the rat model. Cimetidine administration to women in labor to prevent Mendelson's syndrome (aspiration pneumonitis) has not been reported to produce adverse effects on the fetus. An in vitro study of the ability of cimetidine to block the response of the fetal heart to histamine would indicate a potential to impair the fetal stress response.

E. **Docusate (Doss, Colace, and others)** [320,407]. Docusate is often taken in pregnancy, either as a single agent or in a component of prenatal vitamins. Thus first-trimester exposure is common. Contrary to initial beliefs, it is systemically absorbed and has been associated with hepatotoxicity. Retrospective review of its use in pregnancy has not revealed an increased risk for the infants of women who take it.

F. **Metoclopramide (Reglan)** [13,274]. Metoclopramide has been used in early pregnancy for management of nausea and vomiting. In a Russian report, 23 of 24 treated women gave birth to normal children. Metoclopramide also has been used near term for prophylaxis of aspiration pneumonitis; maternal-fetal transfer results in rapid equilibrium between mother and child, with a mean umbilical vein to maternal plasma concentration ratio of 0.6:1.0. Metoclopramide use results in an increase in maternal prolactin and a slight but significant elevation of cord blood thyroid-stimulating hormone.

G. **Sulfasalazine (Azulfidine)** (see **XV**)

XI. **Hormones (See Chap. 25)**

A. **Bromocriptine (Parlodel)** [464]. A survey of the outcome of 1410 pregnancies in 1335 women to whom bromocriptine was given for hyperprolactinemia revealed no increase in the incidence of congenital malformations or pregnancy loss relative to normal populations.

B. **Clomiphene (Clomid)** [1,170]. One review of 159 pregnancies in which clomiphene was taken for induction of ovulation demonstrated a slightly increased risk of malformations (5.4 percent compared with 3.2 percent for controls from Swedish Register data) in 141 births, 7 of which were twins. Not surprisingly, case reports of cleft lip, hypospadias, and imperforate anus have appeared in association with maternal use of clomiphene. Less common birth defects reported after clomiphene use in pregnancy are retinopathy, ovarian dysplasia, and anencephaly.

C. **Danazol (Danocrine)** [66,105,414,489]. A review of the manufacturer's reports of inadvertent danazol exposure in utero in 36 fetuses at 5 days' to 3.5 months' gestation showed that 5 of 14 (36 percent) female fetuses were virilized. No effect was apparent in male infants. Five fetuses were spontaneously aborted, and two were terminated electively. Follow-up of case reports note that pseudohermaphroditism may be accompanied by transient adrenogenital syndrome; this salt-losing adrenal hyperplasia has reverted to normal adrenal function by 1 year of age.

D. **Diethylstibestrol** [11,31,184,278,373,401,441,491]. Diethylstilbestrol (DES) has been implicated as a cause of vaginal adenosis, abnormal vaginal cytology (cervical ectropion or eversion, transverse vaginal or cervical ridges), abnormal uteri, and vaginal adenocarcinoma in female offspring. The risk of clear-cell adenocarcinoma of the vagina is increased and is between 0.014 and 0.140 percent of exposures. Mesonephroma is rarely seen. Increased risks of spontaneous abortion, premature delivery, and ectopic pregnancy in DES daughters with abnormalities of the genitourinary tract have been reported but are not yet validated; the bias of poor obstetric performance in the mothers, leading to DES intake, confounds interpretation of a cause-and-effect relationship. Marked regression of genital anomalies has occurred in many women, and most of those studied have had normal pregnancies and deliveries. Males exposed to DES in utero may show testicular changes (epidydymal cysts, hypoplastic testes, and cryptorchidism in 33 percent versus 10 percent of controls), urethral stenosis, and seminal anomalies at increased frequency (decreased sperm motility and abnormal morphology in 15 to 77 percent versus 5 to 8 percent of controls). The artifact of referral to the reporting urologists must be considered in evaluating these data.

E. **Estrogens** [184,405,498]. The use of estrogens during pregnancy has been associated with masculinization of the female fetus. See **hormonal pregnancy tests** and **oral contraceptives** below for effects of combination therapy (see Chap. 25).

F. **Glucocorticoids** (see **XV**)

G. **Hormonal pregnancy tests** [405,460]. Although the indication for the use of hormonal pregnancy tests has been removed by the Food and Drug Administration, those infants who had been exposed to norethindrone and ethinyl estradiol, norethynodrel and mestranol, or norethindrone alone in the first trimester did not appear to have a statistically higher risk of severe congenital anomalies than a matched control group [475]. Medroxyprogesterone [illegible] as a withdrawl bleeding test, may have an increased relative ri[illegible] alies as high as 2.2 times normal; although data are conflicti[illegible] still be low overall. All progestins carry a risk o[illegible] female fetus; the sensitive time for this expos[illegible] gestation.

H. Hydroxyprogesterone [473]. A review of 150 pregnancies with a history of miscarriage or infertility in which IM hydroxyprogesterone was given from 6 to 8 weeks' gestation through 16 to 18 weeks' gestation failed to prove an adverse effect on physical formation of the fetus or pregnancy outcome.

I. Oral contraceptives [50,260,365,389,402,405,498]. Recent surveys and extensive analysis of the literature indicate that oral contraceptives taken prior to or continued during pregnancy pose either no risk or only a slightly increased risk of nongenital malformations (heart, limb, or CNS). When sex hormones with progestational activity (particularly ethisterone or norethindrone) are continued during pregnancy, virilization of the female external genitalia (clitoral hypertrophy, labioscrotal fusion, penile urethra) may occur. This effect appears to be of low frequency (0.3 to 2.2 percent) after progestogens in general but has been reported to be as high as 18.3 percent after norethindrone, and it also seems to be dose- and time-related. Labioscrotal fusion is exhibited when exposure is prior to the thirteenth week. Phallic enlargement can occur at any stage of development and regresses postnatally. The possibility exists that functional or carcinogenic effects on the exposed fetus may not yet be recognized.

Two recent reports are of particular interest, but the risk cannot be defined. A case report of an infant with transposition of the great vessels who was born after the mother took 120 to 150 combination contraceptive tablets in the first trimester as an abortion attempt is not clearly causative but would strengthen the relation between use and increased risk of truncoclonal defects, which has been inconsistently reported. A syndrome of dysmorphic features (frontal bossing, primary telecanthus, downward-slanting palpebral fissure, broad nasal bridge, pouting lower lip, and square chin) with growth and mental retardation, umbilical eversion, sacral pits, and hypospadias (in males) was noted in 9 of 16 children exposed to sex hormones in the first trimester who were referred for genetic consultation. This has been called a possible embryo/fetal exogenous sex steroid exposure syndrome. The bias of referral is evident here.

J. Thyroid hormones (see **XVII**)

XII. Drugs with obstetric indications

A. Magnesium sulfate (see **VII**)

B. Oxytocin [53,247,415,424]. A newborn whose mother became hyponatremic during oxytocin infusion also became hyponatremic and developed seizures. With correction of the sodium deficit, the seizures ceased and the infant was neurologically normal on follow-up examination (see Chap. 24). Although retrospective analyses have indicated that the risk of hyperbilirubinemia might be higher after use of oxytocin, one prospective study failed to demonstrate a significant influence. Unfortunately, this study did not measure serum bilirubin level in all infants, only those in whom jaundice was seen (see Chap. 15).

C. Prostaglandins [247]. No anomalies have been reported in humans, but these agents are usually given close to term. Comparative studies of neonatal hyperbilirubinemia have shown a lower risk in infants whose mothers were given prostaglandins, rather than oxytocin, to induce labor.

D. Terbutaline (see **XIV**)

XIII. Psychotherapeutic agents

A. Antianxiety drugs

1. Benzodiazepines [4,120,140,210,211,213,340,370,382,400,408,459,493]

a. Clorazepate ingestion in the first trimester has been associated with a child born with multiple congenital anomalies in one case report ...togenital malformations, shortening of the thigh, bifid foot with ...omalies, and lung, bowel, and kidney abnormalities [340].

...**ium)** can be found in fetal plasma in amounts equal to ...as soon as 2 minutes after injection, but generally ...lightly less in the fetus. Diazepam-active me... ...in the fetal liver, particularly with chronic

PO dosing. Maternal-fetal distribution equilibrium is seen 5 to 10 minutes after IV injection. Fetal heart rate beat-to-beat variability is suppressed as soon as 2 minutes after injection; this effect may persist for approximately 1 hour. Significant depression of neonatal neurobehavior is unlikely to be seen in the healthy term infant when the mother has received less than 30 mg in labor. Diazepam use in the first trimester was thought to be associated with an increased risk of cleft lip, with and without cleft palate (frequency as high as 0.4 percent), but this association has been disproved. Neonatal withdrawal symptoms have been described after chronic use during pregnancy [120,140,211,370,382,400,408] (see Chap. 2).

c. **Lorazepam** given IV for induction of anesthesia is found in similar concentrations in maternal and fetal blood at delivery. The fetal cord plasma level rarely exceeds that of the mother, but the drug will persist in plasma for as long as 10 days. Full-term babies may experience a delay in establishing feeding after the mother is given PO lorazepam, but low Apgar scores, poor suck, respiratory depression, and poor temperature control have been observed after IM use. Preterm newborns were more likely to be adversely affected or to show these signs. Notably, the mothers of the infants observed had fulminating hypertension, which may have affected infant outcome [211,213,493].

d. **Oxazepam** levels rise to exceed maternal concentrations by as much as 35 percent by 3 hours after PO dose, and this relationship is sustained for at least a day. The conjugated metabolite of oxazepam does not accumulate in the fetus, despite delayed elimination of the parent drug. Apgar scores have generally been observed to be good [210,459].

2. **Hydroxyzine** [359]. Withdrawal symptoms have been described in newborns after administration of extremely high doses (600 mg per day) during pregnancy for control of itching (see Chap. 2).

B. **Haloperidol (Haldol)** [228]. A single case report notes a child afflicted with phocomelia in association with maternal ingestion of haloperidol. This adverse effect has not been seen in other treated pregnancies.

C. **Lithium** [2,131,322,404,487]. Although the risk of a rare congenital defect of the heart valve (Ebstein's anomaly) is increased in children born to women taking lithium, the risk remains very low (2.8 percent estimate). A small review of lithium use in pregnancy revealed that 18 of 166 children were abnormal; this risk of 10.8 percent malformation cannot be taken as absolute because of the small numbers. It has been stated that echocardiography can detect Ebstein's anomaly prior to 20 weeks' gestation. Neonatal intoxication (hypotonia, respiratory depression) has been seen after maternal use in late pregnancy. In one case, neonatal intoxication was followed by persistent pulmonary hypertension.

D. **Phenothiazines** [45,101,126,366,411,426]. Despite the demonstration of teratogenicity and postnatal growth retardation in rats, reviews of up to 1209 pregnancies have failed to demonstrate increased risk in humans. A study of first-trimester use in 316 pregnancies indicated a relatively increased risk of anomalies in the treated group compared with a control group; however, the incidence of anomalies in the control group (1.6 percent) was somewhat smaller than normal. A syndrome of functional small colon, which is diagnosed and treatable by meglumine diatrizoate (Gastrografin) enema, has been described after maternal use of chlorpromazine and benztropine, with and without thiothixene, doxepin, and biperiden, presumably due to the anticholinergic properties of these agents. A withdrawal reaction also has been described (see Chap. 2), as well as extrapyramidal reactions in the newborn.

E. **Tricyclic antidepressants** [17,24,198,420,471,485]. There is no stror
dence of an increased risk of malformations in children born aft
tricyclic antidepressant use. Case reports of limb redu
anomalies (including cleft palate and exencephalia)

diaphragmatic hernia have appeared. In addition to a withdrawal syndrome (see Chap. 2), urinary retention has been observed in infants born to treated women.

XIV. Respiratory drugs

A. Antiasthmatic medications [465]. Except for neonatal hypoglycemia due to beta agonists and thyroid suppression due to iodides, little risk has been associated with the use of antiasthmatic drugs during pregnancy. The possibility of unrecognized adverse drug effects on the fetus should be weighed against the known hazards of maternal hypoxia and acidosis for the fetus.

1. **Cromolyn sodium (Intal)** [442]. Information from the manufacturer, who does not recommend the use of cromolyn during pregnancy, reveals 474 reports of its use during all or part of gestation. Abnormalities were seen in 14 cases, including CNS and gastrointestinal malformations and limb anomalies. These small numbers would not appear to indicate an increased risk of defects associated with the use of cromolyn.
2. **Terbutaline and other beta agonists** [18,314,432,451,506]. Evaluation of the safety of beta-sympathomimetic agents (hexoprenaline, isoproterenol, isoxsuprine, ritodrine, albuterol, and terbutaline) is confounded by the morbidity of prematurity when their use for labor suppression is unsuccessful. Short-term adverse effects have included hypoglycemia secondary to maternal hyperglycemia and glycogenolysis. The incidence has been estimated at 15 percent and is not consistently observed to be more frequent than in age-matched control infants; it is more common when the fetus is also exposed to steroids. Fetal metabolic acidosis may occur due to increased lactic acid, but no change in oxygen tension is expected. Isolated placental perfusion studies have estimated the placental transfer of ritodrine to be 16 percent, compared with 12 percent for albuterol. The clearance of norepinephrine to the placenta is approximately two-thirds that of ritodrine. Although fetal tachycardia has been noted in association with the use of beta-sympathomimetic agents, the relatively low amount of these drugs passed to the fetus raises questions about a direct effect and may question the risk of maternal hypotension. Animal studies have not demonstrated an adverse effect on fetal brain development or on the electroencephalogram. Although administration of large doses to animals in early pregnancy has been associated with increased risks of cleft lip and palate, no adverse effect has been reported after use of these agents for relief of bronchospasm in early human pregnancy.
3. **Theophylline (including aminophylline)** [14,195,241]. No increased risk of anomalies has been associated with the use of theophylline in pregnancy. At delivery, theophylline is usually present in equal amounts in maternal and cord serum, although higher neonatal values may be found when heel-stick sampling is performed (mean value of 1.83 μg/ml, higher 30 to 60 minutes after delivery). Transient tachycardia and jitteriness have been reported in infants with serum levels in excess of 10 μg/ml, but no adverse effect on heart rate or Apgar score has been seen for theophylline-exposed newborns in general. In one infant who displayed vomiting, jitteriness, and opisthotonus, the level at delivery was 9.2 μg/ml. Since subsequent levels were not determined until 56 hours later, it is difficult to ascribe this to drug toxicity by means of redistribution. An apneic spell was seen in a term infant whose mother had taken a combination theophylline and sympathomimetic tablet during pregnancy. The [illegible]ord theophylline level was 14.9 μg/ml, and the first spell occurred only [illegible]rs later. The authors postulated that this was a theophylline with-[illegible] but pneumograms were persistently abnormal, suggesting [illegible]nea.

[illegible]**tiemetics and antipruritics)** [317]

[illegible]e retrospective study that included a very [illegible]in which brompheniramine was used indi-[illegible]r malformation. The overall risk would still be expected to be quite low, but the statistical method does not allow precise prediction.

2. **Chlorpheniramine, chlorpromazine, diphenhydramine, diphenylpyraline, prochlorperazine, promethazine, trimeprazine, and triprolidine.** Several large retrospective studies have shown that mothers who consumed these antihistamines and antiemetics produced infants with fewer anomalies than mothers who did not receive these medications. Withdrawal syndromes have been seen for both antihistamines and phenothiazines (see Chap. 2).
3. **Cyclizine, chlorcyclizine, and meclizine.** Early reports of numerous anomalies (in animal studies and case reports) in infants whose mothers received these drugs have not been substantiated by larger, more controlled studies.
4. **Terfenidine** [153]. Doses of 300 mg/kg per day were not teratogenic in rats or rabbits but were often lethal to rabbits. No evidence of mutagenicity or carcinogenicity potential was observed. For rats that remained on the drug after weaning and were given 300 or 150 mg/kg per day, their offspring had decreased weight gain and survival and decreased weight gain, respectively.

XV. Antirheumatics, anti-inflammatory agents, and immunosuppressants

A. Azathioprine (Imuran) [148,183,360,496]. A review of more than 38 cases of azathioprine use in pregnancy (primarily for management of rejection after renal transplant) did not demonstrate an increased risk of anomalies, even when used throughout pregnancy. A case report of preaxial polydactyly ascribed to azathioprine exposure, despite maternal ingestion of other drugs, has been questioned because of inconsistency of the induction of this disorder in animal models. The major metabolite of azathioprine, 6-mercaptopurine, has occasionally been associated with fetal defects (see **VIII**).

B. Colchicine [505]. Despite characterization of the drug as antispermatogenic and its former use as an abortifacient, there are 11 case reports of conception during colchicine therapy for familial Mediterranean fever. All three treated males fathered normal children. Of eight females who conceived on colchicine, four gave birth to normal infants and only one miscarried. No follow-up has been published on the three who were still pregnant at the time of the report.

C. Cyclosporin A [252]. A women who conceived while taking cyclosporin A, 450 mg daily, was continued on this drug throughout gestation; low urinary estriols were noted from 32 weeks on and were attributed to a low glomerular filtration rate. The drug was detected in cord blood at a concentration of 54 μg/liter at a time when maternal concentration was 86 μg/liter. The child born to this woman was entirely normal, and there is no evidence of teratogenicity in laboratory animals.

D. Glucocorticoids [8,19,20,26,75,97,169,246,263,330,333,360,369,406,449]. The commonly used steroids (betamethasone, dexamethasone, hydrocortisone) have all been demonstrated to cross the placenta or to have active metabolites that do. Despite observations of anomalies in animals (neurologic changes, cleft palate, cellular or organ growth disruption), steroids administered to pregnant women have not been reported to increase the risk of malformation. In a small review of 70 pregnancies in which corticosteroids were used in the management of asthma, no increase in the rate of toxemia, hemorrhage, or malformations was seen. Several studies have noted growth retardation (in women who received steroids for infertility) or increased risk of spontaneous abortion (severely hypertensive mothers) relative to control gravidas with the same disorder.

The use of steroids to enhance fetal lung maturation was not associated with adverse neurobehavioral outcome for the offspring, who were examined at 5 years of age. Antenatal administration has been associated with decreased maternal urinary estriols and serum placental lactogen concentrations in the week after treatment. Neonatal and maternal leukocytosis and neonatal lymphocytopenia (with abnormal chromosomes observed transiently) have been seen. The premature infant is seen to undergo suppression of cortisol secretion for 7 days (by as much as 55 percent), suppression of dehydroepiandrosterone sulfate by 65 percent for 7 days, and suppression of growth hormone by 53 percent, returning to levels higher than controls between 2 and 4 days after betamethasone (see Chap. 13).

E. **Gold** [59,375,379]. Gold is recognized to cross the placenta and to deposit in the fetus after administration of the thiomalate salt (Myochrysine). There are several case reports of normal offspring after use throughout pregnancy and one report of an infant with cleft lip and palate and brain abnormalities.

F. **Nonsteroidal anti-inflammatory agents (ibuprofen, indomethacin, naproxen, and others)** [59,86,90,295,391,397,495]. It has been recommended that pregnant women avoid ingestion of drugs that inhibit prostaglandin synthesis unless there are strong indications, because of the association of their use with premature closure of the ductus arteriosus and persistent pulmonary hypertension in the newborn. CNS damage also has been reported as well as stimulation of fetal respiratory movements in utero. Hemostatic abnormalities have been reported. Anomalies have not been reported after use in early pregnancy or prior to conception.

G. **Penicillamine** [117]. A review of case reports of penicillamine use in pregnancy shows that of 87 patients treated during pregnancy, only 2 infants showed the collagen defect disorders (growth retardation, lax skin, poor healing, vein fragility, varicosities, hernias) that had previously been reported. If one excludes the cases of Wilson's disease, in which the penicillamine is presumed to be less available to cross the placenta because of chelation, 2 of 34 infants were affected. It has been suggested that this agent is acceptable for the management of cystinuria and Wilson's disease in pregnancy, but that other agents are preferable for rheumatoid arthritis.

H. **Sulfasalazine (Azulfidine)** [83,266]. Although there are isolated case reports of adverse pregnancy outcomes (hydrocephalus with oral clefts) associated with maternal use of sulfasalazine for the control of inflammatory bowel disease, a review of 287 pregnancies in which the drug was taken did not reveal an increased risk of abnormalities when the drug was used alone or in combination with steroids for ulcerative colitis. In a subgroup of women with Crohn's disease, the use of steroids plus sulfasalazine was associated with a greater incidence of anomalies (congenital deafness, ear defects, or cleft palate). There was no increase in spontaneous abortions or growth retardation in the treated groups.

XVI. **Testing and diagnostic agents**

A. **Methylene blue** [215,280]. The use of methylene blue in pregnancy has been discouraged because of the potential for metabolic disturbances (hemolysis, hyperbilirubinemia, methemoglobinemia) in the newborn when given close to delivery. A woman who inadvertently underwent diagnostic laparoscopy during early gestation ($5\frac{1}{2}$ weeks after last menstrual period) was given methylene blue solution 0.2% by intrauterine injection and gave birth to a normal male at term.

B. **Radiographic contrast media** [27,218,304,376]. Neonatal intestinal opacification has been observed in infants who were exposed in utero to maternally administered Renografin-60 (meglumine diatrizoate with sodium diatrizoate). No harmful effects of the exposure were seen, despite an iodide content of 34.5 gm. Fetal thyroid suppression has been occasionally reported after amniography and bronchography using meglumine diatrizoate and is usually not seen after amniography or renography.

C. **Tuberculin skin testing** [309]. The manufacturer of Aplisol PPD test (Park-Davis, Division of Warner-Lambert Co., Morris Plains, NJ) is unaware of any specific studies indicating its safety for use during pregnancy. There are no data to suggest any particular problem associated with its use.

XVII. **Thyroid medications** (see also Chap. 1, Thyroid Disorders)

A. **Antithyroid agents (propylthiouracil/methimazole/carbimazole)** [55,56,70, 185,289, 311]. Fetal growth retardation has been reported in association with both the need for and use of these agents in pregnancy. Both hyper- and hypothyroidism have been reported in infants born to women treated with antithyroid agents. The risk of abnormal neonatal thyroid function may be partly related to the etiology of the mother's disorder, but hypothyroidism appears to be fairly uncommon when minimum doses are used. The combination of thyroid hormone with antithyroid drugs has been discouraged, since it may increase the maternal dose requirement, thereby increasing fetal risk. The incidence of neonatal goiter after the use of these agents has been estimated at 1 to 5 percent. Propylthiouracil is the preferred agent, because it blocks peripheral conversion of T_4 to T_3. Case reports of scalp defects occurring in association with methimazole use in pregnancy should be evaluated based on the strong heritable nature of this defect. A recommendation exists that the mother should be maintained on as low a dose of propylthiouracil as is tolerated, preferably less than 100 mg daily. Congenital hypothyroidism appears to be unlikely at a dose less than 300 mg daily. A controlled study of the intellectual development of children exposed to propylthiouracil in utero did not reveal any adverse effect up to 28 years of age.

B. Iodides [55,63,123,144]. Goiter can occur in the fetus with maternal ingestion of as little as 12 mg of iodine daily. These goiters tend to be larger than those seen with propylthiouracil, and although they regress with time, they may obstruct the airway. Mental retardation has been reported in association with maternal iodine use.

C. Radioactive iodine-131 [133,374,484]. **Therapeutic** doses of iodine-131 are contraindicated in pregnancy because of fetal radiation exposure and thyroid destruction. When a pregnant woman is inadvertently exposed to 10 mCi of iodine-131, the total-body radiation exposure is approximately 5 rads. The gonadal dose is 0.30 to 0.45 rad/mCi of drug. Persistent chromosomal changes have been observed in the leukocytes of patients who have received the drug. The fetal radiation exposure is relatively greater than the mother's.

Congenital hypothyroidism has been reported, and carcinogenic potential should be considered. Observations of radiation exposure in victims of the atomic bomb have shown that microcephaly was most common when exposure occurred at 7 to 15 weeks' gestation; growth and development also were delayed. Long-term effects were generally correlated with a dose above 50 rads. It has been stated that the dose of both iodide and radiation from **diagnostic** iodine-131 exposure during pregnancy need to be a concern. If the therapeutic dose is given and pregnancy is identified within a week, however, the use of 300 mg propylthiouracil daily for 7 days has been recommended to block recycling of iodine-131 in the fetal gland.

D. Thyroid hormones [185,221,276,363,472]. Thyroid hormones cross the placenta only with difficulty. For this reason, where there is a desire to use them therapeutically, as in known fetal hypothyroidism or in an attempt to hasten fetal lung maturation, they have been administered into either fetal muscle or amniotic fluid. Administration of thyroid hormones to the mother receiving antithyroid drugs does not decrease the risk of congenital hypothyroidism and may result in the need to use a higher dose of antithyroid drug.

XVIII. Toxins and environmental agents

A. Fluoride [118,225]. A retrospective study of 492 children whose mothers were given sodium fluoride tablets in addition to drinking fluoridated water revealed, at a 4- to 9-year evaluation, that prenatal fluoride use was associated with a 90 percent reduction in decay incidence compared with control siblings. There were more caries-free children in the treated group, and birth weights and lengths were greater in the treated group; in addition, more term pregnancies were seen in the treated group. A 1976 review of 1,387,027 births in a fluoridated community did not detect an increased rate of malformations. This was also the finding of a similar study in an Alabama community.

B. Hexachlorophene [172]. Hexachlorophene is transferred to the fetus. A retrospective survey of 460 neonates born to Swedish hospital workers revealed a 5.4 percent malformation rate compared with 0 percent in 233 controls. The small size of the study and the abnormally low incidence of malformations in the control group makes one unable to evaluate these data; no specific defect was seen with increased frequency. The workers washed with hexachlorophene soap 10 to 60 times daily.

C. **Herbicides (Agent Orange, dioxin, paraquat, 2,4,5-T)** [46,174,312,436,455, 461]. Despite great public concern regarding the public health risk of **Agent Orange** (of which 2,4,5-tetrachlorophenoxyacetic acid is a component and 2,3,7,8-tetrachlorodibenzoparadioxin a contaminant), retrospective analysis of reproductive histories of the families of these herbicide sprayers or manufacturing workers did not reveal an increased risk of spontaneous abortion, stillbirth, or anomalies. There are studies of births in sprayed areas of New Zealand (in which increased risk of talipes malformation was seen) and in a community where a chemical plant explosion occurred (in which increased miscarriages and malformations were reported). Because of known animal teratogenicity and fetotoxicity, careful review of the known exposures is needed. A woman who ingested paraquat as a suicide attempt at 20 weeks' gestation underwent gastric decontamination and diuretic therapy. Serum levels were 0.1 percent of toxic. The infant was normal, born at term, and well clinically at 3-year follow-up.

D. **Lead** [214,259,325]. Lead crosses the placenta and is found in the fetus in amounts equal to or exceeding maternal concentrations. An infant who was exposed to high levels of lead in utero, owing to maternal paint-chip pica, had elevated numbers of leukocytes with chromosomal breaks at 3 weeks, 6 weeks, and 3 months of age. Physical and neurologic examination at 18 months of age was within normal limits. The mother had been treated in the eighth month of pregnancy with calcium disodium edetate (EDTA). Radiographs showed metaphysitis, submetaphyseal lucencies, and sclerosis of the shafts of the long bones. Women who have occupations exposing them to lead show a higher incidence of sterility and spontaneous abortion than other women. An infant was reported to have neurologic defects and intrauterine and postnatal growth retardation after maternal ingestion of lead through moonshine alcohol; the etiology of the infant's problems was not clearly an effect of lead.

E. **Methylmercury** [6,197,227,272]. The Minamata syndrome of mercury poisoning involves cerebral palsy, skull deformities, abortion, stillbirth, and neonatal death. One survey of 29 mother-infant pairs with mercury exposure correlated normalcy in offspring with maternal hair concentrations less than 25 ppm, whereas two severely affected children had mothers with peak hair contents of 165 and 209 ppm. Signs and symptoms of mercury poisoning were more frequent in the group with the highest hair mercury levels (90 to 394 ppm). There was no significant difference in the frequency of abnormalities in children whose mothers had hair levels of 0 to 11 ppm versus 12 to 85 ppm. Head circumference in offspring did not correlate with maternal hair level. Maternal symptoms did not correlate with fetal abnormality; mercury readily crosses the placenta and is retained in the fetus for a long period of time. One review of fetal risk associated with maternal exposure to mercury has recommended that women of child-bearing age limit their fish consumption to 350 gm per week and avoid exposure (1) to mercury vapor concentration greater than 0.01 mg/m^3, (2) to inorganic or phenylmercuric compounds greater than 0.02 mg/m^3, or (3) to any methylmercury. Ethanol use may increase the risk of mercury toxicity.

F. **Organic solvents** [192,421]. A report of an increased risk of CNS defects among children of women exposed to organic solvents has been criticized for poor matching of controls and cases with regard to social variables known to be associated with congenital CNS defects.

G. **Polychlorinated biphenyls (PCBs)** [226,378]. Most studies show that exposure to PCBs in utero causes slow growth, altered immune function, and slowed development, although usual tests for teratogenesis in animals are negative. Yusho disease—the "cola-colored baby" syndrome of dark skin, eye disease, severe acne (chloracne), and growth retardation—was reported after ingestion of cooking oil contaminated with this by-product of the electrical industry. Similar accidents have occurred worldwide, with the additional recognition of an abnormal black pigmentation of the nose. No clear relationship between maternal dose and symptoms or fetopathy has been found; cord blood levels tend to be 24 percent of maternal concentrations. Follow-up of Japanese children has shown that growth disturbance tended to disappear a few years following end of exposure, but that residual pigmentation, apathy, and "soft" neurologic signs were common.

H. **Polyvinyl chloride, vinyl chloride** [179,468]. Hungarian epidemiologic studies note the higher incidence of chromosomal aberrations in workers exposed to **polyvinyl chloride** but disagree about whether or not the risk of congenital malformations is increased for the offspring of those exposed. Increased stillbirth rates and numbers of spontaneous abortions also have been reported. The data are not conclusive. Ecologic studies of communities where **vinyl chloride** is produced appear to indicate an increased risk of neural tube defects in these areas, compared with statewide controls. Case-control studies, however, suggest that the relative risk is likely to be less than 2.3 times normal but is still too small to define precisely. The methodology of studies indicating an increased risk of spontaneous abortion have been criticized; larger studies are needed.

XIX. **Vaccines, sera, and toxoids.** The consequences of intrauterine infection can be subtle and inapparent at birth, only to manifest later. Theoretically, some vaccinations might harm the fetus despite the absence of adverse effects on the mother.

A. **Bacillus Calmette-Guerin (BCG) vaccine** [362,463]. This vaccine should be avoided during pregnancy.

B. **Cholera vaccine** [362,463]. No malformations have been associated with first-trimester vaccination. Risk of intrauterine fetal death increased with third-trimester infection with cholera.

C. **Diphtheria** [362,463]. Diphtheria antitoxin should be avoided during pregnancy; however, no adverse effects have been observed.

D. **Hepatitis B vaccine.** The Centers for Disease Control do not consider pregnancy to be a contraindication in situations in which this vaccine is indicated.

E. **Influenza virus vaccine** [362,463]. Use of this vaccine has been associated with some malformations, but it is not clear that this association represents an increased risk.

F. **Measles virus vaccine** [250,362,431,463]. Most adult women are immune to measles (roseola); if not, they should be vaccinated when traveling to developing areas. Immunoglobulin is considered a safer prophylactic measure in pregnancy than is measles vaccine. A 10-fold greater incidence of neural tube tumors and malignancies has been noted in the offspring of vaccinated women in one study.

G. **Meningococcal vaccine** [65]. When mixed vaccine containing polysaccharides of meningococcus groups A and C was administered to 91 pregnant women during an epidemic in Brazil, there was evidence of passive transfer of antibody, but it was inconsistent. The presence of antibodies in the mother did not guarantee that they would be present in the infant. When present, the antibody transferred to the babies lasted 2 to 5 months. No adverse outcomes were reported, even in those infants of mothers vaccinated in the first trimester (among the 21 women for whom complete information was collected).

H. **Mumps virus vaccine** [116,199,250,362,463]. Most adult women are immune to mumps. The risk of vaccination is unknown. Vaccine virus is capable of infecting the placenta, but fetal infection has not been shown. Although there is no evidence of a teratogenic effect of the mumps virus, it is suggested that the vaccine be avoided in pregnancy. One case of bladder exstrophy has been reported after exposure to the vaccine in the first trimester.

I. **Pertussis vaccine** [463]. Hyperthermia leading to abortion may occur after vaccination; however, pertussis vaccine should not be given to patients over 6 years old.

J. **Poliomyelitis vaccine** [358,362,463]. There are some reports of congenital anomalies, abortion, and stillbirth, but the clinical risk is believed to be low. A twofold increase in malignancies in offspring of vaccinated mothers has been reported. Adults should be given killed polio vaccine if they are to be immunized.

K. **Rabies vaccine** [250,362,463,474]. Allergic and neurologic side effects have been observed in the offspring of mothers given this vaccine. A mother who developed clinical rabies during pregnancy produced a child with growth retardation and astigmatism. One case report of prophylaxis during the third trimester with duck embryo vaccine showed no growth or developmental anomaly. Another woman vaccinated at 34 weeks' gestation, after a bat bite, was given rabies immunoglobulin and then human diploid rabies vaccine repeatedly; her child was born at term and was developmentally normal at 1 year of age.

L. **Rubella virus vaccine** [138,250,357,362,463,469]. Rubella virus has been isolated from placental and fetal tissues. Although it is recommended that vaccination be avoided during pregnancy, infants of vaccinated women do not appear to be at a higher risk for anomalies (see Chap. 12).

M. **Tetanus toxoid** [362,463]. No adverse effects have been reported. The vaccine confers immunity to the fetus (see Chap. 12).

N. **Yellow fever vaccine** [250,362,463]. Vaccination is indicated only if the woman is traveling to an endemic area; it should be avoided in the first trimester. There is little information available. No adverse effects have been reported.

XX. Vitamins

A. **Vitamin A** [35]. Vitamin A is known to be a teratogen in animals. Anomalies (e.g., malformed genital system, obstructive salt-losing nephropathy, neural tube defects) have been described in humans after excessive doses of vitamin A and after use of isotretinoin (Accutane) [see **isotretinoin** (retinoic acid)]. Because of the widespread use of these agents in prenatal vitamins, the risk for exposure to vitamin A is difficult to define. Dosage in excess of the recommended daily allowance for pregnancy should be avoided (see **XXI**).

B. **Vitamin B_6 (pyridoxine).** Pyridoxine dependence has been seen in infants of mothers using excessively high doses. Use in the first trimester, as a component of the antiemetic drug Bendectin, has not been associated with an increase in the overall risk of congenital malformations.

C. **Vitamin D** [142,168,390]. There are conflicting reports of supravalvular aortic stenosis associated with infantile hypercalcemia related to altered vitamin D metabolism. When 25-hydroxycholecalciferol is administered to the mother, cord blood levels average about 81 percent of maternal values; higher fetal-to-maternal ratios (to 1.08:1.00) have been seen with low maternal levels.

D. **Vitamin K** [94,371]. The rate and extent of transfer of vitamin K across the placenta have not been adequately examined. Large doses given to the mother just before delivery or to the infant soon after birth may produce jaundice by hemolysis, by competition for bilirubin metabolism, or by direct hepatotoxicity. Prenatal use of vitamin K has been suggested for pregnant women being treated with anticonvulsants (especially phenytoin) as prophylaxis against drug-induced clotting factor deficiency (see **V**) (see Chap. 17).

XXI. Uncategorized agents

A. **Isotretinoin (Accutane)** [47,244,345,439]. Isotretinoin is a potent human teratogen. Several reports of spontaneous abortion and a range of birth defects exist. Isotretinoin produces a characteristic pattern of malformations, i.e., craniofacial, cardiac, thymic, and central nervous system (see **XX**).

B. **Oral antidiabetic agents** [201,409]. Two small studies have indicated a higher incidence of death in infants of chlorpropamide-treated women when compared with tolbutamide- or insulin-treated women. Although congenital malformations have been reported, the increase in congenital anomalies associated with poor diabetic control makes these reports difficult to ascribe to a drug effect. Transient neonatal thrombocytopenia and neonatal hypoglycemia have been reported with maternal tolbutamide use; the etiology was not investigated and the effect was attributed to the drug. These agents are not considered drugs of choice for diabetes in pregnancy (see Chap. 1).

C. **Parenteral nutrition solutions** [436,462,483]. The use of total parenteral nutrition (TPN) in the third trimester has not been associated with any problems for the fetus. One woman who was maintained on dextrose/Synthamin/Intralipid solutions from conception through gestation delivered a normal child who had decreased weight for length.

D. **Spermatocides** [196,202,292,323,355]. Although a preliminary study appeared to indicate an increased risk of congenital malformations among children whose mothers had used a spermatocide in the 10 months prior to conception, subsequent studies have not confirmed an increased risk or have had uninterpretable results because of limitations in study design. At present, spermatocides are not known to increase the risk of birth defects.

E. **Tretinoin (Retin-A).** Reproduction studies in rats (using 50 times the usual human dose) showed no harm to the fetus. There was a slightly higher incidence of ossified skull bones in some rats. Normal application of Retin-A should provide minimal amounts of vitamin A to be absorbed. Retin-A should be used in pregnancy only if clearly needed.

XXII. **Drugs to be avoided in patients with glucose-6-phosphate dehydrogenase (G-6-PD) deficiency** [136,233,285,435]:

acetanilid
antimalarials
antipyrine
ascorbic acid
aspirin
chloramphenicol
dimercaprol
fava beans
furazolidone
mestranol
methylene blue
nalidixic acid
naphthalene
nitrofurantoin
nitrofurazone
phenacetin
phenylhydrazine
quinidine
sulfonamides
trinitrotoluene
vitamin K

References

1. Algren, M. *Acta. Obstet. Gynaecol. Scand.* 55: 371, 1976.
2. Allan, L. D. *Lancet* 2: 875, 1982.
3. Allen, R. W. *J.A.M.A.* 244: 1464, 1980.
4. American Academy of Pediatrics, Committee on Drugs. *Pediatrics* 69: 241, 1982.
5. American Academy of Pediatrics, Committee on Drugs. *Pediatrics* 63: 331, 1979.
6. Amin Zaki, L. *Am. J. Dis. Child.* 133: 172, 1979.
7. Anand, S. *Science* 218: 493, 1982.
8. Anderson, G. *Am. J. Obstet. Gynecol.* 140: 699, 1981.
9. Anderson, J. B. *Acta Paediatr. Scand.* 59: 659, 1970.
10. Anderson, R. C. *J. Pediatr.* 89: 318, 1976.
11. Antoniolo, D. A. *Am. J. Obstet. Gynecol.* 137: 847, 1980.
12. Armstrong, J. G. *Ann. Intern. Med.* 61: 106, 1964.
13. Arvela, P. *Eur. J. Clin. Pharmacol.* 24: 345, 1983.
14. Arwood, L. L. *Pediatrics* 63: 844, 1979.
15. Aswog, V. F. *Nord. Med.* 83: 498, 1970.
16. Attkin, G. W. *J. Obstet. Gynecol. Br. Comm.* 69: 677, 1962.
17. Australian Drug Evaluation Committee. *Med. J. Aust.* 1: 768, 1973.
18. Ayromlooi, J. *Pediatr. Pharmacol.* 1: 321, 1981.
19. Ballard, P. L. *J. Pediatr.* 101: 468, 1982.
20. Ballard, P. L. *Pediatr. Res.* 14: 122, 1980.
21. Barber, H. R. *Obstet. Gynecol.* 58: 41S, 1981.

22. Bardy, A. H. *Br. Med. J.* 283: 515, 1981.
23. Barrier, G. *Clin. Obstet. Gynaecol.* 9: 351, 1982.
24. Barson, A. J. *Br. Med. J.* 2: 45, 1972.
25. Baskin, C. G. *Cardiology* 65: 222, 1980.
26. Beck, J. C. *Clin. Obstet. Gynecol.* 23: 93, 1980.
27. Becroft, D. M. A. *Arch. Dis. Child.* 55: 213, 1980.
28. Beermann, B. *Gynecol. Obstet. Invest.* 2: 45, 1980.
29. Belsey, E. M. *Br. J. Obstet. Gynaecol.* 88: 398, 1981.
30. Benawra, R. *J. Pediatr.* 96: 1069, 1980.
31. Berger, M. J. *Obstet. Gynecol.* 55: 254, 1980.
32. Berget, A. *Ugeskr. Laeger.* 134: 2085, 1972.
33. Berglung, F. *J. Urol.* 114: 802, 1975.
34. Bernard, B. *J. Infect. Dis.* 136: 377, 1977.
35. Bernhardt, I. B. *Obstet. Gynecol.* 43: 750, 1974.
36. Bianchetti, G. *Clin. Pharmacol. Ther.* 29: 233, 1981.
37. Bjerkedal, T. *Lancet* 2: 1096, 1982.
38. Blatt, J. *N. Engl. J. Med.* 304: 1121, 1981.
39. Blatt, J. *Am. J. Med.* 69: 828, 1980.
40. Bleyer, W. A. *J.A.M.A.* 235: 626, 1976.
41. Blinick, G. *Am. J. Obstet. Gynecol.* 125: 135, 1976.
42. Bodendorfer, T. W. *Am. J. Obstet. Gynecol.* 135: 490, 1979.
43. Boros, S. J. *Am. J. Obstet. Gynecol.* 129: 111, 1977.
44. Boue, J. *Basic Life Sci.* 4: 317, 1975.
45. Bouquette, C. R. *Teratology* 15: 57, 1976.
46. Bower, C. *Lancet* 2: 1247, 1980.
47. Braur, J. R. *Lancet* 1: 506, 1986.
48. Brazy, J. E. *J. Pediatr.* 100: 265, 1982.
49. Breitfeld-Fox, R. F. *Am. J. Obstet. Gynecol.* 152: 1045, 1985.
50. Briggs, M. H. *Adv. Steroid Biochem. Pharmacol.* 7: 51, 1979.
51. Brodsky, J. B. *Am. J. Obstet. Gynecol.* 138: 1165, 1980.
52. Brook, O. G. *Br. Med. J.* 298: 795, 1989.
53. Buchan, P. C. *Br. Med. J.* 2: 1255, 1979.
54. Burn, J. *J. Pediatr.* 100: 836, 1982.
55. Burrow, G. N. Thyroid Diseases. In G. N. Burrow and T. F. Ferris (Eds.), *Medical Complications During Pregnancy.* Philadelphia: Saunders, 1982. Pp. 187–214.
56. Burrow, G. N. *Yale J. Biol. Med.* 51: 151, 1978.
57. Burstein, Y. *J. Pediatr.* 94: 895, 1979.
58. Byer, A. J. *J.A.M.A.* 247: 3114, 1982.
59. Byron, M. A. *Br. Med. J.* 294: 36, 1987.
60. Campbell, D. E. (Mead Johnson Pharmaceutical Co., Evansville, Ind. 47721). Personal communication, April 15, 1984.
61. Campbell, D. M. *Br. J. Obstet. Gynaecol.* 82: 572, 1975.
62. Carakunshansky, G. *Lancet* 1: 150, 1969.
63. Carswell, F. *Lancet* 1: 1241, 1970.
64. Carswell, W. *J. Obstet. Gynecol.* 81: 472, 1974.
65. Carvalho, A. D. A. *Lancet* 2: 809, 1977.
66. Castro Magana, M. *Am. J. Dis. Child.* 135: 1032, 1981.
67. Chapman, R. M. *Ann. Intern. Med.* 96: 681, 1982.
68. Char, V. C. *J. Pediatr.* 86: 639, 1975.
69. Chasnoff, I. J. *Am. J. Dis. Child.* 135: 968, 1981.
70. Check, J. H. *Obstet. Gynecol.* 60: 122, 1982.
71. Cohen, E. N. *J. Am. Dent. Assoc.* 90: 1291, 1975.
72. Cohen, E. N. *Anesthesiology* 41: 317, 1974.
73. Cohn, E. H. *Gynecol. Invest.* 7: 57, 1976.
74. Colbert, N. *Nouv. Presse Med.* 9: 175, 1980.
75. Collaborative Group on Antenatal Steroid Therapy. *J. Pediatr.* 104: 259, 1984.
76. Connaughton, J. F., Jr. *Am. J. Obstet. Gynecol.* 129: 679, 1977.
77. Conover, B., et al. *Ann. Intern. Med.* 109: 927, 1988.
78. Corby, D. G. *Pediatrics* 62(Suppl. No. 5): 930, November, 1978.

79. Cordero, J. F. *J.A.M.A.* 245: 2307, 1981.
80. Cotrill, C. M. *J. Pediatr.* 81: 812, 1977.
81. Council on Scientific Affairs. *J.A.M.A.* 249: 2517, 1983.
82. Crane, C. H. *J.A.M.A.* 165: 1517, 1957.
83. Crazi, A. *Arch. Intern. Med.* 140: 1674, 1980.
84. Creatsas, G. *J. Perinat. Med.* 8: 13, 1980.
85. Crombie, D. L. *Br. Med. J.* 5720: 178, 1970.
86. Csaba, I. F. *J. Pediatr.* 92: 484, 1978.
87. Dailey, P. A. *Anesthesiology* 57: A391, 1982.
88. Dailey, P. A. *Clin. Perinatol.* 9: 191, 1982.
89. D'Alauro, F. *Obstet. Gynecol.* 66: 639, 1985.
90. Dalens, B. *Arch. Fr. Pediatr.* 38: 261, 1981.
91. Dalens, B. *J. Pediatr.* 97: 332, 1980.
92. Dansky, L., et al. Maternal Epilepsy and Congenital Malformations: Correlation with Maternal Plasma Anticonvulsant Levels During Pregnancy. In D. Janz (Ed.), *Epilepsy, Pregnancy and the Child.* New York: Raven Press, 1982.
93. Dara, P. *Cancer* 47: 845, 1981.
94. DeBlay, M. F. *Lancet* 1: 1247, 1982.
95. Dekel, A. *Eur. J. Obstet. Gynecol. Reprod. Biol.* 10: 303, 1980.
96. Desmond, M. M. *J. Pediatr.* 80: 190, 1972.
97. Devoe, L. D. *Am. J. Obstet. Gynecol.* 135: 473, 1979.
98. Diamond, I. *Pediatrics* 25: 85, 1960.
99. Divers, W. A. *Am. J. Obstet. Gynecol.* 141: 625, 1982.
100. Donald, P. R. *S. Afr. Med. J.* 60: 316, 1981.
101. Donaldson, G. L. *Acta Paediatr. Scand.* 71: 335, 1982.
102. Doney, K. C. *Cancer Treat. Rep.* 63: 369, 1979.
103. Dow, E. G. *Lancet* 2: 984, 1970.
104. Dubois, M. *J. Clin. Pharmacol.* 21: 477, 1981.
105. Duck, S. C. *Fertil. Steril.* 35: 230, 1981.
106. Dumesic, D. A. *N. Engl. J. Med.* 307: 1128, 1982.
107. Dumez, T. *Br. Med. J.* 283: 1077, 1981.
108. Duminy, P. C. *S. Afr. Med. J.* 60: 805, 1981.
109. Dunn, H. G. *Can. J. Public Health* 68: 43, 1977.
110. Dunn, P. M. *J. Obstet. Gynaecol. Br. Comm.* 71: 128, 1964.
111. Durie, B. G. M. *Arch. Intern. Med.* 137: 90, 1977.
112. Duval, J. *Nouv. Presse Med.* 1: 1419, 1972.
113. Ebstein, M. *Pediatrics* 75: 732, 1985.
114. Editorial. *Br. Med. J.* 283: 515, 1981.
115. Elek, E. *Int. J. Clin. Pharmacol. Ther. Toxicol.* 63: 223, 1972.
116. Emanuel, T. *Lancet* 2: 156, 1971.
117. Endres, W. *Klin. Wochenshcr.* 59: 535, 1981.
118. Erickson, D. *J. Am. Dent. Assoc.* 93: 981, 1976.
119. Erkkola, R. *Acta Obstet. Gynaecol. Scand.* 61: 31, 1982.
120. Erkkola, R. *Acta Obstet. Gynaecol. Scand.* 52: 167, 1973.
121. Eskenazi, B. *Am. J. Obstet. Gynecol.* 144: 919, 1982.
122. Essein, E. E. *Clin. Chem.* 28: 1148, 1982.
123. Etling, M. *Obstet. Gynecol.* 53: 376, 1979.
124. Evens, R. P. *Pediatrics* 666: 329, 1980.
125. Fabro, S. *N. Engl. J. Med.* 300: 1280, 1979.
126. Falterman, C. G. *J. Pediatr.* 97: 308, 1980.
127. Fantel, A. G. *Teratology* 26: 17, 1982.
128. Feldman, G. L. *Am. J. Dis. Child.* 131: 1389, 1977.
129. Feldman, R. *South Med. J.* 52: 1415, 1959.
130. Ferstandig, L. I. *Acta Anaesthiol. Scand. (Suppl.)* 75: 38, 1982.
131. Filtenborg, J. A. *Eur. J. Pediatr.* 138: 321, 1982.
132. Finnegan, L. P. *Ann. N.Y. Acad. Sci.* 362: 136, 1981.
133. Fisher, D. A. *J. Pediatr.* 62: 132, 1963.
134. Flaherty, J. F. *Am. J. Obstet. Gynecol.* 146: 760, 1983.
135. Food and Drug Administration. *F.D.A. Drug Bull.* 11: 1, 1981.

136. Forfar, J. G. *Clin. Pharmacol. Ther.* 14: 632, 1973.
137. Fortunato, S. J. *Am. J. Obstet. Gynecol.* 160: 759, 1989.
138. Fox, J. P. *J.A.M.A.* 246: 1444, 1981.
139. Fried, P. A. *Neurobehav. Toxicol. Teratol.* 4: 451, 1982.
140. Friedman, E. A. *Obstet. Gynecol.* 34: 82, 1969.
141. Friedman, J. M. *J. Pediatr.* 101: 232, 1982.
142. Friedman, W. F. *Pediatrics* 43: 12, 1969.
143. Friis, B. *Arch. Dis. Child.* 52: 239, 1977.
144. Galina, M. P. *N. Engl. J. Med.* 267: 1124, 1977.
145. Gallery, E. D. M. *Br. Med. J.* 1: 1591, 1979.
146. Gant, N. F. *Am. J. Obstet. Gynecol.* 123: 159, 1975.
147. Garrett, G. J. *Clin. Oncol.* 3: 145, 1977.
148. Gebhardt, D. O. E. *Obstet. Gynecol.* 59: 270, 1982.
149. Gelehrter, T. D. *J. Pediatr.* 77: 1065, 1970.
150. Genot, M. T. *J. Oral Med.* 25: 75, 1970.
151. Ghisan, F. K. *Am. J. Obstet. Gynecol.* 142: 922, 1982.
152. Gibson, G. T. *Med. J. Aust.* 1: 410, 1981.
153. Gibson, J. P. *Apzreimittelforsch.* 32: 1179, 1988.
154. Gililland, J. *Obstet. Gynecol. Surv.* 38: 6, 1983.
155. Ginsburg, C. M. *J. Pediatr.* 91: 988, 1977.
156. Glade, G. *Am. J. Dis. Child.* 134: 87, 1980.
157. Goetz, R. L. *J. Pediatr.* 84: 887, 1974.
158. Golden, N. L. *Pediatrics* 65: 16, 1980.
159. Goldman, A. S. *Clin. Perinatol.* 6: 203, 1979.
160. Goodlin, R. C. *Am. J. Obstet. Gynecol.* 129: 845, 1977.
161. Goodlin, R. C. *Obstet. Gynecol.* 48: 117, 1976.
162. Goyan, J. E. *F.D.A. Press Release.* Washington, D.C., P80-36:3, 1980.
163. Granstrom, M. L., Bardy, A. H., and Hiilesmaa, V. K. Prolonged Feeding Difficulties of Infants of Primidone Mothers During Neonatal Period: Preliminary Results from the Prospective Helsinki Study. In D. Janz (Ed.), *Pregnancy, Epilepsy and the Child.* New York: Raven Press, 1982. Pp. 357–358.
164. Greaves, W. L., et al. *Rev. Infect. Dis.* 4(Suppl. No. 1): 5857, 1982.
165. Green, K. W. *Am. J. Obstet. Gynecol.* 146: 29, 1983.
166. Greenberg, L. H. *J.A.M.A.* 188: 423, 1964.
167. Greenland, S. *Am. J. Obstet. Gynecol.* 143: 408, 1982.
168. Gupta, M. M. *Postgrad. Med. J.* 58: 408, 1982.
169. Hagler, S. *Am. J. Dis. Child.* 106: 96, 1963.
170. Halal, F. *Can. Med. Assoc. J.* 133: 1159, 1980.
171. Hall, J. G. *Am. J. Med.* 68: 122, 1980.
172. Halling, H. *Ann. N.Y. Acad. Sci.* 320: 426, 1979.
173. Hankey, G. J., et al. *Neurology* 37: 1534, 1987.
174. Hanley, J. A. *Science* 212: 349, 1981.
175. Hanson, J. W. *J. Pediatr.* 92: 457, 1978.
176. Harley, J. D. *Lancet* 1: 472, 1964.
177. Harrigan, J. T. *N. Engl. J. Med.* 304: 1527, 1981.
178. Hart, C. W. *Arch. Otolaryngol.* 80: 407, 1964.
179. Hatch, M. *Environ. Health Perspect.* 41: 195, 1981.
180. Hay, D. *Br. J. Obstet. Gynaecol.* 85: 299, 1978.
181. Hays, D. P. *Drug Intell. Clin. Pharm.* 15: 444, 1981.
182. Hecht, F. *Lancet* 2: 1087, 1968.
183. Henahen, J. *J.A.M.A.* 249: 2287, 1983.
184. Herbst, A. L. *Obstet. Gynecol.* 58(Suppl. No. 5): 35S, November, 1981.
185. Herbst, A. L. *Obstet. Gynecol.* 21: 543, 1963.
186. Hilesman, V. K. *Lancet* 2: 165, 1981.
187. Hill, L. M. *Obstet. Gynecol.* 54: 366, 1979.
188. Hingson, R. *Am. J. Obstet. Gynecol.* 144: 959, 1982.
189. Ho, P. C. *Aust. N.Z. J. Obstet. Gynaecol.* 20: 24, 1980.
190. Hodgkinson, R. *J. Int. Med. Res.* 7: 244, 1979.
191. Hoff, W. V. *Lancet* 1: 1020, 1982.

192. Holmberg, P. C. *Am. J. Ind. Med.* 1: 167, 1980.
193. Holmes, G. E. *Cancer* 31: 1317, 1978.
194. Horning, S. J. *N. Engl. J. Med.* 304: 1377, 1981.
195. Horowitz, D. A. *Am. J. Dis. Child.* 136: 73, 1982.
196. Huggins, G. *Contraception* 25: 219, 1982.
197. Hursh, J. B. *J. Pharmacol. Exp. Ther.* 214: 3, 1980.
198. Idanpaan Heikkila, J. *Lancet* 1: 282, 1973.
199. Immunization Practices Advisory Committee, Centers for Disease Control. *M.M.W.R.* 31: 617, 1982.
200. Jacobs, C. *Ann. Intern. Med.* 95: 669, 1981.
201. Jackson, W. P. U. *Diabetes* 11(Supp. 1): 98, 1962.
202. Jick, H. *J.A.M.A.* 245: 1329, 1981.
203. Jirakulsomchok, S. *Brain Res. Bull.* 8: 45, 1982.
204. Jochimsen, R. P. *J.A.M.A.* 245: 1660, 1981.
205. Jones, H. M. R. *Br. J. Clin. Pharmacol.* 8: 433, 1979.
206. Jones, R. T. *Obstet. Gynecol.* 54: 477, 1979.
207. Jung, A. L. *Am. J. Dis. Child.* 134: 419, 1980.
208. Kafetzis, D. A. *J. Antimicrob. Chemother.* 6(Suppl. A): 135, 1980.
209. Kalter, H. *N. Engl. J. Med.* 308: 424, 1983.
210. Kangas, I. *Eur. J. Clin. Pharmacol.* 17: 301, 1980.
211. Kanto, J. H. *Drugs* 23: 354, 1982.
212. Kanto, J. *Acta Anaesthiol. Scand.* 25: 85, 1981.
213. Kanto, J. *Acta Pharmacol. Toxicol. (Copenh.)* 47: 130, 1980.
214. Karlog, O. *Acta Pharmacol.* 15: 8, 1958.
215. Katz, Z. *N. Engl. J. Med.* 304: 1427, 1981.
216. Kauffman, R. E. *Pediatr. Res.* 9: 104, 1975.
217. Kauffman, R. E., Azarnoff, D. L., and Morris, J. A. Placental Transfer and Fetal Urinary Excretion of Gentamicin: Comparison Between an Animal Model and the Human Fetus. In P. L. Morselli, S. Garattini, and F. Sereni (Eds.), *Basic and Therapeutic Aspects of Perinatal Pharmacology.* New York: Raven Press, 1975. Pp. 75–81.
218. Kelleher, J. *A.J.R.* 132: 63, 1979.
219. Kerenyi, T. D. *Lancet* 2: 393, 1980.
220. Kivado, I. *Br. J. Anaesth.* 49: 1017, 1977.
221. Klein, A. H. *J. Clin. Endocrinol. Metab.* 47: 1034, 1978.
222. Kleinman, C. S., et al. *J.C.U.* 13: 265, 1985.
223. Knill Jones, R. P. *Lancet* 1: 1326, 1972.
224. Knott, P. D., et al. *Lancet* 1: 451, 1989.
225. Knox, E. G. *Community Med.* 21: 190, 1980.
226. Kodama, H. *Arch. Environ. Health* 35: 97, 1980.
227. Koos, V. J. *Am. J. Obstet. Gynecol.* 126: 390, 1976.
228. Kopelman, A. E. *J.A.M.A.* 231: 62, 1975.
229. Kopelman, A. E. *Pediatrics* 55: 888, 1975.
230. Kort, K. I. *S. Afr. Med. J.* 60: 578, 1981.
231. Koup, J. R. *Epilepsia* 19: 535, 1978.
232. Kousseff, B. G. *Pediatrics* 70: 328, 1982.
233. Kraybill, E. N. *Am. J. Obstet. Gynecol.* 138: 793, 1980.
234. Kreft Jais, C. *Br. Med. J.* 296: 421, 1988.
235. Kreutner, A. K., et al. *Am. J. Obstet. Gynecol.* 140: 895, 1981.
236. Kuhnert, B. R. *Am. J. Obstet. Gynecol.* 133: 909, 1979.
237. Kuhnert, B. R. *Clin. Pharmacol. Ther.* 26: 213, 1979.
238. Kuhnz, W. *Pediatr. Pharmacol.* 3: 199, 1983.
239. Kunelis, C. T. *Am. J. Med.* 38: 359, 1967.
240. Kurshid, M. *Lancet* 2: 534, 1978.
241. Labovitz, E. *J.A.M.A.* 247: 786, 1982.
242. Lagrew, D. C. *J.A.M.A.* 252: 2058, 1984.
243. L'Allemand, D. *J. Pediatr.* 102: 935, 1983.
244. Lammer, E. J. *N. Engl. J. Med.* 313: 837, 1985.
245. Lamming, D. *Br. J. Clin. Pharmacol.* 9: 217S, 1979.

246. Lange, A. P. *Acta Obstet. Gynaecol. Scand.* 59:111, 1980.
247. Lange, E. P. *Lancet* 1: 991, 1982.
248. Lavde, P. M. *Teratology* 21: 105, 1980.
249. Leonard, R. F. *N. Engl. J. Med.* 299: 84, 1978.
250. Levine, M. M. *Lancet* 2: 34, 1974.
251. Levy, G. *Pediatrics* 55: 818, 1975.
252. Lewis, G. J. *Br. Med. J. (Clin. Res.)* 286: 603, 1983.
253. Lewis, P. E. *Gynecol. Invest.* 8: 46, 1977.
254. Liedholm, H. *Eur. J. Clin. Pharmacol.* 21: 417, 1982.
255. Lillyman, J. S. *Cancer* 40: 1300, 1977.
256. Lima, J. J. *Pediatrics* 61: 491, 1978.
257. Linn, S. *N. Engl. J. Med.* 306: 141, 1982.
258. Lippert, V. T. H. *Arzneim. Forsch. Drug Res.* 29: 1172, 1979.
259. Longo, L. D. *Am. J. Obstet. Gynecol.* 137: 162, 1980.
260. Lorber, C. A. *Fertil. Steril.* 31: 21, 1979.
261. Lowenthal, R. M. *Aust. N.Z. J. Med.* 8: 431, 1978.
262. Lundborg, P. *Br. J. Clin. Pharmacol.* 12: 598, 1981.
263. MacArthur, B. A. *Pediatrics* 68: 38, 1981.
264. MacArthur, C. *Br. J. Obstet. Gynecol.* 95: 551, 1988.
265. MacAulay, M. A. *Am. J. Obstet. Gynecol.* 115: 58, 1973.
266. Magadam, M. *Gastroenterology* 80: 72, 1981.
267. Mahalik, M. P. *J. Pharm. Sci.* 69: 703, 1980.
268. Main, E. K. *J.A.M.A.* 249: 3207, 1983.
269. Margolis, S. *Ann. Ophthalmol.* 12: 1378, 1980.
270. Margulis, E. *Am. J. Obstet. Gynecol.* 148: 340, 1984.
271. Marradi, P. *Nouv. Rev. Fr. Hematol.* 24: 75, 1982.
272. Marsh, D. O. *Ann. Neurol.* 7: 348, 1980.
273. Martinez, G. *Neurology* 23: 381, 1973.
274. Martynshin, M. Y. A. *Akush. Ginekol. (Sofiia)* 57: 44, 1981.
275. Marx. G. F. *Anesthetist* 25: 318, 1976.
276. Mashiach, S. *J. Perinat. Med.* 7: 161, 1979.
277. Matthews, J. H. *N. Engl. J. Med.* 303: 1235, 1981.
278. Mattingly, R. F. *Am. J. Obstet. Gynecol.* 126: 543, 1976.
279. McCoy, M. J. *Am. J. Obstet. Gynecol.* 137: 739, 1980.
280. McEnerey, J. K. *Obstet. Gynecol.* 61(Suppl. No. 3): 35S, March, 1983.
281. McGowan, W. A. W. *J. R. Soc. Med.* 72: 902, 1979.
282. McKeen, E. *Lancet* 2: 590, 1979.
283. McKinna, A. J. *Can. J. Ophthalmol.* 1: 261, 1966.
284. Mennuti, M. T. *Obstet. Gynecol.* 46: 194, 1975.
285. Metzer, W. C. *J. Pediatr.* 85: 565, 1975.
286. Meyer, M. B. *Am. J. Epidemiol.* 103: 464, 1976.
287. Meyer, M. B. *Am. J. Epidemiol.* 100: 443, 1975.
288. Michael, A. *Br. J. Clin. Pharmacol.* 8: 211S, 1979.
289. Milham, S. *Teratology* 5: 125, 1972.
290. Miller, H. C. *Am. J. Obstet. Gynecol.* 125: 55, 1976.
291. Miller, R. D. *Br. J. Anaesth.* 54: 161, 1962.
292. Mills, J. I. *J.A.M.A.* 248: 2146, 1982.
293. Misrahy, G. A. *Anesthesiology* 24: 198, 1963.
294. Moar, V. A. *Br. J. Obstet. Gynecol.* 85: 933, 1978.
295. Mogilner, B. M. *Acta Obstet. Gynecol. Scand.* 61: 183, 1982.
296. Molinatti, G. M. *Minerva Ginecol.* 31: 239, 1980.
297. Monistat Product Monograph, Ortho Pharmaceutical Corporation, Raritan, N.J. 08869, 1983.
298. Monnet, P. *Rev. Tuberc. Pneumol.* 31: 845, 1967.
299. Moore, A. L. *Fundam. Appl. Toxicol.* 3: 560, 1983.
300. Moreno, H. *Cancer* 40: 988, 1977.
301. Morgan, D. J. *Dev. Pharmacol. Ther.* 5: 136, 1982.
302. Morris, M. B. *Am. J. Obstet. Gynecol.* 140: 607, 1981.
303. Morrison, J. *Am. J. Obstet. Gynecol.* 145: 1132, 1983.

304. Morrison, J. C. *Obstet. Gynecol.* 42: 99, 1973.
305. Morrow, R. J. *Am. J. Obstet. Gynecol.* 159: 1069, 1988.
306. Morrow, S. *Tex. Rep. Biol. Med.* 26: 567, 1968.
307. Morselli, P. L. *Eur. J. Clin. Pharmacol.* 18: 25, 1980.
308. Moyer, R. (Janssen Pharmaceutica, Piscataway, N.J. 08854). Personal communication, November 20, 1981.
309. Mueller, R. D. (Parke-Davis, Morris Plains, N.J. 07950). Personal communication, April 13, 1981.
310. Mulley, B. A. *J. Clin. Pharmacol.* 4: 213, 1979.
311. Mussay, R. D. *Mayo Clin. Proc.* 14: 205, 1938.
312. Musson, F. A. *Postgrad. Med. J.* 58: 731, 1982.
313. Myhre, S. A. *J. Pediatr.* 99: 160, 1981.
314. Nandakumaran, M. *Dev. Pharmacol. Ther.* 4: 71, 1982.
315. Nau, H. *J. Pharmacol. Exp. Ther.* 219: 768, 1981.
316. Nau, H. *Eur. J. Clin. Pharmacol.* 18: 31, 1980.
317. Nelson, M. M. *Br. Med. J.* 1: 523, 1971.
318. Newcomb, M. *J.A.M.A.* 139: 2691, 1978.
319. Nicholson, H. O. *J. Obstet. Gynaecol. Br. Comm.* 75: 307, 1968.
320. Nishimura, H., and Tanimura, T. *Clinical Aspects of the Teratogenicity of Drugs.* Amsterdam: Elsevier, 1976.
321. Niwa, S. *Med. Media* 14: 307, 1968.
322. Nora, J. J. *Lancet* 2: 594, 1974.
323. Oakley, G. P. *J.A.M.A.* 247: 2405, 1982.
324. Oakley, G. P., Jr. Causal Inference in Teratology. In R. H. Schwartz and S. J. Yaffe (Eds.), *Drug and Chemical Risks to the Fetus and Newborn* (*Progress in Clinical and Biological Research,* Vol 36). New York: Liss, 1980.
325. Oazi, Q. H. *Hum. Genet.* 53: 201, 1980.
326. O'Donnell, R. *Acta Haematol. (Basel)* 61: 298, 1979.
327. O'Hare, M. F. *Br. J. Clin. Pharmacol.* 87: 390, 1980.
328. Onnen, I. *Eur. J. Clin. Pharmacol.* 15: 443, 1979.
329. Ortega, J. *Cancer* 40: 2829, 1977.
330. Osathonaondh, R. *J. Pediatr.* 90: 617, 1977.
331. Ostrea, E. M., Jr. *J. Pediatr.* 94: 292, 1979.
332. Ostrea, E. M. *J. Pediatr.* 88: 642, 1976.
333. Otero, L. *Pediatrics* 68: 778, 1981.
334. Ouellette, E. *N. Engl. J. Med.* 297: 528, 1977.
335. Ounsted, M. K. *Br. J. Obstet. Gynaecol.* 87: 19, 1980.
336. Owen, J. *Am. J. Obstet. Gynecol.* 158: 1169, 1988.
337. Padeletti, L. *Int. J. Clin. Pharmacol. Biopharmacol.* 17: 82, 1979.
338. Page, H. B. *Ann. N.Y. Acad. Sci.* 191: 123, 1971.
339. Parsons, W. D. *Can. Med. Assoc. J.* 127: 377, 1982.
340. Patel, D. A. *J.A.M.A.* 244: 135, 1980.
341. Pawlinger, F. *Ann. Intern. Med.* 74: 1012, 1971.
342. Pecorari, D. *Acta Biomed. Ateneo Parmense* 40: 2, 1969.
343. Perry, J. E. *Tex. Rep. Biol. Med.* 25: 265, 1967.
344. Perry, J. E. *Tex. Rep. Biol. Med.* 25: 270, 1967.
345. Personal communication, Ortho Pharmaceutical Corporation, 1989.
346. Peterson, W. F. *Am. J. Obstet. Gynecol.* 94: 343, 1966.
347. Phelan, M. C. *N. Engl. J. Med.* 307: 99, 1982.
348. Philipson, A. *Am. J. Obstet. Gynecol.* 142: 823, 1982.
349. Philipson, A. *Acta Obstet. Gynaecol. Scand.* 60: 121, 1981.
350. Philipson, A. *N. Engl. J. Med.* 5: 1152, 1966.
351. Philpot, C. R. *Med. J. Aust.* 2: 1005, 1972.
352. Piepho, R. W. *Am. J. Cardiol.* 49: 525, 1982.
353. Pipkin, F. B. *Lancet* 1: 1256, 1980.
354. Pittman, K. A., et al. *Am. J. Obstet. Gynecol.* 138: 797, 1980.
355. Polednak, A. P. *Teratology* 26: 27, 1982.
356. Potworoska, M. *Pol. Med. J.* 5: 1152, 1966.
357. Preblud, S. R. *J.A.M.A.* 246: 1413, 1981.

358. Prem, K. A., et al. *Second International Conference on Live Poliovirus Vaccines*. Washington: WHO Scientific Publications, 50: 207, 1960.
359. Prenner, B. M. *Am. J. Dis. Child.* 131: 529, 1977.
360. Price, H. V. *Transplantation* 21: 294, 1976.
361. Pruyn, S. C. *Am. J. Obstet. Gynecol.* 135: 485, 1979.
362. Pulkkinen, M. O. *Am. J. Obstet. Gynecol.* 115: 1153, 1973.
363. Raiti, S. *N. Engl. J. Med.* 277: 456, 1967.
364. Rating, D. *Acta Paediatr. Scand.* 71: 301, 1982.
365. Redline, R. W. *Am. J. Obstet. Gynecol.* 141: 468, 1981.
366. Redmond, G. P. *Pediatr. Pharmacol.* 1: 153, 1980.
367. Refstad, S. O. *Br. J. Anaesth.* 52: 265, 1980.
368. Reid, D. W. *Can. Med. Assoc. J.* 112: 67, 1975.
369. Reinisch, J. M. *Science* 202: 436, 1978.
370. Rementeria, J. L. *J. Pediatr.* 90: 123, 1977.
371. Reynolds, J. W. *Clin. Obstet. Gynecol.* 17: 95, 1974.
372. Riley, A. J. *Br. J. Clin. Pharmacol.* 8: 53S, 1979.
373. Robboy, S. J. National Institutes of Health Publication No. 80-2049. Washington: NIH, 1980.
374. Robertson, J. S. *J. Nucl. Med.* 17: 826, 1976.
375. Rocker, I. *Lancet* 2: 1246, 1976.
376. Rodesch, F. *Am. J. Obstet. Gynecol.* 126: 723, 1976.
377. Roe, F. J. C. *Surgery* 93: 158, 1983.
378. Rogan, W. J. *Teratology* 26: 259, 1982.
379. Rogers, J. G. *Aust. Paediatr. J.* 16: 194, 1980.
380. Rogers, M. C. *N. Engl. J. Med.* 287: 1010, 1972.
381. Rosen, T. S. *J. Pediatr.* 101: 192, 1982.
382. Rosenberg, L. *N. Engl. J. Med.* 309: 1282, 1983.
383. Rosenberg, L. *J.A.M.A.* 247: 1429, 1982.
384. Rosett, H. L. *Obstet. Gynecol.* 57: 1, 1981.
385. Rosner, M. A. *Am. J. Obstet. Gynecol.* 144: 23, 1982.
386. Ross, J. B. *Arch. Dermatol.* 109: 573, 1974.
387. Ross, S. *J.A.M.A.* 142: 1361, 1950.
388. Rotblatt, M. D. *Drug Intell. Clin. Pharm.* 17: 187, 1983.
389. Rothman, K. J. *Am. J. Epidemiol.* 109: 433, 1979.
390. Rowe, R. D. *Pediatrics* 43: 1, 1969.
391. Rubaltelli, F. F. *J. Pediatr.* 94: 161, 1979.
392. Rubin, P. C. *Br. J. Clin. Pharmacol.* 16: 543, 1983.
393. Rubin, P. C. *Br. J. Clin. Pharmacol.* 16: 659, 1983.
394. Rubin, P. C. *N. Engl. J. Med.* 305: 1323, 1981.
395. Rudd, N. L. *J. Pediatr.* 94: 835, 1979.
396. Rudolph, A. M. *Arch. Intern. Med.* 141: 358, 1981.
397. Rudolph, A. R. *Obstet. Gynecol.* 58(Suppl. No. 5): 63S, November, 1981.
398. Rumack, C. M. *Obstet. Gynecol.* 58(Suppl. No. 5): 52S, November, 1981.
399. Ruo, P. *Med. J. Aust.* 1: 558, 1962.
400. Safra, M. J. *Lancet* 2: 478, 1975.
401. Sandberg, E. *Am. J. Obstet. Gynecol.* 140: 194, 1981.
402. Savolainen, E. *Am. J. Obstet. Gynecol.* 140: 521, 1981.
403. Schafer, A. I. *Arch. Intern. Med.* 141: 514, 1981.
404. Schou, M. *Br. Med. J.* 2: 135, 1973.
405. Schardein, J. L. *Teratology* 22: 251, 1980.
406. Schatz, M. *J.A.M.A.* 233: 804, 1975.
407. Schenkel, B. *J. Reprod. Med.* 12: 27, 1974.
408. Scher, J. *J. Obstet. Gynaecol. Br. Comm.* 79: 635, 1972.
409. Schiff, D. *J. Pediatr.* 77: 457, 1970.
410. Schire, I. *Lancet* 1: 174, 1963.
411. Schneerson, J. M. *Tubercle* 60: 167, 1979.
412. Schreiner, C. M. *J. Histochem. Cytochem.* 29: 1213, 1981.
413. Schubiger, G. *Ann. Intern. Med.* 108: 215, 1988.

414. Schwartz, B. *Am. J. Dis. Child.* 136: 474, 1982.
415. Schwartz, R. H. *Br. Med. J.* 2: 152, 1978.
416. Scott, W. C. *J.A.M.A.* 142: 1331, 1950.
417. Scott, W. J. *Teratology* 24: 37, 1981.
418. Shah, N. S. *Toxicol. Appl. Pharmacol.* 53: 279, 1980.
419. Shaxted, E. *J. Curr. Med. Res. Opin.* 6: 70, 1979.
420. Shearer, W. T. *J. Pediatr.* 81: 571, 1972.
421. Sheikh, K. *Lancet* 2: 963, 1979.
422. Simila, S. *Arch. Dis. Child.* 55: 985, 1980.
423. Simon, R. *Cancer* 45: 2890, 1980.
424. Singh, S. *Arch. Dis. Child.* 54: 400, 1979.
425. Singlas, E. *Nouv. Presse Med.* 11: 373, 1982.
426. Slone, D. *Am. J. Obstet. Gynecol.* 128: 486, 1977.
427. Smith, A. H. *Arch. Environ. Health* 37: 197, 1982.
428. Smith, M. J. *Br. Med. J.* 284: 1234, 1982.
429. Snider, D. E. *Am. Rev. Respir. Dis.* 122: 65, 1980.
430. Synder, S. W. *Anesthesiology* 51: 563, 1979.
431. Sonntag, A. C. *Clin. Obstet. Gynecol.* 18: 199, 1975.
432. Souney, P. F. *Clin. Pharmacol.* 2: 29, 1983.
433. Spence, A. A. *J.A.M.A.* 238: 955, 1977.
434. Stadler, G. E. *J.A.M.A.* 217: 214, 1971.
435. Stanbury, J. B., Wyngaarden, J. B., and Frederickson, D. S. (Eds.). *The Metabolic Basis of Inherited Disease,* 5th Ed. New York: McGraw-Hill, 1983.
436. Stegink, L. D. *Prog. Food Nutr. Sci.* 5: 265, 1981.
437. Stenshener, M. A. *Am. J. Obstet. Gynecol.* 118: 104, 1974.
438. Stephens, J. D. *Am. J. Obstet. Gynecol.* 137: 747, 1980.
439. Stern, R. S. *J. Am. Acad. Dermatol.* 10: 851, 1984.
440. Stevenson, R. E. *J.A.M.A.* 243: 1549, 1980.
441. Stillman, R. J. *Am. J. Obstet. Gynecol.* 142: 905, 1982.
442. P. Stoddard (Fisons Corporation, Bedford, Mass. 01730). Personal communication, March 9, 1983.
443. Strauss, A. A. *Pediatrics* 68: 550, 1981.
444. Streissguth, A. P. *Dev. Pharmacol. Ther.* 5: 21, 1982.
445. Streissguth, A. P. *Science* 209: 353, 1980.
446. Strigl, R. *J. Perinat. Med.* 9: 235, 1981.
447. Strigl, R. *Geburtshilfe Frauenheilkd.* 40: 496, 1980.
448. Stuart, M. J. *N. Engl. J. Med.* 307: 909, 1982.
449. Suraínder, S. V. *Obstet. Gynecol.* 57: 124, 1981.
450. Surgeon General's Advisory on Alcohol and Pregnancy. *F.D.A. Drug Bull.* 11: 2, 1981.
451. Svenningsen, N. W. *Acta Obstet. Gynaecol. Scand. (Suppl.)* 296: 28, 1982.
452. Takese, Z. *Asian Med. J.* 11: 370, 1968.
453. Tennes, K. *Am. J. Obstet. Gynecol.* 138: 274, 1980.
454. Thomas, C. R. *Obstet. Gynecol.* 50: 607, 1977.
455. Thomas, H. F. *Nature* 295: 276, 1980.
456. Thorley, K. J. *Br. Med. J.* 285: 1116, 1982.
457. Thorley, K. J. *Br. J. Clin. Pharmacol.* 12: 725, 1981.
458. Tobias, J. S. *Lancet* 1: 776, 1980.
459. Tomson, G. *Clin. Pharmacol. Ther.* 25: 74, 1979.
460. Torfs, C. P. *Am. J. Epidemiol.* 113: 563, 1981.
461. Townsend, J. C. *Am. J. Epidemiol.* 115: 695, 1982.
462. Tresadern, J. C. *Br. Med. J.* 286: 602, 1983.
463. Tuchmann-Duplessis, H. *Drug Effects on the Fetus.* Acton, Mass.: Publishing Sciences Group, 1975.
464. Turkalj, I. *J.A.M.A.* 247: 1589, 1982.
465. Turner, E. S. *Ann. Intern. Med.* 6: 905, 1980.
466. Tyson, H. K. *J. Pediatr.* 85: 684, 1974.
467. Ullberg, S. *Nature* 227: 1257, 1970.

468. Ungvary, G. *Acta Morphol. Acad. Sci. Hung.* 28: 159, 1980.
469. United States Department of Health and Human Services. *M.M.W.R.* 31: 479, 1982.
470. Valenzuela, G. *Am. J. Obstet. Gynecol.* 143: 718, 1982.
471. Van Blerk, A. *Int. J. Gynaecol. Obstet.* 17: 401, 1980.
472. Van Herle, A. J. *J. Clin. Endocrinol. Metab.* 40: 474, 1975.
473. Varma, T. R. *Int. J. Gynecol. Obstet.* 20: 13, 1982.
474. Varner, M. W. *Am. J. Obstet. Gynecol.* 148: 717, 1982.
475. Vert, P. *Eur. J. Clin. Pharmacol.* 22: 39, 1982.
476. Vladimiroff, H. W. *Br. J. Obstet. Gynaecol.* 82: 221, 1975.
477. Vorherr, H. *J.A.M.A.* 244: 2628, 1980.
478. Wagner, V. M. *Lancet* 2: 98, 1980.
479. Walden, P. A. M. *Lancet* 2: 1241, 1979.
480. Walson, P. D. *Pediatr. Pharmacol.* 2: 341, 1982.
481. Ward, R. M. *Pediatr. Clin. North Am.* Maternal-Placental-Fetal Unit: unique Problems of Pharmacological Study. 36: 1075, 1989.
482. Wareham, G. F. *J.A.M.A.* 240: 251, 1976.
483. Webb, G. A. *Am. J. Obstet. Gynecol.* 137: 263, 1980.
484. Weijer, D. L. *J. Can. Assoc. Radiol.* 11: 50, 1960.
485. Webster, P. A. C. *Lancet* 2: 318, 1973.
486. Weinstein, A. J. *Am. J. Obstet. Gynecol.* 124: 688, 1976.
487. Weinstein, M. R. *Am. J. Psychol.* 132: 529, 1975.
488. Weiss, C. F. *N. Engl. J. Med.* 262: 787, 1960.
489. Wentz, A. C. *Ann. Intern. Med.* 96: 672, 1982.
490. Wharton, R. S. *Anesthesiology* 51: 532, 1979.
491. Whitehead, E. D. *J. Urol.* 125: 47, 1981.
492. Whitelaw, A. G. L. *Br. Med. J.* 283: 471, 1981.
493. Whitelaw, A. G. L. *Br. Med. J.* 282: 1106, 1981.
494. Widerlov, E. *N. Engl. J. Med.* 303: 335, 1980.
495. Wilkinson, A. R. *Lancet* 2: 591, 1980.
496. Williamson, R. A. *Obstet. Gynecol.* 58: 247, 1981.
497. Wilson, A. L. *Drug Intell. Clin. Pharm.* 15: 21, 1981.
498. Wilson, J. G. *Am. J. Obstet. Gynecol.* 141: 567, 1981.
499. Wolleman, M. *Agents Actions* 9: 29, 1979.
500. Young, D. S. *Clin. Chem.* 21: 294D, 1975.
501. Yurth, D. A. *Clin. Perinatol.* 9: 13, 1982.
502. Zackai, E. H. *J. Pediatr.* 87: 280, 1975.
503. Zagoraycki, M. T. *Obstet. Gynecol. Surv.* 39: 134, 1984.
504. Zellweger, H. *Lancet* 2: 1066, 1967.
505. Zemer, D. *N. Engl. J. Med.* 294: 170, 1976.
506. Zmora, E. *Dev. Pharmacol. Ther.* 5: 76, 1982.
507. Zuckerman, B. *N. Engl. J. Med.* 320: 762, 1989.
508. Zulli, P. *Lancet* 2: 945, 1978.

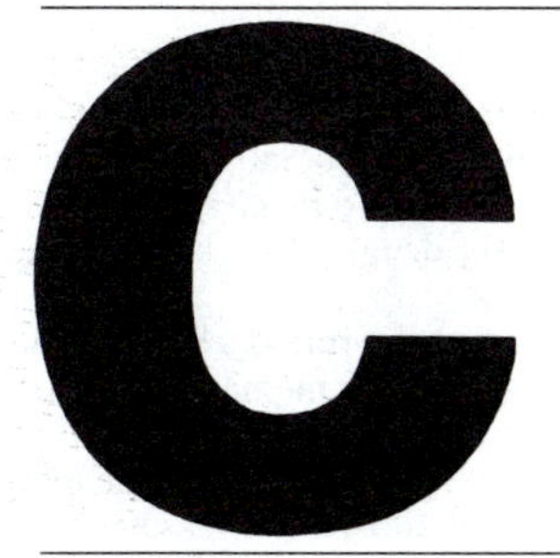

Drug Use by Nursing Mothers

Celeste M. Marx and
Cheryl A. Stoukides

Background

Breast-feeding is the preferred method of infant feeding. At present, 75 percent of women delivering at Brigham & Women's Hospital choose to breast-feed. One factor influencing this decision is the need for medication(s) by the mother. It has been recognized for many years that drugs taken by the nursing mother can have adverse effects on her infant. Despite numerous reports of measurement of drugs in milk and reviews of these data, there is little agreement about which drugs should be absolutely avoided during nursing or which drugs, if needed by the mother, contraindicate breast-feeding. During the past 5 years, the problem has grown even more complex, since both the quantity and the quality of data on the drug excretion in milk have increased. Recent revelations include the following:

1. Some drugs are now known to have been erroneously classified as "not excreted" owing to insensitive or invalid assay procedures or improper study designs.
2. Many agents have been recognized to have been previously prohibited for nursing mothers based on speculations about their effects rather than on actual clinical experience. This misconception was frequently perpetuated in review articles.
3. A few medications previously regarded as contraindicated are now considered compatible with nursing, with the stipulation that the infant receive careful follow-up.
4. Excretion of a drug in milk does not in itself contraindicate breast-feeding. Most agents are inefficiently passed to the child after distribution to maternal tissues and after partial elimination by the mother. The risk of drug toxicity (excessive drug effect) should be judged on the basis of the following:
   a. The inherent toxicity of the drug (therapeutic index).
   b. The actual magnitude of drug ingested by the infant rather than a relationship between maternal serum levels and milk concentrations.
   c. Knowledge of newborn and older infants' pharmacokinetic characteristics for distribution and elimination of this dose.
   d. Experience with the infants' sensitivity to the drug, with regard to therapeutic effects, side effects, and adverse effects, particularly the premature or ill baby who requires other medications.
   e. The duration of potential use by the mother, e.g., a few days postpartum (such as antibiotics) or chronically (such as anticonvulsants).
   f. Clinical experience with the use, particularly chronically, by nursing mothers, with observations of adverse effects on lactation.

All these factors must be considered when deciding whether or not to recommend disrupting the nursing relationship for required maternal drug therapy. Published experience generally notes problems that have occurred in infants of treated mothers. These known risks are presented in the tables that follow. Unfortunately, extensive publication of uncomplicated nursing during therapy does not exist. Where anecdotal experience is significant, it is noted. Information regarding delayed effects of even low-dose exposures during this sensitive time of development is lacking for most agents. This limitation of current scientific information regarding long-term safety should be presented to parents who are considering breast-feeding during treatment with drugs that have no known contraindication.

Short-term safety also should be evaluated based on the infant's history and likelihood of exposure to the drug. For some chronically taken medications, the infant has been exposed as a fetus in utero; the magnitude of exposure is generally much less when the infant is nursing. The risk then is not a new one, but merely is continued and likely lessened. The risk is avoidable if the mother chooses not to breast-feed. However, the decision regarding a short period of breast-feeding should be made (1) in consideration of the factors determining toxicity (noted previously), (2) the importance of breast-feeding to the parent(s), (3) other factors that might make nursing detrimental to maternal health, (4) the availability of pediatric follow-up, and (5) reliability of the parents for monitoring adverse effects.

To assist in achieving safe nursing during drug use, parameters to be monitored are presented (see Table C-1). In general, measurements of milk levels are unnecessary. Infant exposure and differentiation of suspected toxicity can be made from infant serum level determinations where these are meaningful.

The data presented are drawn from the published experience. In order to standardize disparate information, reported milk levels are stated and infant exposure is estimated and compared with recommended newborn dosage of the drug. When the newborn dose is not known, the predicted exposure can be compared with the adult or child weight-corrected (per kilogram) dosage, indicated by an asterisk (*). The accuracy of all dosage estimates is greatly limited by the quality of the data on milk concentrations. Some of these data are taken from single case reports or single-dose studies. Chronic administration, particularly to mothers with impaired elimination processes, can result in greater exposure through accumulation. Therefore, an attempt has been made to err on the side of overestimating infant dosage (1) by assuming a generous newborn milk intake of 200 ml/kg per day and (2) by calculating as if reported milk concentrations were continuously maintained throughout the dosing interval. These estimates must not be taken as absolute doses and should not be relied on for treatment.

When known, the recommended amount of time to withhold nursing after taking contraindicated agents is given. The mother should be encouraged to express milk to maintain supply until it is determined that she will remain on the drug long-term. In general, it is not practical to alter feeding schedules to avoid exposure of the baby to a drug in the mother's milk. Because infants naturally nurse very frequently, every 1½ to 3 hours, exposure is avoided by taking the drug after nursing only for agents that are extremely rapidly absorbed and eliminated. For most drugs, a peak concentration occurs at the next feeding or more. Unless the alteration in feeding is very carefully planned, the result is only slightly less drug exposure, a frustrated mother and baby, and a compromised milk supply.

When a drug is known to cause problems during nursing, alternative therapies should be considered by the mother's physician. To aid in this decision, the tables that follow present data in various therapeutic categories:

Table C-1: Analgesics and anti-inflammatory agents
Table C-2: Anti-infective agents (including antibiotics, antituberculars, and antimalarials)
Table C-3: Cardiovascular drugs
Table C-4: Sedative hypnotics
Table C-5: Anticonvulsants
Table C-6: Gastrointestinal medications
Table C-7: Respiratory medications
Table C-8: Endocrine medications
Table C-9: Agents with gynecologic indication
Table C-10: Diagnostic agents

Table C-11: Drugs of abuse or social use
Table C-12: Antineoplastic agents
Table C-13: Miscellaneous agents

Methods to measure drugs in breast milk are improving, and new data on the clinical experience of drug use by nursing mothers continue to be reported. This will cause changes in recommendations in the use of drugs by nursing mothers. The American Academy of Pediatrics Committee on Drugs has recently published a statement on Transfer of Drugs and Other Chemicals into Human Milk [5]. Physicians should review all up-to-date information before making a decision on whether or not to allow nursing when a mother is on a required medication. We have a Drug Information Center at the Brigham & Women's Hospital that keeps up-to-date information on drug use in breast milk.
In summary, it is rarely possible to delcare a drug absolutely prohibited or safe for the nursing infant. The benefits of nursing and the potential and known risks should be discussed with the parent(s), and a safe plan should be developed for each individual case. A recent review of this subject (Berlin, C. M. Drugs and Chemicals: Exposure of the Nursing Mother) is found *Ped. Clin. No. Amer.* 3:1089, 1989.

Anti-Infective Agents

Most anti-infective agents are present only in very small amounts in the mother's milk; toxicity is therefore unlikely, but there is the potential for non-dose-related adverse effects. Those to monitor are indicated in Table C-2. Some agents are not systemically available when taken orally with milk and may exert a local action. Thus there is a potential for altered bowel flora and diarrhea (a change from the **infant's** normal stooling pattern). Allergic reactions, such as rash or fever, are also potential effects. These reactions probably are rare, owing to the lack of reported cases despite the frequent use of these agents by nursing mothers. This first exposusre by means of milk may sensitize the infant, like a first prescription, leading to the possibility of allergic reactions with the next exposure.

Anticonvulsants

Although the use of anticonvulsants during nursing has not been associated with many reports of even minor adverse effects, their safety, in long-term follow-up, remains largely unstudied. Their long-term safety is a concern because of the potential anti-intellectual effects of these drugs. For many patients, exposure during nursing is not a new risk, but one continued from pregnancy, at a lower level. The risk is avoidable, however. If the mother chooses to breast-feed (after understanding the unknown nature of the risk), the physician should monitor growth and development and specific side effects of each agent. If excessive drug effect is believed to be present, there is no need to check milk levels; infant serum levels provide the necessary information about toxicity.

Drugs of Abuse or Social Use

It is difficult to provide reliable recommendations for practitioners seeking information about the presence of these agents in milk. Purity and actual drug taken are unknown in most cases. Abstinence is always desirable. If the mother will not avoid these drugs, she should reconsider her decision to breast-feed (see also Chap. 2).

Table C-1. Analgesics and anti-inflammatory agents[a]

Agent	Maternal dose	Reported milk levels	Estimated newborn intake	Predicted % of newborn therapeutic dose	Reported adverse reactions and cautions	References
Acetaminophen	500–650 mg PO	1–15 μg/ml	0.2–3.0 mg/kg/day	0.05–0.70	No need to withhold nursing; exposure is largely avoided if dosed after feeding.	19,24,61
Aspirin	650 mg PO	1.1–42.6 μg/ml salicylate	0.2–8.5 mg/kg/day	0.06–25.00	Substantial exposure is possible with mothers taking rheumatoid doses (3–5 gm day); the effect of aspirin on platelets and its role in Reyes syndrome as well as reports of metabolic acidosis in infants whose mothers were on rheumatoid doses suggest that aspirin should not be used by breast-feeding mothers.	18,39,61
Butorphanol (Stadol)	1–2 mg IM or 8 mg PO	4 ng/ml	0.8 μg/kg/day	1[b]	No reported adverse effects; rapidly eliminated; dose after feedings to minimize exposure.	41

Diclofenac (Voltaren)	50 mg × 1 100 mg QD × 7d	"Not detected" <1 μg/ml	2–5 μg/kg/day	Not used	Probably safe for breast-feeding infants; however, presence of 4 metabolites in human milk not established.	186
Flurbifrofen (Ansaid)	50 mg qid × 9 doses	"Not detected" <1 μg/ml	—	Not used	Probably safe in breast-feeding; prolonged half of drug makes more extensive studies necessary.	183
Ibuprofen (Motrin)	600 mg q6h PO	"Not found" (<1 μg/ml)	<0.2 mg/kg/day	<0.5[b]	No reports of adverse effects in nursed infants; ibuprofen does not enter milk in significant quantities; breast-feed with no problems.	37,161,199
Indomethacin	200 mg PO daily	0.2–4.0 μg/ml	40–800 μg/kg/day	66–133	Potentially large dose; case report of seizures in nursed infant; choose alternative agent.	52
Naproxen (Naprosyn, Anaprox)	375 mg bid PO	0.55 μg/ml	110 μg/kg/day or less	Not used	Small quantities pass into milk; effects on infants unknown; probably safe while breast-feeding.	82
Piroxicam (Feldene)	20 mg qd × 4 mos.; 40 mg × 2d, then 20 mg × 5d	0.05–0.22 μg/ml	10–44 μg/kg/day	Not used	Isolated case reports; drug not detected in serum of infant whose mother took the drug for 4 months while breast-feeding; Probably safe short term.	153

[a]See introduction to table on page 671.
[b]Compared with adult corrected dose.

Table C-1. (continued)

Agent	Maternal dose	Reported milk levels	Estimated newborn intake	Predicted % of newborn therapeutic dose	Reported adverse reactions and cautions	References
Narcotics						
Codeine	60 mg PO	"Traces," 179 µg/ml	35.8–91.0 µg/kg/day	1.5	Poor data on narcotic excretion, but extensive anecdotal experience without serious adverse effect; at high dose, monitor for sedation; sedation from narcotics is reversible with naloxone, but this may cause acute withdrawal symptoms; it is best to let the drug wear off	61,77
Hydromorphone (Dilaudid)	Not studied	Not studied	Unknown	Unknown		
Meperidine (Demerol)	Not reported	<1 µg/ml	<200 µg/kg/day	<3.3		150

				kg	at 20 mg daily or less; use may mask onset of very likely (90 percent) withdrawal and delay it until after discharge from hospital, in uncontrolled setting; long-term effect of continued methadone exposure in very high risk group (for delayed neurodevelopment and sudden infant death syndrome) not studied but of great concern; use maternal desire to nurse to motivate detoxification during infant withdrawal period; mother must express milk to build supply; most feel it is best to limit the duration of exposure and thus not nurse (see Chap. 2).	
Morphine	From 60 mg codeine	<6 μg/ml	<1.2 mg/kg/day	<20		61,107,197
Oxycodone (Tylox, Percocet-5, Percodan)	Not studied	Not studied	Unknown	Not used		
Propoxyphene (Darvon)	65 mg q4h PO	90.4–709.0 ng/ml propoxyphene 169–1691 ng/ml norpropoxyphene	18–142 μg/kg/day 34–338 μg/kg/day norpropoxyphene	<0.3[b]	—	107

[b]Compared with adult corrected dose.

Table C-2. Anti-infective agents[a]

Agent	Maternal dose	Reported milk levels	Estimated newborn intake	Predicted % of newborn therapeutic dose	Reported adverse reactions and cautions	References
Acyclovir	200 mg 5 × d × 5d	1.06–1.26 μg/ml	1.0 mg/day		The amount of drug the infant is exposed to in breast milk is low. Doses up to 75 mg/kg/day have been used in neonates with no toxicity. However, acyclovir interferes with peripheral blood lymphocytes, and the effects on the infant's immune system have not been studied. Use of acyclovir while breast-feeding provides a low "theoretical" risk.	112
Amoxicillin	1 gm PO	0.81 ± 0.33 μg/ml	162 ± 66 μg/kg/day	0.18[b]	Minimum exposure; may "flavor" milk; monitor for rash, diarrhea, spitting up (very uncommon).	89,120
Ampicillin	500 mg q6h	0.014–1.0 μg/ml	2.8–200.0 μg/kg/day	0.14–0.40		
Carbenicillin	1 gm parenterally	0.265 μg/ml	53 μg/kg/day	0.03	Miniscule amount; not well absorbed from infant's gastrointestinal tract; nurse as planned.	150
First-Generation Cephalosporins						
Cefadroxil	1 gm PO	0.10–1.64 μg/ml	20–328 μg/kg/day	Not used	Small amount present; therapeutic dose not known for infant; monitor for rash	89

Cefazolin	2 gm IV 500 mg IM tid	1.5 μg/ml None detected	300 μg/kg/day	0.9	Exposure to these agents is very small compared with therapeutic doses; monitor for rash or diarrhea.	208
Cephalexin	500 mg PO 1 gm PO	5.00 ± 0.23 μg/ml 0.2–0.5 μg/ml	0.04–1.00 mg/kg/day	0.04–0.40		89,141,150
Cephradine	500 mg × 4d	0.63–0.68	≤0.102 μg/kg/day			140
Cephalothin	1 gm IV	0.27–0.47 μg/ml	54–94 μg/kg/day	0.05–0.09	—	89
Cephapirin	1 gm IV	0.12–0.64 μg/ml	24–128 μg/kg/day	0.25–25.0		89
Second-Generation Cephalosporin						
Cefoxitin	Usual doses	<0.5–1.0 μg/ml	<100–200 μg/kg/day	—	Compared with the adult weight-corrected dosage, the excreted dose is very small even for those agents for which the newborn dose is not known; use of these agents is probably compatible with nursing; monitor infant for any side effects specific to each drug.	124
Third-Generation Cephalosporins						
Cefotaxine	1 gm IV	<0.16–0.52 μg/ml	<50–104 μg/kg/day	0.1–0.2		90,212
Ceftazidime	2 gm q8h × 5d	4.9 ± 2.7 μg/ml	98 ± 54 μg/kg/day	—		26
Ceftizoxime	1 gm IM	0.2 μg/ml	40 μg/kg/day	—		123
Ceftriaxone	1 gm IM or IV	0.3–0.7 μg/ml	60–140 μg/kg/day	0.05–0.09		87

[a]See introduction to table on 671.
[b]Compared with adult corrected dose.

Table C-2. (continued)

Agent	Maternal dose	Reported milk levels	Estimated newborn intake	Predicted % of newborn therapeutic dose	Reported adverse reactions and cautions	References
Ciprofloxacin	750 mg × 3 doses ciprofloxacin 400 mg × 3 doses perfloxacin 400 mg × 3 doses ofloxacin	Various	Not studied	Not used	Ciprofloxacin has been shown to cause arthropathy and cartilage erosion in juvenile animals. Quinolones are distributed into breast milk in high levels. Due to potential risks, nursing should be suspended.	67
Chloramphenicol (Chloromycetin)	250–500 mg PO q6h	0.26–26.00 μg/ml	52–500 μg/kg/day		Although nonspecific method (measures inactive metabolite) use may explain high reported milk levels, it is best to avoid nursing during and for at least 12 hours after stopping this drug; risks include bone marrow suppression (see Appendix A).	70,71,181

Clindamycin (Cleocin)	600 mg IV qid 150 mg PO bid	0.7–3.8 μg/ml 0.3–0.5 μg/ml	148–760 μg/kg/day 60–100 μg/kg/day	1.0–4.7	Case report of one infant who developed bloody stools when mother took clindamycin; no relationship to the drug could be established. Probably safe to breast-feed.	129,182,189
Cycloserine	250 mg qid	6–19 μg/ml	1.2–3.8 mg/kg/day	Not used	No reported adverse effects from use during nursing.	184
Dicloxacillin	Not studied	Not studied	Unknown	Unknown	No reported adverse effects; has been used for treatment of mastitis without stopping nursing. Has been used in infants without problems.	
Doxycycline	200 mg, then 100 mg	0.38–0.77 μg/ml	76–154 μg/kg/day	Not used	See tetracyclines.	172
Erythromycin	400 mg q8h	0.3–6.2 μg/ml	30–124 μg/kg/day	0.10–0.25	No reported adverse effects with animal data.	112
Ethambutol	15 mg/kg/day PO	1.4–4.6 μg/ml	280–920 μg/kg/day	1.0–3.6	Despite small dose, potential for ophthalmic toxicity (macular degeneration); no reported adverse effects, but avoid.	184
Gentamicin	80 mg IM	0.003–0.157 μg/ml	0.6–47.1 μg/kg/day	0.012–0.900	No need to restrict nursing; aminoglycosides are usually very poorly absorbed from bowel.	82
Hydroxychloroquine	400 mg hs daily	0.85–1.46 μg/ml	0.11 (author's estimate)–0.29 mg/kg/day	Not used	**Avoid:** Plaquenil is potentially retinotoxic and bone marrow toxic; substantial amount of drug may be passed to infant.	145

Table C-2. (continued)

Agent	Maternal dose	Reported milk levels	Estimated newborn intake	Predicted % of newborn therapeutic dose	Reported adverse reactions and cautions	References
Isoniazid (INH)	5–10 mg/kg PO 300 mg/day	1–12 μg/ml 16.6 μg/ml with 3.8 μg/ml acetylisoniazid	0.2–3.3 mg/kg/day	6.3–25.0	Will not provide reliable dosing for infant needing isoniazid therapy; some consider isoniazid contraindicated for nursing infant due to anti-DNA effect and thus avoid nursing. There is not much evidence of toxicity when used in the newborn at doses of 10 mg/kg/day. If baby is nursed, monitor for anemia, rash, and hepatitis.	20,167,184,207 see Ch. 12
Methenamine:						15
Hiprex	1 gm PO	71.4 μmol/liter	50–100 μg/kg/day	0.07–0.60[b]	Monitor infant for hematuria and albuminuria with chronic use.	
Mandelamine	12 gm, then 300 mg/day	0.2–1.1 μg/ml	44–280 μg/kg/day	—	No reported adverse effects.	
Metronidazole (Flagyl)	2 gm dose PO 1 gm rectally	1–56 μg/ml Up to 25 μg/ml	0.2–11.2 mg/kg/day Up to 5 mg/kg/day	1.3–75.0	Despite lack of reports of adverse effect, drug is contraindicated for nursing due to potential carcinogenicity; withhold mother's milk for at least 12 hours (48 is best) after last dose.	56

Minocycline	200 mg PO	0.8 μg/ml	36–160 μg/kg/day	Not used	See tetracyclines.	34
Naladixic acid	1 gm qid	4 μg/ml	800 μg/kg/day	Not used	Do not breast-feed in G-6-PD-deficient infant. A case of hemolytic anemia in a non-G-6-PD-deficient child has been described. The risk to a non-G-6-PD-deficient infant may be regarded as minimal.	14
Nitrofurantoin	100 mg qid	0.3–0.5 μg/ml	60–100 μg/kg/day	Not used	Infants who are G-6-PD-deficient can develop hemolytic anemia.	79,204
Norfloxacin	Not studied	Not studied	Not studied	Not used	See precautions for ciprofloxacin.	67
Nystatin	Not reported	Not found	Unknown	Unknown	Even if present, not absorbed orally; nurse as planned.	205
Oxacillin or nafcillin	1 gm oxacillin	Not found	Unknown	Unknown	Anecdotal experience in nursing mothers without report of adverse effects; drug frequently used in newborns with only rare hepatitis or leukopenia.	
Paromomycin	Not studied	Not studied	Not studied	Not used	An aminoglycoside antibiotic that is usually poorly absorbed from the GI tract. Probably the agent of choice in treating giardiasis while breast-feeding, given the potential risk of alternate agents.	105

[b]Compared with adult corrected dose.

Table C-2. (continued)

Agent	Maternal dose	Reported milk levels	Estimated newborn intake	Predicted % of newborn therapeutic dose	Reported adverse reactions and cautions	References
Penicillin	100,000–600,000 units benzathine IM 2.4 million units procaine	60–162 units/liter	12–192 units/kg/day	0.005–0.400	Miniscule dose; extensive neonatal use without problems.	61,173,209
Pyrimethamine	50–75 mg PO	3.1–3.3 μg/ml	620–660 μg/kg/day	62–66	Despite substantial dose present in milk, cannot be expected to provide therapeutic dose to infant less than 6 months old who has malaria.	40
Rifampin	450 mg PO dose 600 mg PO dose	3.4–4.9 μg/ml 10–30 μg/ml	0.68–0.98 mg/kg/day 2–6 mg/kg/day	6.8–60.0	No reported adverse effects; if used, monitor liver function; may color breast milk.	114
Streptomycin	1 gm IM	0.3–1.3 μg/ml	0.06–0.26 mg/kg/day	0.3–1.3	Not orally absorbed from normal bowel; no reported adverse effects.	64

Sulfamethoxazole (Gantanol)	Unknown	Not studied	Unknown	Unknown	Highly protein bound sulfas can displace bilirubin from albumin and increase risk of kernicterus without changing serum bilirubin. Acceptable for term infants over 3 weeks old if not G-6-PD-deficient.	55,96
Sulfisoxazole (Gantrisin)	1 gm q6h PO	Not specified	18 ± 8.4 mg/day recovered in milk	33–50		
Tetracyclines	500 mg qid PO 1.5–2.5 gm/day PO 275 mg/day PO as hydrochloride	0.43–8.0 μg/ml	0.09–1.60 μg/kg/day	Not used	The potential for tooth staining and altered bone growth appear to be minimal. Due to the small quantity of drug passing into the milk, the drug should generally be avoided in children, but probably poses no risk to the breast fed infant whose mother takes a short course of therapy.	163
Ticarcillin	5 gm tid	2–2.5 mg/μl	1.2 mg/day		Not absorbed when taken orally. May alter intestinal flora.	206
Tobramycin	80 mg IM	0–0.6 μg/ml	0–120 μg/kg/day	0–2.4	See gentacimin.	194
Trimethoprim (Proloprim, Trimpex; also in Bactrim, Septra)	160 mg bid–tid PO	1.2–5.5 μg/ml	0.2–1.1 μg/kg/day	Not used	No reports of adverse effects; preferred to sulfa-containing combinations (Bactrim, Septra) when nursing newborn; monitor for rash and anemia.	9

Table C-2. (continued)

Agent	Maternal dose	Reported milk levels	Estimated newborn intake	Predicted % of newborn therapeutic dose	Reported adverse reactions and cautions	References
Vancomycin	Not studied	Not studied	Unknown	Unknown	Do not restrict nursing; drug is not absorbed from intact gastrointestinal tract.	
Vermox (Mebendazole)	15 mg/kg (to sheep and cows)	<0.005–0.430 μg/ml	<1–86 μg/kg/day	Not used	Case report of a nursing mother whose lactation decreased after 3 days of Mebendazole and then stopped completely after 1 week; the patient had also taken 7 days of Metronidazole prior to Mebendazole. The authors conclude that the halt in lactation was due to Mebendazole. From animal work, mebendazole is expected to be present in human milk; withhold nursing for 48 hours after last dose.	37,143

Agent	Maternal dose	Reported milk levels	Estimated newborn intake	Predicted % of newborn therapeutic dose	Reported adverse reactions and cautions	References
Antiarrhythmic Agents						
Amiodarone	400 mg daily	2.8–16.4 μg/ml	0.56–3.28 mg/kg/day	8–50	This constitutes a low therapeutic dose; amiodarone should be avoided during nursing, or an alternative agent tried before stopping nursing.	136
		With 1.1–6.5 μg/ml	0.2–1.3 mg/kg/day			
Digoxin	0.25 mg daily 0.75 mg daily	0.2–0.9 ng/ml 1.9 ng/ml	40–180 ng/kg/day 380 ng/kg/day	0.06–0.30	Insignificant dose passed to baby; monitor for excessive spitting up, diarrhea, and abnormal heart rate; no value in checking digoxin level in baby (positive in unexposed infants).	63,125
Mexelitine	200 mg tid 250 mg tid	300–959 ng/ml Not measured	60–192 μg/kg/day Not measured	0.6–2.4[b]	Suboptimal growth and failure to feed seen in first 2 weeks of infant breast-feeding. At 8 to 10 months infants had normal neuro exam and EEG. Neurologic side effects include seizures, nausea, and vomiting; until neonatal pharmacology is studied, avoid nursing when mexelitine is used.	116,127
Procainamide	500 mg qid	5.4 μg/ml procainamide 3.5 μg/ml *N*-acteyl-procainamide	1.08 mg/kg/day 0.7 mg/kg/day *N*-acetyl-procainamide	2.2	When the mother has therapeutic blood levels, the baby may be exposed to therapeutic effects; mother and infant should have serum levels, blood count, heart rate, vomiting, and rashes monitored.	158

[a]See introduction to table on page 671.
[b]Compared with adult corrected dose.

Table C-3. (continued)

Agent	Maternal dose	Reported milk levels	Estimated newborn intake	Predicted % of newborn therapeutic dose	Reported adverse reactions and cautions	References
Quinidine	600 mg tid PO	6.4–8.2 μg/ml	1.3–1.6 mg/kg/day	3.5–10.0	Relatively large dose passed to infant; monitor rash, anemias, widening of QRS on electrocardiogram, and arrhythmias; may be best to avoid chronic use due to risk of optic neuritis.	74
Anticoagulants [51]						
Heparin	Not studied	Not studied	Unknown	Unknown	Very large molecule not expected to be excreted or orally absorbed; nurse as planned.	150
Warfarin (Coumadin)	5–12 mg daily	Not detectable (<25 mg/ml)	<5 μg/kg/day	Not used	Excretion and effect on infant has been well studied; do not restrict nursing; only most conservative would verify normal infant prothrombin time after 2 weeks of therapy.	114,130
Antihypertensives						
Beta Blockers:						
Acebutolol	0.2–1.2 gm/day	Acebutolol, 65–1545 ng/ml Diacetolol, <1–6640 ng/ml	—	Not used	Signs of beta blockade in 1 of 7 breast-fed infants. The infant may receive significant amounts of acebutolol if maternal dose is >400 mg/day or in decreased renal function. (see also atenolol)	35

Atenolol (Tenormin)	50–100 mg PO daily	0.40–6.35 μmol/liter	0.08–1.27 μmol/kg/day	Not used	There are reports of two infants with no adverse effects. There is one report of infant who acquired toxic concentrations while breast-feeding and showed signs of beta blockade (hypotension, bradycardia). Acebutolol and Atenolol are secreted in milk to a greater degree than propranolol; therefore, accumulation is expected in milk.	117,177
Labetalol	600–1200 mg/day	129–662 μg/ml	—	—	No adverse effects seen in infants. One infant had a plasma labetolol concentration equal to mother's (another was lower). No consistent milk plasma ratios reported; therefore, no conclusions for safety in breast-feeding drawn.	126
Metoprolol	50–100 mg bid PO	0.38–2.58 μmol/liter	76–516 mmol/kg/day	Not used		104,118
Nadolol	80 mg PO daily 20 mg PO daily	161.9 ng/ml 146–440 ng/ml	29–88 μg/kg/day	Not used	Of these beta-blockers, propranolol has been used most without reported adverse effect; monitor growth and development.	32,48
Propranolol	Up to 160 mg PO	10–150 ng/ml	2–30 μg/kg/day	0.5–3.0		13,94
Other antihypertensives:						
Captopril (Capoten)	100 mg PO tid	4.7 ± 0.7 ng/ml	0.94 ± 0.14 ng/ml	0.1	Minimal exposure, but pharmacology in newborns is unstudied; alternative agents preferred.	47
Clonidine (Catapres)	0.2 mg bid	<0.05–1.24 ng/ml	<10–248 ng/kg/day	Up to 10	Potentially retinotoxic; avoid while nursing.	131

Table C-3. (continued)

Agent	Maternal dose	Reported milk levels	Estimated newborn intake	Predicted % of newborn therapeutic dose	Reported adverse reactions and cautions	References
Guanethidine (Ismelin)	Not stated	Negligible	Unknown; probably microgram quantity	Unknown	No reported adverse effects in nursing infants.	150
Hydralazine	50 mg PO tid	762–1263 nmol/liter	0.034 mg/kg/day	0.3–3.0	No reports of adverse effects in many nursed infants; do not restrict for short-term therapy; if long-term, monitor allergic and autoimmune reactions.	117
Methyldopa (Aldomet)	250 mg bid–500 mg qid	0.07–1.36 μg/ml	14–272 μg/kg/day	0.04–2.70	Extensive anecdotal experience without reported adverse effects; potential for hemolysis and elevated liver enzymes; monitor infant for decreased respiration and blood pressure.	87,214
	250–500 mg	0.2–1.14 μg/ml (mean values)	855 μg/d (estimated with 1-gm dose)		—	
Minoxidil	5 mg bid × 2 months	0.3–41.7 ng/ml (0.5–3.4 glucuronide conjugate)		Not used	No adverse effects were seen in infant after 2-month exposure to minoxidil in breast milk. This single case report does not guarantee safety.	202
Prazosin (Minipress)	5 mg tid	5–18 ng/ml	1.0–3.6 μg/kg/day	1–4[b]	Minimal passage; no reported adverse effects.	131

Diuretics (Use not contraindicated if mother is well hydrated.)						
Acetazolamide	500 mg bid	1.3–2.1 μg/ml	0.6 mg	—	Low levels excreted into breast milk. No adverse effects seen in infant. Monitor for sedation.	185
Chlorothiazide (Diuril)	500 mg PO	1 μg/ml	0.2 mg/kg/day	0.4–1.0	No reported adverse effects; may decrease milk flow initially; flow improves with continued use; potential to increase bilirubin only at very high dose.	139
Chlorthalidone (Hygroton)	50 mg PO daily	90–860 ng/ml	18–174 μg/kg/day	0.75–7.50[b]	Shorter-acting diuretics preferred; no reported adverse effects.	144
Furosemide (Lasix)	Not studied	Not studied	Unknown	Unknown	Exposure likely very small and poorly absorbed; may decrease milk flow at first dose or if mother becomes fluid depleted; monitor infant's fluid output.	
Hydrochlorothiazide	50 mg PO daily	<50–120 ng/ml	<10–24 μg/kg/day	<0.02–0.12	No reported adverse effects; may decrease milk flow initially; flow improves with continued use; potential to increase bilirubin only at very high dose.	139
Spironolactone	25 mg bid	47–104 ng/ml	9.4–20.8 μg/kg/day	0.31–1.04	No reported adverse effects; some express concern over potential carcinogenicity of this agent.	157
Triamterine with hydrochlorothiazide	Not studied	Not studied	Unknown	Not used	Limited anecdotal experience; no reported adverse effects (see hydrochlorothiazide).	

[b]Compared with adult corrected dose.

Table C-3. (continued)

Agent	Maternal dose	Reported milk levels	Estimated newborn intake	Predicted % of newborn therapeutic dose	Reported adverse reactions and cautions	References
Calcium-Channel Blockers						
Diltiazem	60 mg qid × 4d	<50–200 ng/ml	Unknown		Single case report; infant not fed during study. Drug passes into milk at comparable concentrations to other calcium-channel blockers. More information needed before safety established.	151
Nifedipine	30 mg q8 × 48 h 20 mg q8 × 48 h 10 mg q8 × 36 h	4.90–53.35 ng/ml 3.19–16.35 ng/ml <0.1–12.89 ng/ml	7.5 μg/kg/day	>5	Study only of excretion into milk. Infant not exposed to milk. Levels of drug in breast milk are low and probably pose little risk to breast-feeding infant. Delaying breast-feeding 3 to 4 hours after dose significantly decreases exposure of infant to drug.	54
Nitrendipine	10 mg bid × 5d	Average 355 ng	1.7 μg/day	—	Study of excretion in milk. Effect on infant is unknown. Levels in breast milk are low.	215
Verapamil	80 mg tid 320 mg daily	<20–40 ng/ml <300 ng/ml	<4–8 μg/kg/day <60 μg/kg/day	<0.8–10.0	Dose passed is small; if nursing elected, monitor blood pressure, electrocardiogram, and for signs of heart failure and vomiting.	6,46

Table C-4. Sedatives and hypnotics

Agent	Maternal dose	Reported milk levels	Estimated newborn intake	Predicted % of newborn therapeutic dose	Reported adverse reactions and cautions	References
Sedative-Hypnotics						
Alprazolam	Not studied	Not studied	Not studied	—	No published data. Since it is probably excreted in breast milk, use same precautions as diazepam.	
Butabarbital	8 mg PO bid	0.37 μg/ml	74 μg/kg/day	Not used	See pentobarbital.	218
Chloral hydrate	1.33 gm rectally	0–15 μg/ml	0–3 mg/kg/day	0–15	Sedation reported in infant of mother given "hypnotic dose"; long history of use in children; mother should avoid alcohol when taking this drug; monitor sedation, rash.	21
Diazepam (Valium)	5–10 mg tid PO	17–100 ng/ml and more (plus 19–85 ng/ml desmethyl-diazepam active metabolite)	>3.4–20.0 μg/kg/day plus active metabolite	1–6 or more	Infant sedation, lethargy, and weight loss reported with chronic high-dose (30 mg/day) use; higher milk levels may cause accumulation in infant due to basicity and long persistence in body; single dose probably acceptable for nursing mothers.	31,42,59
Flurazepam (Dalmane)	Not reported	Not found	Unknown	Not used	Although very early report stated Dalmane "not found," it is probably present in low levels; chronic use should be avoided; accumulation may occur; monitor sedation.	207
Glutethimide (Doriden)	500 mg PO	3 ng/ml	600 ng/kg/day	Not used	Agents with greater safety margin and experience in infants preferred.	45

Table C-4. (continued)

Agent	Maternal dose	Reported milk levels	Estimated newborn intake	Predicted % of newborn therapeutic dose	Reported adverse reactions and cautions	References
Lorazepam (Ativan)	3–5 mg	8–9 ng/ml			As with other benzodiazepines, occasional doses may be safe. Long-term effects unknown.	193
Pentobarbital (Nembutal) (see phenobarbital)	100 mg PO daily	0.17 μg/ml	34 μg/kg/day	Not used	Barbiturates with long duration of action (pentobarbital, secobarbital) may accumulate in infant with chronic use; occasional doses acceptable for nursing mothers; shortest-acting sedative preferred to induce sleep; barbiturates can induce metabolism of endogenous compounds.	218
Secobarbital (Seconal)	Present	Unknown	Unknown	Not used		
Thiopental (Pentothal)	1.125 gm IV	20 μg/ml	4 μg/kg/day	Not used		
Antipsychotic Drugs						
Chlorpromazine (Thorazine)	Up to 1200 mg/day PO	Up to 290 ng/ml	1.4–58.0 μg/kg/day	0.05–0.26	Sedation reported in infants of chlorpromazine-treated	217
	Maternal serum level 16–52 ng/ml	7–98 ng/ml			mothers; several babies who nursed on chlorpromazine were developmentally normal at age 5. Although the amounts of Haldol excreted in breast milk are low, adverse effects in developing CNS may occur. Avoid use. For other agents, no follow-up is available; the drug has often been received in utero in much	25

					higher amounts; nursing is therefore not a new risk, but a continued one; if the baby is nursed, monitor sedation, dystonia, liver enzymes, and growth and development.	
Haloperidol (Haldol)	5 mg bid PO 12 mg daily PO 30 mg daily PO	2.6–23.5 ng/ml 2 ng/ml 5 ng/ml	0.1–1.0 μg/kg/day	1.3–10.0[b]		192,213
Mesoridazine (Serentil)	Not reported	Reportedly present	Unknown	Not used		150
Prochlorperazine (Compazine)	Not reported	Reportedly present	Unknown	Not used		150
Thioridazine (Mellaril)	Not reported	Reportedly present	Unknown	Not used		8
Trifluoperazine (Stelazine)	Not reported	Reportedly present	Unknown	Not used		101
Lithium	600–1200 mg/day	0.12–0.60 mEq/liter	24–120 μEq/kg/day	Not used	Reports of serum level in infant equal to one-third of the mother's; considered to be contraindicated; may be safest to avoid nursing during lithium therapy owing to infant's susceptibility to fluid and sodium imbalance, which would increase lithium toxicity, and owing to lack of follow-up.	170,177,200

Table C-4. (continued)

Agent	Maternal dose	Reported milk levels	Estimated newborn intake	Predicted % of newborn therapeutic dose	Reported adverse reactions and cautions	References
MAO Inhibitor Antidepressants						
Phenelzine (Nardil)	Not studied	Not studied	Unknown	Not used	It is not known whether these agents get into the milk of nursing mothers. Agents should be used with **caution** owing to potential both to suppress milk production and for hypertensive crisis with tyramine exposure.	150
Tranylcypromine (Parnate)	Not stated	"Too low to affect child"	Unknown	Not used		78
Stimulants						
Amphetamines	Not reported	Not measured	Unknown	Unknown	No stimulation or insomnia observed in 103 infants whose nursing mothers received low-dose amphetamine for depression. In cases of nursing mothers abusing amphetamines, poor sleep patterns and irritability are seen in the infants.	10
Caffeine	1 cup of coffee 36–336 mg as 146 mg as coffee	8.2 μg/ml Up to 7.17 μg/ml 0.82 ± 0.29 μg/ml	1.6 mg/kg/day 0.01–1.64 mg/day (author's estimate)	8–30 per cup of coffee or more	Although a single cup of normal-strength coffee (or similar-dose drug) would not produce therapeutic serum levels in term infants, newborns or premature babies can experience caffeine effect (agitation, insomnia, gastrointestinal distress) with high or repeated dosage; moderation in intake is advised.	16,59,73

Tricyclic Antidepressants						
Amitriptyline (Elavil, others)	100 mg/day PO	135–151 ng/ml plus 52–59 ng/ml nortriptyline	27–30 μg/kg/day	Not used	There is no information about usual dose or safety in the newborn; because early studies were not able to detect antidepressants in milk, many babies have been nursed without reported problems; no information on long-term safety is available for these children; the very small amounts of drug present in breast milk are much less than fetuses experience in treated pregnancies; consider whether risk is new or continued; generally, nursing is not contraindicated; monitor growth and development.	11
	25–50 mg/day PO	"Not detectable" (<100 ng/ml	<40 μg/kg/day			
Amoxapine (Asendin)	250 mg/day PO	<20 ng/ml plus active metabolite	<4 μg/kg/day plus metabolite	Not used		66
Desipramine (Norpramin, others)	200 mg/day Imipramine	17–35 ng/ml (estimate)	3.4–7.0 μg/kg/day	Not used		
Doxepin (Adapin)	10 mg/day, then 25 mg tid	7–29 μg/ml Doxepin 7–11 μg/ml DDP[a]	14 μg 7 μg	—	No adverse effects noted in one case; may cause sedation; should be used with **caution** due to increased risk of sedation.	99,132
	150 mg h.s. × 8 mos.	35–68 μg/ml Doxepin 65–131 μg/ml DDP	71 μg 131 μg	—		
Imipramine (Tofranil)	200 mg/day PO	12–29 ng/ml (estimate)	2.4–5.8 μg/kg/day (predicted)	Not used	Imipramine enters milk in low concentrations. Agent is probably safe to use while breast-feeding.	188
Nortriptyline (Pamelor, others)	25 mg PO	"Not detected"; seen after amitriptyline	Unknown	Not used	Not detected in serum of breast-fed infants. Chronic exposure risk unknown.	7

[a]DDP = *n*-desmethyldoxepin.

Table C-5. Anticonvulsants [125]

Agent	Maternal dose	Reported milk levels	Estimated newborn intake	Predicted % of newborn therapeutic dose	Reported adverse reactions and cautions	References
Carbamazepine (Tegretol)	8 mg/kg/day 3–22 mg/kg/day	0.3–3.5 μg/ml 0.85–3.00 μg/ml plus 0.15–0.80 μg/ml epoxide metabolite	60–700 μg/kg/day plus epoxide	Not used (0.6–7.0 child's dose/kg[a])	Probably safe while breast-feeding; infant exposure may be low; monitor infant for bone marrow suppression; sedation, poor feeding, serum levels to 4.7 mg/liter accumulate.	92,106,149, 164,217
Ethosuximide (Zarontin)	250 mg bid	18.5–68.5 μg/ml	3.7–13.9 mg/kg/day	Not used (10–69 of child's dose/kg[a])	Because of rare occurrence of bone marrow depression and gastrointestinal upset, must weigh benefit of nursing against potential risks of use; no reported adverse effects despite reported infant serum levels of 24–30% of maternal level; ascertain that mother still requires drug.	92,103,165, 218
Phenobarbital	30 mg qid (short term) 100–200 mg/day (qs to produce maternal serum level of 19.3 μg/ml)	1–3 μg/ml 1–33 μg/ml	0.2–0.6 mg/kg/day 0.2–6.6 mg/kg/day	4–100	Sedation reported; may be best to avoid if the mother is receiving anticonvulsant or hypnotic dosage (100–200) mg/day); sedative dosage for preeclampsia, given short-term, does not contraindicate nursing except for sick or very premature babies; can alter hepatic metabolism; monitor sedation, sucking pattern, and rashes.	92,106,218

Phenytoin (Dilantin)	200–400 mg/day	[illegible] µg/ml	0.1–1.2 mg/kg/day	2–[illegible]	Risk to the breast-feeding infant appears to be low; few adverse effects reported (methemoglobinemia and cyanosis in one infant, gastrointestinal distress in another). Highest exposure to drug through milk is still lower than therapeutic daily doses in infants (10 mg/kg). Monitor growth and development.	92,190,218
Primidone (Mysoline)	Not reported 5.8–8.5 mg/kg/day	0.1–4.5 µg/ml 0.4–8.2 µg/ml primidone 0.9–2.9 µg/ml PEMA 0.8–4.3 µg/ml phenobarbital	20–900 µg/kg/day 0.08–1.60 mg/kg/day primidone 0.18–0.60 mg/kg/day PEMA 0.16–0.80 mg/kg/day phenobarbital	Unknown	Can cause irritability; avoid or monitor same as for phenobarbital (which is a primidone metabolite).	92,106,218
Valproic acid (Depakene)	250 mg bid PO 9.5–31.0 mg/kg/day PO Not reported	0.17–0.47 µg/ml 0.034–5.400 µg/ml 3.3–8.3 µg/ml	34–94 µg/kg/day 0.007–1.100 mg/kg/day 0.7–1.7 mg/kg/day	0.05–11.30	There have been no adverse effects in infants exposed to breast milk of mothers on valproic acid. Pharmacologic experience in neonates is limited; potential adverse effects include hepatitis and hemorrhagic pancreatitis. If woman treated during pregnancy decides to nurse, monitor the infant's liver enzymes, bleeding time, platelet count (during protracted nursing), and serum level if toxicity is suspected by gastrointestinal distress or oversedation (especially in high doses).	1,49,146, 218

[a]Compared with adult weight-corrected dose.

Table C-6. Gastrointestinal medications[a]

Agent	Maternal dose	Reported milk levels	Estimated newborn intake	Predicted % of newborn therapeutic dose	Reported adverse reactions and cautions	References
H_2 Antagonists						
Cimetidine (Tagamet)	200 mg tid plus 400 mg hs × 3 days	4.88–6.00 μg/ml	0.96–1.20 mg/kg/day	2.0–2.5	Dose small despite relative concentration in milk; however, considered **contraindicated** because of potential antiendocrine effects.	187
Ranitidine	150 mg × 4	993–2610 ng/ml	Not established	Not used		98
Laxatives	Aloin (15 mg)	Detected	Not calculated	Not used	Associated with increased infant bowel motility; alternative agents preferred.	201
	Cascara fluid extract (4 ml)	Not reported	Unknown			
	Dulcolax (tablet or suppository; usual therapeutic doses)	Not studied	Unknown	Not used	No report of adverse effect on infant, despite considerable anecdoctal use.	
	Milk of magnesia	Not reported	Unknown	Not used	Reported to have no effect on infant.	201
	Mineral oil (15 ml)	Not reported	Unknown	—	—	

	Phenolphthalein (30–800 mg)	Not reported	Not calculated	—	—	
	Rhubarb syrup (10 ml)	Not reported	Unknown	—	—	
	Senna fluid extract (4 ml)	Not detected	Unknown	—	Probably does not affect infants bowel function; probably safe while breast-feeding.	180,201,211
	Senokot (100 mg or 1 tsp)	Not detected	Unknown	—	—	
Metoclopramide	10 mg tid	52–157 ng/ml	10.4–31.4 μg/kg/day	10–31	Small dose; monitor sedation and dystonia; enhances lactation; should probably be avoided while breast-feeding.	97
Neomycin	Not studied	Not studied	Unknown	Unknown	No reported adverse effects; poor oral absorption predicted for both mother and baby.	
Sulfasalazine	1–3 gm daily	0.5–2.5 μg/ml 0–35 μg/ml total sulfapyridine 0–38 μg/ml free sulfapyridine	0.1–0.5 mg/kg/day 0–7 mg/kg/day 0–8 mg/kg/day	Not used (0.1–0.8 of child's dose/kg[b])	Considered compatible with nursing, as sulfapyridine does not displace bilirubin extensively; no reported adverse effects; monitor for rashes, hemolytic anemia, and leukopenia.	84

[a]When deciding whether or not to advise nursing by women taking these drugs, consider potential detriment of nursing to the mother's nutritional status.
[b]Compared with adult weight-corrected dose.

Table C-7. Respiratory medications

Agent	Maternal dose	Reported milk levels	Estimated newborn intake	Predicted % of newborn therapeutic dose	Reported adverse reactions and cautions	References
Antihistamines						
Brompheniramine (Dimetane)	Not studied	Not studied	Unknown	Not used	Reports of agitation when taken in combination with decongestant (brompheniramine/ isoephedrine); no other documented adverse effects on infant or milk supply; use short-acting agents (chlorpheniramine, diphenhydramine) if possible; monitor sedation, feeding.	3
Chlorpheniramine (Chlor-Trimeton)	Not studied	Not studied	Unknown	Not used		
Cyprophetadine (Periactin)	Not studied	Not studied	Unknown	Not used		
Diphenhydramine (Benadryl)	Not studied	Not studied	Unknown	Unknown	Probably present in small amounts. No adverse effects reported with considerable anecdotal use. Monitor newborn for sedation or agitation.	150
Loratidine	40 mg	29.2 ng/ml loratidine 16 ng/ml descarbo-ethoxyloratidine	7.3–26.0 μg/day	—	Small amounts of loratidine get into breast milk. No reports of infant exposure exist. May wish to use alternate agent.	72
Bronchodilators						
Albuterol (Proventil, Ventolin)	Not studied	Not studied	Unknown		No reported adverse effects; use of inhaled forms, rather than oral, can limit maternal systemic absorption and minimize infant exposure when the mother requires a bronchodilator.	
Isoproterenol (Iso-Medihaler, Isuprel)	Not studied	Not studied	Unknown			

(Alupent)						
Terbutaline (Brethine, Bricanyl)	2.5–5.0 mg tid	2.4–4.6 ng/ml	0.5–0.9 μg/kg/day	0.2–1.4 of adult dose/kg	Generally well tolerated; monitor for tachycardia and agitation if mother takes terbutaline chronically.	29,122
Decongestants						
Ephedrine Phenylpropanolamine Pseudoephedrine	Not reported	No quantitative data	Unknown	Not used	Report of agitated infant with oral therapy; use of topical (nasal) preparations may decrease systemic absorption and minimize infant exposure; of oral forms, pseudophedrine would be expected to cause the least excitation and is probably the agent of choice while breast-feeding.	3
Prednisone	10 mg/day	26.7 ng/ml prednisone with 6.1 ng/ml prednisolone	5.3 μg/kg/day prednisone; 1.2 μg/kg/day prednisolone	0.3	At 80 mg/day the infant receives <0.1 percent of dose, which corresponds to <10 percent of endogenous cortisol production. Breast-feeding is safer at doses of 20 mg 1 to 2 times a day. At higher doses, limit exposure to infant by feeding 4 hours after the dose.	95,137,154,174
	20 mg/day	41.5 ng/ml (mean) prednisone with 14.5 ng/ml prednisolone	8.3 μg/kg/day prednisone; 2.9 μg/kg/day prednisolone	0.6		
	10–80 mg/day short- and long-term use	30–317 ng/ml	6 μg/kg			
Theophylline (or aminophylline)	200 mg qid	2–4 μg/ml	0.4–0.8 mg/kg/day	6.7–20.0	Theophylline is usually well tolerated; monitor digestive intolerance, agitation, heart rate; infant serum level may be checked after 1 week of therapy if mother takes theophylline chronically; reasonable for mother to avoid excessive coffee or tea ingestion during therapy.	17,219

Table C-8. Endocrine medications

Agent	Maternal dose	Reported milk levels	Estimated newborn intake	Predicted % of newborn therapeutic dose	Reported adverse reactions and cautions	References
Antithyroid Agents						
Carbimazole	40 mg PO (equals 24.5 mg methimazole) 5–15 mg (3.3–10 mg methimazole)	100–200 μg methimazole/ml	20–40 μg/ methimazole/ml	Not used (7–14 of adult dose/kg)	All breast-feeding infants had normal thyroid function. At small doses, breast-feeding with carbimazole (methimazole) is probably safe. Infant thyroid function **must** be monitored frequently. Avoid breast-feeding if possible.	85 85,195
Methimazole (Tapazole)	2.5 mg bid	22–70 ng/ml	4.4–14.0 μg/kg/day	Not used (1.5–5.0 of adult dose/kg)	Avoid breast-feeding if possible.	
Propylthiouracil (PTU)	200–600 mg/day	500–700 ng/ml	100–140 μg/kg/day	Not used (1.2–5.0 of adult dose/kg)	PTU is the preferred agent; passes into breast milk less freely than methimazole because it is ionized and highly protein bound. Although exposure to these antithyroid drugs in milk is probably too low to affect thyroid function, serious side effects (bone marrow suppression, rashes) can occur; monitor growth and development, thyroid function, and blood count.	43,91,109, 134

(saturated solution of potassium iodide, vaginal povidone-iodine)		excreted in milk over 3 days			and goiter due to thyroid suppression may be seen; use as expectorant or antithyroid agent should be avoided while nursing.	
Iodine-131	100 mCi	39 nCi at 6 h 1.3–2.0 nCi at 24 h	0.3–8.0 μCi/kg/day 0.26–7.80 μCi/kg/day	Not used	**Contraindicated** during nursing; nursing may be restarted 2 days after a test dose, but must be delayed for 2 weeks after antithyroid therapy.	77,93,155
Iodine-125	—				Same as I-131	
Thyroid Hormones[a]						
Thyroxine (T_4)	—	<5–8 ng/ml T_3	<1.0–1.6 μg/kg/day T_3	18–50	Because thyroid hormone is naturally found in untreated mother's milk, use should not contraindicate nursing; it would be expected that women treated to euthyroid state would have only normal milk levels; this is yet unstudied; should not rely on nursing to treat known hypothyroid infant; some express concern that nursing could mask neonatal hypothyroidism; breast-feeding does not interfere with testing first week of life, but thereafter, both T_4 and thyroid-stimulating hormone should be measured.	203
Triiodothyronine (T_3)	—	<5–13 ng/ml T_4	<1.0–2.6 μg/kg/day T_4			

[a]Normal milk content: euthyroid woman.

Table C-8. (continued)

Agent	Maternal dose	Reported milk levels	Estimated newborn intake	Predicted % of newborn therapeutic dose	Reported adverse reactions and cautions	References
Steroids, adrenal (see Table C-7, Prednisone)						
Steroids, sex (see Table C-9, Oral contraceptives)						
Tolbutamide (Orinase)	500 mg PO	3–18 μg/ml	0.6–3.6 μg/kg/day	Not used	Despite lack of reported adverse effect, considered **contraindicated** due to available alternatives (diet, insulin) which would not affect baby. Diabinese is also reported to be excreted in breast milk.	142

Table C-9. Agents with gynecologic indication

Agent	Maternal dose	Reported milk levels	Estimated newborn intake	Predicted % of newborn therapeutic dose	Reported adverse reactions and cautions	References
Bromocriptine (Parlodel)	2.5 mg bid and more	Not studied	Unknown	Not used	Contraindicated; suppresses lactation.	50
Magnesium sulfate ($MgSO_4$)	1–2 gm/h by infusion after 2–10 gm loading dose	60% of concurrent serum level; normal by 12–14 hours after end of dose infusion	If full milk volume produced during infusion: 16 mg/kg/day or (usually much) less	300 normal maintenance intake or less during infusion	Unless mother produces full milk volume during magnesium sulfate infusion, newborn intake is likely to be insignificant; for women still on infusion, document presence of bowel sounds in baby (sign of hypermagnesemia from in utero exposure); and bowel movements until 24 hours after the end of infusion; formula often has more magnesium than milk from treated mothers.	44,130
Methylergonovine (Methergine)	0.25 mg	<0.5–1.3 ng/ml	<100–260 ng/kg/day	<5 of adult dose/kg	Does not suppress lactation; earlier crude ergot preparations were associated with infant ergotism, vomiting, diarrhea, weak pulse, and unstable blood pressure; no similar adverse effects reported from considerable use of methylergonovine; monitor baby for potential toxicity during use.	58,60

Table C-9. (continued)

Agent	Maternal dose	Reported milk levels	Estimated newborn intake	Predicted % of newborn therapeutic dose	Reported adverse reactions and cautions	References
Oral contraceptives	Combination	Estrogen content not significantly different from that of untreated women; progestogen present but does not appear to accumulate	Unknown	Not used	No change in quantity of milk if started after the immediate postpartum period; quality of milk not clearly demonstrated to be altered; long-term safety unknown; breast enlargement in infant (exposed to large estrogen dose) reported; does not contraindicate nursing; choose lowest effective combination dose and monitor the infant's weight gain.	4,5,68,121
Oxytocin	Not reported	Too large to be excreted (presumably)	Unknown	Not used	May enhance letdown reflex; no reported adverse effects.	218

Agent	Maternal dose	Reported milk levels	Estimated newborn intake	Predicted % of newborn therapeutic dose	Reported adverse reactions and cautions	References
Diatrizoate (Hypaque, Reno-M 60)	Not studied	Not studied	Unknown	Unknown	No reported adverse effects, despite considerable use as agent for IV pyelography in postpartum period; rapidly excreted by mother; see comment for iopanoic acid.	
Gallium-67	3 mCi	70 nCi/ml at 96 and 120 hours postdose	Approximately 14 μCi/kg/day	Unknown	Radioactivity persists for more than 5 days after maternal dose; resume nursing after 2 weeks.	111,198
Iodine-125	See Table C-8					
Iodine-131	See Table C-8					
Iopanoic acid (Telepaque)	Not reported	3–11 mg iodide/ "feeding" at 5–19 hours postdose (peak)	120–440 mg/kg/day	Unknown	Very high iodide intake; if available to infant, may suppress thyroid function or cause allergic reactions or rash.	76
Metrizamide	5 gm into subarachnoid space	1.7–214.0 μg/ml	1 mg over 48 hours after single dose	0.02 of total subarachnoid dose; (1.4 of adult dose/kg)	Not likely to affect infant unless he or she is allergic.	80,81
Technetium	4–20 mCi	Radioactivity present at 300–500% of plasma level at 17 and 20 hours postdose	Unknown	Unknown	Two studies indicate that infant would be exposed to no excessive radioactivity if nursing began 48 hours after a 20-mCi dose to the mother or 24 hours after a 4-mCi dose.	159,160

Table C-11. Drugs of abuse or social use. The Committee on Drugs of the American Academy of Pediatrics strongly feels that nursing mothers should not use any of these compounds [5]. (See Ch. 2)

Agent	Maternal dose	Reported milk levels	Estimated newborn intake	Predicted % of newborn therapeutic dose	Reported adverse reactions and cautions	References
Amphetamines (see Table C-4)						
Cocaine	(1) 0.5 gm in a 4-h period	Not studied but probably present (lipid soluble)	Unknown	Not given	(1) Report of infant with cocaine intoxication following ingestion of mother's milk. Infant became irritable, tremulous, tachycardic, with vomiting and diarrhea. Effects seen for $>$24 hours.	38
	(2) Topically applied for nipple soreness				(2) Report of an infant in status epilepticus 3 hours after feeding from nipple that had cocaine topically applied.	36
					Drug may remain in milk up to 60 hours after mother uses the drug.	
					Mothers using cocaine	

Ethanol (alcohol)	0.6–1.0 gm/kg (3 or 4 cocktails, glasses of wine, or bottles of beer)	800–5600 μg/ml	0.16–1.12 gm/kg/day	16–112 (or less)	Sedation is likely only with high maternal blood levels seen with either acute very high dose exposure or chronic use; pseudo-Cushing's syndrome seen after intake of more than seven 12-oz cans of beer plus other alcohol daily; infant drunkenness reported with intake of 750 ml port wine daily; high dosage (1 gm/kg) can inhibit letdown and impair lactation; hypoprothrombinemia with bleeding has been seen in infants of nursing Chinese alcoholics. New evidence suggests delayed motor development in infants being nursed by mother drinking ethanol.	22,23,75, 100,119, 218
Heroin	2–45 mg daily	Not measured	Unknown, but probably variable	Not given	May delay onset of withdrawal until after discharge from hospital and allow it to occur in uncontrolled setting; chaotic lifestyle of heroin user is generally incompatible with commitment to nurse.	41,63

Table C-11. (continued)

Agent	Maternal dose	Reported milk levels	Estimated newborn intake	Predicted % of newborn therapeutic dose	Reported adverse reactions and cautions	References
Nicotine (smoking)					Symptoms reported are vomiting, diarrhea, tachycardia, and irritability.	128
Tetrahydrocannabinol (THC in marijuana)	1–7 pipes/day	60–340 ng/ml plus metabolites	12–68 μg/kg/day	Not given	Encourage abstinence; no reported adverse effects, but may persist in milk for days after exposure; concentrated in milk with use. Infants studied 1 to 2 years after the milk exposure showed no adverse effects. More long-term studies needed.	156,196
Lysergic diethylamide (LSD)	Not studied	Not studied	Unknown	Not given	No reported experience; may persist in body long after exposure; may be sold as "speed"; encourage abstinence or discourage nursing.	
Phencyclidine (PCP, angel dust)	Not studied	Not studied	Unknown	Not given	—	

Table C-12. Antineoplastic agents

Agent	Maternal dose	Reported milk levels	Estimated newborn intake	Predicted % of newborn therapeutic dose	Reported adverse reactions and cautions	References
Any agent					Due to potential toxicity and carcinogenicity, no antineoplastic agents are considered safe while breast-feeding.	2,30,86,216

Table C-13. Miscellaneous agents

Agent	Maternal dose	Reported milk levels	Estimated newborn intake	Predicted % of newborn therapeutic dose	Reported adverse reactions and cautions	References
Anticholinergics						
Atropine	Not stated	<1 μg/ml	<200 μg/kg/day	—	Potential inhibitory effect on lactation and risk of infant atropine poisoning are unsubstantiated. Because these drugs have been considered prohibited for nursing mothers, experience is limited; avoid if possible. Infants are more susceptible to anticholinergic effects.	7
Propantheline	Not stated	"Not excreted" according to manufacturer	Unknown	—		
Scopolamine	Not stated	Reportedly present	Unknown	—		
Azathioprine (imuran)	75–125 mg daily	Not found (<0.6 μg/ml)	<120 μg/kg/day	Not used	Despite nondetection, azathioprine is **contraindicated** due to inherent toxicity and potential carcinogenicity.	148
Ergonovine (Wygraine, Cafegot)	200 μg PO	Not measured	Unknown	Not used	Ergots may decrease lactation; infant ergotism (vomiting, diarrhea, weak pulse, unstable blood pressure, or seizures) was common in one 1934 study of mothers using a crude ergot preparation; while the occasional use of small doses of purer ergots has not been associated with infant toxicity, it has been **contraindicated** to nurse during their use; this may have biased the experience; for	64,179
Ergot alkaloid extract	Unknown	Not measured	Unknown	Not used		

					postpartum bleeding, see Table C-9, Methylergonovine. When managing migraines that require high (1 mg), repeated doses, it is considered **contraindicated** to nurse; during hiatus, the mother should express milk to fight the antilactation effect; because of slow and erratic absorption, must avoid nursing for at least 48 hours after dose; alternative palliative analgesics (narcotics) may allow a woman to continue to breast-feed, if she wishes.	
Isotretinoin	Not studied	Not studied	Not used	Not used	No studies of isotretinoin in breast milk are reported. Since vitamin A is excreted in breast milk, isotretinoin is probably also excreted. The manufacturer advises against breast-feeding.	172
Gold thiomalate	50 mg/week IM	0.022 μg/ml	4.4 μg/kg/day	Not used (2.3 of adult dose/kg)	Considered **contraindicated** due to potential for adverse effects on liver and kidneys and severe rashes.	27,165
Mepenzolate (Cantil)	Not stated	"Not excreted"	Unknown	Not used	No reported adverse effects; monitor sedation.	129
Methocarbemol (Robaxin)	Not stated	"Traces" present	Unknown	Not used	—	129
Baclofen	20 mg	0.052–0.68 μg/ml (mean values)		Not used	Single case report, low dose, single dose, effects of feeding infant not reported. Although low concentrations attained, more long-term and high-dose studies needed.	57

Table C-13. (continued)

Agent	Maternal dose	Reported milk levels	Estimated newborn intake	Predicted % of newborn therapeutic dose	Reported adverse reactions and cautions	References
Quinine sulfate	600–1300 mg PO	0.4–1.6 μg/ml	80–320 μg/kg/day	Not used (0.8–3.0 of adult dose/kg)	No reported adverse effects, but should be avoided due to potential adverse effects on the retinal vasculature.	
RhoGam or other gamma globulin	Not reported	Not reported	Unknown	Not given	It is believed that antibodies present in milk would be inactivated in infant's stomach; compatible with nursing.	99
Rubella vaccine	Not reported	See comment	Unknown	Unknown	Live virus has been found in milk after vaccination with previously used vaccine strain (HPV-77) and is likely to be present with the RA 27/3 strain; there are few reported adverse effects, despite common vaccination of susceptible women in the early puerperium; only one case of clinical rubella was reported in a 13-day-old infant after maternal vaccination with HPV-77 on the first postpartum day; there is considerable controversy about whether or not this is vaccine related; at present, vaccination of the mother is considered compatible with nursing.	34,110, 113,115

References

1. Alexander, R. W. *Arch. Dis. Child.* 54: 240, 1979.
2. Amato, D. *Med. J. Aust.* 1: 383, 1977.
3. American Academy of Pediatrics, Committee on Drugs. *Pediatrics* 72: 375, 1983.
4. American Academy of Pediatrics, Committee on Drugs. *Pediatrics* 68: 138, 1981.
5. American Academy of Pediatrics, Committee on Drugs. *Pediatrics* 84: 924, 1989.
6. Anderson, H. J. *Eur. J. Clin. Pharmacol.* 25: 279, 1983.
7. Anderson, P. O. *Drug Intell. Clin. Pharm.* 11: 208, 1977.
8. Arais, I. *J.A.M.A.* 218: 746, 1971.
9. Arnaud, R. *Quest Med.* 25: 959, 1972.
10. Ayd, F. E. (Ed.). *Int. Drug Ther. Newsletter* 8: 33, 1973.
11. Bader, T. F. *Am. J. Psychiatry* 137: 855, 1980.
12. Baier, R., et al. Piperacillin Concentrations in Milk and Serum from Lactating Women (Abstract). In *Abstracts of the 1982 International Congress of Antimicrobial Agents and Chemotherapy.* Boston, 1982. P.227.
13. Bauer, J. H. *Am. J. Cardiol.* 43: 860, 1979.
14. Belton, E. M. *Lancet* 2: 691, 1965.
15. Berger, H. *Am. J. Dis. Child.* 61: 256, 1941.
16. Berlin, C. M., Jr. *Pediatrics* 73: 59, 1984.
17. Berlin, C. M., Jr. *Semin. Perinatol.* 5: 389, 1981.
18. Berlin, C. M., Jr. *Clin. Pharmacol. Ther.* 27: 245, 1980.
19. Berlin, C. M., Jr. *Pediatr. Pharmacol.* 1: 135, 1980.
20. Berlin, C. M., Jr. *Fed. Proc.* 38: 426, 1979.
21. Bernstine, J. B. *J. Obstet. Gynaecol. Br. Comm.* 63: 228, 1956.
22. Binkiewicz, A. *J. Pediatr.* 93: 956, 1978.
23. Bisdom, C. J. W. *Maandshrift voor Kindergeneeskunde* 6: 332, 1937.
24. Bitzen, P. O. *Eur. J. Clin. Pharmacol.* 20: 123, 1981.
25. Blacker, K. H. *Am. J. Psychiatry* 119: 178, 1962.
26. Blanco, J. D. *Antimicrob. Agents Chemother.* 23: 479, 1983.
27. Blau, S. P. *Arthritis Rheum.* 16: 777, 1973.
28. Blinick, G. *Am. J. Obstet. Gynecol.* 121: 617, 1975.
29. Boreus, L. O. *Br. J. Clin. Pharmacol.* 13: 731, 1982.
30. Bounameaux, Y. *Ann. Soc. Belg. Med. Trop.* 44: 381, 1964.
31. Brandt, R. *Arzneim. Forsch. Drug Res.* 26: 454, 1976.
32. Breitfeld-Fox, R. F. *Am. J. Obstet. Gynecol.* 152: 1045, 1985.
33. Brogden, R. N. *Drugs* 9: 251, 1975.
34. Buimovici-Klein, E. *J. Pediatr.* 91: 939, 1977.
35. Buotroy, M. J., et al. *Eur. J. Clin. Pharmacol.* 30: 737, 1986.
36. Chaney, N., et al. *J. Pediatr.* 112: 134, 1988.
37. Chapin, S. *Adv. Drug React. Bull.* 1: 255, 1982.
38. Chasnoff, I. J., et al. *Pediatrics* 80: 836, 1987.
39. Clark, J. H. *Clin. Pediatr.* 20: 53, 1981.
40. Clyde, D. R. *East Afr. Med. J.* 37: 659, 1960.
41. Cobrinik, R. W. *Pediatrics* 24: 288, 1959.
42. Cole, A. P. *Arch. Dis. Child.* 50: 741, 1975.
43. Cooper, D. S. *N. Engl. J. Med.* 311: 1353, 1984.
44. Cruikshank, D. P. *Am. J. Obstet. Gynecol.* 143: 685, 1982.
45. Curry, S. H. *Clin. Pharmacol. Ther.* 12: 849, 1971.
46. DeSwiet, M. *Br. Med. J.* 1: 288, 1984.
47. Devlin, R. G. *J. Clin. Pharmacol.* 21: 110, 1981.
48. Devlin, R. G. *Br. J. Clin. Pharmacol.* 12: 393, 1981.
49. Dickenson, R. G. *J. Pediatr.* 94: 832, 1979.
50. Duchesne, C. *Obstet. Gynecol.* 57: 464, 1981.
51. Eckstein, H. B. *Lancet* 1: 672, 1970.
52. Eeg-Olofsson, O. *Lancet* 2: 216, 1978.
53. Egan, P. C. *Cancer Treat. Rep.* 69: 1387, 1985.
54. Ehrenkranz, R. *J. Pediatr.* 114: 478, 1989.

55. Elliott, G. T. *J. Pediatr.* 99: 171, 1981.
56. Ericson, H. S. *Obstet. Gynecol.* 57: 49, 1981.
57. Eriksson, G. *Scand. J. Clin. Lab. Invest.* 41: 185, 1981.
58. Erkkola, R. *Int. J. Clin. Pharmacol. Biopharm.* 16: 579, 1978.
59. Erkkola, R. *Lancet* 1: 1235, 1972.
60. Ferris, A. J. (Sandoz Pharmaceuticals, East Hanover, N.J. 07936). Personal communication, July 22, 1981.
61. Findlay, J. W. A. *Clin. Pharmacol. Ther.* 29: 625, 1981.
62. Finley, J. P. *J. Pediatr.* 93: 339, 1979.
63. Finnegan, L. P. *Contemp. Drug Probl.* 1: 795, 1972.
64. Fomina, P. I. *Arch. Gynecol.* 157: 275, 1934.
65. Fujimori, H. *J. Jpn. Obstet. Gynecol. Soc.* 4: 133, 1957.
66. Gelenberg, J. *J. Nerv. Ment. Dis.* 135: 1483, 1979.
67. Giamerellou, H. *Am. J. Med.* 87: 495, 1989.
68. Greene, H. J. *Am. J. Obstet. Gynecol.* 51: 732, 1946.
69. Guiloff, E., et al. *Am. J. Obstet. Gynecol.* 118: 42, 1974.
70. Havelka, J. *Excerpta Med.* 27: 258, 1972.
71. Havelka, J. *Chemotherapy* 13: 204, 1968.
72. Hilbert, J., et al. *J. Clin. Pharmacol.* 28: 234, 1988.
73. Hildebrandt, R. *Pediatr. Pharmacol.* 3: 237, 1983.
74. Hill, L. M. *Obstet. Gynecol.* 54: 366, 1979.
75. Hoh, T. K. *Singapore Med. J.* 10: 43, 1969.
76. Holmdahl, K., II. *Acta Radiol.* 45: 305, 1955.
77. Honour, A. J. *Clin. Sci.* 11: 447, 1952.
78. Horning, M. G. *Mod. Probl. Paediatr.* 178: 135, 1973.
79. Hosbach, R. E. *J.A.M.A.* 202: 1057, 1967.
80. Ilett, K. F. *Br. J. Radiol.* 54: 537, 1981.
81. Ilett, K. F. *Clin. Exp. Pharmacol. Physiol.* 8: 672, 1981.
82. Ito, T. *Jpn. J. Antibiot.* 23: 298, 1970.
83. Jamali, F. *Drug Intell. Clin. Pharm.* 17: 910, 1983.
84. Janerot, G. *Scand. J. Gastroenterol.* 14: 869, 1979.
85. Johanse, K. *Eur. J. Clin. Pharmacol.* 23: 339, 1982.
86. Johns, D. G. *Am. J. Obstet. Gynecol.* 112: 978, 1972.
87. Jones, H. M. R. *Br. J. Clin. Pharmacol.* 6: 432, 1978.
88. Kafetzis, D. A. *Antimicrob. Agents Chemother.* 23: 870, 1983.
89. Kafetzis, D. A. *Acta Paediatr. Scand.* 70: 285, 1981.
90. Kafetzis, D. A. *J. Antimicrob. Chemother.* 6(S): 135, 1980.
91. Kampmann, J. P. *Lancet* 1: 736, 1980.
92. Kaneko, S. *Br. J. Clin. Pharmacol.* 7: 624, 1979.
93. Karjalainen, P. *Acta Obstet. Gynaecol. Scand.* 50: 357, 1971.
94. Karlberg, B. *Acta Pharmacol. Toxicol. (Copenh.)* 43: 222, 1974.
95. Katz, F. H. *N. Engl. J. Med.* 293: 1154, 1975.
96. Kaufman, R. E. *J. Pediatr.* 97: 639, 1980.
97. Kauppila, H. *Eur. J. Clin. Pharmacol.* 25: 819, 1983.
98. Kearns, G. L., et al. *Clin. Pharmacol.* 4: 322, 1985.
99. Kemp, J., et al. *Br. J. Clin. Pharmacol.* 20: 497, 1985.
100. Kesaniemi, Y. A. *Obstet. Gynecol. Br. Comm.* 81: 84, 1974.
101. Knowles, J. *J. Pediatr.* 66: 1068, 1965.
102. Kok, T. *Lancet* 1: 914, 1982.
103. Koup, J. R. *Epilepsia* 19: 535, 1978.
104. Krause, W. *Eur. J. Clin. Pharmacol.* 22: 53, 1982.
105. Kreutner, A. K., et al. *Am. J. Obstet. Gynecol.* 140: 895, 1981.
106. Kuhnz, W. *Pediatr. Pharmacol.* 3: 199, 1983.
107. Kunka, R. L. *Clin. Pharmacol. Ther.* 35: 675, 1984.
108. Kwit, N. T. *Am. J. Dis. Child.* 49: 900, 1935.
109. Lamberg, B. A., et al. *Clin. Endocrinol.* 21: 81, 1984.
110. Landes, R. D. *J. Pediatr.* 97: 465, 1980.
111. Larson, S. M. *J.A.M.A.* 218: 257, 1971.
112. Lau, R. J., et al. *Obstet. Gynecol.* 69: 468, 1987.

113. Lawrence, R. A. *Breast-Feeding: A Guide for the Medical Profession*. St. Louis: Mosby, 1980. Pp. 157–171.
114. Lenzi, E. *Atti Accad. Lancisiana Roma* 13(Suppl. 1): 87, 1969.
115. Lerman, S. J. *J. Pediatr.* 97: 668, 1981.
116. Lewis, A. M. *Postgrad. Med. J.* 57: 546, 1981.
117. Liedholm, H. *Eur. J. Clin. Pharmacol.* 21: 417, 1982.
118. Liedholm, H. *Eur. J. Clin. Pharmacol.* 20: 229, 1981.
119. Little, R. E. *N. Engl. J. Med.* 321: 425, 1989.
120. Lohmeyer, L. Z. *Geburtshilfe Gynakol.* 164: 184, 1965.
121. Lonnerdal, B., et al. *Am. J. Clin. Nutr.* 33: 816, 1980.
122. Lonnerholm, G. *Br. J. Clin. Pharmacol.* 13: 729, 1982.
123. Lou, M. A., et al. Penetration of Celtizoxime in Human Breast Milk, Several Body Fluids and Tissues (Abstract). In *Abstracts of the 1982 International Congress of Antimicrobial Agents and Chemotherapy*. Boston, 1982. P. 203.
124. Lou, M. A., et al. *Rev. Infect. Dis.* 6: 5816, 1984.
125. Loughnan, P. M. *J. Pediatr.* 92: 1019, 1978.
126. Lunell, N. O. *Eur. J. Clin. Pharmacol.* 28: 597, 1985.
127. Lownes, H. E., et al. *Am. J. Obstet. Gynecol.* 157: 446, 1987.
128. Luck, W. *Eur. J. Pediatr.* 17: 1055, 1987.
129. Mann, C. F. *Pediatrics* 66: 1930, 1980.
130. Marx, C. M., Scavone, J. S., and Epstein, M. E. Magnesium concentration of human milk after MA magnesium sulfate treatment for preeclampsia. *Submitted for publication.*
131. Marx, C. M. Unpublished observation, 1981.
132. Matheson, I. *Lancet* 2: 1124, 1985.
133. Maurer, E. *M.M.W.* 75: 249, 1928.
134. McDougall, et al. *Clin. Nucl. Med.* 11: 249, 1986.
135. McKenna, R. *J. Pediatr.* 103: 325, 1983.
136. McKenna, W. J. *Am. J. Cardiol.* 51: 1231, 1983.
137. McKenzie, S. A. *Arch. Dis. Child.* 50: 894, 1975.
138. Meyer, L. J. *Am. J. Obstet. Gynecol.* 158: 586, 1988.
139. Miller, R. E. *J. Pediatr.* 105: 789, 1982.
140. Mishler, T. W., et al. *J. Reprod. Med.* 21: 130, 1978.
141. Mizuno, S., et al. *Proceedings of a Symposium on Cephalexin*. London: Royal Society of Medicine, 1969. P. 49.
142. Moiel, R. H. *Clin. Pediatr. (Phila.)* 8: 480, 1967.
143. Moyer, R. (Janssen Pharmaceutica, Piscataway, N.J. 08854). Personal communication, November 20, 1981.
144. Mulley, B. A. *Eur. J. Clin. Pharmacol.* 13: 129, 1978.
145. Nation, R. L. *Br. J. Clin. Pharmacol.* 17: 368, 1983.
146. Nau, H. *J. Pharmacol. Exp. Ther.* 29: 768, 1981.
147. Nau, H. *Eur. J. Clin. Pharmacol.* 18: 31, 1980.
148. Nelson, D., and Bugge, C. Imuran metabolites in baby's and mother's blood and breast milk. (Unpublished data on file at Burroughs Wellcome Company, Research Triangle Park, N.C. 27709). Personal communication with J. Pelkey, January 25, 1982.
149. Niebyl, J. *Obstet. Gynecol.* 53: 139, 1979.
150. O'Brien, T. E. *Am. J. Hosp. Pharm.* 31: 844, 1974.
151. Okada, M., et al. *N. Engl. J. Med.* 312: 992, 1985.
152. Orme, M. L. *Br. Med. J.* 1: 1564, 1977.
153. Ostensen, M. *Eur. J. Clin. Pharmacol.* 25: 829, 1983.
154. Ost, L., et al. *J. Pediatr.* 106: 1008, 1985.
155. Palmer, K. E. *Br. J. Radiol.* 52: 672, 1979.
156. Perez-Reyes, M. *N. Engl. J. Med.* 307: 819, 1982.
157. Phelps, D. L. *J. Pharm. Sci.* 66: 1203, 1977.
158. Pittard, W. B., III. *J. Pediatr.* 51: 1231, 1983.
159. Pittard, W. B., III. *Pediatrics* 70: 321, 1982.
160. Pittard, W. B., III. *J. Pediatr.* 94: 605, 1979.
161. Pittman, K. A. *Am. J. Obstet. Gynecol.* 138: 797, 1980.

162. Ponstellon, D. C. *J.A.M.A.* 247: 463, 1982.
163. Posner, A. C. *Antibiot. Annu.* 2: 594, 1954–1955.
164. Pynnonen, S. *Lancet* 1: 563, 1975.
165. Rane, A. *J. Clin. Pharmacol.* 12: 855, 1981.
166. Rao, T. S. *New Zealand Med. J.* 96: 589, 1983.
167. Rees, J. A. *Practitioner* 217: 686, 1976.
168. Ricci, G. *Rasse Int. Clin. Ter.* 209: 53, 1954–1955.
169. Riley, A. J., Crowley, P., and Harrison, C. Transfer of Ranitidine to Biological Fluids: Milk and Semen. In J. J. Misiewicz and K. G. Wormsley (Eds.), *The Clinical Use of Ranitidine.* Oxford: Medicine Publishing, 1981. Pp. 78–81.
170. Riordan, J. *Am. J. Nurs.* 84: 328, 1984.
171. Ritchie, J. M., et al. Local Anesthesics. In A. G. Goodman-Gilman, L. Goodman and A. Gilman (Eds.), *The Pharmacologic Basis of Therapeutics,* 6th Ed. New York: Macmillan, 1980. P. 300.
172. Roche Laboratories Product Information, Accutane, 1988.
173. Rozansky, R. *J. Lab. Clin. Med.* 34: 497, 1973.
174. Sagraves, R. *Drug Intell. Clin. Pharm.* 14: 484, 1981.
175. Sanders, S. W. *Ann. Intern. Med.* 96: 465, 1982.
176. Schilf, E. *Arch. Gynaekol.* 134: 201, 1928.
177. Schimmel, M. S., et al. *J. Pediatr.* 114: 446, 1989.
178. Schutt, J. C. (Parke-Davis, Division of Warner-Lambert Company, Morris Plains, N.J. 07950). Personal communication, January 16, 1981.
179. Shane, J. M. *Am. J. Obstet. Gynecol.* 120: 129, 1974.
180. Shelton, M. G., et al. *S. Afr. Med. J.* 57: 78, 1980.
181. Smadel, J. E. *J. Clin. Invest.* 28: 1196, 1949.
182. Smith, J. A. *Can. Med. Assoc. J.* 112: 806, 1975.
183. Smith, I. J., et al. *J. Clin. Pharmacol.* 29: 174, 1989.
184. Snyder, D. R., Jr. *Arch. Intern. Med.* 144: 589, 1984.
185. Soderman, P. *Br. J. Clin. Pharmacol.* 17: 599, 1984.
186. Solufi, A., et al. In H. Kass (Ed.), *Voltaren: New Findings.* Vienna: Hans Huber, 1982. P. 19.
187. Somogyi, A. *Br. J. Clin. Pharmacol.* 7: 627, 1979.
188. Sovner, R. *Am. J. Psychiatry* 136: 451, 1979.
189. Steen, B. *Br. J. Clin. Pharmacol.* 13: 661, 1982.
190. Steen, B. *Ther. Drug Monit.* 4: 331, 1982.
191. Steiner, E. *Eur. J. Clin. Pharmacol.* 27: 123, 1984.
192. Stewart, R. B. *Am. J. Psychiatry* 137: 849, 1980.
193. Summerfield, R. J., et al. *Br. J. Anesth.* 57: 1043, 1985.
194. Tahase, Z. *Chemotherapy* 23: 1399, 1975.
195. Tegler, L. *Lancet* 2: 591, 1980.
196. Tennesk, et al. *Natl. Inst. Drug Abuse Res. Monogr. Serv.* 59: 48, 1985.
197. Terwilliger, W. G. *Surg. Gynecol. Obstet.* 58: 823, 1934.
198. Tobin, R. E. *J. Nucl. Med.* 17: 1055, 1976.
199. Townsend, R. J. *Am. J. Obstet. Gynecol.* 149: 184, 1984.
200. Tunnesen, W. J. *J. Pediatr.* 81: 804, 1972.
201. Tyson, R. M. *J. Pediatr.* 11: 824, 1937.
202. Valdivieso, A., et al. *Ann. Intern. Med.* 102: 135, 1985.
203. Varma, S. K. *J. Pediatr.* 93: 803, 1978.
204. Varsano, I. *J. Pediatr.* 82: 886, 1973.
205. Von Kobyletzki, D. Z. *Geburtshilfe Gynakol.* 161: 292, 1964.
206. Von Kobyletzki, D. Z. *Infection* 11: 144, 1983.
207. Vorherr, H. *Postgrad. Med.* 56: 97, 1974.
208. Voshioka, H. *J. Pediatr.* 94: 151, 1979.
209. Wagner, J. G. *Biopharmaceutics and Relevant Pharmacokinetics.* Hamilton, Ill.: Drug Intelligence Publications, 1971. Pp. 392–394.
210. Weibert, R. T. *Clin. Pharmacol.* 1: 457, 1982.
211. Werthmann, M. W. *Med. Annu.* 42: 4, 1973.
212. Whalen, J. J. (Merck Sharp and Dohme, Division of Merck and Co., Inc., West Point, Pa. 19486). Personal communication, March 31, 1981.

213. Whalley, L. J. *Br. Med. J.* 282: 1746, 1981.
214. White, W. B., et al. *Clin. Pharmacol. Ther.* 37: 387, 1985.
215. White, W. B., et al. *Eur. J. Clin. Pharmacol.* 36: 531, 1989.
216. Wiernik, P. H. *Lancet* 1: 912, 1971.
217. Wiles, O. H. *Br. J. Clin. Pharmacol.* 5: 272, 1978.
218. Wilson, J. T. *Clin. Pharmacokinet.* 5: 1, 1980.
219. Yurchak, A. M. *Pediatrics* 57: 520, 1976.

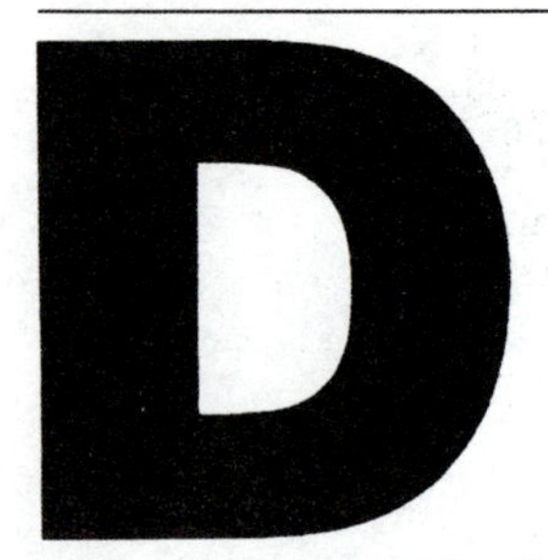

Normal Blood Chemistry Values in the Newborn

Table D-1. Normal blood chemistry values in cord blood and capillary blood of full-term infants (by time after birth; average values are given first, and the range of values is in parentheses)

		Infant's blood			
Determination	Cord blood	1–12 hours	12–24 hours	24–48 hours	48–72 hours
Sodium (mEq/liter)	147 (126–166)	143 (124–156)	145 (132–159)	148 (134–160)	149 (139–162)
Potassium (mEq/liter)	7.8 (5.6–12)	6.4 (5.3–7.3)	6.3 (5.3–8.9)	6.0 (5.2–7.3)	5.9 (5.0–7.7)
Chloride (mEq/liter)	103 (98–110)	100.7 (90–111)	103 (87–114)	102 (92–114)	103 (93–112)
Calcium (mg/dl)	9.3 (8.2–11.1)	8.4 (7.3–9.2)	7.8 (6.9–9.4)	8.0 (6.1–9.9)	7.9 (5.9–9.7)
Phosphorus (mg/dl)	5.6 (3.7–8.1)	6.1 (3.5–8.6)	5.7 (2.9–8.1)	5.9 (3.0–8.7)	5.8 (2.8–7.6)
Blood urea (mg/dl)	29 (21–40)	27 (8–34)	33 (9–63)	32 (13–77)	31 (13–68)
Total protein (gm/dl)	6.1 (4.8–7.3)	6.6 (5.6–8.5)	6.6 (5.8–8.2)	6.9 (5.9–8.2)	7.2 (6.0–8.5)
Blood glucose (mg/dl)	73 (45–96)	63 (40–97)	63 (42–104)	56 (30–91)	59 (40–90)
Lactate (m*M*/liter)	2–3	2	—	—	—

Source: P. T. Acharya and W. W. Payne, Blood chemistry of normal full-term infants in the first 48 hours of life. *Arch. Dis. Child.* 40: 430, 1965.

Table D-2. Normal blood chemistry values in low-birth-weight infants (capillary blood, first day)

Determination	Weight of infant			
	< 1000 gm	1001–1500 gm	1501–2000 gm	2001–2500 gm
Sodium (mEq/liter)	138	133	135	134
Potassium (mEq/liter)	6.4	6.0	5.4	5.6
Chloride (mEq/liter)	100	101	105	104
Total carbon dioxide (mEq/liter)	19	20	20	20
Blood urea (mg/dl)	22	21	16	16
Total protein (gm/dl)	4.8	4.8	5.2	5.3

Source: J. B. Pincus et al., A study of plasma values of sodium, potassium, chloride, carbon dioxide tension, urea and the protein base binding power, pH and hematocrit in prematures on the first day of life. *Pediatrics* 18: 39, 1956.

Table D-3. Other blood chemistry values

Liver function tests		
Ammonia (μg/dl)	14–65	
Alkaline phosphatase (mU/ml)		
Infants	100–150	
Children	50–125	
Lactic acid dehydrogenase (LAD) (mU/ml)	<84	
Serum glutamic oxaloacetic transaminase (SGOT) (mU/ml) [now called aspantate aminotransferase (AST)]	Usually ≤54; may be normal ≤100 on the first 2 days of life	
Serum glutamic pyruvate transaminase (SGPT) (mU/ml) [now called alanine aminotransferase (ALT)]	<29	
Cholesterol (mg/dl)		
Premature, cord blood	67 (47–98)	
Full-term, cord blood	67 (45–98)	
Full-term, newborn infant	85 (45–167)	
Infant, 3 days to 1 year	130 (69–174)	
Copper (μg/dl), 0–6 months	<70	
Creatinine (mg/dl)		
Premature (26–36 weeks' gestational age)		
0–10 days	1.3 (0.8–1.8)	
1–3 months	0.6 (0.2–0.95)	
Term infants	0.6 (0.2–0.9)	
Creatinine phosphokinase, term infants (units/liter)	**Cord blood**	**24 hours**
Skeletal muscle isoenzyme (MM)	126 (48–250)	406 (140–950)
Cardiac isoenzyme (MB)	3 (0–26)	19 (0–97)
Brain isoenzyme (BB)	29 (0–78)	14 (0–93)
Total	157 (80–288)	439 (192–1079)

Table D-3. (continued)

Free fatty acids (mEq/dl)* in newborn	90 ± 47
Magnesium (mEq/liter)	1.5–2.5
Osmolarity (mOsmol/liter)	270–290
Phenylalanine (mg/dl)	
Newborn	Up to 4
Older child	0.8–1.8
Zinc (μg/dl)	77–137

*This value depends on the fasting level.

Sources: J. B. Alpers (Ed.), *Clinical Laboratories Handbook Childrens Hospital,* 6th Ed. Stow, Ohio: Lexi-Comp, 1988–1989; G. B. Avery (Ed.), *Neonatology.* Philadelphia: Lippincott, 1987; B. S. Stonestreet and W. Oh, Plasma creatinine levels in low-birth-weight infants during the first three months of life. *Pediatrics* 61: 788, 1978; and T. M. Sutton et al., Serum levels of creatinine phosphokinase in normal and stressed neonates. *Mayo Clin. Proc.* 56: 150, 1981.

Table D-4. Blood chemistry values in premature infants (birth weight 1500–1750 gm)

Determination	Age 1 week		Age 3 weeks		Age 5 weeks		Age 7 weeks	
	Mean	Range	Mean	Range	Mean	Range	Mean	Range
Sodium (mEq/liter)	139.6	133–146	136.3	129–142	136.8	133–148	137.2	133–142
Potassium (mEq/liter)	5.6	4.6–6.7	5.8	4.5–7.1	5.5	4.5–6.6	5.7	4.6–7.1
Chloride (mEq/liter)	108.2	100–117	108.3	102–116	107.0	100–115	107.0	101–115
Carbon dioxide (mM/liter)	20.3	13.8–27.1	18.4	12.4–26.2	20.4	12.5–26.1	20.6	13.7–26.9
Calcium (mg/dl)	9.2	6.1–11.6	9.6	8.1–11.0	9.4	8.6–10.5	9.5	8.6–10.8
Phosphorus (mg/dl)	7.6	5.4–10.9	7.5	6.2–8.7	7.0	5.6–7.9	6.8	4.2–8.2
Blood urea nitrogen (mg/dl)	9.3	3.1–25.5	13.3	2.1–31.4	13.3	2.0–26.5	13.4	2.5–30.5
Total protein (gm/dl)	5.49	4.40–6.26	5.38	4.28–6.70	4.98	4.14–6.90	4.93	4.02–5.86
Albumin (gm/dl)	3.85	3.28–4.50	3.92	3.16–5.26	3.73	3.20–4.34	3.89	3.40–4.60
Globulin (gm/dl)	1.58	0.88–2.20	1.44	0.62–2.90	1.17	0.48–1.48	1.12	0.50–2.60

Source: J. L. Thomas and T. Reichelderfer, Premature infants: Analysis of serum during the first seven weeks. *Clin. Chem.* 14: 272, 1968.

Table D-5. Normal hematologic values during the first 12 weeks of life in the term infant as determined by an electronic cell counter (see Chap. 16)

Age	Hb (gm/dl) ± S.D.	RBC × 10^6 ± S.D.	Hct % ± S.D.	MCV cuμ ± S.D.	MCHC % ± S.D.	Retic. % ± S.D.
Days						
1	19.0 ± 2.2	5.14 ± 0.7	61 ± 7.4	119 ± 9.4	31.6 ± 1.9	3.2 ± 1.4
2	19.0 ± 1.9	5.15 ± 0.8	60 ± 6.4	115 ± 7.0	31.6 ± 1.4	3.2 ± 1.3
3	18.7 ± 3.4	5.11 ± 0.7	62 ± 9.3	116 ± 5.3	31.1 ± 2.8	2.8 ± 1.7
4	18.6 ± 2.1	5.00 ± 0.6	57 ± 8.1	114 ± 7.5	32.6 ± 1.5	1.8 ± 1.1
5	17.6 ± 1.1	4.97 ± 0.4	57 ± 7.3	114 ± 8.9	30.9 ± 2.2	1.2 ± 0.2
6	17.4 ± 2.2	5.00 ± 0.7	54 ± 7.2	113 ± 10.0	32.2 ± 1.6	0.6 ± 0.2
7	17.9 ± 2.5	4.86 ± 0.6	56 ± 9.4	118 ± 11.2	32.0 ± 1.6	0.5 ± 0.4
Weeks						
1–2	17.3 ± 2.3	4.80 ± 0.8	54 ± 8.3	112 ± 19.0	32.1 ± 2.9	0.5 ± 0.3
2–3	15.6 ± 2.6	4.20 ± 0.6	46 ± 7.3	111 ± 8.2	33.9 ± 1.9	0.8 ± 0.6
3–4	14.2 ± 2.1	4.00 ± 0.6	43 ± 5.7	105 ± 7.5	33.5 ± 1.6	0.6 ± 0.3
4–5	12.7 ± 1.6	3.60 ± 0.4	36 ± 4.8	101 ± 8.1	34.9 ± 1.6	0.9 ± 0.8
5–6	11.9 ± 1.5	3.55 ± 0.2	36 ± 6.2	102 ± 10.2	34.1 ± 2.9	1.0 ± 0.7
6–7	12.0 ± 1.5	3.40 ± 0.4	36 ± 4.8	105 ± 12.0	33.8 ± 2.3	1.2 ± 0.7
7–8	11.1 ± 1.1	3.40 ± 0.4	33 ± 3.7	100 ± 13.0	33.7 ± 2.6	1.5 ± 0.7
8–9	10.7 ± 0.9	3.40 ± 0.5	31 ± 2.5	93 ± 12.0	34.1 ± 2.2	1.8 ± 1.0
9–10	11.2 ± 0.9	3.60 ± 0.3	32 ± 2.7	91 ± 9.3	34.3 ± 2.9	1.2 ± 0.6
10–11	11.4 ± 0.9	3.70 ± 0.4	34 ± 2.1	91 ± 7.7	33.2 ± 2.4	1.2 ± 0.7
11–12	11.3 ± 0.9	3.70 ± 0.3	33 ± 3.3	88 ± 7.9	34.8 ± 2.2	0.7 ± 0.3

Key: Hb = hemoglobin; S.D. = standard deviation; RBC = red blood count; Hct = hematocrit; MCV = mean corpuscular volume; MCHC = mean corpuscular hemoglobin concentration; Retic. = reticulocyte.

Source: Y. Matoth, R. Zaizov, and I. Varsano, Postnatal changes in some red cell parameters. *Acta Paediatr. Scand.* 60: 317, 1971.

Table D-6. The white blood cell count and the differential count during the first 2 weeks of life

Age	Leukocytes	Neutrophils			Eosinophils	Basophils	Lymphocytes	Monocytes
		Total	Segmented	Band				
Birth								
Mean	18,000	11,000	9400	1600	400	100	5500	1050
Range	9.0–30.0	6.0–26.0			20–850	0–640	2.0–11.0	0.4–3.1
Mean %		61	52	9	2.2	0.6	31	5.8
7 Days								
Mean	12,000	5500	4700	830	500	50	5000	1100
Range	5.0–21.0	1.5–10.0			70–1100	0–250	2.0–17.0	0.3–2.7
Mean %		45	39	6	4.1	0.4	41	9.1
14 Days								
Mean	11,400	4500	3900	630	350	50	5500	1000
Range	5.0–20.0	1.0–9.5			70–1000	0–230	2.0–17.0	0.2–2.4
Mean %		40	34	5.5	3.1	0.4	48	8.8

Source: F. A. Oski and J. L. Naiman, *Hematologic Problems in the Newborn*, 3d Ed. Philadelphia: Saunders, 1982.

Table D-7. Hematologic values in low-birth-weight infants

Size of infant	Determination	Age of infant: 1–3 Days	4–7 Days	2 Weeks	4 Weeks	6 Weeks	8 Weeks
Birth weight less than 1200 gm	Hemoglobin	15.6	16.4	15.5	11.3	8.5	7.8
	Reticulocytes as % of RBC	8.4	3.9	1.9	4.1	5.4	6.1
	Platelets	148,000 ± 61,000	163,000 ± 69,000	162,000	158,000	210,000	212,000
	Leukocytes	14,800 ± 10,200	12,200 ± 7000	15,800	13,200	10,800	9900
	Segmented neutrophils	46	32	41	28	23	23
	Band neutrophils	10.7	9.7	8.0	5.9	5.8	4.4
	Juvenile neutrophils	2.0	3.9	5.3	3.6	2.6	2.0
	Lymphocytes	32	43	39	55	61	65
	Monocytes	5	7	5	4	6	3
	Eosinophils	0.4	6.2	1.0	3.7	2.0	3.8
	Nucleated RBC as % of total RBC	16.7	1.1	0.1	1.0	2.7	2.0
Birth weight 1200–1500 gm	Hemoglobin	20.0	18.0	17.1	12.0	9.1	8.3
	Reticulocytes as % of RBC	2.7	1.2	0.9	1.0	2.2	2.7
	Platelets	151,000 ± 35,000	134,000 ± 49,000	153,000	189,000	212,000	244,000
	Leukocytes	10,800 ± 4000	8900 ± 2900	14,300	11,000	10,500	9100
	Segmented neutrophils	47	31	33	26	20	25
	Band neutrophils	11.9	10.5	5.9	3.0	1.4	2.1
	Juvenile neutrophils	5.1	2.4	2.7	1.8	1.7	1.6
	Lymphocytes	34	48	52	59	69	64
	Monocytes	3	6	3	4	5	5
	Eosinophils	1.3	2.2	2.5	5.1	2.6	2.3
	Nucleated RBC as % of total RBC	19.8	0.8	0	0.4	1.4	1.0

Key: RBC = red blood count.
Source: J. A. Wolff and A. N. Goodfellow, Hematopoiesis in premature infants: With consideration of the effect of iron and animal-protein factors. *Pediatrics* 16: 753, 1955, and F. A. Oski and J. L. Naiman, *Hematologic Problems in the Newborn*, 3d Ed. Philadelphia: Saunders, 1982.

Index

Index